Second Edition

Textbook of
Anatomy and
Physiology

for Paramedics and Health Professionals

Indu Khurana MD
Dean-cum-Principal
World College of Medical Sciences and Research
Jhajjar, Haryana, India
Former Professor and Head
Department of Physiology
Pt BD Sharma Postgraduate Institute of Medical Sciences
Rohtak, Haryana, India

Arushi Khurana MD
Fellow, Hematology-Oncology
Massey Cancer Center
Virginia Commonwealth University
Richmond, VA

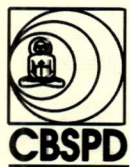

CBSPD

CBS Publishers & Distributors Pvt Ltd

New Delhi • Bengaluru • Chennai • Kochi • Kolkata • Lucknow • Mumbai
Gujarat • Hyderabad • Jharkhand • Nagpur • Patna • Pune • Uttarakhand

Second Edition

Textbook of Anatomy and Physiology

for Paramedics and Health Professionals

ISBN: 978-93-5466-209-6

Copyright © Publisher

Second Edition 2022
Reprint 2026
First Edition 2009
Reprint 2010, 2014, 2015, 2017, 2019

Published by Satish Kumar Jain and produced by Varun Jain for

CBS Publishers & Distributors Pvt Ltd

4819/XI Prahlad Street, 24 Ansari Road, Daryaganj, New Delhi 110 002, India
Ph: 011-23289259, 23266838   Website: www.cbspd.com   e-mail: delhi@cbspd.com
Corporate Office: 204 FIE, Industrial Area, Patparganj, Delhi 110 092, India
Ph: 011-49344934   Fax: 011-49344935
                        e-mail: publishing@cbspd.com; publicity@cbspd.com

Branches

- Bengaluru: Seema House 2975, 17th Cross, KR Road, Banasankari 2nd Stage, Bengaluru 560 070, Karnataka, India
  Ph: +91-80-26771678/79   Fax: +91-80-26771680   e-mail: bangalore@cbspd.com
- Chennai: No.18/8B, Subbarayan Street, Shenoy Nagar, Chennai 600 030, Tamil Nadu, India
  Ph: +91-44-42032115, 26681266   e-mail: chennai@cbspd.com
- Kochi: 42/1325, 1326, Power House Road, Opposite KSEB, Power House, Ernakulum 682018, Kochi, Kerala, India
  Ph: +91-484-4059061–67   Fax: +91-484-4059065   e-mail: kochi@cbspd.com
- Kolkata: 147, Hind Ceramics Compound, 1st Floor, Nilgunj Road, Belghoria, Kolkata 700056, West Bengal, India
  Ph: +91-33-25330055/56   e-mail: kolkata@cbspd.com
- Lucknow: Basement, Khushuma Complex, 7 Meerabai Marg (behind Jawahar Bhawan), Lucknow 226001, UP, India
  Ph: +91-522-4000032   e-mail: tiwari.lucknow@cbspd.com
- Mumbai: PWD Shed, Gala No. 25/26, Ramchandra Bhatt Marg, Next JJ Hospital Gate No. 2, Opp. Union Bank of India, Noorbaug, Mumbai 400009, Maharashtra, India
  Ph: +91-22-66661880/89   e-mail: mumbai@cbspd.com

Representatives

- Gujarat   0-9879558667
- Nagpur   0-8692091830
- Uttarakhand   0-9716462459
- Hyderabad   0-9885175004
- Patna   0-9334159340
- Jharkhand   0-9811541605
- Pune   0-9664372571

Printed at Magic International Pvt. Ltd., Greater Noida, UP, India

Preface to the Third Edition

The Third edition of *Textbook of Applied Anatomy and Physiology for BSc Nursing* has been thoroughly revised and updated in such a way that it meets the requisite goal of curriculum recommended by the Indian Nursing Council. The text provides a thorough yet concise exposition of fundamental aspects of human Anatomy and Physiology. The text matter is aimed at providing an insight into how the human body is structured, how it works and how the abnormalities of the structures and functions cause diseases. The text has been arranged into ten sections, and each section has been subdivided into various chapters.

Salient Features of the Third Edition:

- Thoroughly revised and updated text, retaining its well accepted style of organization in ten sections.
- To further upgrade the book, many new figures, tables and flowcharts have been added.
- A brief review given in the beginning of each section, highlights the topics covered.
- Chapter outline given in the beginning of each chapter provides clear layout of the text included.
- Text in each chapter has been organized in such a way that the students can easily understand, retain and reproduce it.
- Various levels of headings, subheadings, boldface and italics given in the text will be helpful for quick revision of the subject.
- The text is illustrated with plenty of diagrams. The illustrations mostly include clear line diagrams providing vivid and lucid details.
- Relevant anatomical aspects of various structures in each chapter have been illustrated with high quality colored diagrams and histology plates which is quite useful to students in conceptualizing the subject.
- In order to emphasize the applied clinical significance of Anatomy and Physiology, the relevant clinical aspects have been covered adequately in each chapter and properly highlighted.
- Based on basic concepts of Anatomy and Physiology, the relevant nursing implications and applications are adequately covered.
- Additional important information in the form of 'Important to know' has been highlighted.
- For self-assessment, the subjective questionnaire and multiple choice questions are given at the end of each chapter.

Indu Khurana
Arushi Khurana
N Gurukripa Kowlgi

Preface to the First Edition

A sound knowledge of anatomy and physiology of the human body is most essential for all the health science graduate students. An effort has been made in this Textbook of Anatomy and Physiology to provide the essential matter in a thorough yet concise manner. The book has been written primarily for the students of nursing and other allied health sciences to help them understand the fundamental of the subject. Material provided is aimed at providing an insight into how the body is structured and how it functions and how the alterations in normal structure and functioning result in disease. To achieve this aim, the text matter on pure and applied aspects of human anatomy and physiology has been skillfully intermingled and presented in an adorned form. Care has been taken to include the material as per syLabi prescribed by Council for Nursing and Council for Other Allied Health Sciences. It is hoped, the book will be useful in laying a strong foundation for health science graduate students.

The book has been organized in twelve sections and each section has been subdivided into various chapters. Section 1 is devoted to general anatomy and physiology and the rest eleven sections describe the human body system by system.

Salient Features:

- The text has been organized in such a way that the students can easily understand, retain and reproduce it. Various levels of headings, subheadings, bold face and italics given in the text will be helpful in quick revision of the text.
- A brief list of contents given in the beginning of each chapter provides a clear layout of the text.
- The exposition of the text is such that an average student will not find any difficulty in conceptulizing it.
- The text has been well illustrated with a high quality clear line diagrams which provide vivid and lucid details.
- To further enhance the lucidity of the book, the text and figures are presented in an attractive color format
- To emphasize the clinical significance of anatomy and physiology, the relevant applied aspects have been covered adequately in each chapter.
- The important information has been highlighted with the help of plenty of tables and flowcharts.

An arduous task like this is never possible without the unending blessings of teachers and parents, to whom we shall ever remain indebted. We wish to express gratitude to our esteemed teachers Prof. Inderbir Singh and Prof. P.I. Singh for their valuable guidance.

We acknowledge, with profound gratitude, the contribution of Professor AK Khurana who has not only guided and helped us during each and every step of preparation of this book, but has also authored a chapter on Anatomy and Physiology of Eye and Vision. We also wish to express our gratitude to Dr (Mrs) Sushma Sood, Professor & Head, Department of Physiology and Professor SS Sangwan, Director, PGIMS, Rohtak for providing an excellent academic and working atmosphere.

It is our special pleasure to acknowledge with gratitude the most assured cooperation and skill of M/s CBS Publishers & Distributors in general and Mr SK Jain, Managing Director, and Mr Vinod Jain, Production Director, in particular. Dr Aashima and Dr Saurav deserve a special slot in the preface for their artistic touch which we feel has provided a considerable beauty to this book.

Mr YN Arjuna and Mr Dharmvir from CBS Publishers need a special appreciation for their generous help. Ventures like this are never entirely free from human errors, some inaccuracies, ambiguities and typographical mistakes. We would, therefore, welcome feedback and suggestions from teachers and students for further improvement of the book.

Indu Khurana
Arushi Khurana

Acknowledgments

This Third edition of the *Textbook of Applied Anatomy and Physiology for BSc Nursing* has come into the readers' hand because of the feedback, active criticism, suggestions and generous help of many faculty members and students. I owe sincere thanks to them all. Those who need special mention include Dr Arushi Khurana, MD, Faculty, Medical Oncology Services, and Dr N Gurukripa Kowlgi, MD, Faculty, Department of Cardiology, Mayo Clinic College of Medicine and Science, Rochester, Minnesota, USA who as co-authors have been very helpful in updating the text, especially the clinical aspects.

I wish to express indebtedness to my husband Dr AK Khurana MS, FAICO, CTO (London), Professor and Head, Department of Ophthalmology, SGT Medical College, Hospital and Research Institute, Gurugram, and former Senior Professor and Head, Regional Institute of Ophthalmology, Postgraduate Institute of Medical Sciences (PGIMS), Rohtak for contributing text on 'Physiology of Vision for this book. My son, Dr Aruj K Khurana, DNB, FICO, FVRS, Assistant Professor, Vitreo-Retinal Services, Dr Bhawna Piplani Khurana, MS, DNB, FICO, FNN, FRCS, Associate Professor, Department of Ophthalmology, SGT Medical College Hospital and Research, Gurugram, Haryana, and my grandchildren Agastya, Abhinaman and Amyra, need to be complimented for keeping me energized by their never ending love and affection.

I also thank Shri Manmohan Singh Chawla, Managing Trustee; Ms Madhupreet Chawla, Chairperson; Shri Ram Bahadur Rai, Chancellor; Professor Sham Singla, Advisor; Professor OP Kalra, Vice Chancellor; Professor Gen. SPS Kochar, Dean FHMS; Dr Shobha Baroor, Professor Emeritus, Chief Advisor IJHSC; and Shri. GL Khanna, Head HR Department; SGT University, for providing atmosphere conducive to such academic activities.

I would like to thank **Mr Satish Kumar Jain** (Chairman) and **Mr Varun Jain** (Managing Director), M/s CBS Publishers and Distributors Pvt Ltd for providing me the platform in bringing out the book. I have no words to describe the role, efforts, inputs and initiatives undertaken by **Mr Bhupesh Aarora**, Sr. Vice President – Publishing and Marketing (Health Sciences Division) for helping and motivating me.

I sincerely thank the entire CBS team for bringing out the book with utmost care and attractive presentation. I would like to thank Ms Nitasha Arora (Publishing Head and Content Strategist – Medical and Nursing), and Dr Anju Dhir (Product Manager cum Commissioning Editor – Medical) for their editorial support. I would also extend my thanks to Mr Shivendu Bhushan Pandey (Sr. Manager and Team Lead), Mr Ashutosh Pathak (Sr. Proofreader cum Team Coordinator) and all the production team members for devoting laborious hours in designing and typesetting the book.

Sincere efforts have been made to verify the correctness of the text. However, in spite of best efforts some inaccuracies, ambiguities and typographical mistakes are likely to be noticed by the readers. Therefore, feedback and suggestions from the teachers and students are invited for improving the future edition. Feedback received will be highly appreciated and duly acknowledged.

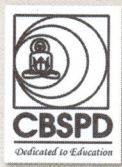

CBS Nursing Knowledge Tree

Extends its Tribute to

Florence Nightingale

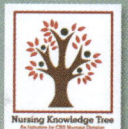

"

> *For glorifying the role of women as nurses,*
> *For holding the title of " The Lady with the Lamp,"*
> *For working tirelessly for humanity—*
> *Florence Nightingale will always be*
> *remembered for her*
> *selfless and memorable services to the*
> *human race.*

"

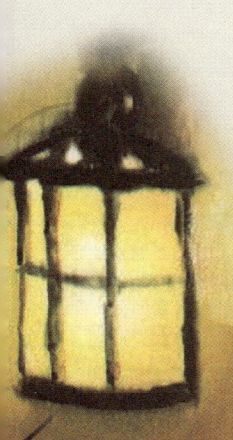

Florence Nightingale
(May 1820 – August 1910)

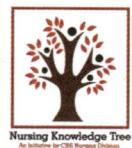

Nursing Knowledge Tree

An Initiative by CBS Nursing Division

"Coming together is a beginning. Keeping together is progress. Working together is success."

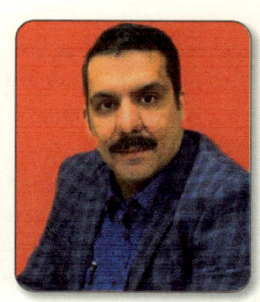

It gives us immense pleasure to share with you that Nursing Knowledge Tree—An initiative by CBS Nursing Division, has successful established itself in the field of nursing as we have been standing as a strong contender by sharing approximately 50% of market share. This growth could not have been possible without your invaluable contribution as our reader, author, reviewer, contributor and recommender, and your outstanding support for the growth of our titles as a whole. Before I enunciate in detail, I would like to thank each and every Clinical Nurse, Academician and Nursing Student for the phenomenal support during the COVID-19 pandemic. It is all your support that instilled a sense of responsibility in us and provided us with strength and motivation to survive under the worst circumstances of the pandemic.

The last two years were the most crucial phase when the entire world stood still due to adversity of COVID-19. The normal life was in turmoil, and people had no idea what would be their next step and how long this crisis would persist. In the midst of all, a few things which nobody could stop is 'Change', which is inevitable. During the last two years, we have done a lot of innovations and put our best efforts in implementing those innovations to bring quality education and make sure that every person should have access to best possible education.

It is worth mentioning that with all your support we have made some remarkable innovations in the field of nursing education, which are:

1. More quality books by the top Authors from the top institutes
2. Entered into Nursing EdTech Segment with NNL App (Nursing Next Live Application)
3. NN Social
4. Phygital Books
5. Social Media Presence
6. Built Strong Community (Faculty/Student Ambassador Program)

As a publisher, we have been contributing to the field of Medical Sciences, Nursing and Allied Sciences and have many established titles in the market. Tradition is carrying forward the legacy of the old pattern and approach in the contemporary time. We broke the boundary of being a traditional publisher through innovations and changes. As far as publishing industry is concerned, we are the first to enter the **Nursing EdTech** with the Launch of **Nursing Next Live App.**

Through Nursing Next Live, we made possible the reach of quality education from Jammu and Kashmir to Kanyakumari and from Gujarat to Arunachal Pradesh.

We started with the mission:

"We are bringing Learning to the People Instead People are going for the Learning."

When pandemic halted everything, the future seemed to be doomed, Nursing Next Live made it possible for the Nursing Professionals across the nation to keep continuing their learning and helped them to achieve their dream career.

In a step toward strengthening the Nursing Segment, we have melded the four important pillars—Print, Digital, Nursing Professionals and Social Media—to work in a homogenized manner for the better future of the nursing education through:

NN Social, a community of 20K+ professionals, is an initiative of Nursing Next Live as India's knowledge-sharing network platform for the nursing segment. Nursing Next Social is curated with the aim to bring all the nursing faculty members across the nation closer and together on a single platform. Through **NN Social**, we aim to connect the sharp minds across the nation to use their knowledge for the better future of Nursing Profession. With NN Social **India's top-notch societies, like TNAI, SOCN, NTA, KINS, etc. are associated with us.** Apart from this, NN Social has a strong network of 100+ authors, 500+ reviewers and contributors. They all are dedicated and committed as we are, toward imparting quality nursing education.

In the era of digitalization, to make study interactive and convenient, we have conceptualized the idea of **Hybrid Edition of the books**. In this series, our many bestselling titles are available in the hybrid form. This hybrid learning is a blended learning wherein printed booklets are thoughtfully integrated with the digital support to reconceptualize the learning method in a more interactive manner with added values to knowledge. Hybrid edition is an endeavor to facilitate the next level of preparation for any nursing competitive exams through quality content, flexibility, customization and engaging interactive learning experiences.

We have also increased our **social media presence** through meaningful and innovative ideas and are committed to assist the nursing professionals in gaining and sharing the knowledge. We have taken the initiative to learn from the experience of the others and started **NNL Talks**. It is a platform where every nursing professional who has done exceptionally well in his/her career, toppers of any Nursing Exams and those who manage themselves in all the odds and stand firm and determined and succeed in his/her life, can share the success journey. We aim to motivate, educate and encourage the nursing professionals through various activities and posts on our social media platform.

Whatever initiative we take, we always make sure that it is for a noble cause of promoting the quality education accessible to everyone.

Today we can say this with confidence, we "CBS Publishers and NNL" have an edge over all other Indian and International Publishers. Our Approach, Vision, Mission, Concept, Content, Reach, Ideas all have a single goal that is better nursing education can lead to a better healthcare system.

Long way to go…. Together!

Looking forward to invite more young and experienced minds who can join us as Authors, Reviewers, Contributors, and Faculties and accomplish our mission of providing quality nursing education to all.

With Best Wishes
Mr Bhupesh Aarora
Sr. Vice President – Publishing and Marketing
(Health Sciences Division)

Special Features of the Book

Chapter Outline gives a glimpse of the content covered in the Chapter.

CHAPTER OUTLINE

The Cell
- Cell Membrane
- Cytoplasm
- Nucleus
- Cell Cycle

Intercellular Junctions
- Tight Junction

- Adherens Junction
- Gap Junction

Transport of Substances Across Cell Membranes
- Passive Transport
- Active Transport
- Vesicular Transport

- Other Transport Processes

Membrane Potential
- Genesis of Membrane Potential

CLINICAL ASPECTS

Clinical Aspects boxes are used to highlight the clinical aspects in the form of cases for better understanding of practical application

Abnormalities of Carbohydrate Digestion and Absorption

Congenital lactose intolerance: It refers to a condition in which lactose (milk sugar) cannot be digested due to congenital deficiency of enzyme lactase.

- The undigested lactose acts as osmotic particles and draws excessive fluids into intestine resulting in *diarrhea*.
- The diarrhea so produced can lead to life-threatening dehydration and electrolyte imbalance.
- Avoidance of milk and milk products prevents the symptoms from developing if the infant can be fed by synthetic milk containing sucrose instead of lactose.

Secondary lactase deficiency occurring in adults is very common. It produces intestinal distension, diarrhea and flatulence. For adults, it is usually not a problem, as they can easily avoid milk and milk products.

Nursing Implications and Applications have been highlighted at respective places from clinical practical point of view.

NURSING IMPLICATIONS AND APPLICATIONS

Prevention and Treatment of Bed Sores

Nursing care is very important for prevention of bed sores in bed ridden patients. Bed sores can be prevented by opting following five tips.

1. *Proper hydration and nutrition* is crucial for preventing bed sores. When the internal body is well taken care of, the skin will be less prone to sores and any resulting infection. Therefore, nourishing the patient with good healthy protein rich diet and hydration can help.
2. *Exercise*. It is very important for bed ridden patients to perform movements, so that air flow can occur to every part of the body. The attending nurse should help in doing movements of the body in such patients and preventing bed sores.
3. *Repositioning* Frequent repositioning the patient (once in every two hours) and checking of pressure points for development of bed sore is also important point for nursing care to bedridden patients.
4. *Extra-cushioning* by putting extra pillows under high pressure points such as tail-bone and shoulders can improve air flow.

IMPORTANT TO KNOW

Serum

Plasma from which fibrinogen and clotting factors (II, V and VIII) have been removed is called serum. Serum is formed when the blood is allowed to clot in a test tube and clot is retracted. Serum has a higher serotonin (5HT) content because of the breakdown of platelets during clotting.

Important to Know boxes have been added to provide additional important information.

Histology plates at relevant places have been added for an integrated study approach.

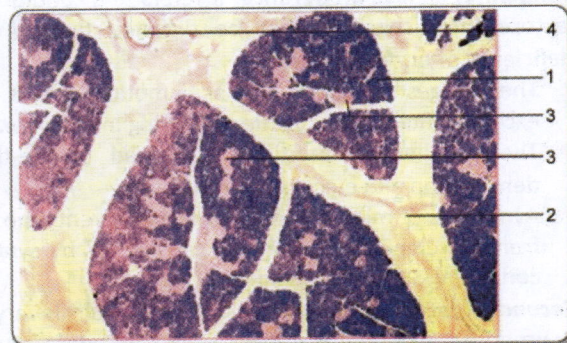

Histology Plate 3.1-2:

The photomicrograph of parotid gland shows, serous acini (1) connective tissue septa, (2) divides it into lobules, (3) intercalated duct, (4) intralobular duct

TABLE 4.2-4: Distribution of blood flow to various organs of the body during resting and maximum activity conditions

Organs	Blood flow per organ (mL/min)		Blood flow (mL/100 g/min)	
	At rest	During maximum activity	At rest	During maximum activity
Heart	250	1200	80	400
Brain	750	2100	55	150
Liver	1500	3000	58	120
Skeletal muscles	150	1800	4	70
Kidney	1200	1400	400	450
Skin	200	3500	8	150

Numerous **Tables** summarizing important information have been included wherever necessary.

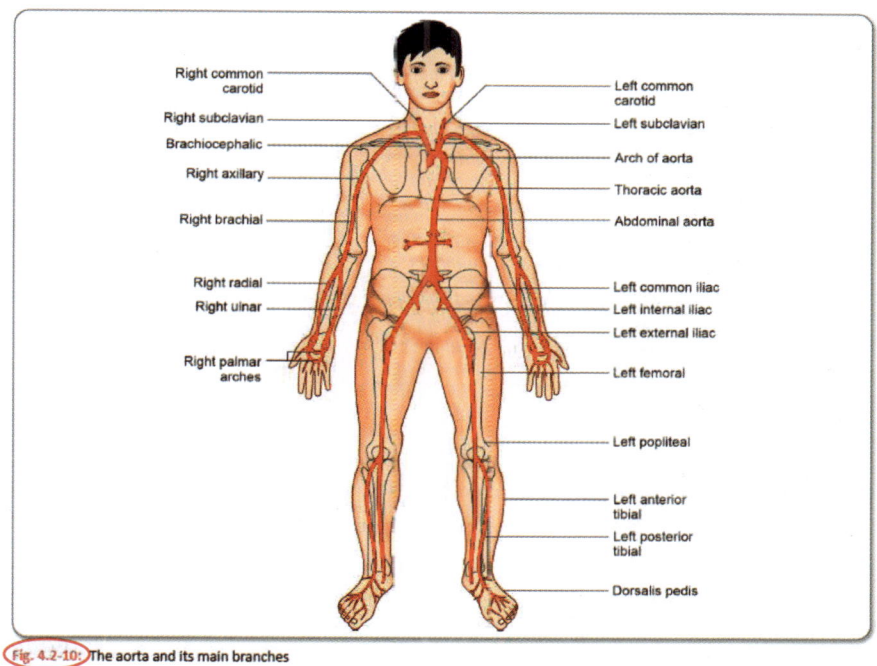

Fig. 4.2-10: The aorta and its main branches

Number of illustrations have been complimented with text which can easily be reproduce.

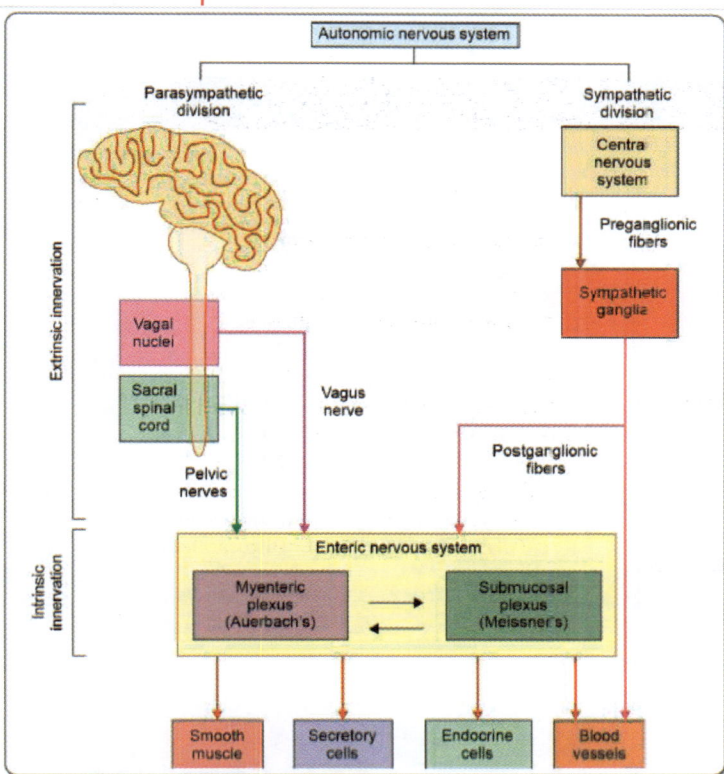

Fig. 3.1-4: Schematic illustration of the innervation of gut

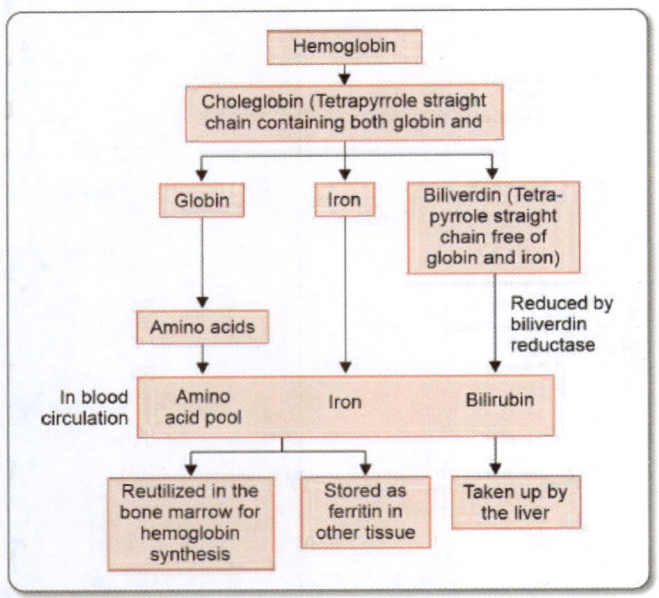

Fig. 4.1-8: Fate of hemoglobin

Numerous **Flowcharts** are supplemented with the text to make concept more clear to understand.

At the end of chapters, **Assess Yourself** section is given which contains variety of subjective and multiple choice questions to help you attain mastery over the subject.

ASSESS YOURSELF

Short and Long Answer Questions

1. **Define the following:**
   - Atom
   - Molecule
   - Element
   - Atomic weight
   - Atomic number
2. **Discuss briefly the significance of following in the human body:**
   - Carbohydrates
   - Proteins
   - Lipids
3. **What are essential amino acids? List them.**
4. **Describe types of enzymes and their role in human body.**

Multiple Choice Questions

1. **The atomic weight of oxygen is:**
   a. 16   b. 12
   c. 11   d. 8
2. **The atomic number of sodium is:**
   a. 1   b. 4
   c. 8   d. 11
3. **The pH of blood is:**
   a. 5.7   b. 6.4
   c. 7   d. 7.4
4. **Cane sugar is:**
   a. Monosaccharide   b. Disaccharide
   c. Polysaccharide   d. Oligosaccharide

Applied Anatomy

Placement: I Semester

Theory: 3 Credits (60 hours)

Unit	Time (hrs)	Learning Outcomes	Content	Teaching/ Learning Activities	Assessment Methods
I	8 (T)	• Define the terms relative to the anatomical position • Describe the anatomical planes • Define and describe the terms used to describe movements • Organization of human body and structure of cell, tissues membranes and glands • Describe the types of cartilage • Compare and contrast the features of skeletal, smooth and cardiac muscle	**Introduction to Anatomical Terms and Organization of the Human Body** • Introduction to anatomical terms relative to position—anterior, ventral, posterior dorsal, superior, inferior, median, lateral, proximal, distal, superficial, deep, prone, supine, palmar and plantar • Anatomical planes (axial/ transverse/ horizontal, sagittal/vertical plane and coronal/ frontal/oblique plane) • Movements (flexion, extension, abduction, adduction, medial rotation, lateral rotation, inversion, eversion, supination, pronation, plantar flexion, dorsal flexion and circumduction • Cell structure, cell division • Tissue—definition, types, characteristics, classification, location • Membrane, glands—classification and structure • Identify major surface and bony landmarks in each body region, organization of human body • Hyaline, fibro cartilage, elastic cartilage • Features of skeletal, smooth and cardiac muscle • Application and implication in nursing	• Lecture cum discussion • Use of models • Video demonstration • Use of microscopic slides • Lecture cum discussion • Video/slides • Anatomical Torso	• Quiz • MCQ • Short answer
II	6 (T)	• Describe the structure of respiratory system • Identify the muscles of respiration and examine their contribution to the mechanism of breathing	**The Respiratory System** • Structure of the organs of respiration • Muscles of respiration • Application and implication in nursing	• Lecture cum discussion • Models • Video/slides	• Short answer • Objective type
III	6 (T)	Describe the structure of digestive system	**The Digestive System** • Structure of alimentary canal and accessory organs of digestion • Application and implications in nursing	• Lecture cum discussion • Video/slides • Anatomical Torso	• Short answer • Objective type

Contd...

Unit	Time (hrs)	Learning Outcomes	Content	Teaching/ Learning Activities	Assessment Methods
IV	6 (T)	Describe the structure of circulatory and lymphatic system	**The Circulatory and Lymphatic System** • Structure of blood components, blood vessels—arterial and venous system • Position of heart relative to the associated structures • Chambers of heart, layers of heart • Heart valves, coronary arteries • Nerve and blood supply to heart • Lymphatic tissue • Veins used for IV injections • Application and implication in nursing	• Lecture • Models • Video/slides	• Short answer • MCQ
V	4 (T)	Identify the major endocrine glands and describe the structure of endocrine glands	**The Endocrine System** Structure of hypothalamus, pineal gland, pituitary gland, thyroid, parathyroid, thymus, pancreas and adrenal glands	• Lecture • Models/charts	• Short answer • Objective type
VI	4 (T)	Describe the structure of various sensory organs	**The Sensory Organs** • Structure of skin, eye, ear, nose and tongue • Application and implications in nursing	• Lecture • Explain with video/ models/charts	• Short answer • MCQ
VII	10 (T)	• Describe anatomical position and structure of bones and joints • Identify major bones that make up the axial and appendicular skeleton • Classify the joints • Identify the application and implications in nursing • Describe the structure of muscle • Apply the knowledge in performing nursing procedures/skills	**The Musculoskeletal System:** **The Skeletal System** • Anatomical positions • Bones—types, structure, growth and ossification • Axial and appendicular skeleton • Joints—classification, major joints and structure • Application and implications in nursing **The Muscular System** • Types and structure of muscles • Muscle groups—muscles of the head, neck, thorax, abdomen, pelvis, upper limb and lower limbs • Principal muscles—deltoid, biceps, triceps, respiratory, abdominal, pelvic floor, pelvic floor muscles, gluteal muscles and vastus lateralis • Major muscles involved in nursing procedures	• Review—discussion • Lecture • Discussions • Explain using charts, skeleton and loose bones and torso • Identifying muscles involved in nursing procedures in lab	• Short answer • Objective type
VIII	5 (T)	Describe the structure of renal system	**The Renal System** • Structure of kidney, ureters, bladder, urethra • Application and implication in nursing	• Lecture • Models/charts	• MCQ • Short answer
IX	5 (T)	Describe the structure of reproductive system	**The Reproductive System** • Structure of male reproductive organs • Structure of female reproductive organs • Structure of breast	• Lecture • Models/charts	• MCQ • Short answer

Contd...

Unit	Time (hrs)	Learning Outcomes	Content	Teaching/ Learning Activities	Assessment Methods
X	6 (T)	• Describe the structure of nervous system including the distribution of the nerves, nerve plexuses • Describe the ventricular system	**The Nervous System** • Review structure of neurons • CNS, ANS and PNS (central, autonomic and peripheral) • Structure of brain, spinal cord, cranial nerves, spinal nerves, peripheral nerves, functional areas of cerebral cortex • Ventricular system—formation, circulation, and drainage • Application and implication in nursing	• Lecture • Explain with models • Video slides	• MCQ • Short answer

Applied Physiology

Placement: I Semester

Theory: 3 Credits (60 hours)

Unit	Time (Hrs)	Learning Outcomes	Content	Teaching/ Learning Activities	Assessment Methods
I	4 (T)	Describe the physiology of cell, tissues membranes and glands	**General Physiology—Basic Concepts** • Cell physiology including transportation across cell membrane • Body fluid compartments, distribution of total body fluid, intracellular and extracellular compartments, major electrolytes and maintenance of homeostasis • Cell cycle • Tissue—formation, repair • Membranes and glands—functions • Application and implication in nursing	• Review—discussion • Lecture cum discussion • Video demonstrations	• Quiz • MCQ • Short answer
II	6 (T)	• Describe the physiology and mechanism of respiration • Identify the muscles of respiration and examine their contribution to the mechanism of breathing	**Respiratory System** • Functions of respiratory organs • Physiology of respiration • Pulmonary circulation—functional features • Pulmonary ventilation, exchange of gases • Carriage of oxygen and carbon dioxide, exchange of gases in tissue • Regulation of respiration • Hypoxia, cyanosis, dyspnea, periodic breathing • Respiratory changes during exercise • Application and implication in nursing	• Lecture • Video slides	• Essay • Short answer • MCQ
III	8 (T)	Describe the functions of digestive system	**Digestive System** • Functions of the organs of digestive tract • Saliva—composition, regulation of secretion and functions of saliva • Composition and function of gastric juice, mechanism and regulation of gastric secretion	• Lecture cum discussion • Video slides	• Essay • Short answer • MCQ

Contd…

Unit	Time (Hrs)	Learning Outcomes	Content	Teaching/ Learning Activities	Assessment Methods
			• Composition of pancreatic juice, function, regulation of pancreatic secretion • Functions of liver, gallbladder and pancreas • Composition of bile and function • Secretion and function of small and large intestine • Movements of alimentary tract • Digestion in mouth, stomach, small intestine, large intestine, absorption of food • Application and implications in nursing		
IV	6 (T)	Explain the functions of the heart, and physiology of circulation	**Circulatory and Lymphatic System** • Functions of heart, conduction system, cardiac cycle, stroke volume and cardiac output • Blood pressure and pulse • Circulation—principles, factors influencing blood pressure, pulse • Coronary circulation, pulmonary and systemic circulation • Heart rate—regulation of heart rate • Normal value and variations • Cardiovascular homeostasis in exercise and posture • Application and implication in nursing	• Lecture • Discussion • Video/slides	• Short answer • MCQ
V	5 (T)	Describe the composition and functions of blood	**Blood** • Blood—functions, physical characteristics • Formation of blood cells • Erythropoiesis—functions of RBC, RBC life cycle • WBC—types, functions • Platelets—function and production of platelets • Clotting mechanism of blood, clotting time, bleeding time, PTT • Hemostasis—role of vasoconstriction, platelet plug formation in hemostasis, coagulation factors, intrinsic and extrinsic pathways of coagulation • Blood groups and types • Functions of reticuloendothelial system, immunity • Application in nursing	• Lecture • Discussion • Videos	• Essay • Short answer • MCQ
VI	5 (T)	Identify the major endocrine glands and describe their functions	**The Endocrine System** • Functions and hormones of pineal gland, pituitary gland, thyroid, parathyroid, thymus, pancreas and adrenal glands. • Other hormones • Alterations in disease • Application and implication in nursing	• Lecture • Explain using charts	• Short answer • MCQ

Contd…

Unit	Time (Hrs)	Learning Outcomes	Content	Teaching/ Learning Activities	Assessment Methods
VII	4 (T)	Describe the structure of various sensory organs	**The Sensory Organs** • Functions of skin • Vision, hearing, taste and smell • Errors of refraction, aging changes • Application and implications in nursing	• Lecture • Video	• Short answer • MCQ
VIII	6 (T)	Describe the functions of bones, joints, various types of muscles its special properties and nerves supplying them	**Musculoskeletal System** • Bones—functions, movements of bones of axial and appendicular skeleton, Bone healing • Joints and joint movements • Alteration of joint disease • Properties and functions of skeletal muscles—mechanism of muscle contraction • Structure and properties of cardiac muscles and smooth muscles • Application and implication in nursing	• Lecture • Discussion • Video presentation	• Structured essay • Short answer • MCQ
IX	4 (T)	Describe the physiology of renal system	**Renal System** • Functions of kidney in maintaining homeostasis • GFR • Functions of ureters, bladder and urethra • Micturition • Regulation of renal function • Application and implication in nursing	• Lecture • Charts and models	• Short answer • MCQ
X	4 (T)	Describe the structure of reproductive system	**The Reproductive System** • Female reproductive system—menstrual cycle, function and hormones of ovary, oogenesis, fertilization, implantation, functions of breast • Male reproductive system—spermatogenesis, hormones and its functions, semen • Application and implication in providing nursing care	• Lecture • Explain using charts, models, specimens	• Short answer • MCQ
XI	8 (T)	Describe the functions of brain, physiology of nerve stimulus, reflexes, cranial and spinal nerves	**Nervous System** • Overview of nervous system • Review of types, structure and functions of neurons • Nerve impulse • Review functions of brain—medulla, pons, cerebrum, cerebellum • Sensory and motor nervous system • Peripheral nervous system • Autonomic nervous system • Limbic system and higher mental functions—hippocampus, thalamus, hypothalamus • Vestibular apparatus • Functions of cranial nerves	• Lecture cum discussion • Video slides	• Brief structured essays • Short answer • MCQ • Critical reflection

Contd...

Unit	Time (Hrs)	Learning Outcomes	Content	Teaching/ Learning Activities	Assessment Methods
			• Autonomic functions • Physiology of pain-somatic, visceral and referred • Reflexes • CSF formation, composition, circulation of CSF, blood brain barrier and blood CSF barrier • Application and implication in nursing		

Contents

Section

I

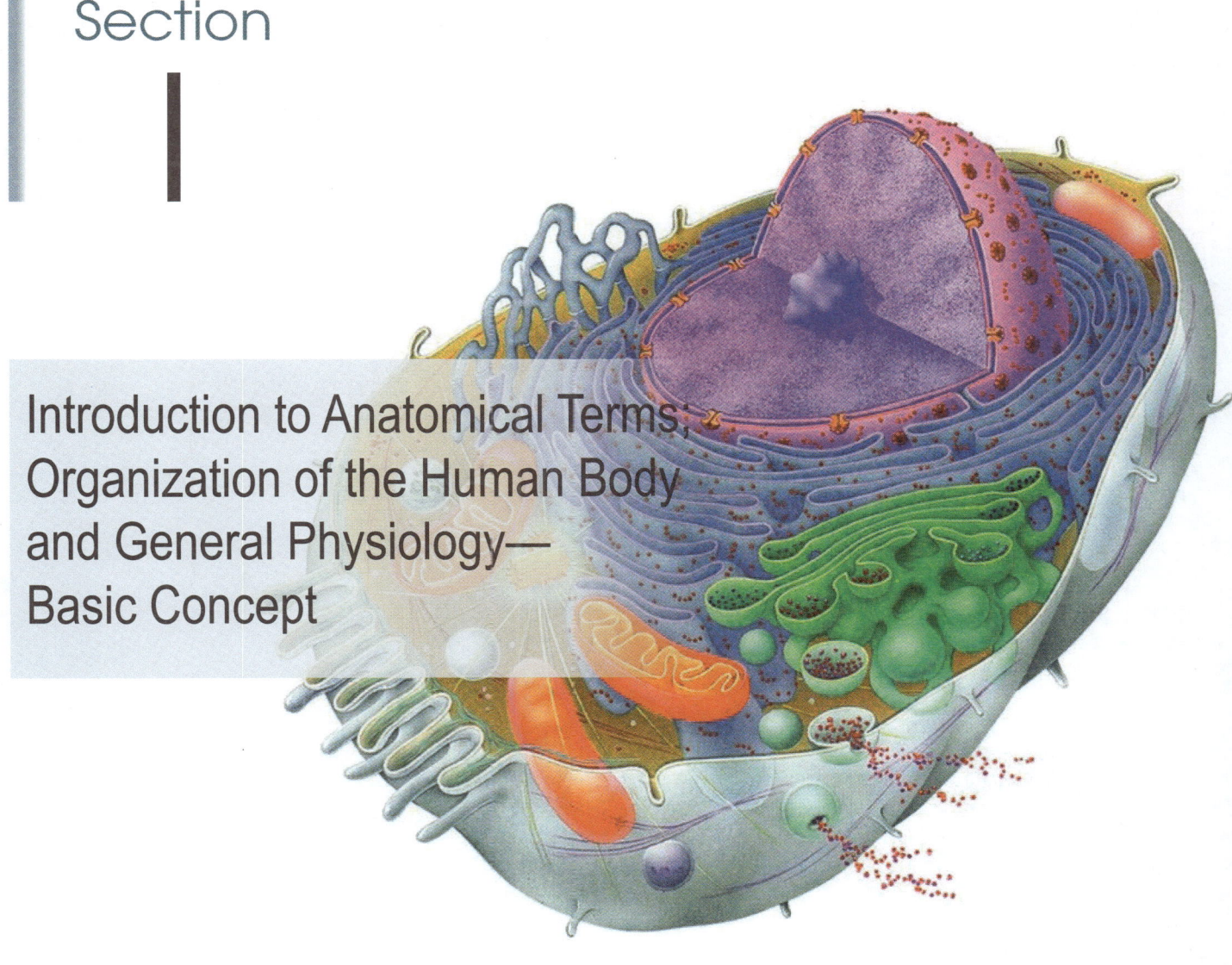

Introduction to Anatomical Terms, Organization of the Human Body and General Physiology— Basic Concept

Section Outline

Introduction to Anatomical and Physiological Terms and Organization of Human Body

ANATOMY AND PHYSIOLOGY: DEFINITIONS

Anatomy and physiology are two branches of science that help us to understand various parts of the body and their functions.

ANATOMY

Anatomy is the branch of biology which deals with the study of structure of the body. It has the following subdivisions:

Gross anatomy is the macroscopic structure of body parts that can be seen with the unaided eyes. It can be studied using either of the following two approaches:
- *Systemic anatomy:* Study of the different systems of body, e.g., cardiovascular system, respiratory system.
- *Regional anatomy:* Study of the specific region of the body, e.g., chest or abdomen.

Comparative anatomy is the study of similarities and differences in the structure of body parts of various species of animals.

Surface anatomy or topographic anatomy is the study of deeper parts of the body in relation to the skin surface. It is helpful in clinical practice and surgical operations.

Developmental anatomy or embryology refers to the study of development of animal body from the one cell stage to the period of growth and development before birth.

Histology is the study of minute structure of body parts that can only be seen with the aid of a microscope, and therefore, is often called *microscopic anatomy* or *microanatomy*.

Radiographic anatomy is the study of deeper organs by plain and contrast radiography and by other imaging techniques like CT (computed tomography) scan or and MRI (magnetic resonance imaging).

PHYSIOLOGY

Physiology, in simple terms, refers to the study of normal functioning of the living structures. The human physiology is concerned with the way various systems of the human body function and the way each contributes to the functions of the body as a whole. In other words, the human physiology is concerned with specific characteristics and mechanisms of the human body that make it a living being and the mechanisms which help in adaptation and homeostasis which are the two fundamental features of life. The term "physiology" includes following subdivisions:

General physiology this term envisages the general concepts and principles that are basic to the functions of all systems.

Systemic physiology deals with the functioning of different systems of the body, e.g., respiratory physiology includes different physiological aspects of respiration.

Cell physiology is the study of individual cells themselves, as they live out on a small scale all the activities that characterize larger organisms.

LEVELS OF STRUCTURAL COMPLEXITY

From smallest to the largest, there are 6 levels of structural organization of the human body (Figs 1.1-1A to F). They are:

Chemical level. This is the most basic level and includes atoms (the smallest unit of matter) and molecules (formed by joining of 2 or more atoms). Atoms like carbon, oxygen, hydrogen, calcium, etc. are essential for maintenance of life. Important molecules found in the human body are deoxyribonucleic acid (DNA), glucose, etc.

Cellular level. Various molecules combine to form the basic structural and functional unit of an organism, the cell. Various important cells in the body are epithelial cells, muscle cells,

nerve cells (nervous), osteoblasts (to bone forming cells), etc. Each cell has become specialized to carry out a particular function according to various needs of the body.

Tissue level. The cells with similar structure and functions combine together as a group to form a tissue. For example, muscle cells combine to form muscle tissue that performs a particular function.

Organ level. Multiple tissues combine together to form a particular organ, that has a recognizable shape and performs a specific function. For example, heart, stomach, liver, brain, lungs, etc.

System level. A number of organs and tissues together form a system that contributes to one or more survival needs of the body. For example, digestive system, nervous system, etc.

Organism level. The human body consists of several systems that work harmoniously and interdependently to carry out specific functions.

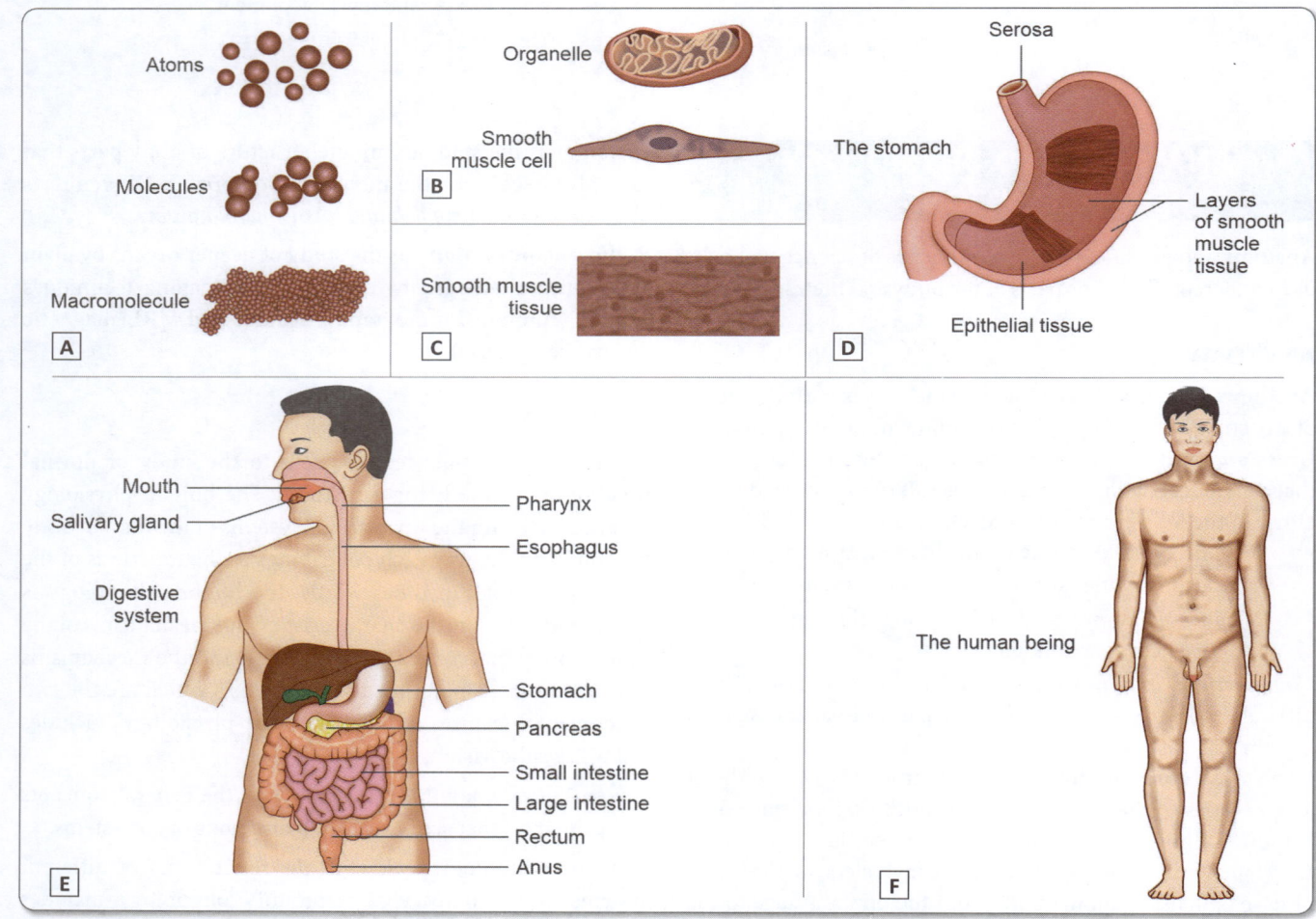

Figs 1.1-1A to F: Levels of structural organization of the human body; A. Chemical level; B. Cellular level; C. Tissue level; D. Organ level; E. Organ-system level; F. Organism level

REGIONAL ORGANIZATION OF HUMAN BODY AND ANATOMICAL TERMS

ANATOMICAL REGIONS AND CAVITIES OF THE BODY

Anatomical regions

For convenience of anatomical description, the human body can be divided into following regions (Fig. 1.1-2):

- Head and neck region
- Thorax
- Abdomen and pelvis
- Upper and lower extremities (limbs)

Cavities of human body

The organs that make up different systems of the body are contained in five cavities (Fig. 1.1-3):

- Cranial cavity
- Vertebral cavity
- Thoracic cavity
- Abdominal cavity
- Pelvic cavity

Head and Neck Region and Cranial Cavity

Head is the uppermost part of the body.

Face is the part of the head which includes the regions of forehead, eyes, nose, cheeks and chin.

Cranial cavity refers to that part of the head, which is bounded by the bones of skull and contains the brain.

Neck is that part of the body, which connects the head with the trunk. Trunk refers to combined thorax and abdomen.

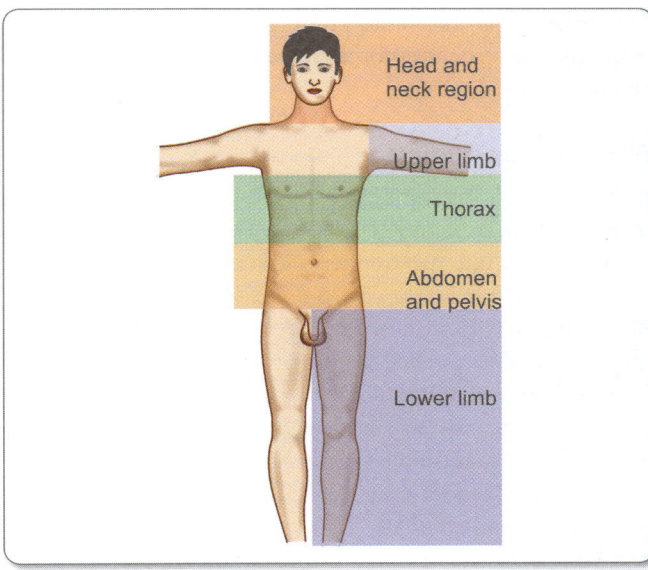

Fig. 1.1-2: Regions of the body

Thorax or Thoracic Cavity

Thorax refers to the chest, which is a cage formed by a bony framework and supporting muscles. This bony cage is also called thoracic cavity. It contains:

- Lungs, trachea and bronchi
- Heart and major blood vessels
- Esophagus
- Lymph vessels and lymph nodes
- Nerves

The thoracic cavity is divided into right and left cavities, each containing one lung.

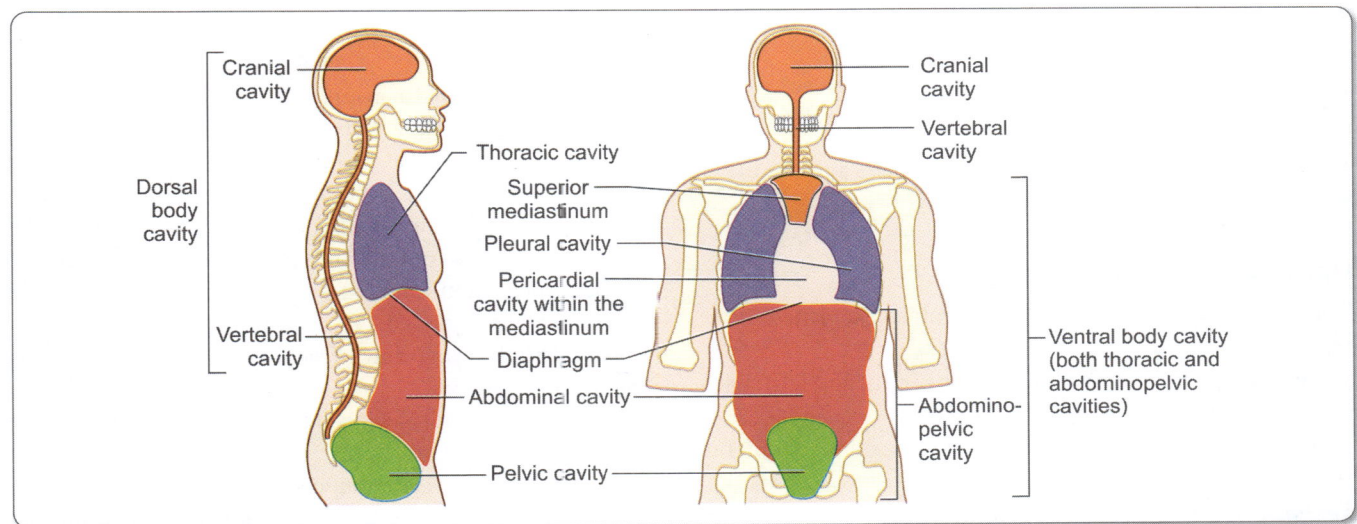

Fig. 1.1-3: Cavities of the human body

Mediastinum is the name given to the space between the lungs and the structures found there such as heart, esophagus and blood vessels.

Abdomen and Pelvis

Abdomen is the anatomical term used for the region of the trunk, which lies below the thorax. The region of abdomen can be divided into two cavities—abdominal cavity and pelvic cavity.

Abdominal cavity. It is separated from thoracic cavity by a muscular structure called diaphragm.

Contents. The abdominal cavity contains several organs of vital importance to body, such as:

- Stomach, small and large intestines
- Liver, gallbladder, pancreas and spleen
- Kidneys and adrenals
- Vessels, nerves, lymphatics and lymph nodes.

Regions. The abdominal cavity can be divided into following nine regions (Fig. 1.1-4) which facilitate the description of the positions of the organs and structures it contains:

- Right hypochondriac region (1)
- Epigastric region (2)
- Left hypochondriac region (3)
- Right lumbar region (4)
- Umbilical region (5)
- Left lumbar region (6)
- Right iliac fossa (7)
- Hypogastric region (8)
- Left iliac fossa (9)

Pelvic cavity. It refers to a funnel-shaped cavity, which extends from the lower end of the abdominal cavity. It is bounded by pelvic bones.

The contents of pelvic cavity include:

- Sigmoid colon, rectum and anus
- Some loops of small intestine
- Urinary bladder, lower parts of the ureters and urethra
- Some organs of reproductive system

Upper and Lower Extremities

The upper and lower extremities or limbs are attached to the trunk.

Upper limbs. There are two upper limbs (right and left). Each upper limb or upper extremity consists of:

Arm. The region of upper limb, which extends from the shoulder to elbow.

Forearm. The region between elbow and wrist.

Wrist. The area between forearm and hand.

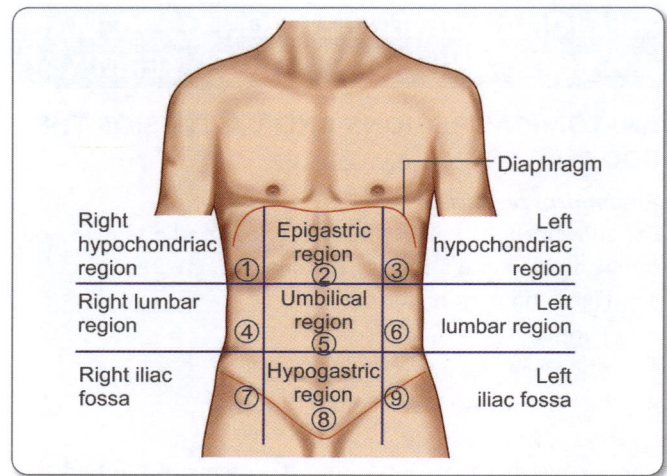

Fig. 1.1-4: Abdominal regions

Hand. It is the distal part of the upper limb which comprises the palm and digits (fingers and thumb).

Lower limbs. There are two lower limbs (right and left). Each lower limb or lower extremity consists of:

Thigh: The region between hip and knee joint.

Leg: The region between knee joint and ankle.

Ankle: The junction between the leg and foot.

Foot: The distal most part of lower limb which comprises the sole and digits (toes).

ANATOMICAL TERMS

For precise anatomical description of the mutual relationship between various structures of the body, following special anatomical terms are used.

Body Positions

Anatomical position. To ensure accuracy and consistency, all anatomical descriptions are made in relation to the anatomical position. The anatomical position refers to the position of body in which a person is presumed to be standing upright, with the head facing forward, the arms held by the sides of the body with the palms of the hands facing forward and the feet together. The anatomical names for specific body regions are also indicated in Figures 1.1-5A and B.

Supine position. Lying down (recumbent) position with the face directed upwards.

Prone position. Lying down (recumbent) position with the face directed downwards.

Lithotomy position. Lying supine with the buttocks at the edge of the table, the hips and knees fully flexed, and the feet strapped in position (Fig. 1.1-6).

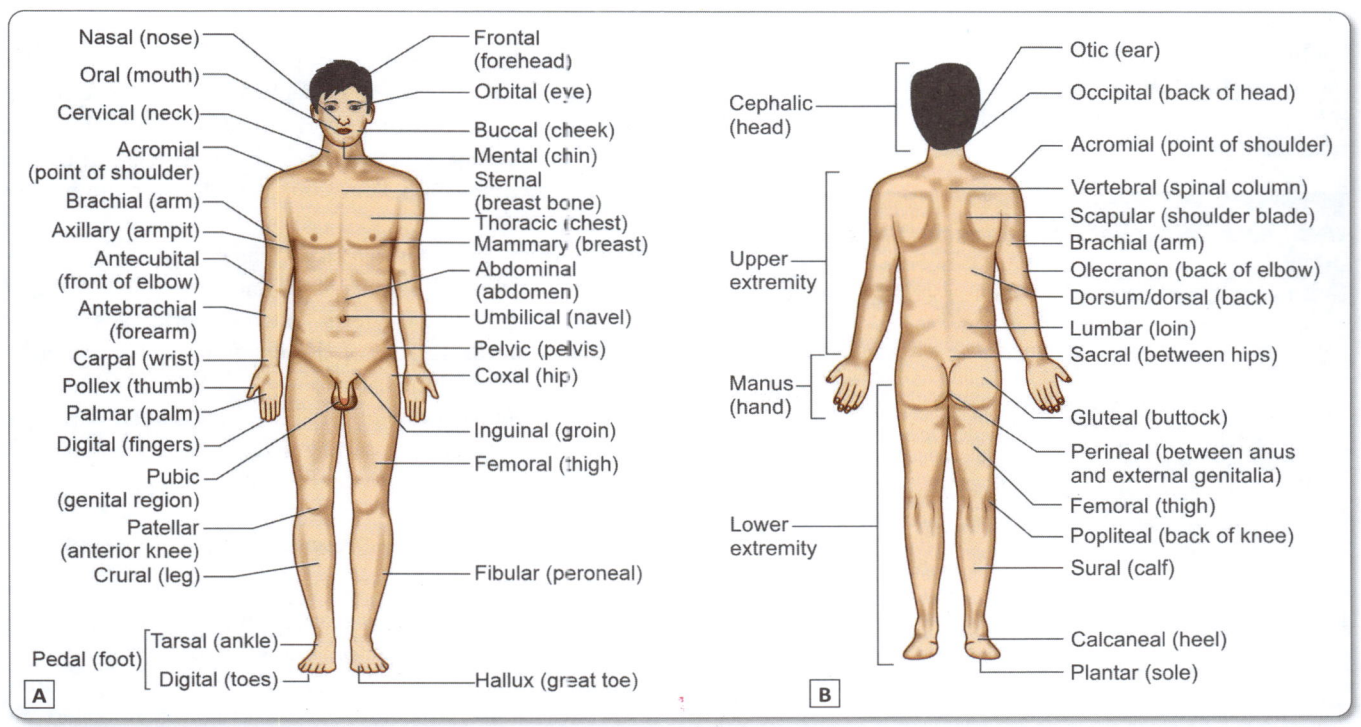

Figs 1.1-5A and B: Anatomical position: A. Anterior view; B. Posterior view. The anatomical names are indicated for specific body regions

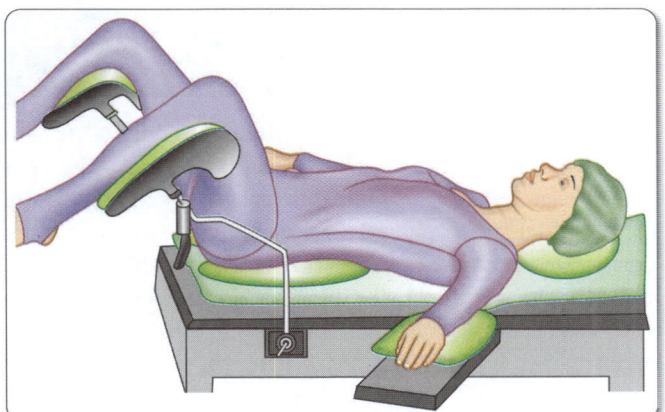

Fig. 1.1-6: Lithotomy position

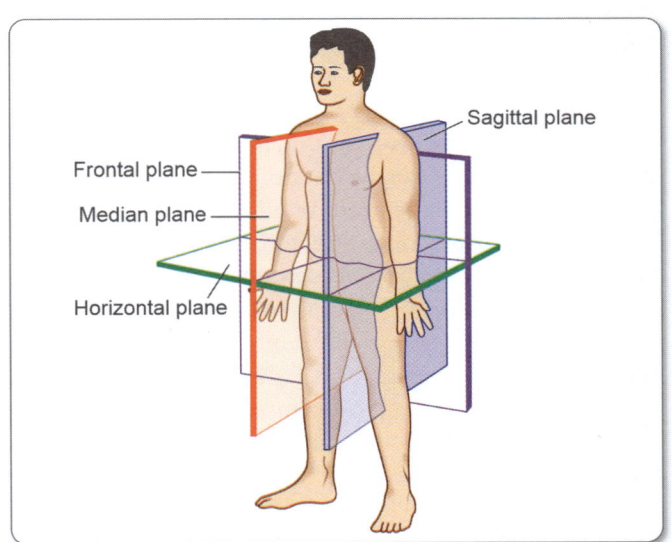

Fig. 1.1-7: Anatomical planes of reference

Anatomical Planes

Anatomical planes, to describe positions of the body, are (Fig. 1.1-7):

Median plane. Median or mid sagittal plane refers to the plane which passes longitudinally through midline when the body is in anatomical position. The median plane thus divides the body into two equal right and left halves.

Paramedian or sagittal planes. They refer to those planes which pass vertically through the body either to the right or left of the median plane and are parallel to the latter.

Coronal or frontal plane. It refers to the plane which is placed at right angle to the median plane and divides the body into anterior (ventral) and posterior (dorsal) parts.

Horizontal plane. It refers to the plane which passes horizontally across the body (i.e., at right angles to both the sagittal and coronal planes) and divides the body into upper and lower parts.

Transverse plane. Transverse plane passes at right angle to the longitudinal axis of the structure concerned. Thus, a transverse section through an artery is not necessarily horizontal. A transverse section through the hand is horizontal, whereas a transverse section through the foot is coronal.

NURSING IMPLICATIONS AND APPLICATIONS

- Directional terms are used in comparison of anatomical structures, which are useful in understanding the movements of body parts.
- The planes are important for knowing the structure of internal body organs from different body angles. Therefore, sagittal, coronal and horizontal planes are extensively used in imaging techniques like; CT scan (Computerized tomography), MRI (Magnetic resonance imaging) and ultrasonography.
- For treatment purpose planes are quite useful for surgeons to locate and remove the tumor growth without damaging the near by healthy tissues.

Paired Directional Terms

Paired directional terms used in anatomy are as follows:

Medial versus lateral. The term "medial" is used to describe a structure which is near to the median plane as compared to other structure. For example, the heart is medial to the lung. While the term "lateral" is used for a structure which is away from the median plane. For example, the lungs are lateral to the heart.

Anterior (ventral) versus posterior (dorsal). The term "anterior" or "ventral" is used to describe the position of a structure which lies near the front of the body. For example, the sternum is anterior to heart. While the term "posterior" or "dorsal" is used to describe a structure which lies near back of the body. For example, heart is posterior to the sternum.

Superior versus inferior. Structure located near the head is called superior. For example, skull is superior to scapula. While a structure located farther from the head is labeled inferior. For example, scapulae are inferior to the skull. While referring to structures in the trunk, the term *cranial* (towards the head) is sometimes used instead of superior; and the term *caudal* (towards the tail) in place of inferior.

Superficial versus deep. The term "superficial" is used for the structure which is placed toward the body surface, and the term "deep" is used for the structure which is placed inner to the surface.

Ipsilateral versus contralateral. The term "ipsilateral" is used to denote the structures of the same side and "contralateral" to denote the structures of the opposite side.

Special Terms Used for Limbs

Proximal versus distal: The term "proximal" is used for the attached end of a limb. For example, in the upper limb the humerous bone is proximal to radial bone. While the term "distal" is used for the structure which is away from the attached end of the limb. For example, in the lower limb, tibia is distal to femur.

Flexor versus extensor surface: Flexor surface refers to anterior surface of the upper limb and posterior surface of the lower limb. While the term "extensor surface" is used to describe posterior surface of the upper limbs and anterior surface of the lower limbs.

Palmar or volar versus plantar: The term "palmar" pertains to (toward) the palm of the hand and the term "plantar" pertains to (toward) the sole of the foot.

Terms Used for Hollow Organs

Interior versus exterior: The term "interior" is used to describe inner of the hollow organs, while the term "exterior" is used to describe the outer of hollow organs.

Invagination versus evagination: The term "invagination" refers to inward protusion, while "evagination" refers to outward protusion.

FUNCTIONAL ORGANIZATION OF THE HUMAN BODY

The human body is actually composed of about 100 trillion cells organized in different functional structures. The cells with similar features constitute different tissues and the tissues combine to form organs and organs combine to form a system. For convenience of description, the human body can be considered to be functionally organized into various systems.

INTEGUMENTARY SYSTEM (FIG. 1.1-8)

Integumentary system comprises skin and its appendages. Skin is the outermost covering of the human body. Its appendages include hairs, nails, sebacious glands and sweat glands. In addition to providing mechanical protection to the underlying tissues, the skin performs the following important functions:

- It acts as a physical barrier against entry of micro-organisms and other substances.
- It prevents loss of water from the body.
- It is a very important sensory organ, containing receptors for touch and related sensations.
- It plays an important role in regulating body temperature.

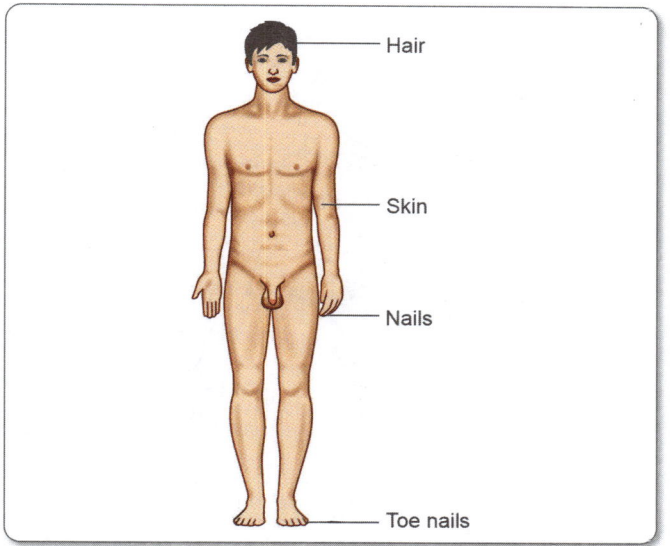

Fig. 1.1-8: Integumentary system

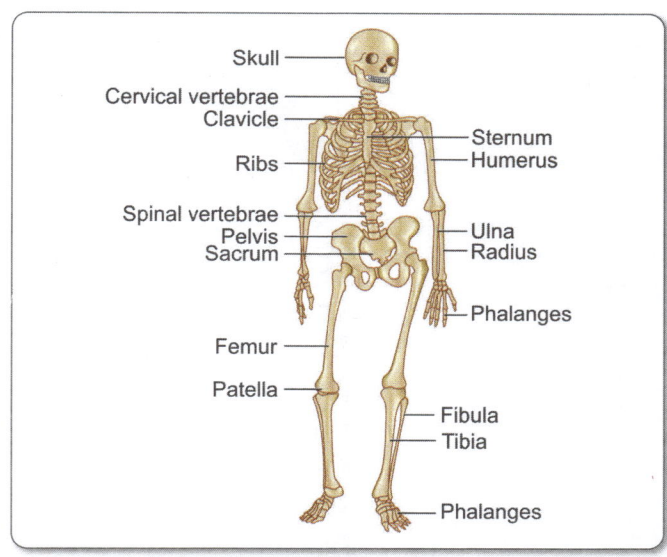

Fig. 1.1-9: Skeletal system

SKELETAL SYSTEM (FIG. 1.1-9)

The basic framework of the body is provided by a large number of bones that collectively form the skeleton. At joints, the bones are united to each other by fibrous bands called ligaments. In addition to the bones and joints, the skeletal system also includes the cartilages present in the body.

MUSCULAR SYSTEM (FIG. 1.1-10)

Overlying and usually attached to the bones are various muscles. Muscles are composed of many elongated cells called muscle fibers which are able to contract and relax. Three distinct types of muscles can be identified which are skeletal muscles, smooth muscles and cardiac muscles.

NERVOUS SYSTEM (FIG. 1.1-11)

The nervous system is made up, predominantly, of tissue that has the special property of being able to conduct impulses rapidly from one part of the body to another. The specialized cells that constitute the functional units of the nervous system are called neurons. The nervous system may be divided into: (i) the central nervous system, made up of brain and spinal cord, and (ii) the peripheral nervous system, consisting of the peripheral nerves and the ganglia associated with them.

CARDIOVASCULAR SYSTEM (FIG. 1.1-12)

The cardiovascular system consists of the heart and the blood vessels. The blood vessels that take blood from the heart to various tissues are called arteries. The smallest arteries are called arterioles. Arterioles open into a network of capillaries

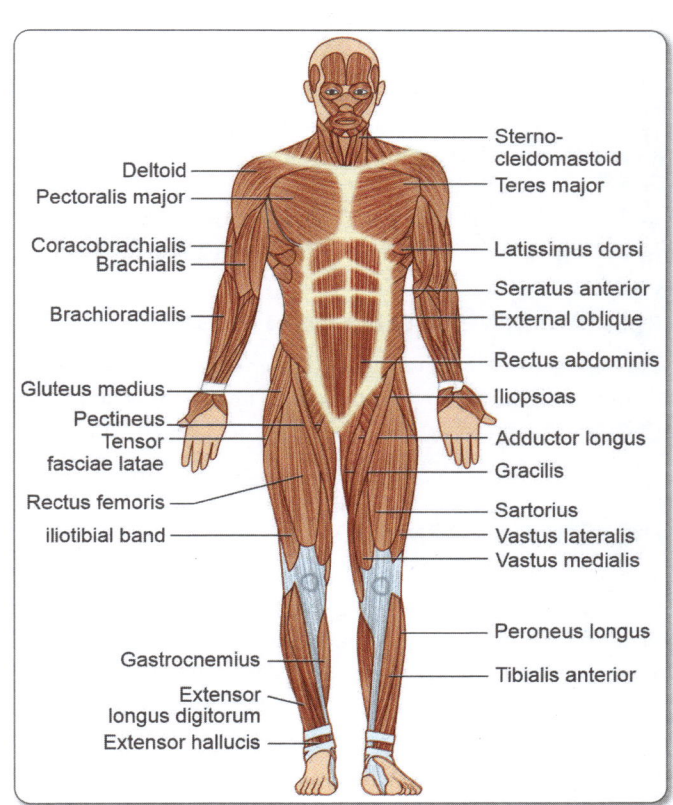

Fig. 1.1-10: Muscular system

that perfuse the tissues. Exchange of various substances between the blood and the tissues takes place through the walls of capillaries. In some situations, capillaries are replaced by slightly different vessels called sinusoids. Blood from

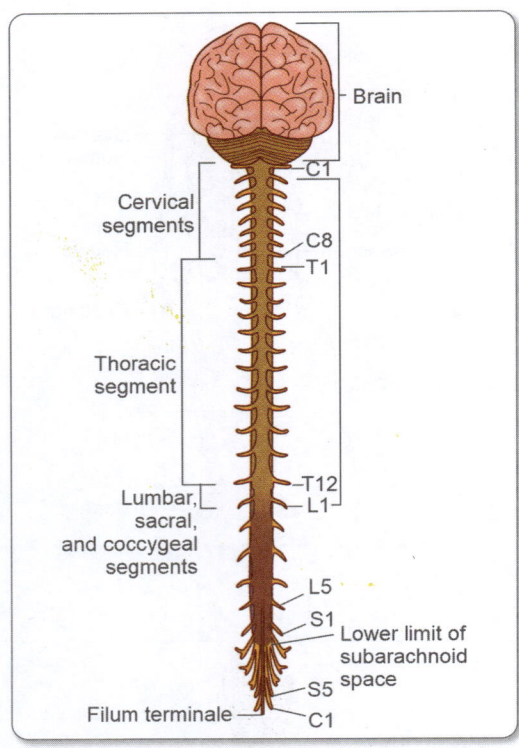

Fig. 1.1-11: Nervous system

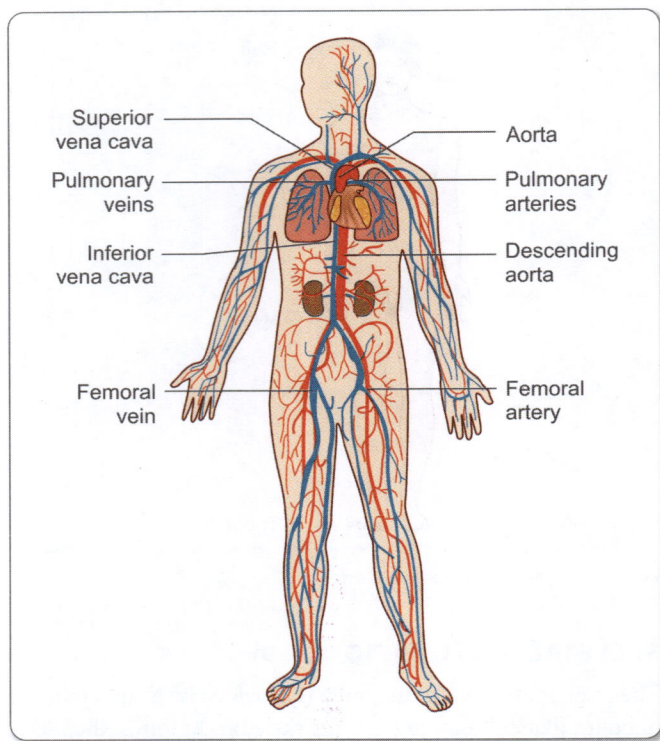

Fig. 1.1-12: Cardiovascular system

capillaries (or from sinusoids) is collected by small venules which join to form veins. The veins return blood to the heart.

RESPIRATORY SYSTEM (FIG. 1.1-13)

The respiratory system consists of the lungs and the passages through which air reaches them. The passages are nasal cavities, the pharynx, the trachea, the bronchi and their intrapulmonary continuations.

DIGESTIVE SYSTEM (FIG. 1.1-14)

The digestive or the so-called alimentary system includes all those structures that are concerned with eating, and with the digestion and absorption of food. The system consists of an alimentary canal which starts at the mouth and ends at the anus. The alimentary canal includes the oral cavity, pharynx, esophagus, stomach, small intestine and large intestine. Other structures included in the digestive system are the liver, the gallbladder and the pancreas.

EXCRETORY SYSTEM (FIG. 1.1-15)

Excretion is the removal of waste products of metabolism from the body. Egestion (or defecation) is the removal of undigested food from the gut and is not regarded as excretion

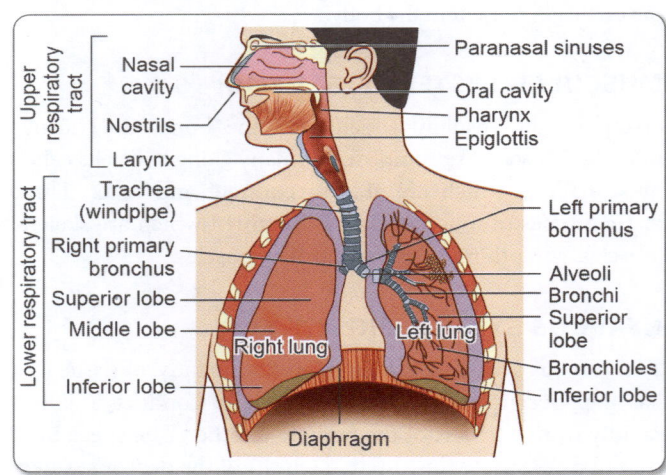

Fig. 1.1-13: Respiratory system

because the material taken into the gut through the mouth is not made by the body itself. The organs forming excretory system are the kidney, the ureters, the bladder and the urethra.

REPRODUCTIVE SYSTEM (FIGS 1.1-16A AND B)

Reproduction is the production of a new generation of individuals of the same species. It involves the transmission

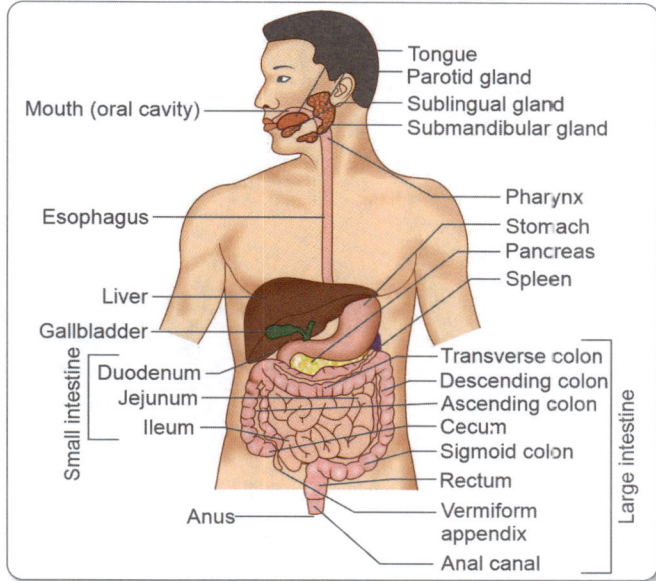

Fig. 1.1-14: Digestive system

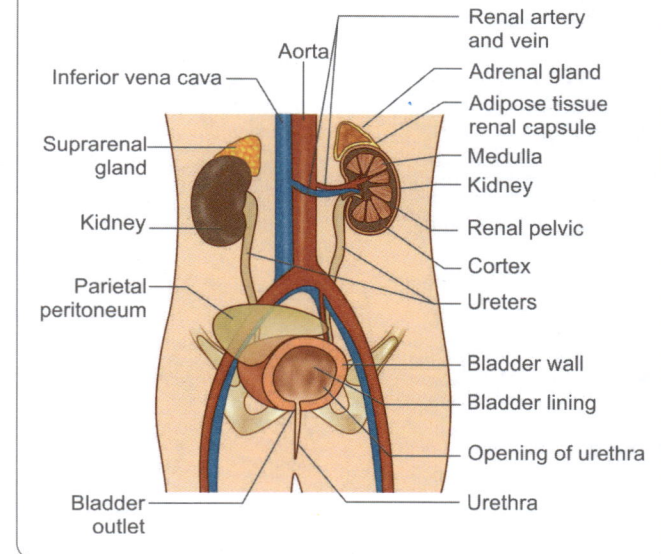

Fig. 1.1-15: Excretory system

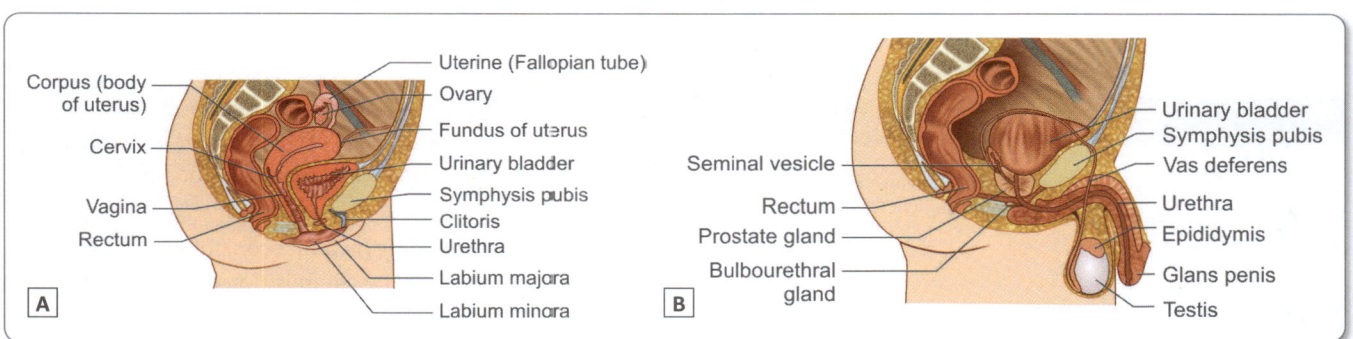

Figs 1.16A and B: Reproductive system: A. Female; B. Male

of genetic material from one generation to the next. The male reproductive organs are the testis, the epididymis, the ductus deferens, and the seminal vesicles (which are paired), and the prostate, the male urethra and the penis (which are unpaired). The female reproductive organs are the right and left ovaries and uterine tubes, the uterus, the vagina, the external genitalia and the mammary glands.

ENDOCRINE SYSTEM (FIG. 1.1-17)

Endocrine tissue is made up essentially of cells that produce secretions which are poured directly into blood. The secretions of the endocrine cells are called hormones. Some organs are entirely endocrine in function. They are referred to as endocrine glands (or ductless glands).Those traditionally included under this heading are the hypophysis

cerebri (pituitary gland), the pineal gland, the thyroid gland, the parathyroid glands, and the suprarenal (adrenal) glands. Groups of endocrine cells may be present in the organs that have other functions. These include the islets of Langerhans of pancreas, the interstitial cells of the testis, the follicles and corpora lutea of the ovaries. Hormones are also produced by some cells in the kidney, the thymus and the placenta. Some workers describe the liver as being partly an endocrine gland.

LYMPHATIC SYSTEM (FIG. 1.1-18)

The lymphatic system consists of lymph vessels, lymph (a tissue fluid that contains material drained from tissue spaces, including plasma proteins and sometimes bacteria), spleen, thymus, lymph nodes and tonsils. The lymphatic system provides sites for formation and maturation of lymphocytes.

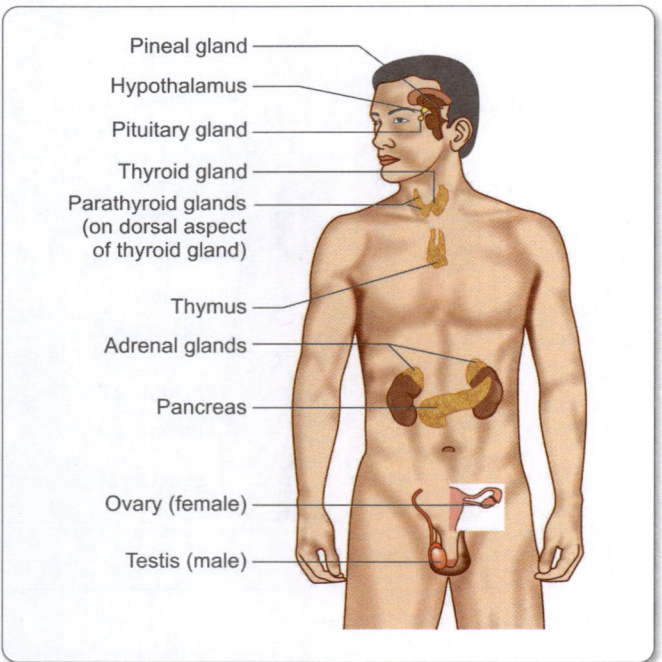

Fig. 1.1-17: Endocrine system

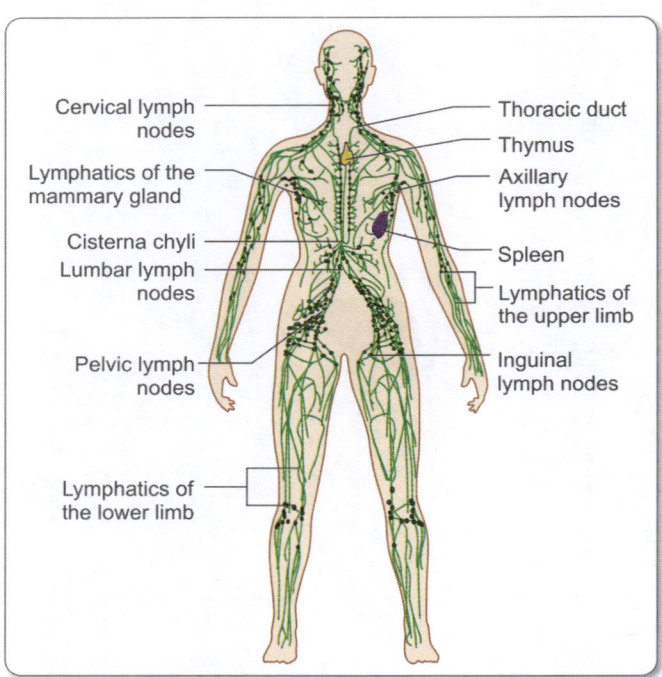

Fig. 1.1-18: Lymphatic system

BODY COMPOSITION

The normal body of an average adult male is composed of water (60%), minerals electrolytes (7%), protein and related substances (18%), and fat (15%).

TOTAL BODY WATER

Water is the principal and essential constituent of the human body. The total body water is about 10% less in a normal young adult female (average 50%) than that in average adult male (60%) due to relatively greater amount of adipose tissue in the females. In both sexes, the value tends to decrease with age.

Body Fluid Compartments

The total body water is distributed into two main compartments of the body fluids separated from each other by membranes freely permeable to water (Fig. 1.1-19, Table 1.1-1):

Intracellular fluid compartment. The intracellular fluid (ICF) compartment comprises about 40% of the body weight, the bulk of which is contained in the muscles.

Extracellular fluid compartment. The extracellular fluid (ECF) compartment constitutes about 20% of the body weight. The ECF compartment comprises the following:

Plasma. It is the fluid portion of the blood (*intravascular fluid*) and comprises about 5% of the body weight (i.e., 25% of the ECF). On an average, out of 5 liters of total blood volume, 3.5 liters is plasma.

Interstitial fluid including lymph. It constitutes major portion (about 3/4) of the ECF. The composition of interstitial fluid is the same as that of plasma, except it has little protein. Thus, interstitial fluid is an ultrafiltrate of plasma.

Transcellular fluid. It is the fluid contained in the secretions of the secretory cells and cavities of the body, e.g., saliva, sweat, bile, cerebrospinal fluid (CSF), intraocular fluids (aqueous humor and vitreous humor), pericardial fluid, fluid present between the layers (pleura, peritoneum and synovial membrane), lacrimal fluid and luminal fluids of the gut, thyroid and cochlea.

Mesenchymal tissue fluid. The mesenchymal tissues such as dense connective tissue, cartilage and bones contain about 6% of the body water.

The interstitial fluid, transcellular fluid and mesenchymal tissue fluid combinedly form the 75% of ECF.

The normal distribution of total body water in the fluid compartments is kept constant by two opposing sets of forces—osmotic and hydrostatic pressure.

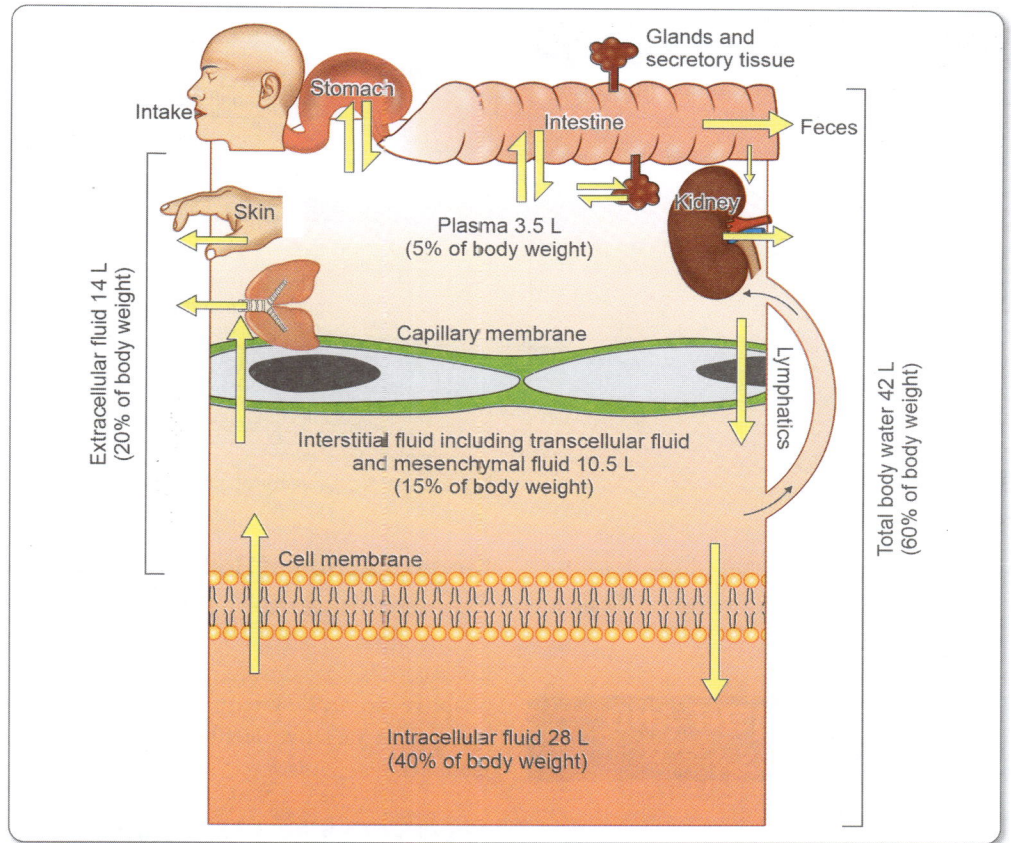

Fig. 1.1-19: Distribution of total body water in different compartments. Arrows indicate fluid movement

TABLE 1.1-1: Distribution of total body water in a normal 70 kg person

Compartment	Volume (L)	Percentage	
		Body weight	Body water
Total body water (TBW)	42	60	100
Intracellular fluid (ICF)	28	40	67
Extracellular fluid (ECF)	14	20	33
Plasma (25% of ECF)	3.5	05	08
Interstitial fluid, transcellular fluid and mesenchymal tissue fluid (75% of ECF)	10.5	15	25

BODY ELECTROLYTES

The electrolytes constitute about 7% of the total body weight. The distribution of electrolytes in various compartments differs markedly. Table 1.1-2 shows the distribution of electrolytes in two major compartments of body fluid—the extracellular fluid (ECF), and the intracellular fluid (ICF).

From Table 1.1-2, it may be noted that in the ICF, the main cations are K^+ and Mg^{2+}, and the main anions are PO_4^{3-} and proteins. While in ECF, the predominant cation is Na^+ and the principal anions are Cl^- and HCO_3^-. Besides these, a small proportion of non-diffusible proteins, nutrients and metabolites such as glucose and urea are also present in ECF.

IMPORTANT TO KNOW

It is important to note that:
- Essentially all of the body K^+ is in the exchangeable pool.
- Only 65–70% of the body Na^+ is exchangeable.
- Almost all of the body Ca^{2+} and Mg^{2+} are non-exchangeable.
- Only the exchangeable solutes are osmotically active.

Functions of Electrolytes

- Electrolytes are the main solutes in the body fluids for maintenance of acid-base balance.
- Electrolytes maintain the proper osmolality and volume of body fluids.

14   **Textbook of Applied Anatomy and Physiology for Nurses**

Section I ◉ Introduction to Anatomical Terms; Organization of the Human Body...

TABLE 1.1-2: Distribution of ions in the ECF and ICF (values are in mEq/L of H_2O)

Ion	Extracellular fluid (ECF)	Intracellular fluid (ICF)
Cations		
Na^+	142	14
K^+	5.5	150
Ca^{2+}	5	<1
Mg^{2+}	3	58
Anions		
Cl^-	103	4
HCO_3^-	28	10
PO_4^{3-}	4	75
Protein	1 g/dL	5 g/dL

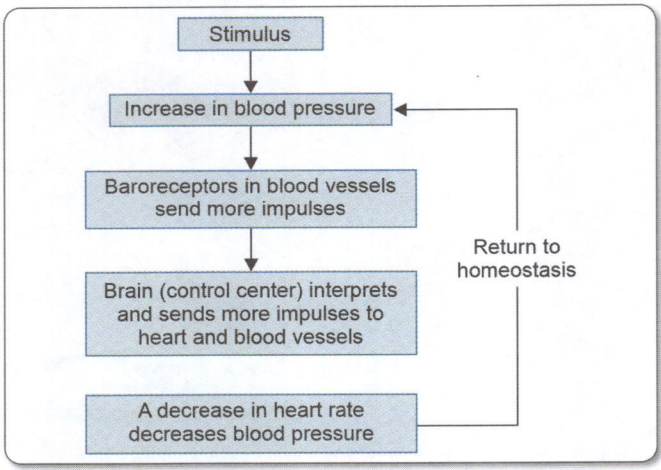

Fig. 1.1-20 Negative feedback mechanism

- The concentration of certain electrolytes determines their specific physiologic functions, e.g., the effect of calcium ions on neuromuscular excitability.

INTERNAL ENVIRONMENT AND HOMEOSTASIS

INTERNAL ENVIRONMENT

Claude Bernard (1813–1878), the great French physiologist, introduced the term "internal environment" of the body or the *milieu interieur* for the ECF of the body. He said so since all the body cells essentially depend upon the ECF for maintenance of cellular life. Cells are capable of living, growing and performing their special functions so long as the proper concentration of oxygen, glucose, different ions, amino acids, fatty substances and other constituents are available in the internal environment.

HOMEOSTASIS

Homeostasis, a term introduced by WB Cannon, refers to the mechanism by which the constancy of the internal environment is maintained and ensured. For this purpose, living membranes with varying permeabilities such as vascular endothelium and cell membrane play important role.

Factors involved in the maintenance of internal environment can be summarized as:
- Maintenance of pH of ECF (acid-base balance)
- Regulation of temperature
- Maintenance of water and electrolyte balance
- Supply of nutrients, oxygen, enzymes and hormones
- Removal of metabolic and other waste products

Mode of Action of Homeostatic Control System

The homeostasis is a complex phenomenon. The mode of operation of all the systems, which are involved in the homeostasis, is through 'feedback' mechanism and the adaptive control system. Feedback mechanism is of two types—the negative feedback mechanism and the positive feedback mechanism.

Negative Feedback Mechanism

Most control systems of the body act by negative feedback. That is, in general if the activity of a particular system is increased or decreased, a control system initiates a negative feedback, which consists of a series of changes that return the activity toward normal.

Examples of a feedback mechanism
- When the blood pressure suddenly rises or lowers, it initiates a series of reactions that tries to bring the blood pressure to normal levels (Fig. 1.1-20).
- When thyroxine secretion is more, it inhibits the secretion of thyroid stimulating hormone (TSH) from pituitary so that thyroxine is not secreted from the thyroid gland.

Positive Feedback Mechanism

Positive feedback is better known as a vicious circle. Usually, it is harmful and in some instances, even death can occur due to positive feedback. For example, as shown in Fig. 1.1-21, when a person has suddenly bled 2L of blood, a vicious circle of progressive weakening of the heart is set which ultimately causes death.

Sometimes positive feedback can serve useful purposes under the following circumstances:

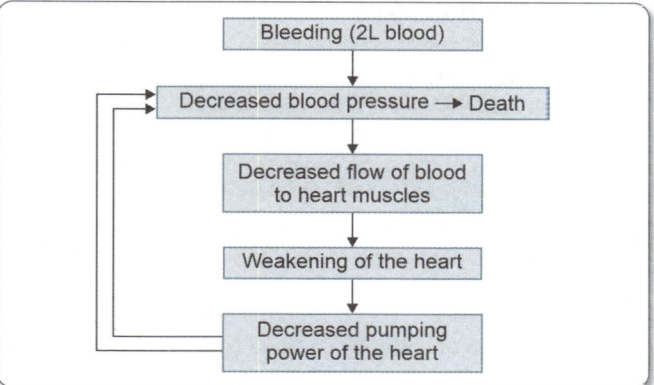

Fig. 1.1-21: How a positive feedback mechanism can cause death

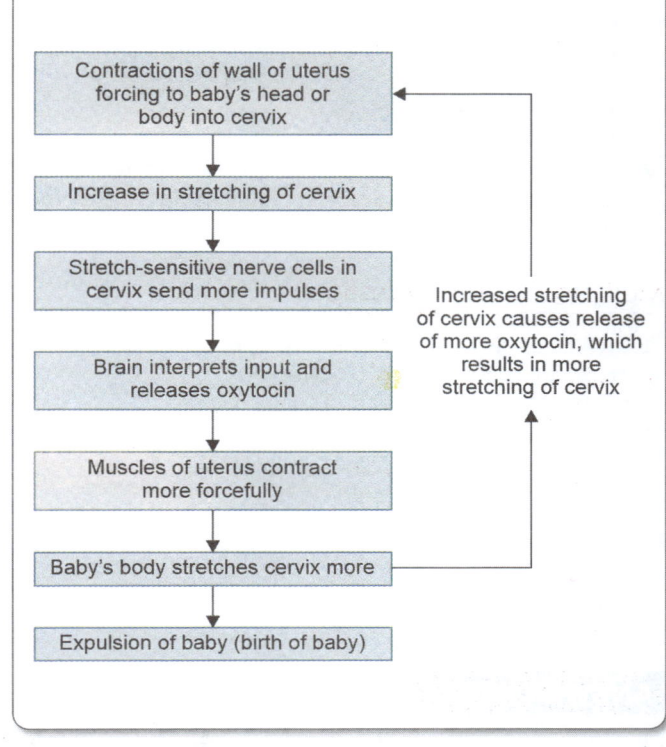

Fig. 1.1-22 Positive feedback mechanism

- Clot formation following rupture of vessels is accelerated by vicious cycle of thrombin formation. This stops the bleeding.
- Child birth during labor is facilitated by progressively increasing uterine contractions due to positive feedback from stretching of cervix by head of the baby (Fig. 1.1-22).
- Generation of nerve signals by the vicious cycle of progressive leakage of Na^+ ions from the channels set up following the stimulation of membrane of nerve fiber is due to the positive feedback.

Adaptive Control System

Adaptive control system refers to a delayed type of negative feedback mechanism. This is seen in nervous system. For example, when some movements of the body occur very rapidly, there is not enough time for nerve signals to travel from the peripheral parts of the body all the way to the brain and then back to the periphery again in time to control the movements. Under such circumstances, brain uses a principle called feed-forward control to cause the required muscle contraction, which is retrospectively conveyed to the brain by the sensory nerve signals from the moving part. If the movement performed is found incorrect, then the brain corrects the feed-forward signals that it sends to the muscle the next time the movement is required. Such a correction made by successive retrospective feedback mechanism is called adaptive control.

ASSESS YOURSELF

Short and Long Answer Questions

1. **Define the following terms:**
   - Gross anatomy
   - Surface anatomy
   - Developmental anatomy
   - Histology
   - Radiographic anatomy
   - General physiology
   - Systemic physiology
2. **Describe briefly the chemical level of human body.**
3. **What are different anatomical regions of abdomen?**
4. **What are the contents of:**
   - Thoracic cavity
   - Abdominal cavity
   - Pelvic cavity
5. **Describe the following terms:**
   - Medial and lateral
   - Ipsilateral and contralateral
   - Pronation and supination
   - Adduction and abduction

6. **Write short notes on:**
   - Body composition
   - Total body water and its distribution in various body fluid compartments
   - Feedback mechanism
   - Homeostasis
7. **Write a note on distribution of electrolytes in the extracellular and intracellular compartments and their significance.**

Multiple Choice Questions

1. **Which of the following is located in mediastinum?**
   a. Heart   b. Liver
   c. Uterus   d. Urinary bladder
2. **The system that removes carbon dioxide from the body is:**
   a. Skin   b. Cardiovascular
   c. Respiratory   d. Urinary
3. **Which is not a feature of anatomical position?**
   a. Erect standing   b. Pronated forearms
   c. Feet together   d. Eyes looking forward

4. **True about adduction is:**
   a. Movement toward central axis
   b. Movement away from central axis
   c. Approximation of two ventral surfaces
   d. Approximation of two dorsal surfaces
5. **The position of forearms in anatomical position:**
   a. Midprone   b. Pronated
   c. Supinated   d. Abducted
6. **The plane at right angle to the long axis of body is a:**
   a. Horizontal plane   b. Sagittal plane
   c. Coronal plane   d. Frontal plane
7. **The main ion of extracellular fluid is:**
   a. Na^+
   b. K^+
   c. Mg^{2+}
   d. PO_4^-
8. **The concentration of K^+ in the extracellular fluid is:**
   a. 142 mEq/L
   b. 152 mEq/L
   c. 58 mEq/L
   d. 5 mEq/L

ANSWER KEY

1.	a	**2.**	c	**3.**	b	**4.**	a	**5.**	a	**6.**	c	**7.**	a	**8.**	d

Introduction to Chemistry of Life

INTRODUCTION

In Chapter 1.1, under levels of structural organization, we learnt that the lowest levels of organization are atoms and molecules. The study of anatomy and physiology depends on understanding some concepts of biochemistry, the chemistry of life. This also includes the study of several groups of molecules that have unique properties contributing to the assembly of various structures of the human body and helping in powering various processes necessary for life.

Before we continue to explore the unique chemistry of life, it is important to understand what these biomolecules are comprised of.

ATOMS

All forms of matter are made up of small building blocks called chemical elements. An element is a substance that cannot be split into a simpler substance by ordinary chemical means. There are 117 elements recognized now, out of which 92 are naturally occurring in the earth. Atoms are the smallest unit of matter that retain the characteristics of an element. An element consists of one type of atoms, e.g., hydrogen, oxygen, nitrogen, etc.

A compound contains 2 or more types of atoms. For example, water (H_2O) contains atoms of hydrogen (H) and oxygen (O).

There are a variety of compounds that make up the human body and they are primarily composed of 4 elements—carbon, hydrogen, oxygen and nitrogen. The other important elements are sodium, potassium, calcium, sulfur, iron and phosphorus.

STRUCTURE OF AN ATOM

An atom consists of a small nucleus in the center containing neutrons (that carry no electrical charge) and protons (that carry positive electrical charge), enveloped by a cloud of negatively charged particles called electrons.

Although it is hard to predict the exact positions of the electrons, specific groups of electrons move about within certain regions around the nucleus, called electron shells and are depicted as simple circles around the nucleus. The electron shell can hold only a specific number of electrons. The first shell, which is the closest to the nucleus, cannot hold more than 2 electrons.

Further shells can also hold only a specific number of electrons. For example, second shell can hold only 8, third shell can hold only 18 and so on (Fig. 1.2-1).

Because an atom contains equal number of protons and electrons, it carries no net charge.

ATOMIC NUMBER AND ATOMIC WEIGHT

Atomic Number

Atomic number is the number of protons in the nucleus of an atom. Atoms of different elements have different atomic numbers because the number of protons is different in the nucleus of every atom.

For example, hydrogen has 1 proton in its nucleus, carbon has 4, oxygen has 8 and sodium has 11. Therefore, the atomic number of hydrogen is 1, carbon is 4, oxygen is 8 and sodium is 11. The atomic structures of these elements are given in Figure 1.2-2.

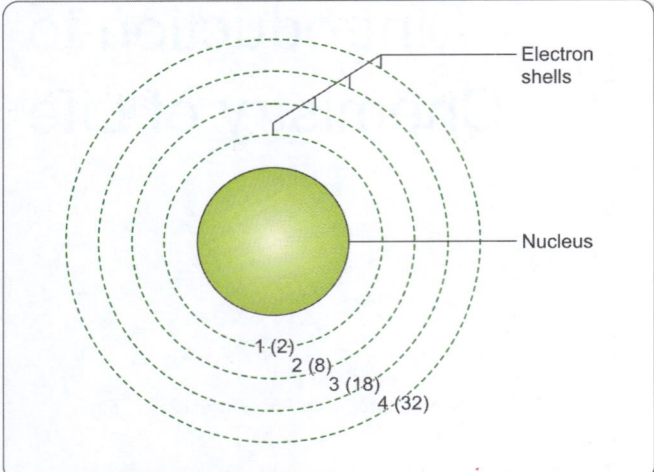

Fig. 1.2-1: Structure of an atom

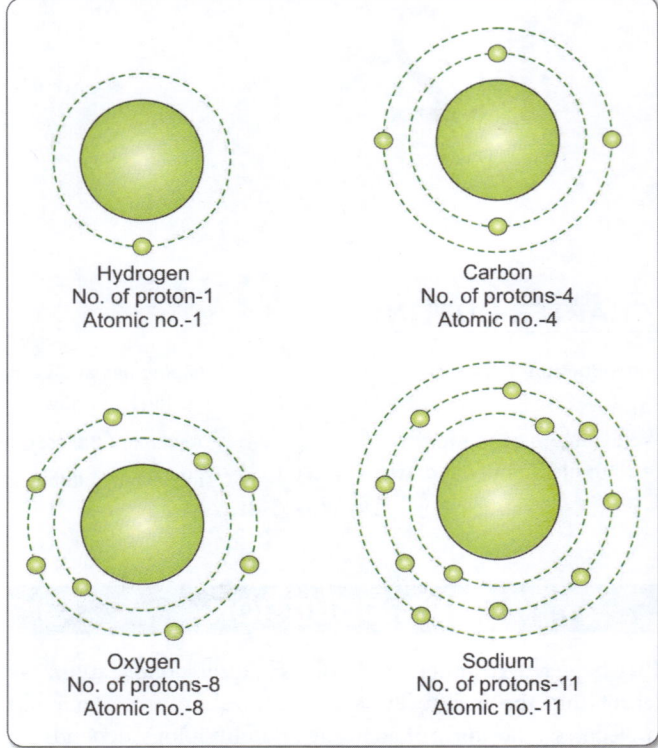

Fig. 1.2-2: Atomic structures of the elements: hydrogen, carbon, oxygen and sodium

The Atomic Weight

The atomic weight of an element is the sum of protons and neutrons in the atomic nucleus. For example, the atomic weight of oxygen is 16 (8 neutrons + 8 protons) and sodium is 23 (11 protons + 12 neutrons). When the atom does not contain stable number of electrons in the outer shell, it becomes reactive and will either share, donate or receive electrons to gain stability. This leads to the formation of innumerable substances present in the world.

IMPORTANT TO KNOW

Isotopes

Isotopes are the atoms of a chemical element with different number of neutrons in the nucleus. Thus, they share the same atomic number but different atomic weight. Different number of neutrons does not affect the electrical activity of the element. For example, Carbon has 3 isotopes: Carbon-12, Carbon-13 and Carbon-14 with no. of protons being 6 in all of them and no. of neutrons being 6, 7 and 8, respectively.

The atomic weight of an element is actually the average atomic weight of all its atoms. Therefore, the actual atomic weight of carbon is 12.011.

MOLECULES AND COMPOUNDS

A molecule is formed when 2 or more atoms join together chemically. The atoms can be of the same element or different elements. A compound is formed by atoms of 2 different elements. Hence, all compounds are molecules, but not all molecules are compounds. For example, a molecule of oxygen contains 2 atoms of oxygen as it is depicted as O_2. Water (H_2O) and carbon dioxide (CO_2) are compounds as they contain atoms of 2 different elements.

IONIC AND COVALENT BONDS

Atoms are joined together by a chemical bond that can be either ionic or covalent bond.

Ionic bonds are formed when one element transfers the electrons to the other and becomes positively and negatively charged, respectively, making the two stick together because of this mutually attractive charge. For example, sodium chloride is held together by an ionic bond (Fig. 1.2-3).

Covalent bonds are formed between two or more elements, when they share their electrons with each other. Most molecules are formed because of this bond. Covalent bond is strong and more stable than ionic bond. For example, water is formed by covalent bond between hydrogen and oxygen. The outer shell of hydrogen contains just one electron and that of oxygen contains only 6. For hydrogen to get stable, it needs one more electron and for oxygen to get stable, it need 2 electrons. Hence, oxygen shares electrons with 2 hydrogen atoms and forms a stable compound, water (Fig. 1.2-4).

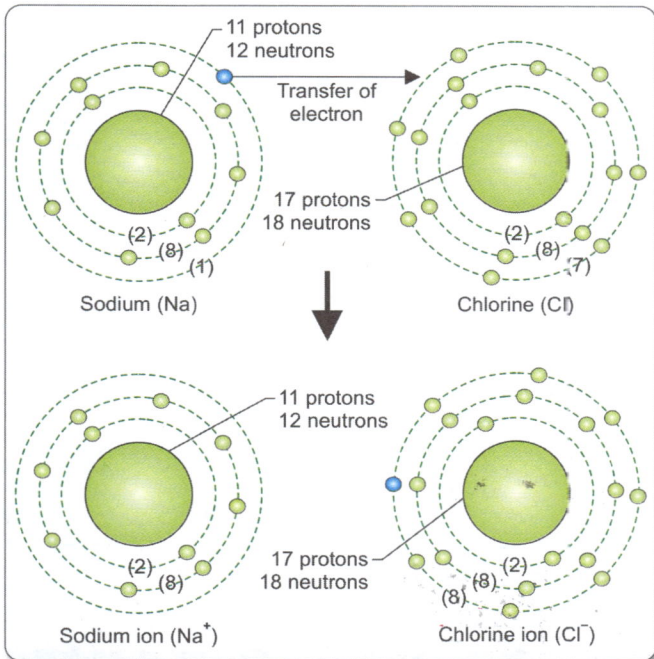

Fig. 1.2-3: Ionic bond between sodium and chlorine

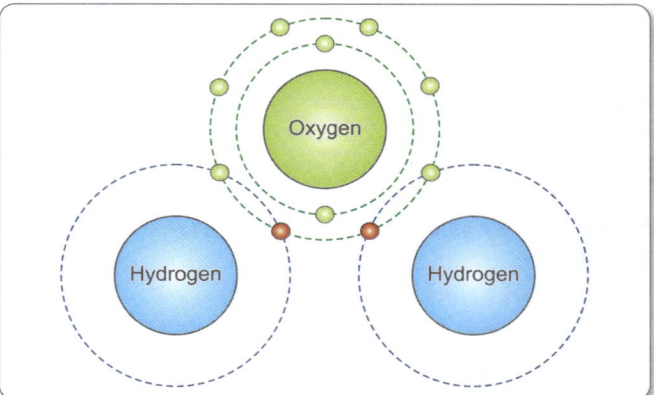

Fig. 1.2-4: Covalent bond between hydrogen and oxygen to form water molecule

as 7 that depicts the neutral nature of a fluid. pH of pure water is 7.

IMPORTANT TO KNOW

Water (H_2O) is considered to be a neutral molecule as it gives out one H^+ and one OH^- that balance out each other.

The values below 7 are considered to be acidic and above 7 are alkaline.

The pH values of important body fluids are enlisted in Table 1.2-1.

TABLE 1.2-1: pH of body fluids	
Body fluids	**pH value**
Cerebrospinal fluid	7.349
Blood	7.39
Lymph	7.4
Synovial fluid	7.434
Saliva	6.4
Gastric juice	1.92–2.59
Bile	7.15–7.5
Feces	7.15
Urine	5.7
Sweat	4–6.8

IMPORTANT TO KNOW

Electrolytes

Electrolytes are the substances which when dissolved in water conduct electricity. They are usually ionic compounds like sodium chloride: They form an important constituent of the body as they help in:

● Muscular and nervous activity by conducting electricity
● Keeping body fluids in their compartments by exerting osmotic pressure and resist pH changes in body fluids.
● Other important electrolytes found in the body are potassium (K^+), calcium (Ca^{2+}), bicarbonate (HCO_3^-) and phosphate (PO_4^3) (For details *refer to* page 13).

ACIDS AND BASES: CONCEPT OF pH

The biochemical processes of life produce or consume hydrogen ions (H^+) and the living cells are highly sensitive to the changes in H^+ concentration. pH is the measuring system, used as an indicator of acidity or alkalinity of a fluid based on the concentration of H^+ ions.

● An acidic substance releases H^+ ions when in a solution and an alkaline or basic substance accepts H^+ and releases hydroxyl (OH^-) ions.
● The acidic and alkaline nature of a fluid is determined through pH scale. It measures from 0 to 14, with midpoint

IMPORTANT BIOLOGICAL MOLECULES

CARBOHYDRATES

Carbohydrates are the most abundant biological molecules containing C, H and O, which are combined in the ratio of 2 : 1. Depending upon the number of monomer units present in a molecule, carbohydrates are classified as monosaccharides, disaccharides, oligosaccharides and polysaccharides.

Monosaccharides

Monosaccharides are simple sugars, which can join in several ways to form di-, oligo- and polysaccharides. According to the number of carbon atoms, monosaccharides are designated as trioses, tetroses, pentoses, and hexoses.

Hexoses contain six carbon atoms, Such as:
- Glucose (an aldohexose) and fructose (a ketohexose).
- Glucose, commonly known as dextrose, is used as a source of energy in the body. Galactose is a constituent of milk sugar lactose. Fructose is a constituent of the common sugar sucrose.

Monosaccharides of biological importance are exhibited in Figure 1.2-5.

Disaccharides

Disaccharides consist of two similar or dissimilar monosaccharides which are linked together by a glycosidic bond. These include: Maltose, lactose and sucrose.

Note: Sucrose, also known as invert sugar, is the most abundant disaccharide, which is found in plants. It is also referred to as table sugar or cane sugar. It is hydrolyzed to its mono-saccharides, i.e., glucose and fructose by the intestinal enzyme sucrase, which is also referred to as invertase (Fig. 1.2-6).

Polysaccharides

These are polymers of a large number (usually more than ten) of monosaccharides, which are linked together by glycosidic bonds. The polysaccharides are present in the following forms:
- Starch
- Glycogen
- Cellulose (plant polysaccharide)

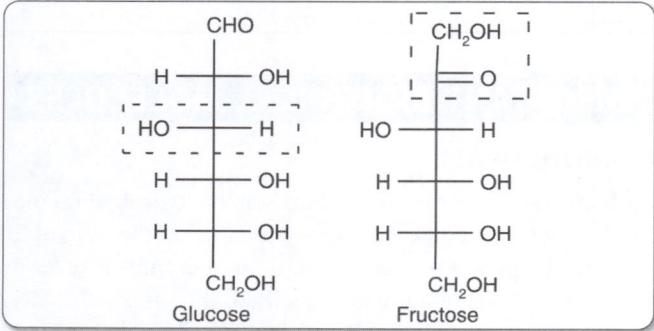

Fig. 1.2-5: Structure of glucose and fructose

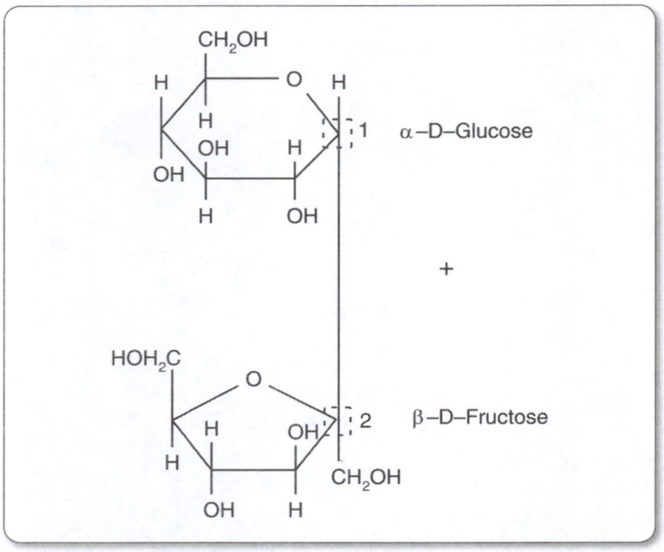

Fig. 1.2-6: Structure of sucrose

LIPIDS

Lipid is a heterogeneous group of hydrophobic organic molecules found in cells. Lipids exhibit greater structural variability and are classified into three groups as simple lipids, compound lipids and derived lipids.

Simple lipids are esters of fatty acids with alcohol. These include neutral fats, oils and waxes.

Neutral fats and oils are the mixtures of triacylglycerols (triglycerides) whose fatty acid composition may vary with source. They differ only in that fats are solid, while oils are liquid at room temperature.

Compound fats in addition to fatty acids and alcohol, compound lipids also contain an amphipathic group. For example, lipids conjugated with phosphoric acid are called phospholipids. They are obtained after hydrolysis of simple and compound lipids. They include fatty acids, glycerol, etc.

Fatty acids are the carboxylic acids with a long hydrocarbon side chain which may be saturated or unsaturated with one or more double bonds.

Chapter 1.2 ⊙ Introduction to Chemistry of Life   21

Section I ⊙ Introduction to Anatomical Terms; Organization of the Human Body...

Triacylglycerols (also called triglycerides) or neutral fats are fatty acid triesters of glycerol (glycerin), which is a trihydric alcohol.

Glycerol with one molecule of fatty acid is called monoacylglycerol, with two molecules of fatty acids, a diacylglycerol and with three molecules of fatty acids, a triacylglycerol.

Phospholipids are a heterogeneous group of compounds, which contain one or more phosphoric acid residues and a polar group that may be a nitrogenous base, an amino acid or a polyhydroxy-alcohol. In addition, they also contain one or two long chain fatty acids.

Steroids, the most common steroid is cholesterol. Cholesterol is the most abundant steroid found in animals.

Because of the presence of the OH group, cholesterol is called a steroid alcohol (sterol). Due to the presence of this group, cholesterol can form an ester with a long chain fatty acid and form cholesterol esters.

NURSING IMPLICATIONS AND APPLICATIONS

Significance of Lipids

- Triacylglycerol stored in adipose tissue releases free fatty acids during fasting and starvation.
- They are the structural components of biomembranes (phospholipids and cholesterol).
- They also act as metabolic regulators (steroid hormones and prostaglandins).
- They act as surfactants, detergents and emulsifying agents (amphipathic lipids).
- They act as electric insulators in myelin sheath of nervous system.
- They provide insulation against changes in external temperature (subcutaneous fat).
- They give shape and contour to the body.
- They protect internal organs by providing a cushioning effect (pads of fat)—loss of these fat pad lead to visceroptosis.
- They help in absorption of fat soluble vitamins (A, D, E and K).
- They improve taste and palatability of food.

PROTEINS AND AMINO ACIDS

Proteins

Protein is a class of natural products, which contains nitrogen. It is well known that proteins are the center of action in biological processes and are essential structural components of a cell. They are most abundant and functionally diverse molecules present in all living systems.

Amino Acids

All proteins are polymers of small units called amino acids. Though a large number of amino acids have been described in nature, only 20 are commonly found as constituents of mammalian proteins. Amino acids are also called building blocks of proteins.

When several amino acids are linked together, they form polypeptides and proteins. Each polypeptide has a free α-amino group on the left hand side of the peptide chain. This end of the protein chain is referred to as N-terminal (amino terminal) end:

- Amino acids are important dietary sources of nitrogen.
- They are used in protein biosynthesis.
- Glucogenic amino acids, e.g., alanine, serve as a source of energy.
- Some of the amino acids are also used in the biosynthesis of various specialized products. For example—Aromatic amino acids are the precursors of thyroid hormones, catecholamines and melanin.

Amino acids are of two types:

1. Essential amino acids
2. Nonessential amino acids

Essential Amino Acids

All amino acids that cannot be synthesized in the body and are to be essentially included in the diet are called indispensable or essential amino acids. There are eight amino acids which are essential for adult human beings. These are as follows:

- Methionine
- Threonine
- Tryptophan
- Valine
- Isoleucine
- Leucine
- Phenylalanine
- Lysine

Nonessential Amino Acids

Remaining all the amino acids that can be synthesized by a normal human being and are not dietary essential are called non-essential amino acids.

NURSING IMPLICATIONS AND APPLICATIONS

Significance of Proteins

With respect to their biological importance, proteins are divided into several groups.

Structural Proteins. Some of the proteins, e.g., collagens (found in bone and cartilage), keratins (found in hair and nail), etc., form an essential part of particular structures within the body.

Enzymes. Some of the proteins, such as pepsin, catalyze biological reactions and act as enzymes.

Hormones. Some of the proteins act as hormones, e.g., insulin. They regulate metabolic processes within the body.

Transport proteins. Some of the proteins, e.g., hemoglobin, ceruloplasmin, etc., serve as carriers for the transport of certain substances within the body and are called transport proteins.

Receptors. Proteins, such as hormone receptors, act as receptors for certain hormones and play an important role in signal transduction.

Storage Proteins. Some of the proteins bind to a substance for its storage in different tissues in the body, e.g., ferritin for the storage of Fe^{3+}.

Antibodies. Proteins, such as γ-globulin, act as antibodies and provide immunity.

Enzymes

Enzymes are organic molecules that are produced in living organisms and increase the rate of a biochemical reaction without being utilized in the overall process. An enzyme increases the rate of a chemical reaction by lowering its free energy barrier that separates a substrate (reactant) from the product. The enzymes are classified as:

Intracellular Enzymes

The enzymes which are produced within the cell of a particular tissue and function there only. Such enzymes are called intracellular enzymes, e.g., enzymes of the glycolysis, citric acid cycle, fatty acid synthesis, etc.

Extracellular Enzymes

There are certain enzymes which are produced by the cells of a particular tissue from where they are liberated but function in some other tissues. Such enzymes are called extracellular enzymes, e.g., proteolytic enzymes such as trypsin, chymotrypsin, etc.

Most of the enzymes are secreted in their active form called zymase. Some of the enzymes, however, are secreted in their inactive form called proenzyme or zymogen. After it comes in contact with certain activating agent, the proenzyme undergoes some modifications and is converted to active enzyme (zymase). e.g., gastric juice contains pepsin which is secreted as pepsinogen (a zymogen). Pepsinogen is changed to its active form pepsin by the H^+ of the gastric juice.

ASSESS YOURSELF

Short and Long Answer Questions

1. **Define the following:**
   - Atom
   - Molecule
   - Element
   - Atomic weight
   - Atomic number
2. **Discuss briefly the significance of following in the human body:**
   - Carbohydrates
   - Proteins
   - Lipids
3. **What are essential amino acids? List them.**
4. **Describe types of enzymes and their role in human body.**

Multiple Choice Questions

1. **The atomic weight of oxygen is:**
   a. 16   b. 12
   c. 11   d. 8
2. **The atomic number of sodium is:**
   a. 1   b. 4
   c. 8   d. 11
3. **The pH of blood is:**
   a. 5.7   b. 6.4
   c. 7   d. 7.4
4. **Cane sugar is:**
   a. Monosaccharide   b. Disaccharide
   c. Polysaccharide   d. Oligosaccharide

5. **Which of the following is neutral fat?**
   a. Alcohol
   b. Esters of fatty acids
   c. Triglycerides
   d. Glycerol
6. **Which of the following is not the function of lipids?**
   a. Provides insulation against change of environmental temperature
   b. Source of energy
   c. Help in absorption of vitamin K
   d. Help in protein synthesis
7. **Which of the following is not an essential amino acid?**
   a. Creatinine
   b. Methionin
   c. Leucine
   d. Phenylalanine

8. **Which of the following is a transport protein?**
   a. Ferritin
   b. Ceruloplasmin
   c. Gamma globulins
   d. Transducin
9. **Which of the following is an example of proteolytic enzyme?**
   a. Secretin
   b. Chymotrypsin
   c. Gastrin
   d. Cholecystokinin

ANSWER KEY

| 1. a | 2. d | 3. d | 4. b | 5. c | 6. d | 7. a | 8. b |
| 9. b |

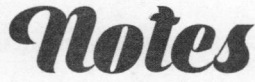

The Cell Physiology

THE CELL

The cell is the smallest structural and functional unit of the body. The human body contains about 100 trillion cells. Different types of cells of the body possess features, which distinguish one type from the other and are specially adapted to form one or few particular functions, e.g., the red blood cells transport oxygen from lungs to the tissues, muscle cell is specialized for the function of contraction, the intestinal mucosal cells specialized for absorption of foodstuffs and so on. However, most mammalian cells have an overall common structure and certain basic characteristics, which are described here. A typical cell (Fig. 1.3-1) as seen by the light microscope consists of three basic components:

1. Cell membrane
2. Cytoplasm
3. Nucleus.

CELL MEMBRANE

Cell membrane or the plasma membrane is the protective semipermeable sheath, enveloping the cell body. It separates the contents of cell from the external environment and controls exchange of materials between the fluid outside the cell (extracellular fluid) and the fluid inside the cell (intracellular fluid). A detailed knowledge the its structure (Fig. 1.3-1) is essential for understanding the cell functions.

Structure

Electron microscopy has shown that cell membrane/or plasma membrane has a *trilayer* structure having total thickness of 7–10 nm (70–100 Å). The three layers consist of *two electron dense layers* separated by an *electron lucent layer* (clear zone). Biochemically, the cell membrane is composed of complex mixture of lipids (40%), proteins (55%) and carbohydrates (5%).

A few hypotheses have been proposed to explain the distribution of various biochemical components in the cell membrane. The most important hypothesis is the fluid mosaic model of Singer and Nicolson.

Fluid Mosaic Model of Membrane Structure

In 1972, Singer and Nicolson put forward the fluid mosaic model of membrane structure (Fig. 1.3-2), which is presently the most accepted structure. The structure of the cell membrane based on this model has been described below.

Phospholipid bilayer

It is the basic continuous structure forming the cell membrane. The phospholipids are present in fluid form. This fluidity makes the membrane quite flexible and thus allows the cells to undergo considerable changes in the shape without disruption of structural integrity.

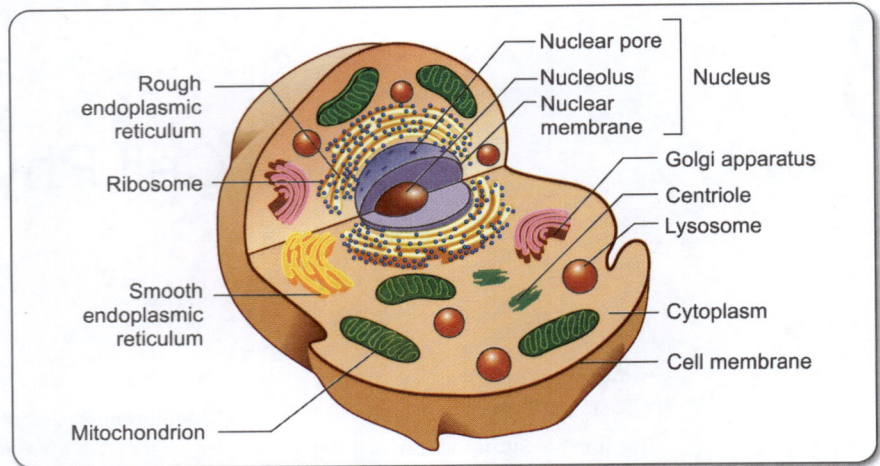

Fig. 1.3-1: Structure of a typical cell showing various organelles

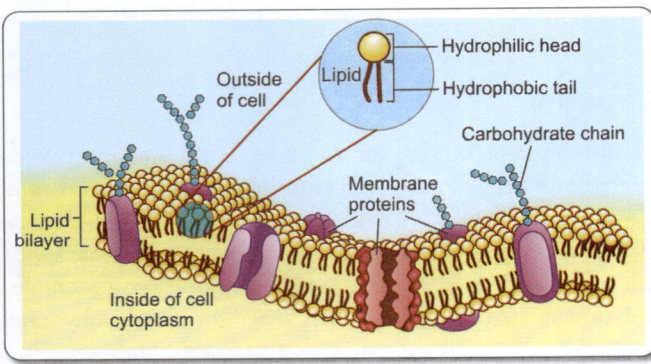

Fig. 1.3-2: Fluid mosaic model of cell membrane

Each lipid molecule in the lipid bilayer of the cell membrane primarily consists of phospholipid, cholesterol and glycolipids. The lipid molecule is of clothespin shape and consists of a *head end* and a *tail end.*

The head end or the globular end is positively, charged and quite soluble in water (i.e., *polar* or *hydrophilic).*

The tail end is quite insoluble in water (*nonpolar* or *hydrophobic).* These lipid molecules are arranged as bilayer in such a way that their nonpolar hydrophobic tail ends are directed toward the center of the membrane, whereas their polar hydrophilic head ends are directed outward on either side of the membrane (Fig. 1.3-2). In this way, head ends of molecules face the aqueous phase, i.e. extracellular fluid on outside and the intracellular fluid (cytoplasm) on inner side.

The protein molecules

They are present as a discontinuous mosaic of globular proteins, which float about in the fluid phospholipid bilayer forming a *fluid mosaic pattern.* Two types of proteins recognized in the cell membrane are:

1. *Peripheral proteins.* These are present peripheral to the lipid bilayer both inside and outside to it.

Intrinsic proteins. These are located in the inner surface of the lipid bilayer and serve mainly as enzymes.

Extrinsic or surface proteins. These are the proteins located on the outer surface of the lipid bilayer. Some of these proteins serve as *cell adhesion molecules* (CAM) that anchor cells to neighboring cells and to the basal lamina.

2. *Integral proteins or transmembrane proteins.* These are the proteins, which extend into the lipid bilayer. The integral proteins, on the basis of functions they serve, are:
* Channel proteins
* Carrier proteins
* Receptor proteins
* Antigens
* Pumps.

Functions of protein

* Proteins act as carrier proteins to facilitate the transportation of certain molecules across the membranes.
* They also serve as receptors for binding hormones.
* They help in transport of water and water-soluble ions across the cell membrane.
* They act as pumps in active transportation of substances against their concentration gradients e.g. sodium-potassium adenosine triphosphatase (ATPase) pump.
* They also act as cell adhesions molecules (CAM) that are responsible for the specific growth, shape and differentiation of cells.
* Some of them also act as enzymes.

The carbohydrates

The carbohydrates in the cell membrane are attached either to the proteins (glycoproteins) or the lipids (glycolipids). Throughout the surface of cell membrane, the carbohydrate molecules form a thin loose covering called *glycocalyx*.

Functions of cell membrane carbohydrates

- Being negatively charged, the carbohydrate molecules of the cell membrane do not allow the negatively charged particles to move out of the cell.
- The glycocalyx helps in tight fixation of the cells with one another.
- Some of the carbohydrate molecules also serve as receptors.

Functions of Cell Membrane

The cell membrane performs the following functions:
- It protects the organelles in cytoplasm.
- The selective permeability of the cell membrane helps in acting as a barrier to harmful substances.
- It helps in absorbing nutrients.
- It helps in maintaining the shape and size of cells.

CYTOPLASM

Cytoplasm is an aqueous substance (cytosol) containing a variety of cell organelles and other structures. The structures dispersed in the cytoplasm can be broadly divided into three groups—organelles, cytoplasmic inclusion bodies, and cytoskeleton.

Organelles

The organelles are the permanent components of the cells, which are bounded by limiting membrane and contain enzymes; hence they participate in the cellular metabolic activity. These include the mitochondria, the endoplasmic reticulum, ribosomes, the Golgi apparatus, peroxisomes, centrosomes and centriole.

Mitochondria (Fig. 1.3-3)

These are oval structures and more numerous in metabolically active cells. The mitochondria consists of two layers of the membrane and the matrix.

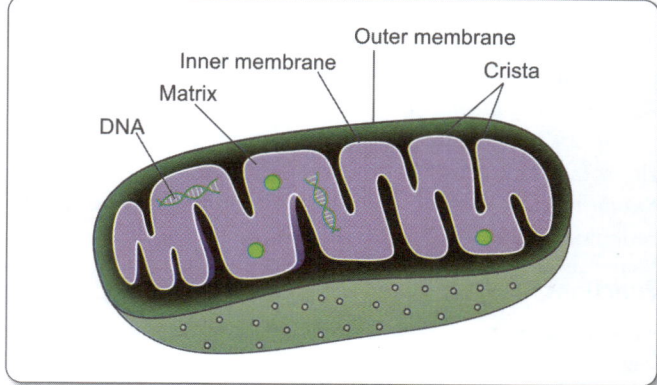

Fig. 1.3-3: Mitochondrion

Membrane the outer membrane is smooth and inner is folded into incomplete septa called cristae.

Matrix of the mitochondria contains enzymes required in Krebs' cycle by which products of carbohydrate, fat and protein metabolism are oxidized to produce energy which is stored in the form of adenosine triphosphate (ATP).

Functions

The functions of mitochondria are:
- They are major sites for aerobic respiration.
- In addition to their role as power generating units, the mitochondria may have a role in synthesizing proteins since they also possess DNA and ribosomes.

Endoplasmic Reticulum (Fig. 1.3-4)

Endoplasmic reticulum is a system of flattened, membrane-bound vesicles and tubules called *cisternae*. It is continuous with the outer membrane of the nuclear envelope and Golgi

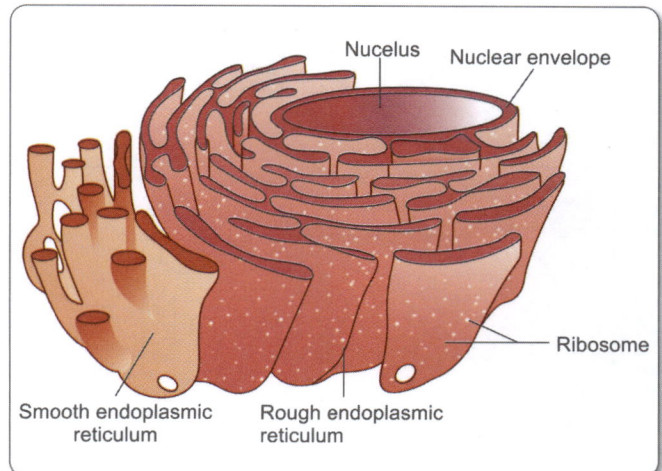

Fig. 1.3-4: Endoplasmic reticulum

apparatus. Morphologically, two types of endoplasmic reticulum can be identified—rough or granular and smooth or agranular.

Rough endoplasmic reticulum. The rough endoplasmic reticulum is characterized by the presence of a number of ribosomes on its surface.

Smooth endoplasmic reticulum. Smooth endoplasmic reticulum is devoid of ribosomes on its surface.

Functions

Rough endoplasmic reticulum is especially well developed in cells active in protein synthesis.

Smooth endoplasmic reticulum is a site of lipid and steroid synthesis. In the skeletal and cardiac muscles, smooth endoplasmic reticulum is modified to form sarcoplasmic reticulum, which is involved in the release and sequestration of calcium ions during muscular contraction.

Golgi Apparatus (Fig. 1.3-5)

The Golgi apparatus or complex is a collection of membranous vesicles, sacs or tubules, generally located close to the nucleus. It is continuous with the endoplasmic reticulum. Golgi apparatus is particularly well developed in exocrine glandular cells.

Functions

The main functions of Golgi apparatus are as follows:
- Synthesis of carbohydrates and complex proteins.
- Packaging of proteins synthesized in the rough endoplasmic reticulum into vesicles.

Ribosomes

Ribosomes are spherical particles which contain 80–85% of the cell's RNA. They may be present in the cytosol as free or inbound form. Slightly smaller forms of ribosomes are also found in mitochondria.

Functions

They are the site of protein synthesis. They synthesize all transmembrane proteins, secreted proteins and most proteins that are stored in Golgi apparatus, lysosomes and endosomes.

Lysosomes

Lysosomes are rounded to oval membrane-bound organelles containing powerful lysosomal digestive (hydrolytic) enzymes. They are formed by the Golgi apparatus.

Functions

Lysosomes are particularly abundant in cells involved in phagocytic activity, e.g. neutrophils and macrophages.

Peroxisomes

Peroxisomes, also known as microbodies, are spherical structures enclosed by a single layer of unit membrane. These are predominantly present in hepatocytes and tubular epithelial cells. They essentially contain two types of enzymes:
1. *Oxidases*, which are active in oxidation of lipid; and
2. *Catalases*, which act on hydrogen peroxide to liberate oxygen.

Centrosome

The centrosome consists of two short cylindrical structures called centrioles. It is situated near the center of the cell close to the nucleus.

Functions

The centrioles are responsible for movement of chromosomes during cell division.

Cytoplasmic Inclusions Bodies

The cytoplasmic inclusions are the temporary components of certain cells. A few examples of cytoplasmic inclusions are:
- Lipid droplets
- Glycogen
- Proteins as secretory granules
- Melanin pigment
- Lipofuscin.

Cytoskeleton

The cytoskeleton is a complex network of fibers that maintains the structure of the cell and allows it to change shape and move. It primarily consists of microtubules, intermediate filaments and microfilaments along with proteins which anchor and tie them together.

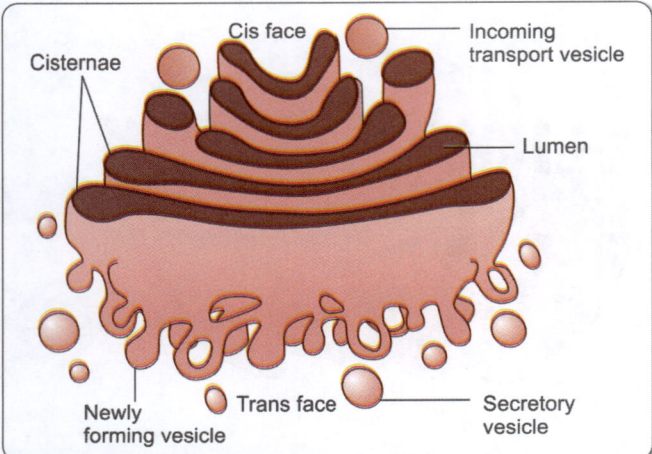

Fig. 1.3-5: Golgi apparatus

Chapter 1.3 ⊙ The Cell Physiology   29

Section I ⊙ Introduction to Anatomical Terms; Organization of the Human Body...

Microtubules

Microtubules are long hollow tubular structures without limiting membrane and are about 25 nm in diameter.

They are made up of tubulin and are involved in movement of organelles within the cell, movement of chromosomes during cell division and movement of cell extensions like cilia, flagella and microvilli.

Intermediate Filaments

Intermediate filaments are filamentous structures about 10 nm in diameter. Some of these filaments connect the nuclear membrane to the cell membrane. Their main function is to mechanically integrate the cell organelles within the cytoplasm.

Microfilaments

Microfilaments are long solid filamentous structures having a diameter of 6–8 nm. These are made up of contractile proteins, actin and myosin. Actin is the most abundant protein in the mammalian cell. It attaches to various parts of cytoskeleton by other proteins (anchor proteins). In the skeletal muscle, presence of actin and myosin filaments is responsible for their contractile property.

Cell extensions

Three types of cell extensions are seen that present as a projection from the cell surface

1. *Microvilli.* Microvilli are tiny projections that cover the exposed surface of certain cells like absorptive cells lining the small intestine. They help in increasing the surface area and in intestines, maximize the absorption of nutrients.

2. *Cilia.* Cilia occurs as small hair-like projections from the free surface of some cells. They move in coordination, and help in moving substances like fluid, mucus or small solid object along the surface.

3. *Flagella.* Flagella is a long whip-like projection, forming the tail of spermatozoa, helping them to propel through female reproductive tract.

NURSING IMPLICATIONS AND APPLICATIONS

Kartagener's syndrome or immotile cilia syndrome is a genetic disorder leading to defects in the structure and functions of cilia. This leads to frequent respiratory infections, frequent ear infection, chromic nasal congestion and infertility.

NUCLEUS (FIG. 1.3-6)

Nucleus is present in all the eukaryotic cells. It controls all the cellular activities including reproduction of the cell.

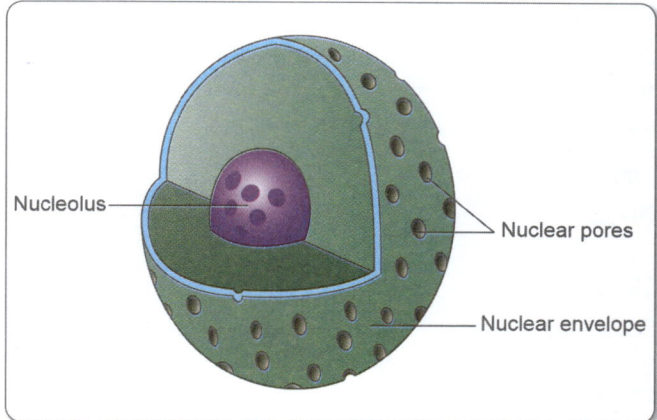

Fig. 1.3-6: Nucleus

Structure

The nucleus consists of an outer nuclear membrane enclosing nucleoplasm and nucleoli.

Nuclear Membrane

The nuclear membrane is double-layered porous structure having a 40–70 nm wide space called *perinuclear cistern*, which is continuous with the lumen of endoplasmic reticulum. The outer layer of the nuclear membrane is continuous with endoplasmic reticulum.

Functions

The exchange of materials between nucleoplasm and cytoplasm occurs through nuclear membrane.

Nucleoplasm

The nucleoplasm or the nuclear matrix is a gel-like ground substance containing large quantity of genetic material in the form of deoxyribonucleic acid (DNA). When a cell is not dividing, the nucleoplasm appears as dark-staining thread-like material called nuclear *chromatin*. During cell division, the chromatin material is converted into rod-shaped structures, the chromosomes. There are 46 chromosomes (23 pairs) in all the dividing cells of the body except the gamete (sex cells), which contain only 23 chromosomes (haploid number). Each chromosome is composed of two chromatids connected at the centromere to form 'X' configuration having variation of the location of centromere. The chromosomes are composed of three components: DNA, ribonucleic acid (RNA), and other nuclear proteins. The nuclear DNA carries the genetic information, which is passed via RNA into the cytoplasm for synthesis of proteins of similar composition.

Nucleolus

The nucleus may contain one or more rounded bodies called nucleoli. The nucleoli are more common in growing cells or in cells actively synthesizing proteins.

Functions

The nucleoli are the site of synthesis of ribosomal RNA.

CELL CYCLE

Cell multiplication is an essential feature of development and growth. In human body most of the cells divide by process of mitosis, but the gametes divide by meiosis.

Cell cycle is a series of stages through which a cell passes and consists of the following stages (Fig. 1.3-7).

Interphase

Interphase refers to the period between the two cell cycles and it includes the following phases:

G1 or first gap phase. This is the longest phase and involves an increase in size and volume of the cell. Sometimes cells do not continue the cell cycle and enter a resting phase, during which they carry out their specific functions, e.g. secretion, and absorption.

S phase or synthesis phase. This phase includes replication of chromosomes to form two identical copies of DNA.

G2 or second gap phase. This phase includes further growth and preparation for cell division.

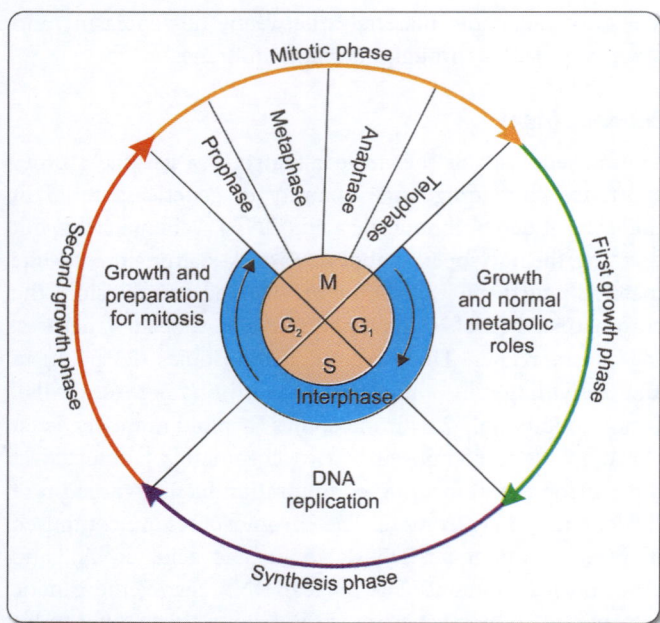

Fig. 1.3-7: Cell cycle

Mitosis (Figs 1.3-8A to E)

This stage leads to formation of two identical daughter cells. It is divided into four stages.

1. *Prophase.* This is usually longest phase. In this stage:

- The chromatin condenses into discrete chromosomes. Each of the 46 chromosomes pair up with its copy (now termed chromatid).
- The sister chromatids join with each other at the centromere.
- The mitotic spindle (formed by microtubules) and 2 centrioles appear at this stage and the centrioles migrate to opposite ends of the cell due to lengthening of microtubules.
- The nuclear envelop disappears in this stage.

2. *Metaphase.* It includes the alignment of the chromatids on the center of the spindle attached by their centromeres.

3. *Anaphase.* In this phase:

- The centromeres split into two, and spindle fibers pull the daughter centromeres toward opposite poles.
- Then the separated chromatids become independent chromosomes.
- Thus at this stage cell possess 46 pairs of chromosomes.

4. *Telophase.* The spindle fibers degenerate and the chromosomes uncoil. The nuclear envelope is also reformed in this stage. After telophase, the cell undergoes cytokinesis.

5. *Cytokinesis.* The cell membrane constricts in the mid region between the poles leading to division of the cytosol, intercellular organelles and form two identical daughter cells.

Meiosis

Meiosis (meio=to reduce) is a form of cell division in which the chromosome number is halved-being diploid (2n) to haploid (n). Like mitosis; it involves DNA replication once during interphase of the parent cell, but this is followed by two consecutive nuclear divisions and cell divisions, known as **meiosis I** (the first meiotic division) and **meiosis II** (the second meiotic division). Thus, a single diploid cell gives rise to four haploid cells.

Meiosis occurs during the formation of sperms and ova (gametogenesis).

Meiosis I

The phases of meiosis I are as follows Fig. 1.3-9:

1. *Prophase I.* Involves exchange between maternal and paternal chromatids by the process of crossing over Fig. 1.3-9A.

- In this stage, the homologous chromosomes pair up and each pair is referred to as **bivalent**.

Chapter 1.3 ⊙ The Cell Physiology   31

Section I ⊙ Introduction to Anatomical Terms; Organization of the Human Body...

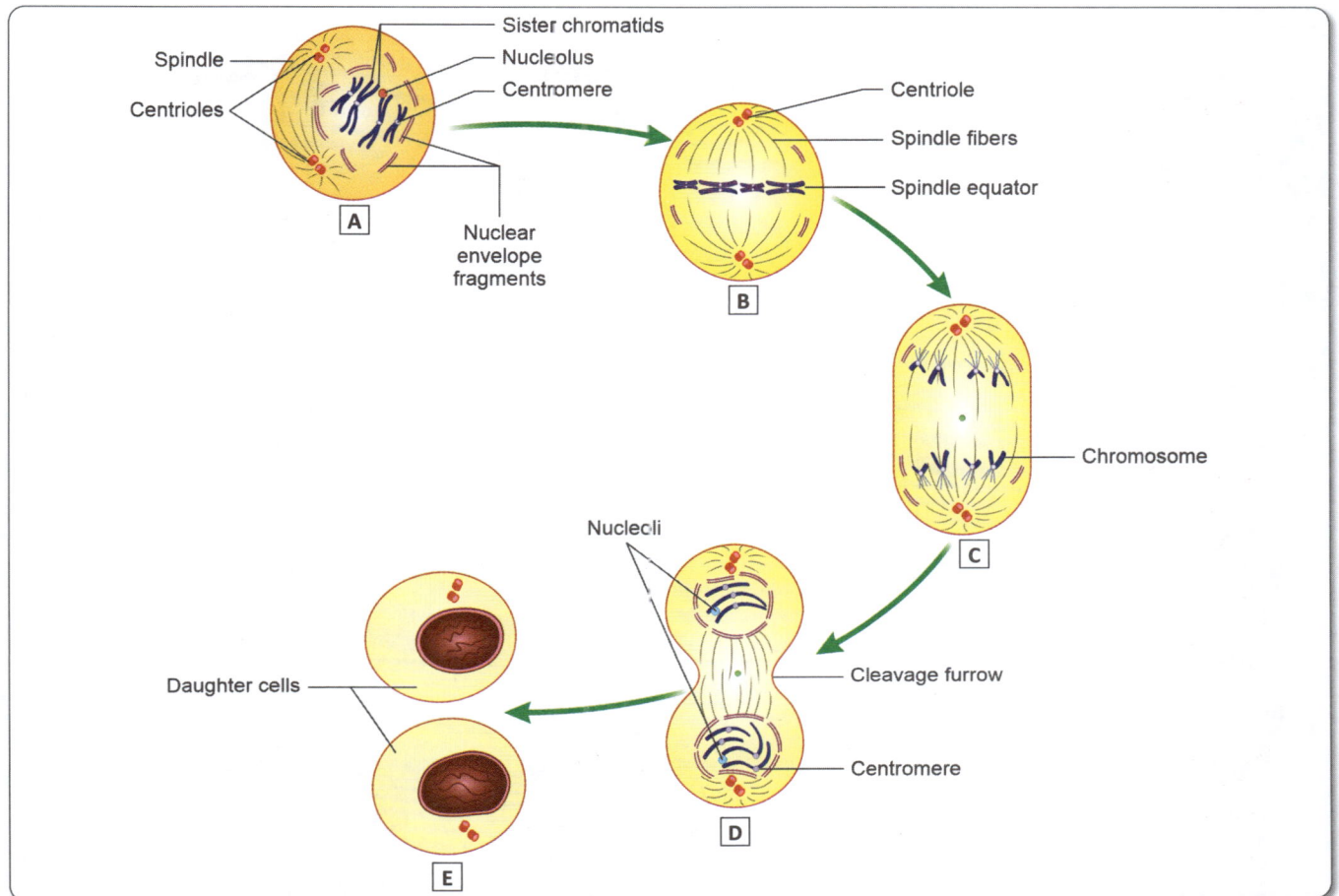

Figs 1.3-8A to E: Phases of mitosis: A. Prophase; B. Metaphase; C. Anaphase; D. Telophase; E. Cytokinesis

- One of the pair comes from male parent and one from the female parent. Later, the two chromatids of each chromosome separate, and is now represented by four chromatids called a tetrad.
- Then crossing over occurs, whereby one or both chromatids of the paternal chromosome cross over to exchange genetic material with those from the maternal
- The site of cross over is called chiasmata. The crossing over results: Genes from paternal chromosome swap with genes from the maternal chromosomes leading to a new gene combination of the resulting chromatids.

Toward the end of this stage, the reorganized chromosomes begin to move apart. Each bivalent can now be seen to contain four chromatids linked by a common centromere.

2. *Metaphase I.* The bivalents become arranged around the equator of the spindle, attached by their centromeres Fig. 1.3-9B.

3. *Anaphase I.* Spindle fibers pull homologous chromosomes, centromeres first, toward the opposite poles of the spindle (unlike in mitosis, there is no splitting of the centromeres). This separates the chromosome into two haploid sets, one set at each end of the spindle Fig. 1.3-9C.

4. *Telophase I.* The telophase is similar to that in mitosis Fig. 1.3-9D.

- The homologous chromosomes which have reached the opposite poles of the cell uncoil and lengthen to form chromatin again, losing the ability to be seen clearly.
- The spindle fibers usually disappear.
- A nuclear envelope reforms around the chromosomes at each pole.

Cytokinesis then occurs and two daugher cells are formed. Thus, at the end of meiosis I each daughter cell contains 23 chromosomes (n), each consisting of two chromatids.

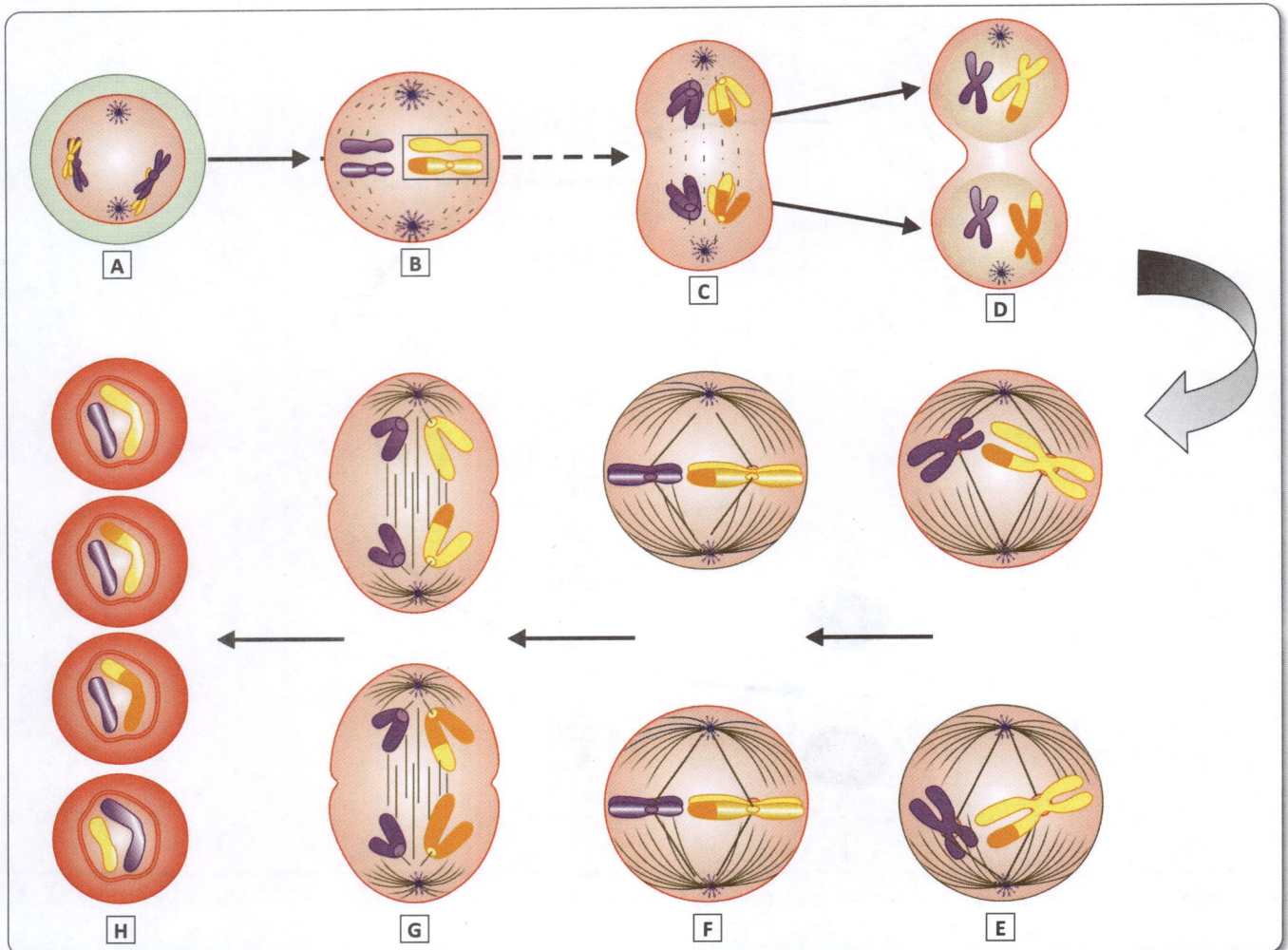

Figs 1.3-9A to H: Phases of meiosis: A. Prophase I; B. Metaphase I; C. Anaphase I; D. Telophase I; E. Prophase II; F. Metaphase II; G. Anaphase II; H. Prophase II

Meiosis II

Phases of meiosis II are as follows:

1. *Interphase II.* There is a transient interphase II after meiosis I. This differs from the usual interphase in which no chromosome replication occurs (since the daughter cells after meiosis I already possess two chromatids each).

2. *Prophase II.* **metaphase II, anaphase II, telophase II and cytokinesis** are similar to the phases of mitosis in which the pair of chromatids (bivalents) linked at their centromere become aligned at the metaphase plate and then drawn into separate daughter cells following replication of the centromeric DNA 1.3-9E-H).

Unlike mitosis, because of the crossing over has occurred during meiosis I, the daughter cells are not identical in genetic content. Further daughter cells at the end of meiosis II contain chromosomes (n), each consisting of a simple chromatid Figs 1.3-9E to H.

The biologically significant difference between mitosis and meiosis are really between meiosis I. Meiosis II is almost identical to mitosis Table 1.3-1 summarizes the comparison of mitosis and meiosis I.

INTERCELLULAR JUNCTIONS

The cell membranes of the neighboring cells are connected with one another through the *intercellular junctions* or the junctional complexes, which are of three types (Fig. 1.3-10).

TABLE 1.3-1: Comparison between mitosis and meiosis I

Stages	Mitosis	Meiosis I
Prophase	• Homologous chromosomes remain separate • No formation of chromatids • No crossing over	• Homologous chromosomes pair up • Formation of chromatids • Crossing over may occur
Metaphase	Pairs of chromatids line up at the equator	Pairs of chromosomes line up at the equator
Anaphase	• Centromere divide • Chromatids separate • Separated chromatids are identical	• Centromere do not divide • Whole chromosomes separate • Separated chromosomes may not be identical due to crossing over
Telophase	• Same number of chromosomes present in daughter cells • Both homologous chromosomes present in daughter cells are diploid	• Half the number of chromosomes in the daughter cells • Only one of each pair of homologous chromosomes is present in daughter cells
Occurrence	• May occur in haploid, diploid or polyploidy cells • Occurs in the formation of somatic (body) cells	• Only occurs in diploid or polyploidy cells • Occurs only in sex cells gametes

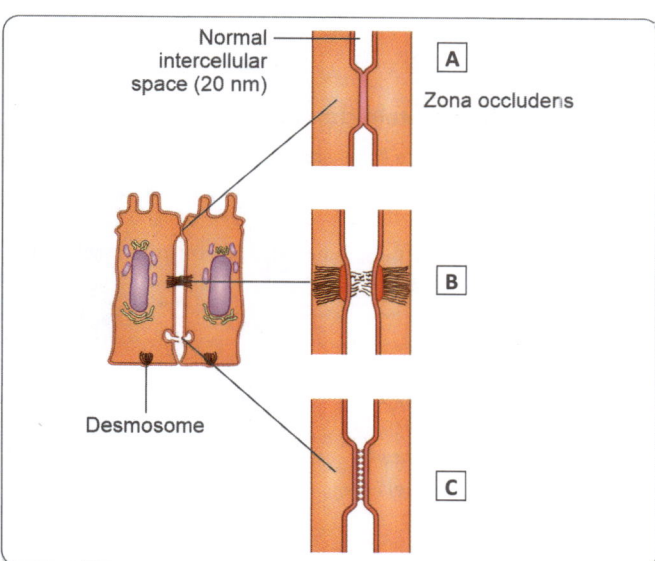

Figs 1.3-10A to C: Schematic diagram of a cell to show various intercellular junctions: A. Tight junction; B. Adherens junction; C. Gap junction

TIGHT JUNCTION

This is also called *zonula occludens* or the *occluding zone (Fig. 1.3-10A)*. In this type of intercellular junction, the outer layer of the cell membrane of the neighboring cells fuse with each other, thus obliterating the space between the cells. Such junctions form a barrier to the movement of ions and other solutes from one cell to another.

ADHERENS JUNCTION

This is also called *zonula adherens*. In this type of junction, cell membrane of the adjacent cells are separated by a 15–20 nm wide space, which is at focal places obliterated by the dense accumulation of the proteins at the cell surface. Bundles of intermediate filaments project from the intercellular junctional areas and radiate into the cytoplasm. This holds the adjacent cells at these focal places. These are of two types:

1. *Desmosomes* are the adherens junctions, where thickened focal areas are formed on both the apposing cell membranes (Fig. 1.3-10B).

2. *Hemidesmosomes* are the adherens junctions, where focal thickening is seen only on the membrane of one of the two adjacent cells.

GAP JUNCTION

Gap junctions or the nexus are the channels on the lateral surfaces of the two adjacent cells through which the molecules are exchanged between the cells (Fig. 1.3-10C). Gap junctions serve the following functions:

- These permit the intercellular passage of glucose, amino acids, ions and other substances, which have a molecular weight of about 1000.
- These permit rapid propagation of electrical potential changes from one cell to another as seen in cardiac muscle and other smooth muscle cells.
- These help in the exchange of chemical messengers between the cells.

TRANSPORT OF SUBSTANCES ACROSS CELL MEMBRANES

The physiological activities of a cell depend upon the substances, like nutrients, oxygen and water, which must be transported into the cell, and at the same time metabolic waste must be transported out of the cell. Various processes involved in the transport of substances across the cell membrane may be grouped as under:

- Passive transport
- Active transport
- Vesicular transport

PASSIVE TRANSPORT

Passive transport refers to the mechanism of transport of substances along the gradient without expenditure of any energy. This process is also called *downhill movement*. It depends upon the physical factors like concentration gradient, electrical gradient and pressure gradient. The passive transport mechanisms operating at the cell membrane level are diffusion and osmosis.

Diffusion

Diffusion refers to passive transport of molecules from areas of higher concentration to areas of lower concentration. Diffusion through cell membrane is of two subtypes, called simple diffusion and facilitated diffusion.

Simple Diffusion

In simple diffusion, transport of atoms or molecules occurs from one place to another due to their random movement. Due to constant random movement, the molecules collide with each other and also strike with the cell membrane. The frequency of collision and the probability of striking to the cell membrane will be higher on the side of the membrane having higher concentration of that particular molecule. In this process, there occurs a net flux of the molecules from the areas of high concentration to areas of low concentration. The net movement of the molecules ceases when the concentration of molecules equals, and there occurs a condition of *diffusional equilibrium.* Quantitatively, the net movement of the molecules across a permeable membrane, where only simple diffusion occurring, is expressed by *Fick's Law of Diffusion,* which states that rate of diffusion (J) is directly proportional to the difference in the concentration of the substance in two regions (concentration gradient, i.e. $C_1 - C_2$) and cross-sectional area (A) and inversely proportional to the distance to be traveled (thickness of the membrane, i.e. T).

$$\text{Thus:} \qquad J = D \frac{A(C_1 - C_2)}{T}$$

where D is the diffusion coefficient.

The diffusion of molecules across the biological membranes differs depending upon the lipid solubility, water solubility, type of electrical charge and size of the molecules.

Further, selective permeability of the semipermeable cell membrane also affects the diffusion of different molecules. How the different molecules diffuse across a cell membrane is discussed below.

Simple diffusion of lipid soluble substances through the cell membrane

The rate of diffusion through the lipid bilayer of the cell membrane is directly proportional to the solubility of a substance in lipids. Therefore, molecules of oxygen, nitrogen, carbon dioxide, alcohol, steroid hormones and weak organic acids and bases, being lipid soluble, diffuse very rapidly through the lipid bilayer of the cell membrane (Fig. 1.3-11).

Simple diffusion of water and other lipid insoluble molecules through the cell membrane

Astonishingly, water and other lipid insoluble substances can also pass easily through the cell membrane. It has been shown that it is possible due to the presence of the so-called *protein channels.*

Diffusion through protein channels

The protein channels are tube-shaped channels, which extend in the cell membrane from the extracellular to the intracellular ends (Fig. 1.3-11).

The protein channels have been equipped with the following characteristics:

- Selective permeability
- Gating mechanism.

Selective permeability of protein channels

The protein channels are highly selective, i.e., each channel can permit only one types of ion to pass through it. Examples of some selective channels are:

- Sodium channels
- Potassium channels.

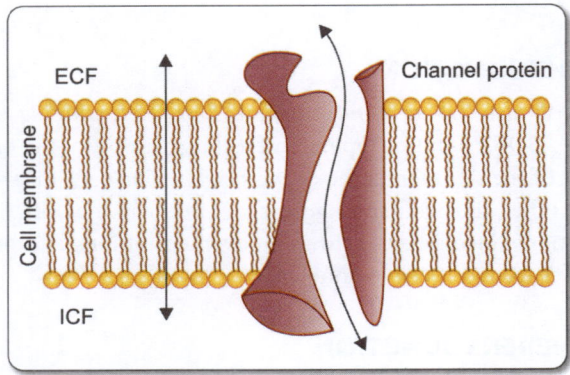

Fig. 1.3-11: Simple diffusion

Gating mechanism in protein channels

Some protein channels are continuously open, whereas most others are 'gated'. This gating mechanism is a means of controlling the permeability of the channels. The opening and closing of gates are controlled by three principal ways:

1. **Voltage-gated channels.** These respond to the electrical potential across the cell membrane. Sodium and potassium channels are voltage-gated channels. In the case of sodium channels, the gates are located at the outer end of the channels (Fig. 1.3-12A) and these remain tightly closed. When the inside of cell membrane loses its negative charge, the sodium channel gates open and there occurs a tremendous inflow of sodium ions. This is the basis of occurrence of action potentials in nerves that are responsible for nerve signals.

In the case of potassium channels, the gates are located at inner end of the channel (Fig. 1.3-12B) and they too open when inside of the cell membrane loses its negative charge. The opening of potassium channel gates is partly responsible for terminating the action potential.

2. **Ligand-gated channels.** Gates of these channels open when some other chemical molecule binds with the gate proteins. That is why this is also called *chemical gating*.

One of the most important examples of ligand channel gating is the effect of acetylcholine on the so-called *acetylcholine channels*. This gate plays an important role in transmission of nerve signals from one nerve cell to another and from nerve cells to muscle cells.

3. **Mechanical-gated channels.** Some protein channels are opened by mechanical stretch. These mechano-sensitive channels play an important role in cell movements.

Facilitated Diffusion

The water-soluble substances having larger molecules such as glucose cannot diffuse through the protein channels by simple diffusion. Such substances diffuse through the cell membrane with the help of some carrier proteins. Therefore, this type of diffusion is called *facilitated* or the *carrier-mediated diffusion*.

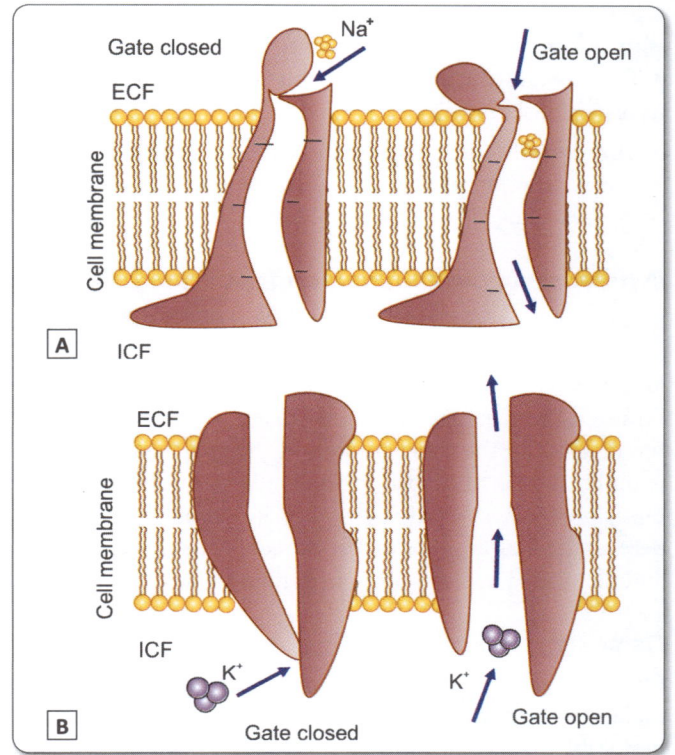

Figs 1.3-12A and B: Voltage-gated sodium channels: A. and potassium channels B.

There are many types of carrier proteins in the cell membrane, each type having binding sites that are specific for a particular substance. Among the most important substances that cross cell membranes by facilitated diffusion are *glucose* and most of the *amino acids*.

Types of Carrier Protein Systems

Three types of carrier protein systems are known (Figs 1.3-13A to C):

1. **Uniport.** In this system, the carrier proteins transport only one type of molecules.

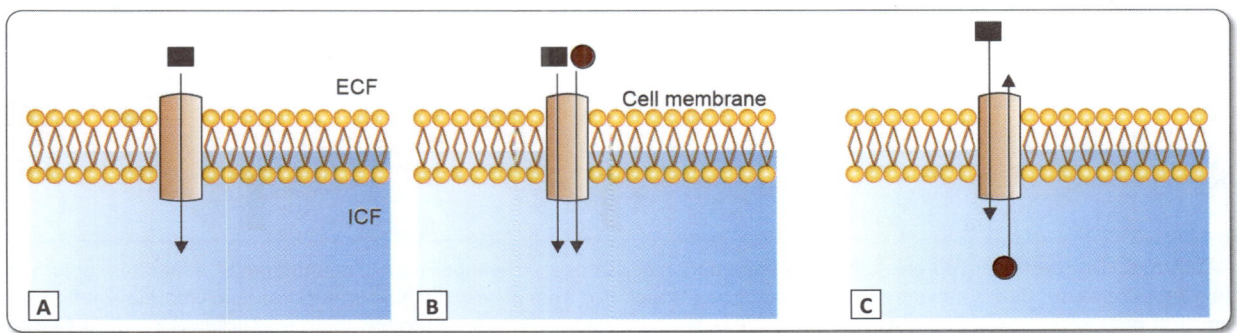

Figs 1.3-13A to C: Various types of carrier protein systems. A. Uniport; B. Symport; C. Antiport

2. *Symport.* In this system, transport of one substance is linked with transfer of another substance. For example, facilitated diffusion of glucose in the renal tubular cells is linked with the transport of sodium.

3. *Antiport.* In this system, the carrier proteins exchange one substance for another. For example, Na^+-K^+ exchange or Na^+-H^+ exchange in the renal tubules.

Differences between Simple and Facilitated Diffusion

Specificity. The carrier proteins are highly specific for different molecules.

Saturation. As shown in Figures 1.3-14A and B, in simple diffusion the rate of diffusion increases proportionately with the increase in the concentration of the substance and there is no limit to it. However, in facilitated diffusion the rate of diffusion reaches a limit. This is called *saturation* point and here all the binding sites on the carrier proteins are occupied and the system operates at its maximum capacity.

Osmosis

Osmosis refers to diffusion of water or any other solvent molecules through a semipermeable membrane, (i.e., membrane permeable to solvent but not to the solute) from a solution containing lower concentration of solutes toward the solution containing higher concentration of solutes. Figure 1.3-15A shows osmosis across a selective permeable membrane. When a sodium chloride solution is placed on one side of the membrane and water on the other side (Fig. 1.3-15A), net movement of water occurs from the pure water into the sodium chloride solution (Fig. 1.3-15B).

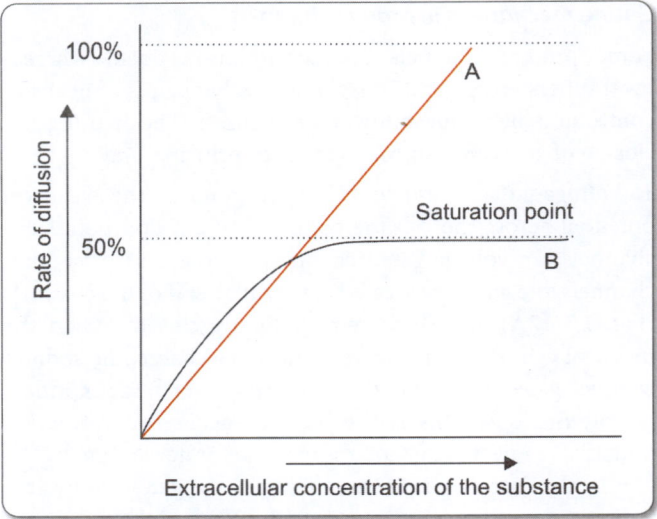

Fig. 1.3-14A and B: Effect of concentration of substance on rate of diffusion in: A. Simple diffusion; and B. Facilitated diffusion

Osmotic Pressure

Osmotic pressure refers to the minimum pressure which when applied on the side of higher solute concentration prevents the osmosis. Figure 1.3-15C shows that when appropriate pressure is applied, the net diffusion of water into the sodium chloride solution is prevented.

The osmotic pressure in the body fluids refers to the pressure exerted by the solutes dissolved in water or other solvents. The osmotic pressure exerted by the colloidal substances in the body is called *colloidal osmotic pressure.* The colloidal osmotic pressure

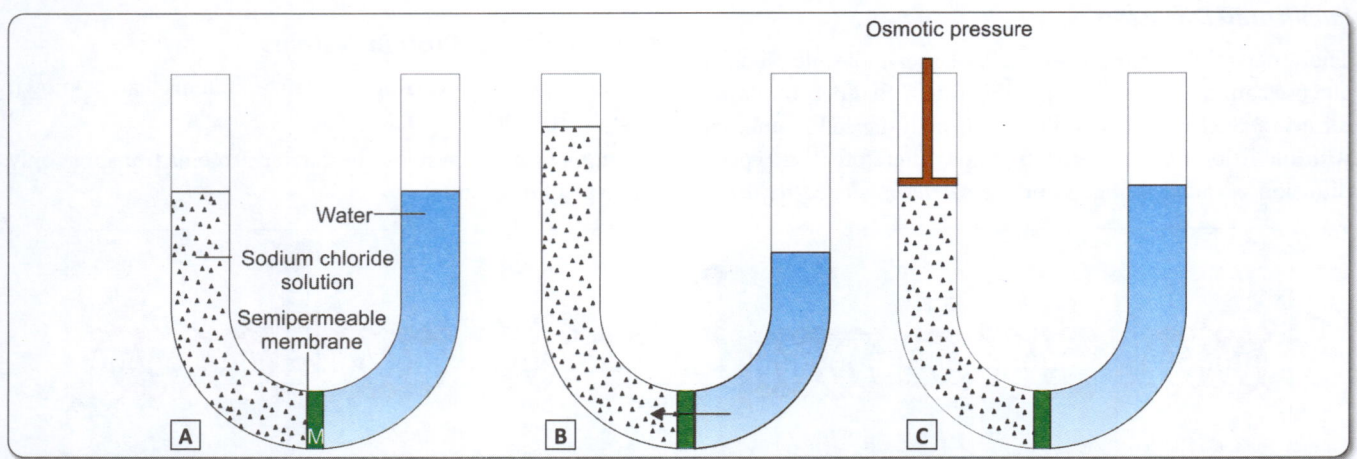

Figs 1.3-15A to C: Diagrammatic representation of phenomenon of osmosis: A. Semipermeable membrane 'M' separates sodium chloride solution from pure water; B. Net movement of water occurs through (M) from pure water side into the sodium chloride solution side; and C. Demonstration of osmotic pressure (net movement of water from pure water side to sodium chloride solution is prevented by applying appropriate pressure on the solution side)

due to plasma colloids (proteins) is called *oncotic pressure*. The osmotic pressure depends upon the number of molecules or ions dissolved in a solution.

Osmole, Osmolality and Osmolarity

Osmole is the unit used in place of grams to express the concentration in terms of number of osmotically active particles in a given solution. One osmole is equal to the molecular weight of a substance in grams divided by the number of freely moving particles liberated in solution by each molecule. Thus:

- A molar solution of glucose contains 1 mole and exerts osmotic pressure of 1 atmosphere
- A molar solution of NaCl contains 2 osmoles (1 mole of Na^+ and 1 mole of Cl^-) and exerts osmotic pressure of 2 atmospheres
- A molar solution of $CaCl_2$ contains 3 osmoles (1 mole of Ca^{2+} and 2 moles of Cl^-) and thus, exerts osmotic pressure of 3 atmospheres.
- One milliosmole (mOsm) is 1/1000 of an osmole.

Osmolality of a solution refers to the number of osmotically active particles (osmoles) per kilogram (kg) of a solution.

Osmolarity refers to the number of osmoles per liter (L) of a solution. Therefore, osmolarity is affected by the volume of the various solutes in the solution and the temperature, while the osmolality is not. The osmotic pressure is determined by the osmolality and not the osmolarity.

Tonicity of Fluids

In clinical practice, the word tonicity always refers to tonicity of a solution with respect to that of plasma (290 mOsm). In other words, it is the red blood cell (RBC) membrane across, which the tonicity is tested. Thus:

Isotonic fluids are those, which have osmolality similar to plasma. RBCs neither shrink nor swell in such solution (Fig. 1.3-16A). A solution of 0.9% NaCl is isotonic with plasma.

Hypertonic fluids have osmolality higher than the plasma. The RBCs shrink in such solutions by losing water by osmosis (Fig. 1.3-16B).

Hypotonic fluids are those whose osmolality is lower than that of plasma. The RBCs swell up in hypotonic solutions by gaining water by osmosis (Fig. 1.3-16C).

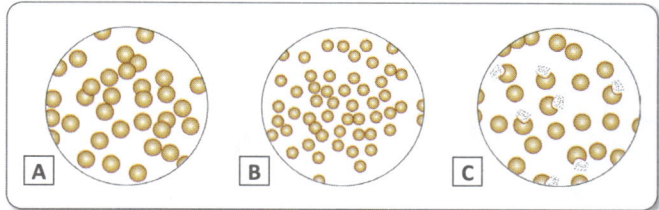

Figs 1.3-16A to C: Tonicity of fluids: A. Isotonic fluid (0.9% NaCl) has osmolarity similar to plasma, RBCs neither shrink nor swell in it; B. Hypertonic fluid (2% NaCl) has osmolarity higher than plasma, RBCs shrink in it; and C. Hypotonic fluid (0.3% NaCl) has osmolarity lower than plasma, RBCs swell in it

ACTIVE TRANSPORT

Active transport refers to the mechanism of transport of substances against the chemical and/or electrical gradient. Active transport involves expenditure of energy which is liberated by breakdown of high energy compounds like ATP. This process is also called *uphill movement*.

The active transport is of two types:

1. Primary active transport
2. Secondary active transport

Primary Active Transport Processes

In primary active transport process, the energy is derived directly from the breakdown of adenosine triphosphate (ATP) or some other high-energy phosphate compound. Some of the important pumps involved in the primary active transport processes are:

- Sodium-potassium pump
- Calcium pump
- Potassium-hydrogen pump.

Sodium-potassium Pump

Sodium-potassium (Na^+-K^+) pump is present in all the cells of the body.

Structure of Na^+-K^+ pump (Fig. 1.3-17A)

The carrier protein involved in Na^+-K^+ pump is a complex consisting of two separate protein units, a larger α subunit, and a smaller β subunit. The α subunit is mainly concerned with Na^+-K^+ transport. It has got the following binding sites:

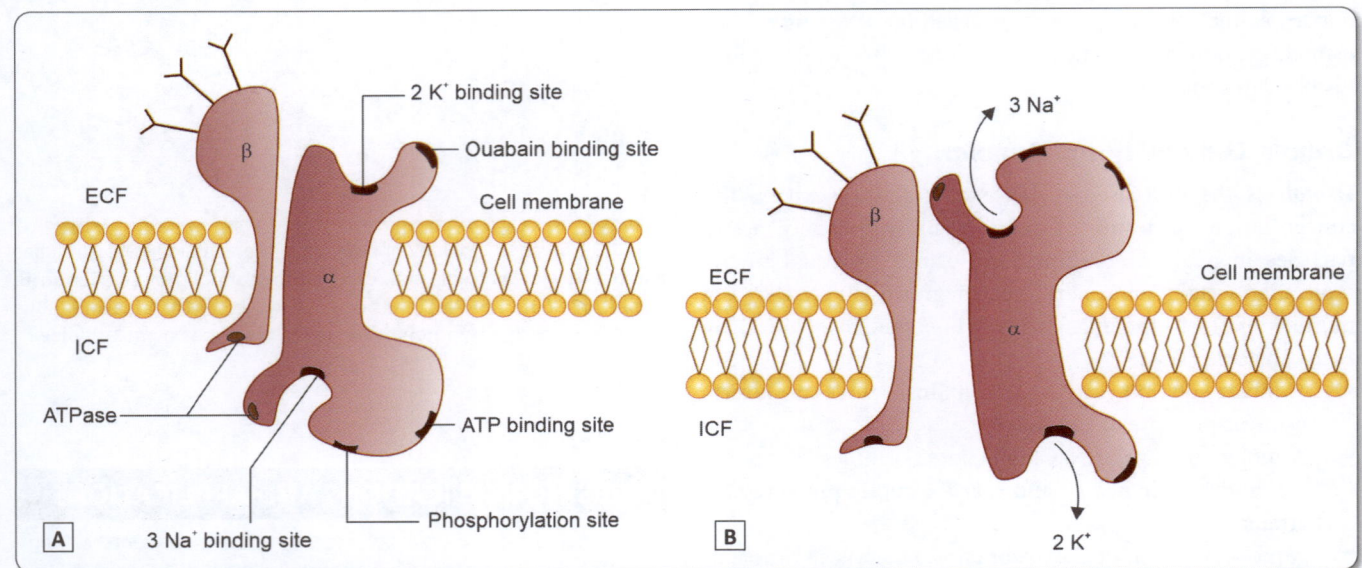

Figs 1.3-17A and B: Sodium-potassium ATPase pump: A. Structure; and B. Mechanism of operation

- Three intracellular sites, one each for binding sodium ions ($3Na^+$) and ATP, and one phosphorylation site
- Two extracellular sites, one each for binding potassium ions ($2K^+$) and ouabain.

Mechanism of operation of Na⁺-K⁺ pump (Fig. 1.3-17B)

The functioning of $Na^+–K^+$ pump involves the use of enzyme ATPase. The enzyme ATPase is activated when 3 sodium ions and 1 ATP molecule bind to their respective binding sites. The activated ATPase catalyzes the hydrolysis of ATP to adenosine diphosphate (ADP) and liberates a high-energy phosphate bond of energy (phosphorylation). The energy so liberated is believed to cause a conformational change in the carrier protein molecule extruding sodium into the extracellular fluid. This is followed by binding of two potassium ions to the receptor site on extracellular surface of the carrier protein and dephosphorylation of α subunit, which returns to its previous conformation, releasing potassium into the cytoplasm.

Functions of Na⁺-K⁺ pump

This pump is responsible for maintaining the Na^+ and K^+ concentration differences across the cell membrane and for establishing a negative electrical potential inside the cells.

Calcium Pump

The calcium pump forms another important active transport mechanism. Like Na^+-K^+ pump, it also operates through a carrier protein, which has ATPase activity. The calcium pump helps in maintaining extremely low concentration of calcium in the intracellular fluid [10,000 times less than the (extracellular fluid)].

Potassium-hydrogen Pump

The primary active transport system of hydrogen ion also operates through ATPase (K^+-H^+ ATPase) activity. These are present at the following two places in the human body:
1. Parietal cells of gastric glands
2. Renal tubules.

Secondary Active Transport

In secondary active transport processes, the energy is derived secondarily from the energy, which has been stored in the form of ionic concentration differences between the two sides of a membrane, created in the first place by primary active transport. The secondary active transport of substance may occur in the form of sodium co-transport or sodium counter-transport.

Sodium Co-transport

The carrier protein here acts as symport, i.e. transports some other substance along with the sodium. Substances carried by sodium co-transport include glucose, amino acids, chloride and iodine.

Sodium co-transport of glucose

The glucose is transported into most cells against large concentration gradient. As shown in Figure 1.3-18A, the carrier protein has two receptor sites on the outer surface, one for sodium and other for glucose. The special feature of the carrier protein is that the conformational change in it occurs only when both the sodium and glucose molecules are attached to it. Due to conformational change in the carrier

Chapter 1.3 ⊙ The Cell Physiology   39

Section I ⊙ Introduction to Anatomical Terms; Organization of the Human Body...

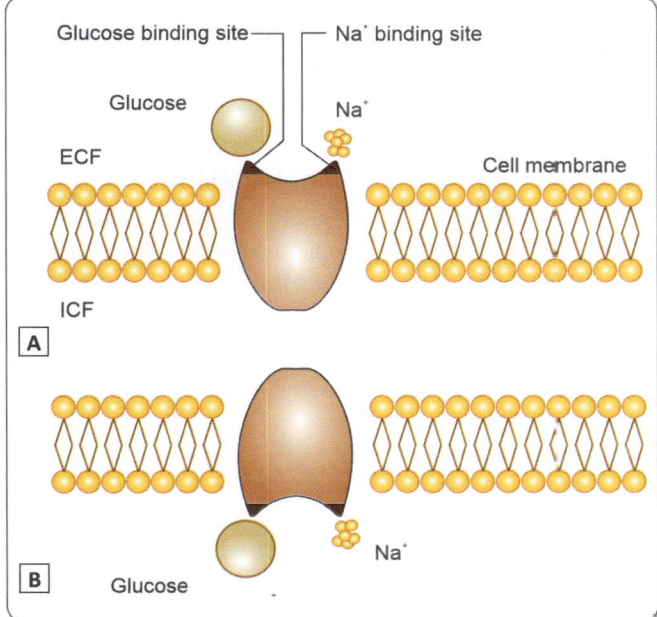

Figs 1.3-18A and B: Postulated mechanism of sodium co-transport of glucose (secondary active transport): A. Carrier protein has two receptor sites, one for sodium and one for glucose; and B. Conformational change in carrier proteins causes transport of both glucose and sodium inside the cell simultaneously

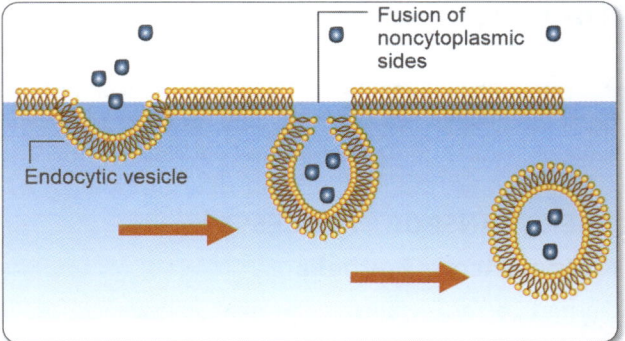

Fig. 1.3-19: Endocytosis

protein, both the sodium and the glucose are transported simultaneously inside the cell (Fig. 1.3-18B). The co-transport of glucose occurs during its absorption from the intestine into the blood and during the reabsorption of glucose from renal tubule in the blood.

Sodium co-transport of amino acids

It occurs especially in the epithelial cells of intestinal tract and renal tubules during absorption of the amino acids into the blood.

Sodium Counter-transport

The carrier protein involved here acts as *antiport*, i.e. sodium ion is exchanged for some other substance. Some of the sodium counter-transport mechanisms occurring in the body are:
- Sodium-calcium counter-transport
- Sodium-hydrogen counter-transport

VESICULAR TRANSPORT

Vesicular transport mechanisms are involved in the transport of macromolecules such as large protein molecules which can neither pass through the cell membrane by diffusion

nor by active transport mechanisms. The vesicular transport mechanisms include endocytosis, exocytosis and transcytosis.

Endocytosis

Endocytosis is the process in which the substance is transported into the cell by infolding of the cell membrane around the substance and internalizing it (Fig. 1.3-19).
- Pinocytosis is a similar process like endocytosis used for absorption of fluid or other small molecules.
- Phagocytosis is a process like endocytosis in which a cell engulfs a foreign particle (e.g. bacteria).

Exocytosis

Exocytosis (Fig. 1.3-20) is reverse of endocytosis, i.e. by this process the substances are expelled from the cell without passing through the cell membrane. In this process, the substances which are to be extruded are collected in the form of granules or vesicles that move toward the cell membrane. Their membranes then fuse to the cell membrane. The area of fusion breaks down releasing the contents to the exterior and leaving the cell membrane intact. Release of hormones and enzymes by secretory cells of the body occurs by exocytosis.

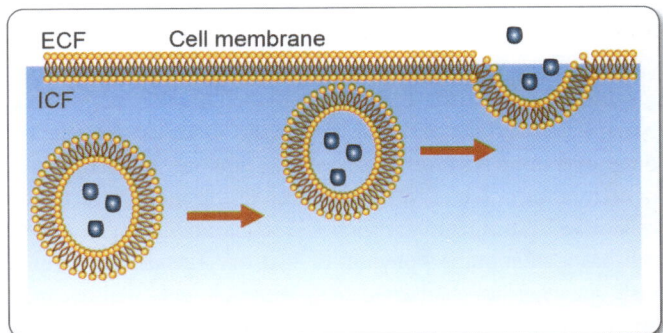

Fig. 1.3-20: Exocytosis

Transcytosis

Vesicular transport within the cell is called transcytosis or cytopemisis. It is quite similar to exocytosis and endocytosis. Three basic steps involved in this process are: vesicle formation, vesicle transportation, and docking in the cell.

OTHER TRANSPORT PROCESSES

Transport Across Epithelia

Transport across epithelia involves movement of the substances from one side of the epithelium to the other. The transepithelial transport occurs in body cavities lined by continuous sheet of cells such as in gastrointestinal tract, renal tubules, pulmonary airways and other structures. Transport across epithelia may occur in two ways:
1. Transport through the cells proper.
2. Transport across the tight junction.

Ultrafiltration

When a solution of protein and salt is separated from plain water or a less concentrated salt solution by a membrane permeable to salt and water and not to the protein, there will be a net movement of water on the protein side by diffusion and a movement of salt away from the protein side. This process is called *dialysis*.

It refers to occurrence of dialysis under hydrostatic pressure. Ultrafiltration is occurring at the capillary level in the body. The capillary blood is under hydrostatic pressure. The pressure is 35 mm Hg near the arteriolar end and gradually declines to 12 mm Hg near the venous end of the capillary. Through the capillaries, there occurs ultrafiltration of all the constituents of the plasma except the proteins into the interstitial spaces. Ultrafiltration plays important role in the formation of body fluids. For details refer to Chapter 4.2 page 217.

MEMBRANE POTENTIAL

There exists a potential difference across the membrane of all living cells with the inside being negative in relation to the outside. This potential difference is named *membrane potential*, because the cations and anions arrange themselves along the outer and inner surfaces of the cell membrane. The magnitude of membrane potential varies from cell to cell and in a particular cell, varies according to its functional status. For example, a nerve cell has a membrane potential of –70 mV (inside negative) at rest, but when it gets excited the membrane potential becomes about +30 mV (inside positive). The membrane potential at rest is called *resting membrane potential* or resting transmembrane potential or simply resting potential. The term rest does not imply that cell is metabolically quiescent but that it is not undergoing any electrical change. The membrane potential measured during excited state of the cell is called *action potential.*

GENESIS OF MEMBRANE POTENTIAL

Membrane potential is basically due to unequal distribution of ions across the cell membrane, which in turn results due to the combined effect of various forces acting on the ions. The factors involved in genesis of membrane potential which need elaboration are:

- Selective permeability of the cell membrane
- Gibbs-Donnan equilibrium
- Nernst equation
- Sodium-potassium ATPase pump.

Selective Permeability of the Cell Membrane

The cell membrane is selectively permeable, that is, to some ions it is freely permeable, to others impermeable and to some others it has variable permeability as:

- Ions like Na^+, K^+, Cl^- and HCO_3^- are diffusible ions. The cell membrane is freely permeable to K^+ and Cl^- and moderately permeable to Na^+.
- The cell membrane is practically impermeable to intracellular proteins and organic phosphate, which are negatively charged ions.
- Presence of gated channels in the cell membrane is responsible for the variable permeability of certain ions in different circumstances.

Gibbs-Donnan Membrane Equilibrium

According to Gibbs-Donnan membrane equilibrium, when 2 ionized solutions are separated by a semipermeable membrane, at equilibrium:

- Each solution shall be electrically neutral, i.e. total charges on cations will be equal to total charges on anions.
- The product of diffusible ions on one side of the membrane will be equal to product of diffusible ions on the other side of the membrane.

Since the intracellular fluid (ICF) contains non-diffusible anions like proteins and organic phosphate, so, according to Gibbs-Donnan equilibrium, there should be an asymmetrical distribution of diffusible ions across the cell membrane.

Nernst Equation

The asymmetrical distribution of diffusible ions across the cell membrane in the form of excess diffusible cations inside due to Gibbs-Donnan equilibrium (as explained above) results in concentration gradient. As a result of this, diffusible cations (K^+) will try to diffuse back into the ECF from ICF, but it is counteracted by the electrical gradient, which will be created due to the presence of non-diffusible anions inside the cell. Thus an equilibrium will be reached between the concentration gradient and the electrical gradient resulting in diffusion potential (equilibrium potential) across the cell membrane. The magnitude of this equilibrium potential can be determined by Nernst equation as:

$$E_{(m)} = \pm 61 \log \frac{(\text{Conc})_i}{(\text{Conc})_o}$$

The equilibrium potential (E_m) for some of the important ions in the mammalian spinal motor neuron calculated from the simplified Nernst equation is shown in Table 1.3-2.

TABLE 1.3-2: Equilibrium potential (E_m) for important ions in a mammalian spinal motor neuron

Ion	Concentration (in mmol/L of H_2O)		Equilibrium potential (in mV)
	Outside the cell	Inside the cell	
Na^+	150	15	+60
K^+	5.5	150	−90
Cl^-	125	9	−70

Role of Na^+-K^+ ATPase Pump

The role of Na^+-K^+ ATPase lies in building the concentration gradient. It serves to pump back the Na^+ that diffuses into the cell and K^+ that diffuses out of the cell. The Na^+-K^+ pump is potentially electrogenic, since it pumps out $3Na^+$ ions for $2K^+$ ions.

ASSESS YOURSELF

Short and Long Answer Questions

1. **Write brief notes on the functions of:**
   - Mitochondria
   - Lysosomes
   - Ribosomes
   - Endoplasmic reticulum
2. **Describe briefly:**
   - About structure and functions of cell membrane.
   - Mechanism of action of Na^+– K^+ ATPase
3. **Define the following terms:**
   - Diffusion
   - Osmosis
   - Active transport
   - Tonicity
4. **Write short notes on:**
   - Tight junction
   - Osmolality
   - Sodium–Potassium ATPase
   - Membrane potential
5. **Differentiate between:**
   - Simple and facilitated diffusion
   - Active and passive transport
   - Endocytosis and exocytosis
   - Hypertonic and hypotonic fluid

Multiple Choice Questions

1. **The intrinsic proteins mainly act as:**
   a. Antigens   b. Receptors
   c. Enzymes   d. Cell adhesion molecules

2. **The main function of Golgi apparatus is:**
   a. Synthesis of complex proteins
   b. Secretion of digestive enzymes
   c. Formation of endoplasmic reticulum
   d. Source of energy
3. **The true statement for peroxisomes:**
   a. Contain catalase
   b. Main site for protein synthesis
   c. Involved in antibody synthesis
   d. Mainly present in adipose tissues
4. **Which of the following belongs to inclusion bodies:**
   a. Microfilaments   b. Ribosomes
   c. Melanin pigment   d. Microfilaments
5. **The longest phase of mitosis cell division is:**
   a. Interphase   b. Prophase
   c. Metaphase   d. Anaphase
6. **The gap junctions are mainly present in:**
   a. Skeletal muscle   b. Cardiac muscle
   c. Nervous tissue   d. Adipose tissue
7. **Through the cell membrane which is transported by simple diffusion:**
   a. Oxygen
   b. Sodium ions
   c. Calcium
   d. Proteins
8. **Microtubules are not present in:**
   a. Micronvilli
   b. Flagella
   c. Cilia
   d. Centriole

9. **The true statement for meiosis:**
   a. Occurs both in gametes and somatic cells
   b. At the end two daughter cells are formed
   c. Replication of DNA occurs in interphase
   d. Crossing over of genetic material occurs in cytokinesis

10. **The statement not true for Sodium-potassium pump:**
    a. Maintains $Na^+ - K^+$ concentration difference across the cell membrane
    b. Establishes membrane potential
    c. It is a carrier protein
    d. It has three extracellular sites and two intracellular sites

11. **Which of the following transported by sodium Co-transport mechanism:**
    a. Steroids
    b. Alcohol
    c. Glucose
    d. Proteins

12. **The change in RBCs when kept in hypertonic saline:**
    a. No change in size and shape
    b. RBCs become large and swollen
    c. RBCs become small and crenated
    d. RBCs burst

13. **Which of the following is an example of primary active transport:**
    a. Sodium co-transport
    b. Sodium- Potassium pump
    c. Sodium counter transport
    d. Transport of water

14. **$Na^+ - K^+$ pump is an example of:**
    a. Primary active transport
    b. Secondary active transport
    c. Co-transport
    d. G protein–mediated transport

ANSWER KEY

1.	c	2.	a	3.	a	4.	c	5.	b	6.	b	7.	a	8.	a
9.	c	10.	d	11.	c	12.	c	13.	b	14.	a				

Tissues, Glands and Membranes

TISSUES

DEFINITION AND CLASSIFICATION

Body organs are made of many tissues. Tissues are collections of cells performing the same function and having almost similar structure.

Adult tissues are classified into four major groups (each having subdivisions):
1. Epithelial tissue or epithelium
2. Connective tissue
3. Muscle tissue (described in Chapter 7.4)
4. Nervous tissue (described in Chapter 10.1)

Epithelial Tissue

Epithelial tissue or epithelium consists of a single layer or multiple layers of cells, which are closely packed without any intercellular space. The cells usually lie on a basement membrane, which is an inert connective tissue. Epithelial tissue does not have blood supply of its own and it depends upon the diffusion from the underlying vascularized tissues for their nutrition.

Location

Epithelium lines or covers the external and internal surfaces of the human body organs as below:
- Lines outer surface of the body, i.e., skin.
- Forms the mucosa of the luminal surfaces of the cavities within the body such as in gastrointestinal tract (GIT), urinary tract, blood vessels, heart chambers, uterus, etc.
- Epithelial tissue also lines the ducts and secretory elements of glands (which develop as outgrowths from epithelium-lined surfaces).

Functions

Protection. It protects against injuries, bacteria and chemical agents.

Secretion. The epithelium lining the glandular tissue secretes different juices and enzymes.

Excretion. Epithelium performs excretory function in kidneys and skin.

Absorption. The intestinal epithelium plays vital role in absorption of digested food.

Lubrication. The mesothelial cells lining the serous cavities help in lubrication, e.g. in pleural cavity.

Sensory function. For example, as taste buds and organ of Corti (neuroepithelium).

Classification

Epithelium is of the following types:
i. Simple epithelium
- Simple squamous epithelium
- Simple cuboidal epithelium
- Simple columnar epithelium
- Simple columnar ciliated epithelium
- Pseudostratified columnar epithelium

ii. Compound or stratified epithelium
- Stratified squamous epithelium
- Stratified columnar epithelium
- Stratified columnar ciliated epithelium
- Transitional epithelium

Simple epithelium

Simple epithelium refers to a cellular sheet formed of single layer of cells. According to the shape of constituting cells the different types of simple epithelium are described here.

Squamous epithelium

Structure. Squamous epithelium is composed of single layer of flat cells resting on the basement membrane with flattened nuclei. The cells are closely packed like flat stones, so also called pavement epithelium (Figs 1.4-1A to D Histology Plate 1.4-1).

Functions and location. Squamous epithelium forms thin smooth surface for easy diffusion of fluid and gases of the following structures:

- Endothelium of heart, blood vessels and lymph vessels
- Alveoli of the lung
- Bowman's capsule of kidney
- Endothelium of cornea
- Mesothelium of serous membranes such as pleura, pericardium and peritoneum which facilitate the movement of viscera.

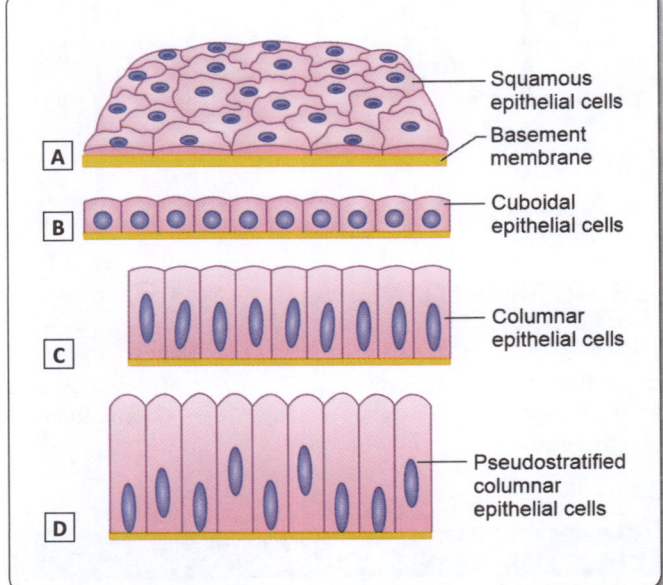

Figs 1.4-1A to D: Types of simple epithelium: A. Squamous; B. Cuboidal; C. Columnar; and D. Pseudostratified

Histology Plate 1.4-1: Squamous Epithelium

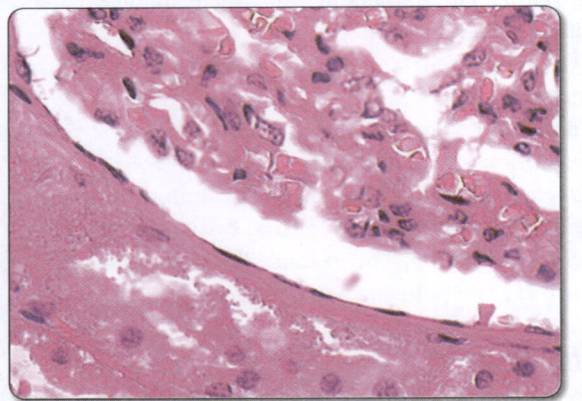

A portion of a renal corpuscle and adjacent renal tubules are shown. The glomerulus and renal corpuscle contains endothelium, simple squamous cells that constitute the capillary.

Cuboidal epithelium

Structure. Simple cuboidal epithelium is composed of a single layer of cubical cells resting on the basement membrane. Nucleus in the cuboidal cells is rounded and centrally placed (Fig. 1.4-1B and Histology Plate 1.4-2).

Functions and location. Cuboidal epithelium is actively involved in secretion, absorption and excretion, and also

provides limited protection to the organ as a covering. It is present in the following locations:

- Lining of the thyroid follicles
- Lining of the tubules of the kidneys
- Lining of the acini and small ducts of glands
- Germinal epithelium of ovary.

Histology Plate 1.4-2: Cuboidal Epithelium

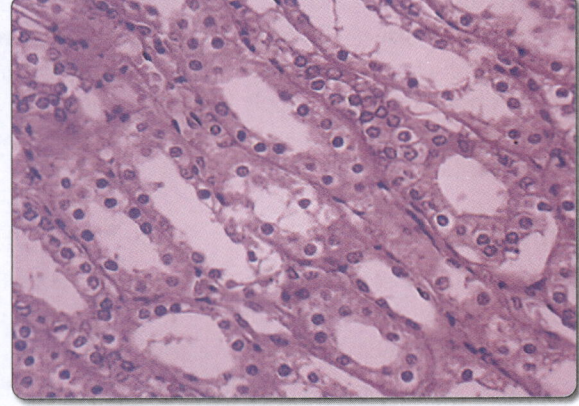

The renal tubules surrounding the renal corpuscles are portions of proximal and distal tubules lined with a simple cuboidal epithelium.

Chapter 1.4 ⊙ Tissues, Glands and Membranes   45

Section I ⊙ Introduction to Anatomical Terms; Organization of the Human Body...

Columnar epithelium

Structure. Columnar epithelium is composed of a single layer of tall columnar cells resting on basement membrane. Nucleus of columnar cells is oval and is placed centrally or toward base (Fig. 1.4-1C and Histology Plate 1.4-3).

Functions and location. Columnar epithelium is mainly concerned with secretion, absorption and protection. It is present in the following areas:

- Gastrointestinal tract and its glands
- Gallbladder, common bile duct and pancreatic duct.

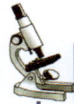

Histology Plate 1.4-3: Columnar Epithelium

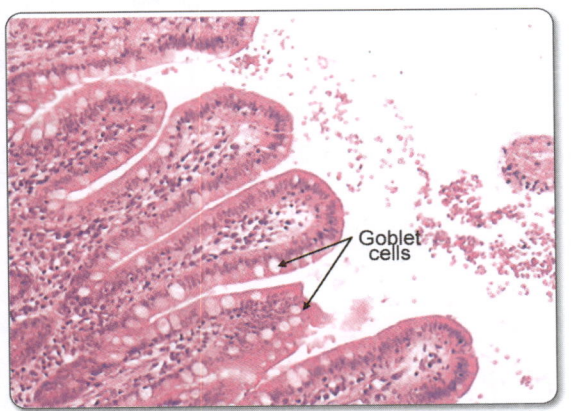

Goblet cells

The finger-like villi of the intestinal mucosa are shown. Note that the epithelial lining of the villi is interrupted by pale-staining, mucus-secreting goblet cells.

Columnar ciliated epithelium

Structure. The columnar ciliated epithelium is composed of simple columnar cells, the free surfaces of which bear a large number of cilia. Nucleus in these cells is oval and placed toward base.

Functions and location. These cells are protective in function. The wave-like movement of the cilia pushes the contents of the tubes, which they line, in one direction. Ciliated epithelium is found lining in the:

- Respiratory passages, i.e., trachea and its branches
- Uterine tubes
- Outer or bony part of Eustachian tube
- Central canal of spinal cord and brain ventricles.

Pseudostratified columnar epithelium

Structure. Pseudostratified columnar epithelium consists of single layer of tall columnar cells of different heights. All the cells rest on the basement membrane but some cells are small in size and do not reach the surface. Thus, their nuclei appear at different levels forming false rows, hence named pseudostratified epithelium (Fig. 1.4-1D and Histology Plate 1.4-4).

Functions and location. Pseudostratified columnar epithelium is protective and secretory in function. Three different types of pseudostratified columnar epithelia are located as below:

1. *Pseudostratified columnar ciliated epithelium with goblet cells (with motile cilia) is found lining the:*

- Upper respiratory passages such as nasal air sinuses, nasopharynx, part of larynx, trachea and bronchi
- Inner or cartilaginous part of Eustachian tube
- Lacrimal sac

2. *Pseudostratified columnar ciliated epithelium* (with microvilli or stereocilia) is only present in the epididymis.

3. *Pseudostratified columnar non-ciliated epithelium is present in:*

- Upper part of ductus deferens
- Large ducts of salivary glands
- Male urethra (penile part).

Histology Plate 1.4-4: Pseudostratified Columnar Epithelium

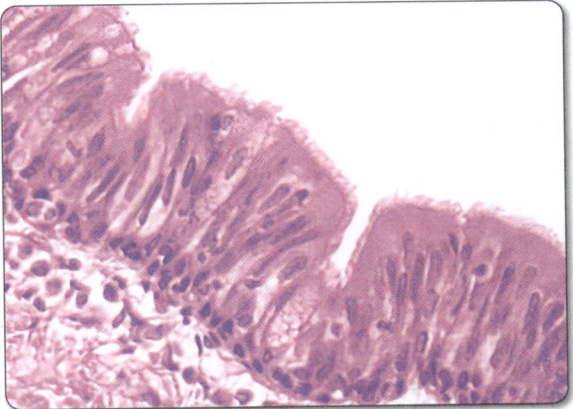

The nasal mucosa is seen to be lined by a ciliated, pseudostratified columnar epithelium. Although the nuclei of the epithelium are at different levels, all cells make contact with the basement membrane, hence the term pseudostratified columnar epithelium.

Compound or stratified epithelium

Compound or stratified epithelium refers to the cellular sheet formed of several layers of cells of various shapes. The

46 | **Textbook of Applied Anatomy and Physiology for Nurses**

Section I ⊙ Introduction to Anatomical Terms; Organization of the Human Body...

superficial layers of stratified epithelium grow up from the basal layer. Different types of stratified epithelia are described below.

Stratified squamous epithelium

Structure. Stratified squamous epithelium consists of multiple layers of cells of different shapes arranged as follows (Fig. 1.4-2A and Histology Plate 1.4-5).

Basal cells or the deepest cells are columnar in shape and rest on a clear wavy basement membrane.

Intermediate layers are formed of polygonal cells with desmosomes anchoring them to each other between their cell boundaries.

Superficial layers are of flat squamous cells which may be nucleated or non-nucleated.

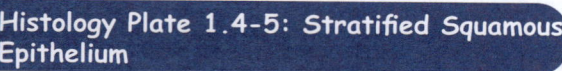

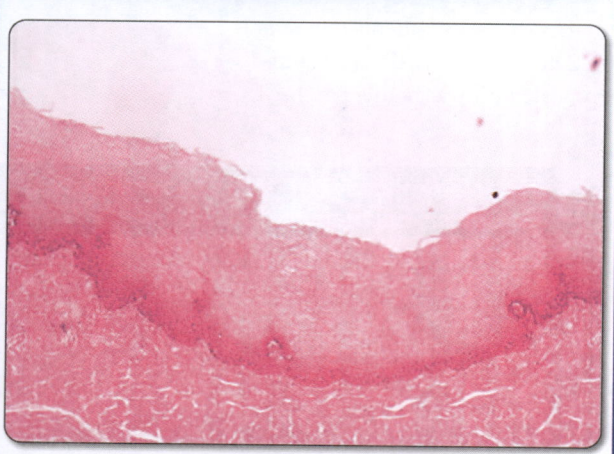

A portion of the wall of the esophagus is shown. Note the lumen at the top, the stratified squamous non-keratinized epithelium of the mucosa and the underlying connective tissue of the submucosa.

Types: Stratified squamous epithelium is of two types:

1. *Non-keratinized squamous epithelium.* In this epithelium all cells are living and have nuclei up to the surface. This is found on following wet surfaces that may be subject to wear and tear but are protected from drying:
- *Eye.* Cornea and exposed part of conjunctiva.
- *Gastrointestinal tract.* Oral cavity, i.e., inner surface of lips, tongue, gums, palatine tonsils, oropharynx, esophagus and middle part of anal canal.
- *Genitourinary tract.* Vagina, and terminal parts of male and female urethra.

2. *Keratinized squamous epithelium:* The surface layer of this epithelium consists of dead cells which have lost their nuclei and the protein keratin has been added to them (Fig. 1.4-2B). This tough layer of dead cells protects and prevents drying of underlying cells. This is found in the following areas:
- Epidermis of skin
- Tip of filiform papillae of tongue
- Hair and nails.

Stratified columnar epithelium

Structure. It is formed of multiple layers (less in number than stratified squamous epithelium). Superficial cells are columnar in type (Fig. 1.4-2B).

Location and function. Stratified columnar epithelium is rare epithelium seen in the ducts of some glands.

Transitional epithelium

Structure. Transitional epithelium is composed of several layers of cells arranged classically in three strata (Fig. 1.4-2C and Histology Plate 1.4-6):

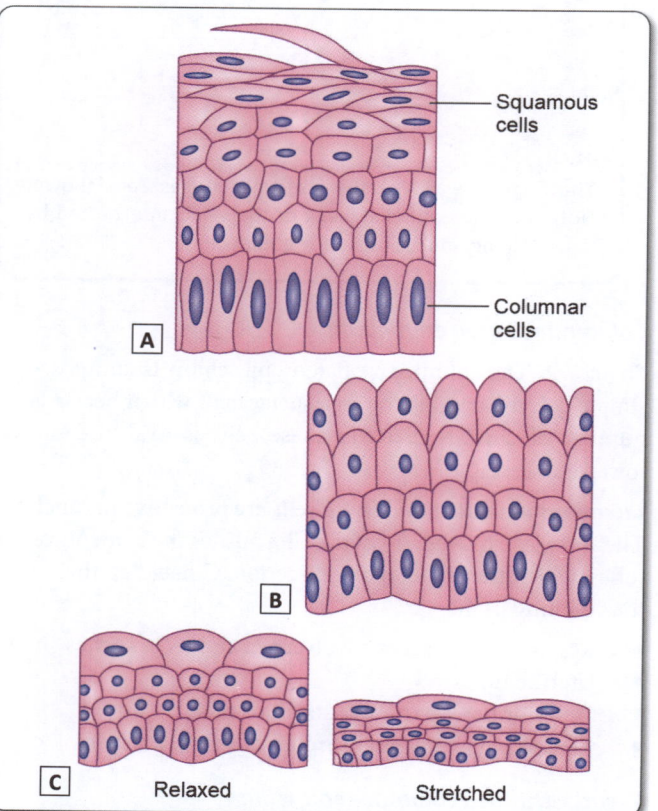

Figs 1.4-2A to C: Types of compound or stratified epithelium: A. Squamous; B. Columnar; C. Transitional (relaxed and stretched)

Histology Plate 1.4-6: Transitional Epithelium

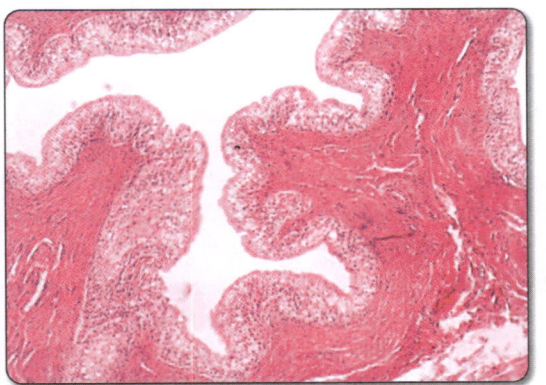

The wall of the urinary bladder is shown. The transitional epithelium of the mucosa is seen interposed between the lumen and the muscular wall of the bladder.

- *Superficial layer* is formed by large polyhedral umbrella-like cells.
- *Intermediate layers* are made up of pear-shaped cells; the tip is directed toward membrane.
- *Basal cell layer* is formed of high cuboidal cells.

Location and function. Transitional epithelium is found in the renal pelvis and calyces, the ureter, the urinary bladder, and part of the urethra. Because of this distribution it is also called *urothelium.*

In the urinary bladder, the transitional epithelium allows the stretching when the bladder fills with urine. When stretched, it is not damaged and appears to be thinner with cells becoming flattened and rounded (Fig. 1.4-2C).

Connective Tissue

General Considerations

The term connective tissue is applied to a tissue which connects one tissue or organ with other tissues or organs.

Structure of connective tissue in general

Connective tissue, in general, is formed of cells and matrix.

Cells. The cells forming the connective tissue differ in different types of connective tissues. The peculiar feature of all connective tissues is that the cells are more widely separated from each other than those forming the epithelium.

Matrix. The matrix refers to the intercellular substance. The matrix is present in considerably large amount in all the connective tissues. The structure of matrix varies in different types of connective tissues.

Types of connective tissues

Depending upon the type of cells and nature of matrix the connective tissue is of the following types:

- Connective tissue proper (described below)
- Skeletal (supporting) connective tissue, i.e., bone and cartilage (for details see Chapter 7.1).
- Fluid connective tissue, i.e., blood and lymph (for details see Chapter 4.1 & 4.3).

Connective Tissue Proper

Definition and functions

Connective tissue proper is in fact the connective tissue in real sense which serves the following functions:

Connects the various tissues and organs of the body with each other. Thus the connective tissue fills the interstices between more specialized elements and serves to hold them together.

Supports the tissues and organs of the body by providing a framework.

Protects the tissues and organs by withstanding internal as well as external mechanical stresses. It also defends the body from invasion by microorganisms.

Structure of connective tissue proper

Depending upon the structure the connective tissue proper is of various types (which are described later). In general, the connective tissue proper is composed of:

- Cells
- Matrix, i.e., intercellular substance which includes fibers and ground substance.

A. Cells of connective tissue proper

As mentioned earlier the connective tissue proper is found in all organs supporting the specialized tissues. The different types of cells of connective tissue proper are:

- Fibroblasts and fibrocytes
- Fat cells
- Plasma cells
- Mast cells
- Macrophages (histiocytes)
- Leukocytes
- Pigment cells
- Mesenchyme cells.

1. *Fibroblasts and fibrocytes.* Fibroblasts on maturation change to fibrocytes.

Structure. Fibroblasts are flat, branched (irregular) cells with multiple processes (Fig. 1.4-3A). Cytoplasm of these cells is deeply basophilic and rich in RNA, granular endoplasmic reticulum and Golgi apparatus.

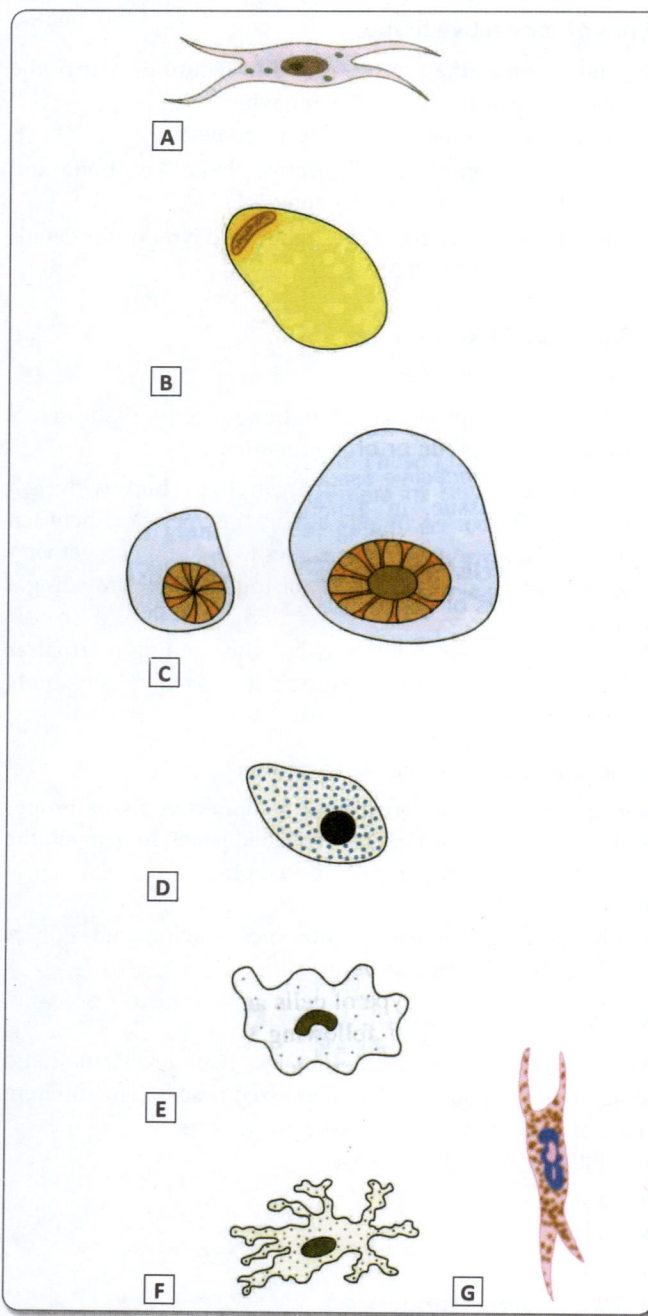

Figs 1.4-3A to G: Cells of connective tissue proper: A. Fibroblast; B. Fat cell; C. Plasma cell; D. Mast cell; E. Macrophage; F. Pigment cell with pigment granules and G. Mesenchyme cell

Function. Fibroblasts are responsible for formation of both the collagen and elastic fibers as well as ground substance of the matrix. These cells are particularly active in tissue repair (wound healing) where they may bind together the cut surfaces of wounds to form granulation tissue.

2. *Fat cells* also known as *adipocytes* may be found singly or in groups.
Structure. Fat cells are large ovoid with peripheral nucleus (signet ring appearance) (Fig. 1.4-3B). They vary in size and shape depending upon the amount of fat they contain.
Function. They store fat and are especially abundant in adipose tissue.

3. *Plasma cells.* These are ovoid or rounded in shape. Chromatin in the nucleus is arranged in radiating manner giving the appearance of *cartwheel shape* (Fig. 1.4-3C). Their cytoplasm contains *Russell bodies* (immunoglobulin granules). These cells play important role in defence mechanism.

4. *Mast cells.* These cells are present in loose connective tissue. They are usually present in groups around the blood vessels.
Structure. Mast cells are oval or rounded in shape similar to basophil leukocytes. Their cytoplasm is filled with large basophilic granules which are precursor of histamine (Fig. 1.4-3D).
Functions. These cells produce histamine and heparin which are released when the cells are damaged by disease or injury. Histamine is involved in local and general inflammatory reactions.

5. *Macrophages* or histiocytes form the part of macrophage system of the body.
Structure. Macrophages are irregular, usually branched with multiple processes (Fig. 1.4-3E), but may be elongated or spindle-shaped. Their cytoplasm is basophilic and may be granular or vacuolated.
Function. They form important part of body's defence mechanism as they are actively phagocytic, engulfing worn-out leucocytes (which die in the process of destroying bacteria), bacteria and foreign bodies.

6. *Leukocytes,* i.e., white blood cells, particularly lymphocytes, are normally found in a small number in healthy connective tissue. Their number increases in chronic infections when they play an important role in tissue defence.

7. *Pigment cells.* They are particularly found in the connective tissue of skin, and uveal tissue of eye.
Structure. They are small stellate-shaped cells with many branching processes. Their cytoplasm contains numerous pigment granules (Fig. 1.4-3F).
Function. These cells protect the skin against the harmful effects of sun rays.

8. *Mesenchyme cells.* These are undifferentiated cells and can give rise to all varieties of connective tissue cells.
Structure. They are small stellate-shaped cells with large oval nucleus (Fig. 1.4-3G).
In adult connective tissue, they are arranged along blood vessels. They develop into endothelial cells lining the blood capillaries.

CONNECTIVE TISSUE FIBERS

The adult connective tissue contains three types of fibers:

1. Collagen fibers
2. Elastic fibers
3. Reticular fibers

1. Collagen fibers. Their characteristic features are:

- Colorless, strong fibers arranged in bundles (Fig. 1.4-4A).
- Flexible but nonextensible.
- Formed of a protein tropocollagen which can be transformed into gelatin on boiling.
- Found in all types of connective tissue but are specially abundant in skin, dense connective tissue, tendons, ligaments, aponeurosis and meninges of the brain.
- Abnormal conditions include deficient formation in scurvy due to vitamin C deficiency and excessive production and abnormal organization in rheumatoid arthritis.

2. Elastic fibers. Characteristic features are:

- Very elastic, yellowish branched fibers which run singly and not in bundles (Fig. 1.4-4B)
- Formed of the protein tropoelastin which is resistant to boiling.
- Found in ligamentum nuchae, ligamentum flavum, walls of large arteries and lining of nerve cells.

3. Reticular fibers are types of collagen fibers having the following features (Fig. 1.4-4C):

- Thin branching fibers arranged in a net-like framework called reticulum.
- Found in glandular organs, lymphoid tissue, spleen and liver.

Ground Substance of Matrix of Connective Tissue

- It is an amorphous material in which are embedded the cells and fibers of connective tissue.
- It contains a number of proteoglycans which are composed of glycosaminoglycans (GAGs) linked to specific polypeptide chains. The proteoglycans bind water and provide resilience to connective tissue.
- It is synthesized by fibroblasts, osteoblasts, chondroblasts, and smooth muscle cells.

Types of connective tissue proper

Depending upon the relative amount of fibers, cells and matrix the connective tissue proper is of the following types:

- Loose (or areolar) connective tissue
- Dense connective tissue
- Reticular connective tissue
- Adipose connective tissue
- Pigmented connective tissue.

1. Loose (Areolar) connective tissue

Structural characteristics of loose (areolar) connective tissue include (Fig. 1.4-5 and Histology Plate 1.4-7):

- *Matrix* is semisolid and contains loose, irregularly arranged collagen and elastic fibers in the amorphous ground substance.
- *Cells* embedded in the matrix include fibroblasts, some fat cells, mast cells and macrophages. Cells are widely separated by the fibers.

Location. Areolar connective tissue is widely distributed all over the body. It is present mainly:

- Under the skin
- In between the muscles

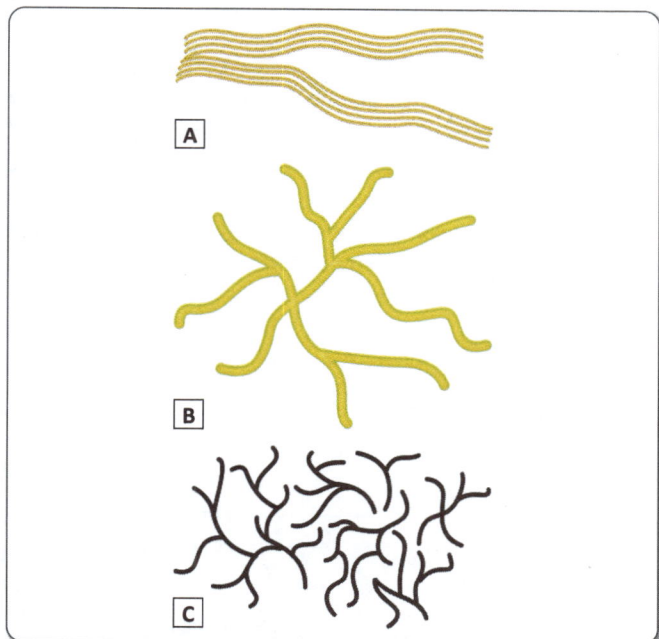

Figs 1.4-4A to C: Fibers of connective tissue proper: A. Collagen fibers; B. Elastic fibers; C. Reticular fibers

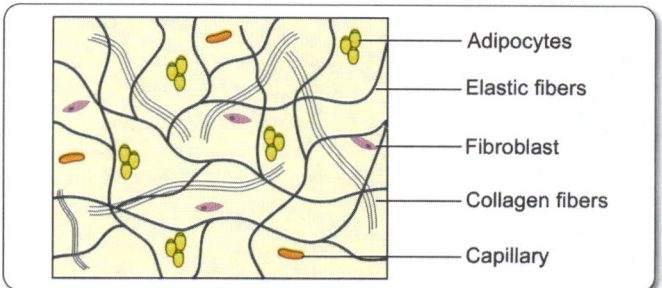

Adipocytes

Elastic fibers

Fibroblast

Collagen fibers

Capillary

Fig. 1.4-5: Loose (areolar) connective tissue

Histology Plate 1.4-7: Loose (Areolar) Connective Tissue

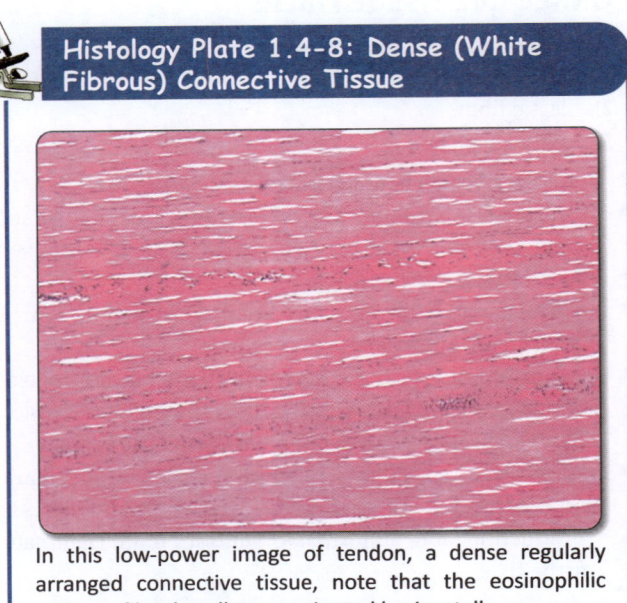

A whole mount of mesentery prepared with an elastic stain is shown. Even at magnification, the fibrous nature of this loose connective tissue is evident.

Histology Plate 1.4-8: Dense (White Fibrous) Connective Tissue

In this low-power image of tendon, a dense regularly arranged connective tissue, note that the eosinophilic collagen fiber bundles are oriented horizontally.

* In stroma of most of the organs
* Below the mucous membranes
* Around the vessels and nerves
* In serous membranes
* In glands supporting secretory cells.

Functions. Areolar connective tissue provides elasticity and tensile strength to almost every part of the body.

2. Dense (white fibrous) connective tissue

Structure. It is formed mainly by closely packed bundles of collagen tissue with very little ground substance. Cells (fibrocytes) are few in number and are found lying in rows between the bundles of fibers.

Location. Dense connective tissue is of two types, regular and irregular. The dense regular (Fig. 1.4-6 and Histology Plate 1.4-8)

(white fibrous) connective tissue is present in tendons, ligaments and aponeurosis. The dense irregular connective tissue is present in dermis, periosteum, perichondrium and capsule and stroma of some organs and glands, dura mater and sclera of the eyeball.

Functions. Dense connective tissue connects (supports) and forms tough covering to the various organs.

3. Reticular onnective tissue

Structure. It is made up mainly of stellate-shaped reticular cells and fibrillar network of reticular fibers (Fig. 1.4-7 and Histology Plate 1.4-9). The reticular fibers are thin immature collagen fibers.

Location. Reticular connective tissue is present in the stroma of bone marrow, spleen, lymph nodes, thymus, liver, testis, ovary, and endocrine glands.

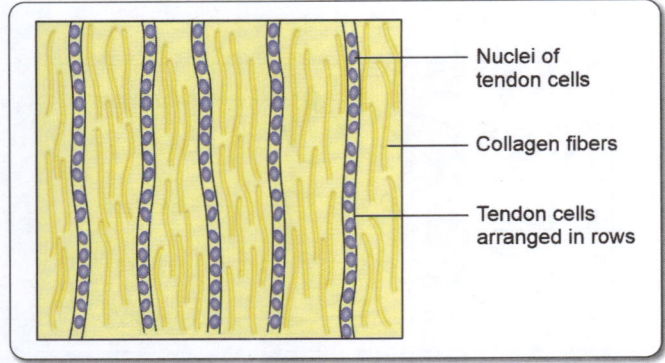

Fig. 1.4-6: Dense connective tissue

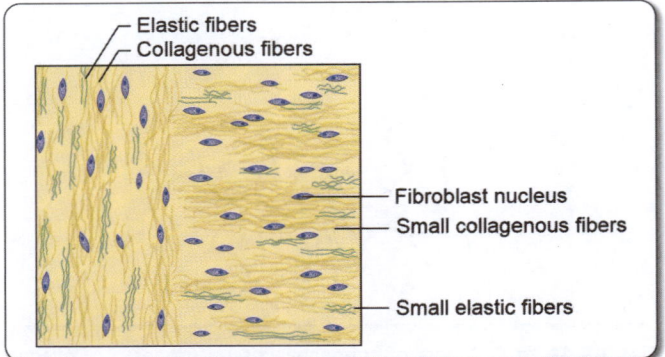

Fig. 1.4-7: Reticular connective tissue

Histology Plate 1.4-9: Reticular Connective Tissue

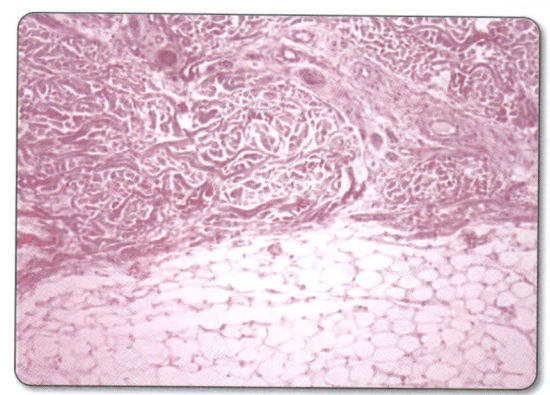

A low-power image of a lymph node stained using silver impregnation methods reveals the delicate reticular fiber network of this lymphoid structure. The capsule is at upper right with several lymphoid nodules beneath.

Histology Plate 1.4-10: Adipose Connective Tissue

At high magnification, the interface of the dermis and hypodermis reveals a patch of adipose tissue. The adipose cells have the appearance of a honey comb network.

Function. The reticular connective tissue forms a network in the background of organs and glands.

4. Adipose connective tissue

Adipose connective tissue is of two types: white and brown.

1. *White adipose connective tissue.* It is mainly composed of large fat cells (more than 100 microns in diameter), each containing a single large globule of non-pigmented fat, in a matrix of areolar tissue (Fig. 1.4-8 and Histology Plate 1.4-10). *Location and functions.* In well-nourished adults it makes up 20–25% of the body weight. It is present between muscle fibers and under the skin in superficial fascia where it acts as thermal insulator.

- It is present around the kidneys and eyeballs where it provides a supporting cushion.
- In the abdominal wall, mesentery and abdomen as fat storage.

2. *Brown adipose tissue.* It is made up of small fat cells which are filled with many droplets of pigmented fat. It appears brown because it is rich in cytochrome pigments. It has more extensive capillary network than white adipose tissue.

Location and function. Brown adipose tissue is mainly present in the newborn and persists for few months after birth. It acts as *heat generator* and protects the infant from cold after birth. It is located in interscapular region, axillary region, and mediastinal region.

IMPORTANT TO KNOW

It is important to note that adipose connective tissue is not present in the eyelids, penis, labia minora, clitoris, nipples and scrotum.

5. Pigmented connective tissue

Structure. It is similar to loose areolar connective tissue with a large number of pigment cells.

Location. It is present in the vascular layer of the eyeballs (iris, ciliary body and choroid) and in the skin.

NURSING IMPLICATIONS AND APPLICATIONS

Connective tissue disorders (CTDs) affect the main proteins that are responsible for the strength and integrity of all of the organs, vessels, skin and bones. CTDs are caused by specific genetic mutations that adversely affect the main building blocks of the human body: fibrillin, collagen, and elastin protein molecules.

- Many patients with a CTD have no symptoms until their 20s or 30s. Easy bruising, hyperflexibility, and orthopedic issues in a very young child may signal an elevated risk for a CTD.
- Some CTDs are associated with characteristic facial, skeletal, eye and skin features.

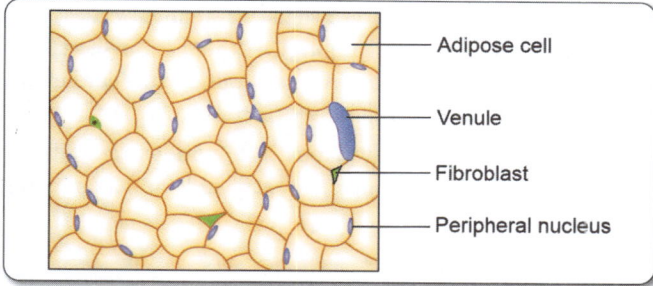

Fig. 1.4-8: White adipose tissue

- Adipose cell
- Venule
- Fibroblast
- Peripheral nucleus

FORMATION AND REGENERATION OF BODY TISSUES

Formation

The body tissues are formed from the embryonic mesenchyme. The mesenchyme is also known as embryonic connective tissue, consisting of loosely arranged mesenchymal cells, which are derived from two sources; mesoderm cells and neural crest cells. The mesenchyme lies between the ectoderm and mesoderm, and also between mesoderm and endoderm.

Mesoderm

The characteristic feature of mesenchymal cells in ability to proliferate and differentiate into other type of cells, which in turn give rise to different kind of tissues (Fig. 1.4-4) as under:

Chondroblasts proliferate into chondrocytes, which are cartilage forming cells.

Osteoblasts are bone forming cells. In the area of bone formation mesenchyme begins to differentiate into osteoblasts which proliferate into osteocytes depositing matrix or intracellular substance to form osteoid or probone.

Cells of connective tissue. The mesenchyme cells also differentiate into various types of connective tissue cells such as fibroblasts, histeocytes, mast cells, plasma cells and fat cells.

Blood forming cells. Some mesenchyme cells form precursors of various blood cells such as hemocytoblast and lymphoblasts.

Vascular endothelial cells are also formed by the differentiation of mesenchyme cells, which form the endothelial lining of the blood vessels and heart.

Myoblasts are differentiated mesenchyme cells for formation of muscle tissue.

Ectoderm

Ectoderm forms the epithelium of the nervous tissue (brain and spinal cord). The neuroectoderm forms the ganglia and medulla of adrenal glands.

Endoderm

Endoderm forms the epithelium of gastrointestinal tract (GIT), liver, pancreas and gallbladder.

Regeneration

After birth, growth and development is a continuous process up to adulthood. Regeneration process plays the primary role in restoration of damaged tissue after tissue injury. Regeneration or repair of injured part of the body occurs in four stages as under:

(i) Hemostasis or stoppage of bleeding after injury. Platelets and other coagulation factors play an important role in stoppage of bleeding.

(ii) Inflammatory phase. Inflammation is a protective tissue reaction by the substances released due to injury. The inflammation phase begins at the time of injury and lasts for up to 4–5 days. In the inflammatory phase two types of reactions occur:

1. *Vascular reaction.* There is vasodilation of local blood vessels and leakage of fluid into the interstitial space.
2. *Cellular reaction.* In this phase, there is migration of white blood cells into the injury site.

(iii) Proliferative phase. It begins after 3 days of injury and overlaps with inflammatory phase

(iv) Remodeling phase. Healing occurs under this phase.

Apoptosis

Apoptosis refers to programmed cell death (PCD), which occurs under genetic control. The cells own genes that play vital role in its demise, therefore it is also called "cell suicide". Apoptosis is very important during the development of fetus as well as in adulthood.

During development apoptosis is responsible for sexual differentiation, i.e., formation of male and female genital organs and also formation of fingers and toes in the fetus.

In adulthood in females apoptosis is responsible for cyclic endometrial changes during menstrual cycle.

GLANDS

Epithelial cells which are specialized to produce secretion constitute the glandular epithelium or the so-called glands.

TYPES OF GLANDS

Glands can be classified in different ways:

A. According to Number of Constituting Cells

Unicellular glands. These are made of a single cell. These glands are interspersed amongst other (non-secretory) epithelial cells. For example, *goblet cells* found in the epithelium lining the intestine and respiratory tract.

Multicellular glands. Most glands in the body are made up of multiple cells. For example, sweat glands and mammary glands.

B. According to the Nature of Secretion

Mucus-secreting glands, e.g. goblet cells and sublingual salivary gland.

Serous glands, e.g. parotid gland.

Mixed or seromucous glands, e.g. submandibular gland.

Watery secretion glands, e.g. sweat glands.

Waxy secretion glands, e.g. ceruminous glands of ear.

Fatty secretion glands, e.g. sebaceous glands.

Cellular secretory glands, e.g. testis and ovary.

C. According to Mode of Pouring the Secretion

Endocrine or ductless glands pour their secretion directly into the blood. Examples of endocrine glands are thyroid, parathyroid, pituitary, suprarenal, pineal body, and islets of Langerhans of pancreas.

Endocrine glands are usually arranged in cords or in clumps that are intimately related to a rich network of blood capillaries or sinusoids. In some cases (for example, thyroid gland) the cells may form rounded follicles. Endocrine cells and their blood vessels are supported by delicate connective tissue, and are usually surrounded by a capsule.

Exocrine glands. These glands pour their secretion onto the epithelial surface directly or through the ducts. Examples of exocrine glands are salivary glands, sweat glands and sebaceous glands.

Mixed glands. These glands have features of both endocrine and exocrine glands. For example, pancreas, testis and ovary have both types of glandular tissues.

D. According to Manner of Secretion (Figs 1.4-9A to C)

Merocrine glands produce their secretion by exocytosis, i.e., the secretory cells remain intact. Most glands such as pituitary, pancreas, etc. are merocrine glands.

Apocrine glands lose apical portion of the secretory cells along with the secretory product, as in axillary sweat glands and mammary glands.

Holocrine glands discharge the entire cell with secretion, e.g. sebaceous glands of skin.

CLASSIFICATION OF EXOCRINE GLANDS

Depending upon the shape of secretory part and their ducts the multicellular exocrine glands can be classified as below:

A. Simple Glands (Figs 1.4-10A to E)

These have a single duct in which all the secretory cells pour their secretion. Depending upon the arrangement of secretory cells the simple glands may be tubular, alveolar or tubuloalveolar:

Simple tubular glands. The tube-shaped simple glands may be:
- *Straight*, e.g. intestinal glands (crypts of Lieberkühn).
- *Coiled*, e.g. sweat glands of skin.
- *Branched*, e.g. glands of stomach and uterus.

Simple alveolar glands. These glands have a single duct and the secretory cells are arranged in the form of flask-shaped structures called alveoli. For example, sebaceous glands and tarsal glands.

Simple tubuloalveolar glands. These glands have tubular as well as alveolar arrangement of secretory cells.

B. Compound Glands (Figs 1.4-10F to H)

These glands are composed of a number of groups of secretory cells, each group discharging into its own duct. The ducts from each group of secretory cells unite to form large ducts that ultimately drain on the epithelial surface. Depending upon the arrangement of secretory cells (like that of simple glands) the compound glands may also be:

Compound tubular glands, e.g. kidney and testis

Compound alveolar glands, e.g. mammary glands

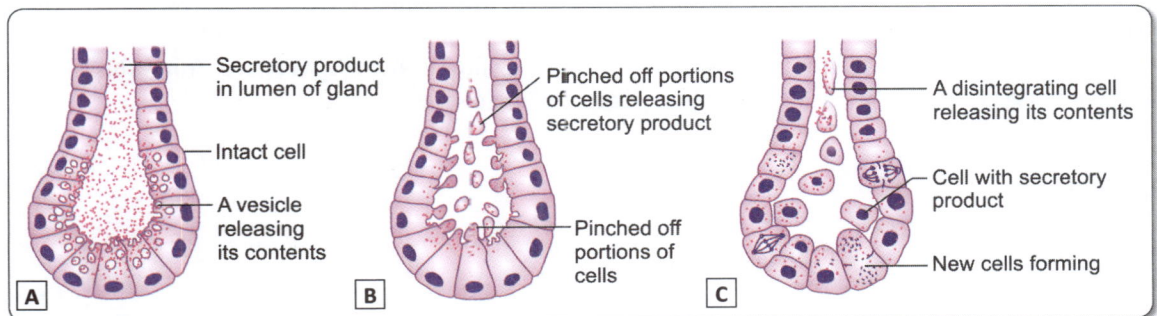

Figs 1.4-9A to C: Types of glands according to manner of secretion: A. Merocrine gland; B. Apocrine gland; C. Holocrine gland

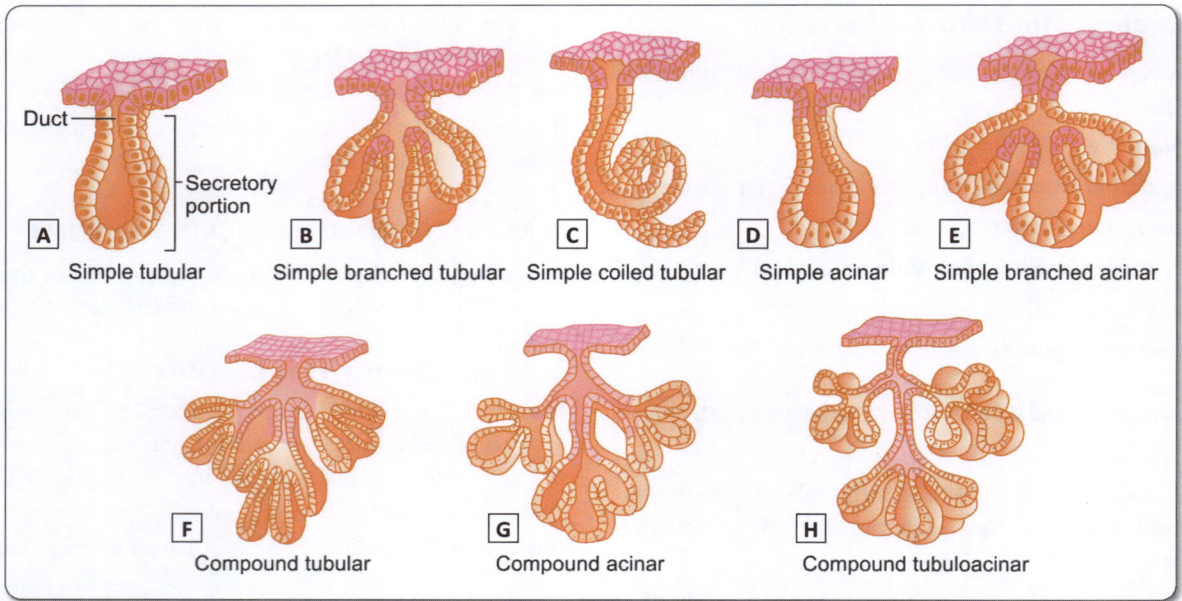

Figs 1.4-10A to H: Types of exocrine glands

Compound tubuloalveolar glands, e.g. pancreas, prostate, and salivary glands.

MEMBRANES

There are two important types of membranes present in human body
1. Epithelial membranes
2. Synovial membrane

Epithelial Membranes

Epithelial membranes are formed of sheets of epithelial tissue and supporting connective tissue. The internal structures and cavities are lined by epithelial membranes.

Mucous Membrane

Mucous membrane is the moist lining of alimentary, respiratory and genitourinary tracts. Some of the epithelial cells on the membrane surface produce a secretion called, mucus that protects the membrane from drying and any injuries. In respiratory tract, mucus helps in trapping the inhaled particles, and then, preventing them from entering the alveoli of the lungs.

Serous Membrane

Serous membrane secretes serous fluid. It consists of a double layered loose areolar connective tissue. One of the layers lines the cavity (parietal layer) and the other layer lines the organ (visceral layer). The layers are separated by the serous fluid that enables the organ to glide freely within the cavity without being damaged by friction. There are three sites where serous membranes are found:
1. The pleura (around the lungs)
2. The pericardium (around the heart)
3. The peritoneum (surrounding abdominal organs)

Synovial Membranes

This membrane lines the cavities of moveable joints and surrounds tendons, e.g. over the wrist joint. It consists of areolar connective tissue and elastic fibers.

Synovial fluid is secreted from this membrane that lubricates the joints.

Chapter 1.4 ◉ Tissues, Glands and Membranes   55

Section I ◉ Introduction to Anatomical Terms; Organization of the Human Body...

ASSESS YOURSELF

Short and Long Answer Questions

1. **Describe briefly the following types of tissues and their functions:**
   - Stratified sequamous epithelium
   - Simple ciliated epithelium
   - Pseudostratified columnar epithelium
   - Transitional epithelium
2. **Discuss in brief the classification of glands with examples.**
3. **What are different types of membranes? Describe their characteristic features, give example of each.**

Multiple Choice Questions

1. **Simple cuboidal epithelial lining is present in:**
   a. Gall bladder
   b. Ducts of exocrine glands
   c. Trachea
   d. Urinary bladder
2. **Simple squamous epithelium lining mainly present in:**
   a. Kidney tubules
   b. Lung alveoli
   c. Thyroid follicles
   d. Gastrointestinal tract
3. **The epithelial lining of thyroid follicles is by:**
   a. Columnar ciliated
   b. Columnar
   c. Simple cuboidal
   d. Pseudostratified
4. **The large ducts of the glands are lined by which epithelium:**
   a. Stratified squamous
   b. Pseudostratified non-ciliated columnar
   c. Transitional
   d. Stratified columnar

5. **Bone and cartilage are examples of which tissue:**
   a. Connective tissue proper
   b. Supporting connective tissue
   c. Fluid connective tissue
   d. Alveolar connective tissue
6. **The true statement about collagen fibers:**
   a. Formed by protein tropoelastin
   b. Present in glandular tissue
   c. Extensible
   d. Mainly present in the skin
7. **The main function of white adipose tissues is:**
   a. Acts as support by forming tough covering
   b. Provides elasticity and tensile strength
   c. Acts as thermal insulator
   d. Acts as heat generator
8. **The sebaceous glands secrete which type of secretion:**
   a. Watery
   b. Serous
   c. Waxy
   d. Oily
9. **Which of the following is example of holocrine gland:**
   a. Sweat gland
   b. Sebacious gland
   c. Pituitary gland
   d. Gastric glalnd
10. **The synovial membrane is present in:**
    a. Pleura
    b. Lung alveoli
    c. Peritoneum
    d. Joint cavity

ANSWER KEY

| 1. | b | 2. | b | 3. | c | 4. | b | 5. | a | 6. | d | 7. | c | 8. | d |
| 9. | b | 10. | d | | | | | | | | | | | | |

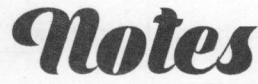

Section

II

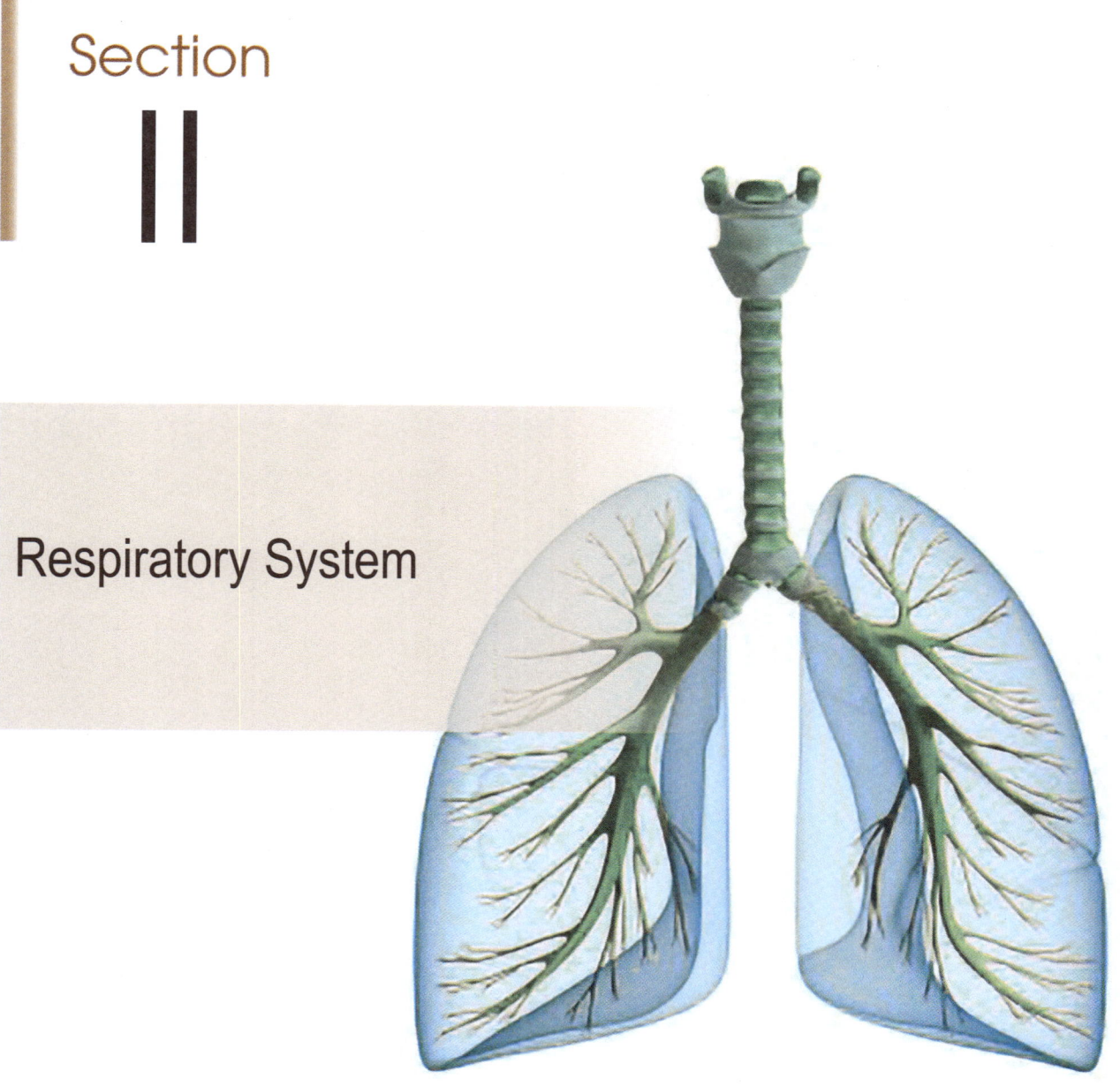

Respiratory System

Section Outline

Anatomy, Organization and Functions of Respiratory System

RESPIRATORY PASSAGES

The chief organs of the respiratory system are right and left *lungs*. The oxygen contained in the atmospheric air reaches the lungs by passing through a series of *respiratory passages*, which also serve for removal of CO_2 from the alveoli to the atmosphere. The respiratory system also includes a pump that ventilates the lung. This pump consists of the chest wall and respiratory muscles.

The respiratory passages include (Fig. 2.1-1):
- Nose and nasal cavities
- Pharynx
- Larynx
- Tracheobronchial tree

NOSE AND NASAL CAVITY

The nose is a special organ of the sense of smell, but it also serves as a passageway for air going to and from the lungs.

Shape and Structure

The external nose is a projection of the face with a free tip. It is composed of a triangular framework of bone and cartilage, covered by skin and lined by mucous membrane.

Nostrils (Anterior Nares)

These are two oval openings on the undersurface of the nose. The anterior nares open into the right and left nasal cavities. These openings are guarded by numerous internal hairs that help to prevent the entrance of relatively coarse particles sometimes present in the air.

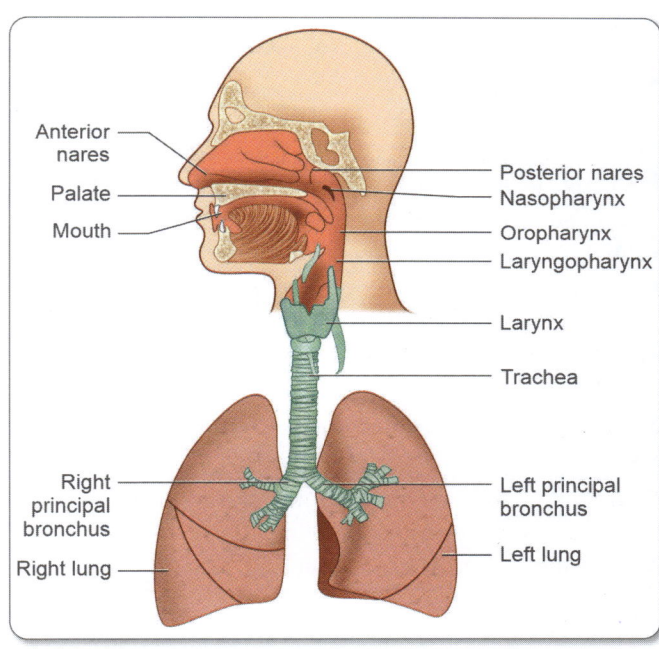

Fig. 2.1-1: The air passages

Nasal Cavity

The nasal cavity is divided into two parts (right and left) by the nasal septum. The nasal cavity extends from the anterior nares (nostrils) to the posterior nares (the choanae), through which it opens into the nasopharynx.

Boundaries of Nasal Cavity

The bony and cartilaginous framework of each half of the nasal cavity forms its (Fig. 2.1-2):

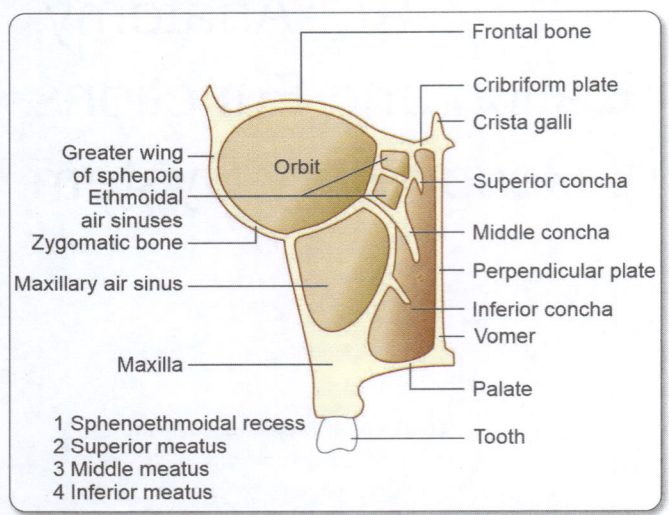

Fig. 2.1-2: Schematic coronal section through nasal cavity to show bony framework of its walls

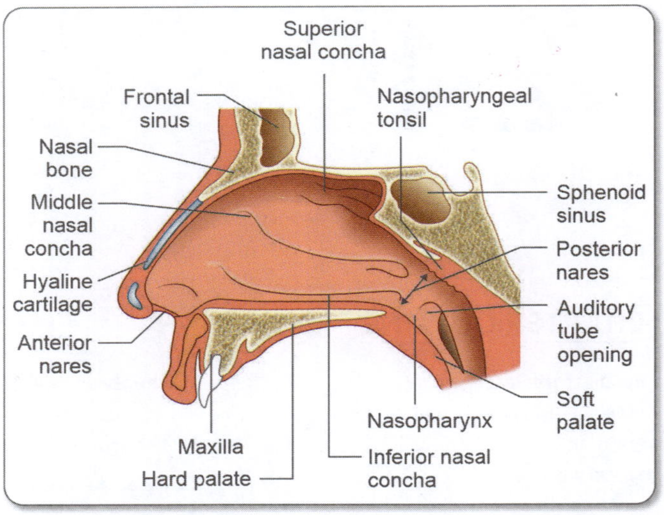

- Roof
- Floor
- Medial wall
- Lateral wall.

Roof. Roof of the nose is very narrow about 1 cm in breadth posteriorly and about 6 cm long. It is formed anteriorly by the cartilage and posteriorly by nasal and ethmoid bones. The middle part of the roof is formed by cribriform plate of ethmoid bone which separates it from the cranial cavity.

Floor. Floor of nasal cavity is constituted by hard palate which separates it from the mouth. The hard palate is formed by palatine process of maxilla (anterior 2/3rd) and palatine bone (posterior 1/3rd).

Medial wall. Nasal septum (medial wall) divides the nasal cavity into right and left halves. It is made up of two parts:

Bony part, is posterior and is formed by the vomer bone and perpendicular plate of ethmoid bone.

Cartilaginous part, is anterior and is formed by the septal cartilage.

Fig. 2.1-3: Features of lateral wall of nasal cavity

Lateral wall. The bony framework of lateral wall is formed by the maxilla, the ethmoid bone and inferior conchae. On interior view of nasal cavity, the lateral wall of nasal cavity presents the following features.

Vestibule (Fig. 2.1-3). It is the lowest part of the lateral wall just above the anterior nares. It is lined by skin of the nose and is characterized by presence of long hair (vibrissae) (Fig. 2.1-3).

Conchae. These are three shelf-like projections called superior, middle and inferior conchae (Fig. 2.1-3). Each concha has a core of exceedingly light spongy bone covered by thick mucosa.

Meatuses. The conchae divide the nasal cavity into three spaces called the meatuses. These are:

- *Superior meatus* is the space below and in front of superior concha. The posterior ethmoidal air cells open into the superior meatus by one or more orifices (Fig. 2.1-4).
- *Middle meatus* is the space below and in front of middle concha. The frontal sinus, middle ethmoidal sinus and maxillary sinus open into this space (Fig. 2.1-4).

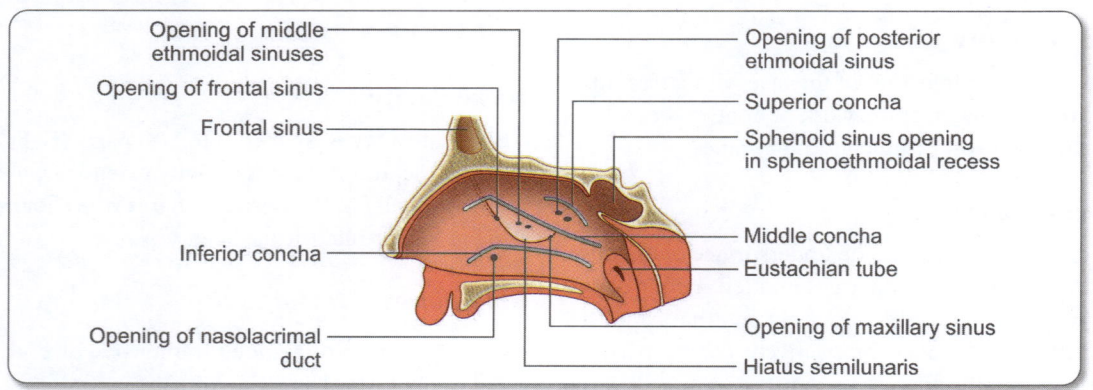

Fig. 2.1-4: Lateral wall of nasal cavity with turbinate removed, showing the openings of various paranasal sinuses

- *Inferior meatus* is the space below the inferior concha. The nasolacrimal duct, which drains the lacrimal sac opens in its anterior part (Fig. 2.1-4).

Lining of the Nasal Cavity

At the entrance the vestibule of the nasal cavity is lined with thick stratified squamous epithelium (skin) containing sebaceous glands and numerous coarse hairs.

Middle or respiratory portion of nasal cavity is lined by ciliated pseudostratified columnar epithelium which contains mucus-secreting goblet cells.

Upper or olfactory region, which includes the superior concha and adjacent part of nasal septum, is lined by neuroepithelium (olfactory epithelium) containing olfactory cells, (which are the receptors for smell), basal cells in the epithelial lining and Bowman's glands in the lamina propria (Histology Plate 2.1-1).

The nasal mucosa, which is highly vascular, is continuous externally with the skin and internally with the mucous membrane lining the paranasal sinuses and nasopharynx.

Respiratory Functions of Nasal Cavity

The nasal cavity is the first organ of respiration. It subserves the following respiratory functions:

Warming the air. Thick and highly vascular mucosa of nasal cavity warms the air to the body temperature.

Humidification of the air to 100% saturation is caused when the air passes over the moist mucosa.

Filtration of air. The hairs at the entrance to the nostrils and the cilia of the epithelium serve as filters to remove the particles which may be present in the air. The tortuous path between the turbinates also helps in filtering the air—The particles are deposited at the bends where they adhere to the mucous membrane of nasal cavity.

PHARYNX

The pharynx is a median passage that is common to gastrointestinal tract (GIT) and respiratory system. It is about 12–14 cm long and connects the mouth to the esophagus.

Parts of Pharynx

It is divisible, from above downward, into three parts (Fig. 2.1-5):

1. Nasopharynx or nasal part of the pharynx into which nasal cavity opens through the posterior nares (choanae).

2. Oropharynx or oral part of the pharynx which is continuous with the posterior end of oral cavity. It lies below the nasopharynx separated from it incompletely by the soft palate. The communication between the nasopharynx and the oropharynx is called the *pharyngeal isthmus.*

3. Laryngopharynx or the laryngeal part of the pharynx is continuous in front with larynx and below with esophagus.

Histology Plate 2.1-1: Nasal Mucosa

The photomicrograph shows olfactory mucosa having olfactory cells (1) and basal cells (3) in the olfactory epithelium (2) Bowman's glands (4) can be seen in lamina propria

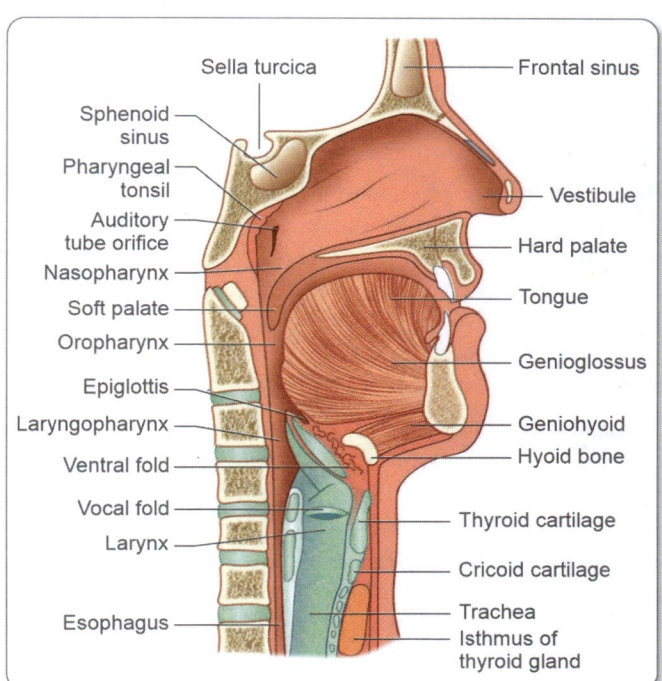

Fig. 2.1-5: Sagittal section of nose, mouth and pharynx

Structure of Pharynx

The pharyngeal wall consists of four layers:

1. *Mucous coat* lining is as below:

Nasopharynx is lined by ciliated columnar epithelium, which is continuous with lining of nasal cavity.

Oropharynx and laryngopharynx are lined by stratified squamous epithelium, which is continuous with the lining of the mouth and esophagus.

2. *Fibrous coat* is formed by the *pharyngobasilar fascia* which really is a dense thickening of submucosa. It is thicker in the nasopharynx, where there is little muscle, and becomes thinner toward the lower end, where the muscle layer is thick.

3. *Muscle coat* is made of striped muscles which are in two layers:

i. Outer circular layer is formed by superior, middle and inferior constrictor muscles.

ii. Inner longitudinal layer is formed by stylo-pharyngeus, salpingopharyngeus and palato-pharyngeus muscles.

4. *Areolar coat* is formed by the *bucopharyngeous* fascia. It is an inconspicuous layer.

Nerve Supply and Blood Supply of Pharynx

Nerve supply. All the muscles of pharynx are supplied by the pharyngeal plexus except stylopharyngeus, which is supplied by the glossopharyngeal nerve.

Pharyngeal plexus is formed by:

- Pharyngeal branch of vagus nerve carrying motor fibers for the muscles
- Pharyngeal branch of glossopharyngeal nerve carrying sensory impulses from the mucosa
- Pharyngeal branch of superior cervical ganglion carrying sympathetic vasoconstrictor fibers for vessels of pharynx.

Blood supply of the pharynx consists of:

Arterial supply is from the branches of facial, lingual, maxillary and ascending pharyngeal arteries.

Venous blood drains into facial veins and internal jugular veins.

Functions of Pharynx

Passageway for air. Air from the nasal cavities enters the nasopharynx and passes down through the oropharynx and laryngopharynx to larynx. From the mouth the air can directly pass to oropharynx.

Warming and humidification of air occur while passing through the pharynx, as like nasal cavities, its mucosa is also vascular and moist.

Passage and taste of food. The oropharynx serves as a passages for food, and some taste buds present here take part in taste sensation.

Role in hearing. The opening of eustachian tubes present in the nasopharynx equalizes the air pressure on tympanic membrane and thus plays important role in hearing.

Role in defense mechanism. Lymphoid tissue present in the pharyngeal and laryngeal tonsils takes part in defense mechanism of the body.

Role of speech. Pharynx along with the paranasal sinuses work as sound resonator and help to give voice its individual characteristics.

NURSING IMPLICATIONS AND APPLICATIONS

Pharyngitis or more commonly known as sore throat, can be classified as acute and chronic.

- *Acute pharyngitis* is usually caused by viral infection. The signs and symptoms include fever, reddening of pharyngeal membrane, swollen and painful tonsils.
- *Chronic pharyngitis* mainly occurs in people working in dusty atmosphere, using excess of alcohol and tobacco. The signs are constant irritation of throat, cough and collection of mucous.

LARYNX

It is a hollow organ for respiration and phonation (voice box). It is continuous above with laryngopharynx and below with trachea. It is about 5 cm in length, 4 cm in width and 3.5 cm in its anteroposterior diameter. It lies in the middle of the anterior part of neck opposite fourth, fifth and sixth cervical vertebrae.

Structure

The larynx is made of:

- Mucous membrane
- Cartilages
- Ligaments and membranes
- Muscles of larynx.

Mucous Membrane

The larynx is made of rigid framework of cartilage, ligaments and muscles. These structures are covered on the inside by mucous membrane that is continuous above with that of the laryngeal part of pharynx and below with that of the trachea.

Cartilages of Larynx

There are nine cartilages (3 single and 3 sets of paired cartilages) of larynx (Figs 2.1-6A to C).

Single cartilages are:

Thyroid cartilage. It is the largest cartilage of larynx. It resembles a shield and rests on cricoid. It consists of two plates

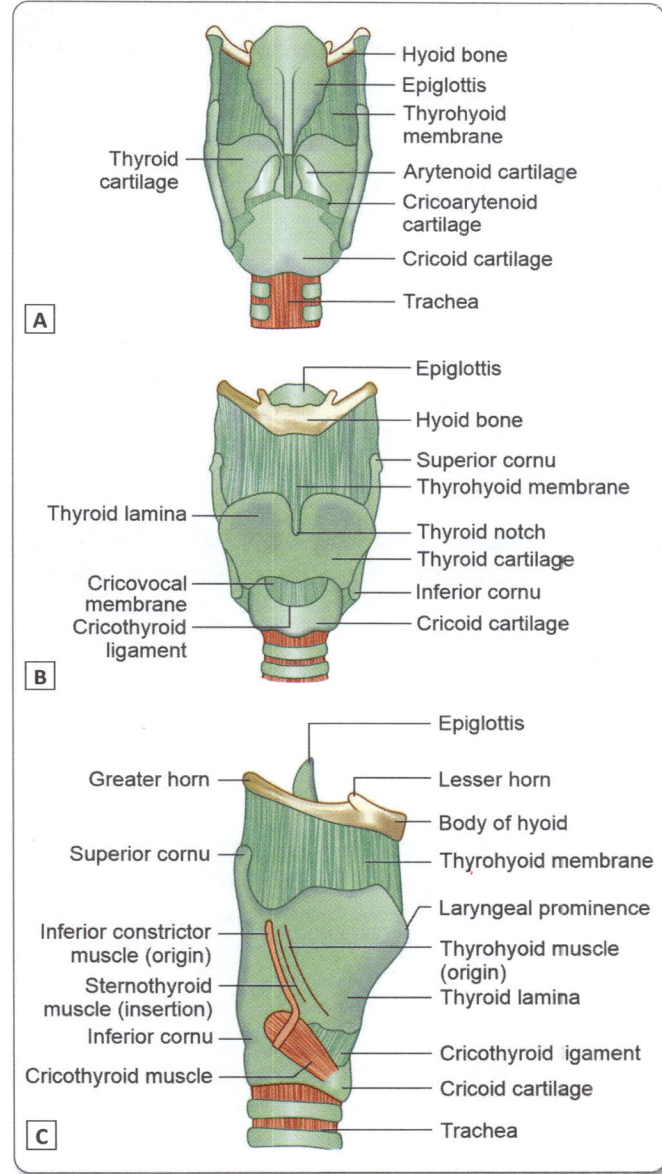

Figs 2.1-6A to C: Cartilages of larynx: A. Anterior view; B. Posterior view; and C. Lateral view

(laminae) joined at acute angle in midline forming laryngeal prominence (Adam's apple).

Cricoid cartilage. It is shaped like a signet ring with a broad lamina posteriorly and a narrow arch anteriorly. The anterior part (arch) lies below the thyroid cartilage and its posterior part (broad lamina) extends upward into the interval between the laminae of thyroid cartilage.

Epiglottic cartilage. It is tongue- or leaf-shaped, having a broad upper part, and a narrow lower end. Its lower narrow end is attached by thyroepiglottic ligament to the back of thyroid angle. Its upper broad end is free and rounded. In this way it guards the inlet of larynx.

Paired cartilages are:

Arytenoid cartilages. These are pyramid-shaped cartilages, which rest on the upper border of posterior lamina of cricoid cartilage (Fig. 2.1-6B).

Corniculate cartilages. These are small conical nodules of elastic cartilage which are placed on either side above the apex of arytenoid cartilages.

Cuneiform cartilages. These are small elongated pieces of elastic cartilages present within the aryepiglottic fold.

Ligaments and Membranes of Larynx

Various ligaments and membranes attach the cartilages of larynx to each other and to the hyoid bone above and to the tracheal ring below. Some important ligaments and membranes are (Figs 2.1-6A to C):

Thyroid membrane connects the upper border of thyroid cartilage with the body and greater corner of hyoid bone.

Anterior cricothyroid ligament connects the lower border of thyroid cartilage to the arch of cricoid cartilage (Fig. 2.1-6A).

Cricotracheal ligament connects the lower margin of cricoid cartilage to the trachea.

Thyroepiglottic ligament connects thyroid cartilage to epiglottic cartilage.

Muscles of the Larynx

The muscles of larynx are divided into extrinsic and intrinsic muscles:

Extrinsic muscles of larynx connect cartilages of larynx with the surrounding bones. These muscles raise or lower the larynx as a whole during deglutition. These include sternothyroid, thyrohyoid, sternohyoid, omohyoid and some pharyngeal muscles.

Intrinsic muscles. There are various intrinsic muscles, which are confined to the larynx. Various actions of different intrinsic muscles of larynx are:

- Increase or decrease in the tension of vocal cords
- Abducts or adducts the vocal cords
- Opening or closing the glottis
- Opening and closing of the inlet of larynx.

Cavity (Interior) of Larynx

The cavity (interior) of larynx is lined by mucous membrane and is divided into three parts by two pairs of upper vestibular and lower vocal folds lying approximately anteroposteriorly

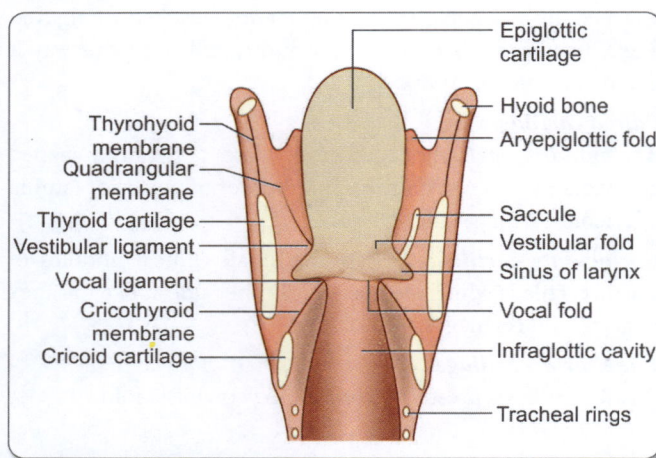

Fig. 2.1-7: Coronal section of larynx viewed from behind showing three parts of the cavity of larynx

and projecting into the cavity of larynx. The three parts from above downward are (Fig. 2.1-7):

1. Vestibule. It is the upper part of laryngeal cavity which extends from its inlet to the vestibular folds. *Vestibular folds* the right and left vestibular folds are formed by the *vestibular ligaments* formed by bundle of fibers at lower free edge of a quadrangular membrane. These are directed downward and medially.

2. Ventricle or sinus. It is the middle part of laryngeal cavity which is limited above by the vestibular folds and below by vocal folds. *Vocal folds* are formed by the vocal ligament lined by mucosa. These are directed upward and medially. The space between the right and left vocal folds is called *rima glottidis*.

3. Infraglottic cavity. It is the lower part of laryngeal cavity which lies below the vocal folds. Inferiorly, it widens and becomes continuous with the trachea.

Functions of Larynx

Phonation, i.e., production of vocal sounds is the main function of the larynx. Sound is characterized by pitch, volume and resonance.

- *Pitch* of voice depends upon the length and tightness of vocal cords.
- *Volume* of voice depends upon the force with which the vocal cords vibrate.
- *Resonance* and tone of the voice are determined by the shape of mouth, position of tongue and lips and air in the paranasal sinuses.

Protection of lower respiratory tract during deglutition is caused by closure of respiratory passages by the hinged epiglottis. This allows the food to pass into esophagus and prevents it from entering the respiratory passages.

TRACHEOBRONCHIAL TREE

The tracheobronchial tree consists of:
- Trachea
- Bronchi
- Branches of bronchi.

TRACHEA

Trachea, or windpipe, is a flexible, cylindrical tube about 2.5 cm in diameter and 12.5 cm in length. It extends downwards from the lower end of larynx (at the level of 6th cervical vertebra) down into the thoracic cavity up to the upper border of thoracic vertebra, where it divides into two bronchi, one for each lung (Fig. 2.1-8). In the thoracic cavity trachea lies in front of the esophagus.

NURSING IMPLICATIONS AND APPLICATIONS

Carina (Latin *keel*) of the trachea is a sensitive area. When patient is made to lie on her/his left side, secretions from right bronchial tree flow toward the carina due to the effect of gravity. This stimulates the cough reflex and sputum is brought out. This is called *postural drainage*.

BRONCHI

The right and left principal bronchi, into which the trachea divides, differ slightly—the right bronchus being shorter wider, and more vertical in direction than left. The right bronchus enters the right lung and ends by dividing into

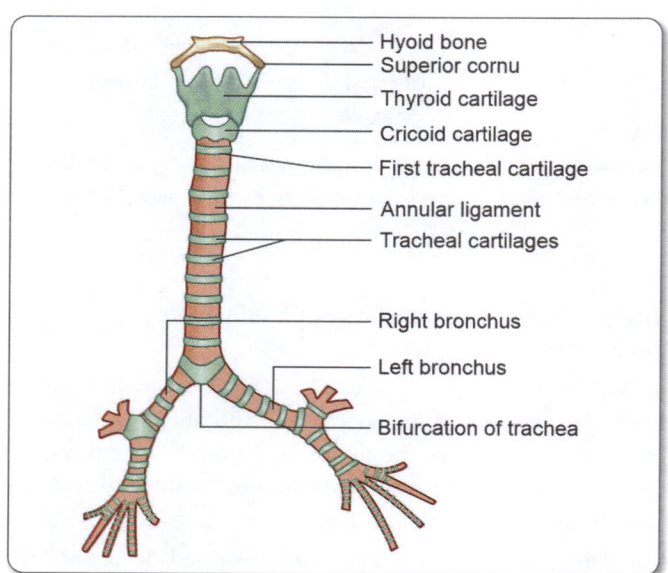

Fig. 2.1-8: Trachea and its main branches

three *lobar bronchi*—superior, middle and inferior, while the left bronchus ends by dividing into two lobar bronchi—superior and inferior, corresponding to two lobes of left lung (Fig. 2.1-8).

Organization of Tracheobronchial Tree

The air passages between trachea and alveoli divide 23 times to form the extensive tracheobronchial tree (Fig. 2.1-9). These multiple divisions greatly increase the total cross-sectional area of the airway from 2.5 cm² in the trachea to 11,800 cm² in the alveoli. Consequently, the velocity of air flow in the small airway declines to very low values. The 23 generation divisions of tracheobronchial tree have been numbered as:

The trachea is designated as generation zero.

The principal bronchi right and left which are two major divisions of trachea constitute the first generation.

Lobar bronchi, which are divisions of the principal bronchus, form the 2nd generation.

Segmental bronchi, which are further divisions of each lobar bronchus, forms the 3rd generation. Each segmental bronchus divides into several generations of branches that ultimately end in very small tubes called *bronchioles*.

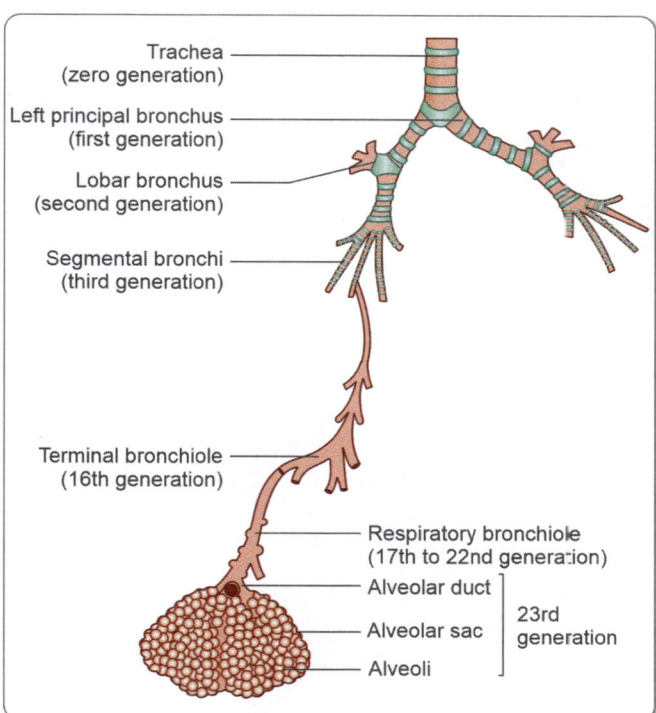

Fig. 2.1-9: The tracheobronchial tree

Terminal bronchiole is the name given to 16th generation of the divisions. Up to this generation of division no exchange of gases is possible.

Respiratory bronchiole is the name given to 17th to 22nd generation of divisions. These are labeled as respiratory bronchioles because some exchange of gases is possible in these tubes.

Alveolar ducts end in the alveoli or the alveolar sacs which form the 23rd generation division. It is here that most of the O₂ and CO₂ exchange occurs.

Zones of Respiratory Passages

Thus, from the functional point of view the tracheobronchial tree can be divided into two major zones:

1. *Conducting zone* of the air passages is formed by the first 16 generations of passages and it only transports gases from and to the exterior. Thus, conducting zone starts from trachea and extends up to terminal bronchioles. Since no exchange of gases is possible here, so starting from nose to the terminal brochioles forms the so-called *dead space* which has a total capacity of approximately 150 mL.

2. *Respiratory zone.* The remaining 7 generations of tracheobronchial tree which includes the respiratory bronchioles, alveolar ducts and alveoli form the respiratory zone, where exchange of gases occurs. Its volume is approximately 4 L.

Histological Features of Tracheobronchial Tree

Cartilaginous rings are present in trachea and initial bronchi of few generations. These are absent in terminal bronchioles and respiratory bronchioles. The cartilaginous rings of trachea are incomplete on their posterior aspect. This allows some contraction of trachea but tracheal lumen cannot be completely obliterated easily.

Smooth muscles. Ends of cartilaginous rings of trachea are approximated by transverse smooth muscle fibers. In terminal bronchioles, they are present in large amount and form a sphincter. Smooth muscles are not present in alveoli.

Epithelial lining in trachea and large bronchi is columnar and becomes cuboidal in bronchioles and simple squamous in alveoli. The epithelial cells of tracheobronchial tree are ciliated (Histology plate-2.1-2). Cilia are absent in alveoli. Efficiency of ciliated cells of trachea and bronchi in propelling mucus and waste products is of higher order. Cilia are not influenced by nerve impulses. The mucus-secreting goblet cells and deep serous glands are present in trachea and bronchi but are absent in bronchioles and alveoli.

Histology Plate 2.1-2: Trachea

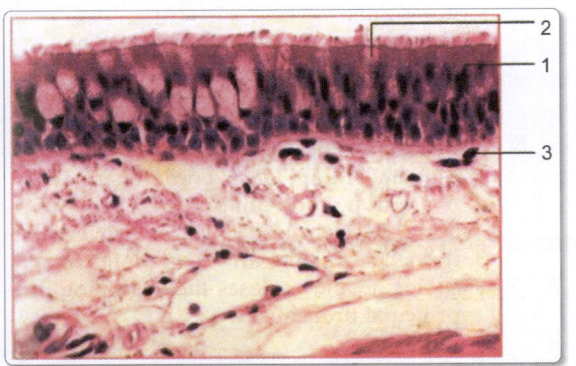

The photomicrograph of trachea has been shown. Trachea in lined by pseudostratified columnar ciliated epithelium (1) with goblet cells (2). Lamina propria (3) and also contains tracheal glands

LUNGS AND PLEURA

LUNGS

Gross Anatomy

The right and left lungs (pulmones) are soft spongy, cone-shaped organs that lie in the corresponding halves of the thoracic cavity enclosed in a sac, the pleura. They are separated from each other by the mediastinal structures including the heart, the trachea, the esophagus, great vessels, lymph nodes, lymph vessels and nerves.

External Features

Each lung can be described to present the following external features: An apex, base, costal surface, medial surface and anterior, posterior and inferior borders (Figs 2.1-10A to C).

Apex refers to narrow upper end of the lung which is rounded and projects into the root of neck, about 2.5 cm above the level of middle third of clavicle.

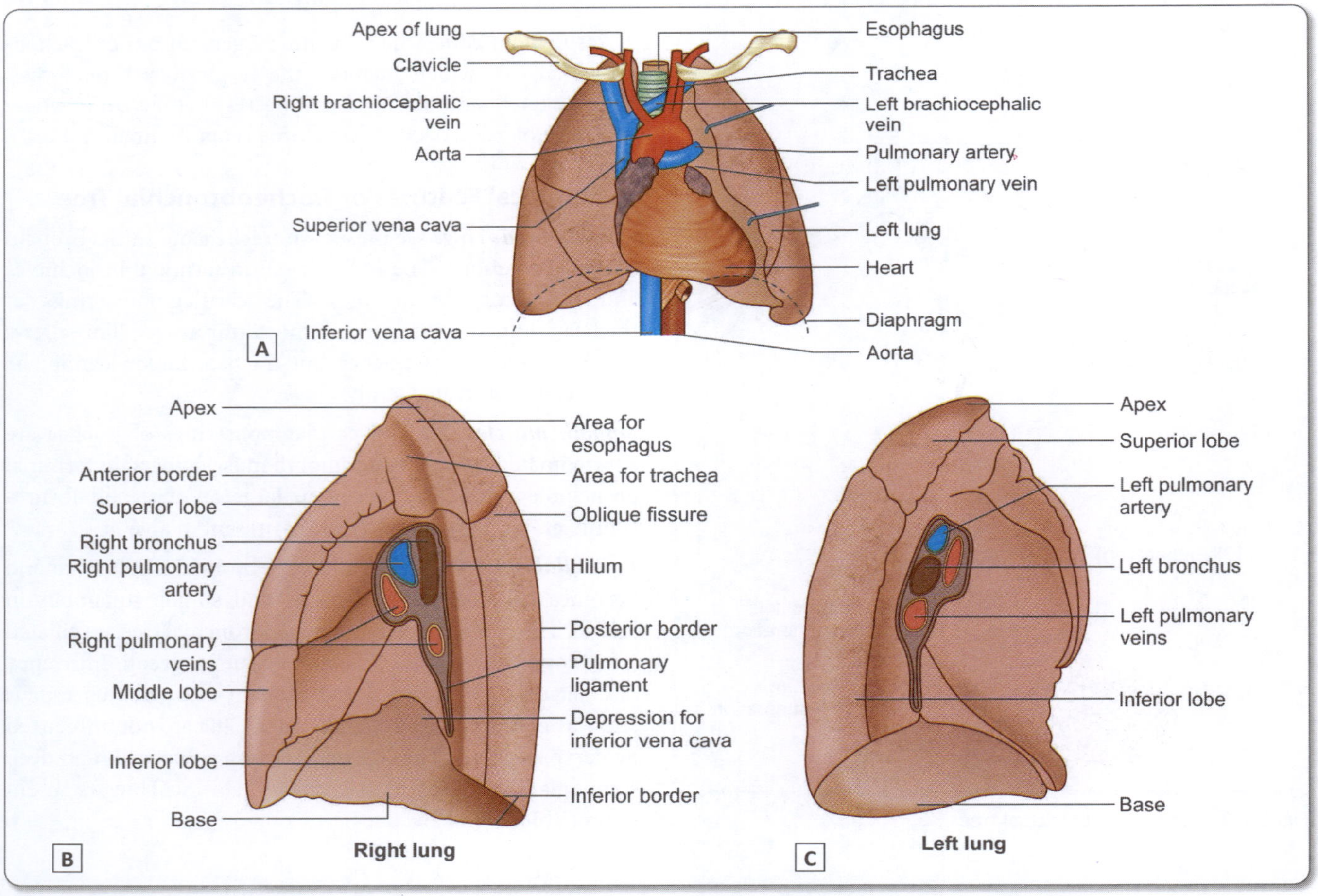

A

Apex of lung — Clavicle — Right brachiocephalic vein — Aorta — Superior vena cava — Inferior vena cava

Esophagus — Trachea — Left brachiocephalic vein — Pulmonary artery — Left pulmonary vein — Left lung — Heart — Diaphragm — Aorta

B

Apex — Anterior border — Superior lobe — Right bronchus — Right pulmonary artery — Right pulmonary veins — Middle lobe — Inferior lobe — Base

Area for esophagus — Area for trachea — Oblique fissure — Hilum — Posterior border — Pulmonary ligament — Depression for inferior vena cava — Inferior border

Right lung

C

Apex — Superior lobe — Left pulmonary artery — Left bronchus — Left pulmonary veins — Inferior lobe — Base

Left lung

Figs 2.1-10A to C: Gross features of the lungs: A. Front view; B. Medial view of right lung; C. Medial view of left lung

Base refers to the broader inferior surface of the lung, which is concave to fit over the convex portion of diaphragm.

Costal surface, also called lateral or outer surface of the lung, is convex and is closely associated with structures of thoracic wall which include the costal cartilages, the ribs and the intercostal muscles.

Medial surface is concave and associated with mediastinal structures. It presents the following features:

Hilum is a vertical triangular notch in the medial surface of each lung, which gives passage to the structures forming *root of the lung*, i.e., primary bronchus, pulmonary artery and vein, bronchial arteries and veins, plexuses of nerves, lymphatics and lymph nodes. Structures forming root of the lung are covered by pleura and connect the lung to the trachea and heart.

Cardiac impression is a deep concavity on the medial surface of lung just below and in front of the hilum where the heart lies. It is larger and deeper on the left than on the right lung, because the heart projects farther to the left side.

Borders of the lung. The costal surface meets the medial surface in front at the *anterior border* and behind at the *posterior border*. The costal and medial surfaces meet below with the base at the *inferior border*.

Fissures and Lobes of the Lungs

Right lung is divided into the following three lobes by the oblique and horizontal fissures (Fig. 2.1-10B):

1. Superior lobe   3. Inferior lobe.
2. Middle lobe

Left lung is smaller than the right due to inclination of the heart to left side. It contains only the oblique fissure which divides it into two lobes (Fig. 2.1-10C):

1. Superior lobe   2. Inferior lobe.

Respiratory Parenchyma

Each respiratory unit consists of one respiratory bronchiole which opens into a number of alveolar ducts, and each alveolar duct in turn opens into number of alveoli. The two lungs contain about 300 million alveoli. Each alveolus has a diameter of about 0.2 μm. The alveoli are surrounded by pulmonary capillaries. The total area of the alveolar walls in contact with capillaries in both the lungs is about 70 m².

Microscopic Structure of Alveolus (Fig. 2.1-11 and Histology Plate 2.1-3)

Each alveolus is lined by two types of epithelial cells:

1. Type I cells (pneumocyte I) are flat cells with large cytoplasmic extensions and are the primary lining cells.

2. Type II cells (pneumocyte II or granular pneumocytes) are thicker and contain numerous lamellar inclusion bodies. These cells secrete *surfactant*.

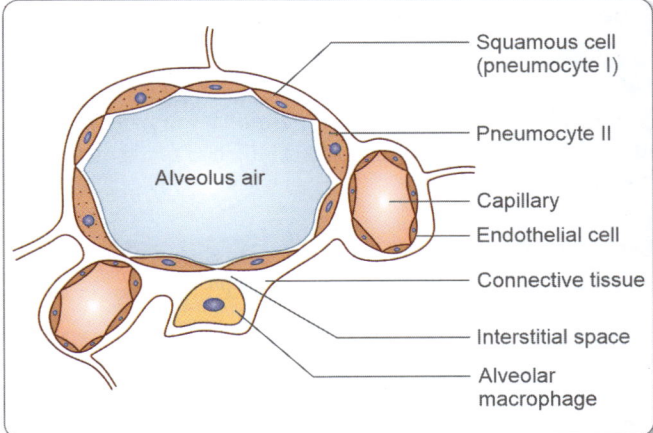

Fig. 2.1-11: Microscopic structure of alveolus

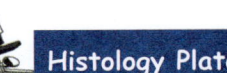

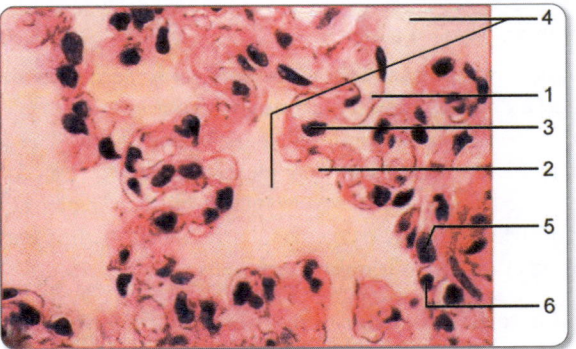

Histology Plate 2.1-3: Alveolus

The photomicrograph of alveolus (4) show. In between two alveoli, lies the interalveolar septum (1), Capillary (2), Type II pneumocyte (3), alveolar macrophage (5), and type I pneumocyte (6) are also seen.

IMPORTANT TO KNOW

The alveolar wall also contains:
- Other *special type of epithelial cells*
- *Pulmonary alveolar macrophages* (PAM) which are active phagocytic cells
- *Lymphocytes*
- *Plasma cells* which form and secrete immunoglobulins
- *Amine precursor uptake and decarboxylation (APUD) cells* which store and secrete many biologically active peptidases, e.g. vasoactive intestinal peptide (VIP) and substance P, etc.
- *Mast cells* which contain heparin, various lipids, histamine and various proteases that participate in allergic reactions.

Communication between the two alveoli occurs through small pores, called *pores of Kohn*.

Blood Supply

Conducting airway is supplied by systemic blood, whereas respiratory zone of the lung is supplied by deoxygenated (venous) blood coming through pulmonary arteries to lungs. Blood is oxygenated in lungs and is returned to left atrium via pulmonary veins.

Bronchial Circulation

The lungs receive oxygenated blood like other tissues in the body through *bronchial arteries* (two left and one right), which are branches of the descending thoracic aorta. Bronchial blood flow amounts to about 1–2% of total cardiac output. The oxygenated blood in the bronchial arteries supplies the connective tissues, septa and large and small bronchi of the lungs. Because the bronchial blood empties into the pulmonary veins and bypasses the right heart, the bronchial circulation, therefore, constitutes a *physiological shunt*, i.e., a channel that bypasses oxygenation in the lungs.

Pulmonary Circulation

Pulmonary trunk arises from the right ventricle and divides into right and left pulmonary arteries, which convey deoxygenated blood to the right and left lung, respectively. The blood circulates through a capillary plexus intimately related to the walls of alveoli and receives oxygen from the alveolar air. This blood which is now oxygenated is returned to the heart (left atrium) through four pulmonary veins.

Characteristic features of pulmonary circulation

- The pulmonary arteries and their branches are thin-walled and distensible, giving the pulmonary arterial tree a large compliance. The distensibility of pulmonary vessels makes the pulmonary circulation a *low-pressure, low-resistance* and *high-capacitance system.*
- The thickness of the right ventricle and pulmonary artery is approximately one-third of the thickness of left ventricle and aorta, respectively.
- The pulmonary arterioles have very little smooth muscles in their walls. The pulmonary capillaries are larger in diameter than systemic capillaries and have multiple anastomoses.
- The pulmonary capillaries surround the alveoli and are sandwiched between their walls as a result each alveolus seems to be enclosed in a basket of capillaries (Fig. 2.1-12).
- Pulmonary capillary pressure is about 10 mm Hg. Since this pressure is far below the colloid osmotic pressure (25 mm Hg), so a net suction force of 15 mm Hg tends to draw fluid from alveolar interstitial space into the pulmonary capillaries *which keeps the alveoli dry.* However, if the pulmonary capillary hydrostatic pressure

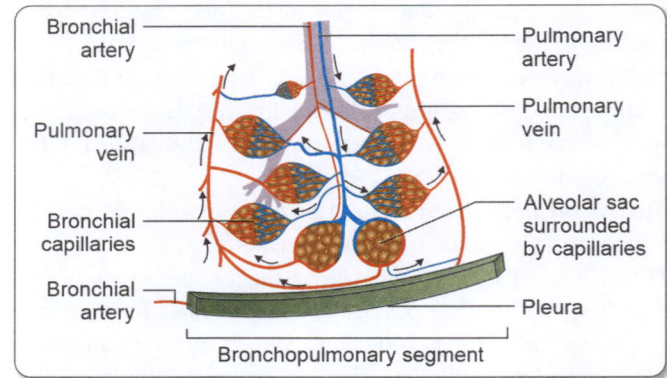

Fig. 2.1-12: Organization of pulmonary circulation

rises above 25 mm Hg fluid can escape into the interstitial space leading to *pulmonary edema.* This can happen during exercise, particularly at high altitude, in left heart failure, mitral stenosis and pulmonary fibrosis, reduce the rate of gas exchange in the lungs. The resultant hypoxia may be fatal.

- Pulmonary vessels contain about 600 mL of blood at rest. Since the pulmonary vessels act as capacitance vessels their blood content can vary from 200 mL to 900 mL. Pulmonary blood volume *decreases* in conditions like standing and *increases* on changing posture from standing to lying.

Lymphatic Circulation

Lungs are richly supplied by lymphatics. Lymphatics are present in the walls of the terminal bronchioles and in all the supportive tissues of the lungs. Particulate matter entering the alveoli during inspiration is removed by way of lymphatic channels. Lymphatics also remove the plasma proteins leaking from the lung capillaries and thus help to prevent the pulmonary edema. The deep lymphatic vessels follow the bronchi and first drain into the *pulmonary nodes* (in the substance of the lungs) and then into *bronchopulmonary nodes.* The superficial lymph vessels lie near the surface of lungs and converge on to bronchopulmonary nodes. From bronchopulmonary node, lymph drains into *tracheobronchial nodes* and from there into the *bronchomediastinal trunk.*

Innervation

Parasympathetic fibers pass through vagus nerve. Their stimulation causes bronchoconstriction and increased bronchial secretion via muscarinic receptors.

Sympathetic nerves supplying the lungs when stimulated cause bronchodilation and decreased bronchial secretion via adrenergic receptors, predominantly β_2.

Afferents from the lungs pass through vagii.

NURSING IMPLICATIONS AND APPLICATIONS

- *Tuberculosis* of lung is one of the most common diseases. A complete course of treatment must be taken under the guidance of a physician.
- *Bronchial asthma* is a common disease of respiratory system. It occurs due to bronchospasm of smooth muscles in the wall of bronchioles. Patient has difficulty especially during expiration. It is accompanied by wheezing. Epinephrine, a sympathomimetic drug, relieves the symptoms.

PLEURA

The pleura is a thin, transparent, moist membrane which lines the lung and walls of thoracic cavity. Thus pleura has two layers which are continuous with each other (Figs 2.1-13A and B).

1. Visceral layer or pulmonary pleura closely covers the lung at the level of fissures, the visceral pleura dips into the fissure and lines the contiguous sides of the lobes. At the level of hilum of lung, the visceral pleura becomes continuous with the part of parietal pleura which covers the structures forming the root of lung (Fig. 2.1-10).

2. Parietal layer of pleura lines the walls of thoracic cavity and becomes continuous with the visceral pleura round the edges of hilum. Parietal pleura can be divided into the following parts (Figs 2.1-13A and B):

Costovertebral pleura refers to that part of parietal pleura which lines the inner aspect of ribs, intercostal spaces, part of inner surface of sternum and the sides of thoracic vertebrae.

Diaphragmatic pleura refers to that part of parietal pleura that lines the convex part of diaphragm coming in contact with the base of lung.

Mediastinal pleura lines the structures of mediastinum coming in contact with medial surface of the lung. The mediastinal pleura extends as a tube around the structures forming root of the lung and becomes continuous with visceral pleura round the edges of hilum.

Pleural Cavity

Pleural cavity refers to the potential space between the visceral and parietal layer of pleura. The two layers of pleura are separated by only a very thin layer of serous fluid which helps these layers to move easily upon each other with respiratory movements of chest wall.

NURSING IMPLICATIONS AND APPLICATIONS

Some Clinical Conditions Associated with the Pleura are as follows:

Pleurisy: The surface of pleura becomes inflamed, friction results, and the sounds produced by this rubbing can be heard through the stethoscope. This causes inflammation of the pleura. It may be dry, but often it is accompanied by collection of fluid in the pleural cavity. The condition is called the pleural effusion. Dry pleurisy is more painful because during inspiration both layers come in contact and there is friction.

Pneumothorax, i.e., collection of air in the pleural cavity occurs following a puncture in the thoracic wall. It also results in collapse of lung. If the puncture in chest wall is closed, the air is gradually absorbed, and the lung resumes its normal position.

Hemothorax: Presence of blood in the pleural cavity.

Hydropneumothorax: Presence of both fluid and air in the pleural cavity.

Empyema: Presence of pus in pleural cavity.

Hydrothorax refers to collection of fluid in the pleural cavity (e.g. as in pleurisy). It results in compression of the lung and possibly collapse of the portion of lung.

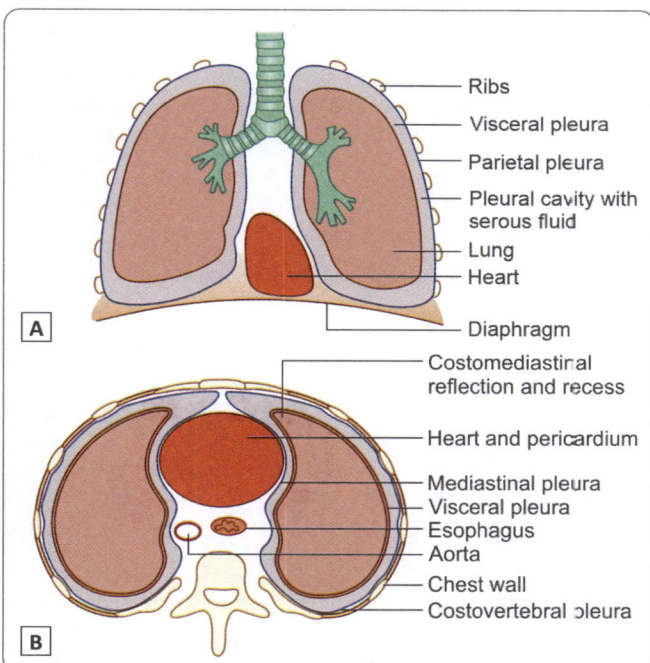

A
- Ribs
- Visceral pleura
- Parietal pleura
- Pleural cavity with serous fluid
- Lung
- Heart
- Diaphragm

B
- Costomediastinal reflection and recess
- Heart and pericardium
- Mediastinal pleura
- Visceral pleura
- Esophagus
- Aorta
- Chest wall
- Costovertebral pleura

Figs 2.1-13A and B: Pleura and pleural cavity: A. As seen in schematic coronal section through the thorax; B. As seen in schematic transverse section through the thorax

FUNCTIONS OF RESPIRATORY SYSTEM

RESPIRATORY FUNCTIONS

The main function of the respiratory system in general and lung in particular is exchange of gases between atmosphere and blood (for details see chapter 2.2).

NONRESPIRATORY FUNCTIONS
Functions Subserved by Lung Defence Mechanisms

Immunoglobulin-A (IgA) secreted in the bronchial secretion protects against respiratory infections.

Ciliary escalator action is an important defence system against air-borne infections. The dust particles in the inhaled air are often laden with bacteria. While passing through the repeatedly branched bronchial tree the dust particles and the bacteria are caught in the mucous layer present at the mucosal surface of respiratory passages and are moved up toward pharynx by the rhythmic upward beating action of cilia (Fig. 2.1-14) and swallowed. Cigarette smoke disturbs the ciliary function.

Pulmonary alveolar macrophages (PAM) play important role in defence system by the following mechanisms:

- Being actively phagocytic cells they ingest the inhaled bacteria and small particles.
- Help in processing inhaled antigens for immunologic attack.
- PAMs secrete substances that attract polymorphonuclear cells to the lungs.

- By some secretions they stimulate granulocyte and monocyte formation in the bone marrow.

Cough reflex. The laryngeal, tracheal, and bronchial mucous membranes contain vagal afferent terminals which act as *irritant receptors.* Stimulation of these receptors by chemical or mechanical stimuli (excessive mucus, inadvertently inhaled foodstuff, etc.) produce a bout of coughing which helps in expulsion of foreign material.

Functions Subserved by Pulmonary Circulation

Reservoir for left ventricle. When left ventricle output becomes transiently greater than systemic venous return, the blood stored in pulmonary circulation helps in maintaining the left ventricular output for few strokes.

Pulmonary circulation acts as a filter and filters out particles from the blood, which may include small fibrin or blood clots, detached cancer cells, fat cells, gas bubbles, agglutinated RBCs, masses of platelets and debris from stored blood.

Removal of fluid from alveoli. Because of low pulmonary hydrostatic pressure, the fluid entering the alveoli is absorbed by the capillaries. This protects the gas exchange function of lungs and opposes transudation of fluid from capillaries to the alveoli.

Role in absorption of drugs. Certain drugs that rapidly pass through the alveolar capillary barrier by diffusion are administered by inhalation, e.g. anesthetic gases, aerosol and other bronchodilators.

Metabolic Functions of Lungs

Surfactant produced in the lungs plays an important role in respiration.

Protein synthesis for maintenance of structural framework.

Conversion of angiotensin I to II is performed by the enzyme angiotensin-converting enzyme (ACE) present in the pulmonary capillary endothelium.

Inactivation partly or completely of many vasoactive substances present in the blood is done by capillary endothelial cells as they pass through pulmonary circulation.

Fibrinolytic mechanism present in the lung lyses clot in the pulmonary vessels.

Storage of hormones and certain biologically active peptides is done in the APUD cells and nerve fibers present in the alveoli. These substances include VIP, substance P, opioid peptides, cholecystokinin- pancreozymin (CCK-PZ) and somatostatin. These substances are later released into the systemic circulation.

Functions Subserved by Respiratory Muscles

Respiratory muscles are also used during laughing and singing.

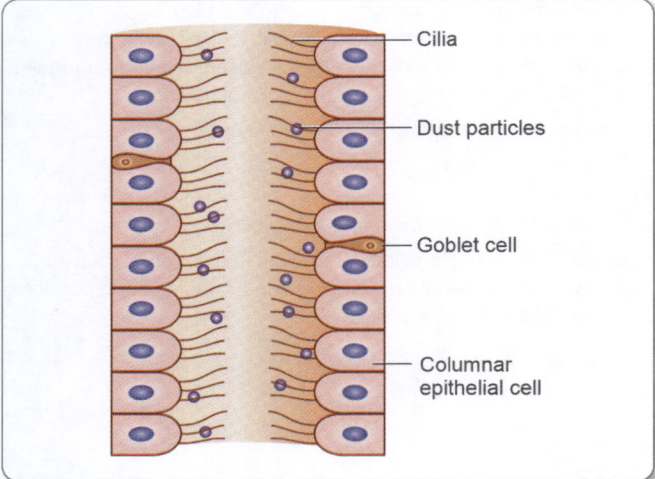

Cilia

Dust particles

Goblet cell

Columnar epithelial cell

Fig. 2.1-14: Ciliary escalator action of the respiratory mucosa

ASSESS YOURSELF

Short and Long Answer Questions

1. **Briefly discuss:**
   i. Functional anatomy of nasal cavity and its functions
   ii. Structure, blood supply, innervations and functions of pharynx
2. **Write notes on:**
   - Functions of larynx
   - Tracheobronchial tree
   - Zones of respiratory passages
   - Features of pulmonary circulation
3. **Write briefly on non-respiratory functions of respiratory system**

Multiple Choice Questions

1. **Which is the component of medial wall of the nasal cavity:**
   a. Vestibule   b. Middle choncha
   c. Vomer bone   d. Maxillary sinus
2. **The mucus secreting cells are present in which part of the nasal cavity:**
   a. Vestibule   b. Respiratory part
   c. Olfactory region   d. Superior choncha
3. **Which is the single cartilage of the larynx:**
   a. Arytenoid
   b. Thyroid
   c. Cuneiform
   d. Corniculate
4. **Which of the following is paired cartilage of the larynx:**
   a. Epiglottic   b. Cricoid
   c. Thyroid   d. Arytenoid

5. **The anterior cricothyroid ligament of larynx connects:**
   a. Upper border of thyroid cartilage to hyoid bone
   b. Lower border of thyroid cartilage to cricoids cartilage
   c. Thyroid cartilage to epiglottic cartilage
   d. Lower margin of cricoids cartilage to trachea
6. **Which is the function of extrinsic muscles of larynx:**
   a. Increase/decrease of tension of vocal cords
   b. Abduct/adduct the vocal cords
   c. Opening/closing of glottis
   d. Raise/lower the larynx during deglutition
7. **The 22nd generation of tracheobroncheal tree is:**
   a. Terminal bronchioles
   b. Segmental bronchi
   c. Alveolar ducts
   d. Respiratory bronchi
8. **The function of type II alveolar cells is:**
   a. Conversion of angiotensinogen I into II
   b. Production of surfactant
   c. Formation of angiotensin converting enzyme
   d. Storage of hormones
9. **The true statement for stimulation of parasympathetic innervations to respiratory system is:**
   a. Causes broncho-dilation
   b. Decreases bronchial secretions
   c. Increases bronchial secretions
   d. Bronchial constriction and decrease secretions
10. **The main function of pulmonary alveolar macrophages is:**
    a. Secrete immuneglobulins
    b. Secrete surfactant
    c. Ingest inhaled bacteria
    d. Secrete angiotensin converting enzyme

ANSWER KEY

1. c	**2.** b	**3.** b	**4.** d	**5.** c	**6.** d	**7.** a	**8.** b
9. c	**10.** c						

Notes

Physiology of Respiration

CHAPTER OUTLINE

INTRODUCTION

The word respiration has been derived from the Latin word *respirare*, which means to *breathe*. The primary role of the respiratory system is to provide O_2 to the tissues for metabolic needs and remove the CO_2 formed by them. An adult body consumes about 250 mL of O_2 and produces about 200 mL of CO_2 per minute. Respiration entails two processes: The external respiration and internal respiration.

The *internal respiration* or tissue respiration refers to utilization of O_2 and production of CO_2 by the tissue.

The *external respiration* includes supply of O_2 to the tissues from the environment and excretion of CO_2 released by the tissues into the atmosphere. The process of external respiration involves three major events:

1. *Pulmonary ventilation*, i.e., exchange of gases between the environment and lungs. It includes mechanics of respiration.

2. *Pulmonary diffusion* refers to transfer of gases from alveoli to the blood by diffusion across the respiratory membrane.

3. *Transport of gases* from the blood to the body cells and back.

PULMONARY VENTILATION

Pulmonary ventilation, as defined above, refers to the process of exchange of gases between the environment and lungs. Inflation and deflation of the lung occurring with each breath ensure this regular exchange of gases. The aspects and concept related to pulmonary ventilation, which need deliberation include:
- Mechanism of breathing
- Pressure and volume changes during respiratory cycle
- Lung volumes and capacities
- Pulmonary elastance and compliance.

MECHANISM OF BREATHING

Pulmonary ventilation is accomplished by two processes:
1. Inspiration
2. Expiration

Inspiration

Inspiration refers to inflow of atmospheric air into the lungs. This obviously occurs when the intrapulmonary pressure falls below the atmospheric air pressure.

It is an active process, normally produced by contraction of the *inspiratory muscles*. During tidal inspiration (quiet breathing) the diaphragm and external intercostal muscles contract and cause increase in all the three dimensions of thoracic cavity.

Role of Diaphragm

In tidal inspiration (quiet breathing) 70–75% of expansion of chest is caused due to contraction of diaphragm. The diaphragm is a dome-shaped, musculotendinous partition between thorax and abdomen. The convexity of this dome is directed toward the thorax. When the diaphragm contracts the following changes occur:

- The dome becomes flattened and the level of diaphragm is lowered *increasing the vertical diameter* of the thoracic cavity (Fig. 2.2-1A). During quiet breathing, the descent of diaphragm is about 1.5 cm and during forced inspiration, it increases to 7 cm.
- The descent of diaphragm causes rise in intra-abdominal pressure which is accommodated by the reciprocal relaxation of the abdominal wall musculature.
- Contraction of diaphragm also lifts the lower ribs causing thoracic expansion laterally and anteriorly (the bucket handle and pump handle effect, respectively) (Figs 2.2-1B and C).

Role of External Intercostal Muscles

When the external intercostal muscles contract, the ribs are elevated causing lateral and anteroposterior enlargement of thoracic cavity due to the socalled bucket handle and pump handle effects, respectively.

Role of Laryngeal Muscles

The abductor muscles of the larynx contract during inspiration pulling the vocal cords apart.

Expiration

Expiration refers to outflow of air from the lungs into the atmosphere. This obviously occurs when the intrapulmonary pressure rises above the atmospheric air pressure. Expiration in quiet breathing is largely a passive phenomenon and is brought about by the:

- Elastic recoil of the lungs
- Decrease in size of the thoracic cavity due to relaxation of diaphragm and external intercostal muscles.

Forced expiration is required when respiration is increased during exercise or in the presence of severe respiratory disease. It is an active process caused by:

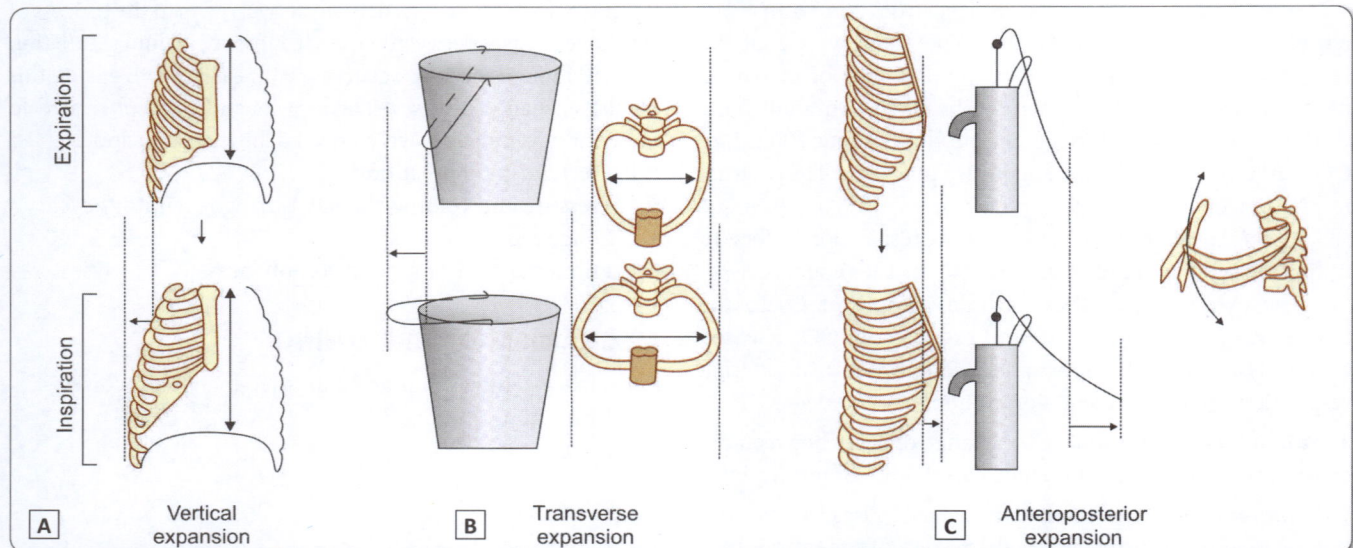

| A | Vertical expansion | B | Transverse expansion | C | Anteroposterior expansion |

Figs 2.2-1A to C: Mechanism of increase in diameter of thoracic cavity: A. Increase in vertical diameter (descent of diaphragm); B. Increase in transverse diameter (bucket handle effect); C. Increase in anteroposterior diameter (pump handle effect)

Contraction of abdominal muscles causes:

- Downward pull on the lower ribs and thus decreases the anteroposterior diameter of the thoracic cavity.
- Fixation of the lower ribs so that internal intercostal muscles act more effectively.

Contraction of the internal intercostal muscles tend to pull all the ribs downward reducing anteroposterior diameter (because of falling of pump handle effect) as well as the transverse diameter (because of action of ribs like falling of bucket handle) of the thoracic cavity.

Pressure and Volume Changes during Respiratory Cycle

Intrapulmonary Pressure Changes during Respiratory Cycle (Fig. 2.2-2)

The movement of air in and out of the lungs depends primarily on the pressure gradient between the alveoli and the atmosphere (i.e., *transairway pressure*). Intrapulmonary or alveolar pressure is the air pressure inside the lung alveoli. Intrapulmonary pressure changes during respiratory cycle are as follows (Fig. 2.2-2):

At end-expiration and end-inspiration, i.e., when the glottis is open and there is no movement of air, pressure in all parts of the respiratory tree are equal to atmospheric pressure, the intrapulmonary pressure is considered to be 0 mm Hg (760 mm Hg atmospheric pressure).

During inspiration in quiet breathing, the pressure in the alveoli decreases to about –1 mm Hg, which is sufficient to suck in about 500 mL of air into the lungs within 2 seconds period of inspiration. At the end-inspiration, the intrapulmonary pressure again becomes zero.

During expiration in quiet breathing, the elastic recoil of the lungs causes the intrapulmonary pressure to swing slightly to the positive side (+1 mm Hg) which forces the 500 mL of inspired air out of the lungs during 2–3 seconds of expiration. At the end-expiration, once again the alveolar pressure regains the atmospheric pressure (0 mm Hg or 760 mm Hg).

Forceful expiration against closed glottis (Valsalva's maneuver) may produce intrapulmonary pressure of as much as 100 mm Hg.

Intrapleural (Pleural) Pressure Changes during Respiratory Cycle

Pleural pressure is the pressure of fluid in the space between the visceral pleura and parietal pleura. Intra-pleural pressure changes during respiratory cycle are as follows (Fig. 2.2-2):

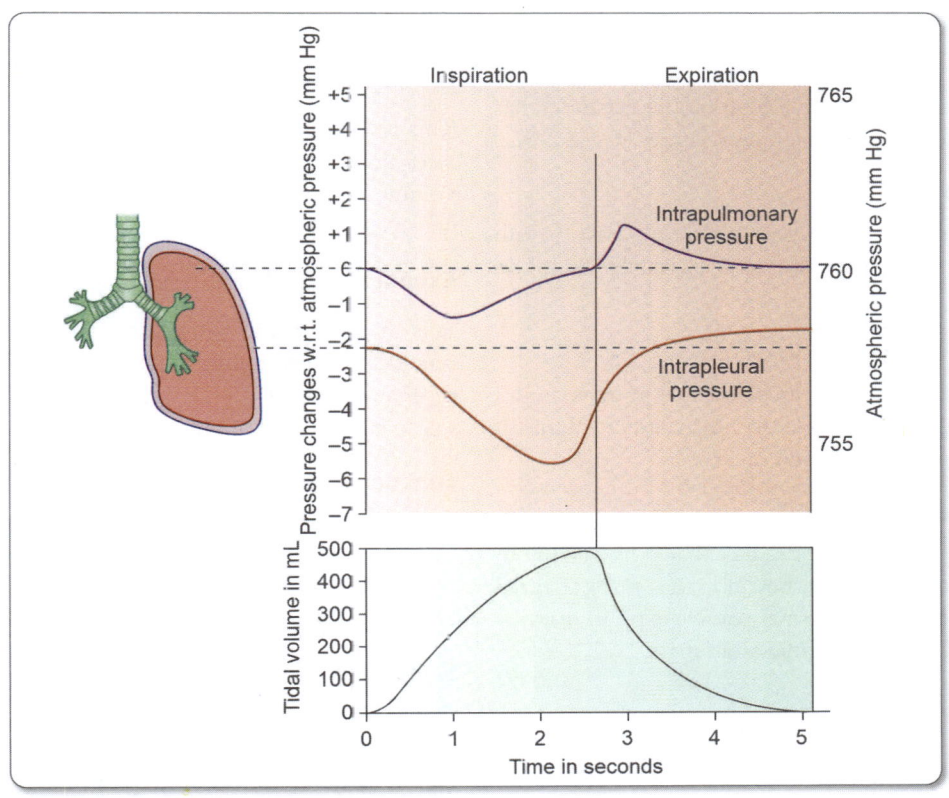

Fig. 2.2-2: Pressure and volume change during respiratory cycle

Normal pleural pressure when the respiratory muscles are completely relaxed and the airways are open, is about –2.5 mm Hg atmospheric pressure. It is the result of balance of two opposite forces, the recoil tendency of the lungs and the recoil tendency of thoracic cage.

During inspiration due to expansion of the chest wall, the pleural pressure becomes still more negative (–6 mm Hg) and pulls the surface of lungs with greater force creating negative intrapulmonary pressure.

At the end of inspiration, the inspiratory muscles relax and the recoiling force of lungs begins to pull the chest wall back to expiratory position. At end-expiratory position where the recoil force of the lungs and recoil force of thoracic cage balance, the pleural pressure returns back to –2.5 mm Hg.

IMPORTANT TO KNOW

Lung Volume Changes during Respiratory Cycle
- *During tidal inspiration*, the volume of air in the lungs increases by 500 mL (tidal volume).
- *During tidal expiration*, the elastic forces compress the gas in the lungs which starts flowing out and at the end of expiration the volume of air in the lungs decreases by 500 mL (Fig. 2.2-2).

Lung Volumes and Capacities

Lung Volumes

The maximum volume to which a lung can be expanded has been divided into four nonoverlapping volumes (Fig. 2.2-3).

Tidal volume (TV)

It is the volume of air inspired or expired with each breath during normal quiet breathing. It is approximately 500 mL in normal adult male.

Inspiratory reserve volume (IRV)

It is the extra volume of air that can be inhaled by a maximum inspiratory effort over and beyond the normal tidal volume. It is about 3000 mL in a normal adult male.

Expiratory reserve volume (ERV)

It is the extra volume of air that can be exhaled by maximum forceful expiration over and beyond the normal tidal volume (i.e. after the end of normal passive expiration). It is approximately 1100 mL in a normal adult male.

Residual volume (RV)

It is the volume of the air that still remains in the lungs after the most forceful expiration. It is about 1200 mL in a normal adult male.

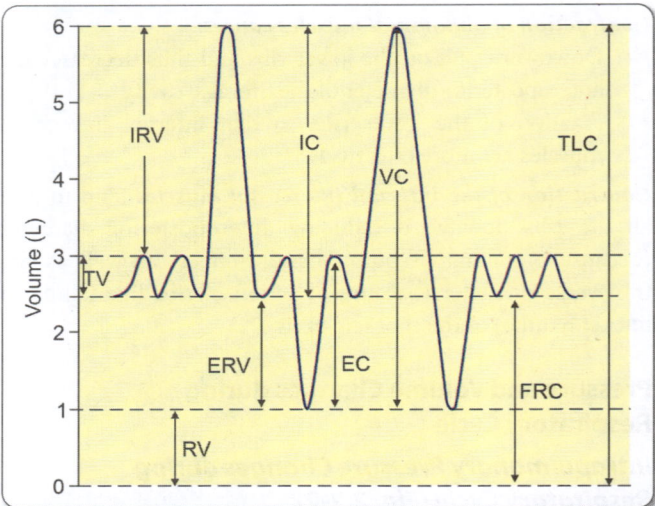

Fig. 2.2-3: A spirogram showing various lung volumes and capacities.

Abbreviations: IRV, inspiratory reserve volume; IC, inspiratory capacity; VC, vital capacity; TLC, total lung capacity; ERV, expiratory reserve volume; EC, expiratory capacity; FRC, functional residual capacity; RV residual volume TV, tidal volume

Lung Capacities

Lung capacities are combination of two or more pulmonary volumes and include the following (Fig. 2.2-3):

Inspiratory capacity (IC)

This is the maximum volume of the air that can be inspired after normal tidal expiration. Therefore, it equals the tidal volume plus inspiratory reserve volume (TV + IRV) and is approximately 3500 mL in a normal adult male.

Expiratory capacity (EC)

It is the maximum volume of air that can be expired after normal tidal inspiration. It equals tidal volume plus expiratory reserve volume (TV + ERV) and is approximately about 1600 mL in a normal adult male.

Functional residual capacity (FRC)

It is the volume of air remaining in the lungs after normal tidal expiration. Therefore, it equals the expiratory reserve volume plus the residual volume (ERV + RV) and is about 2300 mL in a normal adult male.

Significance of functional residual capacity (FRC)

The FRC (RV + ERV) of about 2300 mL represents the air that remains in the lungs most of the time. Even after the most forceful expiration about 1200 mL (residual volume) air is always present in the lungs. This has several advantages:

Continuous exchange of gases is possible due to presence of some air always in the lungs, and thereby concentration of O_2 and CO_2 in blood are maintained constant. Without FRC, pO_2 would have risen to 150 mm Hg during inspiration, and reduced nearly to zero during expiration, which is maintained at about 100 mm Hg due to the FRC.

Breath-holding is made possible due to the FRC.

Dilution of toxic inhaled gases occurs due to the reserve of 2300 mL of air in the lungs (FRC) most of the time.

Load on respiratory mechanism and left ventricle would have been much more if there was no FRC.

Vital Capacity (VC)

This is the maximum amount of air a person can expel from the lungs after the deepest possible inspiration. Therefore, it equals tidal volume plus inspiratory reserve volume plus expiratory reserve volume (TV + IRV + ERV) and is about 4600 mL in a normal adult male. Vital capacity depends on various factors. These include:

Size of the thoracic cavity. VC is more in males (2.6 L/m² body surface area) because of large chest size and more muscle power than females.

Age. In old age VC is decreased due to decrease in elasticity of the lungs.

Strength of respiratory muscles. In swimmers and divers VC is more because of the increased strength of the respiratory muscles.

Gravity. In standing position, VC is more than in sitting and lying position because of:
- Increased size of thoracic cavity in standing (diaphragm moves down)
- Reduced pulmonary blood flow due to decreased venous return.

In pregnancy VC is reduced due to pushing up of diaphragm and reduced capacity of thoracic cavity.

In ascites (accumulation of fluid in the abdominal cavity) VC is reduced due to same reason as in pregnancy.

Pulmonary diseases like pulmonary fibrosis, emphysema, respiratory obstruction, pulmonary edema, pleural effusion and pneumothorax are associated in decreased VC.

Timed Vital Capacity (TVC) or Forced Vital Capacities

Forced vital capacity is the volume of the air that can be expired rapidly with a maximum force following a maximum inspiration. The volume of air expired can be timed by recording

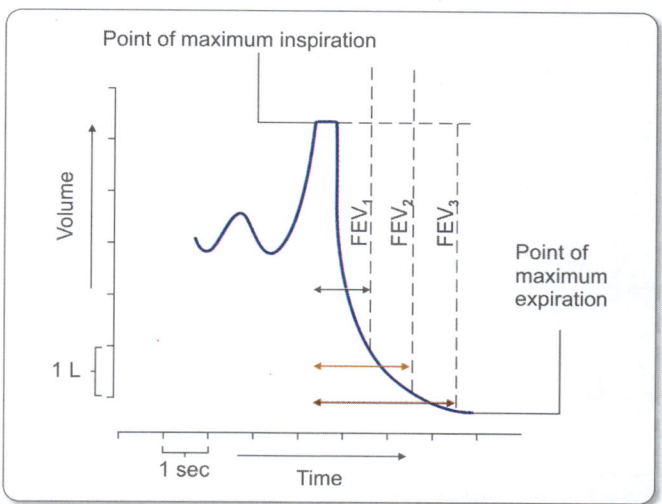

Fig. 2.2-4: Components of timed vital capacity.
Abbreviations: FEV, forced expiratory volume

the vital capacity on a spirograph moving at the known speed. Components of TVC or FVC (Fig. 2.2-4) are:

Forced expiratory volume in 1 sec (FEV₁). It represents the volume expired in the first second of a FVC. $FEV_1\%$ is the per cent of FVC expired in one second (i.e. $FEV_1\% = FEV_1/FVC \times 100$). Normally $FEV_1\%$ is about 80% of the FVC (Fig. 2.2-5A). Estimation of FEV_1 is the most commonly used screening test for airway diseases.

Clinical application. FEV_1 is useful in distinguishing between restrictive and obstructive lung diseases:
- Patients with *restrictive lung disease* (e.g. kyphoscoliosis and ankylosing spondylitis) have a reduced FVC but are able to achieve relatively high flow rates; therefore their $FEV_1\%$ exceeds 80% (Fig. 2.2-5B).
- Patients with *obstructive lung disease* (e.g. bronchial asthma) have low flow rates as a result of high airway resistance. Therefore, their $FEV_1\%$ is abnormally low (Fig. 2.2-5C).

Forced expiratory volume in 2 sec (FEV₂): It represents the volume of air expired in first 2 sec. of FVC; $FEV_2\%$ is about 90% of FVC under normal condition.

Forced expiratory volume in 3 sec. (FEV₃). It represents the volume of air expired in first 3 sec. Normally $FEV_3\%$ is 98–100% of FVC.

Total Lung Capacity (TLC)

It is the volume of air present in the lungs after the maximal inspiration. It equals the vital capacity plus the residual volume (VC + RV) and is about 5800 mL in a normal adult male.

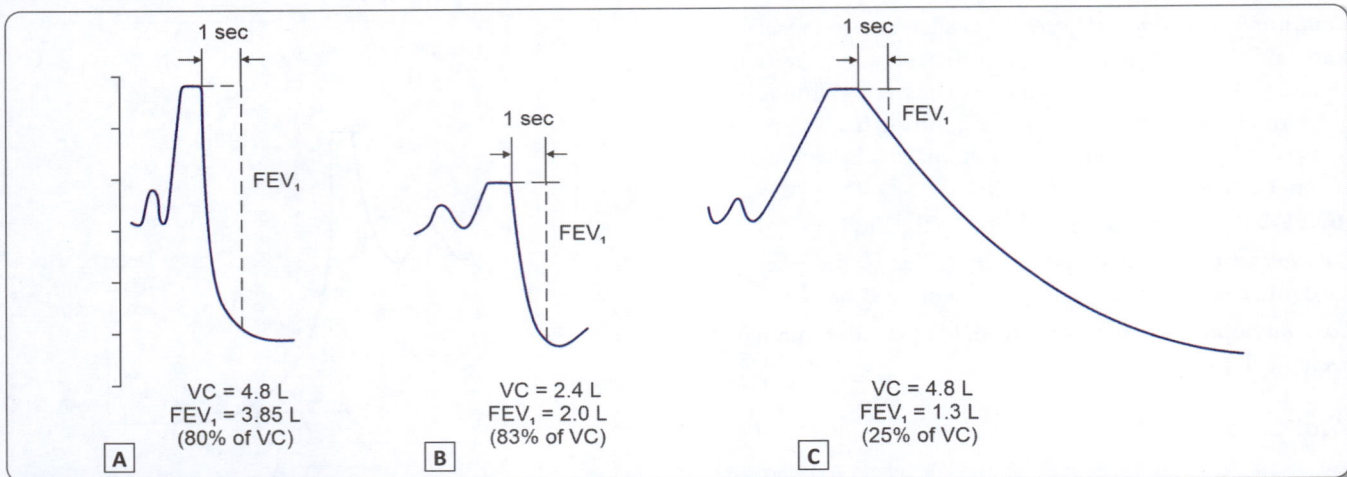

Figs 2.2-5A to C: Forced expiratory volume in first sec (FEV$_1$) component of timed vital capacity. A. In normal subject; B. In a patient with restrictive lung disease; C. In a patient with restrictive lung disease

IMPORTANT TO KNOW

Minute Ventilation (MV) or Pulmonary Ventilation (PV): It is the volume of air inspired or expired per minute. It equals the tidal volume multiplied by respiratory rate (TV × RR). The TV at rest averages 500 mL (0.5 L), and the normal respiratory rate is 12–15 breaths/min; therefore normal minute volume is 6–7.5 L/min.

Maximum breathing capacity (MBC) or maximum voluntary ventilation or maximum ventilation volume (MVV): It is the maximum volume of air that can be ventilated on command during a given interval. Normal adult male can attain a maximum ventilation volume (MVV) of 80–170 L/min (average 100 L/min).

MVV is profoundly reduced in patients with emphysema, airway obstruction and very poor respiratory muscle strength.

Measurement of static lung volumes and capacities

All volumes and capacities except residual volume, functional residual capacity and total lung capacity are recorded by spirometer. Functional residual capacity is determined by nitrogen washout method or helium dilution method and then residual volume and total lung capacity are calculated.

Recording of lung volumes and capacities are the important lung function tests.

PULMONARY ELASTANCE AND COMPLIANCE

Pulmonary Elastance

Elastance refers to *recoil* (retractive) tendency of a structure. Both the thoracic cage and lungs have elastance.

Elastance or recoil tendency of the thoracic cage refers to constant tendency of the thoracic cage to expand (to pop outward). The elastance of the thoracic cage is because of the fact that the chest wall is an elastic structure, which is normally kept partially pulled inward. The elastic property of the thoracic cage is because of the elastic nature of ribs, muscles and tendons.

Elastance of lungs. Elastance or recoil tendency of the lungs refers to the constant tendency of the lungs to collapse. The recoil forces in the lungs are generated by:

Tissue forces. These are due to the presence of many elastic tissues such as smooth muscle, elastic and collagen in the lung parenchyma which are kept under constant stretch in the inflated lungs.

Surface forces. These are generated at the alveolar surface lined by fluid (*alveolar surface tension*) due to which the alveoli become progressively smaller and collapse.

Alveolar Surface Tension

Alveolar surface tension is generated because of the unbalanced attraction of the liquid molecules at the surface of alveolar membrane.

Pulmonary Surfactant

Pulmonary surfactant is a complex mixture of several phospholipids, proteins and ions. It is secreted by type II alveolar epithelial cells (granular pneumocytes). The presence of pulmonary surfactant in the fluid lining the alveoli reduces the surface tension markedly.

NURSING IMPLICATIONS AND APPLICATIONS

Respiratory distress syndrome (RDS) of newborn or the *hyaline membrane disease* occurs in the newborn babies (especially premature) due to inadequate formation of surfactant resulting in an elevated alveolar surface tension. In this condition it is extremely difficult to expand the lungs. Respiratory work is greatly increased and there is inadequate exchange of gases due to alveolar instability, pulmonary edema, and collapse of alveoli (atelectasis) in many areas. This results in severe respiratory insufficiency and the infant may die.

Pulmonary Compliance

- Compliance (C) refers to change in lung volume (ΔV) per unit change in transpulmonary pressure (ΔP), i.e.,

$$C = \frac{\Delta V}{\Delta P}$$

  Transpulmonary pressure is the difference in the pressure between alveolar pressure and pleural pressure.
- Compliance expresses the distensibility (expansibility) of the lung and chest wall.
- Normal value of compliance for the lungs and chest wall combined is 0.13 L/cm of H_2O and for the lung alone it is 0.22 L/cm of H_2O.

PULMONARY DIFFUSION

Pulmonary diffusion refers to transfer of gases from alveoli to capillary blood across the respiratory membrane.

To understand the intricacies of diffusion of gases across the respiratory membrane it is essential to have knowledge about the following related aspects and concepts:

- Pulmonary perfusion, i.e., pulmonary blood flow *Chapter 2.1 see page 68*).
- Physics of gas diffusion and gas partial pressures.
- Alveolar ventilation, i.e., the rate at which new air reaches the gas exchange area of the lungs.
- Alveolar ventilation-perfusion ratio.
- Diffusion of gases through the respiratory membrane.

PHYSICS OF GAS DIFFUSION AND GAS PARTIAL PRESSURES

Some of the important aspects concerning physics of gas diffusion and gas partial pressures are:

Gas Pressure

The gas molecules have a kinetic energy so they are in a continuous random motion. These molecules bounce against each other and/or against the walls of container and exert a pressure. The gas pressure (P) exerted is denoted by the equation:

$$P = \frac{nRT}{V}$$

where

P = Pressure of gas
n = Number of molecules of gas
T = Absolute temperature
V = Volume of gas
R = Gas constant

Partial Pressure

According to *Dalton's law* of partial pressure, the total pressure exerted by a mixture of gases is equal to the sum of the partial pressure of all gases present in the mixture. Thus, the partial pressure (p) refers to the pressure exerted by any one gas present in a mixture of gases. Hence, the partial pressure (p) of a gas can be calculated by multiplying its fractional concentration by the total pressure. For example, environmental air which has atmospheric pressure (at sea level) of about 760 mm Hg is a mixture of 21% oxygen (O_2), and 79% nitrogen (N_2). Therefore, the partial pressure (p) of O_2 and N_2 respectively will be:

$$pO_2 = 760 \times \frac{21}{100} = 160 \text{ mm Hg}$$

$$pN_2 = 760 \times \frac{79}{100} = 600 \text{ mm Hg}$$

Water Vapor Pressure

The atmospheric air entering the respiratory passages during inspiration is humidified by the water vapors from the conducting passages. By the time the atmospheric air reaches the alveoli, it is saturated with water vapors. Thus, in the alveolar air, besides O_2 and N_2, water vapors also exert their partial pressure. Vapor pressure of water is dependent upon its temperature. At body temperature (37°C) the vapor pressure of water in alveolar air is 47 mm Hg.

ALVEOLAR VENTILATION

Alveolar ventilation is the volume of the fresh air, which reaches the gas exchange area of the lung every minute. During inspiration some of the air inhaled never reaches the gas exchange areas but instead fills the non-gas exchange areas (conducting zone) of the respiratory tract called the *dead space*, which is equal to about 150 mL.

During expiration out of 500 mL of tidal volume 150 mL of the alveolar expired air remains in the conducting passages. Therefore, of 500 mL air entering the lungs only

350 mL/breath is the fresh air, which contributes to alveolar ventilation. Thus, alveolar ventilation can be calculated as:

Alveolar ventilation (VA) = Respiratory rate × (Tidal volume – Dead space volume).

With a normal tidal volume of 500 mL, a normal dead space of 150 mL, and a respiratory rate of 12 breaths per minute, alveolar ventilation equals 12 × (500–350), or 4200 mL/min.

ALVEOLAR VENTILATION-PERFUSION RATIO

Alveolar ventilation-perfusion ratio (VA/Q) is the ratio of alveolar ventilation per minute to quantity of blood flow to alveoli per minute. Normally, alveolar ventilation (VA) is 4.2–5.0 L/min, and the pulmonary blood flow (equal to cardiac output) is approximately 5 L/min. So, the normal VA/Q is about 0.84–0.9. At this ratio, maximum oxygenation occurs.

Alveolar Air

Volume of air which is available for exchange of gases in the alveoli per breath is called alveolar air, which is equivalent to tidal volume minus dead space, i.e., (500–150) or 350 mL.

Composition of Alveolar Air

Alveolar air composition is considerably different than that of atmospheric air because of the following reasons:
- Water vapors dilute the other gases in the inspired air.
- Alveolar air is renewed very slowly by atmospheric air.
- Oxygen is constantly being absorbed from the alveolar air.
- Carbon dioxide is constantly diffusing from the pulmonary blood to alveoli.

Composition of Expired Air

As shown in Table 2.2-1, the composition of expired air is different than that of alveolar air. This is because of the fact that the expired air is a combination of dead space air and alveolar air.

DIFFUSION OF GASES THROUGH THE RESPIRATORY MEMBRANE

Respiratory Unit and Respiratory Membrane

Each respiratory unit is composed of a respiratory bronchiole, alveolar ducts, atria and alveoli. There are about 300 million respiratory units in the two lungs. Gas exchange occurs through the membranes of all the structures forming a respiratory unit, not merely in the alveoli themselves.

Respiratory membrane or pulmonary membrane or the alveolocapillary membrane is the name given to the tissues,

TABLE 2.2-1: Composition and partial pressure of gases in atmospheric air, humidified air, alveolar air and expired air

Partial pressure (mm Hg) and concentration (percentage) of various gases				
Gas air	Atmospheric air	Humidified air	Alveolar air	Expired
N_2	597.0 (78.62%)	563.4 (74.09%)	569.0 (74.9%)	566.0 (74.5%)
O_2	159.0 (20.84%)	149.3 (19.67%)	104.0 (13.6%)	120.0 (15.7%)
CO_2	0.3 (0.04%)	0.3 (0.04%)	40.0 (5.3%)	27.0 (3.6%)
H_2O	3.7 (0.5%)	47 (6.20%)	47.0 (6.2%)	47.0 (6.2%)
Total	760.0 (100%)	760 (100%)	760 (100%)	760 (100%)

which separate the capillary blood from the alveolar air. The exchange of gases between the capillary blood and alveolar air requires diffusion through this membrane.

Structure of Respiratory Membrane

It consists of the following layers (Fig. 2.2-6):
- Layer of pulmonary surfactant and fluid lining the alveolus
- Layer of alveolar epithelial cells
- Basement membrane of the alveolar epithelial cells
- A very thin interstitial space between the epithelial and endothelial cells
- Basement membrane of capillary endothelial cells
- Layer of capillary endothelial cells.

Surface area of the total respiratory membrane is about 70 m² in the normal adult.

Diffusion and Equilibration of Gases Across the Respiratory Membrane

Diffusion of O_2

The normal alveolar pO_2 is 104 mm Hg, whereas the blood entering the pulmonary capillary normally has a pO_2 of 40 mm Hg. Pressure gradient therefore is 64 mm Hg in the beginning. After dissolving in the respiratory membrane, the O_2 molecules diffuse into the blood. As O_2 diffuses from alveoli to blood, the pO_2 of blood becomes the same as in alveolar air (104 mm Hg), the gradient becomes zero and no diffusion occurs (Figs 2.2-7A and B). By the time blood passes to one-third of distance in capillary the pO_2 of blood equals that of alveoli.

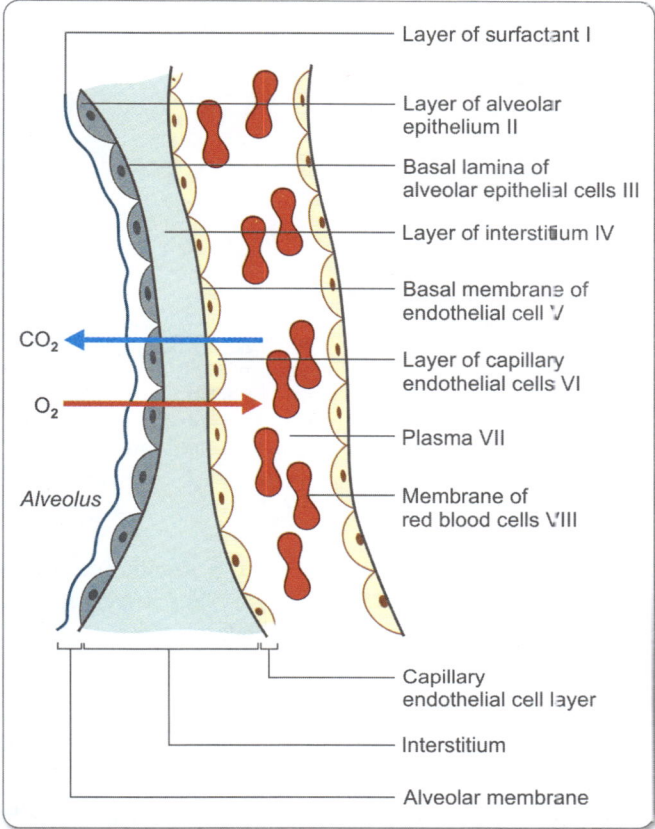

Fig. 2.2-6: Layers of respiratory membrane

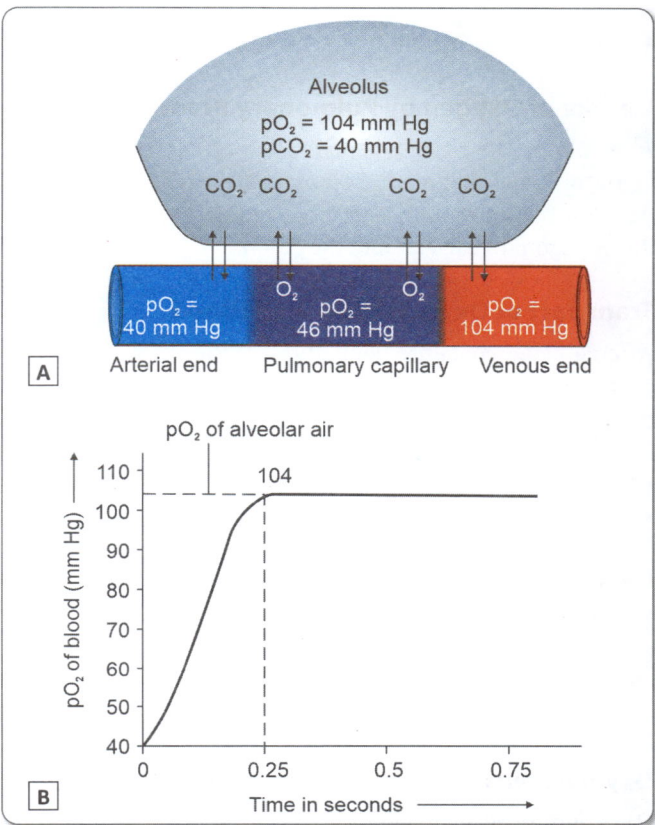

Figs 2.2-7A and B: A. Diffusion of oxygen across respiratory membrane; B. Leading to progressive increase in capillary pO_2

Diffusion of CO_2

It occurs from blood to alveoli because pCO_2 is higher in blood than in alveolar air. The average pCO_2 in the pulmonary capillary blood is 46 mm Hg as opposed to 40 mm Hg in the alveoli. Therefore pressure gradient in the beginning is 6 mm Hg and time integrated pressure gradient calculated for CO_2 (in a manner similar to O_2) across the respiratory membrane is only 1 mm Hg. Although the pressure gradient for CO_2 is only one-tenth of the O_2 diffusion gradient, CO_2 diffuses almost 20 times more rapidly than O_2 because of higher diffusion coefficient.

Effect of Alveolar Ventilation-perfusion Ratio on Pulmonary Gas Exchange

- Optimum gas exchange across the respiratory membrane occurs when the alveolar ventilation-perfusion ratio (VA/Q) is normal, i.e., between 0.8 and 1.
- Both, a decrease as well as an increase, in VA/Q ratio reduce the gas exchange.

IMPORTANT TO KNOW

Diffusion Capacity of Lung

Diffusion capacity (DC) of the lung is quantitative expression of the ability of the respiratory membrane to exchange a gas between the alveoli and the pulmonary blood. It is defined as the volume of gas (V gas) that diffuses through the respiratory membrane of lung each minute for a pressure gradient of 1 mm Hg.

TRANSPORT OF GASES

TRANSPORT OF OXYGEN

Transport of oxygen from the lungs to tissues occurs due to constant circulation of blood and diffusion of O_2 that occurs in the direction of concentration gradient which is represented by O_2 tension (pO_2) differences as given below:
- Alveolar air pO_2: 104 mm Hg
- Arterial blood pO_2: 95 mm Hg

- Venous blood pO_2: 40 mm Hg
- Tissue interstitial fluid pO_2: 40 mm Hg

Uptake of Oxygen by Pulmonary Blood

As mentioned above, pO_2 of pulmonary arterial blood is about 40 mm Hg and that of alveolar air is 104 mm Hg. Therefore, due to this great concentration gradient oxygen readily diffuses from the alveoli into the blood.

Transport of Oxygen in Arterial Blood

Arterial blood contains about 20 mL of O_2 and venous blood about 15 mL of O_2 per 100 mL. Thus, about 5 mL of O_2 is transported per 100 mL of blood from lungs to the tissue cells. Oxygen is transported into the blood in two forms:

- As dissolved form
- In combination with hemoglobin.

Oxygen Transport in Dissolved Form

The solubility of O_2 in water (plasma) is so little that at pO_2 value of 100 mm Hg, out of the 20 mL of O_2 present in 100 mL of blood, only 0.3 mL is in dissolved form and rest is combined with hemoglobin (as oxyhemoglobin).

Oxygen Transport in Combination with Hemoglobin

Oxygenation of hemoglobin. After entering into the blood from the alveolar air, most of the oxygen combines with hemoglobin to form a *loose and reversible* combination. This process is called *oxygenation* (not oxidation) and converts deoxyhemoglobin into oxyhemoglobin. Each molecule of hemoglobin can combine with as many as *four O_2 molecules.*

Oxygen-carrying capacity of hemoglobin. One gram of hemoglobin can bind with maximum of 1.34 mL of O_2. Thus 100 mL of blood with hemoglobin level of 15 gm% can carry 1.34×15, or 20.1 mL of oxygen. Practically 100 mL of the arterial blood carries about 19.8 mL of oxygen out of which about 19.5 mL as oxyhemoglobin and 0.3 mL as dissolved form in plasma.

Oxygen-hemoglobin dissociation curve

Oxygen-hemoglobin dissociation curve refers to the curve obtained when the relation between the pO_2 and the percentage of hemoglobin saturation is plotted (Fig. 2.2-8). The O_2-Hb dissociation curve shows that percentage saturation of hemoglobin increases with the increase in pO_2 of arterial blood. However the relation is not linear but *sigmoid or S-shaped.* Several factors affect the affinity for hemoglobin for O_2 and thus shift the O_2-Hb dissociation curve to either right or left.

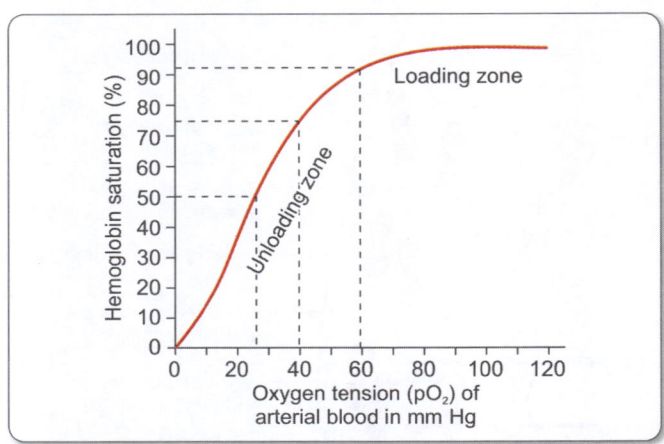

Fig. 2.2-8: Normal oxygen-hemoglobin dissociation curve

Shift to right

Shift to right of O_2-Hb dissociation curve signifies decreased affinity of hemoglobin for O_2 (Fig. 2.2-8). Thus at every level of pO_2, the oxygen saturation of hemoglobin is somewhat lower than the normal curve leading to more offloading of O_2.

Causes: The factors causing right shift are:

An increase in pCO_2 shifts the curve to right, this phenomenon is known as *Bohr's effect* (Fig. 2.2-9A).

A decrease in pH of blood, as occurs in the tissues, also shifts the O_2-Hb dissociation curve to the right.

Effect of temperature. An increase in the temperature of blood shifts the curve to right.

Effect of diphosphoglycerate. The red blood cells are rich in 2, 3-diphosphoglycerate (2, 3-DPG) which is a highly charged anion that binds to β-chain of deoxygenated adult hemoglobin.

$$HbO_2 + 2, 3\text{-}DPG \rightarrow Hb\ 2, 3\text{-}DPG + O_2$$

Thus, an increase in the concentration of 2, 3-DPG decreases the affinity of Hb for O_2 and shifts the normal O_2-Hb dissociation curve to the right. Causes of increased levels of 2, 3-DPG are anemia, exposure to chronic hypoxia at high altitude and certain pulmonary diseases.

Advantages versus disadvantages of right shift are:

- Right shift is advantageous in the tissues where greater O_2 is released from hemoglobin (at the same pO_2).
- However, right shift is disadvantageous in the lungs because (at the same pO_2) blood takes up less oxygen.

Shift to left

Shift to left of O_2-Hb dissociation curve signifies increased affinity of hemoglobin for O_2 (Fig. 2.2-9B). Thus, at every pO_2 level the oxygen saturation of hemoglobin is somewhat greater than in normal curve.

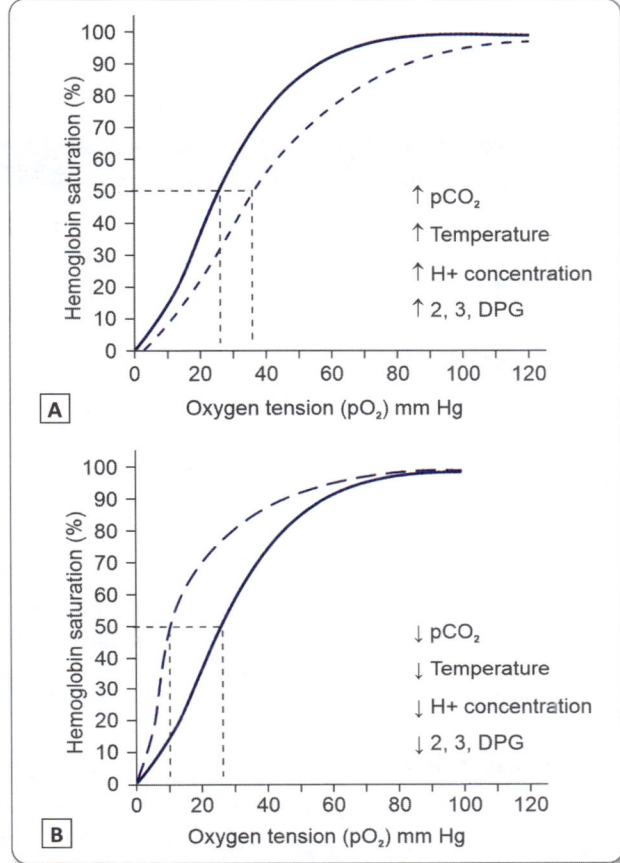

Figs 2.2-9A and B: Right A, and left B, shift of oxygen-hemoglobin dissociation curve

Causes for left shift of the curve are:
• Decreased pCO_2 of blood
• Increased pH of blood
• Decreased temperature
• Fetal hemoglobin.

Advantages versus disadvantages of left shift are:
Left shift of the curve has limited advantage because though it allows greater uptake of O_2 at lungs (at same pO_2), it decreases the release of O_2 to the tissues (at same pO_2).

Effect of carbon monoxide on O_2 transport
• Carbon monoxide (CO) interferes with O_2 transport because it has about 200 times the affinity for hemoglobin as compared to oxygen.
• CO combines with Hb at the same site on its molecule as O_2 and forms the *carboxyhemoglobin*, and thus decreases the functional hemoglobin concentration.

Release of Oxygen in Tissues at Rest
Oxygen Delivery
It represents the amount of O_2 that is presented to body cells per minute. It is equal to the arterial O_2 content multiplied by cardiac output. Since 100 mL of arterial blood at pO_2 of about 100 mm Hg contains about 20 mL of oxygen, thus with a cardiac output of about 5 L/min the normal oxygen delivery to the entire body is about 1 L/min. The oxygen delivery to the tissues decreases with either decrease in arterial O_2 content or decrease in cardiac output.

Oxygen Consumption
When the arterial blood with approximate pO_2 100 mm Hg reaches the tissues with tissue fluid pO_2 40 mm Hg, because of pressure gradient, about 5 mL of O_2 diffuses from the tissue capillaries to the interstitial fluid out of 100 mL of blood (containing ~ 19 mL O_2) every minute. Thus, oxygen consumption of the whole body at rest with a cardiac output of 5 L/min is about $\frac{5 \times 5000}{100}$ or 250 mL of O_2 per minute.

Utilization Coefficient
Utilization coefficient refers to the percentage of oxygen consumed out of oxygen delivered to the tissue, i.e.

$$\text{Coefficient of utilization} = \frac{\text{Oxygen consumed/min}}{\text{Oxygen delivered/min}}$$

So, at rest coefficient of utilization of whole body

$$\frac{250 \text{ mL/min}}{1000 \text{ mL/min}} \times 100 = 25\%$$

TRANSPORT OF CARBON DIOXIDE
Transport of carbon dioxide from tissue cells to the lungs occurs due to *constant circulation* of blood and diffusion of CO_2 that occurs at various sites in the direction of concentration gradient which is represented by CO_2 tension (pCO_2) differences as given below:

• Intracellular pCO_2 : 46 mm Hg
• Interstitial fluid pCO_2 : 45 mm Hg
• Arterial blood pCO_2 : 40 mm Hg
  (in tissue capillaries)
• Venous blood pCO_2 : 45 mm Hg
• Alveolar air pCO_2 : 40 mm Hg

From the above pCO_2 levels, it is clear that:

Diffusion of CO_2 from the cells into the interstitial fluid occurs along a tension gradient of 1 mm Hg.

Diffusion of CO$_2$ in blood. From the interstitial fluid the CO$_2$ diffuses into the capillaries at a tension gradient of 5 mm Hg.

Transport of CO$_2$ in the blood occurs in three forms:

1. In dissolved state (7%)
2. In bicarbonate form (70%)
3. In carbamino compound form (23%).

Release of CO$_2$ in lungs. From the venous blood that is supplied to pulmonary capillaries the CO$_2$ diffuses across the respiratory membrane into the alveoli along a tension gradient of 5 mm Hg.

Carbon dioxide dissociation curve

- Carbon dioxide dissociation curve is obtained by plotting the relationship between pCO$_2$ and total CO$_2$ content of the blood (Fig. 2.2-10).
- The graph shows that relationship between the two is nearly linear over wider range of pCO$_2$ (if compared with O$_2$-Hb dissociation curve, which is sigmoid shaped).

Rate of total CO$_2$ transport

In resting conditions each 100 mL of blood transports about 4 mL of CO$_2$ from the tissues to the lungs. Thus, with an average cardiac output of 5 L/min, a total of (4 × 5000) /100 or 200 mL of CO$_2$ is transported/min.

During exercise the amount of CO$_2$ transported increases depending upon the severity of exercise. In severe exercise, as much as 4 L of CO$_2$ may be transported per minute.

Respiratory quotient

Definition. Respiratory quotient (RQ) refers to the ratio of the rate of CO$_2$ excretion and rate of O$_2$ consumption per minute. It is also called *respiratory exchange ratio*.

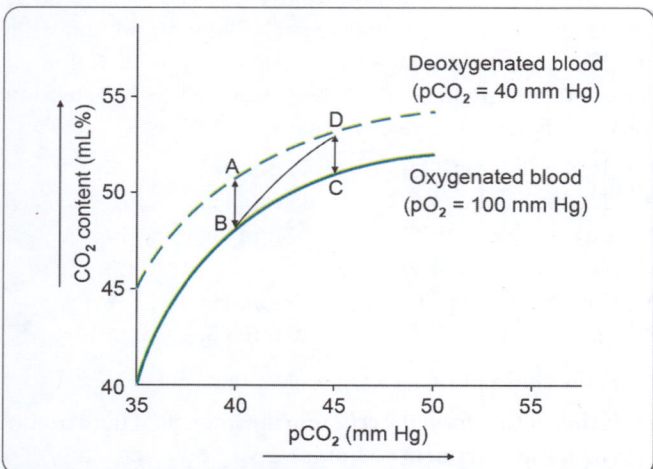

Fig. 2.2-10: Carbon dioxide dissociation curve for oxygenated (solid line) and for deoxygenated blood (dotted line) to demonstrate Haldane's effect

Normal value. Normally, the rate of CO$_2$ excretion is 4 mL/100 mL/min, and rate of O$_2$ consumption is 5 mL/100 mL/min. So, respiratory quotient = 4/5, or 0.8.

REGULATION OF RESPIRATION

Respiration is regulated by a complex integration of neural control mechanisms which are modified by certain respiratory reflexes and chemical control mechanisms.

NEURAL REGULATION OF RESPIRATION

The involuntary neural control system regulates respiration by several groups of neurons situated bilaterally in medulla and pons which include medullary respiratory centers, pontine respiratory centers, and reticular activating system (RAS).

Medullary Respiratory Centers

The medullary respiratory centers include two groups of neurons: the dorsal respiratory group (DRG) and ventral respiratory group (VRG) which generate the basic respiratory rhythm (Fig. 2.2-11A).

Pontine Respiratory Centers

The pontine centers include the apneustic center (APN) and pneumotaxic center (PNC), both of which modify the activity of medullary respiratory centers.

Apneustic center (APN). Refers to a group of inhibitory neurons located bilaterally in the lower part of pons (Figs 2.2-11A and B). It sends signals to neurons of DRG. This increases the tidal volume and duration of inspiration, resulting in a deeper and more prolonged inspiratory effort termed *apneusis*. However, normally the apneustic center is inhibited by impulses carried by the vagus nerves and also by the activity of pneumotaxic center.

Pneumotaxic center (PNC). The pneumotaxic centers are located bilaterally in the upper pons. They inhibit the apneustic center (APN). Therefore, stimulation of PNC shortens inspiration, leading to shallow and more rapid respiratory pattern.

Thus, though rhythm of respiration resides in DRG neurons in medulla, PNC and APN control these neurons to regulate the depth and rate of respiration.

Reticular Activating System

The reticular activating system (RAS) stimulates the respiratory centers to increase respiratory drive. During sleep, RAS activity diminishes, decreasing respiratory drive, which diminishes alveolar ventilation and results in a slight elevation of arterial CO$_2$ tension.

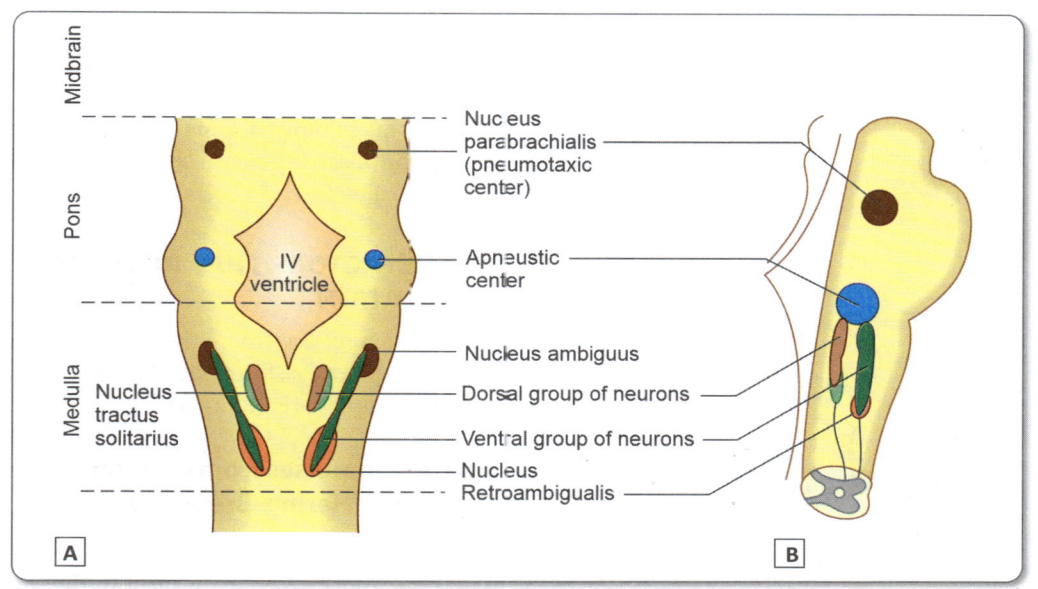

Figs 2.2-11A and B: Medullary and pontine respiratory centers. A. Front view; B. Lateral view

CHEMICAL REGULATION OF RESPIRATION

The chemical factors regulating respiration are pCO_2, pO_2 and pH of blood. These factors influence respiration in such a way that their own blood levels are maintained constant. The chemical mechanism of regulation operates through chemoreceptors.

Chemoreceptors

Chemoreceptors are the sensory nerve endings which are highly sensitive to changes in pCO_2, pO_2 and pH of blood. These are of two types:
1. Peripheral chemoreceptors
2. Central chemoreceptors.

Peripheral Chemoreceptors

Location. Peripheral chemoreceptors include the carotid and aortic bodies (Fig. 2.2-12).
Carotid body is located on either side near the bifurcation of common carotid artery.
Aortic bodies, two or more in number, are located near the arch of aorta.

Functions. The peripheral chemoreceptors respond to lowered pO_2, increased pCO_2 and increased H^+ concentration in the arterial blood. The afferent impulses from the chemoreceptors stimulate the dorsal respiratory group (DRG) neurons, which lead to an increased rate and depth of respiration called *hyperventilation*. The peripheral chemoreceptors are the only sites that detect changes in pO_2.

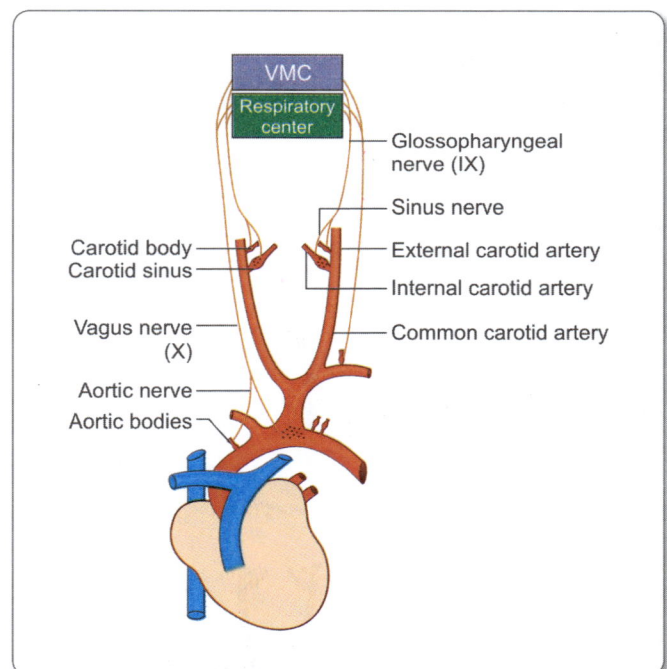

Fig. 2.2-12: Location of carotid and aortic bodies (peripheral chemoreceptors)

Central Chemoreceptors

Location. Central chemoreceptors are the cells (neurons) that lie just beneath the ventral surface of the medulla oblongata and are therefore also called medullary receptors (Figs 2.2-13A and B).

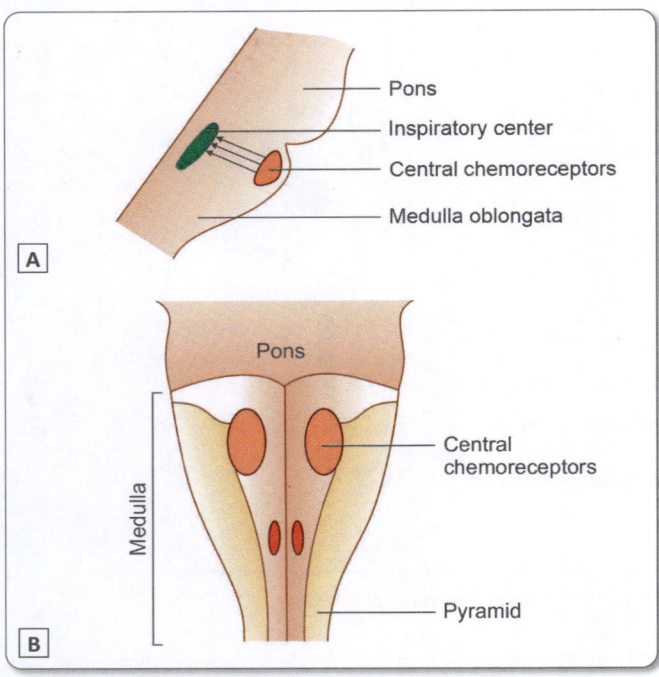

Figs 2.2-13A and B: Location of central chemoreceptors in medulla: A. Lateral view; B. Front view

Stimulation characteristics of central chemoreceptors are:

- They respond to H⁺ concentration in the surrounding interstitial fluid and cerebrospinal fluid.
- The magnitude of stimulation is directly proportional to the local H⁺ concentration, which in turn parallels arterial pCO_2.

OTHER FACTORS THAT INFLUENCE RESPIRATION

Afferent impulses from the receptors other than the chemoreceptors, i.e., from non-chemical receptors include the following impulse (Fig. 2.2-14):

Afferent Impulses from Pulmonary Stretch Receptors (Hering-Breuer Reflex)

The Hering-Breuer inspiratory inhibitory reflex is initiated when the stretch receptors located in the smooth muscles of the bronchi and bronchioles are stimulated by inflation of the lungs. The impulses are then sent through *vagii nerves* to pontomedullary respiratory centers to inhibit respiration. This reflex is weakest in humans. It does not play any regulatory

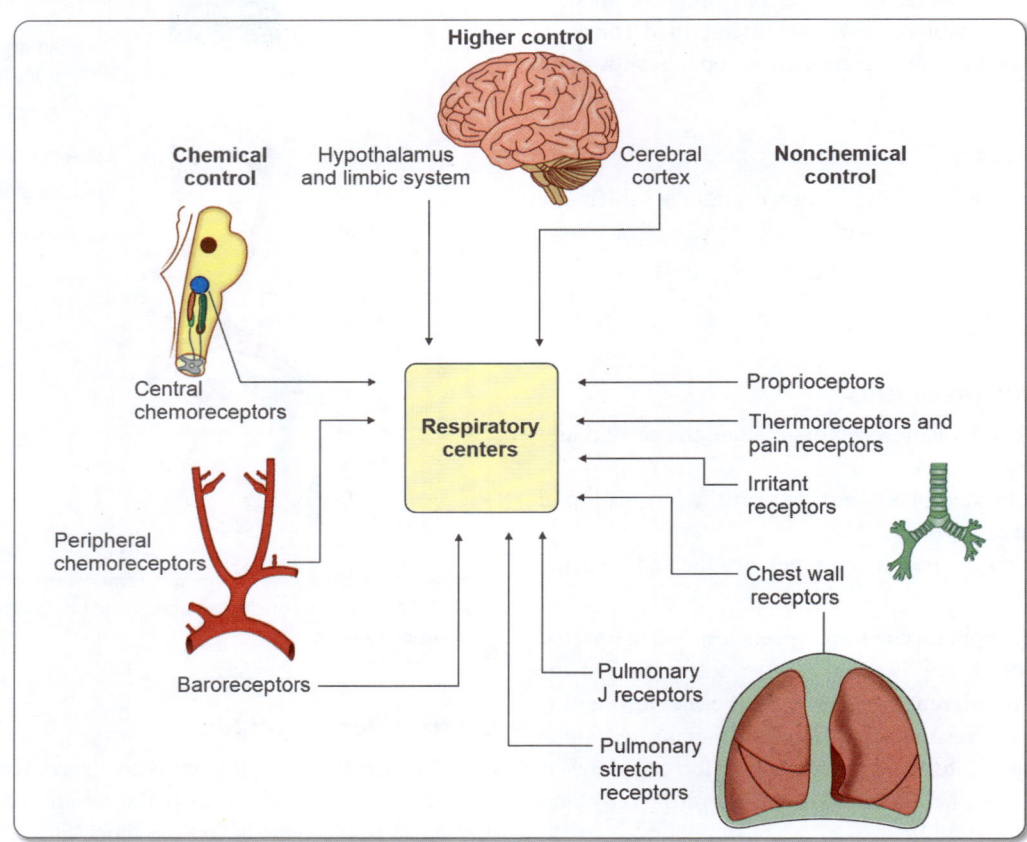

Fig. 2.2-14: Afferent impulses to respiratory centers

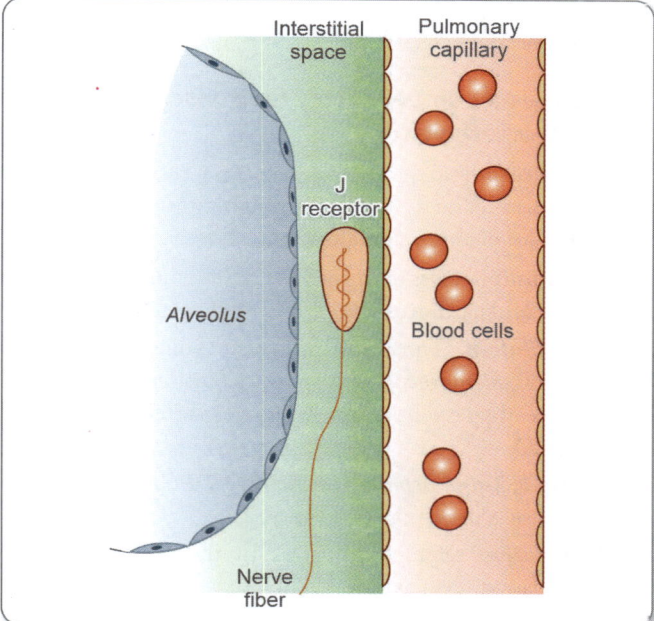

Fig. 2.2-15: Location of J receptors

role in tidal respiration. This reflex is initiated only when the tidal volume is more than 1–1.5 L. Thus, the reflex tends to limit the tidal volume.

Afferent Impulses from J-receptors

Afferent impulses from J-receptors constitute the J-reflex. The J-receptors were discovered by an Indian physiologist AS Paintal in 1954. The name J-receptors (juxtapulmonary capillary receptors) was given to them because of their location very close to the pulmonary capillaries (Fig. 2.2-15).

These receptors are primarily sensitive to increase in the content of interstitial fluid between the capillary endothelium and alveolar epithelium, therefore, they are stimulated in conditions, like pulmonary congestion, pulmonary edema, pneumonia, hyperinflation of lungs and microembolism in pulmonary capillaries.

Afferent Impulses from Proprioceptors

Proprioceptors are the receptors present in the muscles, tendons and joints and are stimulated during change in the position of different parts of the body. This reflex helps in increasing ventilation during exercise. The pediatricians employ this reflex for initiating first breath in the newborn by slapping.

Afferent Impulses from Thermoreceptors

Thermoreceptors are those receptors which are stimulated by a change in the body temperature. When warm receptors are stimulated, the impulses are conveyed to cerebral cortex via somatic afferent nerves. Cerebral cortex in turn stimulates the respiratory centers to produce hyperventilation.

Respiration helps to maintain body temperature, as some amount of heat is lost in the expired air. In dogs, panting is one of the major mechanisms of thermoregulation.

RESPIRATORY ADJUSTMENTS TO STRESSES IN HEALTH

Respiratory adjustments to stresses in health illustrate the integrated operation of the respiratory regulatory mechanisms. The stresses faced by respiration requiring adjustments in day-to-day life include:
- Respiratory adjustments during exercise.
- Respiratory adjustments at high altitude.
- Respiratory adjustments to high atmospheric pressure.

RESPIRATORY ADJUSTMENTS DURING EXERCISE

Exercise is the most frequently faced stress in day-to-day life.

Respiratory Responses to Exercise

Increase in Pulmonary Ventilation

The pulmonary ventilation increases linearly with the increases in intensity of exercise (O_2 consumption) until the anaerobic threshold is reached.

Mechanism of increased pulmonary ventilation

There are several factors which can account for the marked increase in pulmonary ventilation occurring in severe exercise are:

Neural control mechanisms play main role in increasing pulmonary ventilation during exercise.

Chemical mechanism does not play the main role in exercise hyperpnea, as the alveolar and arterial pO_2 and pCO_2 are well maintained during exercise however:

Accentuations of the normal oscillations in pO_2 and pCO_2 synchronous with respiration might stimulate the carotid body chemoreceptors and explains part of exercise hyperpnea. *Acidosis produced due to accumulation of lactic acid* during severe exercise (above the aerobic threshold level) is responsible for increase in pulmonary ventilation.

Increase in Oxygen Uptake in the Lungs

The oxygen uptake by blood in the lungs increases from 250 mL/min at rest to about 4 L/min during heavy exercise. This is made possible by:

- Increased pulmonary perfusion
- Increased alveolar capillary pO_2 gradient
- Increased pulmonary diffusion capacity.

RESPIRATORY ADJUSTMENTS AT HIGH ALTITUDE

At high altitude barometric pressure is low and so the partial pressure of O_2 is also low, however, the amount of O_2 in the atmosphere is same as it is at the sea level. When a person is exposed to high altitude, particularly by rapid ascent, the different systems of the body cannot cope with the lowered O_2 tension and the effects of hypoxia start. The changes in the body at high altitude are produced mainly by:

- Hypoxia produced by low pO_2
- Expansion of gases due to fall in atmospheric pressure.

Hypoxia at High Altitude

The effects of hypoxic hypoxia produced by decreasing pO_2 at high altitude depend upon:

- The level of altitude
- Rate at which hypoxia develops, i.e., hypoxia occurs due to rapid ascent (acute hypoxia) or slow ascent (subacute hypoxia)
- Duration of exposure to hypoxia, i.e., whether short-term stay or long-term stay (chronic hypoxia).

Clinical Syndromes Caused by High Altitude

The three specific entities (clinical syndromes) which produce effects of low pO_2 at high altitude are:

- High altitude pulmonary edema (HAPO),
- Acute mountain sickness
- Chronic mountain sickness.

High altitude pulmonary edema. High altitude pulmonary edema (HAPO) usually occurs as an effect of rapid ascent at high altitude (above 10,000 ft). It is usually seen in individuals who engage in heavy physical work during first 3 –4 days after rapid ascent to high altitude due to sympathetic stimulation caused by hypoxia.

Acute mountain sickness. The characteristics of acute mountain sickness are headache, nausea, vomiting, irritability, insomnia, and breathlessness.

Chronic mountain sickness. Chronic mountain sickness (Monge's disease) occurs in some long-term residents of high altitude who develop extreme polycythemia, cyanosis, malaise, fatigue and exercise intolerance.

Physiological Compensatory Responses to High Altitude Hypoxia

Two types of physiological compensatory responses known to occur in individuals exposed to high altitude hypoxia are accommodation and acclimatization.

Accommodation refers to immediate reflex adjustments of the respiratory and cardiovascular system to hypoxia. These are:

Hyperventilation. Hyperventilation occurs due to stimulation of peripheral chemoreceptors by low O_2 tension in the arterial blood. The hyperventilation improves arterial pO_2 and reduces pCO_2.

Increase in 2, 3-diphosphoglycerate (2, 3-DPG) concentration occurs in RBCs in response to hypoxia.

Acclimatization refers to changes in the body tissues in response to long-term exposure to hypoxia. Following changes occur in the tissues:

Increase in red blood cell count (polycythemia). Occurs due to release of renal erythropoietin. This increase in RBC count leads to:

- Increase in hemoglobin concentration
- Increase in hematocrit value.

Increase in pulmonary ventilation. There is gradual increase in ventilation to an average of above five times as that of normal.

Cardiovascular changes in the form of tachycardia, and increased force of contraction of the heart.

Pulmonary hypertension. It occurs in response to pulmonary vasoconstriction.

Increase in total lung capacity and diffusion capcity of lungs.

Cellular and tissue acclimatization occur by:

- Increase in oxidative enzymes concentration
- Increase in mitochondrial density
- Increase in capillary density.

RESPIRATORY ADJUSTMENTS TO HIGH ATMOSPHERIC PRESSURE

Respiratory adjustments to high atmospheric pressure form a part of physiological problems faced by the body while going under the sea.

Physiological Problems under Depth

If the appropriate preventive measures are not taken, then the individuals working at depth in sea will have to face the following physiological problems:

Physiological Problems due to Effect of High Pressure on Respiratory Gases

Air under high atmospheric pressure is breathed under the sea. At high atmospheric pressure of air the partial pressure of oxygen (pO_2), nitrogen (pN_2) and carbon dioxide (pCO_2) is also increased producing the following physiological problems.

Effects of increased po_2 (oxygen toxicity)

Oxygen toxicity may be acute or chronic.

Acute oxygen toxicity occurs on exposures to four atmosphere pressure of oxygen (pO_2 in lungs about 3000 mm Hg).

1. *Nervous complications of acute oxygen poisoning* include disorientation, dizziness, convulsions and even coma.

2. *Irritation of airways* in the form of nasal congestion, sore throat, substernal discomfort, sneezing, coughing and bronchoconstriction

3. *Pulmonary edema and atelectasis* begin to develop after 12 hours of exposure.

4. *Bronchopneumonia* may be initiated when exposure is continued for >24 hours.

Effects of increased pN_2 (nitrogen narcosis)

Nitrogen narcosis is characterized by:

Euphoric symptoms. The individual becomes jovial and carefree. These are followed by impairment of mental functions and intelligence, individual becomes drowsy and has poor muscular coordination.

Physiological Problems of Ascent

The two physiological problems which occur when an individual ascends back to sea level after sufficient exposure to high atmospheric pressure in the deep sea are:

1. Decompression sickness
2. Air embolism.

Decompression sickness

Decompression sickness is also known as Caisson's disease, dysbarism, compressed air sickness, the bends, and diver's palsy. When the individual ascends rapidly to sea level nitrogen is decompressed and escapes from the tissues at a faster rate. Being gas it forms bubbles while escaping rapidly from the tissues. The gas bubbles block the blood vessels producing tissue ischemia and sometimes the tissue death.

Symptoms produced by escaping gas bubbles constitute the *decompression sickness*. These are:

- *Pain in joints and muscles* of legs or arms
- *Sensation of numbness*, tingling or pricking (paraesthesia) and itching
- *The chokes*—shortness of breath

- *Paralysis* of muscles
- *Coronary ischemia* or myocardial infarction
- *Neurological symptoms* like dizziness and unconsciousness may occur.

Air embolism

Air embolism is another physiological problem which may occur during rapid ascent from a depth below the sea level.

Manifestations of air embolism include chest pain, tachypnea, systemic hypotension and hypoxemia. In severe cases, air emboli may travel to the systemic circulation, block the blood flow to some vital organs and may even result in death.

DISTURBANCES OF RESPIRATION

From the physiological viewpoint, disturbances of respiration can be discussed under the following headings:

- Abnormal respiratory patterns
- Disturbances related to respiratory gases.

ABNORMAL RESPIRATORY PATTERNS

Eupnea refers to normal respiratory pattern, which implies a normal rate, rhythm and depth of respiration. Various abnormal respiratory patterns (Fig. 2.2-16) can be produced by changes in the environment or diseases affecting the respiratory system, cardiovascular system, or brain. The common altered patterns of respiration are:

Tachypnea refers to increase in the rate of respiration.

Bradypnea means decrease in the rate of respiration.

Polypnea is used to denote the rapid but shallow breathing resembling panting in dogs. In this, the rate of respiration is increased but the force does not change significantly.

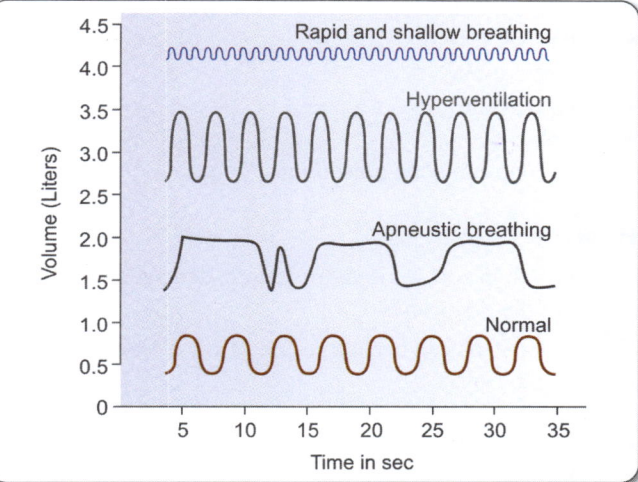

Fig. 2.2-16: Various abnormal respiratory patterns

Hypoventilation term is used to describe a decrease in rate and force of respiration.

Hyperventilation refers to increase in rate as well as force of respiration.

Hyperpnea signifies a marked increase in pulmonary ventilation due to increase in rate and/or force of respiration.

Dyspnea. When hyperpnea involves 4–5 fold increase in pulmonary ventilation, an unpleasant sensation or discomfort is felt. This type of respiration is called dyspnea.

Periodic breathing refers to a respiratory pattern characterized by alternate periods of respiratory activity and apnea.

Apnea refers to temporary cessation of breathing. Depending upon the cause apnea may be of the following types:

- *Voluntary apnea* refers to temporary arrest of breathing due to voluntary control of respiration. It is also called breath-holding.
- *Apnea after hyperventilation* occurs due to reduced stimulation of respiratory center owing to CO_2 wash caused by hyperventilation.
- *Deglutition apnea* occurs reflexly during swallowing (about 0.5 sec). There is closure of glottis (the opening between vocal cords). This effect prevents aspiration of fluid or food into the lungs
- *Breath-holding attacks* are attacks of brief period of apnea which occur in infants and young children and are generally precipitated by emotional distress.
- *Adrenaline apnea* occurs after injection of high doses of adrenaline.
- *Sleep apnea* refers to cessation of breathing for a brief period (10 sec) during sleep in normal individual.

DISTURBANCES RELATED TO RESPIRATORY GASES

Respiratory disturbances related to respiratory gases include:
- Hypoxia
- Hypercapnia
- Hypocapnia
- Asphyxia
- Carbon monoxide poisoning.

Hypoxia

The term hypoxia is used to denote deficiency of oxygen supply at the tissue level.

Causes. Hypoxia can occur because of any one or more of the following defects:
- Decreased oxygen tension (pO_2) of the arterial blood
- Decreased oxygen carrying capacity of the blood
- Decreased rate of blood flow to the tissue
- Decreased utilization of oxygen by tissue cells.

Types. Depending upon the mechanism of occurrence there are four types of hypoxia:
1. Hypoxic hypoxia
2. Anemic hypoxia
3. Stagnant hypoxia
4. Histotoxic hypoxia.

Hypoxic hypoxia occurs due to decreased oxygen tension (pO_2) of the arterial blood, hence also called *arterial hypoxia*. Therefore, in this condition O_2 carrying capacity of blood, rate of blood flow to tissue, and utilization of O_2 by tissues is normal.

Anemic hypoxia occurs due to the decreased O_2 carrying capacity of blood due to decreased hemoglobin content.

Stagnant hypoxia occurs due to decreased blood flow to the tissues so that in spite of normal pO_2 and hemoglobin, adequate O_2 is not delivered to the tissues.

Histotoxic hypoxia occurs due to decreased ability of the tissues themselves to utilize the oxygen. So, strictly speaking, it is not a true hypoxia, because O_2 supply to the tissues is adequate, e.g. as in cyanide poisoning.

Hypercapnia

Hypercapnia refers to increase in arterial pCO_2 (normal value 40 mm Hg). When hypercapnia is the primary problem, it is associated with respiratory acidosis since an increase in CO_2 promptly generates excess H^+ through:

$$H_2O + CO_2 \xrightarrow{\text{Carbonic anhydrase}} H_2CO_3 \rightarrow H^+ + HCO_3^-$$

Causes. Hypercapnia occurs due to:

Defective elimination of CO_2 as occurs in:
- Reduced pulmonary ventilation
- Reduced effective alveolar ventilation

Accidental inhalation of CO_2 in persons working in breweries and refrigeration plants.

Hypocapnia

Hypocapnia, i.e., reduced pCO_2 is usually associated with *respiratory alkalosis*, since decrease in CO_2 promptly drives the following reaction in backward direction, resulting in a decrease in H^+ concentration.

$$H_2O + CO_2 \xleftarrow{\text{Carbonic anhydrase}} H_2CO_3 \leftarrow H^+ + HCO_3^-$$

Causes. Hypocapnia occurs due to hyperventilation.

Asphyxia

Asphyxia refers to a condition in which hypoxia (decreased pO_2) is associated with hypercapnia (increased pCO_2).

Causes. Asphyxia can be general or local.

Local asphyxia occurs due to complete obstruction or ligation of blood vessel.

General asphyxia can be chronic or acute.

- *Chronic asphyxia* may occur in patient with cor pulmonale, i.e., right ventricular failure due to lung diseases.
- *Acute asphyxia* occurs due to sudden blockage in airways. Common causes are strangulation, drowning, acute tracheal obstruction (due to entry of food or due to choking) and paralysis of diaphragm, as in acute poliomyelitis.

Carbon Monoxide Poisoning

Carbon monoxide (CO) is a dangerous gas present in exhaust of gasoline engines, coal mines, gases from deep wells and underground drainage systems.

Toxic effects: Carbon monoxide produces anemic hypoxia and derangement of cellular metabolic system.

ARTIFICIAL RESPIRATION AND CARDIOPULMONARY RESUSCITATION

ARTIFICIAL RESPIRATION

Artificial respiration (AR) alone is required as an emergency life-saving procedure:

When there is sudden stoppage of breathing as seen in:

- Drowning
- Electrocution
- Anesthetic accidents
- Carbon monoxide poisoning
- Strangulation
- Accidents.

IMPORTANT TO KNOW

Artificial respiration may also be needed when breathing is expected to stop gradually as in paralysis of muscles in:
- Poliomyelitis
- Diphtheria
- Ascending paralysis.

It is important to note that the tissues of brain, particularly cerebral cortex, develop irreversible damage if oxygen supply is stopped for 5 minutes. So, the resuscitation must be started quickly without any delay, before the development of cardiac failure.

Methods of Artificial Respiration

Mouth-to-mouth Breathing Method

Mouth-to-mouth breathing (exhaled air ventilation) is very useful because:

- It can be applied quickly without waiting for the availability of any aid.
- It is simple and effective measure of resuscitation.
- It can be applied in all age groups.
- It is the only technique capable of producing adequate ventilation.
- It also works by expanding the lungs.

Procedure of mouth-to-mouth breathing is as:

- To begin with patient's neck is extended by placing one hand under the neck and lifting it and pressing the forehead with the other hand (Fig. 2.2-17A). This prevents the flaccid tongue from falling back into the pharynx.
- Then the patient's nostrils are closed by the thumb and index finger of the hand (Fig. 2.2-17B).
- The resuscitator then takes a deep breath and exhales air into the patient's airway after tightly placing his mouth over patient's mouth, and noting the expansion of the chest at the same time. The volume of the air exhaled must be twice the normal tidal volume. This expands the patient's lungs.
- Then the resuscitator removes his mouth from that of the patient, allowing expiration to occur passively due to the elastic recoil of the lungs and chest (Fig. 2.2-17C).
- The above procedure is repeated 12–16 times per minute till spontaneous breathing returns, or till the patient is shifted to a hospital.

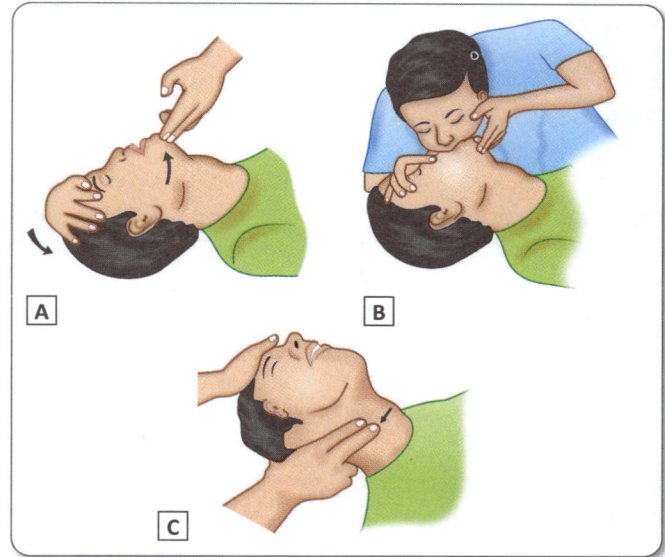

Figs 2.2-17A to C: Mouth-to-mouth breathing: A. The neck is extended by placing one hand under the neck and pressing the forehead with other hand; B. Nostrils are closed with thumb and index finger and resuscitator exhales into the patient's airway by tightly placing his mouth over the patients mouth; C. Allows the patient to exhale passively by unsealing nose and mouth

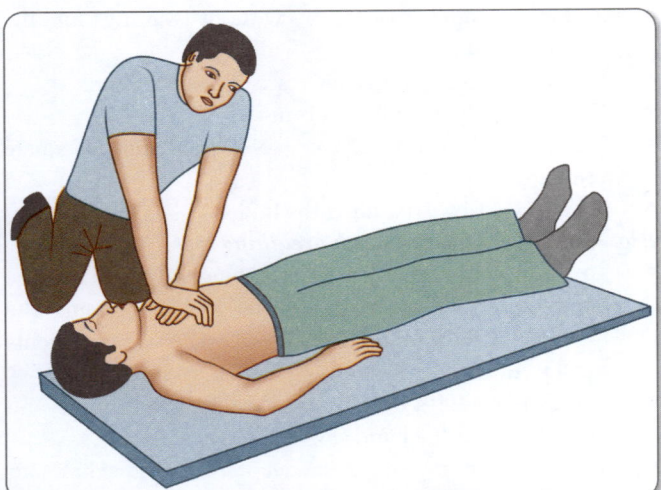

Fig. 2.2-18: Procedure showing external cardiac massage

CARDIOPULMONARY RESUSCITATION

Cardiopulmonary resuscitation (CPR) is required in some patients when heart and respiration both stop. Breathing usually stops before the heart stops, so artificial respiration should be started immediately.

Emergency Plan of Cardiopulmonary Resuscitation

The following plan called ABC of CPR has proved useful in reviving such patients:

A   *Airway care*
B   *Breathing* by artificial respiration (AR) method.
C   *Cardiac massage* is required when carotid pulse cannot be felt (Fig. 2.2-18).

Conventional CPR is performed by 30 chest compression followed by 2 breaths (one cycle). The depth of compression should be minimum 2 inches for adults. For effective CPR rescuer should perform 5 cycles within 2 minutes.

NURSING IMPLICATIONS AND APPLICATIONS

A nurse must know and learn the methods of artificial respiration and cardiopulmonary resuscitation.

PULMONARY FUNCTION TESTS

Pulmonary function tests can be classified into the following groups:

● Ventilatory function tests
● Tests of diffusion
● Tests of ultimate purpose of respiration
● Tests during exercise.

VENTILATORY FUNCTION TESTS

Ventilatory function tests are meant for assessment of the expansion of lungs and chest wall; and for assessment of restrictive and obstructive ventilatory defects. The assessment of ventilatory functions can be accomplished by measurement of various lung volumes and capacities by spirometry.

Spirometry refers to recording of volume changes during various clearly defined breathing maneuvers. It can be performed using a simple spirometer, a modified spirometer called respirometer or computerized spirometer.

Simple spirometer (Fig. 2.2-19) is made of metal. It consists of the following parts:

● *Outer chamber* or container which is filled with water.
● *Floating drum* or a gas bell, with 6 L capacity, floats in the water in an inverted manner. It is attached to a chain which passes over a pulley bearing a balancing weight and a writing needle (pen). The needle (pen) moves with the movement of the floating drum. The floating drum is thus counterpoised and has very little inertia and friction.
● *Inner chamber* is open at the top end which lies above the water level in outer chamber and is connected to a tube at the bottom end. At the end of tube, a mouthpiece is attached through which the subject is made to respire.
● *Kymograph* is a recording drum on which the movements of the needle are recorded.

TESTS OF DIFFUSION

Pulmonary diffusion refers to transfer of gases from alveoli to capillary blood across the respiratory membrane. The

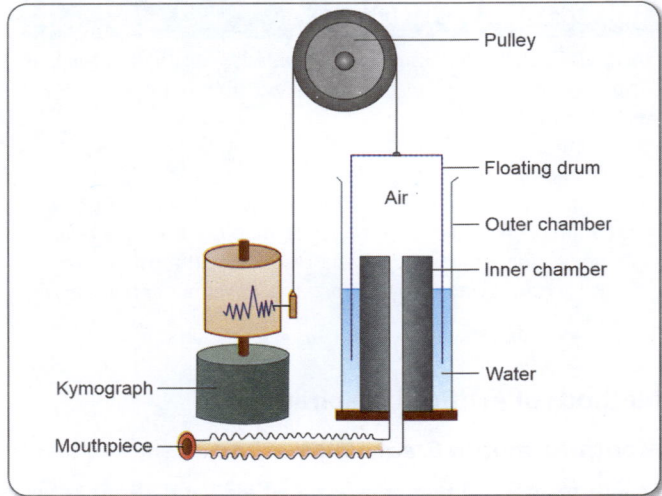

Fig. 2.2-19: Simple spirometer

exchange of gases in the lungs was earlier believed to be dependent merely on the ability of the gases to diffuse across the respiratory membrane. This term led to the use of term *diffusion capacity*. Nowadays, the term *transfer factor*, rather than diffusion capacity, is used.

TESTS OF ULTIMATE PURPOSE OF RESPIRATION

Since the ultimate purpose of respiration is to supply O_2 from atmosphere to tissues and removal of CO_2 from the tissues into the atmosphere; so, the estimation of arterial blood pO_2, pCO_2 and pH (blood gas analysis) are most fundamental of all the pulmonary function tests.

ASSESS YOURSELF

Short and Long Answer Questions

1. **Describe briefly:**
   - Mechanism of tidal respiration
   - Factors affecting vital capacity
   - Transport of oxygen from lungs into the tissues
2. **Define the following:**
   - Functional residual capacity
   - Pulmonary elastance
   - Diffusion capacity
3. **Draw diagram to show:**
   - Hemoglobin–oxygen dissociation curve.
   - Layers of respiratory membrane
4. **Differentiate between;**
   - Intrapleural and intrapulmonary pressure
   - Expired and alveolar air
   - Pulmonary and alveolar ventilation
   - Peripheral and central chemoreceptors
5. **Write notes on:**
   - Surfactant
   - Hypoxia
   - Carbon monoxide poisoning
   - Decompression sickness
   - Oxygen toxicity

Multiple Choice Questions

1. **True statement for role of diaphragm in breathing:**
   a. During expiration dome gets flattened
   b. Descent raises intra-abdominal pressure
   c. Descent raises intrapleural pressure
   d. Descent raises intrapulmonary pressure
2. **The true statement about expiration in quite breathing:**
   a. Intrapulmonary pressure becomes positive
   b. Intrapulmonary pressure becomes negative
   c. Intrapleural pressure is at atmospheric
   d. Intrapleural pressure becomes negative
3. **During tidal expiration there is:**
   a. Contraction of external intercostals muscles
   b. Decrease in thoracic cavity
   c. Relaxation of internal intercostals muscles
   d. Contraction of internal intercostals muscles

4. **Vital capacity is equal to:**
   a. TV + IRV
   b. TV + IRV + ERV
   c. TV + IC
   d. TV + IC + EC
5. **In which of the following condition vital capacity increases:**
   a. Gravity
   b. Old age
   c. In swimmers
   d. Pregnancy
6. **The normal value of FEV_1 is:**
   a. 98–100%
   b. 90%
   c. 80%
   d. 70%
7. **The partial pressure of oxygen (pO_2) of atmospheric air is:**
   a. 600 mm Hg
   b. 160 mm Hg
   c. 47 mm Hg
   d. 4 mm Hg
8. **Hemoglobin–oxygen dissociation curve shifts to the left when:**
   a. Increased pCO_2
   b. Acidic pH
   c. Decrease pO_2
   d. Decrease in body temperature
9. **The peripheral chemoreceptors are most sensitive to:**
   a. Increased pCO_2
   b. Decrease pO_2
   a. H^+ concentration
   b. HCO_3^- concentration
10. **J receptors mainly respond to:**
    a. Increased pCO_2
    b. Decrease pO_2
    c. H^+ concentration
    d. Increased content of interstitial fluid
11. **During exercise, pulmonary ventilation increases because of:**
    a. Hypoxia
    b. Acidosis
    c. Increased pulmonary perfusion
    d. Oxygen debt
12. **At high altitude, hyperventilation occurs due to:**
    a. Increased in level of 2–3 diphosphoglycerate
    b. Polycythemia
    c. Pulmonary hypertension
    d. Increase in oxidative enzymes

13. Which of the following is not the feature of decompression sickness:
    a. Numbness
    b. Myocardial infarction
    c. Pain in joints
    d. Increased total lung capacity

14. Oxygen carrying capacity is low but blood flow to the tissues is normal in:
    a. Anemic hypoxia   b. Hypoxic hypoxia
    c. Histotoxic hypoxia   d. Stagnant hypoxia

15. Asphyxia occurs due to:
    a. Carbon monoxide poisoning
    b. Nitrogen narcosis
    c. Strangulation
    d. Chronic heart failure

16. Which ventilatory function is not done by spirometry:
    a. Vital capacity
    b. Timed vital capacity
    c. Functional residual capacity
    d. Maximum breathing capacity

ANSWER KEY

| 1. | b | 2. | a | 3. | b | 4. | b | 5. | c | 6. | c | 7. | b | 8. | d |
| 9. | b | 10. | d | 11. | b | 12. | a | 13. | d | 14. | a | 15. | c | 16. | c |

Section

III

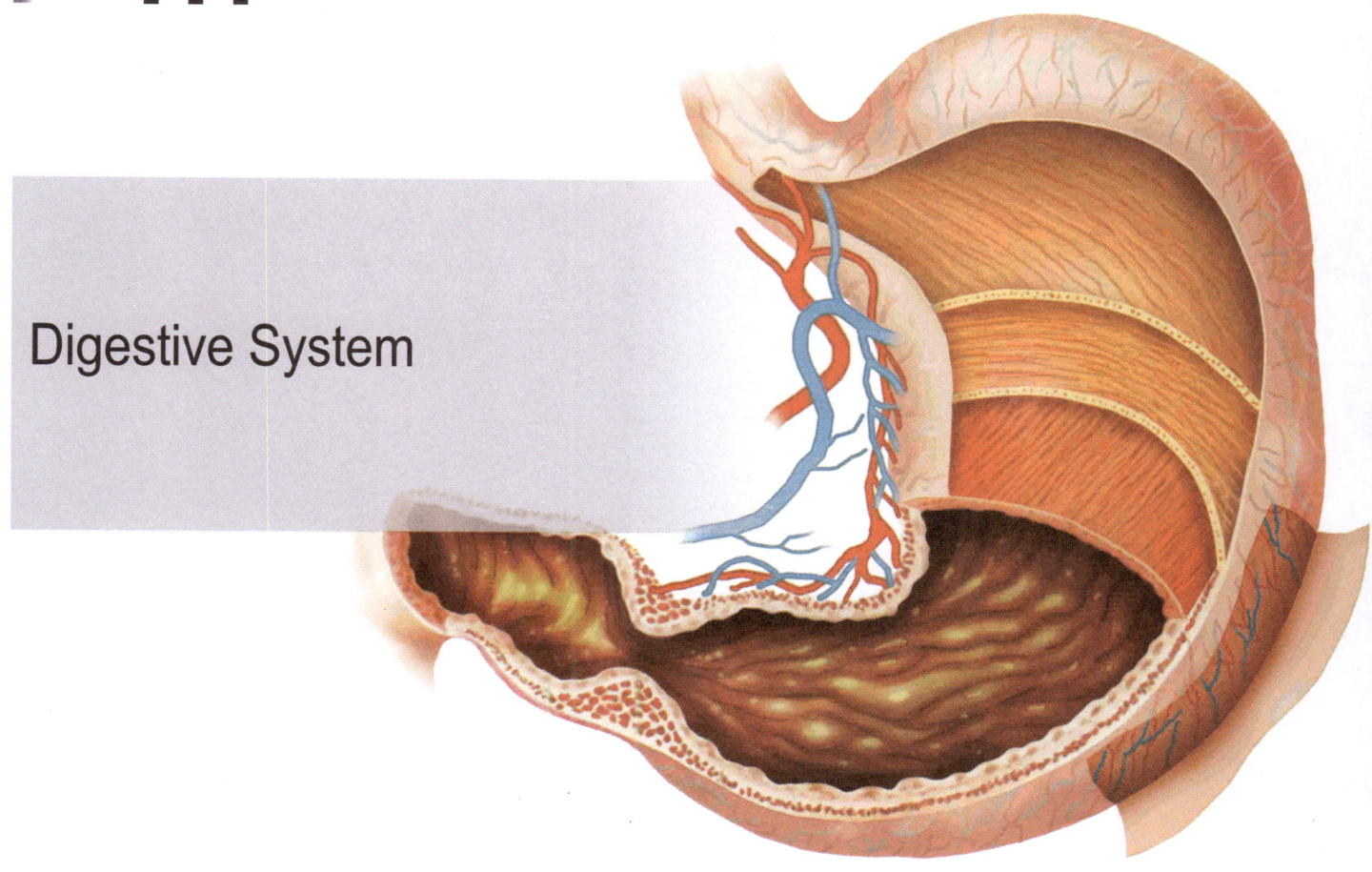

Digestive System

Section Outline

Anatomy and Physiology of Digestive Organs

ORGANIZATION OF DIGESTIVE SYSTEM

Body needs a continual supply of water, electrolytes, and nutrients to sustain life. This function is served by the gastrointestinal or the so-called digestive system. The digestive system comprises gastrointestinal tract (GIT) and accessory organs of digestion like teeth, tongue, salivary glands, liver and exocrine part of pancreas.

PARTS OF GASTROINTESTINAL TRACT

Gastrointestinal tract, also known as alimentary canal, is basically a muscular tube extending from the mouth to the anus (Fig. 3.1-1). At either end, the lumen is continuous with external environment. It measures about 10 m (30 feet) and comprises the following:

Mouth

Mouth is a loosely used term to denote the external opening and for the cavity it leads to. The cavity containing anterior two-thirds of tongue and teeth is the mouth cavity or oral cavity or buccal cavity.

Tongue, in the digestive system, plays two important roles:

- Tells the taste of food
- Helps in chewing and swallowing of the food.

Teeth are accessory organs of digestion which help in chewing the food.

Pharynx

The pharynx is a median passage that is common to the gastrointestinal and respiratory systems.

Esophagus

It is a fibromuscular tube about 25 cm long. At its junction to the pharynx, upper esophageal sphincter is present and at its junction with the stomach, lower esophageal sphincter is present.

Stomach

It is a hollow muscular bag connected to the esophagus at its upper end and to the duodenum at the lower end.

Small Intestine

It is a long tubular structure, which can be divided into three parts:

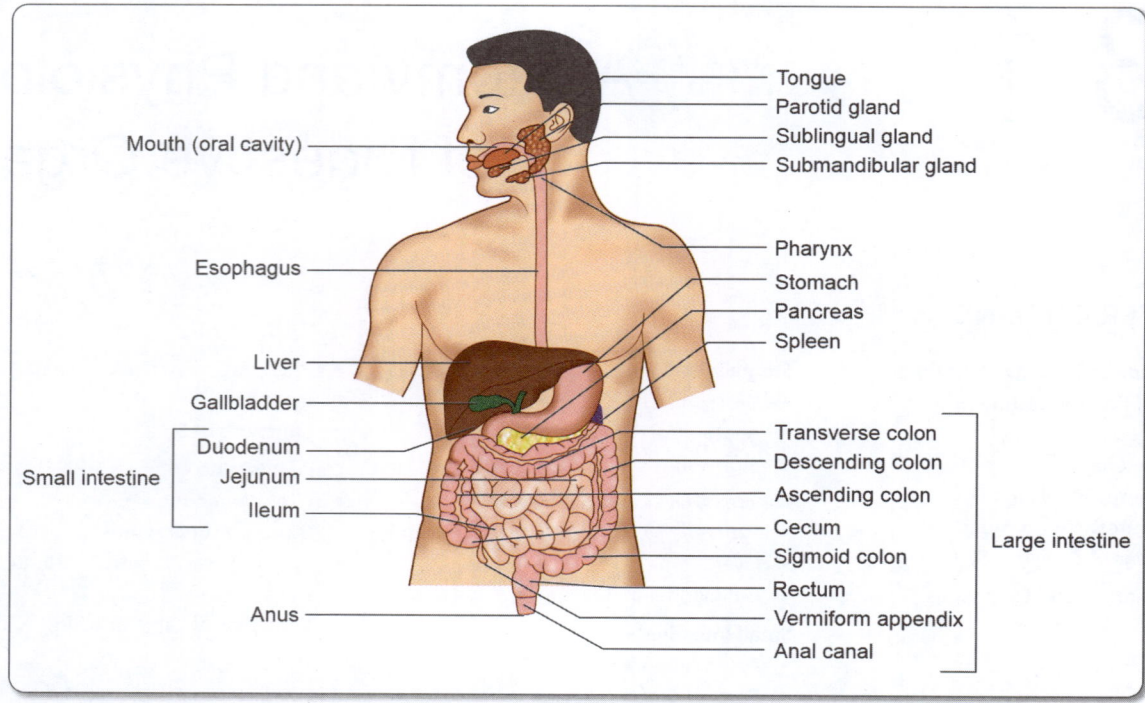

Fig. 3.1-1: The gastrointestinal system

1. *Duodenum* is the first part of small intestine. It is C-shaped and measures about 25 cm in length.

2. *Jejunum,* the middle part of the small intestine, is about 25 m long.

3. *Ileum,* the last part of small intestine, is about 3.5 m long.

Large Intestine

It arches around and encloses the coils of the small intestine and tends to be more fixed than the small intestine. It is divided into the following parts:

- Cecum and appendix
- Colon
- Rectum
- Anal canal

PERITONEUM

Peritoneum refers to serous membrane, which lines the walls of abdominal cavity *(parietal layer)* and also the viscera contained in abdominal and pelvic cavities *(visceral layer)*. The space between the parietal and visceral layers of peritoneum is called the *peritoneal cavity*.

Arrangement of Peritoneum

Abdominal Peritoneum

The arrangement of peritoneum is very complex. For descriptive purpose, the abdominal peritoneum can be considered to have the following arrangements:

Parietal peritoneum lines the walls of the abdominal cavity and covers the *retroperitoneal structures,* e.g., kidneys.

Visceral peritoneum lines the abdominal viscera.

Folds and ligaments of abdominal peritoneum refer to those parts of the peritoneum, which connect the viscera to the abdominal wall or to the other viscera. Some of the important folds and ligaments of peritoneum are (Fig. 3.1-2A):

Lesser omentum. It is a fold of two layers of peritoneum, which extends from the liver above to the lesser curvature of stomach below.

- *Superiorly,* the two layers of peritoneum of lesser omentum are reflected to cover the liver.
- *Inferiorly,* the two layers of peritoneum of lesser omentum separate to cover the anterior and superior surfaces of stomach and upper duodenum.
- *Right free margin* of the lesser omentum is formed by continuity of anterior and posterior layers. The bile duct, the hepatic artery and the portal vein lie within this right free margin of lesser omentum (Fig. 3.1-2B).

Greater omentum. It is a fat-laden, apron-like fold of peritoneum, which hangs from the stomach in front to the intestine. It consists of four layers of peritoneum. At the level of greater curvature of stomach, the layers of peritoneum covering the anterior and posterior surfaces of the stomach meet and continue downward as anterior two layers of the

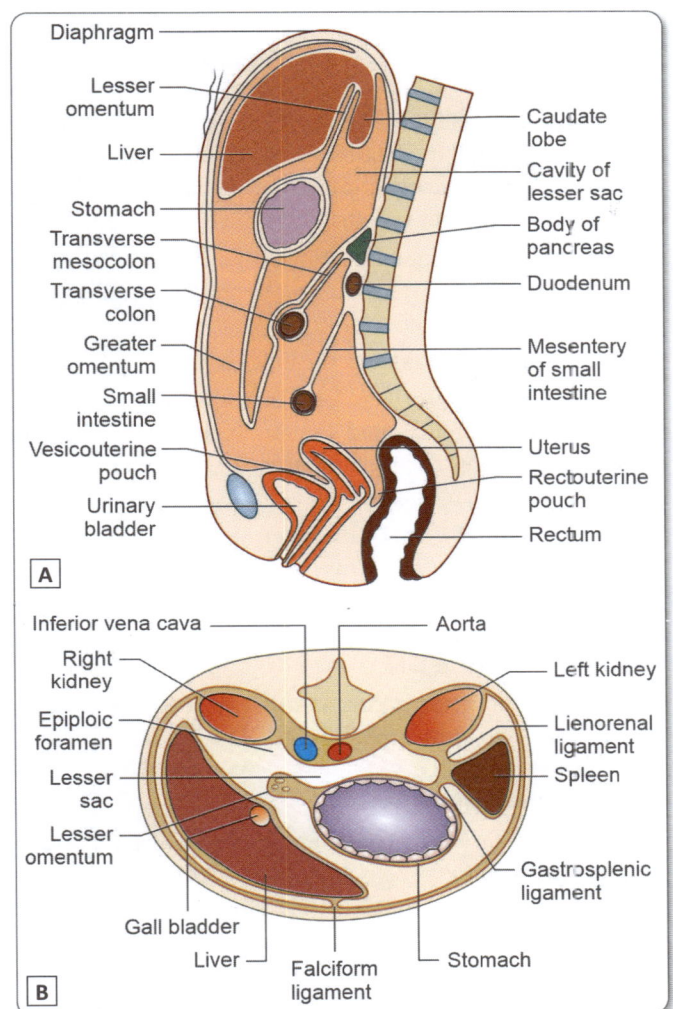

Figs 3.1-2A and B: Arrangement of peritoneum and peritoneal cavity as seen in. A. Schematic sagittal section through abdominal and pelvic cavities; B. Transverse section across the abdomen at the level of epiploic foramen

greater omentum. At the lower end of abdominal cavity, these two layers of peritoneum get folded on themselves to form the posterior two layers of omentum. These extend upward to reach the anterior border of pancreas, where they gain attachment to the posterior abdominal wall.

Mesentery. It refers to the fold of peritoneum that connects the visceral peritoneum covering the small intestine to that covering the posterior abdominal wall. The attachment of mesentery along a short line of insertion on the posterior abdominal wall gives it the appearance of a ruffle or flounce. The mesentery supports the blood vessels and lymph vessels supplying the intestine.

Transverse mesocolon is the fold of peritoneum, which attaches the transverse colon to the posterior abdominal wall.

It lies posterior to the fourth layer of greater omentum (usually fused to it) in its upper part.

Sigmoid mesocolon is the inverted V-shaped fold of peritoneum that connects sigmoid colon to the posterior abdominal and pelvic walls.

Peritoneal folds connecting liver to the abdominal wall include falciform ligament, coronary ligament and the right and left triangular ligaments.

Gastrosplenic ligament is the fold of peritoneum connecting stomach to spleen.

Splenorenal ligament is the fold of peritoneum that connects spleen to the left kidney.

Gastrophrenic ligament refers to the fold of peritoneum, which connects the back of fundus of stomach to the diaphragm. It forms the superior boundary of lesser sac.

Pelvic Peritoneum

The peritoneum in the pelvis is continuous with that of the rest of the abdominal cavity. It covers the front aspect of the rectum. In males, it passes forward over the posterior and upper surfaces of the bladder to become continuous with that on the anterior abdominal wall. In females, it passes from the rectum over the posterior and anterior surfaces of the uterus before reaching the bladder.

Peritoneal Cavity

Peritoneal cavity refers to the space between the visceral and parietal layers of peritoneum. This space contains a thin film of fluid, which allows free movement of the viscera against the abdominal wall and against each other. In males, the peritoneal cavity is a closed sac while in females, the uterine tubes open into the peritoneal cavity. The peritoneal cavity, for descriptive purposes, can be divided into the following parts:

The greater sac refers to the main part of peritoneal cavity, which extends from the roof of abdominal cavity to its floor.

The lesser sac is a fairly large isolated part of the peritoneal cavity, which lies behind the stomach. The lesser sac opens on the right side into the greater sac through an opening called the *epiploic foramen.*

Peritoneal pouches or recesses are isolated areas of peritoneal cavity found in relation to the abdominal and pelvic viscera.

Functions of Peritoneum

- It is a serous membrane, which enables the abdominal contents to glide over each other without friction.
- It forms a partial or complete covering for the abdominal organs.
- It forms ligaments and mesenteries, which help to keep the organs in position.

- The omentum and mesentery contain a considerable amount of fat and act as important fat stores for the body.
- The omentum can move about inside the cavity and in the event of inflammation occurring tends to wrap itself round the affected part of the alimentary tract and prevents the infection from spreading to the rest of the peritoneum.
- It has the power to absorb fluids in large quantities.

GENERAL CHARACTERISTICS OF GASTROINTESTINAL SYSTEM

Structural Characteristics of Gastrointestinal Wall

Different parts of the gastrointestinal tract are specialized for carrying out different functions particularly digestion and absorption, but the basic structural characteristics of the wall of whole gastrointestinal tract are similar. The intestinal wall from inside to outwards consist of the following layers (Fig. 3.1-3):

Mucosa (mucus layer). It is the innermost coat consisting of three layers:

1. *Surface epithelium* lining the luminal surface consists of epithelial cells which vary in type from simple squamous to tall columnar depending upon the function of the part of gastrointestinal tract.

2. *Lamina propria* is composed of loose connective tissue, which contains numerous glands, small blood vessels, lymphatics and nerve fibers.

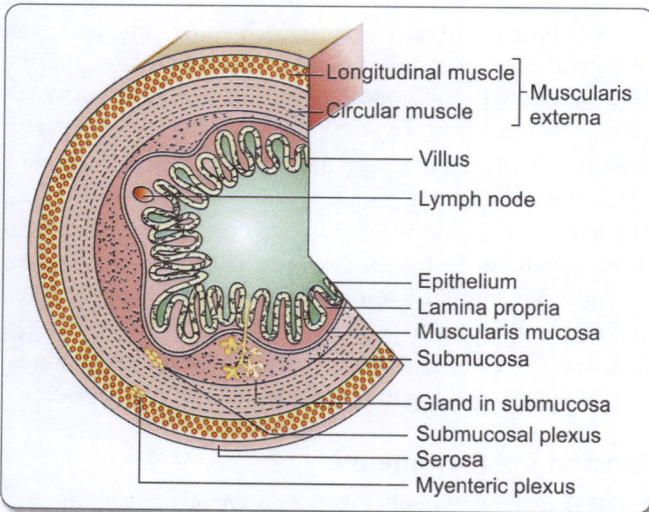

Fig. 3.1-3: Cross-section of the alimentary canal depicting structural characteristics of its wall

3. *Muscularis mucosa* is composed of two thin layers of smooth muscle fibers, which help in localized movements of the mucosa.

Submucosa. This refers to the layer of connective tissue present outside the mucosa. It contains blood vessels, lymphatics and a network of nerve fibers and nerve cells called submucosal nerve plexus (Meissner's plexus).

Muscle coat. It is formed by a thick layer of smooth muscle fibers surrounding the submucosa. The smooth muscle fibers are arranged in two layers:

1. *Circular muscle fibers* form the inner layer.

2. *Longitudinal muscle fibers* form the outer layer.

In between the circular and longitudinal muscle fibers is present an extensive network of nerve cells and fibers named *Auerbach's plexus* (myenteric plexus).

Serosa (serous layer). This is the outermost layer consisting of a layer of connective tissue. This layer helps in the attachment of gut to the surrounding structures.

Innervation of the GIT

The innervation of the gastrointestinal tract (GIT) includes intrinsic and extrinsic system (Fig. 3.1-4).

Intrinsic Innervation

The intrinsic nervous system also called *enteric nervous system* consists of nerve cells and fibers, which originate and are located in the intestinal wall itself. This system supplies the smooth muscles of GIT (i.e., musculature of GIT except upper esophagus and external anal sphincter, which contain striated muscle). This system controls most of the gastrointestinal functions like secretion and motility. The enteric nervous system is composed mainly of two plexuses:

Myenteric plexus or Auerbach's plexus is present in between the circular and longitudinal muscle fibers of muscular coat of the GIT. Stimulation of myenteric plexus causes increase in tone of the gut wall, intensity of rhythmical contractions of gut wall, rate of contraction and velocity of contraction.

Meissner's plexus or submucosal plexus is present in the submucosal layer. It controls the secretory activity and blood flow to the gut.

The Auerbach's and Meissner's plexuses are interconnected with each other and are under the control of parasympathetic and sympathetic components of extrinsic nervous system. In both the plexuses, the axons branch profusely so that stimulation of one region produces a widespread response in the gastrointestinal tract.

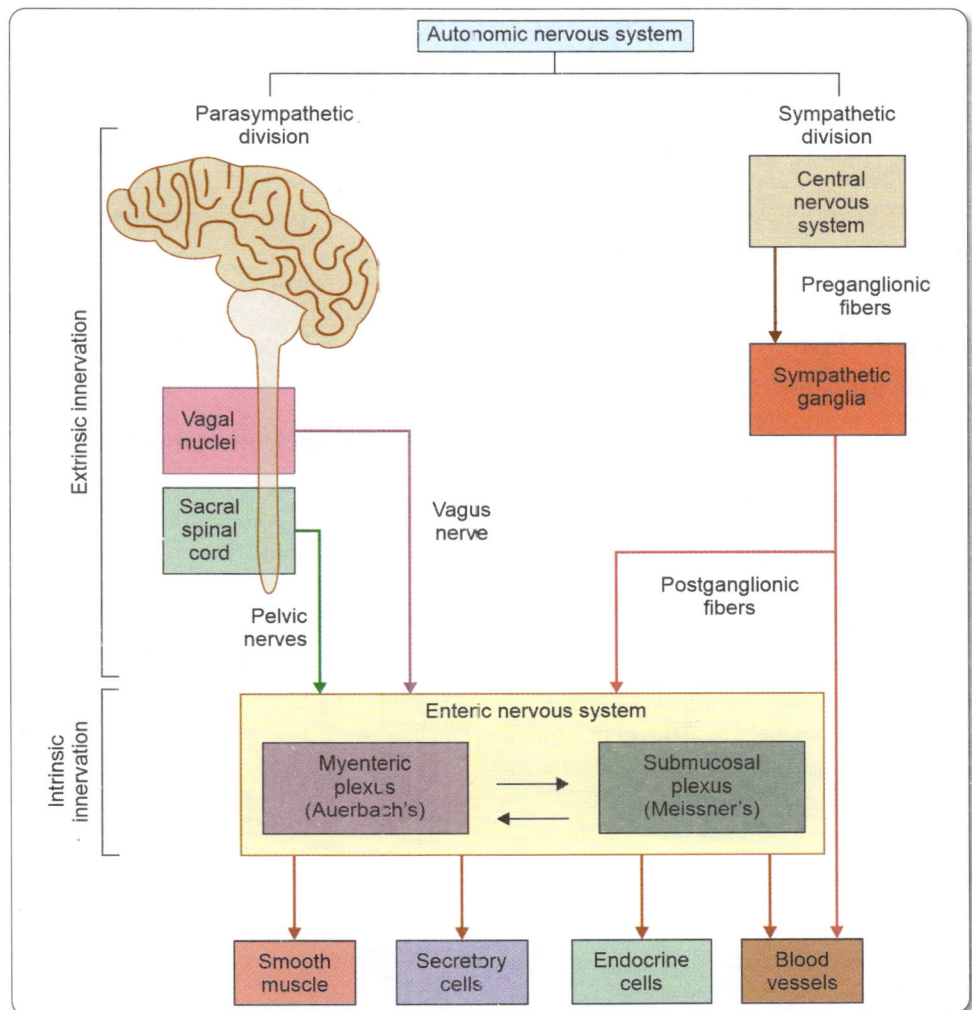

Fig. 3.1-4: Schematic illustration of the innervation of gut

Extrinisic Innervation

The extrinsic system of nerves supplying the gut consists of the parasympathetic and sympathetic components of autonomic nervous system.

Parasympathetic innervation

The parasympathetic supply to the gut is made up of cranial and sacral divisions:

Cranial parasympathetic fibers originate in medulla, come through vagus and supply the esophagus, stomach, small intestine, pancreas and first half of the large intestine. They also make synaptic connections with intramural plexuses.

Sacral parasympathetic fibers originate in sacral spinal cord, pass through pelvic nerves to hypogastric (pelvic) ganglion as a postganglionic fiber, supply the distal half of large intestine and rectum. The sigmoid, rectal and anal regions have an especially rich supply of parasympathetic fibers that function in the defecation reflex.

Functions of parasympathetics. Parasympathetic stimulation causes excitation of all the musculature of gut except the sphincters to which it inhibits. There occurs an increase in gastrointestinal motility and secretory activity.

Sympathetic innervation

The sympathetic fibers to gut arise from eighth thoracic (T_8) to second lumbar (L_2) spinal segments. The sympathetics innervate all portions of the gastrointestinal tract rather than being more extensively supplied to portions near the oral cavity and anus, as is true for parasympathetics.

Functions of sympathetic innervation. Sympathetic stimulation causes:

- Vasoconstriction
- Excitation of ileocecal and internal anal sphincters and smooth muscles of muscularis mucosa throughout (to increase number of folds)
- Inhibition of motility in the gut.

Thus, most of the effects of sympathetic stimulation are opposite to that of parasympathetic stimulation.

Gastrointestinal Blood Flow

The blood supply of the gastrointestinal tract forms part of splanchnic circulation. The main characteristic feature of the gastrointestinal blood flow is that it is *usually proportional to the level of local activity.*

GASTROINTESTINAL HORMONES
General Characteristics

- Gastrointestinal hormones regulate the secretions and even to some extent, the motility of GIT.
- The *glandular cells* secreting gastrointestinal hormones are individually scattered in the epithelium of the stomach and small intestine and not in the form of clusters of cells as in the endocrine glands.
- The luminal surface of glandular cells, when stimulated by various chemicals present in the chyme, releases hormones from the opposite surface into blood capillaries of portal circulation.
- Through portal circulation, the released hormone reaches the target tissue situated in the nearby region of GIT and exhibits physiological actions on the target cells with specific receptors for the hormone. For example, the hormone gastrin, released by G-cells present in mucosa of pyloric part of stomach in response to presence of peptides in chyme, reaches the body of stomach *via* portal circulation and increases the acid secretion as well as motility of the stomach.
- The effects of gastrointestinal hormones persist even after nervous connections between the site of release and the site of action have been severed.

Classification of Gastrointestinal Hormones

The gastrointestinal hormones, based on their physio-anatomical similarities, can be broadly classified into three types:

1. *Gastrin family of hormones* includes:
- Gastrin
- Cholecystokinin-pancreozymin or (CCK-PZ)

2. *Secretin family of hormones* includes:
- Secretin
- Gastric inhibitory polypeptide (GIP)
- Vasoactive intestinal peptide (VIP)
- Glucagon
- Glucagon-like immune reactivity (GLI) or glycentin.

3. *Other gastrointestinal hormones* include:
- Motilin
- Neurotensin
- Substance P
- Gastrin-releasing peptide (GRP)
- Somatostatin.

Actions of Gastrointestinal Hormones

The outline of the action of each gastrointestinal hormone and the stimulus for secretion and site of secretion are given in Table 3.1-1.

FUNCTIONS OF DIGESTIVE SYSTEM

The functions of each part of the GIT are described in the respective sub-headings. However, as introductory remarks to the digestive system, the various functions of GIT are summarized here.

Digestive Functions

The major function of the gastrointestinal system is to transfer nutrients, minerals and water from external environment to the circulating body fluids for distribution to all the body tissues. This function is accomplished by the following processes:

Ingestion of food involves:
- Placing the food into the mouth. Most of the food stuff is taken into mouth as large particles are mainly made of carbohydrates, proteins and fats.
- Chewing the food into smaller pieces is carried out with the help of teeth and jaw muscles. This process is called mastication.
- Lubrication and moistening of the food is done by the saliva.
- Swallowing the food (deglutition) refers to pushing the bolus of food from mouth into the stomach. It is accomplished in three phases: oral phase, pharyngeal phase and esophageal phase.

Digestion of food refers to conversion of complex insoluble large organic molecules (food) into soluble, smaller and simpler molecules, which can be easily absorbed. Digestion of food is accomplished with the help of hydrochloric acid and digestive juices containing various enzymes.

TABLE 3.1-1: Stimuli for secretion, site of action and actions of gastrointestinal hormones

Hormone	Stimuli for secretion	Site of secretion	Actions						
			Gastric secretion	Gastric motility	Pancreatic secretion	Bile secretion	Gallbladder contraction	Small intestine secretion	Small intestine motility
Gastrin	Small peptides, amino acids, gastric distention, vagal stimulation	G cells of gastric antrum	+	+	+	0	0	0	0
Cholecysto-kinin	Small peptides, amino acids, fatty acids	Type I cells of duodenum and jejunum	0	–	+	0	+	0	+
Secretin	Acid in upper intestine Fatty acids	S cells of duodenum	–	0	+	+	0	0	0
Gastric inhibitory polypeptide	Fatty acids, amino acids, oral glucose	Duodenum and jejunum	–	–	0	0	0	+	–
Vasoactive intestinal polypeptide (VIP)	Fatty acids	Jejunum	–	–	0	0	0	0	0
Somatostatin	Acid in stomach	D cells of islets of Langerhans	–	–	–	0	–	0	0

0 (No action), + (stimulatory action) and – (inhibitory action)

Absorption of digested food refers to movement of digested molecules from the lumen of alimentary canal across its epithelial lining to the blood or lymph. The absorbed water, electrolytes and nutrients are carried away to the various tissues by the circulating blood.

Egestion, i.e., excretion of unwanted undigested food by the alimentary canal in the form of feces is called defecation.

Non-digestive Functions

The main non-digestive function of the gastrointestinal system is its role in immune system. The lymphoid tissues in the tonsils, adenoids, and Peyer's patches constitute an important part of body's immune system. These provide both the humoral and cellular immunity which is specially effective against the microorganisms trying to enter the body from the alimentary canal.

MOUTH, PHARYNX AND ESOPHAGUS

MOUTH

Mouth is a loosely used term to denote the external opening and for the cavity it leads to. The cavity containing anterior two-thirds of tongue and teeth is called the mouth cavity or oral cavity or buccal cavity (Figs 3.1-5 and 3.1-6). The oral cavity extends from the lips to the oropharyngeal isthmus, i.e., junction of the mouth with the pharynx. Oral cavity is subdivided into two parts: the vestibule and oral cavity proper.

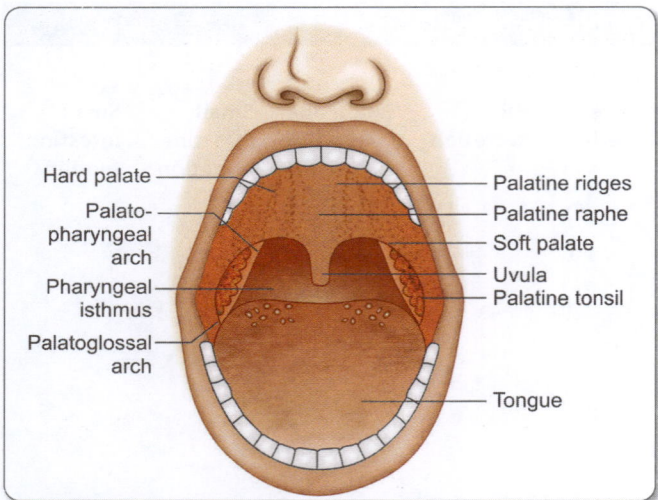

Fig. 3.1-5: Widely open oral fissure to show the mouth cavity

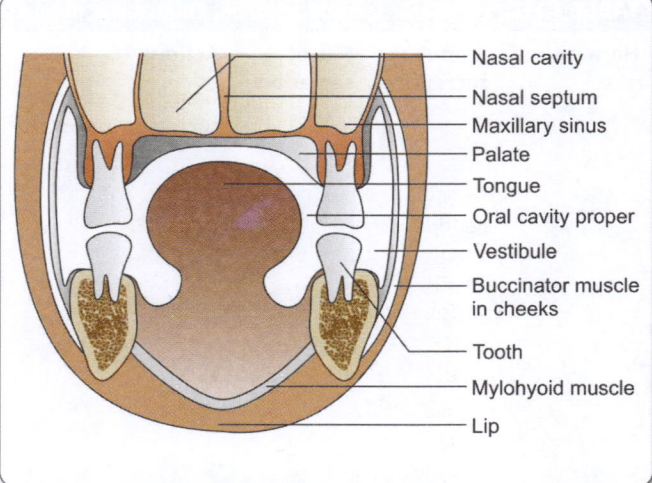

Fig. 3.1-6: Schematic coronal section through oral cavity

Vestibule lies between the lips and cheeks externally and the gums and teeth internally.

Oral cavity proper lies within the alveolar arches, gums and teeth. The roof of the oral cavity is formed by the hard and soft palate.

The floor is mainly formed by tongue and sublingual region of lower jaw.

The Palate

The palate consists of hard and soft palate.

Hard palate, the anterior part of palate, is formed by processes of the maxillae and palatine bones, which are covered by mucus membrane.

Soft palate forms a muscular arch that extends posteriorly. Hanging from the middle of posterior margin of soft palate is a conical structure called the *uvula.*

Tongue

The tongue is a freely movable thick muscular organ covered by mucus membrane. It occupies the floor of the mouth and fills the oral cavity proper when the mouth is closed. The tongue presents the following anatomical features:

Tip of the tongue is its free anterior end, which is directed forward and comes in contact with the incisors.

Body of the tongue is mainly composed of muscles covered by thick mucosa.

Dorsal surface of the tongue is marked by rough projections called *papillae.* These provide friction that is useful in handling the food. These papillae contain taste buds.

Ventral surface of the tongue has a smooth mucosal covering. In the midline, it presents a fold of mucus membrane called

frenulum by which the tongue is anchored to the floor of mouth.

Root of the tongue or the posterior region of tongue is attached to the hyoid bone. The surface of this part of tongue is characterized by presence of rounded masses of lymphatic tissue called *lingual tonsils.*

Histology. The histological structure of tongue is shown in histology plate 3.1-1

Histology Plate 3.1-1: Showing Circumvallate Papilla of Tongue

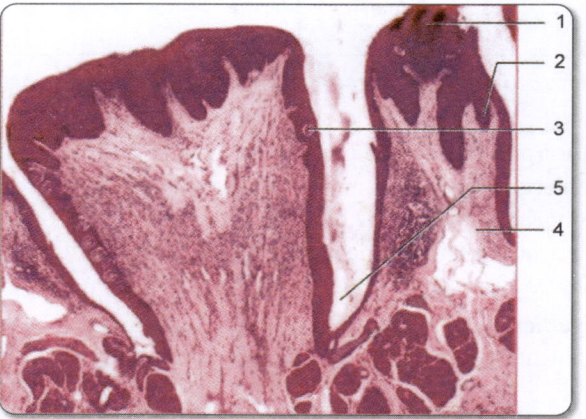

The photomicrograph of circumvallate papilla of tongue is shown. It is covered by stratified squamous epithelium (1). Underlying lamina propria (4) exhibits numerous secondary papillae, (2). Taste buds (3) are present on lateral surface of the papilla. A deep trench (5) surrounds the base of each papilla.

Nerve supply of tongue: facial, glossopharyngeal, vagus and trigeminal nerves

Functions of tongue include:
- Tells the taste of food (special organ of sense of taste)
- Helps in chewing and swallowing of food.
- Helps in speech.

Gums and Teeth

Gums

Gums refer to dense fibrous tissue, covered by a vascular stratified squamous epithelium, which surrounds the neck of teeth and is attached to the alveolar margins of the jaws. The fibrous tissue forming the gums is continuous with the periodontal membrane, which attaches the teeth to their sockets.

The Teeth

The teeth develop in the sockets present in the alveolar processes of the mandible (forming lower jaw) and part of maxillary bone forming upper jaw.

Sets of teeth and time of eruption. There are two sets of teeth:

1. *Deciduous set* (primary or milk teeth) comprises 20 teeth (10 in each jaw). The eruption of milk teeth begins 6 months after birth and is completed by the second year. They start shedding around 6–7 years of age.

2. *Permanent set* comprises 32 teeth that is 8 in each quadrant: 2 incisors, 1 canine, 2 premolar and 3 molar. The dental formula is written as below:

midline

3	2	1	2		2	1	2	3	(Maxilla)
3	2	1	2		2	1	2	3	(Mandible)

Parts of a tooth. Each tooth has three parts (Fig. 3.1-7):

1. *Root* consists of one to three fangs contained in the socket.

2. *Crown* is the part which projects beyond the level of gums.

3. *Neck* is the constricted portion between the root and crown.

Structure of a tooth. Each tooth consists of the following regions:

Pulp cavity occupies the center of a tooth and extends from the root into the crown of the tooth. The cavity is filled by dental pulp consisting of loose fibrous tissue containing nerves, blood vessels and lymphatics, all of which gain access to pulp through the apical foramen.

Dentin or ivory surrounds the pulp cavity and forms the bulk of tooth. It is hard avascular calcified tissue penetrated by minute canals called dentinal tubules. These tubules function as sensory receptors and account for the extreme sensitiveness of dentin to cold, heat, acid and drilling.

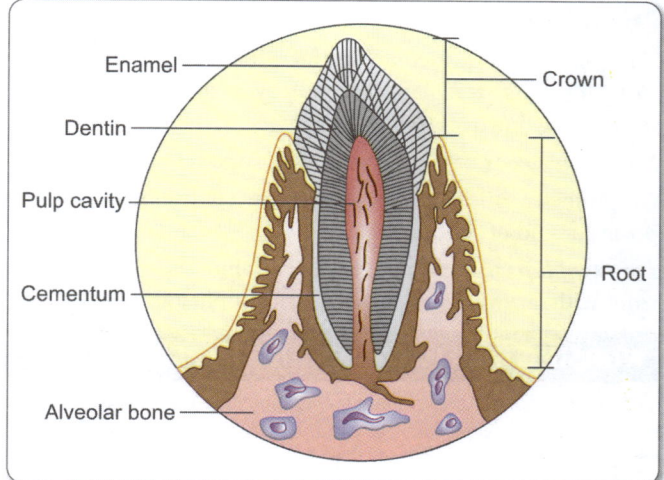

Fig. 3.1-7: Structure and parts of tooth

Enamel is the external layer covering only the dentin of the crown of tooth. It is the hardest substance in the body.

Cementum is bone-like material, which surrounds the dentin in the area of root of tooth. It fastens the tooth into its bony socket.

IMPORTANT TO KNOW

Functions of different types of teeth in chewing:
- *Incisors* provide strong cutting action.
- *Canines* are responsible for tearing action.
- *Premolars and molars* have grinding action.

Fauces

The fauces is the name given to the aperture connecting mouth with the pharynx. The fauces include two arches and palatine tonsils:

Glossopalatine arch (anterior pillar of fauces) extends from the side of uvula to the side of root of tongue.

Pharyngopalatine arch (posterior pillar of fauces) extends from the side of uvula to the side of pharynx.

Palatine Tonsils

Palatine tonsils are two masses of lymphoid tissue situated, one on either side, in the triangular space between the two arches. The tonsils function as lymph nodes.

NURSING IMPLICATIONS AND APPLICATIONS

Unconscious patients or those who are unable to eat food usually have bad breath (halitosis). Therefore, nurses must provide regular mouth care by oral swabbing to cleanse the oral cavity as well as to stimulate salivary secretion for its cleansing and protective action.

PHARYNX

The pharynx is a median passage that is common to the gastrointestinal tract and respiratory system. It is divisible from above downward into three parts:

Nasopharynx or nasal part into which opens the nasal cavities

Oropharynx or oral part, which is continuous with the posterior end of oral cavity

Laryngopharynx or laryngeal part, which is continuous in front with larynx and below with the esophagus.

NURSING IMPLICATIONS AND APPLICATIONS

In certain cases, the nurse has to put the feeding tube into the stomach via nose or mouth. During this procedure, laryngopharynx is the crucial point whereby the tube can be erroneously inserted into the air passage. To avoid this, certain precautionary measures must be ensured for correct placement of the feeding tube including advancing the tube while patient is swallowing.

ESOPHAGUS

The esophagus is a fibromuscular tube, about 25–30 cm long and 25–30 mm wide. It begins at the lower end of the pharynx, behind the trachea and descends in the mediastinum in front of the vertebral column. It passes through the diaphragm at the level of tenth thoracic vertebra, and terminates in the upper or cardiac end of the stomach, about the level of xiphoid process.

Structure

The walls of esophagus are composed of four coats, which from interior to exterior are: mucus coat, submucus tissue, musculature, and fibrous coat (Fig. 3.1-8).

Mucus coat is formed by stratified squamous epithelium. It is arranged in longitudinal folds, which disappear when the esophagus is distended by the passage of food. It is studded with minute papillae and small glands, which secrete mucus to lubricate the canal.

Submucus coat is formed by areolar tissue which serves to connect the mucus coat with the muscular coat and to carry the larger blood vessels and lymph vessles.

Musculature of esophagus has the following characterisitics:

Upper one-third of esophagus including the upper esophageal sphincter is made up of striated muscle that is under the control of vagal fibers emerging from the nucleus ambiguus.

Lower two-third of esophagus including the lower esophageal sphincter is composed of smooth muscle.

Fibrous coat. The external layer of esophagus is made of thin layer of fibrous tissue, which covers the muscular layer.

Upper Esophageal Sphincter

Upper esophageal sphincter (UES) is a true sphincter formed by the cricopharyngeal muscle. The UES is normally contracted tonically and serves to prevent the entry of air into the esophagus during normal respiration. Its tone is maintained by the continual firing of vagal fibers originating from the nucleus ambiguus. The neurotransmitter released by these fibers is acetylcholine (ACh).

The UES opens during swallowing when a rapid peristaltic wave starting in the pharyngeal muscles passes on to esophagus.

Lower Esophageal Sphincter

Lower esophageal sphincter (LES), also known as cardiac sphincter, refers to distal 2 cm of esophagus. Its contractile

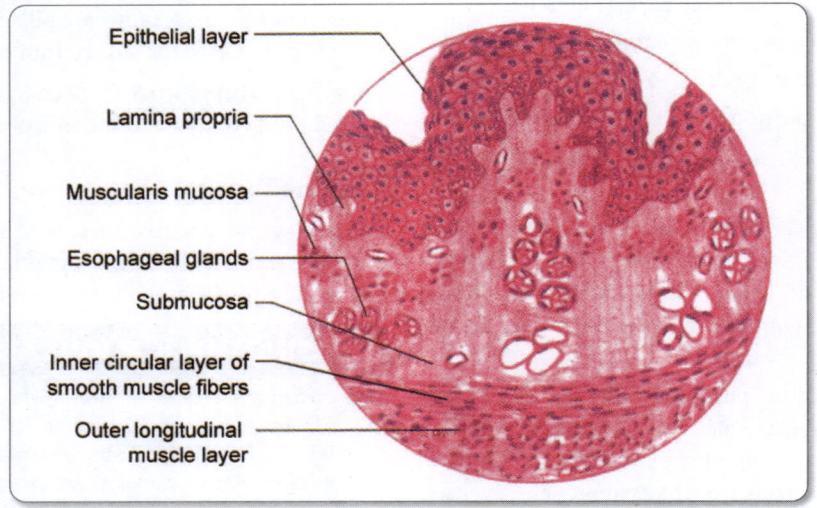

Epithelial layer

Lamina propria

Muscularis mucosa

Esophageal glands

Submucosa

Inner circular layer of smooth muscle fibers

Outer longitudinal muscle layer

Fig. 3.1-8: Histological structure of esophagus

characteristics are quite different from the rest of esophageal smooth muscle (that is why it is called physiological sphincter).

The principal function of LES is to prevent regurgitation of gastric contents (food, gastric juice and air) into the esophagus. When the intragastric pressure is markedly raised (e.g., after a heavy meal or ingestion of carbonated drinks), the resistance of LES is overcome and air escapes into the mouth (belching). The local hormone, gastrin, increases the tone of LES and helps to keep the sphincter more tightly closed during digestion.

NURSING IMPLICATIONS AND APPLICATIONS

During tracheal intubation, doctor usually asks the assisting nurse to apply pressure on the cricoids cartilage of the larynx. By doing so, the esophagus is compressed against vertebral column to prevent regurgitation of gastric contents into the lungs.

PHYSIOLOGICAL ACTIVITIES IN MOUTH, PHARYNX AND ESOPHAGUS

The functioning of digestive system starts from the mouth (oral cavity) and ends at the anus. **Ingestion** of food, a function of mouth, pharynx and esophagus, involves the following processes:

- Placing of food into the mouth
- Mastication, i.e., chewing the food into smaller pieces
- Lubrication of the food with saliva
- Swallowing, i.e., deglutition.

Mastication

Mastication or chewing refers to the process by which the food placed in the mouth is cut and grounded into smaller pieces. It involves:

- Movements of the jaws
- Action of teeth (the incisors provide a strong cutting action, whereas the molars have a grinding action)
- Coordinated movements of the tongue and muscles of the oral cavity.

IMPORTANT TO KNOW

Chewing reflex
Mastication or chewing, though a voluntary act, is coordinated by chewing reflex that facilitates the opening and closing of the jaw. The cycle of opening and closing of the jaw leads to mastication.

Role of tongue. The tongue contributes to the grinding process by positioning the food between the upper and lower teeth.

Muscles of mastication. These include masseter, temporalis, and internal and external pterygoids. Buccinator is an accessory muscle of mastication, which prevents accumulation of food between the cheek and teeth.

Net effect of mastication. The bolus of food becomes a homogenized mixture of small food particles, saliva and mucus, which is easy to swallow and digest.

Lubrication of Food by Saliva

In addition to the chewing, another important physiological activity that takes place in the mouth is lubrication of food by saliva.

Salivary Glands

The saliva is secreted by three pairs of major salivary glands (Fig. 3.1-9).

Parotid glands

Location. Parotid glands are the largest salivary glands (each weighing 20–30 g), located near the angles of jaw.

Acini. The parotid glands are purely serous glands, which secrete watery saliva containing more than 90% water. Parotid glands secrete 25% of the total salivary secretion (which is about 1500 mL/day) (Histology plate 3.1-2).

Ducts. Ducts of the parotid glands open on the inner side of the right and left cheeks and pour their secretions in the vestibule.

Sublingual glands

Location. The sublingual gland is the smallest of the three main salivary glands. It lies just below the mucosa on the floor of mouth. Each gland raises a ridge of mucosa, which starts at the sublingual papilla and runs laterally and backward. The ridge is called the sublingual fold.

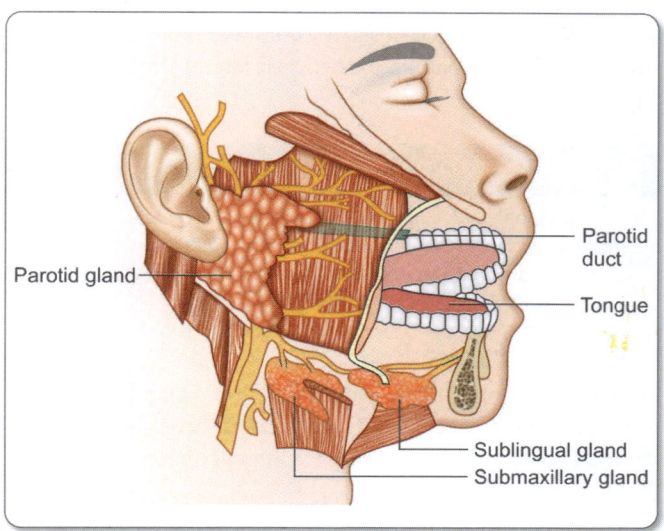

Fig. 3.1-9: Salivary glands and their ducts

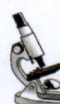

Histology Plate 3.1-2:

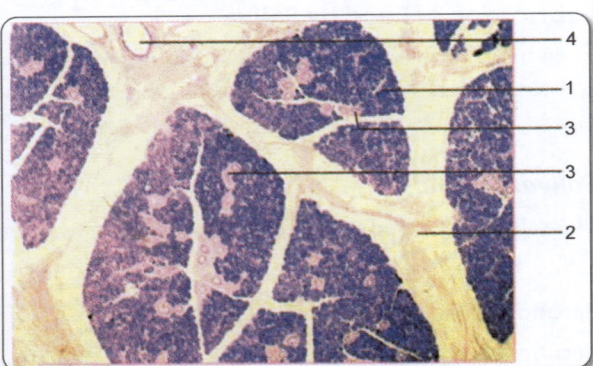

The photomicrograph of parotid gland shows, serous acini (1) connective tissue septa, (2) divides it into lobules, (3) intercalated duct, (4) intralobular duct

Acini. The sublingual gland contains both serous and mucus acini; the latter predominates.

Ducts of sublingual gland are 8–20 in number. Most open into the mouth on the summit of sublingual fold but a few may open into the submandibular duct.

Submandibular glands

Location. The submandibular glands are large salivary glands, which lie (one on each side) partly under cover of the body of the mandible.

Acini. The submandibular gland is composed of a mixture of serous and mucus acini; the former predominates.

Ducts. S-shaped duct of each submandibular gland opens on the sublingual papilla located just lateral to the frenulum lingua.

IMPORTANT TO KNOW

The sublingual and submandibular glands secrete a fluid that contains a higher concentration of proteins and so is more viscous as compared to watery secretion of parotid glands.

Smaller salivary glands

In addition to the three pairs of salivary glands described above, several smaller glands are located throughout the oral cavity. Those in the tongue secrete lingual lipase.

Saliva

Secretion and Composition

Amount. Under normal circumstances, the salivary glands secrete about 500–1500 mL of saliva every day, pH of saliva varies from 6 to 7.4.

Composition. Saliva is composed of *water* 99% and *solids* 1%, which include: Organic substances such as L-amylase (ptyalin), lingual lipase, kallikrein, lysozyme, small amounts of urea, uric acid, cholesterol and mucin. Inorganic substances are Na^+, Cl^-, K^+ and HCO^-_3. Composition of saliva varies with the salivary flow rate.

Phases of Salivary Secretion

Cephalic phase refers to secretion of saliva before entery of food into the mouth. It is caused by a conditioned reflex initiated by the mere sight or smell of food.

Buccal phase refers to secretion of saliva caused by stimulation of buccal receptors by the presence of food in the mouth.

Esophageal phase occurs due to stimulation of salivary glands to a slight degree by the food passing through esophagus.

Gastric phase refers to secretion of saliva by the presence of food in the stomach. It specially occurs when irritant food is present in the stomach (e.g., increased salivation before vomiting).

Intestinal phase refers to salivary secretion caused by presence of irritant food in the upper intestine.

Control of Salivary Secretion

- Salivary secretion is controlled entirely by autonomic nervous system (ANS) reflexes.
- Salivary secretion production is increased by both parasympathetic and sympathetic activity; however, the activity of former is more important.

Functions of Saliva

1. *Protective functions of saliva* include:
- *Dilutes hot and irritant food substances*, thus preventing injury to buccal mucosa.
- *Washes away food particles* that remain in the oral cavity at the end of meal and thus, cleans the oral cavity.
- *Destroys harmful bacteria* in the mouth and thus, minimizes risk of buccal infection and dental caries.
- *Dilutes any hydrochloric acid (HCl) and bile*, which regurgitate into esophagus and mouth.

2. Role in mastication and deglutition is:

- Salivary mucus lubricates the food and buccal mucosa and thus, aids in mastication and swallowing.
- Helps bolus formation by acting as a glue.

3. Digestive functions are:

- *Initial starch digestion* starts by α-amylase (ptyalin) present in the saliva.
- *Initial triglyceride digestion* is caused by lingual lipase present in the saliva.

4. Role in taste sensation. Saliva acts as a solvent for various food stuff. As taste is a chemical sense, the taste receptors respond only to dissolved substances.

5. Role in speech. Salivary mucus lubricates the oral mucosa and thus, aids speech by facilitating movements of lips and tongue.

6. Excretory function. Saliva acts as a vehicle for excretion of certain heavy metals, thiocyanate ions, alcohol and morphine.

7. Role in temperature regulation is as follows:

- During state of dehydration, the salivary secretion is reduced which induces thirst.
- Panting mechanism: In dogs, saliva is evaporated from the surface of tongue to cause evaporative heat loss.

Deglutition (Swallowing)

Deglutition or swallowing refers to passage of food from the oral cavity into the stomach. It comprises three phases:

- Oral phase (voluntary)
- Pharyngeal phase (reflex or involuntary)
- Esophageal phase (reflex or involuntary).

Oral Phase

Oral phase or the first stage of swallowing is a voluntary phase. During this phase, the bolus of food formed after mastication is put over the dorsum of tongue. The tongue forces the bolus into the oropharynx by pushing up and back against the hard palate (Fig. 3.1-10A).

Pharyngeal Phase

Pharyngeal phase or second stage of swallowing is an involuntary phase, i.e., caused by reflex contraction of muscles of pharynx. Deglutition center coordinating the reflex activity is located in the medulla oblongata and lower pons, i.e., in the nucleus of tractus solitarius (NTS) and the nucleus ambiguus.

Events during pharyngeal phase

Events which take place during movement of bolus from the pharynx into the esophagus occur in the following sequence (Figs 3.1-10B to D):

- *Oral cavity is shut off* from the pharynx by the approximation of posterior pillars of the fauces.
- *Nasopharynx is closed* by the upward movement of soft palate, preventing regurgitation of food into the nasal cavities.
- *Palatopharyngeal folds are pulled medially* to make a slit-like opening for food, allowing only properly masticated food to pass through (selective action).
- *Vocal cords* strongly approximate stopping the breathing temporarily (*deglutition apnea*), *larynx* is pulled upward and anteriorly by neck muscles enlarging the opening of esophagus, which is normally a slit and *epiglottis* swings backward to close laryngeal opening. All this guides the food toward the esophagus and prevents its entry into the trachea.
- *Upper esophageal sphincter* (UES), which normally remains contracted tonically opens up and allows the bolus of food to be pushed into the upper part of esophagus by rapid peristaltic contraction wave of pharynx, which also continues in the esophagus.
- Once the bolus of food has passed into the esophagus, cricopharyngeus contracts, vocal cords open up allowing normal breathing to be resumed and the upper esophageal sphincter (UES) once again goes into tonic contraction. The entire process of pharyngeal phase is completed in 1–2 seconds.

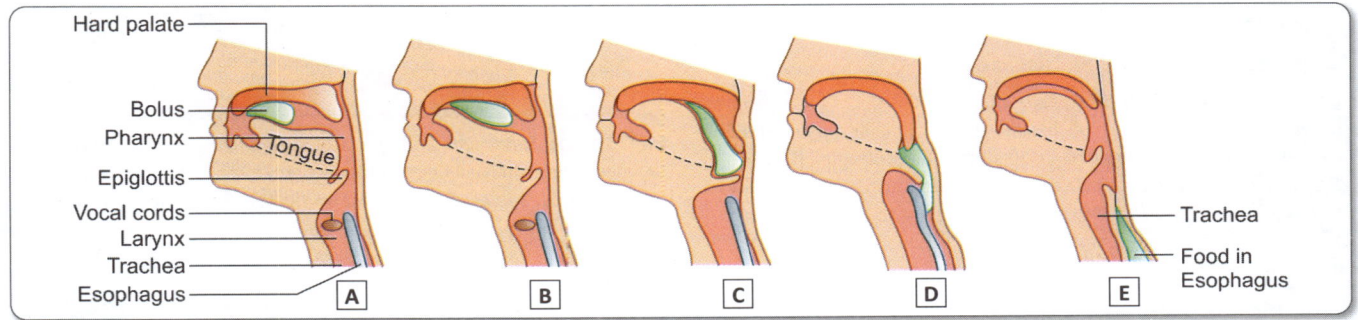

Figs 3.1-10A to E: Phases of swallowing. A. Oral phase; B, C and D. Early, middle and late pharyngeal phases; E. Esophageal phase

Esophageal phase

During esophageal phase, the food bolus is propelled from the upper part of esophagus to the stomach by the esophageal peristalsis and aided by gravity (Fig. 3.1-10E).

IMPORTANT TO KNOW

After the food enters the stomach, the LES contracts to prevent regurgitation of food into the esophagus. With this, the esophageal phase of deglutition is completed.

NURSING IMPLICATIONS AND APPLICATIONS

DISORDERS OF SWALLOWING

Abolition of Deglutition Reflex

Abolition of deglutition reflex causes regurgitation of food into the nose or aspiration into the larynx and trachea. It may occur:
- When IX or X nerve is paralyzed in lesions of medulla
- When pharynx is anesthetized with cocaine (deglutition reflex is abolished temporarily).

Aerophagia

- Aerophagia refers to unavoidable swallowing of air along with the swallowing of food bolus and liquids.
- It usually occurs in nervous individuals having low tone of the upper esophageal sphincter (UES).
- Some of the gases present in the air swallowed are absorbed, partly the air is regurgitated into the oral cavity and out in the atmosphere (belching), and majority of it passes on to the colon and is then expelled as flatus through the anus.

Dysphagia

Dysphagia is a term used to denote difficulty in swallowing due to any cause.

Cardiac Achalasia

- Cardiac achalasia is a neuromuscular disorder of the lower two-third of esophagus characterized by absence of esophageal peristalsis and failure of the lower esophageal sphincter (LES) to relax during swallowing.
- Because of this, food transmission to stomach is impeded. In severe cases, esophagus fails to empty the swallowed food into stomach for several hours.
- Over months and years esophagus becomes enlarged and infected due to long-standing stasis of food.

Gastroesophageal Reflux Disease

Gastroesophageal reflux disease (GERD) refers to a condition in which incompetence of lower esophageal sphincter (LES) causes reflux of acidic gastric contents into esophagus. Reflux of stomach acid causes esophageal pain (heartburn) and may lead to irritation of esophagus or bronchioles (due to aspiration).

STOMACH

GROSS ANATOMY

- Stomach is a J-shaped hollow muscular bag connected to the esophagus at its upper end and to the duodenum at the lower end.
- The *volume* of stomach is 1200–1500 mL, but its *capacity* is greater than 3000 mL.
- The stomach has two curvatures. The concavity of the right inner curve is called *lesser curvature*, and the convexity of the left outer curve is the *greater curvature*. An angle along the lesser curvature is called *incisura angularis* (Fig. 3.1-11).

ANATOMICAL RELATIONS AND PARTS OF STOMACH

Relations (Fig. 3.1-11)

Anteriorly the stomach is related to left lobe of liver and anterior abdominal wall.

Posteriorly the structures related to stomach include: abdominal aorta, pancreas, spleen, left kidney and left adrenal gland (Fig. 3.1-11).

Superiorly the stomach is related to diaphragm, esophagus and left lobe of liver.

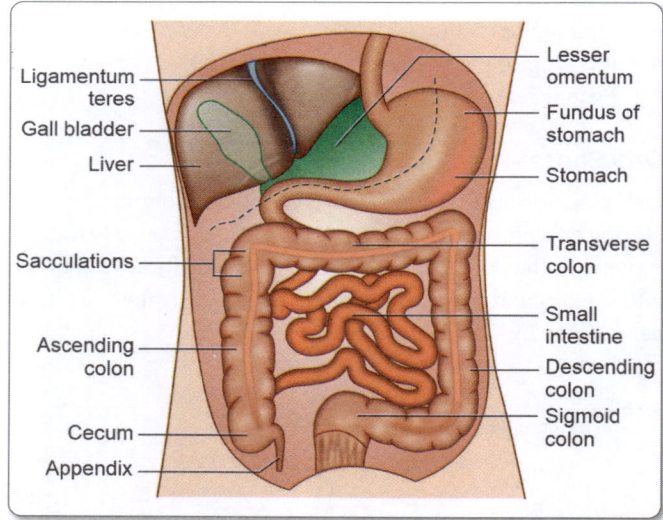

Fig. 3.1-11: Stomach and its associated structures. **Note:** The greater omentum has been removed and liver turned up and to the right to show lesser omentum. The dotted lines show the normal position of liver

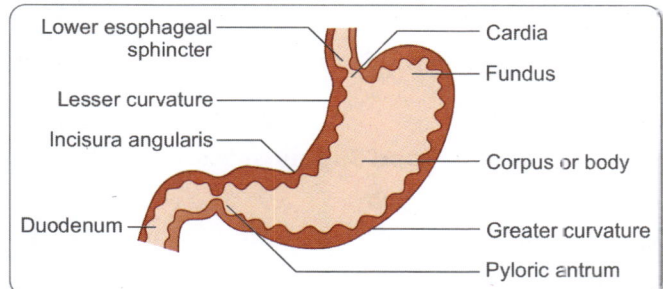

Fig. 3.1-12: Schematic section to depict gross anatomy of stomach

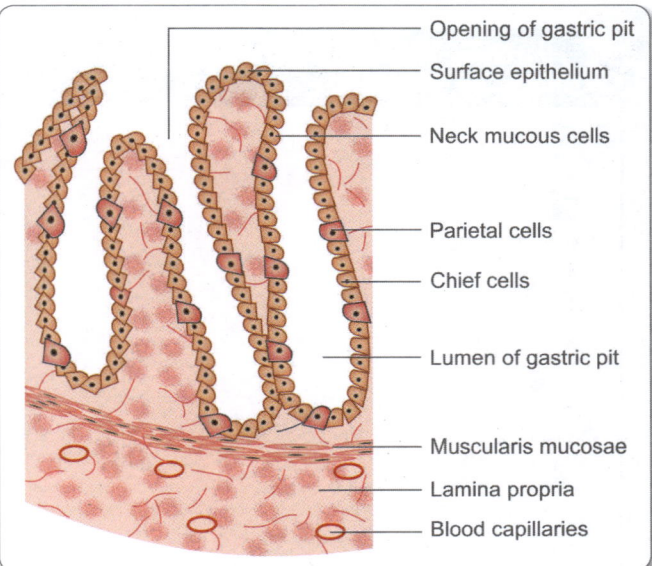

Fig. 3.1-13: Histological features of gastric mucosa

Inferiorly the stomach lies on transverse colon and small intestine.

To the left side of stomach lie diaphragm and spleen.

To the right side of stomach are situated liver and duodenum.

Parts of Stomach

The stomach can be divided into five anatomic regions (Fig. 3.1-12):

Cardia is the narrow conical portion of the stomach immediately distal to the gastroesophageal junction.

Fundus is the dome-shaped proximal portion of the stomach.

Body or corpus is the main part of the stomach that extends up to the incisura angularis.

Pyloric antrum extends from the incisura angularis to the pyloric canal.

Pyloric canal or pylorus is the distal-most one inch long tubular part of stomach.

> ### IMPORTANT TO KNOW
> Anatomically, the antrum and pylorus are continuous and respond to nervous control as a unit. Functionally, first part of duodenum is associated with the pyloric part of stomach.

Structural Characteristics

The gastric wall consists of mucosa, submucosa, muscular coat, and serosa (serous layer) (Histology plate 3.1-3).

Gastric Mucosa

Gross features

- The inner surface of stomach exhibits coarse *rugae*. These infoldings of mucosa and submucosa are most prominent in the proximal stomach.
- The delicate texture of the mucosa is punctured by millions of gastric foveolae or pits, leading to the mucosal glands.

Histological features

Gastric mucosa comprises (Fig. 3.1-13):

Surface foveolar cells are tall columnar mucin-secreting cells, which line the entire gastric mucosa as well as the gastric pits.

Mucus neck cells are present deeper in the gastric pits. These cells are thought to be the progenitors of both the surface epithelium and the cells of gastric glands.

Glandular cells form the gastric glands. There are three types of gastric glands—main gastric glands, cardiac tubular glands, and pyloric (antral) glands.

Gastric glands

Main gastric glands are found in the body and fundus of stomach. These are simple tubular glands (Fig. 3.1-13 and Histology Plate 3.1-3). The alveoli of main gastric glands contain two types of cells:

1. *Chief cells,* also known as peptic or zymogen cells, are basophilic and secrete proteolytic proenzymes, pepsinogen I and II.

2. *Parietal cells* (oxyntic cells) are acidophilic. These secrete *hydrochloric acid* (HCl) and the *intrinsic factor*.

Cardiac tubular glands are found in the mucosa of cardia (a small conical part of the stomach) just around the distal end of esophagus. These secrete *soluble mucus*.

Pyloric (antral) glands are found in the antrum and pylorus region of the stomach. These glands contain two types of cells:

1. *Mucus cells,* which secrete *soluble mucus*

2. *G-cells,* responsible for release of the hormone gastrin.

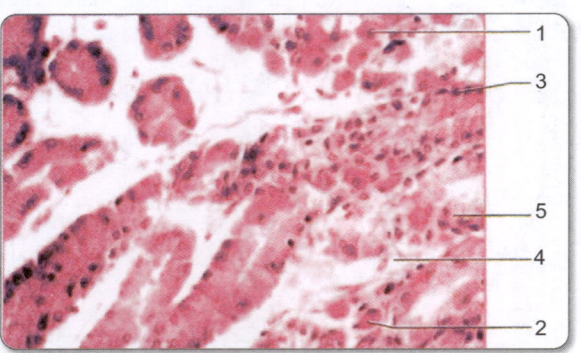

Histology Plate 3.1-3: Showing Fundic Glands of Stomach

Photomicrograph of fundic glands of stomach is shown. Parietal of stomach is shown. Parietal cells (1) are large polyhedral cells with eosinophilic cytoplasmic (2) chief cells (3) are cuboidal cells. Gastric glands (5) and lamina propria (4) are also seen.

Submucus Coat

The submucus coat consists of loose areolar connective tissue connecting the muscular and mucus coats of the stomach.

Musculature of Stomach

Characteristic features of gastric musculature are:

- The muscle coat of stomach has three layers, an outer longitudinal, middle circular, and an inner oblique (Fig. 3.1-14).
- The stomach and duodenum are divided by a thickened circular smooth muscle layer called *pyloric sphincter*.

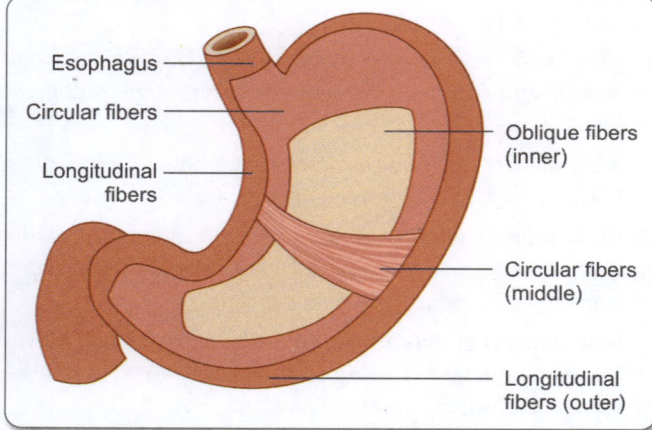

Esophagus

Circular fibers

Longitudinal fibers

Oblique fibers (inner)

Circular fibers (middle)

Longitudinal fibers (outer)

Fig. 3.1-14: Three layers of gastric mucosa

Serous Coat

The serous coat of stomach is a part of the peritoneum which covers the organ.

Innervation and Blood Supply of Stomach

Innervation of Stomach

The stomach is supplied by an intrinsic and an extrinsic system.

Intrinsic innervation comprises two interconnected plexuses:

Myenteric (Auerbach's) plexus, located between the layers of circular and longitudinal muscles of the stomach

Submucosal (Meissner's) plexus, located in the submucosal layer.

The intrinsic innervation is directly responsible for peristalsis and other contractions. Because this system is continuous between the stomach and duodenum, peristalsis in the antrum influences the duodenal bulb.

Extrinsic innervation modifies the coordinated motor activity that arises independently in the intrinsic nervous system. It consists of two components of autonomic nervous system:

Sympathetic innervation comes *via* celiac plexus and *inhibits motility*

Parasympathetic innervation comes *via* the vagus nerve and *stimulates motility*.

Blood Supply of Stomach

The arteries supplying the stomach are derived from the celiac artery and include:

Left gastric artery. It courses along the lesser curvature of the stomach from left to right, distributing branches to both surfaces. It anastomoses with the esophageal arteries and branches of right gastric artery.

Right and left gastroepiploic arteries. They course, respectively, from the right and left side along the greater curvature of the stomach, anastomose with branches of splenic artery and supply blood to the stomach.

The veins draining blood from the stomach include right and left gastroepiploic veins, and several short gastric veins. All of these eventually join the portal vein. A small quantity of the blood is returned to azygos veins instead of portal vein.

Physiological Activities in Stomach

Physiology of Gastric Secretion: Gastric Juice

Composition

Gastric glands secrete about 2–2.5 L of gastric juice in the lumen of stomach per day. It is acidic with a pH varying from 1 to 2. Important constituents of gastric juice are:

- *Water:* 99.45%
- *Solids:* 0.55%, which include:

Electrolytes such as Na^+, K^+, Mg^{2+}, Cl^-, HCO_3^-, HPO_4^{2-} and SO_4^{2-}. The electrolyte content of gastric juice varies with the rate of secretions. At low secretory rates, Na^+ concentration is high and H^+ concentration is low, but as acid secretion increases, Na^+ concentration falls.

Enzymes present in the gastric juice are:
- *Pepsin*
- *Gastric lipase*
- *Gastric gelatinase*
- *Gastric amylase*
- *Lysozyme* and
- *Carbonic anhydrase.*

Mucin or mucus is of two types:

1. *Soluble mucus* secreted by mucus cells of pyloric and cardiac glands

2. *Insoluble mucus* secreted by surface foveolar cells (tall columnar mucin-secreting cells) lining the entire gastric mucosa.

Intrinsic factor is secreted by parietal cells of gastric glands.

Secretion of HCl

Hydrochloric acid (HCl) is secreted by the *parietal cells* (also called oxyntic cells). Gastric glands secrete about 2.5 L of HCl in a day having a pH of approximately 1.0.

Mechanism of HCl secretion

Various theories have been put forward to explain the origin of H^+ of HCl. The hypothesis more widely accepted is shown in (Fig. 3.1-15). Hydrochloric acid is made up of hydrogen (H^+) and chloride ions (Cl^-).

The H^+ ions are believed to be generated inside the parietal cell from metabolic CO_2 and H_2O present in the cell. The enzyme carbonic anhydrase present in abundance in the parietal cells is essential for the secretion.

$$CO_2 + H_2O \xrightarrow[\text{anhydrase}]{\text{carbonic}} H_2CO_3 \longrightarrow H^+ + HCO_3^-$$

Because of the high intracellular negativity, the Cl^- present in the parietal cell is forced out into the lumen of gland through the Cl^- channels located on the apical membrane of the cell.

Functions of HCl

- HCl participates in the breakdown of proteins.
- It provides an optimal pH for the action of pepsin.
- It hinders the growth of pathogenic bacteria.

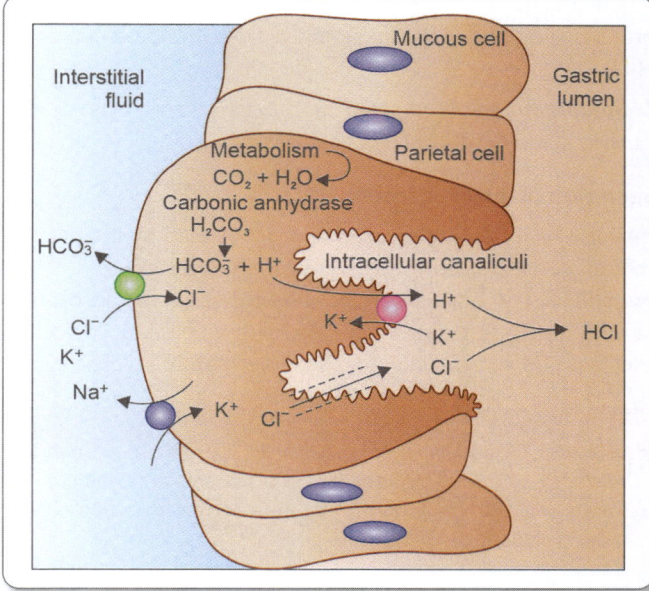

Fig. 3.1-15: Mechanism of HCl secretion in the parietal cells of the stomach

Pepsinogen secretion

- Pepsinogen is an inactive precursor (proenzyme) of pepsin. It is mainly secreted by *chief cells* of the main gastric glands. A small amount of pepsinogen is also secreted by pyloric glands.
- Pepsinogen is synthesized and stored as zymogen granules in the apical region of chief cells.
- Pepsinogen secretion is stimulated by vagal stimulation, gastrin and histamine.
- Pepsinogen is converted to pepsin (the active form) by the action of HCl or preformed pepsin.

$$\text{Pepsinogen} \xrightarrow{\text{HCl}} \text{Pepsin}$$

$$\text{Pepsinogen} \xrightarrow{\text{Pepsin}} \text{Pepsin}$$

Function of pepsinogen

Pepsin, the active form of pepsinogen, is a proteolytic enzyme that begins the process of protein digestion.

Secretion of mucus

Mucus is of two types—insoluble and soluble.

1. *Insoluble mucus* is secreted by the mucussecreting cells lining the entire gastric mucosa. The insoluble mucus is so viscid in nature that it forms a gel-like coat over the mucosa. These cells also secrete bicarbonate ions which make the mucus alkaline with pH of 7, that form an extremely important protective layer saving the stomach from the destruction by HCl.

2. Soluble mucus is secreted by mucus cells of pylorus and cardiac glands.

Secretion of intrinsic factor

Intrinsic factor (IF), a glycoprotein, is secreted by the parietal cells of gastric mucosa, chiefly by those in the fundus.
Functions. The intrinsic factor is essential for the absorption of vitamin B_{12}. It forms a complex with vitamin B_{12}, which is carried to the terminal ileum where the vitamin is absorbed.

> ### CLINICAL ASPECTS
>
> **Deficiency of intrinsic factor** in some patients with idiopathic atrophy of gastric mucosa may cause a serious disorder called pernicious anemia.

Regulation of gastric secretion

Mechanisms regulating the gastric secretion include neural control and chemical control.

Neural control

Neural control over the gastric glands is exerted by local enteric plexus involving cholinergic neurons and impulses from the CNS *via* vagal (extrinsic) innervation.

Vagal stimulation increases the secretion of HCl by parietal cells and pepsin by chief cells. Vagal stimulation increases H^+ secretion by a direct path and an indirect path.

Chemical control

Chemical control on gastric glands is exerted mainly through:

Role of gastrin. Gastrin, a hormone, is secreted by the G-cells into the blood circulation (and not into gastric juice). It reaches the stomach through the arterial circulation and stimulates secretory activity of the parietal cells and chief cells.

Role of histamine. Histamine is released from the enterochromaffin-like (ECL) cells found in the base of the gastric gland. ECL cells bear both gastrin receptors and ACh receptors. They release histamine in response to both circulating gastrin as well as ACh released by vagal fibers. The histamine released stimulates *HCl secretion* from parietal cells by acting on H_2 receptors. H_2 receptor-blocking drugs, such as *cimetidine* and *ranitidine*, inhibit H^+ secretion by blocking the stimulatory effect of histamine.

Role of somatostatin. Somatostatin is secreted by D-cells located adjacent to G-cells or the parietal cells in the gastric glands. Somatostatin inhibits HCl secretion.

Role of low pH (<3) in stomach. Low pH (<3) in the stomach inhibits the secretion of H^+ by parietal cells by a negative feedback mechanism.

Intestinal influences. Chyme containing acid, fats and products of protein digestion when reaches the duodenum, causes the release of several intestinal hormones like secretin, cholecystokinin (CCK) and gastric inhibitory peptide (GIP).

Phases of Gastric Secretion and their Regulation

Meal-related gastric secretion can be divided into three phases (Fig. 3.1-16):
*   Cephalic phase
*   Gastric phase
*   Intestinal phase

Cephalic phase

Cephalic phase of gastric secretion occurs before the entry of food into the stomach.
*   The secretion is *initiated* by the thought, sight, smell or taste of food. Neurogenic signals originate in the cerebral cortex and appetite centers of amygdala or hypothalamus. The impulses are transmitted to dorsal vagal nuclei and from there through vagii to the stomach.
*   Emotions also influence this vagally-mediated gastric secretion. *Anger and hostility* are associated with increased gastric secretion and motility. *Fear and depression* decrease the gastric secretion and motility.

Gastric phase

Gastric phase of gastric secretion occurs when food enters the stomach. The presence of food in the stomach induces gastric secretion by the following mechanisms:
*   *Distension of the body of stomach*
*   *Distension of the antrum* initiates vagally, mediated and local reflexes that result in gastrin release from the antral G-cells. Gastrin release is inhibited when pH becomes low (<3).
*   *Products of partial protein digestion* also stimulate gastrin secretion and this mainly increases secretion of gastric acid.
*   *Low pH* causes increased pepsinogen secretion through local reflexes.

Intestinal phase

Intestinal phase of gastric secretion begins as the chyme begins to empty from the stomach into the duodenum.

In contrast to the excitatory cephalic and gastric influences, the intestinal influence on the gastric secretion is chiefly inhibitory in nature. Intestinal factor inhibits gastric

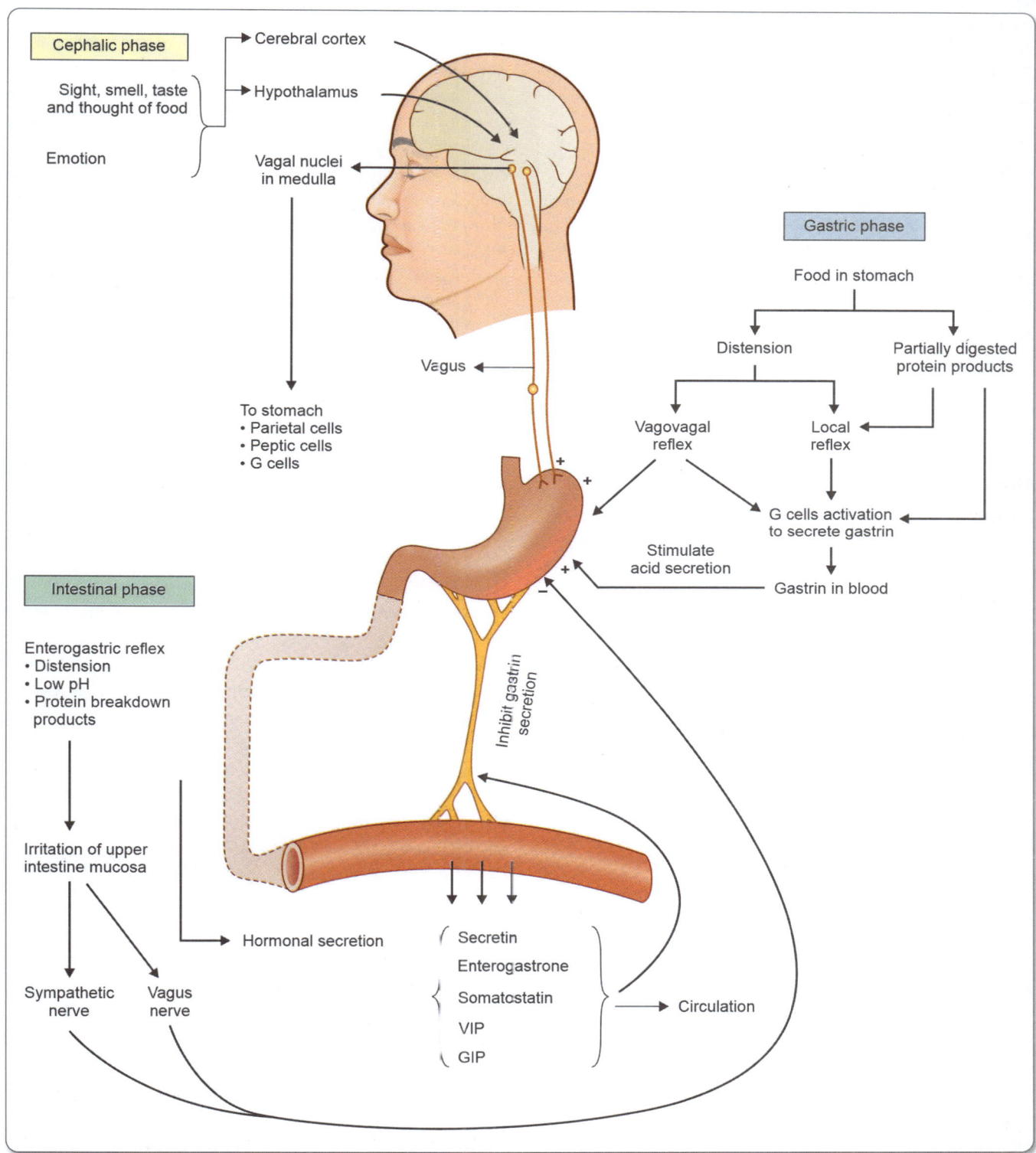

Fig. 3.1-16: Phases and regulation of gastric secretion. VIP, vasoactive intestinal peptide; GIP, gastric inhibitory polypeptide

secretion *by Enterogastric reflex* and through several hormones such as secretin, CCK, GIP, vasoactive intestinal polypeptide (VIP) and somatostatin, which inhibit gastric secretion. The inhibitory influences discussed above help to terminate the gastric secretion when all the food has left stomach.

Physiology of Gastric Motility

The peristaltic activity of the gastric musculature has been given various names depending upon its features and motor function subserved by it. Gastric motility can be described as:

Motility of the empty stomach includes:
- Migrating motor complex
- Hunger contractions

Gastric motility related to meal includes:
- Receptive relaxation
- Mixing peristaltic waves
- Gastric emptying

Motility of Empty Stomach

Migrating motor complex (MMC) is the name given to the peristaltic wave that begins in the esophagus and travels through the entire gastrointestinal tract (migratory motor activity) during interdigestive period.
- The MMCs remove any food remaining in the stomach and intestines during interdigestive period in preparation for the next meal; because of this they have been called the *interdigestive housekeepers.*
- The MMC is abolished immediately after the entry of food in the stomach.

Hunger contractions are the mild peristaltic contractions that occur in the empty stomach, which over a period of hours increase in intensity that MMCs are probably responsible for hunger contractions.

Gastric Motility Related to Meals

Receptive relaxation and accommodation. Storage function of stomach is accomplished by receptive relaxation and accommodation.
- The passage of each bolus of food stimulates the stretch *receptors of oral region* and produces relaxation. By the end of meal, about 1–2 L of food can be accommodated.
- Receptive relaxation is a *vagovagal reflex* initiated by distension of stomach and is synchronized with the primary peristaltic waves in the esophagus.

Mixing peristaltic waves. The presence of food in the caudal region (distal body and antral part) of stomach increases the contractile activity of this part of stomach. This enhanced contractile activity (a combination of peristalsis and retropulsion) is called mixing waves, which mix the food with stomach acid and enzymes and break it into smaller and smaller pieces. When the food is mixed into a pasty consistency, it is called *chyme.*

Gastric emptying. Gastric emptying occurs when the chyme is decomposed into enough small pieces (typically less than 1 mm³) to fit through the pyloric sphincter.
- Gastric emptying results from a progressive wave of forceful contraction which sequentially involves antrum, pylorus (pyloric sphincter) and proximal duodenum; thus, all the three function as a unit.

Functions of Stomach

After studying the physiological activities of stomach, its functions can be summarized as:

Mechanical or motor functions include:
- *Storage of food*
- *Mixing of food*
- *Slow emptying of food* into duodenum occurs to provide proper time for digestion and absorption by small intestine.

Digestive functions. Only a small amount of food is digested in stomach as:

Carbohydrate digestion in the stomach depends on the action of salivary amylase, which remains active until halted by the low pH of stomach.

Protein digestion. About 10% of ingested protein is broken down completely in the stomach. *Gastric pepsin* facilitates later digestion of protein by breaking protein into peptone.

Fat digestion in stomach is minimal due to the restriction of gastric lipase activity to triglycerides containing short chain (<10 carbon) fatty acids.

Absorptive function. Stomach contributes little in absorption function.

Reflex functions. Various reflexes initiated from the stomach are:
- Gastrosalivary reflex
- Gastroileal reflex
- Gastrocolic reflex
- Presence of food in the stomach reflexly stimulates secretion of pancreatic juice and expulsion of bile.

Antiseptic action. HCl present in the gastric juice kills the bacteria and other harmful substances.

NURSING IMPLICATIONS AND APPLICATIONS

Important applied aspects of stomach which need special attention are:
- Gastric mucosal barrier and pathophysiology of peptic ulcer
- Physiology of vomiting

Gastric Mucosal Barrier and Pathophysiology of Peptic Ulcer

Gastric Mucosal Barrier

The gastric mucosal barrier protects the gastric mucosa from damage by intraluminal HCl, i.e., autodigestion. It is created by the following:
- *Mucin secretion:* A thin layer of surface mucus in the stomach and duodenum prevents the direct contact of acid and pepsin-containing fluid with surface epithelial cells.
- *Bicarbonate secretion:* Surface epithelial cells in both the stomach and the duodenum secrete bicarbonate, which creates an essentially pH neutral microenvironment immediately adjacent to the cell surface.
- *Epithelial barrier:* Intercellular tight junctions provide a barrier to the back-diffusion of H$^+$.
- *High mucosal blood flow:* It rapidly carries away any acid that penetrates the cellular lining, and also provides oxygen, bicarbonate, and nutrients to epithelial cells.
- *Prostaglandins* are responsible for maintaining the gastric mucosal barrier.

Pathophysiology of Peptic Ulcer

Peptic ulcer refers to excavation of mucosa of duodenum or pyloric part of stomach caused by the digestive action of gastric juice. Peptic ulcer can be caused by either of two ways:

1. Diminished ability of the gastroduodenal mucosal barrier to protect against the digestive properties of the acid-pepsin complex. Factors that disturb mucosal barrier include:
- *Bacterial infection by Helicobacter pylori.*
- *Other factors* which can disrupt the mucosal barrier are ethyl alcohol, vinegar, bile salts, cigarette smoking and non-steroidal anti-inflammatory drugs (NSAIDs), such as aspirin and ibuprofen.

2. Excessive secretion of gastric acid. Hyperacidity leads to ulcer formation in duodenum and pyloric part of stomach.

Physiologic Basis of Management of Peptic Ulcer

Commonly employed measures for treatment of peptic ulcer are:
- *Antacids.* These form a gel that coats the mucosa and neutralizes the acid.
- *H$_2$-receptor blocking drugs* such as cimetidine.
- *M$_1$-muscarinic receptor blocking drugs* such as atropine.
- *Gastric H$^+$-K$^+$-ATPase inhibiting drugs* such as omeprazole.
- *Bilateral vagotomy combined with resection of gastrin-producing pyloric part of stomach* is performed in very severe cases of duodenal and pyloric ulcers.

Vomiting

Vomiting refers to forceful expulsion of contents from stomach and intestine.

Initiation of Vomiting

Vomiting may be initiated by either activation of vomiting center or by activation of the chemoreceptor trigger zone.

Activation of Vomiting Center

Vomiting center is situated in the reticular formation of medulla oblongata near the vagal nucleus. It may be activated directly or through afferents:
Direct activation of the vomiting center occurs due to injury to the area or by raised intracranial pressure.

Activation of Chemoreceptor Trigger Zone

Chemoreceptor trigger zone (CTZ) is located in the area *postrema* (a V-shaped band of tissue on the lateral walls of fourth ventricle near the obex), which is outside the blood-brain barrier and is, thus, more permeable to many substances.

Efferent Impulses from Vomiting Center and CTZ

Efferent impulses from the vomiting center and CTZ, which give effect to act of vomiting, are transmitted via V, VII, IX, X and XII cranial nerves to upper gastrointestinal tract and through spinal nerves to the muscles of respiration.

PANCREAS, LIVER AND GALLBLADDER

Pancreas, liver and gallbladder are accessory organs of digestive system. It will be worthwhile to know about the physiological role of pancreas, liver and gallbladder in digestive system at this level, because secretions of these organs affect the digestive activities of small intestine.

PANCREAS

Anatomy of Pancreas

The pancreas—an elongated, accessory digestive gland—lies retroperitoneally and transversely across the posterior abdominal wall, posterior to the stomach between the duodenum on the right and spleen on the left (Fig. 3.1-17).

Anatomically, pancreas is divided into four parts: (1) head, (2) neck, (3) body, and (4) tail.

Head. It refers to right enlarged end of pancreas. It lies in the C-shaped space bounded by the duodenum. A projection arising from the lower left part of head is called *uncinate process.*

Neck. Next to the head there is a short somewhat constricted part called the neck.

Body. The neck is continuous with the main part of the pancreas—the body. The neck and body of pancreas are separated from the stomach by lesser sac.

Tail: It refers to the left thin extremity of the pancreas.

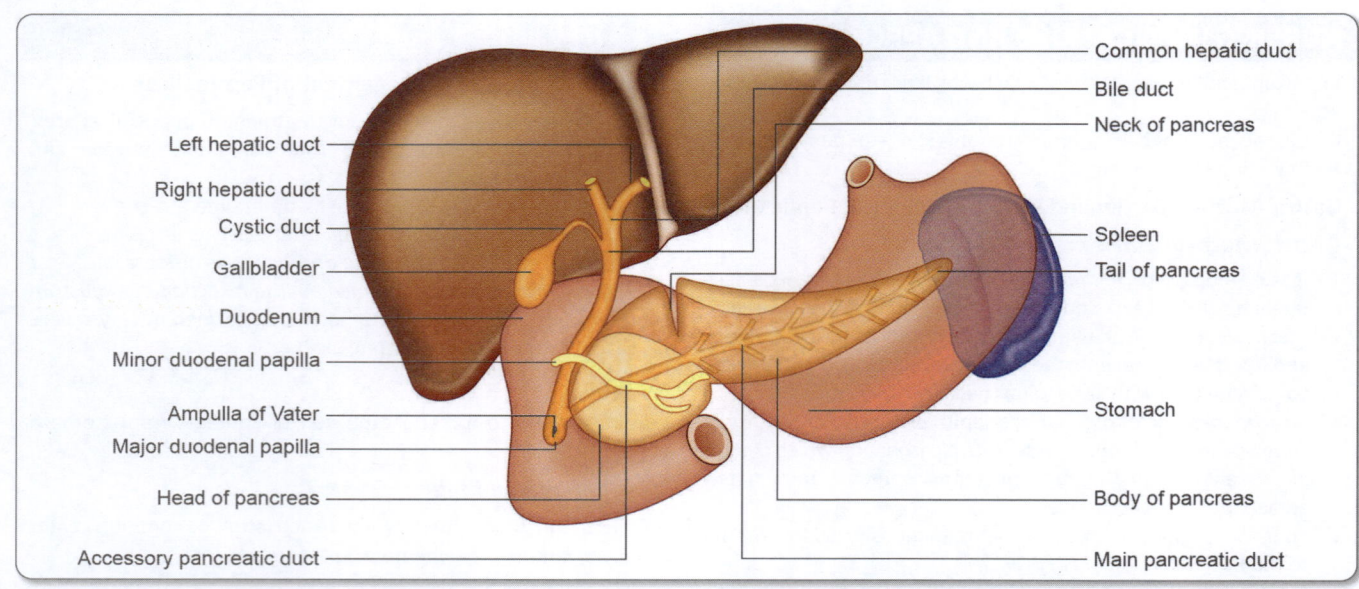

Fig. 3.1-17: Anatomical relations of pancreas, pancreatic duct and extrahepatic biliary system

Physiologically, on the basis of functions performed, the pancreas consists of two parts: (1) Exocrine and (2) endocrine *Exocrine part*, which produces a secretion called pancreatic juice that contains enzymes capable of hydrolyzing proteins, fats and carbohydrates.

Endocrine part of the pancreas, the islets of Langerhans, produces the hormones insulin and glucagon, which play a key role in the carbohydrate metabolism. The endocrine part is discussed in ch. Endocrine system.

Histological and Structural Characteristics of Exocrine Part of Pancreas

The exocrine part of the pancreas is in the form of a serous, compound tubuloalveolar gland, very similar to parotid gland in general structure (Fig. 3.1-18).

Acinar cells lining the alveoli appear triangular in section. Numerous secretory (or zymogen) granules can be demonstrated in the cytoplasm, especially in the apical part of cells.

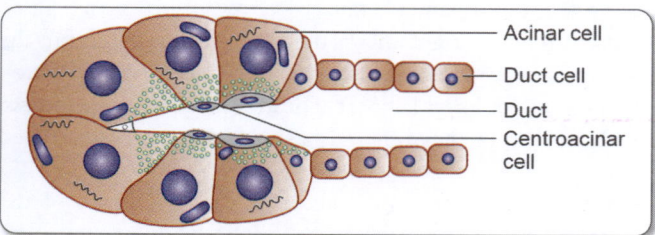

Fig. 3.1-18: Histology of functional unit of exocrine pancreas

The acinar cells produce thick secretion containing numerous enzymes (listed in composition of pancreatic juice).

Centroacinar cells. That are so called because they appear to be located near the center of the acinus (alveolus). These cells really belong to the intercalated ducts which are invaginated into the acinus (Fig. 3.1-18).

Pancreatic Ducts

The intercalated ducts, which receive secretions produced by acini, pass it on to *interlobular ducts*. Ultimately, the pancreatic secretion passes into duodenum through the main pancreatic duct and accessory pancreatic duct.

Main pancreatic duct, also known as duct of Wirsung, begins in the tail and runs the length of the gland, receiving numerous tributaries on the way. It joins the common bile duct to form the ampulla of Vater, which opens into the second part of the duodenum at about its middle on the major duodenal papilla (Fig. 3.1-17). Ampulla of Vater is guarded by the sphincter of Oddi.

Accessory pancreatic duct, also called a duct of Santorini, when present, drains the upper part of the head and then opens into the duodenum about 2 mm above the main duct on the minor duodenal papilla.

Blood Supply

Arterial supply to the pancreas comes from splenic and superior as well as inferior pancreaticoduodenal arteries.

Veins, corresponding to arteries, drain into the portal system.

Lymphatics drain into the lymph nodes situated along the arteries that supply the gland. The efferent vessels ultimately drain into the celiac and superior mesenteric lymph nodes.

Innervation

Nerve supply comes from both sympathetic and parasympathetic (vagi) nerves. Preganglionic vagal fibers synapse with ganglionic cells embedded in the pancreatic tissue. The postganglionic fibers innervate both the acinar cells and smooth muscles of the ducts. Vagal stimulation increases pancreatic juice secretion.

Pancreatic Juice (Secretion)

Properties

- Pancreatic juice is a transparent colorless fluid isotonic with plasma.
- About 1,200–1,500 mL of pancreatic juice is secreted per day.
- Its specific gravity varies from 1.010–1.018.
- Pancreatic juice is markedly alkaline (pH 7.8–8.4), due to very high concentration of HCO_3^- (about 4–5 times that of plasma).

Composition

Pancreatic juice is composed of 99.5% water and 0.5% solids which include organic and inorganic substances.

Organic constituents of pancreatic juice are:

- Enzymes amylase, lipase, protease and trypsin inhibitor and
- Other organic substances present in traces are albumin and globulin.
- Pancreatic enzymes are described with the functions of pancreatic juice.

Inorganic substances present in the pancreatic juice are cations like Na^+, K^+, Ca^{2+}, Mg^{2+}, and Zn^{2+}; and anions such as HCO_3^-, Cl^- and traces of SO_4^{2-} and HPO_4^{2-}. Electrolyte composition varies with rate of secretion.

Functions of Pancreatic Juice

Digestive functions

The pancreatic juice is the major source of digestive enzymes which include:

Pancreatic α amylase is secreted in its active form. Its action on the carbohydrates is like that of salivary amylase.

Pancreatic lipases or lipolytic enzymes include pancreatic lipase, cholesterol ester hydrolase and phospholipase A_2.

Pancreatic proteases or proteolytic enzymes include three endopeptidases (trypsin, chymotrypsin and elastase) and two exopeptidases (carboxypeptidase A and B).

Trypsin. It is the most powerful proteolytic enzyme of the pancreatic juice.

- It hydrolyzes proteins into proteoses and to polypeptides.
- It activates trypsinogen and other pancreatic enzymes.

Chymotrypsin. It hydrolyzes the proteins into small polypeptides.

Elastase. It digests elastin.

Carboxypeptidase A cleaves the carboxyl-terminal amino acids that have aromatic or branched aliphatic side chains.

Carboxypeptidase B cleaves the carboxy-terminal amino acids that have basic side chains.

Nucleases (ribonuclease and deoxyribonuclease) split nucleic acids of ribose and deoxyribose type into nucleotides.

Trypsin inhibitor. If even a small amount of trypsin is released into the pancreas, the resulting chain reaction would produce active enzymes that could digest the pancreas. It is, therefore, not surprising that the pancreas normally contains a trypsin inhibitor, which is secreted by the same cells and at the same time as the pancreatic proenzymes. Trypsin inhibitor protects the pancreas from autodigestion.

For digestive action of pancreatic proteases see page 139

Neutralizing function

Pancreatic juice is highly alkaline due to high concentration of HCO_3^- and neutralizes the gastric HCl in the chyme that enters the duodenum.

Regulation of Pancreatic Secretion

Both, neural and hormonal, mechanisms are involved in the regulation of pancreatic secretion, with the latter playing the predominant role.

Neural regulation is through vagal efferents supplying the exocrine gland of pancreas.

Hormonal regulation is through secretin, CCK, gastrin and somatostatin.

Phases of regulation of pancreatic secretion

The exact role of these regulatory mechanisms in regulation of different phases of pancreatic secretion viz. cephalic phase, gastric phase and intestinal phase is summarized below.

Regulation of cephalic phase. Cephalic phase of pancreatic secretion like that of gastric secretion occurs before the entry of food into the stomach. *Regulation* of this phase is mainly through the reflex vagal stimulation.

Regulation of gastric phase. Gastric phase of pancreatic secretion occurs when stomach is distended by the food. This phase is regulated by *neural control* exerted through vagus and *hormonal control* executed through the hormone gastrin.

Regulation of intestinal phase. The intestinal phase of pancreatic secretion begins when the chyme enters the duodenum and jejunum. It is characterized by marked increase in the secretion of both enzymes and aqueous component of pancreatic juice. This phase is regulated by the hormones, secretin and CCK.

IMPORTANT TO KNOW

Interaction of Nervous and Humoral Regulation

A vagovagal reflex is initiated during intestinal phase of digestion which greatly potentiates the effects of secretin and CCK through the acetylcholine. Thus, vagus stimulation is much more potent in stimulating pancreatic secretions when CCK and secretin are present in the plasma.

NURSING IMPLICATIONS AND APPLICATIONS

Pancreatic disorders:

Acute pancreatitis is an acute inflammatory disease of pancreas, thought to result from autodigestion of pancreatic tissue by the proteolytic enzymes which leak out of the acini and are activated within the pancreas.

Chronic pancreatitis is a chronic inflammation of pancreas which results in slow destruction of the tissue resulting in the deficiency of pancreatic secretions. Patients with extensive destruction of pancreas may develop:

- *Diabetes mellitus* due to pancreatic endocrine deficiency of insulin.
- *Digestive disturbances* due to deficiency of pancreatic enzymes mainly affect the fat metabolism resulting in *steatorrhea,* which is characterized by bulky, foul smelling, pale and greasy stools (due to increase in fecal fat content).

Cystic fibrosis is a disorder of pancreatic secretion. It is caused by a mutation in the cystic fibrosis transmembrane conductance regulator (CFTR) gene. It is associated with a deficiency of pancreatic enzymes resulting in steatorrhea.

LIVER

Gross Anatomy

Liver, the largest gland in the body, weighs approximately 1,500 g.

Location. It is located in the right hypochondriac and epigastric regions and frequently extends in the left hypochondriac area.

Surfaces. The liver has two surfaces. The upper convex surface fits closely into the under surface of the diaphragm. Below the *visceral surface* is concave and fits over the right kidney, the

upper portion of the ascending colon, and the pyloric end of stomach.

Ligaments. The liver is connected to the undersurface of diaphragm and the anterior walls by the ligaments. The falciform ligament, the coronary ligament and right and left triangular ligaments are formed by folds of peritoneum. The ligamentum teres and ligamentum venosum are fibrous cords resulting from the atrophy of left umbilical vein and ductus venosus (which exist in fetal life), respectively.

Lobes: Anatomically, the liver has been divided into *right and left lobes*. Right lobe is much larger and includes caudate lobe and quadrate lobe. Left lobe is much smaller.

- In current terminology, the liver consists of right and left functionally independent parts called the *portal lobes*, that are approximately equal in size (Figs 3.1-19A and B).
- The right and left functional parts of the liver have their own blood supply from the hepatic artery and portal vein and their own venous and biliary drainage.

Liver has got considerable physiological reserve. Even after removal of 80% of liver tissues, all *physiological* functions of liver can be accomplished normally.

The liver possesses considerable *regeneration power*. Original liver mass is restored within 6–8 weeks of removal of up to 3/4th of liver. This occurs due to active mitotic division of the cells.

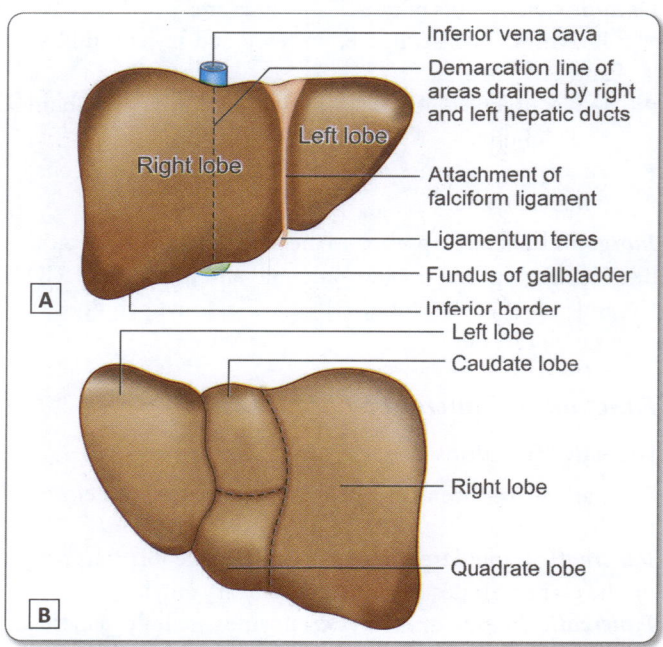

Figs 3.1-19A and B: Gross anatomy of the liver. A. Viewed from front; B. Viewed from behind

Histological and Structural Characteristics

The liver tissue comprises about one lac hexagonal areas that constitute the *hepatic lobules* (Fig. 3.1-20A).

- Each hepatic lobule is made of ramifying columns of hepatic cells (*hepatocytes*) that are arranged in the form of one cell thick plates. Bile canaliculi are present in between the cells. These hepatic cell plates are tunneled by a communicating system of lacunae called *blood sinusoids*. The sinusoids open into a central vein present in the center of each lobule (Fig. 3.1-20B).

- Blood sinusoids are lined by endothelial cells. Few tissue macrophages called *Kupffer cells* are found at regular intervals in between the endothelial cells.

- *Portal triads* are present along the periphery of each lobule.

- *Portal triads* consist of a branch of portal vein, branch of hepatic artery and an interlobular bile duct. Blood from the branch of portal vein and hepatic artery enters the sinusoids which drain into central vein.

- *Concept of portal lobule*, instead of hepatic lobule, has been suggested by some workers. It has been described to consist of adjoining part of three hepatic lobules centerd on a portal triad.

Hepatic Circulation

Liver receives about 1,500 mL blood/min from two sources:

Hepatic artery, which is a branch of celiac trunk, supplies about 20–25% (300–400 mL/min) of total blood, which caters to metabolic requirement of the liver tissue.

Portal vein, which collects blood from the mesenteric and splenic vascular bed, supplies about 75–80% (1,100–1,200 mL/min) of the total blood.

Hepatic vein. The hepatic and portal streams of blood meet in the sinusoids. The various substances produced by liver cells, the waste products and CO_2 are discharged into the sinusoids. The sinusoids drain into the central vein of the lobule. The central veins from different lobules unite to form bigger veins. These veins ultimately form the right and left hepatic veins, which open into the inferior vena cava.

Hepatic Biliary System

Intrahepatic Biliary System

The bile is secreted by liver cells into *bile canaliculi*. These canaliculi have no walls of their own. In fact, the bile canaliculi are the spaces bounded by canalicular surfaces of adjacent hepatic cells. These canaliculi form hexagonal network around the liver cells. At the periphery of a lobule, the canaliculi become continuous with delicate *intralobular ductules*, which in turn become continuous with larger interlobular ductules of portal triads. The *interlobular ductules* are lined by cuboidal epithelium. Some smooth muscle is present in the wall of larger ducts. Ultimately, the larger ducts join to form the *right and left* **hepatic ducts**, which leave the right and left parts of the liver and form part of extrahepatic biliary system.

Extrahepatic Biliary Apparatus

The extrahepatic biliary apparatus consists of gallbladder and the extrahepatic bile ducts (Fig. 3.1-21).

Gallbladder

(*Discussed later for details see page 123*)

Extrahepatic ducts

Hepatic ducts. The right and left hepatic ducts emerge from the right and left lobes of the liver and after a short course join to form *common hepatic duct*, which is about 4 cm long (Fig. 3.1-21).

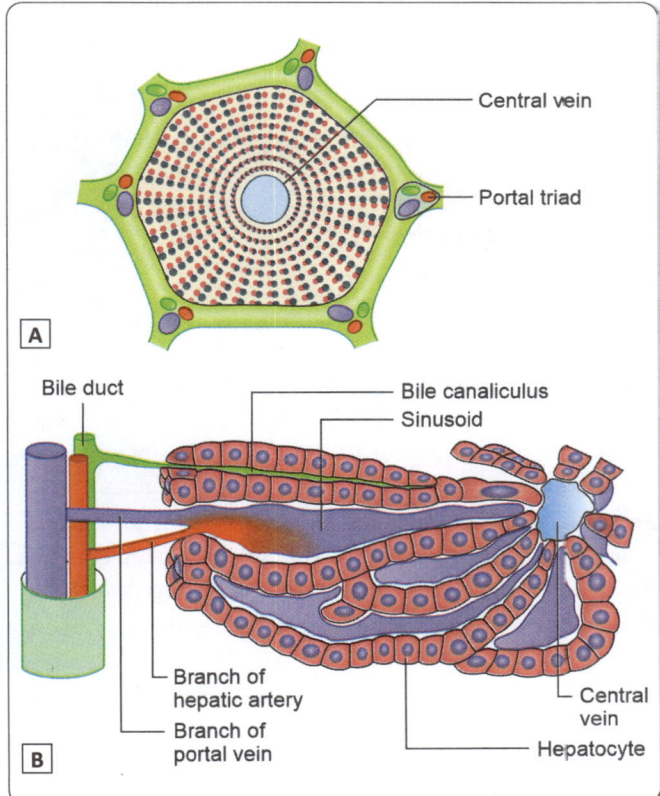

Figs 3.1-20A and B: Histological characteristics of the liver: A. Hexagonal lobule with portal triad; B. Hepatocyte, sinusoid and biliary canaliculi seen under high magnification

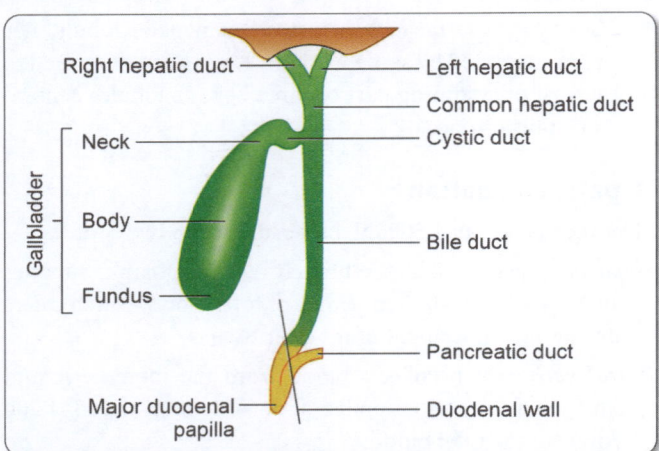

Fig. 3.1-21: Scheme to show the parts of extrahepatic biliary system

Cystic duct. It is also about 4 cm long and connects the neck of gallbladder to the common hepatic duct to form the common bile duct.

Common bile duct (CBD) is about 8 cm long. It joins the pancreatic duct to form the common hepatopancreatic duct, which is otherwise called the ampulla of Vater (Fig. 3.1-21). Ampulla of Vater opens into the duodenum at major duodenal papilla. The terminal parts of bile ducts and ampulla of Vater are surrounded by circular muscle fibers known as sphincter of Oddi, which plays an important role in the storage and release of bile from the gallbladder.

Functions of Liver

Various functions performed by liver are summarized here briefly.

1. Secretory Functions

Liver cells act as exocrine gland and continuously secrete bile, which is important for digestion and absorption of fats.

2. Metabolic Functions

Liver is the key organ and the principal site where the metabolism of carbohydrates, lipids and proteins takes place. Liver is also involved in the metabolism of vitamins and minerals to certain extent.

Role in carbohydrate metabolism. Liver acts as a glucostat in three ways:

1. *Glycogenesis,* i.e., glycogen is formed from glucose and stored in liver.

2. *Glycogenolysis,* i.e., breaking down of liver glycogen to glucose.

3. *Glucogenesis,* i.e., formation of glucose from non-carbohydrate sources such as non-nitrogenous residues of amino acids.

Role in fat metabolism. Both degradation and synthesis of fats take place in liver.

Role in protein metabolism. In man, the protein turnover involves breakdown and resynthesis of 80–100 g of tissue protein per day, and its 50% part (i.e., 40–50 g) occurs in liver.

3. Detoxicating and Protective Functions

- Kupffer cells efficiently remove bacteria and other foreign bodies from portal circulation. This is the blood cleansing action of liver.
- Liver detoxifies certain drugs by either oxidation, or hydrolysis, or reduction or conjugation and excretes out through bile.

4. Storage Functions

- Liver stores glucose (in the form of glycogen), vitamin B_{12}, and vitamin A.
- Liver acts as a blood-iron buffer and iron storage medium. It stores 60% of excess of iron mainly in the form of ferritin and partly as hemosiderin.

5. Excretory Functions

Certain exogenous dyes like bromsulphthalein (BSP) and rose Bengal dye are exclusively excreted through liver cells.

6. Synthesis Function

Liver is the site for synthesis of:

Plasma proteins, especially albumin and to some extent α- and β-globulins.

Some blood coagulation factors. Liver cells are responsible for conversion of pre-prothrombin (inactive) to active prothrombin in the presence of vitamin K. It also produces other clotting factors such as fibrinogen (I), factors V, VII, IX and X.

Enzymes, such as alkaline phosphatase, serum glutamic oxaloacetic transaminase (SGOT), serum glutamic pyruvic transaminase (SGPT), serum isocitrate dehydrogenase (SICD).

Urea. Liver removes ammonia from the body to synthesize urea.

Cholesterol is synthesized from the active acetate.

7. Miscellaneous Functions

Reservoir of blood. Liver acts as reservoir of blood and it stores about 650 mL of blood. It also helps in regulation of blood volume.

Erythropoiesis. Liver is an important site of erythropoiesis in fetal life.

Hormone metabolism. Liver causes:
- *Inactivation* of some hormones such as insulin, glucagon and vasopressin.
- *Reduction and conjugation* of adrenal and gonadal steroid hormones such as cortisol, aldosterone, estrogen and testosterone.
- *Conversion of thyroid hormone*, i.e., tetraiodo-thyronine (T_4) into triiodothyronine (T_3)

Destruction of RBCs also occurs in liver.

Thermal regulation. Liver also helps in thermo-regulation, as it produces large amount of heat.

GALLBLADDER AND BILE

Gallbladder

Gallbladder is a pear-shaped sac lying in gallbladder fossa on the undersurface of liver, where it is held in place by peritoneum, which covers its inferior (or posterior) surface (Fig. 3.1-21). It is about 7–10 cm long, 2.5 cm wide and has a capacity to store about 30–50 mL of bile.

Parts

For descriptive purposes the gallbladder is divided into three parts (Fig. 3.1-21):

Fundus is the lowest globular part, which projects beyond the inferior border of liver and is surrounded all round by peritoneum.

Body is the central part of gallbladder. Its superior (or anterior) surface is in direct contact with the liver.

Neck is the narrow part succeeding the body of gallbladder. The neck becomes continuous with the cystic duct, through which the gallbladder drains into the bile duct.

Functions of Gallbladder

Gallbladder subserves the following functions:

Storage of bile. The bile secreted during interdigestive period is stored in the gallbladder. The gallbladder typically stores 30–50 mL of bile. During meals, the gallbladder contracts and releases its contents into the duodenum.

Concentration of bile. The mucosa of gallbladder is extensively folded and can actively absorb fluid and electrolytes. In this way, the gallbladder bile, in comparison to liver bile, becomes thicker, viscous and darker in color.

Effect on the pH of bile. In the gallbladder, due to rapid absorption of HCO_3^- (mainly), Na^+ and Cl^-, the pH of bile is decreased from 8–8.6 to 7–7.6.

Secretion of mucus. Gallbladder secretes mucin which is added to the bile stored in it. The mucin acts as a lubricant in the intestine for the chyme.

Bile

Formation and Storage of Bile

Bile is a digestive juice formed continuously in the liver. It is formed by the hepatocytes and ductal cells lining the hepatic ducts.
- It is poured into the bile canaliculi from where it ultimately goes to common hepatic duct, which joins with cystic duct to form common bile duct. During interdigestive period, when the sphincter of Oddi is closed, the bile is directed via cystic duct to the gallbladder, where it is stored and concentrated.
- During meals, the sphincter of Oddi is relaxed, and when food reaches the duodenum, there occurs release of CCK, which causes contraction of gallbladder. The bile is then released into the duodenum along with the pancreatic juice through the common opening, ampulla of Vater.

Composition of Bile

The bile is an alkaline juice composed of:
- Water and solids
- Solids include organic and inorganic substances
- Organic substances are bile salts, bile pigments, cholesterol, lecithin, fatty acids and enzyme alkaline phosphatase
- Inorganic substances are Na^+, K^+, Ca^{2+}, HCO_3^- and Cl.

Since the bile is concentrated in the gallbladder, so the concentration of its ingredients in the liver bile and gallbladder bile is bound to differ.

Salient features of the some of the ingredients of bile are described as follows.

Bile salts

Bile salts are sodium and potassium salts of bile acids conjugated with either taurine or glycine.

Enterohepatic circulation of bile salts. Enterohepatic circulation is the recirculation of bile salts from the liver to small intestine and back again (Fig. 3.1-22).
- When the bile salts reach *terminal ileum*, 90–95% of bile salts are reabsorbed into the portal circulation. The liver then extracts the bile salts from the portal blood and secretes them once again into the bile.
- The remaining 5–10% of bile salts are excreted into the feces.

Circulating pool. The total circulating pool of bile salts is approximately 3.6 g. About 4–8 g of bile salts are required

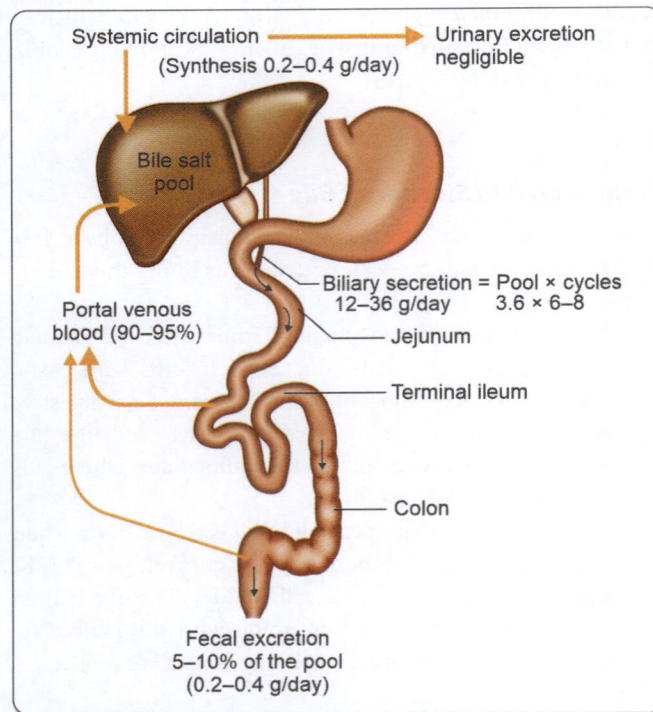

Fig. 3.1-22: Enterohepatic circulation of bile salts

(more if the meal is high in fat) for digestion of fats during each meal; as the total content of bile salts in the body is only 3.6 g, thus most circulate twice during each meal for proper digestion of fats. Consequently, the bile salts usually circulate 6–8 times daily.

Bile pigments

- The two principal bile pigments, *bilirubin* and *biliverdin*, are the other major constituents of bile, which have no digestive function.
- Bile pigments are metabolites of hemoglobin formed in the liver.
- Intestinal bacteria metabolize bilirubin further to urobilinogen, which is responsible for the brown color of stools.

Phospholipids

The phospholipids (primarily lecithins) are, after bile salts, the most abundant organic compound in bile.

Cholesterol

Cholesterol is another important constituent of bile that does not have digestive function. Biliary secretion of cholesterol is important because it is one of the few ways, in which cholesterol stores can be regulated.

Functions of Bile

Functions subserved by the bile poured into the duodenum are because of its constituents (mainly bile salts), which have already been discussed. However, they are compiled and summarized once again:

Digestive function. Bile salts help in digestion of fats by *emulsifying fat drops.*

Absorptive functions. Bile salts help in absorption of fats (by micelle formation) and fat soluble vitamins.

Excretory function. Bile pigments are the major excretory products of the bile. The other substances excreted in bile are heavy metals (e.g., copper and iron), some toxins, some bacteria (e.g., typhoid bacteria), cholesterol, lecithin and alkaline phosphatase.

Laxative action. Bile salts increase the gastrointestinal motility and act as laxative.

Protective action. Bile is a natural detergent. So, it inhibits the growth of certain bacteria in the lumen of intestine.

Choleretic action, i.e., bile salts stimulate the liver to secrete bile.

Maintenance of pH of gastrointestinal tract. Being highly alkaline, the bile juice neutralizes the gastric HCl present in the chyme entering the small intestine. Thus, an optimum pH is maintained for the action of digestive enzymes.

Prevention of gallstone formation. Bile salts keep the cholesterol and lecithin in solution and thus prevents the formation of gallstones. In the absence of bile salts, the cholesterol precipitates along with lecithin and may form gallstones.

Lubricating function. The mucin secreted by gallbladder mucosa into the bile lubricates the chyme in the intestine.

Cholagogue function. Cholagogue is an agent, which increases the release of bile from gallbladder into the intestine. The bile salts perform this function indirectly. The bile salts stimulate the secretion of hormone cholecystokinin, which has got cholagogue action.

Regulation of Bile

The regulation of bile juice released into the duodenum, after the meals, is performed at two levels:
1. Regulation of biliary secretion
2. Regulation of release of bile from the gallbladder.

Regulation of biliary secretion

Secretion of the bile juice is controlled by secretin and vagal stimulation.

Regulation of release of bile juice from gallbladder

Hormonal control. The hormone CCK is the major stimulus for gallbladder contraction and sphincter of Oddi relaxation. When chyme enters the small intestine, *fat and protein digestion products* directly stimulate the secretion of cholecystokinin.

Neural control. Vagal stimulation also causes contraction of gallbladder and relaxation of sphincter of Oddi. Vagal stimulation occurs directly during the cephalic phase of digestion and indirectly via a vagovagal reflex during the gastric phase of digestion.

NURSING IMPLICATIONS AND APPLICATIONS

DISORDERS OF LIVER AND GALLBLADDER

Jaundice or Icterus

Jaundice or icterus refers to yellow discoloration of skin and mucus membrane due to raised levels of bilirubin in the blood.
- *Normal values* of serum bilirubin range between 0.3 and 1 mg%,
- *Jaundice* manifests when serum bilirubin becomes more than 2 mg%.

Types of jaundice. Jaundice is of three types:
1. *Hemolytic jaundice* (pre-hepatic jaundice).
2. *Hepatocellular jaundice* occurs due to damage to hepatocytes, as seen in viral hepatitis, cirrhosis and drug-induced hepatitis.
3. *Obstructive jaundice*, also called post-hepatic jaundice, occurs due to blockage in bile duct either due to stone or any growth (e.g., in carcinoma of head of pancreas).

Cirrhosis of Liver

Cirrhosis of liver refers to an irreversible chronic damage to liver with extensive fibrosis.

Viral Hepatitis

- *Etiology.* Viral hepatitis (inflammation of liver) is caused by hepatitis virus A, B, C, D, E, F or G.
- *Hepatitis-B* is more popular.

Cholecystitis

Cholecystitis refers to inflammation of gallbladder.

Gallstones

Gallstones are formed due to precipitation of cholesterol. Normally, cholesterol is present in soluble form due to a proper ratio of cholesterol and bile salts (1:20–1:30). When this ratio falls below 1:13, the cholesterol is precipitated forming many small crystals.

Liver Function Tests

The liver function tests (LFTs) are the investigations to assess the capacity of the liver to carry any of the functions it performs. Thus, LFTs help in:
- Assessing the extent of functional damage to the liver
- Diagnosing the cause of hepatic insufficiency
- Assessing the progress/regress of the disease.

Tests to Assess Secretory Functions of Liver

Serum bilirubin. The *normal values* are:
- Total serum bilirubin: 0.3–1.0 mg%
- Conjugated bilirubin: 0.1–0.3 mg%
- Unconjugated bilirubin: 0.2–0.7 mg%

Van den Bergh test is specific to identify the increase in serum bilirubin (above reference level). The results of test are interpreted as:
- Normal serum: Negative reaction
- Hemolytic jaundice: Indirect positive reaction
- Obstructive jaundice: Direct positive reaction
- Hepatic jaundice: Biphasic reaction.

Urine bilirubin and bile salts. Normally urine does not contain bilirubin and bile salts. In liver insufficiency, when the serum bilirubin levels increase above 2 mg% the bilirubin is excreted in the urine (*bilirubinuria*).

Urine urobilinogen. In normal individuals, less than 4 mg of urobilinogen is excreted in the urine. In liver insufficiency, initially there occurs mild increase in the daily excretion of urine urobilinogen. However, in later stages, urobilinogen is absent in the urine. This occurs because of the fact that the swollen liver cells block bile canaliculi and prevent excretion of conjugated bilirubin in the bile.

Fecal stercobilinogen. Normal levels 20–25 mg%.
- Increased initially in liver insufficiency producing dark brown stools.
- Decreased in later stages of liver insufficiency producing pale-colored stool.

Fecal fat levels. Normally, 5–6% of total fat intake per day is excreted in the feces.
In liver insufficiency fat excretion in feces increases up to 40–50% of total intake (steatorrhea).

Tests to Assess Metabolic Functions of Liver

Galactose tolerance test. This test is based on the principle that galactose after absorption from the gut gets converted into glycogen in the liver. Therefore, in liver insufficiency, its level in the blood rises.

Blood glucose level. The normal fasting blood glucose level is 70–90 mg%. In hepatic insufficiency, its level decreases.

Blood and urine amino acid levels. Blood and urine amino acid levels are estimated to assess protein metabolism. In liver damage, blood amino acid levels (normal 30–65 mg%) and urine amino acid levels are increased.

Lipid profile. In hepatic insufficiency, lipid profile is affected as abnormalities of serum lipid levels are sensitive but nonspecific indicators.

Tests to Assess Synthesis Functions of Liver

Estimation of plasma proteins

Albumin. Liver cell damage causes hypoalbuminemia (normal 6.4–8.3 g%).

Globulin. Hyperglobulinemia is usually associated with hypoalbuminemia.

A:G ratio. In liver disorder, there occurs reversal of A:G ratio (normal 1.7:1).

Serum levels of liver enzymes

Transaminases. The activity of transaminase like SGPT and SGOT increases in hepatic insufficiency.

Alkaline phosphatase. Alkaline phosphatase is not a liver-specific enzyme, but secreted into the bile. In obstructive jaundice, its level is markedly increased (>30 KA units).

Blood urea. Liver is the main site for urea formation from ammonia. Decreased level of blood urea (normal 20–40 mg%) and raised blood ammonia level (normal 20–80 mg%) occur in liver insufficiency.

Coagulation factors

Factors II, V, VII, IX and X and vitamin K are synthesized by the liver. The integrity and activity of these factors is determined by prothrombin time test (PTT). Prolonged prothrombin time (PT) (normal 10–16 sec) indicates severe liver disease.

Tests to Assess Detoxication Functions of Liver

Bromsulphthalein (BSP) excretion test. BSP is taken up by the liver cells from the blood and detoxified and excreted in the bile. The rate of removal of BSP from the blood depends on the functional efficiency of liver and rate of hepatic blood flow.

Tests to Assess Hepatic Cellular Integrity

Ultrasonography is done to detect diffuse disease of parenchyma of the liver (cirrhosis liver, fatty liver), abscess, cysts, tumors, gallstones and dilatation of biliary system proximal to site of obstruction.

Computed tomography (CT). CT scan has the same diagnostic significance as the ultrasonography except that it can also detect even smaller lesions.

Liver biopsy. This is performed by a special needle passed through intercostal space under local anesthesia to obtain tissue for histopathological examination.

Fine needle aspiration (FNA). Very fine needle is usually guided by ultrasound and material is aspirated for cytological, histopathological and bacteriological examination.

Cholecystography is done to assess the functions and diseases of gallbladder. Nowadays this test is less commonly performed than ultrasonography.

SMALL INTESTINE

GROSS ANATOMY

The small intestine is convoluted tube which extends from the pylorus of stomach to the ileocecal valve, where it joins with cecum, the first part of large intestine. It is about 6–7 m in length.

PARTS OF SMALL INTESTINE

It is divided into three parts: the duodenum, the jejunum and the ileum (Figs 3.1-23A and B).

Duodenum. The first and *shortest* part (25 cm long) of the small intestine is also the *widest* and most fixed part. It is C-shaped and for descriptive purposes is divided into four parts: superior (1st) part, descending (2nd) part, horizontal (3rd) part, and ascending (4th part). Superior part of duodenum is also called *duodenal cap* or bulb. It is the region, which is struck by acidic gastric contents when they pass through pylorus and is a *common site for peptic ulcer*. The bile and pancreatic ducts open by a common hepatopancreatic ampulla of Vater on the posteromedial wall of descending (2nd) part of duodenum.

Jejunum and ileum. Jejunum and ileum form, respectively, the proximal 2/5th and distal 3/5th of the remaining part of small intestine. There is no sharp demarcation between jejunum and ileum. The inner mucosal surfaces of jejunum and ileum, however, can be differentiated from each other.

STRUCTURAL CHARACTERISTICS OF SMALL INTESTINE

Histologically the wall of small intestine is made up of 4 layers, which from within to outwards consist of: mucosa, submucosa, muscle coat and serosa (Figs 3.1-23, 3.1-24 and Histology Plate 3.1-4).

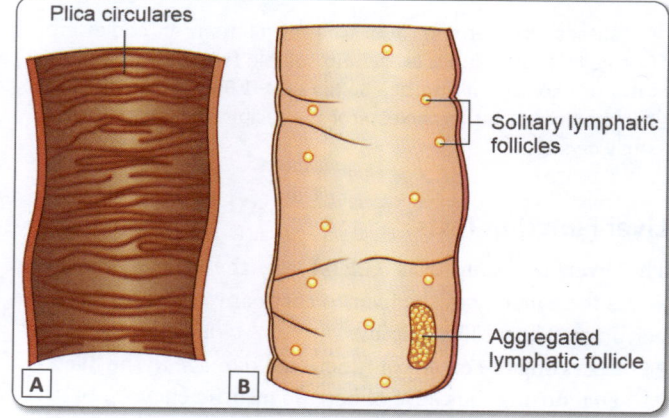

Figs 3.1-23A and B: The mucosal surface of jejunum (A) and ileum (B)

Histology Plate 3.1-4: Duodenum, Jejunum and Ileum

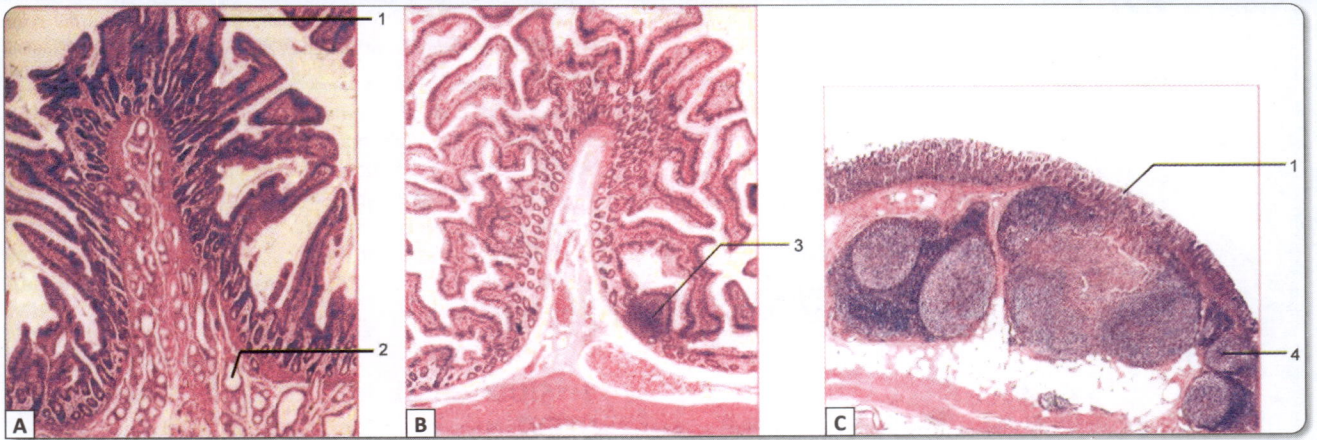

Photomicrographs of duodenum (A) jejunum (B) and ileum (C) are shown. All three are lined by simple columnar epithelium (1). Villi of duodenum are tall, broad and leaf-shaped, while in jejunum and ileum, they have clubbed end and are finger-shaped, respectively. Mucus secreting Brunner's gland (2) in submucosa are a typical feature of duodenum. Jejunum contains large number of lymphatic follicles (3) in lamina propria. Peyer's patches (4) mark the distinction while identifying ileum.

Features of Mucosal Surface of Small Intestine

Although the small intestine is about 6 m long, it has an absorptive area of over 250 m². This larger surface is created by certain characteristic features of the interior, i.e., mucosal surface of the small intestine, which include the following.

Plicae Circulares

The mucosal surface shows numerous circular folds (plicae circulares or valvulae conniventes) (Fig. 3.1-24). Each fold is made up of all layers of the mucosa (lining epithelium, lamina propria, and muscularis mucosa). The submucosa also extends into the fold. The circular folds increase surface area for absorption and also slow down the passage of contents through small intestine, which facilitate absorption.

Villi

Villi are finger-like projections of mucus membrane seen throughout the length of small intestine (Fig. 3.1-24).

Structure. Each villus is covered by a single layer of columnar epithelial cells called enterocytes. The *microvilli* protrude from the surface of intestinal cells. The core of each villus contains (Fig. 3.1-25 and Histology Plate 3.1-5):

- An *arteriole and venule*
- A fine network of *nerves,* which has connections with submucosal and myenteric plexus.

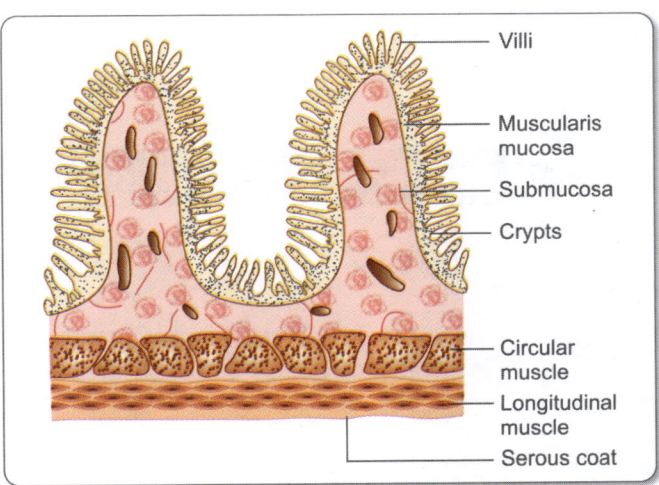

Fig. 3.1-24: Histological structure of small intestine. Note features of plica circulares and villi

Activity. During digestion and absorption, the villi contract quickly with an irregular rhythm and relax slowly. Their muscular fibers serve to pump the lymph from core of villi toward the submucosal lacteals.

Crypts of Lieberkuhn

The crypts of Lieberkühn are single tubular intestinal glands, which invaginate deep into the lamina propria, present

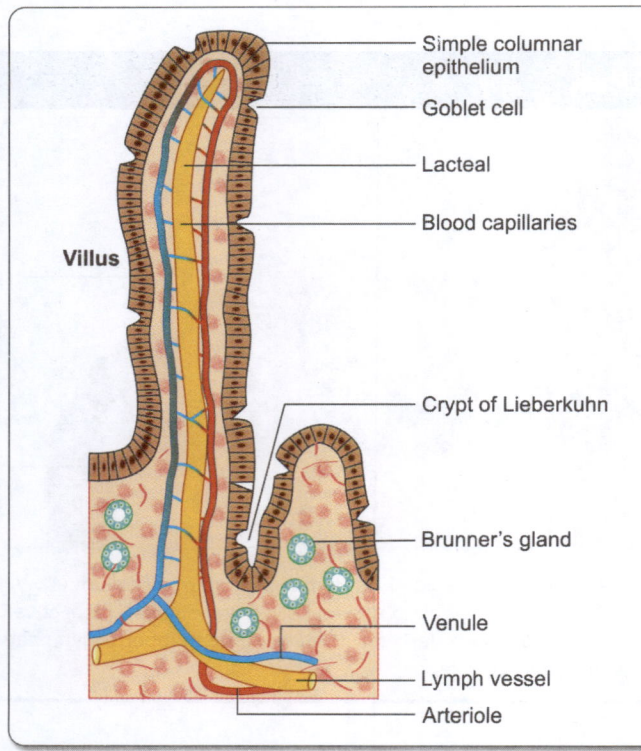

Fig. 3.1-25: Structure of an intestinal villus, crypts of Lieberkuhn and an enterocyte

- Simple columnar epithelium
- Goblet cell
- Lacteal
- Blood capillaries
- Villus
- Crypt of Lieberkuhn
- Brunner's gland
- Venule
- Lymph vessel
- Arteriole

between the villi throughout the length of small intestine (Fig. 3.1-25). These glands are lined by undifferentiated columnar cells and also contain goblet cells, argentaffin cells and Paneth cells.

IMPORTANT TO KNOW

Duodenal glands of Brunner are limited only to the duodenum. These are compound tubuloalveolar glands present in submucosa of duodenum. Their ducts pass through the muscularis mucosa to open into the crypts of Lieberkuhn. They are situated mostly near the pylorus; beyond pylorus their number greatly diminishes. Secretion of these glands contain *mucus and HCO_3^-,* which neutralizes gastric acid entering the duodenum and thus protects its mucosa.

PHYSIOLOGICAL ACTIVITIES IN SMALL INTESTINE

Small Intestinal Secretions

Composition and Formation

The intestinal juice also called *succus entericus* comprises the intestinal secretions which include:

Aqueous component of intestinal juice. Aqueous component of intestinal juice primarily refers to water and electrolytes se-

Histology Plate 3.1-5: Intestinal villus

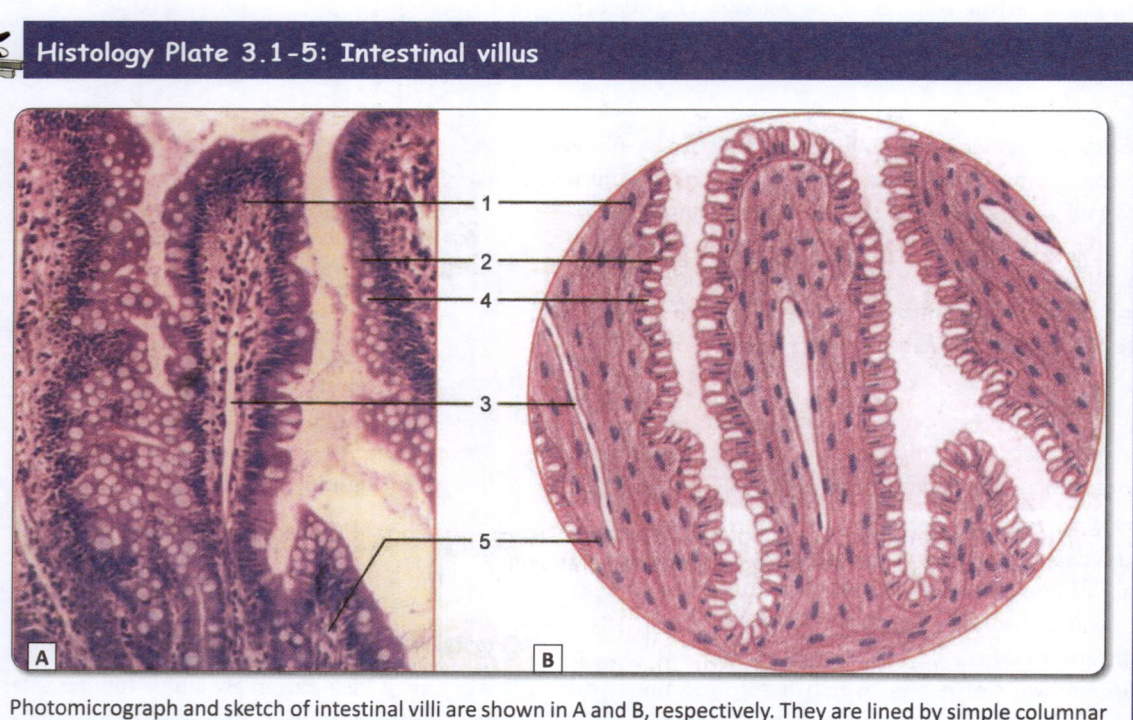

Photomicrograph and sketch of intestinal villi are shown in A and B, respectively. They are lined by simple columnar epithelium (2) with goblet cells (4). Central lacteal (3) is visible in villi (1). Lamina propria (5) is also seen.

creted by the epithelial cells of small intestine, especially those present in the crypts of Lieberkuhn.

Functions. The watery secretion provides a solvent into which the products of digestion are dissolved. This fluid is rapidly reabsorbed by the intestinal villi. Thus, circulation of this fluid from the crypts to the villi supplies a watery vehicle for absorption of foodstuffs from the small intestine.

Intestinal enzymes. Brush border of epithelial cells covering the villi contains a large number of intracellular digestive enzymes. The enzymes, which have been identified in the brush border are:

- *Peptidases* (proteolytic enzymes).
- *Disaccharidases* such as sucrase, maltase and lactase.
- *Intestinal lipases.*
- *Enterokinase* or enteropeptidase.

Mucus. Mucus in the small intestine is secreted by:

- *Brunner's glands*, which secrete thick alkaline mucoid secretion that serves a protective role, preventing HCl and chyme from damaging the duodenal mucosa.
- *Goblet cells* also secrete lot of mucus, which protects the intestinal mucosa and lubricates the chyme.

Regulation of Small Intestinal Secretions

Local stimuli: Mechanical distension of intestinal mucosa by the food or irritation by chemicals, via local myenteric reflexes, increase the volume and total enzyme output of the small intestine; that is why, the greater is the chyme, greater is the secretion of intestinal secretion.

Role of vasoactive intestinal polypeptide (VIP). Though the secretion of the crypts of Lieberkuhn is mainly regulated by the local stimuli, but the local hormone VIP is also reported to increase its secretion.

Secretion of Brunner's gland is increased by:

- Vagus stimulation
- Direct tactile stimulation or irritation of the duodenal mucosa
- Secretin.

Functions of Intestinal Juice

Functions of small intestine are described in Chapter 3.2.

Motility of Small Intestine

Motility of small intestine includes:

- Mixing movements such as segmentation contractions and pendular movements
- Propulsive movements such as peristaltic contractions and peristaltic rush
- Movements of villi
- Motility reflexes.

Mixing Movements

The mixing movements of small intestine are responsible for proper mixing of chyme with digestive juices like pancreatic juice, bile juice and intestinal juice. The mixing movements of small intestine include:

- Segmentation contractions
- Pendular movements.

Segmentation contractions

During segmentation contraction, a section of the small intestine (about 2–5 cm) contracts, sending the intestinal contents (chyme) in both oral and caudal directions. That section of the small intestine then relaxes and the contents move back into that segment. At the same time, the adjoining segment which was relaxed, now contracts (Fig. 3.1-26).

The alternate contracted and relaxed segments give a ring-like appearance resembling the chain of sausages.

Pendular movements

These are small constrictive waves, which sweep forward and backward or upward and downward in pendular fashion. These mixing movements can be noticed only by close observation.

Propulsive Movements

The propulsive movements of small intestine are involved in pushing the chyme toward the aboral end of intestine. These include:

- Peristaltic contractions
- Peristaltic rush.

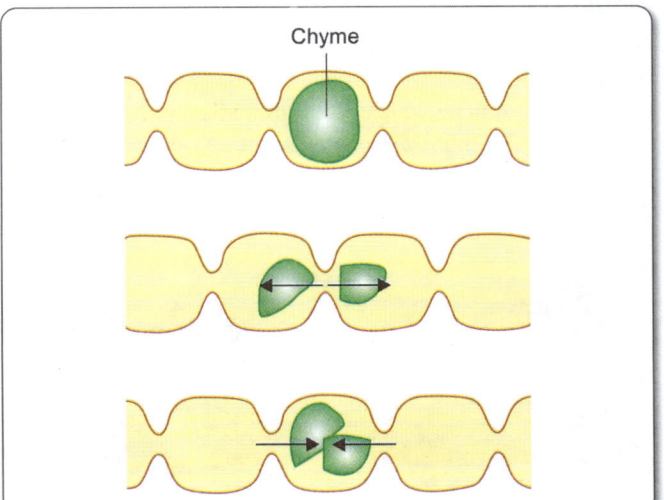

Fig. 3.1-26: Segmentation contractions of small intestine

Peristaltic contractions

Peristalsis refers to a wave of contraction preceded by a wave of relaxation.

IMPORTANT TO KNOW

Law of intestine: The peristaltic waves always travel from the oral end toward the aboral end of the intestine. This phenomenon has been labeled as the *Law of the intestine* by Starling in 1901.

The peristaltic contractions are highly coordinated and typically a peristaltic contraction involves contraction of a segment behind the bolus and simultaneous relaxation of the segment in front of the bolus, causing the chyme to be propelled caudally (Fig. 3.1-27).

Peristaltic rush

Peristaltic rush refers to a very powerful peristaltic contraction which occurs when intestinal mucosa is irritated intensely as in some infectious processes.

Movements of Villi

Movements of villi consist of alternate shortening and elongation of the villi caused by contraction and relaxation of the muscle. *Villikinin*, a hormone secreted from small intestinal mucosa, plays an important role in increasing the movements of villi.

Functions. The surface area of villi is increased during elongation. This helps in absorption of digested foodstuffs from the lumen of intestine.

Initiation. Local nervous reflexes, which occur in response to the presence of chyme in small intestine, initiate the movements of villi.

Motility Reflexes

Gastroileal reflex. Gastroileal reflex refers to marked increase in the peristaltic contractions of ileum associated with relaxation of ileocecal sphincter which occur immediately after the meals. As a result, the intestinal contents are delivered to the large intestine.

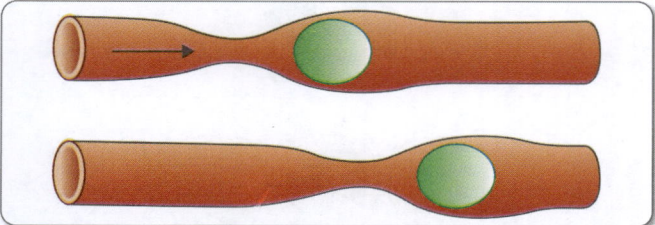

Fig. 3.1-27: Peristaltic contraction moves the food through intestine by pushing bolus ahead of muscle contraction

Intestinointestinal reflex. Intestinointestinal reflex refers to relaxation of smooth muscles of the rest of the small intestine in response to overdistension of one segment of the intestine.

FUNCTIONS OF SMALL INTESTINE

The functions of small intestine can be summarized as:
Mechanical functions. The mixing and propulsive movements of the small intestine help in thorough mixing of chyme with the digestive juices (pancreatic juice, bile juice and succus entericus) and propel it toward the large intestine.

Digestive functions of small intestine are carried out by the digestive enzymes present in the:
- Succus entericus
- Pancreatic enzymes
- Bile.

Absorptive function is accomplished by the huge surface area created by the presence of plicae circulares, villi and microvilli. The end products of digestion of carbohydrates, proteins and fats are absorbed through portal system or through the lymph.

Hormonal functions. The small intestine secretes certain hormones which exert their effect on the secretions and motility of gastrointestinal tract. These hormones include *enterogastrone, secretin* and CCK.

Activator function. The enzyme enterokinase secreted by small intestine activates trypsinogen into trypsin, which in turn activates other enzymes.

Protective function. The mucus secreted into the succus entericus protects the intestinal wall from the gastric acid chyme.

Hydrolytic function. The aqueous component of the succus entericus provides water and thus helps in all the hydrolytic processes of enzymatic reactions of digestion of various food particles.

LARGE INTESTINE

GROSS ANATOMY

The large intestine is a tube about 6 cm in diameter and 150 cm in length. It normally arches around and encloses the coils of small intestine and tends to be more fixed than the small intestine. It extends from the ileum to the anus and is divided into the following parts (Fig. 3.1-28).

Cecum with Appendix

Cecum is a blind-ended sac into which opens the lower end of ileum. The ileocecal junction is guarded by the ileocecal valve, which allows inflow but prevents backflow of intestinal contents.

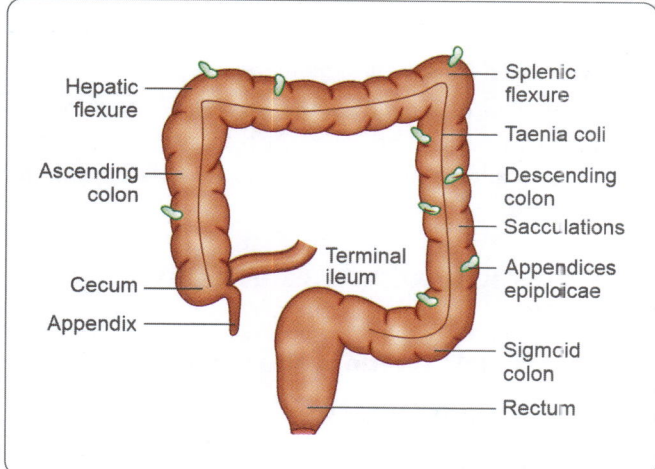

Fig. 3.1-28: Functional organization of the large intestine.
Note: *The labeling of the figure also depicts consistency of fecal contents in its different segments*

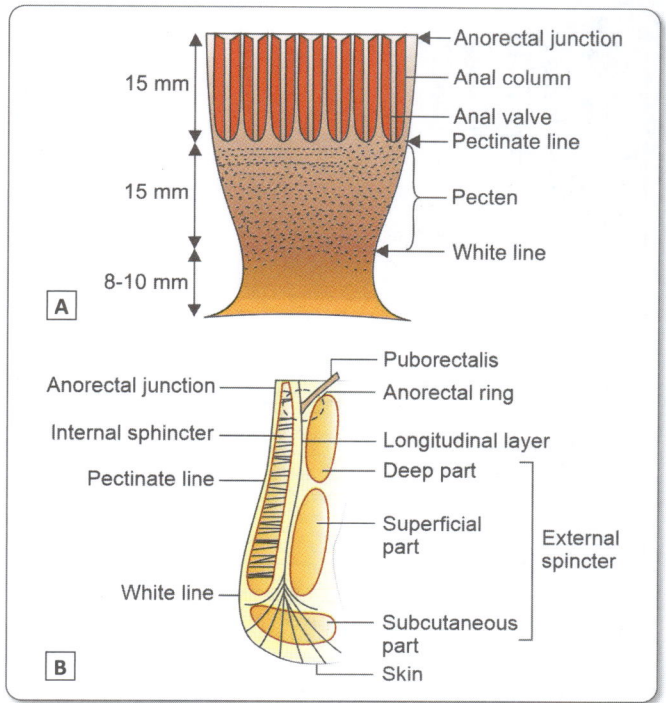

Figs 3.1-29A and B: A. Schematic interior view of the anal canal;
B. Longitudinal section through the anal canal wall to show the anal sphincters and their relation to interior of anal canal.

Appendix is worm-shaped tube that arises from the medial side of cecum which in human being is a vestigial organ.

Colon

The colon, major part of large intestine, can be differentiated from the small intestine by the presence of *haustrations* (a series of sacculations), and *taenia coli* (three bands of thickenings in muscular layer) which run along the length of the colon, approximately equidistant from each other. The colon, although one continuous tube, is subdivided into the ascending, transverse, descending and sigmoid colon.

Ascending colon extends upward from the cecum along the right side of abdomen up to the liver. On reaching the liver, it bends to the left, forming the right hepatic flexure.

Transverse colon extends from the right hepatic flexure to the left splenic flexure and is about 50 cm in length. It is covered by peritoneum all round and is suspended from the posterior abdominal wall by the transverse mesocolon.

Descending colon extends from the left splenic flexure to the pelvic inlet. It is about 25 cm long and ends by becoming continuous with sigmoid colon.

Sigmoid colon begins at the pelvic inlet as continuation of the descending colon and joins the rectum in front of the sacrum.

Rectum

It descends in front of the sacrum to leave the pelvis by piercing the pelvic floor. Here it becomes continuous with anal canal in the perineum. Anteriorly, the rectum is related in the male to the urinary bladder and prostate and in the female to the lower part of uterus and the vagina.

It opens to the exterior through the anus, the opening which is guarded by two sphincters.

Interior of the anal canal is divided into three parts (Figs 3.1-29A and B):

1. Upper part, about 15 mm in length, is characterized by presence of longitudinal mucosal folds, the anal columns.

2. Middle part, about 15 mm in length, is lined by smooth mucosa. It is separated above from the upper part by a wavy line of mucosa the *pectinate* line and below from the lower part by the *white line*.

3. Lower part, about 10 mm in length, is lined by skin.

STRUCTURAL CHARACTERISTICS

Histological structure of large intestines is similar to that described in general with the following special characteristics.

Mucosa of large intestine is characterized by:
- Absence of plicae circulares and villi (as seen in small intestine).
- A large number of simple tubular glands (crypts of Lieberkühn) lined by simple columnar epithelial cells with large number of goblet cells, which secrete mucus (Fig. 3.1-30 and Histology Plate 3.1-6).

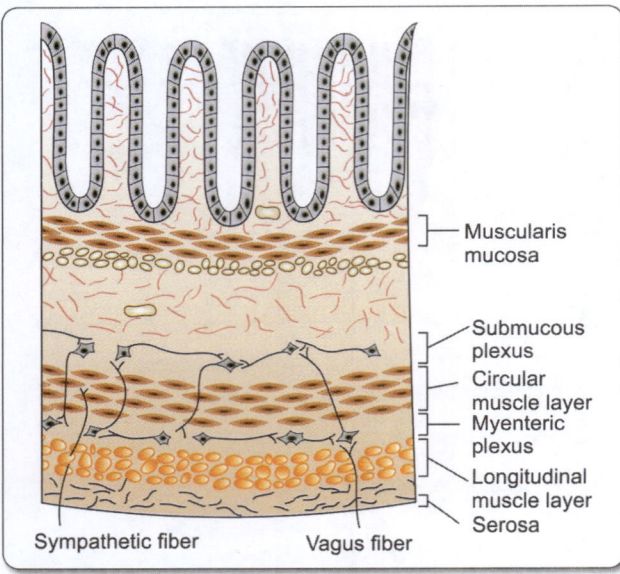

Fig. 3.1-30: Histological structure of the colon

Muscle coat. Longitudinal layer of colon is unusual

- Most of the fibers in it are collected to form three thick bands, the taenia coli which can be seen through the serous layer. A thin layer of longitudinal fibers is present in the intestines between the taenia.

- The taenia coli is shorter in length than other layers of the wall of colon. This results in the production of *sacculations* (also caslled *haustrations*) on the wall of colon.

Serous layer is missing over the posterior aspect of the ascending and descending colon. At places small peritoneal bags of fat, called *appendices epiploicae*, project from the colonic serosa.

PHYSIOLOGICAL ACTIVITIES IN LARGE INTESTINE

Large Intestinal Secretions and Bacterial Activity

Large Intestinal Secretions

- The large intestinal secretions mainly comprise mucus secreted by the goblet cells, and some water and lot of HCO_3^- secreted by glands of Lieberkuhn.

- The mucus lubricates the fecal matter and also protects the mucus membrane of large intestine by preventing the damage caused by mechanical injury or chemical substances.

- The alkaline nature (pH 8.0) of the mucoid secretions of the large intestine is due to the presence of HCO_3^-. It serves to neutralize the acids formed by bacterial action on the fecal matter.

Histology Plate 3.1-6: Colon and Rectum

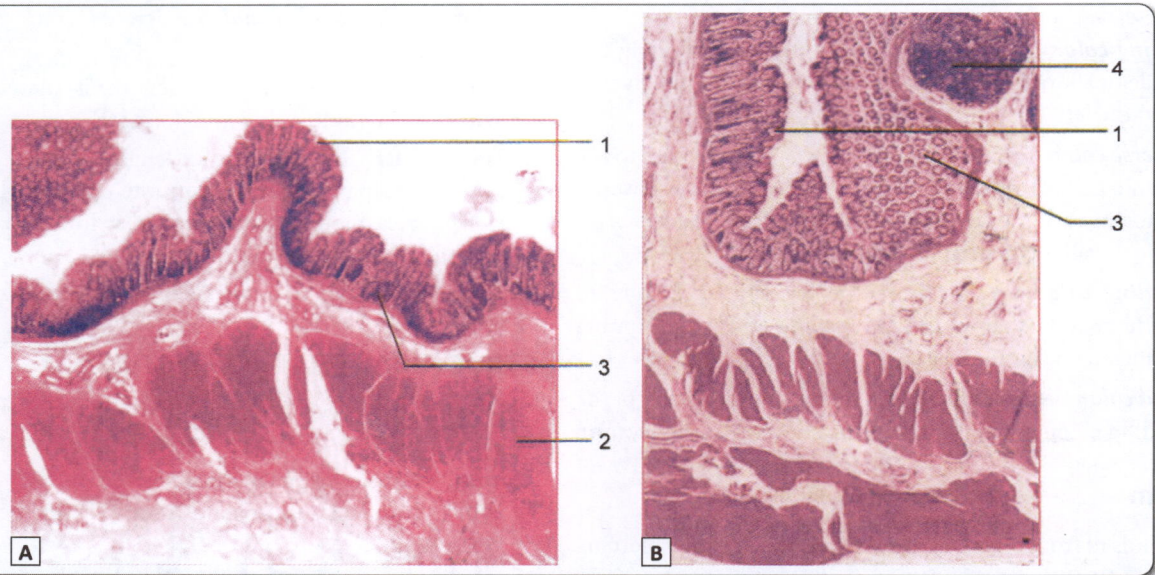

Photomicrographs of colon (A) and rectum (B) are shown. They are lined by simple columnar epithelium with plenty of goblet cells (1), and intestinal glands (3) are seen. The taenia coli (2) can be seen in muscularis externa layer in colon, which are absent in rectum, lymphatic nodule (4) can be seen in rectum.

Intestinal Bacterial Activity

Bacterial flora. At birth, the colon is sterile, but the colonic bacterial flora becomes established early in life and includes:

Harmless bacteria such as *E. coli* and *Enterobacter aerogenes*

Potentially dangerous bacteria such as *Bacteroides fragilis*, various types of cocci and gas gangrene bacilli. These bacteria can cause serious disease in tissues outside the colon.

Intestinal bacterial activities include:

Synthesis of vitamins such as vitamin C, a number of B-complex vitamins and folic acid.

Trophic effects on colonic mucosa. Unabsorbed carbohydrates are converted to short-chain fatty acids by colonic bacteria. Some of the short-chain fatty acids produced have a trophic effect on colonic mucosa.

Play a role in cholesterol metabolism by decreasing plasma cholesterol and low density lipoprotein (LDL) levels.

Motility of Large Intestine

Types of Movements

The different types of movements (most accepted nomenclature) of colon are.

Haustral shuttling

The haustral shuttling or haustral contractions are similar to the segmentation contractions of small intestine, which vigorously mix the contents of colon and by exposing more of the contents to mucosa facilitate absorption.

Peristalsis

Peristalsis is a progressive contractile wave preceded by a wave of relaxation. In the colon, the peristalsis waves are very small pressure waves of prolonged duration.

Function. They propel the contents toward rectum very slowly (5 cm/hour). It can take up to 48 hours for the chyme to traverse the colon.

Mass movements

- The mass movements are special type of peristaltic contractions which are observed in the colon only.
- These occur 3–4 times a day generally after meals and each contraction lasts for about 3 minutes.

NURSING IMPLICATIONS AND APPLICATIONS

Gastrocolic Reflex
Gastrocolic reflex refers to contraction of colon induced by entry of food into the stomach. This reflex results in an urge to defecate after a meal. Because of this, defecation after meals is a rule in children. However, in adults, the bowel training suppresses this reflex.

- The mass movements force the fecal material rapidly in mass down the colon. They also move material into the rectum and rectal distension initiates the defecation reflex.

Defecation

Functional Anatomy

A brief description of functional anatomy of the anal sphincters, which play most important role in the process of defecation needs special emphasis.

Internal or involuntary anal sphincter consists of thickened circular smooth muscles at the pelvic-rectal flexure. It extends from the upper end of anal canal up to the white line. This sphincter relaxes reflexly in response to stimulation of stretch receptors when the rectum is distended.

Innervation of internal anal sphincter is by:

Parasympathetic pelvic splanchnic nerves, which are inhibitory

Sympathetic nerves, which are excitatory.

External or voluntary anal sphincter consists of somatic skeletal muscle fibers innervated by the pudendal nerves. It is divided into deep, superficial and subcutaneous parts.

Characterstic features are:

- It is maintained in a state of tonic contraction.
- Mild to moderate distension of the rectum increases its force of contraction.
- Moderately severe distension of rectum initiates a reflex, which inhibits the discharge of somatic pudendal nerves (which cause tonic contraction) and thus relaxes the internal anal sphincter.
- The external anal sphincter can be voluntarily relaxed, the action which aids the reflex emptying of the distended rectum.

The Act of Defecation

Defecation, the process of excretion of fecal material, involves both voluntary and reflex activity. The events associated with process of defecation proceed as follows:

Distension of rectum. Usually, once or twice a day gastrocolic reflex drives the feces into the rectum which increase the intrarectal pressure passively.

Defecation reflexes. As the rectum starts filling, the resultant rise in the intrarectal pressure stimulates the stretch receptors, and sets up defecation reflexes. As a result there occurs:

- Intensification of colonic peristaltic contraction further raising the intrarectal pressure.
- When the rectal pressure reaches to about 55 mm Hg, there occurs further relaxation of internal and external anal sphincters.

Role of voluntary control on defecation. Once the above described reflex effects are obtained, the voluntary control mechanism depending upon the convenience may or may not allow the act of defecation to occur.

When defecation is not allowed, the voluntary control mechanism maintains the contraction of external anal sphincter (which is composed of skeletal muscle innervated by the pudendal nerves). Soon, the internal anal sphincter also closes and the rectum relaxes to accommodate the fecal matter within it. Once the defecation reflex dies out, it recurs after some hours.

IMPORTANT TO KNOW

When it is convenient to defecate:
- The external anal sphincter is relaxed voluntarily. Thus, both internal and external sphincters are relaxed.
- The intra-abdominal pressure is increased by contraction of abdominal and diaphragmatic muscles (a process of expiring against closed glottis, i.e., Valsalva).
- The smooth muscles of the distal colon and rectum contract forcibly, propelling the fecal matter out of the body through the anal canal.

Feces

Composition

Feces or the fecal matter is derived mainly from the intestinal secretion and partly from the undigested material. The fecal matter consists of:

Water, forms the main bulk of feces (75%), and

Solids, contribute 25% to total fecal matter weight. These include:
- *Inorganic material,* mostly calcium and phosphate
- *Undigested plant fibers,* epithelial cells, dead bacteria, constituents of intestinal secretions including bile pigments, fats and proteins.

pH of stools is slightly acidic (5–7) due to the organic acids formed from carbohydrates by colonic bacteria.

Brown color of stools is due to the pigment *urobilin*, which is formed from oxidation of urobilinogen, which is colorless.

Odor of stools is due to the presence of substances like indole, skatole, mercaptans and hydrogen sulfide. These substances are formed by the action of colonic bacteria on the food.

FUNCTIONS OF LARGE INTESTINE

The functions of large intestine, thus can be summarized as:

Secretory functions. The large intestinal secretion mainly comprises mucin, which helps to lubricate the fecal matter.

The alkaline nature (pH 8) of the secretion serves to neutralize the acids formed by bacterial action on the fecal matter.

Synthesis functions. The bacterial flora of the large intestine synthesizes folic acid, vitamin B_{12} and vitamin K.

Absorptive functions. Absorption of water and electrolytes is the chief function of proximal part of the colon. Organic substances like glucose, alcohol, and some drugs like anesthetic agents, sedatives and steroids can also be absorbed in large intestine. The vitamin K and a number of B complex vitamins which are synthesized in colon by bacterial flora are also absorbed in the large intestine.

Excretory functions. Heavy metals like mercury, lead, bismuth and arsenic are excreted by large intestine through the feces.

NURSING IMPLICATIONS AND APPLICATIONS

APPLIED ASPECTS OF DEFECATION

Defecation in infants: In infants, defecation reflex causes automatic emptying of lower bowel without normal voluntary control on external anal sphincter. The voluntary control of the reflex by higher centers is attained by social training as the child grows.

Defecation in individuals with spinal cord transection: In individuals with spinal cord transection, initially there occurs retention of feces. But defecation reflex returns quickly. However, reflex evacuation occurs automatically, without voluntary control, when the rectal pressure increases to about 55 mm Hg.

Role of dietary fibers: Dietary fibers increase bulk of feces; they play a role in defecation reflex by distending the rectum.
Therapeutic role of dietary fibers: The daily recommended intake of dietary fibers is about 25–35 g/day. High fiber supplements have therapeutic role in the following conditions:
- In constipation
- In spastic colon and diverticular disease
- In diabetes and high cholesterol levels.

DISORDERS OF LARGE INTESTINE MOTILITY

Hirschsprung's disease: Hirschsprung's disease, or the aganglionic megacolon refers to congenital absence of Auerbach's plexus in the wall of rectosigmoid region. This leads to blockage of both the peristalsis and mass contractions at the aganglionic segment. Therefore, the feces pass the aganglionic segment with difficulty and accumulate in the large intestine leading to dilatation of the colon (megacolon).

Constipation: Constipation refers to failure of voiding of feces, which produces discomfort. It results from infrequent mass movement in the colon. As a result, the fecal matter remains in the colon for longer time, so large amount of fluid is absorbed and the feces become hard and dry.

Diarrhea: Diarrhea is a condition, which is characterized by increased frequency of defecation with increased water content of the feces.

ASSESS YOURSELF

Short and Long Answer Questions

1. **Describe briefly:**
   • Structural characteristics of GIT wall
   • Innervation of gut
   • Composition of saliva
   • Composition of gastric secretion
   • Functions of gastric secretion
   • Regulation of gastric secretion
   • Gastric motility
   • Composition of pancreatic secretion
   • Functions of liver
   • Composition of bile

2. **Write short notes on:**
   • Deglutition reflex
   • Cardiac achlasia
   • Gastrin
   • Gastric mucosal barrier
   • Portal triad
   • Bile salts
   • Defecation reflex

Multiple Choice Questions

1. **The fold of peritoneum extending from liver to lesser curvature of the stomach is:**
   a. Greater omentum
   b. Lesser omentum
   c. Mesentery
   d. Coronary ligament

2. **Meissner's plexus is located:**
   a. Between surface epithelium and lamina propria
   b. In submucosa
   c. Between lamina propria and muscularis mucosa
   d. Between circular and longitudinal layers of muscle coat

3. **Choose the correct statement for gut innervations:**
   a. Enteric nervous system supplies the musculature of whole of GIT.
   b. Myenteric plexus is located in the submucosal coat.
   c. Auerbach's plexus is located in the submucosal coat.
   d. Meissner's plexus is present between circular and longitudinal layers of muscle coat.

4. **Stimulation of sympathetic innervations to the gut causes:**
   a. Increase motility
   b. Increase secretion
   c. Increase in blood flow
   d. Inhibition of motility

5. **In the permanent set of teeth, the canines are:**
   a. 4
   b. 8
   c. 12
   d. 16

6. **Which is not the muscle of mastication?**
   a. External pterygoid
   b. Buccinator
   c. Temporalis
   d. Arytenoid

7. **The watery salivary secretion is contributed by which gland?**
   a. Parotid
   b. Submendibular
   c. Sublingual
   d. Smaller salivary glands

8. **The HCL of the gastric secretion is by:**
   a. Chief cells
   b. Parietal cells
   c. Mucous cells
   d. G cells

9. **For chemical control of gastric secretion, the true statement is:**
   a. Gastrin increases activity of parietal cells.
   b. Histamine increases HCl by acting through H_2 receptors.
   c. Low pH increases HCl secretion.
   d. Products of protein digestion inhibit HCl secretion.

10. **The true statement for vomiting center:**
    a. Also called chemoreceptor trigger zone
    b. Located in the pons
    c. Located in area postrema
    d. Stimulated by raised intracranial pressure

11. **The true statement for hepatic blood sinusoids:**
    a. Open into the portal vein
    b. Are lined by hepatocytes
    c. Receive blood from central vein
    d. Drain blood into the central vein

12. **The Brunner's glands are present in which part of the intestines:**
    a. Jejunum
    b. Duodenum
    c. Ileum
    d. Whole of the small intestines

13. **In the small intestines, the mixing of food takes place by:**
    a. Segmentation movements
    b. Peristaltic movements
    c. Villi movements
    d. Propulsive movements

14. **True about external anal sphincter:**
    a. Formed by thickened smooth muscles
    b. Relaxes reflexly by stretch of the wall
    c. The pelvic parasympathetic innervation maintains tonic contraction
    d. Consists of skeletal muscle fibers

15. **Not true about Hirschsprung's disease:**
    a. Occurs due to congenital absence of Auerbach's plexus
    b. Occurs due to congenital absence of Meissner's plexus
    c. Also called megacolon
    d. There is blockage of peristaltic movements

ANSWER KEY

1.	b	2.	b	3.	c	4.	d	5.	a	6.	d	7.	a	8.	b
9.	b	10.	d	11.	d	12.	b	13.	a	14.	d	15.	b		

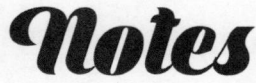
Notes

Digestion and Absorption

INTRODUCTION

The major constituents of food are *carbohydrates*, proteins and *fats (lipids)* which are also referred to as nutrients. They are made of large complex mole unter. Unless these nutrients are digested, they are very large to be absorbed across the small intestinal membrane and cannot be used by the body cells. Hence, digestion refers to the process of breaking down the ingested complex food particles by combinations of the following:

Mechanical digestion, such as mastication in the mouth, churning in the stomach and segmentation in th small intestine (as discussed in Chapter 3.1). In mechanical digestion, large food particles are broken into smaller particles without any chemical reactions.

Chemical digestion that is aided by enzymes which break the chemical bond of the nutrient molecules.

The ultimate aim of digestion is to produce *simple molecules* of nutrients that can be absorbed across the wall of the small intestine.

The simple molecules of nutrients that are absorbed across the membrane of the intestinal villi will be transported into the blood capillaries or lymph capillaries (lacteal) in the villi before they enter the general blood circulation. Henceforth, the dietary sources of the major nutrients chemical digestion and absorption process are discussed briefly.

DIGESTION AND ABSORPTION OF CARBOHYDRATES

Dietary Carbohydrates

Dietary intake of carbohydrates is 250–850 g/day, which represents 50–60% of the diet. Major carbohydrates in the human diet are present in the following forms:

Polysaccharides

These may be present in the following forms:
- *Starch* is the carbohydrate reserve of plants.
- *Glycogen* is available in nonvegetarian diet and so often referred to as animal starch.
- *Cellulose* (plant polysaccharide), which is present in diet in large amounts. But there is no enzyme in the human gastrointestinal tract to digest it.

Oligosaccharides

Based on the number of monosaccharide units present, oligosaccharides are further subdivided into di-, tri-, tetra- and pentasaccharide.

Disaccharides include:
- *Sucrose* (glucose + fructose) also known as table sugar (cane or beet sugar).
- *Lactose* (glucose + galactose) also called milk sugar.
- *Maltose* (glucose + glucose) is a product of starch hydrolysis. It is present in germinating seeds.

Monosaccharides

Monosaccharides consumed mostly in human diet are:
- *Hexoses* such as glucose (in fruits, vegetables and honey), and fructose in fruits.
- *Pentoses* do not occur in free form, but are found in nucleic acid and in certain polysaccharides such as pentosans of fruits and gums.

Digestion of Carbohydrates

The digestion of carbohydrates begins in mouth, continues in stomach but occurs mainly (almost all) in the small intestine.

In the Mouth

Initial starch digestion starts in the mouth by the enzyme α-amylase (ptyalin) present in the saliva which digests cooked starch to maltose.

In the Stomach

In the stomach, there occurs minimal carbohydrates digestive activity: The enzyme α-*amylase* (which enters the stomach with food) activity continues in the stomach for 20–30 minutes till the highly acidic gastric juice mixes with the food and makes it inactive. *The HCl of the gastric juice may hydrolyze some sucrose.*

In the Small Intestine

Pancreatic α-amylase which is present in the pancreatic juice is poured into the duodenum. Its actions on the carbohydrates are much powerful and so it acts on boiled as well as unboiled starch and variety of other carbohydrates except cellulose.

Brush border enzymes of small intestine. The carbohydrate splitting brush border enzymes of small intestine include *dextrinase, maltase, sucrase* and *lactase.* These brush border enzymes digest the oligosaccharides into monosaccharides on the surface of epithelial cells of villi.

End products

- The end products of carbohydrates are monosacch-arides such as glucose, fructose and galactose.
- A little amount of pentoses is the end product of digestion of nucleic acids and partial digestion of pentosans.

Absorption of Carbohydrates

Carbohydrates are absorbed from the gastrointestinal tract in the form of monosaccharides.

Site of Absorption

Most of the monosaccharides are absorbed from the mucosal surface of jejunum and upper ileum.

Mechanism of Absorption

Various monosaccharides are absorbed by the following mechanisms:

- *Glucose* and *galactose* are absorbed by a common *Na+-dependent active transport* system.
- *Fructose* is absorbed by *facilitated diffusion.*
- *Pentoses* are absorbed by simple diffusion.

IMPORTANT TO KNOW

Rate of absorption of monosaccharides is variable, being:
- The fastest with glucose and galactose,
- Intermediate with fructose, and
- The slowest with mannose or pentoses.

FATE OF GLUCOSE IN THE BODY

Storage as Glycogen

About 5% of the total glucose absorbed is stored as glycogen in the liver and muscles.

Catabolism to Produce Energy

About 50–60% of the glucose absorbed is catabolized in the body tissues to produce energy.

Conversion into Fat

About 30–40% of glucose is converted into fat and is stored in the fat depot.

CLINICAL ASPECTS

Abnormalities of Carbohydrate Digestion and Absorption

Congenital lactose intolerance: It refers to a condition in which lactose (milk sugar) cannot be digested due to congenital deficiency of enzyme lactase.
- The undigested lactose acts as osmotic particles and draws excessive fluids into intestine resulting in *diarrhea*.
- The diarrhea so produced can lead to life-threatening dehydration and electrolyte imbalance.
- Avoidance of milk and milk products prevents the symptoms from developing if the infant can be fed by synthetic milk containing sucrose instead of lactose.

Secondary lactase deficiency occurring in adults is very common. It produces intestinal distension, diarrhea and flatulence. For adults, it is usually not a problem, as they can easily avoid milk and milk products.

DIGESTION AND ABSORPTION OF PROTEINS

Sources of Proteins

The proteins that are digested and absorbed in the gastrointestinal tract come from two sources: exogenous and endogenous.

Exogenous (Dietary) Proteins

- *Daily requirement* of dietary proteins for adults is 0.5–0.7 g/kg body weight and for children (1–3 years), it is 4 g/kg.

- *Sources of dietary proteins* with high biological value are meat, fish, eggs, cheese and other milk products. Soybeans, wheat and various types of pulses are also rich sources of proteins.
- The dietary proteins are made of long chains of amino acids bound together by peptide linkages.

Endogenous Proteins

Endogenous proteins, totaling 30–50 g/day, are the proteins which reach the intestine through various gastrointestinal secretions and those which are present in the desquamated epithelial cells of the gut.

Digestion of Proteins

Proteins are digested by the proteolytic enzymes to amino acids and small polypeptides before they are absorbed. Digestion of proteins does not occur in the mouth as there are no proteolytic enzymes in the saliva. Digestion of proteins, thus, begins in the stomach and is completed in the small intestine.

In the Stomach

Pepsin, secreted by chief cells of the main gastric glands in an inactive form (pepsinogen), is responsible for digesting about 10–15% proteins entering the gastrointestinal tract.

- Pepsinogen is converted into pepsin (active form) by the action of HCl or preformed pepsin.
- Pepsin splits proteins into proteases, peptones and polypeptides (Fig. 3.2-1).

In the Small Intestine

In the small intestine, the proteins are digested by the pancreatic proteases, brush border peptidases and intracellular peptidases.

Pancreatic proteases or proteolytic enzymes of pancreas play a major role in protein digestion.

- *Pancreatic proteases* digest the proteins and split them into dipeptides, tripeptides and small polypeptides, which are further digested by brush border peptidases (Fig. 3.2-1).
- Some of the dipeptides and tripeptides are absorbed directly into the epithelial cells of mucosa of small intestine and are further digested by intracellular enzymes into amino acids.

Brush border peptidases include aminopeptidases, dipeptidases, tripeptidases, nuclease and related enzymes. These enzymes continue the digestive process begun by the pancreatic proteases, eventually converting the proteins to small polypeptides and amino acids (Fig. 3.2-1).

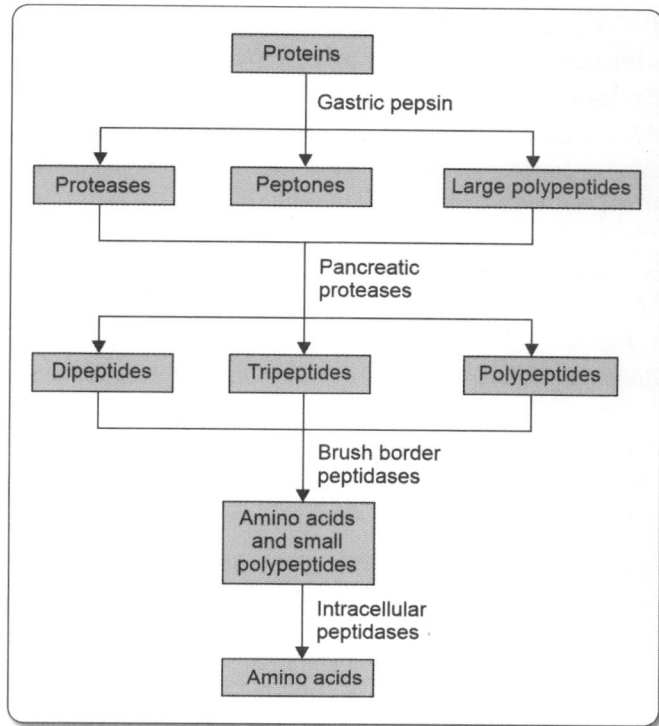

Fig. 3.2-1: Steps of digestion of proteins

Intracellular peptidases are the proteolytic enzymes present in the cytosol of epithelial cells of small intestine. Within minutes, these digest the last dipeptides and tripeptides into amino acids, which then enter the blood.

Digestion of Nucleic Acid and Nucleoproteins

Nucleic acid and nucleoproteins are found in abundance in the food stuff such as liver, kidney, pancreas, yeast, etc.

In the stomach, HCl hydrolyzes the nucleoproteins, removing proteins, which are digested together with other proteins as described above.

In the small intestine, free nucleic acids are digested by the pancreatic enzymes and brush border enzymes.

Pancreatic enzymes, such as ribonuclease and deoxyribonuclease in the duodenum digest free nucleic acids into nucleotides and nucleosides.

Brush border enzymes, such as nucleases, nucleoti-dases and nucleosidases, convert nucleotides and nucleosides into pentoses (purine and pyrimidine).

End products

The protein digestion, which starts in the stomach, is completed in the enterocyte of small intestine. The end products of protein digestion are amino acids.

Absorption of Proteins

Mechanisms of Absorption into the Intestinal Epithelial Cells

The end products of protein digestion (amino acids, dipeptides and tripeptides) are absorbed through the luminal membrane of the epithelial cells of small intestine. Known mechanisms of absorption are:

Na$^+$-dependent active transport mechanism. The levo amino acids, dipeptides and tripeptides are absorbed by a Na$^+$-dependent active transport mechanism.

Simple diffusion. The dextro-amino acids are absorbed solely by passive diffusion.

Endocytosis. Small amounts of larger polypeptides are absorbed by endocytosis. Proteins absorbed by endocytosis usually excite immunological/allergic reaction.

> **IMPORTANT TO KNOW**
>
> In newborn infants, immunoglobulins present in the colostrum are absorbed in the intestinal mucosa by endocytosis and impart passive immunity to child.

Further Digestion in the Epithelial Cells

Once amino acids and polypeptides are absorbed into the intestinal epithelial cells, the intracellular peptidases break the remaining linkages of tripeptides, and dipeptides causing release of amino acids.

Transport of Amino Acids into Blood Capillaries

From inside the epithelial cells, amino acids are transported into the interstitial space across the basolateral membrane of the cells by facilitated or simple diffusion. From the interstitium, amino acids enter the capillaries of villus by simple diffusion, and then *via* portal vein they reach the liver and general circulation.

DIGESTION AND ABSORPTION OF FATS

Dietary Fats

Dietary fat is of both vegetable and animal origin. Mostly, it is in the form of neutral fat (triglycerides). It also includes small amounts of phospholipids, cholesterol, some free fatty acids, lecithin and cholesterol esters.

Daily intake of fats in the diet varies widely from about 25 to 160 g.

Digestion of Fats

Site of Digestion

Although lipolytic enzymes are secreted in the mouth (*lingual lipase*) and stomach (*gastric lipase*), their action is so insignificant that practically digestion of all the dietary fats occurs in the small intestine. Under normal conditions, gastric lipase is soon inactivated by gastric juice (at pH 2.5).

Mechanism of Digestion of Fats

Emulsification of fat by bile salts. There is no chemical reaction, but the large lipid globules are merely dispersed into tiny droplets to increase surface area (Figs 3.2-2A and B).

Hydrolysis of fat by pancreatic and intestinal lipolytic enzymes. The chemical reaction catalyzed by lipase hastens the breaking down of long-chain fat molecules to monoglycerides and fatty acids (Fig. 3.2-3).

Acceleration of fat digestion by micelle formation. Micelles are the fats clustered together with bile salts to form fat droplets which are smaller than the emulsion droplets.

Absorption of Fats

Most of the fat absorption occurs in the duodenum; almost all the digested lipids are totally absorbed by the time the chyme reaches the mid jejunum. Absorption of fats is accomplished by the following steps.

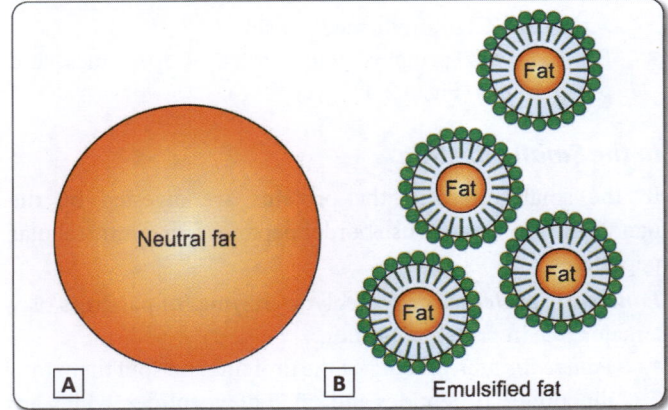

Figs 3.2-2A and B: Emulsification of fats by bile salts: A. A large fat particle; B. Small fat particles surrounded by the bile salts.

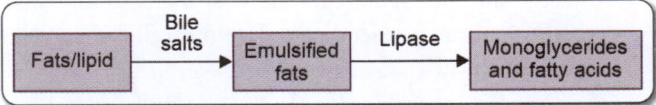

Fig. 3.2-3: Summary of fat digestion

Transportation as Micelles to the Brush Border Membrane

The bile salt micelle acts as a transport vehicle for the products of fat digestion.

Diffusion of Lipids Across the Enterocyte Cell Membrane

Once the micelle comes in contact with the cell membrane, the monoglycerides, free fatty acids, cholesterol and fat soluble vitamins (being soluble in the cell membrane) diffuse passively at a rapid speed through the enterocyte cell membrane to the interior of the cell, leaving bile salts in the intestinal lumen.

The bile salts released from micelle after diffusion of their associated lipids are absorbed in the terminal ileum by a Na^+-dependent active transport process.

Transport of Lipids from Inside the Enterocytes to the Interstitial Space

Once inside the cell, the end products of fat digestion enter the interstitium by two mechanisms:

1. Diffusion across the basal border of enterocyte. The small chain fatty acids are able to diffuse across the basal border of enterocytes to enter the interstitium.

2. Formation and excretion of chylomicrons from enterocytes by exocytosis. The large chain fatty acids, cholesterol and lysophosphatides enter the smooth endoplasmic reticulum, where they are reconstituted.

The reformed lipids coalesce to form small lipid droplets (about 1 nm in diameter) called chylomicrons. The chylomicrons are then excreted into the interstitium by *exocytosis* from the basolateral membrane of enterocyte. Covering of β-lipoproteins is essential for the exocytosis to occur.

Transport of Lipids into Circulation

After exiting the enterocytes (i.e., in the interstitium), the chylomicrons merge into larger droplets. From the interstitium, the lipids diffuse into the *lacteals*, from which they enter the lymphatic circulation and via thoracic duct gain access to the blood circulation.

CLINICAL ASPECTS

Lipid Malabsorption

Lipid malabsorption is much more common than carbohydrate and protein malabsorption.

Causes of lipid malabsorption include:
- Deficiency of pancreatic lipase in certain pancreatic diseases
- Bile deficiency in disorders of liver and gallbladder.

Steatorrhea, i.e., increased amount of fat in the stools, is common manifestation of fat malabsorption.

NURSING IMPLICATIONS AND APPLICATIONS

Serum Lipid Profile

Lipids are present as lipoprotein complexes. Depending upon the density, the lipoproteins are of the following types:
- Very low density lipoproteins (VLDLs); density is <1.060.
- Low density lipoproteins (LDLs).
- High density lipoproteins (HDLs); density is 1.060–1.200.

Normal Values
- Serum triglycerides: 30–150 mg%
- Serum cholesterol: 150–240 mg%
- Serum phospholipids: 150–300 mg%
- Serum free fatty acids (FFA or NEFA = 10–30 mg%).

ABSORPTION OF WATER, ELECTROLYTES MINERALS AND VITAMINS

Water Absorption

Water Balance in the GIT

- The gastrointestinal tract receives about 9 L of water per day which includes about 2 L of ingested water and about 7 L contained in salivary, gastric, biliary, pancreatic and intestinal secretions (Table 3.2-1).
- The gastrointestinal tract absorbs about 8.8 L of water (about 95% of total water received) per day. About 60% of absorption occurs in jejunum, 20–25% in ileum and 10–15% in colon (Table 3.2-1).
- The gastrointestinal tract excretes about 0.2 L of water in the feces per day.

Mechanism of Water Absorption

In general, water is absorbed passively and iso-osmotically across the gastrointestinal mucosa following the osmotic gradient created by the active absorption of electrolytes and nutrients.

TABLE 3.2-1: Daily water balance in gastrointestinal tract

Input (in L)	Absorption (in L)	Fecal excretion (in L)
Water ingested: 2	Jejunum (60%) : 5.5	0.2
Water in GIT secretions: 7	Ileum (25%) : 2.0	
• Saliva: 1.5	Colon (10–15%): 1.3	
• Gastric juice: 2.5		
• Bile: 0.75		
• Pancreatic juice: 0.75		
• Intestinal juice: 1.5		
TOTAL 9	8.8	0.2

Absorption of Sodium

Sodium Balance in GIT

Gastrointestinal tract receives about 40 g of sodium per day, out of which about 10 g is ingested with food and about 30 g is contained in the gastrointestinal secretions. All of it is reabsorbed.

Site of Absorption

Though sodium can be reabsorbed in the entire length of the intestine, but maximum absorption occurs in the jejunum.

Absorption of Calcium

Body Calcium

Calcium is the most abundant mineral in the body. The total content of calcium in an adult man is about 1–1.5 kg of which about 99% is present in the bones and teeth. A small amount (10%) found outside the skeletal tissue performs a wide variety of functions.

Dietary Calcium

Best sources of dietary calcium are milk and milk products. Good sources of calcium are beans, leafy vegetables, fish, cabbage and egg yolk.

IMPORTANT TO KNOW

Dietary requirements of calcium are:
- Infants (<1 year): 300–500 mg/day
- Children (1-18 years): 800–1,200 mg/day
- Adult men and women: 800 mg/day
- Women during pregnancy, lactation and menopause: 1,500 mg/day.

Site of Absorption

Most of the ingested calcium is absorbed in the upper small intestine (duodenum and jejunum).

Mechanism of Absorption

Normally, about 75–80% of the daily intake (about 1,000 mg) of calcium is absorbed from the upper small intestine. Most of the calcium is absorbed by an active transport mechanism.

Regulation of Calcium Absorption

Calcium absorption from the small intestine is well regulated to maintain the plasma calcium (*homeostasis of calcium*) levels within a narrow range (9–11 mg%). Vitamin D and parathyroid hormone (PTH) play main role in the regulation of calcium absorption.

Absorption of Iron

Iron is an essential component of hemoglobin.

Daily requirement of Iron varies as:
- Adult male– 5–10 mg/day
- Adult female– 20 mg/day (to compensate menstrual loss)
- Pregnant and lactating female: 40 mg/day.

Sources are meat, fish, spinach, green leafy vegetables and jaggery.

Absorption occurs mainly in the duodenum and upper jejunum.
- Normally about 10% of 15–20 mg iron ingested each day is actually absorbed in healthy adult males. This absorption is more in menstruating women.

Mechanism of Iron Absorption

Mechanism of iron absorption for the purpose of understanding can be described under three headings:

Transport of iron across brush border of enterocyte

In the diet, iron may be present as heme (derived from meat) or non-heme iron.

Absorption of heme iron. Heme iron is the iron present in myoglobin, hemoglobin and related compounds. From these compounds, the heme is released by proteolytic enzymes in the gut. From the lumen, the heme is transported inside the enterocyte across the brush border membrane by a *heme transport* protein. Inside the cell, the ferrous iron (Fe^{2+}) is released from the heme by the enzyme hemeoxygenase.

Absorption of non-heme iron. Most of the dietary non-heme iron is present in ferric form (Fe^{3+}), whereas iron can be absorbed more efficiently in ferrous form (Fe^{2+}).
- Iron has got tendency to form insoluble complexes with dietary phytates, phosphates and dietary fibers. Gastric hydrochloric acid tends to break insoluble iron complex apart and thus, facilitates iron absorption.
- Ferrous iron (Fe^{2+}) is transported across the brush border by the *iron transport protein* or *receptors* present on the cell membrane (Fig. 3.2-4). Once inside the enterocyte, fate of non-heme ferrous iron is same as that of heme iron.

Fate of Iron in the Enterocyte

As shown in Figure 3.2-4, in the cytosol of enterocyte, the free ferrous iron (Fe^{2+}) has two fates:
1. A part of Fe^{2+}, depending upon the body's require-ment, is actively transported across the basolateral membranes of the enterocytes into the interstitium, from where it enters the blood.

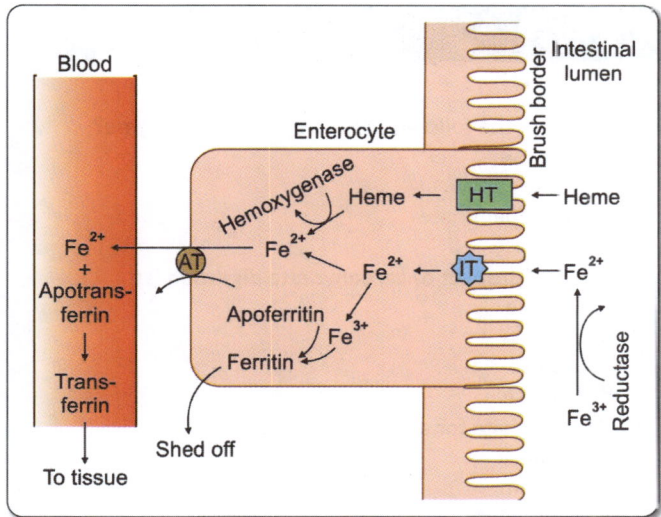

Fig. 3.2-4: Absorption of iron. Heme is carried across brush border of enterocyte by heme transport protein (HT) and Fe^{2+} of non-heme iron by iron transport protein (IT). Inside the enterocyte, some iron binds to ferritin and some across basolateral membrane by active transport process. In the blood, iron binds to the transport protein transferrin (TF)

2. Rest of the ferrous iron is oxidized to ferric form and bound to apoferritin forming ferritin. It is difficult to release iron from this storage form, and in general the ferritin stays in the enterocyte until the cell is sloughed off at the tip of villus.

Transport of Iron in the Blood

Normally, the iron absorbed into the blood binds with a *apotransferrin* to form the *transferrin* and is transported in this form in the plasma.

Mucosal block theory of absorption

This theory states that iron absorption is increased when body iron stores are depleted or when erythropoiesis is increased, and decreased under the reverse conditions.

- As compared to normal conditions, in iron deficiency states a larger percentage of dietary iron enters the circulation and smaller amount forms ferritin in the epithelial cells.
- In the presence of iron overload, more ferritin is formed in the enterocytes and shed with these cells in the stools.

NURSING IMPLICATIONS AND APPLICATIONS

Iron deficiency anemia is the most common nutritional deficiency anemia. It is much more common in women between 20 and 40 years of age than in men and in growing children. The common causes of iron deficiency anemia are:

- Milk fed infants.
- Increase loss of blood in conditions like excessive menstruation, peptic ulcer.
- Increase, demand of iron as in menstruating and lactating female.
- Decreases absorption of iron as in achlorhydria and malabsorption diseases.

ABSORPTION OF VITAMINS

Vitamins are substances of high biological significance and are essential for normal health. The vitamins are named after the letters of the alphabets and are divided into two gorps.

1. *Fats soluble vitamins* which include vitamin A, D, E and K

2. *Water soluble vitamins* are vitamin C and B complex which include.

- Thiamine (β_1)
- Riboflavin (β_2)
- Nicotinic acid (β_3) or niacin
- Pantothenic acid (β_5)
- Pyridoxine (β_6)
- Cyanocobalamin (β_{12})
- Biotin (β_7)
- Folic acid (β_9)

Absorption of Fat Soluble Vitamins

Fat soluble vitamins (A, D, E and K) become part of micelle formed by bile salts and are absorbed along with other lipids in the upper part of small intestine.

The absorption of fat soluble vitamins is deficient if fat absorption is depressed because of lack of pancreatic enzymes or if bile is excluded from the intestine by obstruction of bile duct.

Absorption of Water Soluble Vitamins

Most vitamins are absorbed in the upper part of small intestine (jejunum) except vitamin B_{12} which is absorbed in the ileum.

ASSESS YOURSELF

Short and Long Answer Questions

1. **Discuss digestion and absorption of:**
   - Carbohydrates
   - Proteins
   - Fats
2. **Write notes on:**
   - Pancreatic enzymes
   - Calcium absorption
   - Steatorrhea
   - Lipid profile
   - Lactose intolerance

Multiple Choice Questions

1. **Which of the following is oligosaccharide?**
   - a. Cellulose
   - b. Lactose
   - c. Pentoses
   - d. Glycogen

2. **Which of the following is a brush border enzyme?**
   - a. Amylase
   - b. Lipase
   - c. Aminopeptidase
   - d. Nuclease
3. **The end product of carbohydrate digestion is:**
   - a. Glucose
   - b. Fructose
   - c. Lactose
   - d. Maltose
4. **The main site for absorption of carbohydrates is:**
   - a. Stomach
   - b. Jejunum
   - c. Duodenum
   - d. Colon

ANSWER KEY

| **1.** | b | **2.** | c | **3.** | a | **4.** | b |

Section
IV

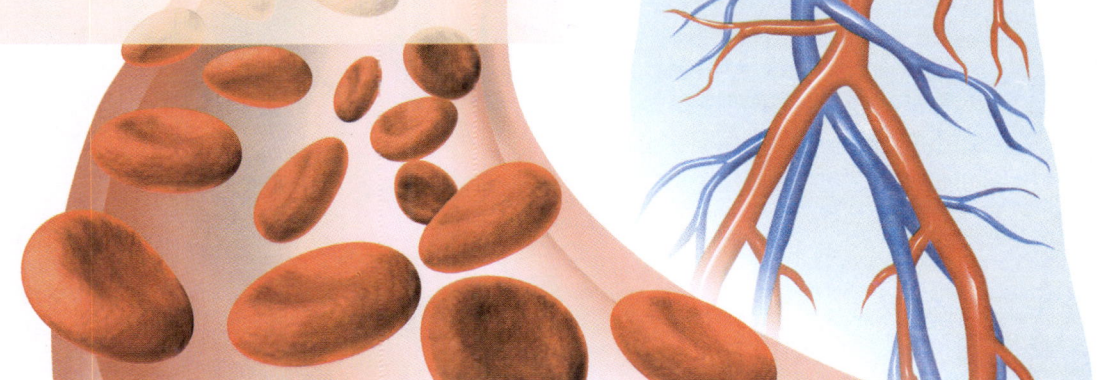

Blood Circulatory and Lymphatic System

BLOOD

Blood is a fluid connective tissue which transports substances from one part of the body to another. It provides nutrients and hormones to the tissues and removes their waste products. Blood, confined in the cardiovascular system, constitutes a major part of the extracellular fluid of the body. Some of the important physical characteristics of blood are:

Color of the blood is opaque red due to the pigment hemoglobin in the RBCs. The arterial blood is bright red and venous blood is dark red in color.

Volume of blood in an average adult is about 5–6 L (8% of the body weight or 80 mL/kg body weight).

Viscosity of blood is five times more than that of water.

Specific gravity of blood is 1.050–1.060. Specific gravity of RBC is greater (1.090) than that of plasma (1.030).

pH of blood is about 7.4 (ranges from 7.38 to 7.42), i.e., it is alkaline in nature. In acidosis, pH of blood falls below 7.38 and in alkalosis pH is more than 7.42.

COMPOSITION

Blood is composed of two main components, plasma and cellular elements.

Plasma constitutes about 55% of the blood volume. It is a clear straw-colored fluid portion of blood. **Plasma proteins**, an important constituent of plasma, form about 7% of its volume.

Cellular elements of blood are about 45% of the total blood volume and constitute the so called packed cell volume (PCV). Blood cells are:

- Erythrocytes or red blood cells (5 million/mm^3)
- Leucocytes or white blood cells (4000–11000/mm^3)
- Platelets or thrombocytes (1.5–4 lac/mm^3)

FUNCTIONS OF BLOOD

Nutritive function. Blood carries the nutritive substances like glucose, amino acids, fatty acids, vitamins, electrolytes and others from the gut to the tissues where they are utilized.

Respiratory function. Blood picks up oxygen from the lungs and delivers it to the various tissues. Most important function of the blood is the uninterrupted delivery of O_2 to heart and brain. It also carries away CO_2 from the tissues to the lungs from where it is expelled out in the expired air.

Excretory function. Blood transports various metabolic waste products such as urea, uric acid and creatinine to excretory organs (kidney, skin, intestine and lungs) for their disposal.

Transport function. The various hormones produced by endocrine glands, the biological enzymes and antibodies are transported by the blood to the target tissue to modulate metabolic process.

Protective function. Blood plays an important role in the defence mechanism of the body:

- Neutrophils and monocytes engulf the micro-organisms entering the body by phagocytosis.
- Lymphocytes and gamma globulins initiate immune response.
- Eosinophils accomplish detoxification, disintegration and removal of foreign proteins.

Homeostatic function. Blood plays an important role in maintaining the internal environment of the body (homeostatic function):

- The water content of blood is freely interchangeable with the interstitial fluid and helps in maintaining the water and electrolyte balance of the body.
- Plasma proteins and hemoglobin act as buffers and help in maintaining the acid-base balance and pH of the body fluids.

Maintenance of body temperature. Blood plays an important role in regulation of the body temperature.

Storage function. Blood serves as a readymade source of substances stored in it (such as glucose, water, proteins, and electrolytes for use in emergency conditions like starvation, fluid loss and electrolyte loss).

PLASMA

Plasma is the clear straw-colored fluid (with dissolved solid substances) portion of the blood minus its cellular elements. It constitutes about 55% of the blood volume.

COMPOSITION

Plasma contains the following constituents:

Water. Water is the main constituent of plasma forming 91% of it.

Solids. The solids dissolved in the plasma constitute a total of 9% of the plasma. The solid constituents of plasma are as follows:

- *Plasma proteins* form 7% of the solids in plasma.
- *Other organic molecules* which form 1% of the solids include carbohydrates, fats, non-protein nitrogenous (NPN) substances, hormones, enzymes and antibodies.
- *Inorganic substances* which constitute 1% of the solids in plasma include sodium, potassium, calcium, magnesium, chloride, iodide, iron, phosphates and copper.

Gases present in the plasma are oxygen, carbon dioxide and nitrogen.

IMPORTANT TO KNOW

Serum

Plasma from which fibrinogen and clotting factors (II, V and VIII) have been removed is called serum. Serum is formed when the blood is allowed to clot in a test tube and clot is retracted. Serum has a higher serotonin (5HT) content because of the breakdown of platelets during clotting.

PLASMA PROTEINS

Classification of Plasma Proteins

Plasma proteins form the major solid constituent of the plasma. The total plasma protein concentration is 7.4 g% (ranges from 6.4 to 8.3 g%). The major forms of plasma proteins are (Figs 4.1-1A and B):

Albumin (4.8 g%)

Globulins (2.3 g%) include:

- Alpha 1 (α_1) globulin
- Alpha 2 (α_2) globulin
- Beta (β) globulin
- Gamma (γ) globulin

Fibrinogen (0.3 g%).

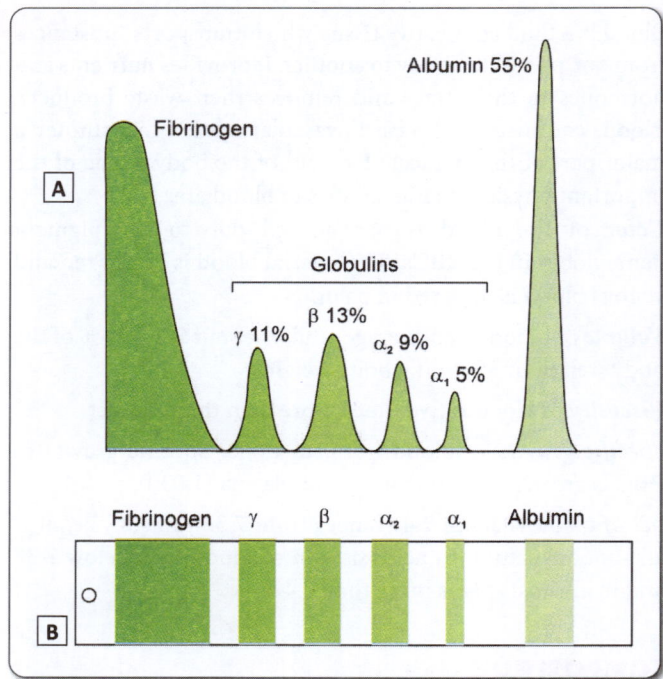

Figs 4.1-1A and B: Paper electrophoresis showing: A. Bands of different plasma proteins; B. Relative amount of plasma proteins

Features of Individual Fraction of Plasma Proteins

Albumin

Plasma levels are 4.8 g% (range 3–5 g%).
Molecular weight of albumin is 69,000.
Synthesized in liver.
Half-life is about 10 days.

Globulins

Plasma levels are 2.3 g% (range 2–3 g%).
Molecular weight varies from 90,000 to 15,600.
Types include alpha 1, alpha 2, beta 1, beta 2 and gamma globulins.

IMPORTANT TO KNOW

Forms of globulins are as follows:
Glycoproteins consist of carbohydrates and protein
Lipoproteins consist of alpha 2 globulin and lipids. It has got the following subtypes:
- High density lipoproteins (HDL)
- Low density lipoproteins (LDL)
- Very low density lipoproteins (VLDL)
- Chylomicrons (CM).

Transferrin has the specific property of iron binding and thus, helps in its transport and storage.
Haptoglobin forms stable complexes with free hemoglobin.
Ceruloplasmin binds with copper and helps in its transport and storage.
Fetunin is a growth promoting protein seen in infants and newborn.
Immunoglobulins are gamma globulins, which play role in immunity.
Angiotensinogen is alpha 2 globulin.
Hemagglutinins are antibodies against the red blood cell antigens.

Fibrinogen

Plasma levels are 0.3 g%.
Molecular weight varies from 4,00,000 to 5,00,000.
Synthesized in the liver.
Functions as a clotting protein.

Prothrombin

Plasma levels are 40 mg%.
Molecular weight is 68,000.
Synthesized in the liver. Synthesis is promoted by vitamin K.

Functions of Plasma Proteins

Exert osmotic pressure. The protein molecules are unable to pass across the capillary membrane and consequently exert colloid osmotic pressure of about 25 mm Hg on the capillary membrane. About 70–80% of the osmotic pressure is contributed by the albumin fraction. The colloid osmotic pressure plays an important role in exchange of water between the blood and tissue fluid.

Contribution to blood viscosity. Fibrinogen and globulins are significant contributors to blood viscosity because of their asymmetrical shape.

Role in coagulation of blood. The fibrinogen, prothrombin and other coagulation proteins present in the plasma play an important role in the coagulation of blood.

Role in defence mechanism of the body. The gamma globulins are antibodies, which play an important role in the immune system meant for defence of the body against the microorganisms.

Role in maintaining acid-base balance of the body. Plasma proteins act as buffers and contribute to about 15% of the buffering capacity of blood. Because of their amphoteric nature, plasma proteins can combine with acids and bases.

Transport function. Plasma proteins combine easily with many substances and play an essential role in their transport. The substances transported by plasma proteins are carbon dioxide, thyroxine, cortisol, vitamin A, D and E, vitamin B_{12}, bilirubin, drugs, calcium, copper, and free hemoglobin.

Role as reserve proteins. Plasma proteins serve as reserve proteins and are utilized by the body tissues during conditions, like fasting, inadequate protein intake.

Role in suspension stability of red blood cells. Suspension stability refers to the property of red blood cells by virtue of which they remain uniformly suspended in the blood. Globulins and fibrinogen accelerate this property.

Fibrinolytic function. The enzymes of fibrinolytic system digest the intravascular clot (thrombus) and thus save from the disastrous effects of thrombosis.

Role in genetic information. Many plasma proteins exhibit *polymorphism*. Polymorphism is a Mendelian trait that exists in the population with differing prevalence. They serve as valuable tool for the studies of population genetics. Plasma proteins that show polymorphism are haptoglobin, transferrin, ceruloplasmin and immunoglobulins.

Synthesis of Plasma Proteins

Site of Synthesis

In adults, plasma proteins are synthesized as described below:
- The albumin and fibrinogen are synthesized mostly by reticuloendothelial cells of the liver.
- Alpha and beta globulins are synthesized by the liver, spleen, and bone marrow.

- Gamma globulins are synthesized by B lymphocytes. Dietary proteins play an important role in synthesis of plasma proteins.

Physiological Variations

In infants, the total protein level is low (about 5.5 g%) due to low gamma globulins.

In old age, there is a tendency for the albumin level to fall and the total globulin level to rise.

In pregnancy, during first six months, the albumin and globulin levels decrease while the fibrinogen level increases.

CLINICAL ASPECTS

ABNORMALITIES OF PLASMA PROTEIN LEVELS

Hypoproteinemia refers to generalized decrease in the levels of plasma proteins.

Causes of hypoproteinemia include the following:
- Dietary deficiency
- Malabsorption syndrome
- Liver diseases
- Renal diseases
- Hemorrhage and extensive burns
- Hereditary analbuminemia
- Congenital afibrinogenemia

Effects of hypoproteinemia. Low levels of plasma proteins are associated with a decrease in the plasma osmotic pressure which causes water retention and edema of the body tissue.

Hyperproteinemia, i.e., increase in the plasma protein levels is seen in the following conditions:

Acute inflammatory conditions which are associated with increased synthesis of acute phase proteins which include C-reactive proteins.

Reversal of normal A/G ratio. The normal albumin: globulin (A/G) ratio (1.7:1) is reversed:
- When albumin synthesis is decreased as occurs in liver diseases (globulin levels being normal because many globulins are synthesized by B lymphocytes).

RED BLOOD CELLS

FUNCTIONAL MORPHOLOGY

The red blood cells (mature erythrocytes) form one of the important constituents of the cellular elements of the blood. Each red blood cell (RBC) like any other cell in the body is bounded by a *cell membrane* but is *non-nucleated* and lacks the usual cell organelles. The cytoplasm of the RBC contains a special pigmented protein called the *hemoglobin* which forms 90% of the weight of erythrocyte. The red color of the RBCs and thus of the blood is due to the presence of hemoglobin.

NORMAL SIZE, SHAPE AND COUNTS OF RBCS

Normal Size

- *Diameter* of each RBC is 7.2 μm (range 6.9–7.4 μm)
- *Thickness* in the periphery is 2 μm and in the center 1 μm
- *Surface area* of each RBC is about 120–140 μm²
- *Volume* is about 80 μm³ (range 78–86 μm³).

Normal Shape

The red blood cells are circular, biconcave discs (Figs 4.1-2A and B).

Advantages of biconcave shape are:
- It renders the red cells quite flexible so that they can pass through capillaries whose minimum diameter is 3.5 μm (Fig. 4.1-3).
- The biconcavity provides greater surface area as compared to volume which allows considerable alterations in the cell volume. Thus, the RBC can withstand considerable changes of osmotic pressure. In this way, the RBCs can resist hemolysis to certain extent when placed in hypotonic solution.

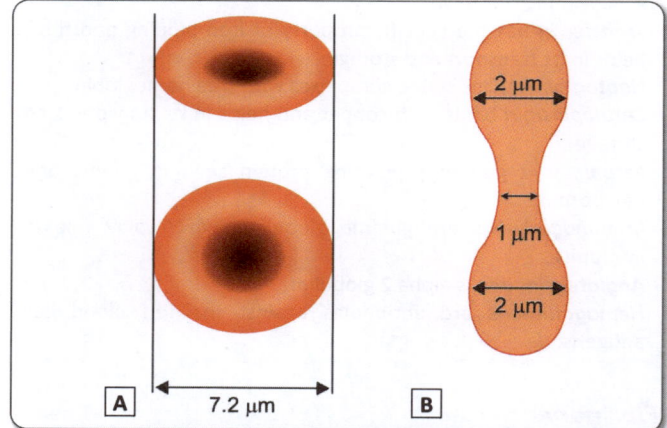

Figs 4.1-2A and B: Size and shape of a normal red blood cell: A. Biconcave disc (diameter 7.2 μm); B. Thickness (2 μm at the periphery and 1 μm in the center)

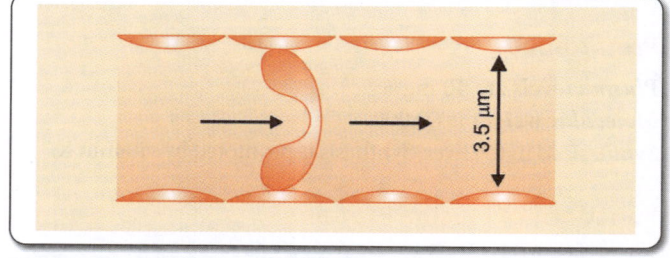

Fig. 4.1-3: Showing how flexibility of red blood cell allows it to pass through smaller capillaries (diameter 3.5 μm).

- Greater surface area allows easy exchange of O_2 and CO_2 and rapid diffusion of other substances.

Normal Counts

- *At birth*, normal RBC count is 6–7 million/mm³.
- *In adult males*, the normal count varies from 5 million/mm³ to 6.5 million/mm³ (average 5.5 million/mm³).
- *In females*, it varies from 4.5 million/mm³ to 5.5 million/mm³ (average 4.8 million/mm³).
- *Clinically*, a count of 5 million/mm³ is considered 100%.

CLINICAL ASPECTS

Abnormalities in Counts of RBCs

Polycythemia or pathological increase in RBC count (above 7 million/mm³) is seen in malignancies of bone marrow and conditions associated with chronic hypoxia.

Anemia: In anemia, there may occur marked reduction in the RBC count or the hemoglobin level or both. (For details see page 157).

Packed Cell Volume

Packed cell volume (PCV) refers to the percentage of the cellular elements (RBCs, WBCs and platelets) in the whole blood. Since the volume of WBCs and platelets is very less, so for all practical purposes the PCV is considered equivalent to the volume of packed red cells (VPRC) or the so called *hematocrit value*. The normal values of PCV in males is about 45% and in females about 42%. The PCV is increased in polycythemia and decreased in anemia.

Rouleaux Formation and Erythrocyte Sedimentation Rate

Rouleaux Formation

- Rouleaux formation refers to the tendency of RBCs to pile one over the other like a pile of coins (Figs 4.1-4A and B).

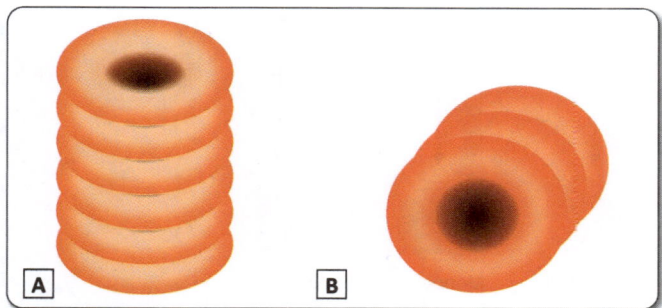

Figs 4.1-4A and B: Rouleaux formation.

- The discoid shape and protein coating of red cells play major role in rouleaux formation. Rouleaux formation does not occur in normal circulation under physiological conditions, as the moving cells show little or no tendency to adhere.
- This is a reversible phenomenon, but it promotes sedimentation of RBCs. It should not be confused with agglutination where the cells are irreversibly clumped.
- Albumin decreases the rouleaux formation, while fibrinogen, globulin and other products of tissue destruction increase rouleaux formation.

Erythrocyte Sedimentation Rate

Erythrocyte sedimentation rate (ESR) is the rate at which the red blood cells sediment (settle down) when the blood containing an anticoagulant is allowed to stand in a vertically placed tube. It is expressed in millimeter at the end of first hour.

CLINICAL ASPECTS

Clinical Significance of ESR

- *Normal values* of ESR by Westergren's method in males vary from 3 mm to 7 mm and in females from 5 mm to 9 mm in first hour.
- Values of ESR are raised in a large number of pathological conditions, so it has got no specific diagnostic value. However, raised levels of ESR do suggest presence of some chronic inflammatory condition in the body.
- Estimation of ESR is more useful as a *prognostic test*, i.e., to judge the progress of the disease in patients under treatment.

FORMATION OF RED BLOOD CELLS

Formation of red blood cells is a part of the process of development of blood cells (RBCs, WBCs and platelets) called *hemopoiesis* which includes:

- Erythropoiesis, i.e., development of RBCs
- Leucopoiesis, i.e., development of WBCs
- Thrombopoiesis or megakaryocytopoiesis, i.e., development of platelets.

Sites of Hemopoiesis

In the first two months of gestation, the *yolk sac* is the main site of hemopoiesis.

From third month of gestation, liver and spleen become the main sites of blood formation.

From 20th week of gestation, hemopoiesis begins in the bone marrow.

At birth (in normal full-term), almost whole of the hemopoiesis occurs in the bone marrow.

In young children, active hemopoietic bone marrow is found in both axial skeleton and bones of extremities. The active hemopoietic bone marrow is red in color due to marked cellularity and hence is called *red bone marrow*. However, during this period, there occurs a progressive fatty replacement throughout the long bones converting red bone marrow into the so called *yellow bone marrow*.

In adults, hemopoietic (red) bone marrow is confined to *axial skeleton* (skull, vertebrae, sternum, ribs, sacrum and pelvis) and *proximal ends of long bones* (humerus, femur and tibia). Even in these hemopoietic areas, about 50% the bone marrow consists of fat.

Blood Cell Precursors

Stem Cells

The *monophyletic theory* of hemopoiesis is now widely accepted, according to which all blood cells originate from pluripotent multipotent stem cell. Stem cells possess two fundamental properties:

1. *Self-replication*, i.e., stem cells are capable of cell division to give rise to more stem cells, and
2. *Differentiation and commitment*, i.e., the stem cells have ability to differentiate into specialized cells called progenitor cells.

Progenitor cells

The stem cells, after a series of divisions, differentiate into progenitor cells (Fig. 4.1-5):

Pluripotent progenitor cells which can give rise to any type of blood cells

Lymphoid (immune system) stem cells which ultimately develop into lymphocytes

Myeloid (trilineage) stem cells, which later differentiate into three types of cell lines:

1. *Granulocyte-monocyte progenitors* which produce all leucocytes except the lymphocytes
2. *Erythroid progenitors* which produce red blood cells
3. *Megakaryocyte progenitors* which produce platelets.

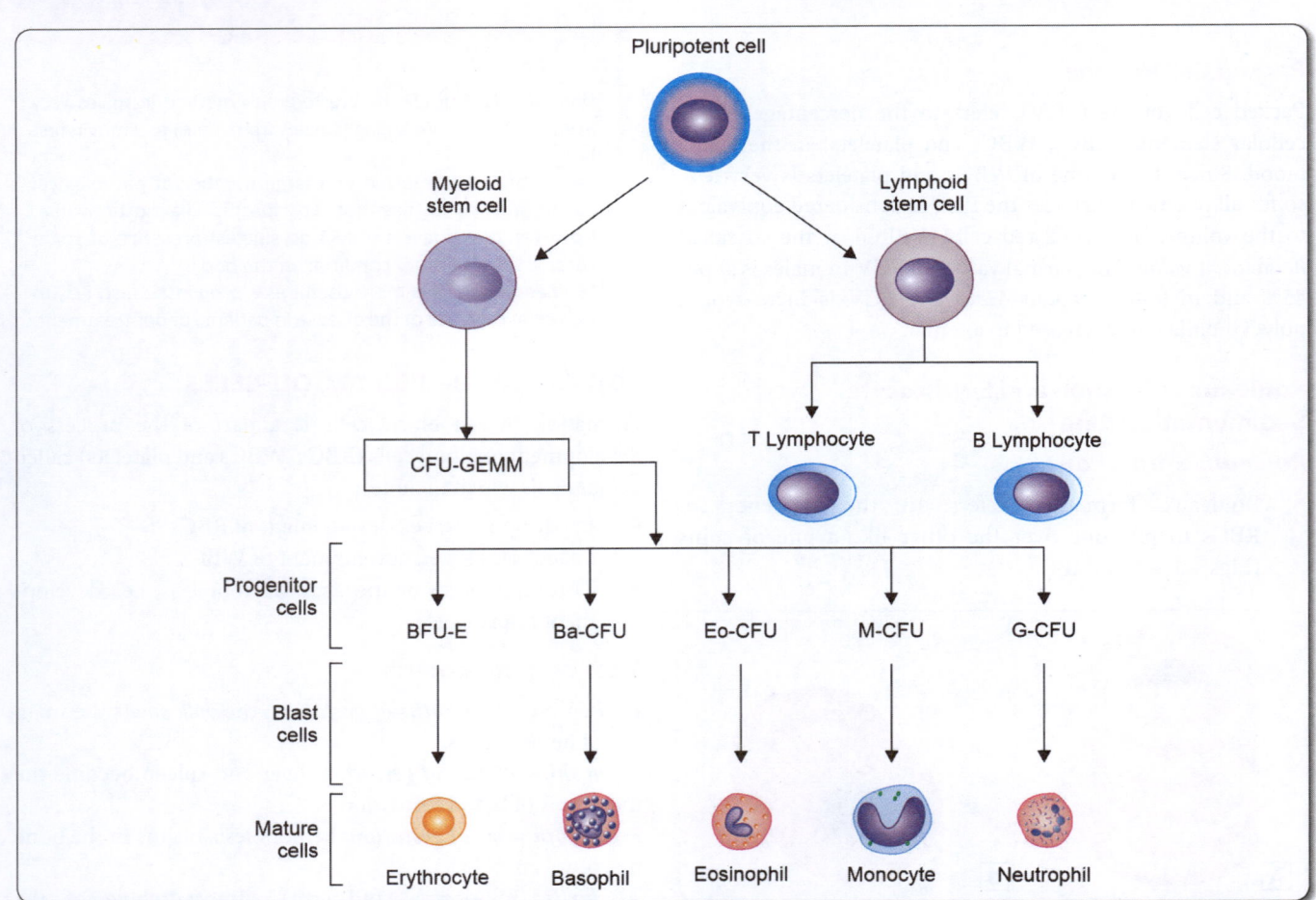

Fig. 4.1-5: Schematic broad outline of hemopoiesis

Abbreviation: BFU-E; burst-forming unit— erythrocyte, CFU; Colony forming units, Ba; basophil, Eo; Eosinophil, M; Monocyte

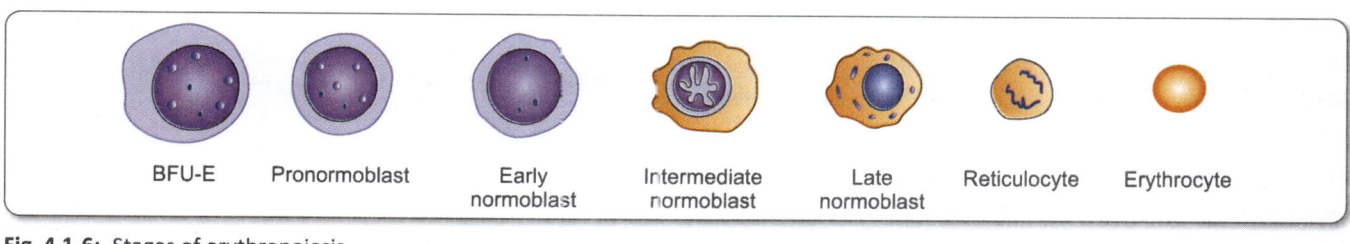

Fig. 4.1-6: Stages of erythropoiesis

Progenitor cells possess ability to give rise to *clones* (group of cells), so they are also called *colony-forming cells* (CFC) or *colony-forming units* (CFU).

The broad outlines of hemopoiesis discussed above are summarized in Figure 4.1-5.

Stages of Erythropoiesis

The red blood cells develop from the burst-forming unit—erythrocyte (BFU-E) and colony-forming unit—erythrocyte (CFU-E) which are derived from the committed progenitor cells.

The different stages of erythropoiesis (Fig. 4.1-6) are as under:

Pronormoblast or proerythroblast is the earliest recognizable cell of the erythroid series seen in the red bone marrow.

Early (basophilic) normoblast (basophilic early erythroblast). The pronormoblast progresses into the early normoblast.

Intermediate (polychromatic) normoblast (poly-chromatic erythroblast). It is the next maturation stage in erythroid series. *Hemoglobin* appears in this stage.

Late (orthochromatic) normoblast (orthochromatic erythroblast) is the last nucleated cell of erythroid series.

Reticulocyte is the last stage in the formation of erythrocytes, that is why it is also called young red cell. Its features are:
- *Size and shape:* The reticulocyte is a flat, disc- shaped, slightly larger (7–7.5 μm) than the mature erythrocytes.
- *Cytoplasm* still contains small amounts of RNA. With supervital stain such as brilliant cresyl blue, the RNA appears in the form of a reticulum (net-like structure). Because of this character the cell is called reticulocyte.
- *Nucleus* is absent.

Summary of Changes Occurring in Cells of Erythroid Series During Maturation

It takes 7 days for the formation and maturation of red blood cells. Various changes which occur during maturation from the stage of pronormoblast to erythrocyte are summarized here:

Size of the cell (from 15 μm to 20 μm of pronormoblast) goes on decreasing with subsequent stages till it reaches about 7 μm.

Nucleus first condenses, then becomes pyknotic and finally disappears at the stage of reticulocyte formation.

Hemoglobin synthesis starts at the stage of intermediate normoblast and then its content increases progressively.

Cytoplasm staining. Initially, before the appearance of hemoglobin the cytoplasm is basophilic. When hemoglobin starts appearing cytoplasm becomes polychromatic, i.e., stained both by acidic and basic dyes. In the stage of late normoblast when hemoglobin synthesis is almost completed, cytoplasm is stained by acidic dye.

Mitosis is seen up to the stage of intermediate normoblast. During these stages, 3–5 cell divisions occur. In this way, each pronormoblast gives rise to 8–320 late normoblasts. From the stage of late normoblast onwards the mitosis ceases and cell only matures.

Regulation of Erythropoiesis

Erythropoietin

Erythropoietin is a hormone which regulates the process of erythropoeisis.

Site of formation. Erythropoietin is mainly produced by the juxtaglomerular apparatus of kidney.

Stimulus for secretion. A certain basal level of the hormone is necessary for the normal rate of erythropoiesis. Whenever, there is hypoxia or decrease in the number of red blood cells (e.g. after hemorrhage or in hemolytic anemia), there occurs a release of renal erythropoietic factor from juxtaglomerular cells of kidney. Renal erythropoietic factor acts on the plasma alpha globulin called erythropoietinogen to form the erythropoietin. Thus the levels of erythropoietin vary with degree of hypoxia or number of circulating red blood cells.

Vitamin B$_{12}$ Folic Acid and Intrinsic Factor of Castle

Role of vitamin B$_{12}$. Vitamin B$_{12}$ (cyanocobalamin), also known as extrinsic factor is essential for maturation of red cells. It is required for the synthesis of DNA and maturation of nucleus and cell.

Intrinsic factor a glycoprotein secreted by parietal cells of gastric mucosa. It is essential for the absorption of vitamin B_{12}.

Folic acid. Folic acid (pteroylglutamic acid) and related compounds, known as folate, play an important role in the synthesis of DNA.

CLINICAL ASPECTS

Deficiency of vitamin B_{12} and folic acid leads to:
- Failure of maturation of nucleus.
- Cells remain large (megaloblasts) and become more fragile causing megaloblastic anemia.

Factors necessary for hemoglobinization. Various factors necessary for hemoglobin formation in the red blood cells are described later. (For details see page 155).

HEMOGLOBIN

The cytoplasm of erythrocytes (red blood cells) contains an *oxygen-binding protein* called hemoglobin. Erythrocyte precursors synthesize hemoglobin, while the mature erythrocytes lose the property of synthesizing hemoglobin.

Normal Blood Hemoglobin

The normal blood hemoglobin/concentration ranges from 16.5 g/dL to 18.5 g/dL.
- *At birth,* the hemoglobin concentration is 23 g/dL.
- *In adult males* the mean blood hemoglobin concentration is 9.5 g/dL (range 14–18 g/dL).
- *In adult females* the mean hemoglobin concentration is 14 g/dL (range 12–15.5 g/dL).

Structure of Hemoglobin (Figs 4.1-7A to D)

Hemoglobin is a globular molecule which consists of the protein *globin* combined with iron-containing pigment called *heme.*

Structure of Globin

The protein globin, present in the hemoglobin, is made of four polypeptide chains. HbA consists of the following four polypeptide chains:

Two α chains, each containing 141 amino acid residues

Two β chains, each containing 146 amino acid residues

Therefore, the normal adult hemoglobin A is written as HbA ($\alpha_2\beta_2$).

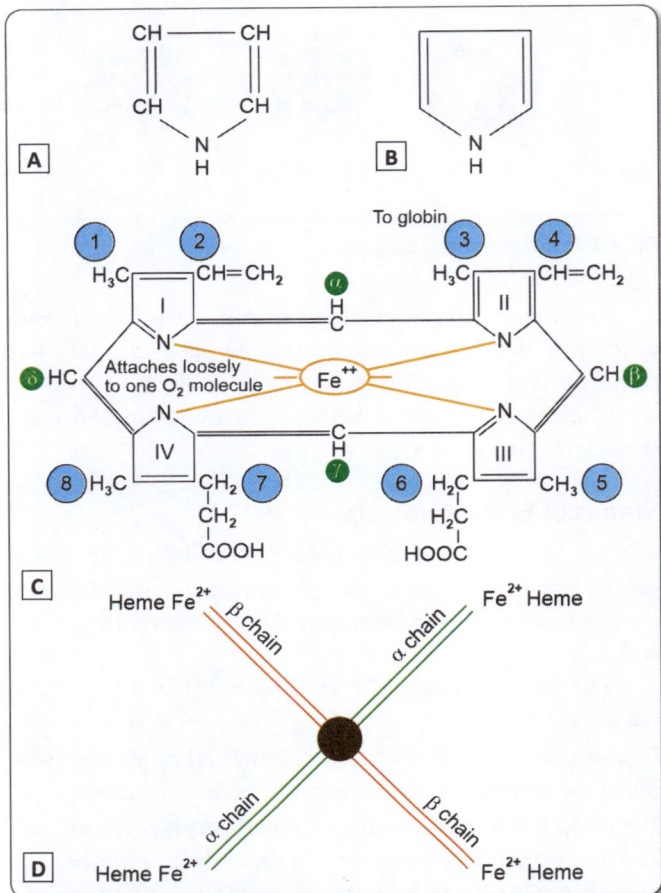

Figs 4.1-7A to D Chemistry of hemoglobin: A. Structure of a pyrrole ring; B. Conventional outline of a pyrrole ring; C. Arrangement of pyrrole rings in one unit of heme (iron protoporphyrin X); D. Arrangement of four units of heme in one molecule of hemoglobin.

Structure of Heme

The heme is a iron-porphyrin complex called *iron-protoporphyrin IX*, i.e., it consists of a porphyrin nucleus and the iron. The iron in the heme is in *ferrous* (Fe^{2+}) form.

One molecule of hemoglobin contains four units of heme, each attached to one of the four polypeptide chains constituting globin (Fig. 4.1-7D). As there are four units of heme in one molecule of hemoglobin, so there are four iron atoms in one molecule of Hb which can carry four molecules (eight atoms) of oxygen.

Functions of Hemoglobin

Transport of O_2 from lungs to tissues. In the lungs, one molecule of O_2 is attached loosely and reversibly at the sixth covalent bond of each iron atom of the hemoglobin to form *oxyhemoglobin* represented as HbO_2:

$$Hb + O_2 \rightarrow HbO_2$$

Deoxygenated (reduced) hemoglobin — Oxygenated hemoglobin

Transport of CO_2 from the tissues to the lungs. Hemoglobin also transports CO_2 from the tissues to the lungs.

It is important to note that CO_2 from the tissues is transported by combining with amino acids of the globin part as shown below and not in combination with Fe^{2+} atom like O_2.

$$R-N\begin{matrix}H\\H\end{matrix} + CO_2 \rightarrow R-N\begin{matrix}H\\COOH\end{matrix}$$

Hemoglobin — Carbaminohemoglobin

Control of pH of the blood. The hemoglobin constitutes the most important acid-base buffer system of blood. Hb has six times the buffering capacity as compared to plasma proteins.

Varieties of Hemoglobin

Various varieties of hemoglobin can be grouped as under:

Physiological Varieties of Hemoglobin
Adult hemoglobin

Adult hemoglobin is of two types.

1. ***Hemoglobin A*** [HbA ($\alpha_2\beta_2$)]: It is the main form of normal adult hemoglobin. As described by Canlier, its globin part consists of two alpha and two beta polypeptide chains.

2. ***Hemoglobin A_2*** [HbA$_2$ ($\alpha_2\delta_2$)]: It is a minor component (about 2.5% of the total Hb) in normal adults. Its globin part consists of two alpha and two delta polypeptide chains.

Fetal hemoglobin

Fetal hemoglobin, or hemoglobin F [HbF $\alpha_2\gamma_2$] as the name indicates refers to the hemoglobin present in the fetal RBCs and gradually disappears 2–3 months after birth. In HbF globin part consists of two alpha and two gamma polypeptide chains (in place of beta chains of HbF).

Special features of HbF are as follows.

1. ***Affinity for oxygen*** in case of HbF more than that of HbA, i.e., it can take more oxygen than HbA at low oxygen pressure.

2. ***Resistance to action of alkalies*** is more in HbF than HbA. This property is used in a photoelectric calorimetric method to estimate HbF in the presence of HbA.

CLINICAL ASPECTS
HEMOGLOBINOPATHIES

Hemoglobinopathies, i.e., abnormal formation of hemoglobin occurs due to disorders of globin synthesis; heme synthesis being normal. Disorders of globin synthesis are of two main types:

1. ***Formation of abnormal polypeptide chains:*** Example of such a disorder is hemoglobin S.
2. ***Suppression of synthesis of polypeptide chain*** of globin as seen in thalassemia.

Synthesis of Hemoglobin

Hemoglobin is synthesized in the cytoplasm of intermediate normoblasts.

Synthesis of Heme

Heme is synthesized in the mitochondria. Succinyl-CoA (derived from the citric acid cycle in mitochondria) and glycine are the starting substances in the synthesis of heme.

Synthesis of Globin

Globin, the protein part of the hemoglobin, is synthesized in ribosomes.

Factors Controlling Hemoglobin Formation

Role of proteins. First class proteins provide amino acids required for synthesis of globin part of the hemoglobin. A low protein intake retards hemoglobin regeneration even in the presence of excess iron.

Role of iron. Iron is necessary for formation of heme part of hemoglobin. In addition to dietary iron, the iron released by degradation of RBCs is also reused for synthesis of hemoglobin.

Role of other metals like:
- *Copper:* Copper is essential for hemoglobin synthesis, as it promotes the absorption, mobilization and utilization of iron.
- *Cobalt:* In some species cobalt increases the production of erythropoietin which in turn stimulates RBC formation.
- *Calcium:* Calcium is reported to help indirectly by conserving iron and its subsequent utilization.

Role of vitamins. Vitamin B_{12}, folic acid, and vitamin C help in synthesis of nucleic acid which in turn is required for the development of RBCs. Vitamin C also helps in absorption of iron from the gut.

Role of bile salts. Presence of bile salts in the intestine is necessary for proper absorption of metals like copper and nickel which in turn are essential factors for synthesis of hemoglobin.

LIFE SPAN AND FATE OF RED BLOOD CELLS

Life Span of Red Blood Cells

Normally, the average life span of red blood cells is 120 days.

Fate of Red Blood Cells

The cell membrane of old RBCs (after about 120 days) becomes more fragile due to decreased NADPH activity. The destruction of red cells occurs mostly in the capillaries of spleen because they have very thin lumen. Because of this, spleen is also called the graveyard of red blood cells. The hemoglobin released after hemolysis of red cells is taken up by the tissue macrophages.

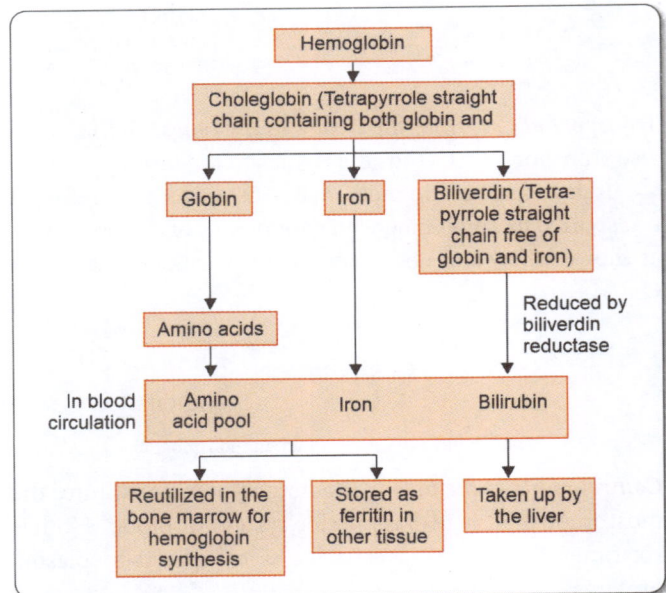

Fig. 4.1-8: Fate of hemoglobin

> **IMPORTANT TO KNOW**
>
> *The tissue macrophage system* (reticuloendothelial system) includes the following phagocytic cells:
> - *In the bone marrow,* these cells form part of the lining of the blood sinuses (littoral cells)
> - *In the liver,* they lie at intervals along the vascular capillaries (Kupffer cells)
> - *In the spleen,* they are found in the pulp
> - *In the lymph nodes,* they line the lymphatic paths.

Fate of hemoglobin (Fig. 4.1-8)

In the macrophages, the heme part of the hemoglobin molecule is altered by oxidation of one of its methine (=CH) bridges. As a result of chemical changes, the globin, iron and biliverdin (tetrapyrrole straight chain free from globin and iron) are formed.

Globin is degraded into amino acids and joins the amino acid pool of plasma and is released.

Iron released into the circulation is:
- Carried into the bone marrow for reutilization, and
- In the other tissues, it combines with apoferritin to form the ferritin (storage form of iron).

Biliverdin (tetrapyrrole straight chain free from globin and iron) is converted into bilirubin (by the enzyme biliverdin reductase) and is released into the blood.

Bilirubin

Bilirubin formation and its fate

As discussed above, the bilirubin is formed in the macrophages. It undergoes the following changes:

Uptake of bilirubin. Macrophages release the bilirubin into circulation. This bilirubin is called free or *unconjugated bilirubin*. It is lipid-soluble which prevents its excretion by the kidneys.

Conjugation of bilirubin. The unconjugated bilirubin (bound to albumin) from the circulation is taken up by the liver. In the hepatic cells, it is conjugated with uridine diphosphate glucuronic acid (UDP-glucuronic acid) making it a water-soluble conjugated *bilirubin*.

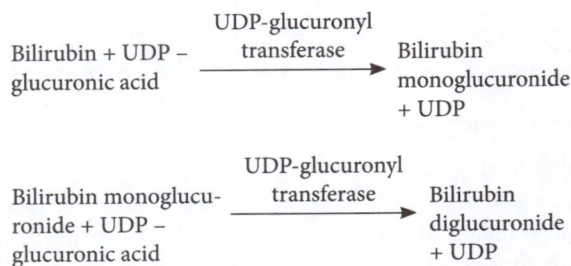

Excretion of bilirubin. The conjugated bilirubin from the hepatic cells is excreted into the bile and enters the intestine. Some of it escapes into general circulation and is excreted by the kidneys in urine as *urine bilirubin*.

Formation and excretion of urobilinogen. The conjugated bilirubin which enters the intestine with the bile is degraded by the intestinal bacteria and bilirubin is converted into the *urobilinogen* (stercobilinogen) which is a colorless compound.
- Some urobilinogen (20%) from the intestine is reabsorbed and goes via the portal system to the liver. From the liver some urobilinogen escapes into general circulation

and some is re-excreted into the bile (enterohepatic circulation).

- From general circulation, the urobilinogen is filtered off by the kidney and is excreted in the urine.

Normal Value

The normal serum bilirubin level ranges from 0.3 mg to 1.0 mg/100 mL.

CLINICAL ASPECTS

JAUNDICE

Jaundice (icterus) refers to the yellow appearance of the skin, sclera and mucous membranes resulting from an increased bilirubin concentration (*hyperbilirubinemia)* in the body fluids. Clinically, jaundice is detectable when the plasma bilirubin exceeds 2–3 mg/100 mL.

Types

Hyperbilirubinemia can result from the following mechanisms:

- *Excessive breakdown* of red blood cells (hemolysis) produces *hemolytic jaundice* or *prehepatic jaundice.*
- *Damage to liver cells* produces hepatic or hepatocellular jaundice.
- *Obstruction to bile duct* produces posthepatic or obstructive jaundice.

Physiological Jaundice of Newborn

Physiological jaundice of newborn is also called neonatal jaundice. It appears within 2–5 days of birth and usually disappears in 2 weeks. Its mechanism of production includes:

- *Excessive destruction of RBCs* occurs in first few days after birth causing increase in serum bilirubin.
- *Hepatic immaturity* in the first few (7–10) days after birth also contributes to increased serum bilirubin.

Prevention and Treatment

Prevention: Neonatal jaundice can be prevented by administration of hepatic microsomal enzyme inducers (e.g. phenobarbital) to the pregnant mother or newborn. The microsomal enzyme inducers increase the activity of glucuronyl transferase in liver.

Treatment: Normal jaundice can be effectively treated by *phototherapy.* Exposure of the skin to white light causes photoisomerization of bilirubin to water-soluble *lumirubin* which can be rapidly excreted in bile without requiring any conjugation.

ANEMIAS

Definition

Anemia is not a single disease but a group of disorders in which hemoglobin concentration of blood is below the normal range for the age and sex of the subject. Therefore anemia is labeled when hemoglobin concentration is less than:

- 13 g/dL in adult males
- 11.5 g/dL in adult females
- 15 g/dL in newborn
- 9.5 g/dL at 3 month of age.

Low RBC count (less than 4 million/mm³) is usually, but not always, associated with low hemoglobin levels in anemia.

Grading of anemia, depending upon the level of hemoglobin, has somewhat arbitrarily been made as:

- Mild anemia—Hb 8–10 g%

- Moderate anemia—Hb 6–8 g%
- Severe anemia—Hb below 6 g%.

Classification

Etiological (Whitby's) Classification

Types of anemia depending upon the causative mechanism are:
Deficiency anemias

- Iron-deficiency anemia
- Megaloblastic anemia (pernicious anemia) due to deficiency of vitamin B_{12}
- Megaloblastic anemia due to deficiency of folic acid
- Protein and vitamin C deficiency can also cause anemia.

Blood loss anemias or hemorrhagic anemias are commonly known and can be:

- *Acute post-hemorrhagic anemia* as in accidents
- *Chronic post-hemorrhagic anemia*

Hemolytic anemias: These are relatively uncommon and occur in conditions associated with increased destruction of red blood cells.

Aplastic anemia: It occurs due to failure of bone marrow to produce RBCs.

Anemia due to chronic diseases: It is seen in tuberculosis, chronic infections, malignancies, chronic lung diseases, etc.

Iron Deficiency Anemia

Iron deficiency anemia is the most common nutritional deficiency disorder present throughout the world, but its prevalence is higher in the developing countries. In India, iron deficiency is the most common cause of anemia. Iron deficiency anemia is much more common:

- In women between 20 and 45 years than in men.
- At periods of active growth in infancy, childhood and adolescence.

Megaloblastic Anemia

Megaloblastic anemias are characterized by abnormally large cells of erythrocyte series. These are caused by defective DNA synthesis due to deficiency of vitamin B_{12} and/or folic acid (folate).

General Clinical Features of Anemia

General clinical manifestations of anemia which occur either due to tissue hypoxia or due to compensatory mechanisms are:

- Generalized muscular weakness
- Pallorness of skin and mucous membranes
- Breathlessness
- Palpitation
- Visual disturbances
- Anorexia, atrophy of papillae on tongue
- In females, menstrual disturbances occur such as amenorrhea and menorrhagia.

WHITE BLOOD CELLS

TYPES OF WHITE BLOOD CELLS AND THEIR COUNTS

The white blood cells (WBCs) or leucocytes are so named since they are colorless in contrast to red color of RBCs. These are nucleated cells and play important role in defence mechanism of the body.

Types

The leucocytes of the peripheral blood are of two main varieties: granulocytes and non-granulocytes.

Granulocytes

The white blood cells with granules in their cytoplasm are called granulocytes. Depending upon the color of granules, granulocytes are further divided into three types (Fig. 4.1-9):

1. Neutrophils
2. Eosinophils
3. Basophils

Agranulocytes

White blood cells which do not contain granules in their cytoplasm are called agranulocytes. These are of two types (Fig. 4.1-9):

1. Lymphocytes
2. Monocytes.

Normal WBC Counts

Total Leucocyte Count

Total leucocyte count (TLC) varies with age as:
Adults. 4000–11000/mm³ of blood.
At birth, in full-term infant: 10,000–25,000/mm³ of blood.
Infants up to 1 year of age: 6,000–16,000/mm³ of blood.

Differential and Absolute Leucocyte Count

Differential leucocyte count (DLC) and absolute count in normal adults is shown in Table 4.1-1.

TABLE 4.1-1: Differential leucocyte count and absolute count in normal adults

WBCs	Differential count (%)	Absolute count (per mm³)
Granulocytes		
• Neutrophils	40–75	2000–7500
• Eosinophils	1–6	40–440
• Basophils	0–1	40–440
Agranulocytes		
• Lymphocytes	20–40	1500–4000
• Monocytes	2–10	500–800

CLINICAL SIGNIFICANCE OF DIFFERENTIAL AND ABSOLUTE COUNTS

The differential leucocyte count (DLC) tells us if there is an increase or decrease in a particular type of leucocyte, because in different diseases one or the other type of cells show an increase or decrease in its numbers. The differential count is done in 100 or 200 cells and tells only a relative increase or decrease in particular variety of cells. DLC alone is not of much importance and so never done as an isolated test, but always it is part of full blood counts including TLC and then calculating absolute count.

VARIATIONS IN WBC COUNT

Leukocytosis

Leukocytosis refers to increase in total WBC count above 11000/mm³.

Physiological Causes of Leucocytosis

Age. In newborn babies up to the age of one year WBC count is higher. At birth WBC count is about 18,000/mm³ which drops gradually to adult level.
Exercise. The WBC count is increased after exercise.
After food intake the WBC count is raised.
Mental stress and emotional conditions like anxiety are associated with raised WBC count.

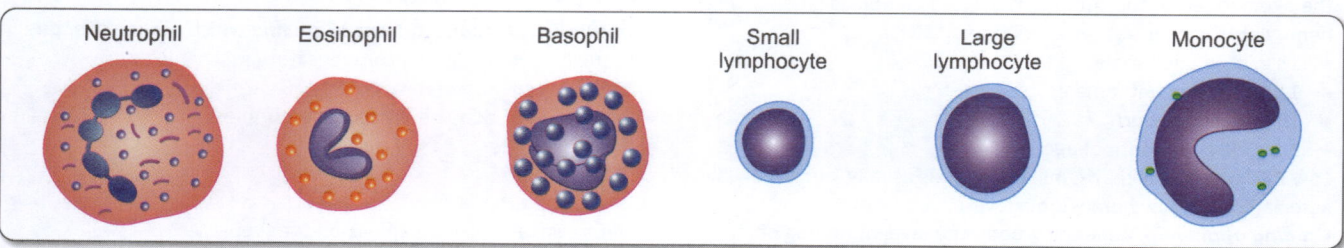

Fig. 4.1-9: Granulocytes and agranulocytes

Pregnancy. At full-term pregnancy WBC count is 12,000–15,000 mm^3.

Exposure to low temperature also causes leucocytosis.

Pathological Causes of Leucocytosis

- Acute bacterial infections especially by pyogenic organisms
- Acute hemorrhage
- Postoperative period
- Burns
- Tuberculosis.

Leucopenia

Leucopenia refers to decrease in the total WBC count below 4000/mm^3.

Causes of Leucopenia

Infections by nonpyogenic bacteria, especially typhoid fever and paratyphoid fever.

Viral infections such as influenza, smallpox, mumps, etc.

Protozoal infections.

Starvation and malnutrition.

Aplasia of bone marrow or bone marrow depression due to:

- Drugs such as chloromycetin and cytotoxic drugs used in malignant diseases.
- Repeated exposure to X-rays or radiations.
- Chemical poisons, like arsenic, dinitrophenol, and antimony.

FORMATION OF WHITE BLOOD CELLS

The process of development and maturation of white blood cells (leucocytes) called leucopoiesis is a part of hemopoiesis (formation of blood cells). All the blood cells develop from the so called pluripotent hemopoietic stem cells (PHSCs). The stem cells after a series of divisions differentiate into progenitor cells which are also called colony-forming units (CFU). (For details see page 152).

The leucopoiesis can be discussed under two headings:

1. Formation of granulocytes (granulopoiesis) and monocytes
2. Formation of lymphocytes (lymphopoiesis).

Formation of Granulocytes and Monocytes

The granulocytes and monocytes are formed in the bone marrow from the colony-forming unit called CFU-GM (colony-forming unit granulocytes and monocytes): The progenitor cells (CFU-GM) forming different cells are further named as:

- CFU-G are neutrophil forming units
- CFU-Eo refers to eosinophil forming units
- CFU-Ba are basophil forming units
- CFU-M refers to monocyte forming units.

The development of granulocytes through various stages is called *myeloid series* and development of monocytes through various stages is called *monocyte-macrophage series.*

Myeloid Series

Some facts about granulopoiesis.

- The cells of myeloid series include myeloblast (most primitive precursor), promyelocytes, myelocytes, metamyelocytes, band forms and segmented granulocyte (mature form).
- The process of granulopoiesis takes about 12 days.
- Granulocytes are formed and stored in the bone marrow. When need arises they are released in circulation. Normally about three times or many granulocytes are stored in the bone marrow as these circulate in the peripheral blood.

Monocyte-macrophage Series (Fig. 4.1-10)

Monocyte macrophage series include monoblast, promonocytes and monocyte.

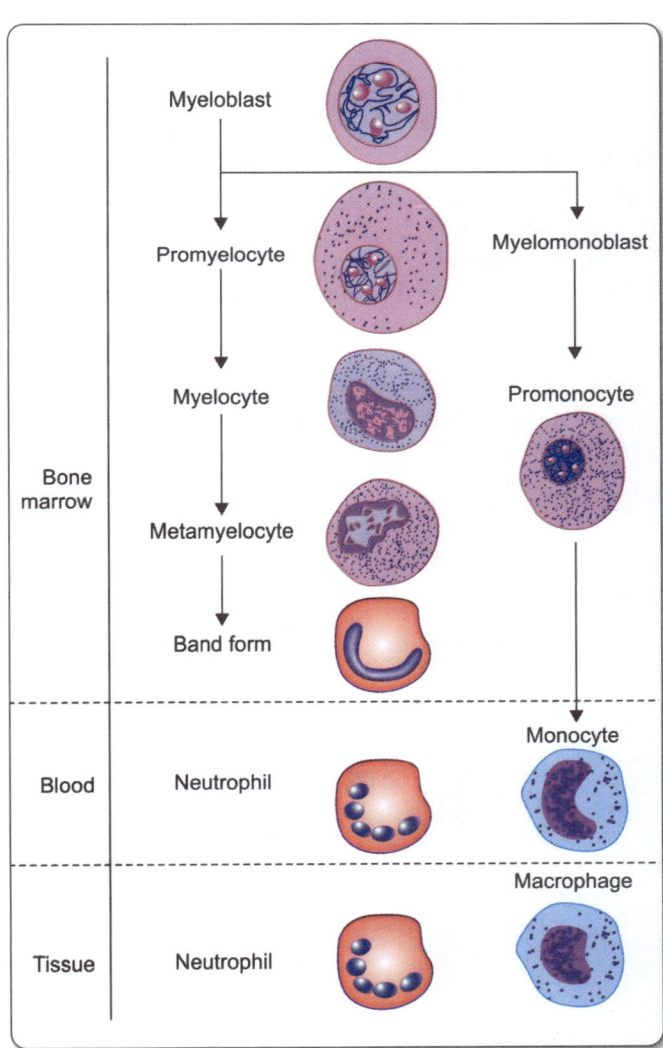

Fig. 4.1-10: Granulopoiesis and features of the cells of myeloid series and monocyte-macrophage series

From the bone marrow, the monocytes migrate into spleen and lymphoid tissues in considerable numbers. The transformed stages of these cells in various tissues are called *tissue macrophages* and form a part of *tissue-macrophage system*, which was previously known as *reticuloendothelial system*.

Formation of Lymphocytes

The lymphocytes are formed from the *lymphocyte stem cells* which are formed from the pluripotent hemopoietic stem cells (PHSC) in the bone marrow (Fig. 4.1-11). The lymphocyte stem cells migrate into thymus and peripheral lymphoid tissues where they proliferate and mature into lymphocytes. The tissues which actively produce lymphocytes from the germinal centers of lymphoid follicles as a response to antigenic stimulation constitute the so called *secondary* or *reactive lymphoid tissue*. It is comprised of the:

- Lymph nodes
- Spleen
- Gut-associated lymphoid tissue (GALT).

Lymphoid Series

The maturation stages of lymphoid series are lymphoblast, prolymphocytes and lymphocyte (Fig. 4.1-11).

Prolymphocytes mature successively into large lymphocyte and small lymphocyte, both of which are found in circulation. Then some lymphocytes enter thymus where they are processed and come out as T lymphocytes. Some lymphocytes are processed in liver (in fetal life) and bone marrow (after birth). These come out as B *lymphocytes.*

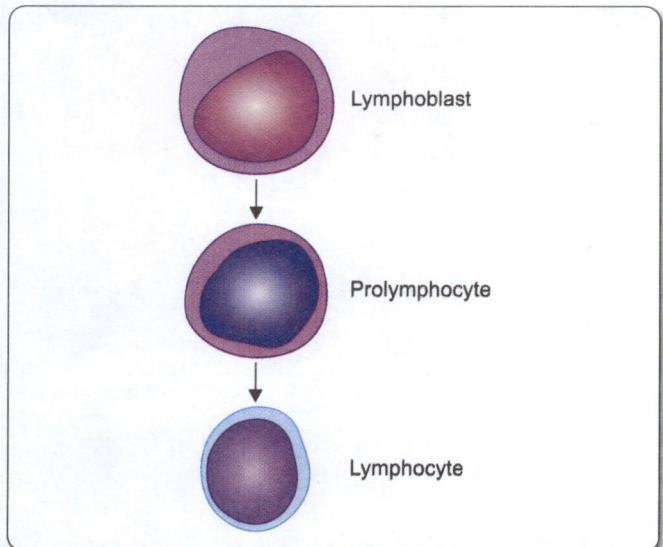

Fig. 4.1-11: Formation of lymphoid series cells.

The word B comes from 'bursa of Fabricius which is the site of B cell processing in birds.

Regulation of Leucopoiesis

The constancy of leucocyte count suggests a feedback mechanism to control their production and release. During tissue injury and inflammation, bacterial toxins, products of injury, etc. cause a great increase in the rate of production and release of leucocytes. Thus, unlike erythropoiesis, the products of dead and dying white cells themselves control leucopoiesis. The substances which stimulate or inhibit the process of leucopoiesis are complex and include the following:

Role of Cytokines

The cytokines which control the formation of different types of granulocytes are called colony stimulating factors (CSFs). The CSFs are glycoproteins formed by monocytes and T-lymphocytes.

Role of Prostaglandins

Prostaglandins formed by monocytes, and possibly some other agents also play role in control of leucopoiesis.

MORPHOLOGY AND FUNCTIONS OF LEUCOCYTE

Morphological features of various types of WBCs as studied under microscope with Leishman's staining and hematoxylin eosin stain are summarized below along with their functions and variations in their counts.

Neutrophils

Morphological features

The polymorphonuclear neutrophils commonly called polymorphs or neutrophils have the following morphological features:

Diameter. Diameter of a neutrophil varies from 10-14 μm.

Nucleus. Nucleus of a mature neutrophil is purple in color and multilobed (2–6 lobes).

Cytoplasm. Cytoplasm of neutrophil is pale bluish in color and full of fine (pinpoint) granules.

- Granules take both acidic and basic stain and look violet-pink in color.

Functions

The neutrophils along with monocytes constitute the first line of defence against the microorganisms, viruses and other injurious agents that enter the body. Neutrophils subserve this role by the following mechanisms:

Phagocytosis. The neutrophils engulf the foreign particles or bacteria and digest them and ultimately may kill them by a process called phagocytosis.

Reaction of inflammation. The neutrophils also release leukotrienes, prostaglandins, thromboxanes, etc. that bring about the reactions of inflammation like vasodilatation and edema.

Febrile response. The neutrophils contain a fever-producing substance called *endogenous pyrogen*, which is an important mediator of febrile response to the bacterial pyrogens.

Eosinophils
Morphological Features
Morphological features of eosinophils are:

Diameter of eosinophils is similar to neutrophils, i.e., 10–14 µm.

Nucleus is purple in color and is bilobed *spectacle-shaped*.

Cytoplasm is acidophilic and appears bright pink in color.
- It contains coarse, deep red staining granules which do not cover the nucleus.
- The granules contain histamine, lysosomal enzymes and eosinophil chemotactic factor of anaphylaxis (ECF-A).

Functions of Eosinophils
Mild phagocytosis. Eosinophils are not very motile and thus have very mild phagocytic activity.

Role in parasitic infestations. They play an important role in the defence mechanism of body, especially in *parasitic infestations.*

Role in allergic reaction. The eosinophils increase in number in allergic conditions like bronchial asthma and hay fever.

Role in immunity. The eosinophils are present in abundance in the mucosa of respiratory tract, gastro-intestinal tract and urinary tract, where they probably provide mucosal immunity.

Basophils
Morphological Features
Diameter of a basophil is similar to neutrophil and eosinophil, i.e., 10–14 µm.

Nucleus of basophil is irregular, may be bilobed or trilobed, and its boundary is not clearly defined because of overcrowding with coarse granules.

Cytoplasm of basophils is slightly basophilic and appears blue. It is full of granules.
- Granules of basophils are very coarse and stain deep purple or blue with basic (methylene) dye.
- They contain heparin, histamine and 5-HT.

Functions
Mild phagocytosis. Basophils have very mild phagocytic function.

Role in allergic reaction. Basophils release histamine, bradykinin, slow reacting substances of anaphylaxis (SRS-A) and serotonin (5HT). These substances, in turn, cause many allergic manifestations.

Role in preventing spread of allergic inflammatory process. Basophils also release eosinophil chemotactic factor that causes eosinophils to migrate toward the inflamed allergic tissue. Eosinophils then phagocytose and destroy antigen-antibody complexes and prevent spread of local inflammatory process.

Release of heparin. Basophils release heparin in the blood which prevents clotting of the blood.

Lymphocytes
Morphological Features
There are two types of lymphocytes large and small having almost similar structure. Morphological features of lymphocytes are:

Diameter. Diameter of large lymphocytes varies from 12 µm to 16 µm and that of small lymphocytes from 7 µm to 10 µm.

Nucleus. Lymphocytes have a large round, single nucleus which almost completely fills the cell. It stains blue very deeply giving *ink-spot appearance*. Nuclear chromatin is coarsely clumped and shapeless.

Cytoplasm. The cytoplasm is scanty, i.e., its amount is always less than that of nucleus. It is seen as crescent of clear light blue color around the nucleus. Cytoplasm does not contain visible granules.

Functional Subtypes
Based on their developmental background, lifespan and functions, the small lymphocytes have been broadly classified into three subtypes:

1. *B lymphocytes,* which are processed in the bone marrow are concerned with the humoral immunity.

2. *T lymphocytes* which are processed in the thymus are concerned with cellular immunity.

3. *Natural killer (NK) cells* are lymphocyte-like cells that nonspecifically kill any cell that is coated with immunoglobulin IgG. This phenomenon is called *antigen-dependent cell-mediated cytotoxicity (ADCC).* Thus NK cells provide *innate immunity.*

Functions

Lymphocytes play important role in immunity. B lymphocytes are responsible for the development of *humoral immunity* also called antibody-mediated immunity (AMI).

T lymphocytes are responsible for the development of *cellular immunity*, also called cell-mediated immunity (CMI) or T cell immunity (For detail see Chapter 4.3).

Monocytes
Morphological Features

Diameter. The monocyte is the largest mature leucocyte in the peripheral blood measuring some 12–20 µm in diameter.

Nucleus. The nucleus of monocyte is large, single and eccentric in position, i.e., present on one side of the cell. It may be notched, or indented, i.e., horseshoe- or kidney-shaped.

Cytoplasm. The cytoplasm is abundant, pale-blue and usually clear (no granules). Sometimes, it may contain fine purple, dust-like granules called *azur granules.*

Functions

Role in defence mechanism. Monocytes along with neutrophils play important role in the body's defence mechanism. Their main function is *phagocytosis.* Monocytes after entering in the tissue get converted to macrophages. They also have ability to engulf large particles such as red blood cells and malarial parasites.

Role in tumor immunity. Monocytes may also kill tumor cells after sensitization by lymphocytes.

Synthesis of biological substances. Monocytes synthesize complement and other biologically important substances.

CLINICAL ASPECTS

VARIATIONS IN COUNTS OF WBCs

Neutrophilia refers to increase in the circulating neutrophil counts (absolute count >10,000/mm³). It is the most common cause of leucocytosis.
Physiological causes of neutrophilia are:
- Newborn babies
- After exercise
- After meals
- Pregnancy, menstruation, parturition and lactation
- Mental stress and emotional stress
- After injection of epinephrine.
Pathological causes of neutrophilia are:
- Acute pyogenic bacterial infections
- Noninfective inflammatory conditions like gout, acute rheumatic fever
Neutropenia: Decrease in neutrophil count is known as neutropenia (absolute count <2500/mm³).
Common causes:
- Typhoid and paratyphoid fever
- Malaria
Eosinophilia refers to increase in the eosinophil count (absolute count >500/mm³).
Causes of eosinophilia are:
- Bronchial asthma and hay fever
- Parasitic infestation, e.g. intestinal worms like hookworm, roundworm and tapeworm
- Skin diseases like urticaria.
Eosinopenia is the decrease in eosinophil count (absolute count <50/mm³). It occurs in stressful conditions.
Basophilia refers to increase in the basophil count (absolute count >100/mm³)
Causes of basophilia are:
- Viral infections, e.g. influenza, smallpox and chicken-pox
- Allergic diseases
- Chronic myeloid leukemia.
Basopenia: Decrease in basophil count is called basopenia.

Lymphocytosis refers to increase in the lymphocyte count (absolute count >4000/mm³).
In healthy infants and young children the lymphocyte count is usually high (about 60% in DLC) while the TLC is normal (relative lymphocytosis).
Pathological causes of lymphocytosis are:
- Chronic infections like tuberculosis, hepatitis and whooping cough
- Viral infections like chickenpox
- Lymphatic leukemia (most common cause of lymphocytes >10,000/mm³).
Lymphopenia or lymphocytopenia refers to decrease in lymphocyte count (absolute count below 1500/mm³).
Causes of lymphopenia are:
- Patients on corticosteroid and immunosuppressive therapy
- Hypoplastic bone marrow
- Acquired immunodeficiency syndrome (AIDS).
Monocytosis: A rise in the blood monocytes above 800/mm³ is termed monocytosis.
Causes of monocytosis are:
- Certain bacterial infections such as tuberculosis, syphilis and subacute bacterial endocarditis.
- Infectious mononucleosis or the so called glandular fever.
- Viral infections
- Protozoal and rickettsial infections, e.g. malaria and kala-azar.
Monocytopenia refers to decrease in the monocyte count. It may be seen in hypoplastic bone marrow.

LEUKEMIAS

Leukemias constitute a group of malignant diseases of the blood in which there occurs an increase in the total WBC count associated with presence of immature WBCs in the peripheral blood. The total WBC count is usually above 50,000/mm³ and may be as high as 100,000–300,000/mm³.
- The proliferation of leukemic cells takes place primarily in the bone marrow and in certain form in the lymphoid tissues.

PLATELETS

STRUCTURE AND COMPOSITION

Platelets (small plates) also known as thrombocytes (thrombo = clot; cytes = cells) have the following features:

Size. Platelets are the smallest blood cells varying in diameter from 2 μm to 4 μm, with an average volume of 5.8 μm^3.

Shape and color. Platelets are colorless, spherical or oval discoid structures.

- *Leishman staining* shows a platelet to consist of faint bluish cytoplasm containing reddish purple granules.
- *Nucleus* is absent in the platelets and therefore, these cannot reproduce.

Electron Microscopic Structure

Under electron microscope, a platelet shows the following structural and compositional characteristics (Fig. 4.1-12):

Cell membrane. It consists of lipids (phospholipids, cholesterol and glycolipids), carbohydrates, proteins and glycoproteins.

Microtubules. Microtubules are made up of proteins called tubulins. These form a compact bundle which is present immediately beneath the platelet membrane. These are responsible for maintenance of discoid shape of circulating platelets.

Cytoplasm. Cytoplasm of the platelets contains:

- *Endoplasmic reticulum and Golgi apparatus:* These structures synthesize various enzymes and store large quantities of calcium.
- *Mitochondria:* These are capable of forming ATP and ADP.

Contractile proteins include actin, myosin and thrombosthenin. Contractile proteins can cause the platelet to contract and are thus responsible for the clot retraction.

Other proteins present in the cytoplasm are:

- Fibrin-stabilizing factor
- Platelet-derived growth factor
- von Willebrand factor

Granules present in the cytoplasm of platelets.

- Contain substances (like phospholipids, triglycerides, cholesterol) ATP, ADP and serotonin (5HT).
- Clotting factors, and platelet-derived growth factor (PDGF).

Enzymes present in the cytoplasm of platelets include adenosine triphosphatase and the enzyme necessary for synthesis of prostaglandins.

PROPERTIES AND FUNCTIONS

Properties of Platelets (Figs 4.1-13A to C)

Adhesiveness. Platelets possess the property of adhesiveness, i.e., when they come in contact with any wet surface or rough surface, these are activated and stick to the surface. Factors responsible for adhesiveness are collagen, thrombin, ADP, thromboxane A$_2$, calcium ions and von Willebrand factor.

Aggregation. Platelets have the property to aggregate, i.e., they stick to each other. This is due to ADP and thromboxane A$_2$.

Agglutination. Clumping together of platelets is called agglutination. This occurs due to the actions of some platelet agglutinins.

Functions of Platelets

When activated, platelets perform the following functions:

Role in hemostasis. Hemostasis refers to spontaneous arrest of bleeding from an injured blood vessel.

Role in clot formation. Platelets play an important role in the formation of the intrinsic prothrombin activator which is responsible for onset of blood clotting.

Role in clot retraction. Contraction of contractile proteins (actin, myosin and thrombosthenin) present in the platelets play an important role in clot retraction.

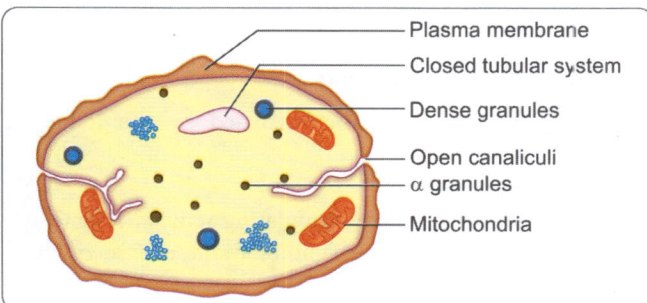

Plasma membrane
Closed tubular system
Dense granules
Open canaliculi
α granules
Mitochondria

Fig. 4.1-12 Structure of a platelet

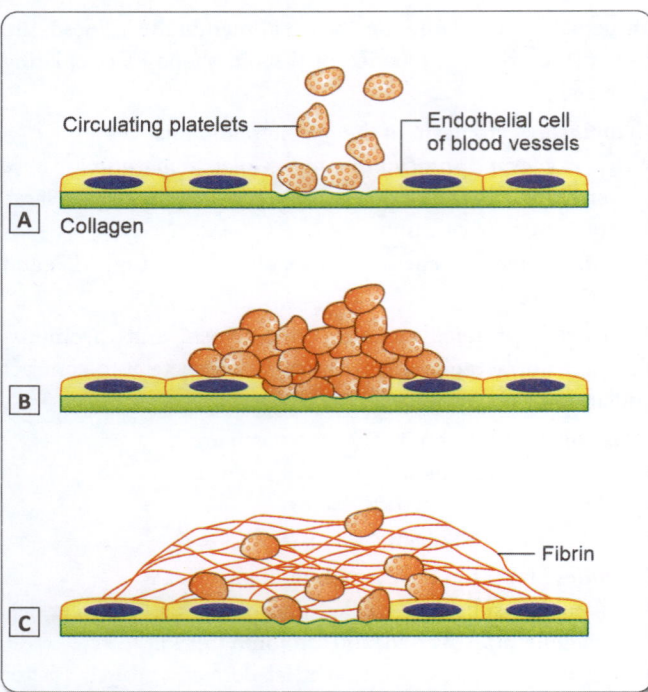

Figs 4.1-13A to C: Properties of platelets: **A.** Adhesiveness; **B.** Aggregation; **C.** Formation of hemostatic plug

Role in repair of injured blood vessels. The platelet-derived growth factor (PDGF) present in the cytoplasm plays an important role in the repair of endothelium of the injured/damaged blood vessels.

Role in defence mechanism. Platelets, due to their property of agglutination, are capable of phagocytosis.

Transport and storage function. The 5HT is stored in the platelets and transported to the site of injury where it is released.

NORMAL COUNT AND VARIATIONS

Normal Count

Normal platelet count ranges from 1,50,000 to 4,50,000/mm³ with an average count of 2.5 lac/mm³.

Physiological Variations

Age. Platelet count is less in infants (1 lac – 2 lac/mm³). Adult levels are reached by 3rd month of age.

Sex. Normally there is no difference in the platelet counts of males and females. However, during menstruation the count is reduced in females.

After meals, the platelet count is slightly increased.

After severe muscular exercise, platelets may increase. *At high altitude*, platelet count is increased.

CLINICAL ASPECTS

THROMBOCYTOSIS

An increase in the number of platelets (more than 4.5 lac/mm³) is called thrombocytosis.

Causes of thrombocytosis: Platelet count is increased:

After splenectomy

After hemorrhage, severe injury, major surgical operation, and parturition

In myeloproliferative disorders such as:

- Chronic myeloid leukemia
- Polycythemia vera
- Myelofibrosis.

THROMBOCYTOPENIA

Decrease in the number of platelets below 1.5 lac/mm³ is called thrombocytopenia.

Causes of thrombocytopenia are:

Idiopathic thrombocytopenic purpura

Bone marrow depression due to:

- Effects of various cytotoxic drugs
- Whole body irradiation
- Hypoplastic and aplastic anemia.

Acute leukemia or secondary deposits of malignancy in the bone marrow.

In infections like smallpox, chickenpox, typhoid and dengue fever.

In hypersplenism

In toxemia, septicemia and uremia.

FORMATION OF PLATELETS

Formation or development of platelets is called *thrombopoiesis*. The platelets are produced in the bone marrow. The pluripotent stem cell destined to form platelets is converted into colony forming units called Meg-CFU, which develop into platelets after passing through various stages Fig. 4.1-14.

Platelets are formed from pseudopodia of megakaryocyte cytoplasm which get detached into the blood stream. Each megakaryocyte may form up to 4000 platelets. The formation of platelets from the stem cell takes about 10 days.

Control of thrombopoiesis

Thrombopoiesis seems to be regulated by the following humoral factors:

- Thrombopoietin
- Megakaryocyte—colony stimulating activity (Meg CSA).

The factors stimulating the synthesis and release of these agents are not yet known.

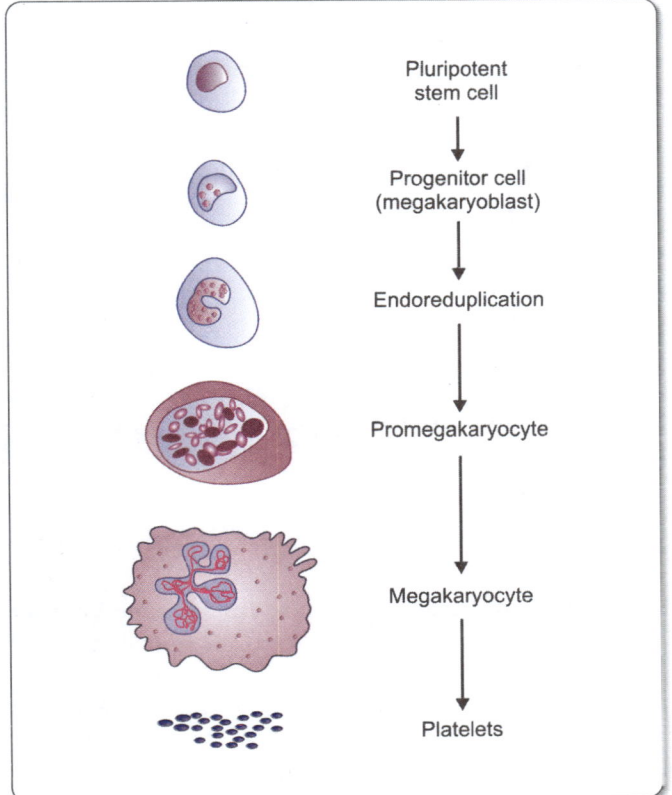

Fig. 4.1-14: Stages of thrombopoiesis

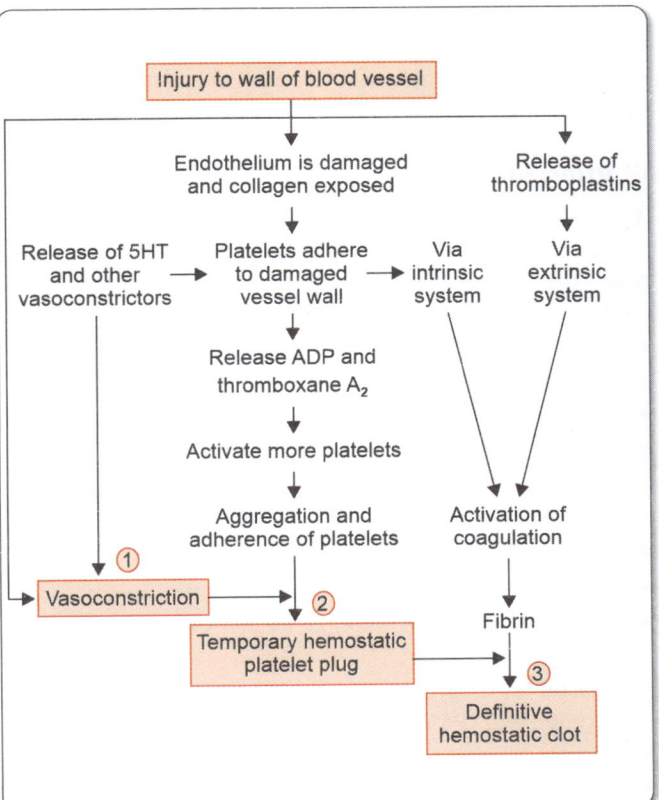

Fig. 4.1-15: Steps of hemostasis

Lifespan and fate of platelets

Lifespan of platelets varies from 8–12 days with an average of 10 days. Platelets are destroyed by tissue macrophage system in spleen. Therefore:

- *Splenomegaly* causes reduction in the platelet count
- *Splenectomy* is followed by an increase in platelet count.

HEMOSTASIS AND BLOOD COAGULATION

HEMOSTASIS

Hemostasis refers to spontaneous arrest or prevention of bleeding from the injured/damaged vessels by the physiological process. It involves three main steps (Fig. 4.1-15).

1. *Vasoconstriction.* Initial vasoconstriction is caused by direct effect of injury on the vascular smooth muscles the following injury to the vessels and due to release 5 HT and other vas constrictors.

2. *Formation of Temporary Hemostatic Plug.* Formation of a temporary hemostatic plug by the platelets at the site of injury involves the following steps:

- Platelet adhesion
- Platelet activation
- Platelet aggregation.

The platelet adherence and aggregation ultimately lead to the formation of platelet plug. At first, it is a fairly loose plug but is successful in blocking the blood loss if the vascular opening is small.

3. *Formation of Definitive Hemostatic Plug.* The temporary platelet plug is converted into the definitive hemostatic plug by the process of clot formation (blood coagulation). Platelets play an important role in the formation of the intrinsic prothrombin activator which is responsible for initiating the process of clot formation.

BLOOD COAGULATION

Blood remains in fluid condition within the blood vessels throughout life. But, when the blood is shed from the blood vessels or collected in a container, it loses its fluidity within a few minutes and gets converted into a jelly-like mass, which is called *clot*. This phenomenon is called *coagulation* or clotting of blood.

Clotting Factors

The process of coagulation essentially involves a stepwise activation of certain substances mostly proteins present in the blood and/or tissue fluids. These substances are called clotting factors and have been given Roman numerals:

- Factor I (Fibrinogen)
- Factor II (Prothrombin)
- Factor III (Thromboplastin)
- Factor IV (Calcium)
- Factor V (Labile factor or proaccelerin or accelerator globulin)
- Factor VI (non-existent)
- Factor VII (Stable factor or proconvertin)
- Factor VIII (antihemophilic factor A (AHF) or anti-hemophilic globulin (AHG))
- Factor IX (Christmas factor or plasma thromboplastic component (PTC or antihemophilic factor B)
- Factor X (Stuart-Prower factor)
- Factor XI (Plasma thromboplastin antecedent, i.e., PTA or antihemophilic factor C)
- Factor XII (Hageman factor or glass factor or contact factor)
- Factor XIII (Fibrin stabilizing factor or fibrinase or Laki-Lorand factor)
- HMW-K (High molecular weight kininogen or Fitzgerald factor)
- Pre-Ka (Prekallikrein or Fletcher factor)
- Ka (Kallikrein)
- PL (Platelet phospholipid).

Mechanism of Coagulation

Normally, blood circulates in the blood vessels and does not clot spontaneously. Clot formation is initiated under the following situations:

- Trauma to the vascular wall and adjacent tissues
- Trauma to blood
- Contact of blood with damaged endothelial cells or collagen or other tissue elements outside the vessel.

The process of coagulation involves a *cascade* of reactions in which activation of one factor leads to activation of next clotting factor (Fig. 4.1-16). This enzyme cascade reaction is also called water fall *sequence*. The process of coagulation can be divided into three main steps:

1. Formation of prothrombin activator
2. Conversion of prothrombin to thrombin
3. Conversion of fibrinogen into fibrin.

Formation of Prothrombin Activator

Two different mechanisms involved in the formation of prothrombin activator are:

- Extrinsic pathway
- Intrinsic pathway

Extrinsic pathway

The extrinsic pathway of formation of prothrombin activator begins with trauma to the vascular wall or the tissues outside the blood vessel. It includes the following three basic steps (Fig. 4.1-16):

1. Release of tissue thromboplastins. The traumatized tissues release several substances which are together known as *tissue thomboplastin (factor III)*.

2. Activation of factor X to form activated factor X. Tissue thromboplastin combines with factor VII (stable factor) to form the tissue thromboplastin-factor VII complex which in the presence of Ca^{2+} activates factor X to form activated factor X (Xa).

3. Effect of activated factor X to form prothrombin activator. The activated factor X along with tissue phospholipids or phospholipids released from platelets, factor V (Labile factor) and Ca^{2+} forms a complex which is called prothrombin activator.

Intrinsic pathway

The intrinsic pathway of formation of prothrombin activator begins in the blood itself the following trauma to blood itself or exposure of blood to collagen in a traumatized vascular wall. The steps of intrinsic pathway are summarized in Figure 4.1-16.

Activation of factor XII. Trauma to blood or exposure to collagen fibers underlying damaged vascular endothelium (or electronegatively charged wettable surface such as glass, in vitro) activates plasma factor XII to form XIIa and initiates the intrinsic pathway. Platelets are also activated.

Activation of factor XI to form XIa is caused by the activated factor XII.

Activation of factor IX to form IXa is in turn caused by the activated factor XI in the presence of Ca^{2+}.

Activation of factor X. Factor IXa in the presence of activated factor VIII, Ca^{2+} and phospholipids (released by activated platelets) activate factor X to form Xa.

Formation of prothrombin activator. The activated factor X along with the phospholipids released by activated platelets,

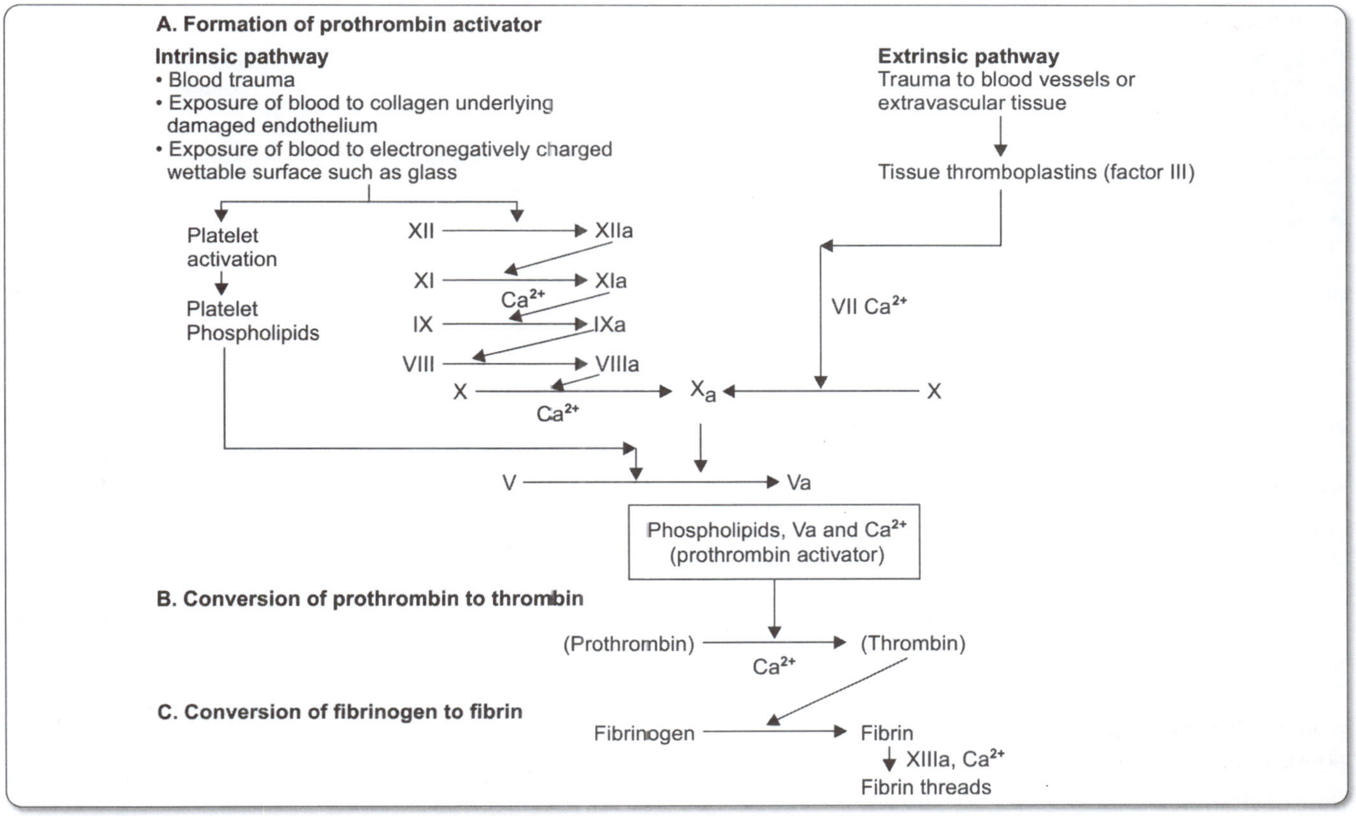

A. Formation of prothrombin activator

Intrinsic pathway
- Blood trauma
- Exposure of blood to collagen underlying damaged endothelium
- Exposure of blood to electronegatively charged wettable surface such as glass

Extrinsic pathway
Trauma to blood vessels or extravascular tissue

Tissue thromboplastins (factor III)

Platelet activation → Platelet Phospholipids

XII → XIIa
XI → XIa
Ca²⁺
IX → IXa
VIII → VIIIa
X → X$_a$
Ca²⁺

VII Ca²⁺

X → X$_a$ ← X

V → Va

Phospholipids, Va and Ca²⁺ (prothrombin activator)

B. Conversion of prothrombin to thrombin

(Prothrombin) → (Thrombin)
Ca²⁺

C. Conversion of fibrinogen to fibrin

Fibrinogen → Fibrin
↓ XIIIa, Ca²⁺
Fibrin threads

Fig. 4.1-16: Mechanism of blood coagulation

activated factor V and Ca²⁺ forms a complex which is called prothrombin activator.

Conversion of Prothrombin to Thrombin

Conversion of prothrombin to thrombin is caused by the prothrombin activator in the presence of Ca²⁺. This occurs at the surface of platelets which form the platelet plug at the site of injury.

Thrombin

Thrombin so formed acts as proteolytic enzyme. It has been estimated that the amount of thrombin produced during clotting of only 1 mL of blood is sufficient to coagulate 3 L of blood.

IMPORTANT TO KNOW

Roles played by thrombin:
- Conversion of fibrinogen to fibrin.
- Positive feedback role of thrombin: It accelerates the rate of formation of prothrombin activator by activating factor VIII, V and XIII.
- It also activates protein-C (which is an anticoagulant).

Conversion of Fibrinogen to Fibrin

Conversion of fibrinogen into fibrin involves three reactions (Fig. 4.1-17):

1. Proteolysis. Thrombin acting as proteolytic enzyme removes four low molecular weight peptide chains from each molecule of fibrinogen to convert it into fibrin monomer.

2. Polymerization. Fibrin monomer polymerizes with another monomer to form *long fibrin* threads which form reticulum of the clot.

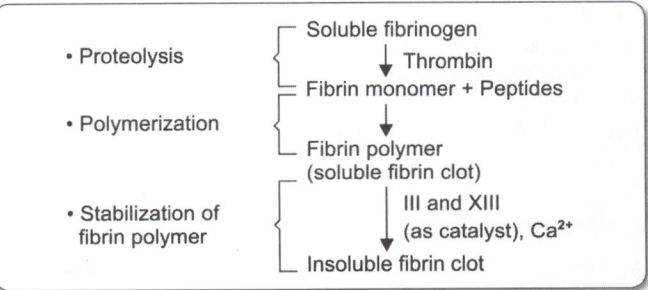

- Proteolysis
  - Soluble fibrinogen
  - ↓ Thrombin
  - Fibrin monomer + Peptides
- Polymerization
  - Fibrin polymer (soluble fibrin clot)
- Stabilization of fibrin polymer
  - III and XIII (as catalyst), Ca²⁺
  - Insoluble fibrin clot

Fig. 4.1-17: Types of reactions involved in conversion of soluble fibrinogen into insoluble fibrin clot

3. *Stabilization of fibrin polymers.* Fibrin stabilizing factor (factor XIII) which is activated by the thrombin to form XIIIa but XIIIa in the presence of Ca^{2+} causes formation of covalent cross linkages between fibrin threads, thus adding tremendous strength to the fibrin meshwork. The fibrin meshwork traps the remaining components of plasma and blood cells to form a solid mass called clot.

The fibrin threads of the clot adhere to damaged surface of blood vessels.

At this juncture, it is important to note that *coagulation is the property of plasma alone.* The RBCs and WBCs do not take part in it. They only become caught up in the meshwork of the clot.

Role of Calcium in Blood Coagulation

From the study of mechanism of blood coagulation, it is quite clear that except for the first two steps in the intrinsic pathway, calcium ions are required for promotion of all the reactions. Therefore in the absence of calcium ions blood clotting will not occur.

Role of Vitamin K, Liver and Blood Vessels in Hemostasis and Coagulation

Role of vitamin K

In the liver, synthesis of the following coagulation factors is dependent upon vitamin K:
- Prothrombin
- Factor VII, IX and X
- Circulatory anticoagulant protein.

CLINICAL ASPECTS

In the deficiency of vitamin K prothrombin time and blood clotting time is prolonged and serious hemorrhages may occur.

CLINICAL ASPECTS

THROMBOSIS
We have studied that physiologically under normal conditions, the circulating blood does not clot and that clotting of blood occurs only extravascularly when a vessel has been injured and bleeding has occurred. However, under certain pathological conditions the intravascular clotting may occur. The intravascular clotting is called *thrombosis* and the clot so formed is called thrombus.

Predisposing Factors
Virchow described three primary events which predispose to thrombus formation (*Virchow's triad*). These are:
- *Endothelial injury* may occur in atherosclerosis.

Role of liver

Liver plays the following significant role in the coagulation mechanism:

Synthesis of procoagulants. It is the site of synthesis of factor V, VII, IX, X, prothrombin and fibrinogen.

Removal of activated procoagulants. Liver also removes the activated procoagulants from the blood.

Synthesis of anticoagulants. Liver also synthesizes anticoagulants like heparin, antithrombin III and protein C.

CLINICAL ASPECTS

Liver failure can cause both:
- *Bleeding disorders* due to hypocoagulability of the blood
- *Uncontrolled extensive clotting* inside the blood vessels where clotting is not only unwanted but dangerous as well.

Role of blood vessels

Endothelium, subendothelial tissue and smooth muscles of the media of the blood vessels in coagulation and hemostasis mechanisms:
- Endothelium secretes von Willebrand's factor (vWF). The plasma vWF initiates platelet aggregation and Hemostasis.
- Tissue factor released by endothelial cells the following trauma initiates the process of extrinsic pathway of clotting mechanism.

Blood Clot Retraction

Within a few minutes after a clot is formed, it begins to contract and usually squeezes out most of the fluid called serum (plasma without fibrinogen and other clotting factors) within 30–60 minutes.

Platelets are essential for clot retraction. The contractile proteins (platelet thrombosthenin, actin and myosin) present in the cytoplasm of platelets cause strong contraction of platelet spicules attached to fibrin fibers.

- *Alterations in flow of blood.* Both in turbulence as well as stasis of blood normal axial flow of blood is disturbed and platelets come in contact with endothelium initiating thrombus formation.
- *Hypercoagulability of blood.*

Effects of Thrombi

Intravascular thrombi may cause:

Ischemia and infarction: Thrombi may decrease or stop the blood supply to part of an organ and cause ischemia which may subsequently result in infarction. For example, myocardial ischemia and infarction.

Contd...

Thromboembolism: The thrombus or its part may get dislodged and be carried along in the blood stream as *embolus* to lodge in a distant vessel. Examples of emboli formation are:
- Pulmonary embolism
- Cerebral embolism

Antihemostatic Mechanisms and Anticoagulants
The factors which balance the tendency of the blood to clot in vivo constitute the *antihemostatic factors*. These can be grouped as:

Factors Preventing Platelet Aggregation
Prostacyclin is an endogenous factor which prevents platelet aggregation by inhibiting the thromboxane A_2 formation (which promotes platelet aggregation).

Circulatory Anticoagulants
The natural anticoagulants circulating in the blood constitute the anticoagulant mechanism of the body.

Fibrinolytic Mechanism
Fibrinolysis refers to the process that brings about the dissolution of fibrin. The important component of the fibrinolytic system is plasmin or fibrinolysin which is present in the blood in an inactive form called plasminogen or profibrinolysin.

Anticoagulants
Anticoagulants refer to the substances which delay or prevent the process of coagulation of blood. Anticoagulants may be divided into endogenous and exogenous anticoagulants.

Endogenous Anticoagulants
Endogenous anticoagulants are those which are present inside the blood naturally:
- Heparin
- Antithrombin III
- Protein C.

Exogenous Anticoagulants
Exogenous anticoagulants are administered from outside or are used in vitro. These include:
Calcium sequesters or decalcifying agents: In vitro, blood clotting sequester (remove) calcium from the blood such as sodium citrate and sodium oxalate, and calcium chelators which bind calcium, e.g. ethylene diaminetetraacetic acid (EDTA).
Vitamin K antagonists: These are used orally and thus can prevent coagulation dicoumarol, and warfarin.
Defibrination substances: Defibrination substances are those which cause destruction of fibrinogen, e.g., *Arvin or ancord.*
Cold: Keeping blood cold (at 5–10°C) can retard the process of coagulation but cannot absolutely prevent it. Because of this reason blood is stored in blood banks at low temperature.

BLEEDING DISORDERS
Bleeding disorders are characterized by spontaneous escape of blood from blood vessels (in the tissues, inside the body cavities or on few surfaces like skin and mucous membrane or persistent and/or excessive bleeding the following minor injuries like tooth extraction, etc.)

Classification of Bleeding Disorders
- Platelet disorders

- Coagulation disorder or defective coagulation mechanism
- *Vascular disorders:* Damage of capillary endothelium (non-thrombocytopenic purpura)

PURPURA
Purpura is a group of bleeding disorders occurring due to various causes. The term purpura is derived from purple-colored petechial hemorrhages and bruises in the skin. The blood that leaks out changes color from red to blue to dark blue and green over a period of time.

Causes and Types of Purpura
Deficiency of platelets (thrombocytopenic purpura): Decrease in the platelet count below 1.5 lac/mm³ is called thrombocytopenia. Thrombocytopenic purpura may be:
Vascular disorders: Bleeding tendencies seen in patients with vascular disorders (damage to capillary endothelium) are referred to as *nonthrombocytopenic purpura*. In all cases of purpura due to vessel wall defects the platelet counts are normal, but bleeding time is prolonged and capillary fragility test is positive.

HEMOPHILIA
Hemophilia is the name given to bleeding disorders occurring due to *hereditary deficiency of coagulation* factor VIII (AHG). It is sex linked recessive disease, therefore affects exclusively to males and females act as carrier (Fig. 4.1-18). It is characterized by bleeding tendencies associated with increased clotting time (CT).

Disseminated Intravascular Coagulation
Disseminated intravascular coagulation (DIC), as the name indicates, refers to the condition when clotting mechanism becomes activated in widespread areas of the circulation.

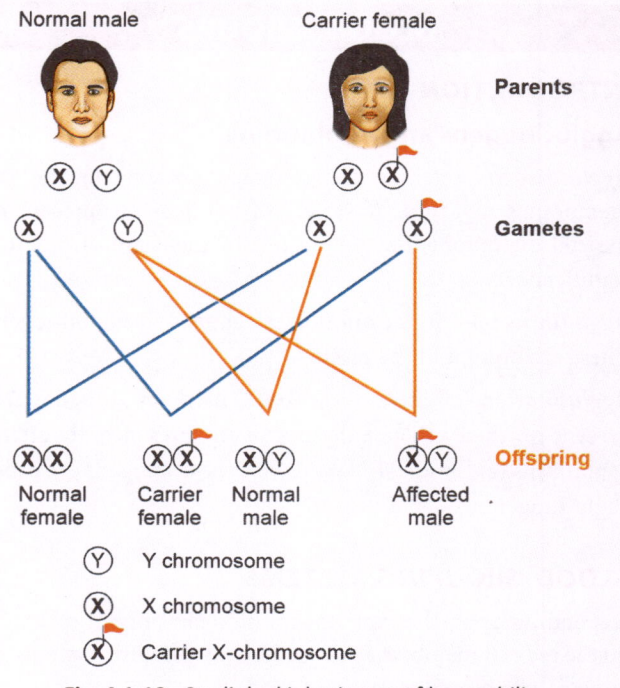

Fig. 4.1-18: Sex linked inheritance of hemophilia

Due to widespread intravascular coagulation there occurs plugging of small vessels with clots resulting into decreased O_2 and nutrient supply to its tissues causing multiple organ damage.

LABORATORY TESTS IN BLEEDING DISORDERS

Bleeding Time (BT)

Bleeding occurs from the skin when it is pricked with a needle, which normally stops of its own within a few minutes. The time lapse between the skin prick and the arrest of bleeding is called *bleeding time* (BT).

- *Normal BT* by Duke's method varies from 1 to 6 minutes. Normal BT indicates that platelet count and their function as well as health of capillaries are normal.
- *Prolonged BT* occurs in purpura, while it is normal in hemophilia.

Platelet Count

It varies from 1.5 lac to 4.5 lac/mm^3 with an average 2.5 lac/mm^3. Platelet count is decreased in primary and secondary thrombocytopenic purpura.

Coagulation time (CT)

Coagulation time (CT) refers to the time taken by the fresh fluid blood to get coagulated demonstrated by formation of fibrin threads. It is an insensitive measure in the assessment of coagulation defects and is abnormally prolonged when the coagulation factors are seriously deficient. The CT is prolonged in hemophilia and other clotting disorders.

BLOOD GROUPS

INTRODUCTION

Agglutinogens and Agglutinins

Agglutinogens refer to the antigens present on the cell membranes of RBCs. A variety of antigens are present on the cell membrane, but only a few of them are of practical significance.

Agglutinins refer to the antibodies against the agglutinogens. These are present in the plasma.

Agglutination of RBCs can be caused by the antigens present on their cell membranes in the presence of suitable agglutinins (antibodies). That is why, these antigens are called agglutinogens.

BLOOD GROUPING SYSTEMS

Depending upon the type of agglutinogen present or absent on the red cell membranes various blood grouping systems are known, which can be classified as:

- The classical ABO blood grouping system
- Rh (CDE) blood grouping system.

Landsteiner's Law

Karl Landsteiner in 1900 framed a law in relation to agglutinogens and agglutinins, which states that:

If an agglutinogen is present on the red cell membrane of an individual, the corresponding agglutinin must be absent in the plasma; and

If an agglutinogen is absent from the cell membrane of RBCs of an individual, the corresponding agglutinin must be present in the plasma.

It is important to note that:

- The Landsteiner law is applicable to ABO blood group system only
- The law is not applicable to other blood group systems, because there are no naturally occurring agglutinins in these systems.

Classical ABO Blood grouping system

A and B Agglutinogens

- The classical ABO blood grouping system is based on the presence of A and B agglutinogens on the cell membrane of RBCs. These are complex oligo-saccharides differing in their terminal sugars.
- The A and B antigens present on the membranes of RBCs are also present in many other tissues like salivary glands, pancreas, kidney, liver, lungs and testis; and also in body fluids, like saliva, semen, and amniotic fluid. The antigens on RBCs membrane are glycolipids, while in the tissues and body fluids they are soluble glycoproteins.

Anti-A and Anti-B Agglutinins

- Anti-A (or α) agglutinin and anti-B (or β) agglutinin refer to the antibody, i.e., which reacts with or acts on the antigen A, and antigen B, respectively.
- The α and β agglutinins are globulins of IgM type and cannot cross the placenta.
- The α and β agglutinins act best at low temperature (5–20°C) and are therefore also called cold antibodies.
- There are two types of α agglutinins: the $α_1$ and α proper.

Types of ABO Blood Groups

Depending upon the presence or absence of A and B agglutinogens and α and β agglutinins there are four types of blood groups:

1. *Blood group A* is characterized by:
- Presence of A agglutinogen and absence of B agglutinogen on the cell membrane of RBC.
- Presence of anti-B (or β) agglutinin and absence of anti-A (or α) agglutinin from the plasma.

- Group A has two subgroups: A_1 and A_2. The α_1-agglutinin agglutinates with subgroup A_1 only, while α-proper agglutinin agglutinates with both A_1 and A_2 subgroups.

2. *Blood group B* is characterized by:
- Presence of B agglutinogen and absence of A agglutinogen on the membrane of RBCs
- Presence of anti-A (or α) agglutinin and absence of anti-B (or β) agglutinin from the plasma.

3. *Blood group AB* is characterized by:
- Presence of both A and B agglutinogens on the cell membrane of RBCs
- Absence of both anti-A (or α) and anti-B or (β) agglutinins from the plasma
- Blood group AB has two subgroups, namely A_1B and A_2B.

4. *Blood group O* is characterized by:
- Absence of both A and B agglutinogens on the red cell membrane
- Presence of both anti-A and anti-B agglutinins in the plasma.

Determination of ABO Blood Groups

The ABO blood group of an individual can be determined by mixing one drop of suspension of his red cells (in isotonic saline) with a drop each of antiserum A (containing α agglutinins) and antiserum B (containing β agglutinins) separately on a glass slide. The antiserum A will cause agglutination (clumping of RBCs having A antigens and antiserum B will cause agglutination of RBCs having B antigens). The blood group of the individual will be shown by the presence of agglutination with one, both or none of the sera (Table 4.1-2 and Fig. 4.1-19).

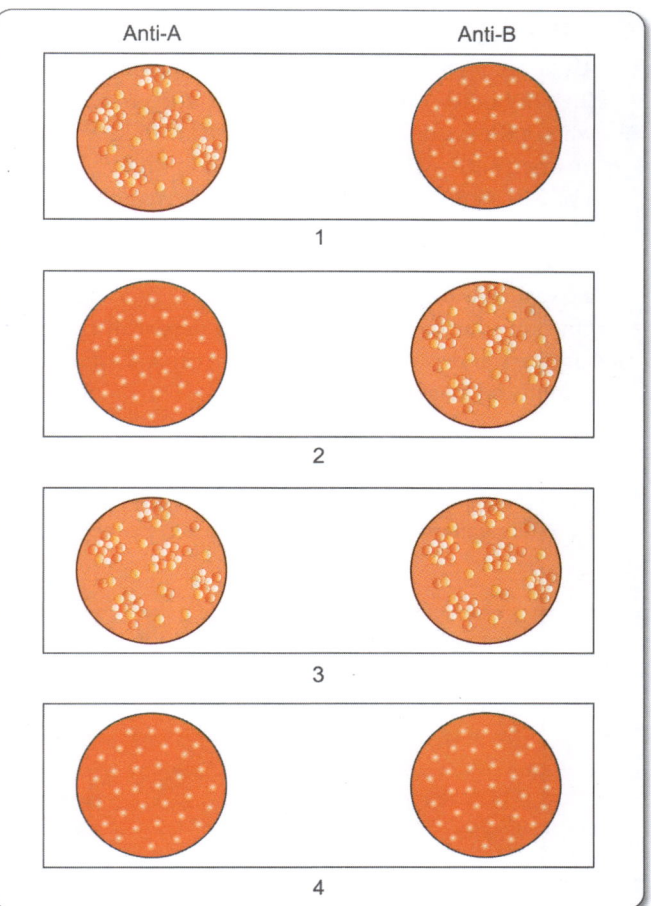

Fig. 4.1-19: Determination of blood groups—the RBCs showing agglutination with antisera are: 1, of blood group 'A' with antisera A; 2, of blood group B with antisera B; 3, of blood group 'AB' with antisera A and B (both); and 4, of blood group 'O' with none.

NURSING IMPLICATIONS AND APPLICATIONS

The antisera A and B are available commercially. For a quick identification, the anti-A serum is tinted blue and anti-B serum is tinted yellow.

TABLE 4.1-2: Determination of blood group of an individual

Blood group of RBC suspension	Agglutination with	
	Antiserum A (containing α agglutinins)	Antiserum B (containing β agglutinins)
A	+	–
B	–	+
AB	+	+
O	–	–

Rh (RHESUS) BLOOD GROUPING SYSTEM

Rh Antigens

- The antigens responsible for this blood grouping system are called Rh antigens or Rh agglutinogens or Rh factor because these were first discovered in the RBCs of rhesus monkeys. Based on the presence of Rh antigen, two types of blood groups are described:
  1. Rh positive blood group
  2. Rh negative blood group.
- Three types of Rh antigens, viz. C, D and E have been recognized. However, D antigen is most common and produces worst transfusion reactions. Therefore, for all practical purposes, the term Rh antigen refers to D antigen.
- Rh antigens are integral membrane proteins. These are *not found* in tissues other than RBCs.

Rh Antibodies

- There are no natural antibodies of Rh antigens.
- Rh antibodies (also called anti-D) are produced only when a Rh –ve individual is transfused with Rh +ve blood or when a Rh –ve mother gives birth to Rh +ve baby (Rh +ve RBCs of fetus enter into the maternal circulation). Rh antibodies are of IgG type and can cross the placenta. Since these react best at body temperature so these are also called warm antibodies.
- Once produced, the Rh antibodies persist in the blood for years and can produce serious reactions during the second transfusion.

Inheritance of Rh Antigens

- The Rh antigen (D antigen) is inherited as dominant gene D. When gene D is absent from a chromosome, its place is occupied by the alternate form (allelomorph) called 'd' Rh gene is inherited from both the parents (father and the mother).
- Rh positive individual may have two genotypes. DD (homozygous) or Dd (heterozygous). Of 85% Rh +ve individuals, about 35% have DD genotype and 50% have Dd genotype.
- The genotype of Rh –ve individual is dd.
- Therefore the genotype (gene composition) of offspring will be:
  - DD, when gene D is carried by both sperm and ovum
  - Dd, when one gamete carries D and other d; and
  - dd, when both the gametes carry gene d.

Inheritance of Rh antigen is summarized in Fig. 4.1-20.

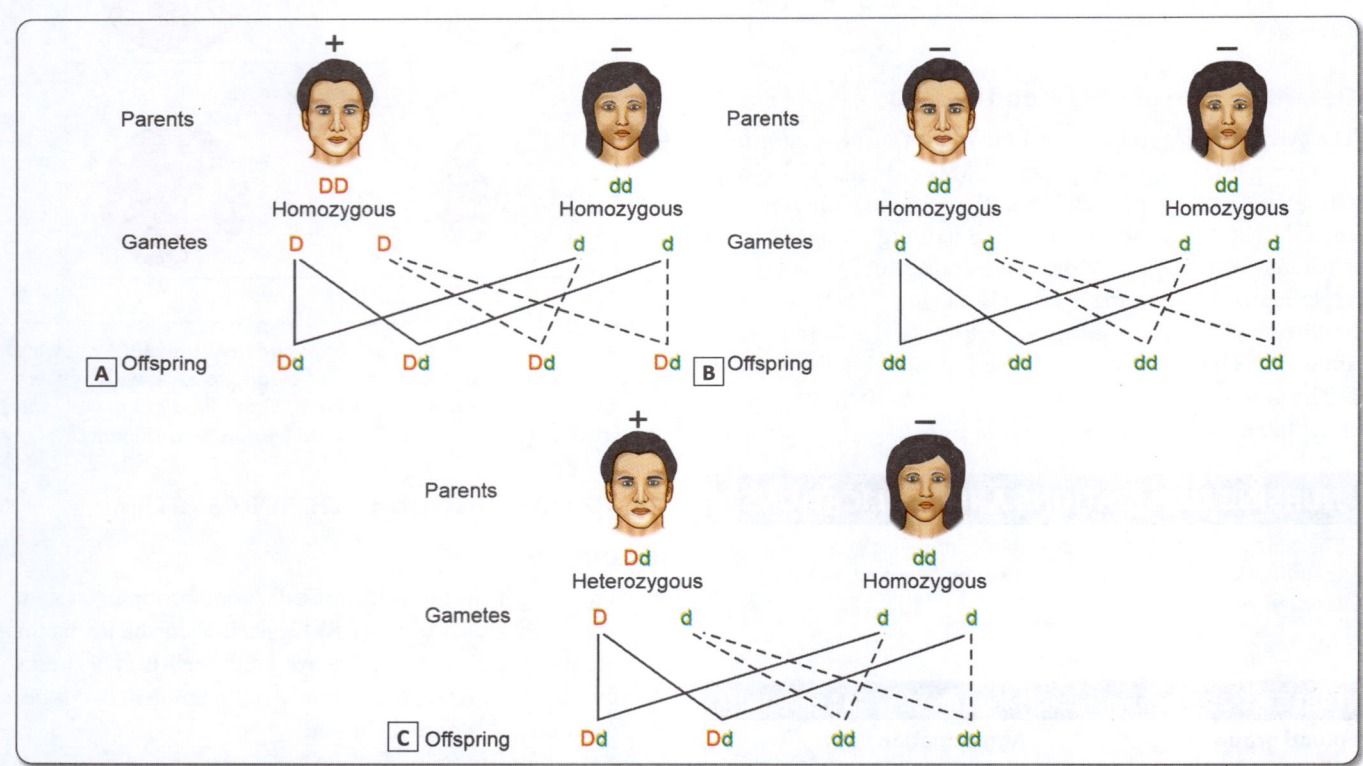

Figs 4.1-20A to C: Inheritance of Rh antigen: A. When father is homozygous Rh +ve and mother is homozygous Rh –ve; then all the offsprings are heterozygous Rh +ve; B. When father and mother both are homozygous Rh –ve then all the offsprings are homozygous Rh –ve; C. When father is heterozygous Rh +ve and mother is homozygous Rh –ve, then 50% of offsprings are Rh +ve (heterozygous) and other 50% are Rh –ve (homozygous)

CLINICAL ASPECTS

HEMOLYTIC DISEASE OF NEWBORN

Hemolytic disease of newborn occurs as a result of incompatibility of Rh blood groups between the mother and fetus.

Mechanism of Hemolytic Disease of Newborn in Rh Incompatibility

Mechanism of development of hemolytic disease of the newborn can be described under the following steps:

Entrance of Rh +ve fetal RBCs into Rh –ve mother's circulation during first pregnancy: When a Rh –ve mother (genotypes dd) bears a Rh +ve child (genotype Dd) with father being Rh +ve (genotype DD or Dd) at the time of delivery the fetal RBCs enter maternal circulation because of severance of umbilical cord. Before delivery, usually the fetal and maternal circulation do not mix. Since no Rh +ve RBCs enter maternal circulation during delivery, so the first child is usually normal.

Production of Rh antibodies (anti-D) in mother: During postpartum period, i.e., within a month after delivery, the mother develops Rh antibodies in her blood. As mentioned earlier, the Rh antibodies are of IgG type and are able to cross the placental barrier. Once formed the Rh antibodies persist for a long period in mother's blood.

Rh incompatibility reaction during second pregnancy: When the Rh –ve mother in the second pregnancy also bears a Rh +ve child, the Rh antibodies present in the mother's blood enter the fetal circulation by crossing the placental barrier and cause agglutination of fetal RBCs leading to hemolytic disease of newborn.

Manifestations of Hemolytic Disease of Newborn

Depending upon the severity the hemolytic disease of newborn may manifest as:

Erythroblastosis fetalis is characterized by:

- *Erythroblastosis*, i.e., appearance of large number of erythroblasts in peripheral blood. It occurs as the hemopoietic tissue of the baby attempts to rapidly replace the hemolyzed RBCs.
- *Anemia* occurs due to excessive hemolysis of RBCs by Rh antibodies. Infant may even die of severe anemia.
- *Icterus gravis neonatorum. Jaundice* may occur within 24 hours of birth due to excessive formation of bilirubin as a result of excessive hemolysis of RBCs.
- *Liver and spleen* are enlarged.

Kernicterus: It is a neurological syndrome occurring in newborns with severe hemolysis. The excessive bilirubin formed may enter the brain tissue as the blood-brain barrier is not well developed in infants and cause damage. The bilirubin mostly affects the basal ganglia producing disturbance of motor activities. It usually develops when serum bilirubin level exceeds 18 mg%.

Hydrops fetalis: The fetus is grossly edematous. It occurs when hemolysis is very severe. Usually there occurs intrauterine death of fetus or if born prematurely or even at term, the infant dies within a few hours.

Prevention and Treatment

Prevention of hemolytic disease of newborn: The hemolytic disease in the newborn during second pregnancy can be prevented by injecting single dose of Rh antibodies (anti-D) in the form of Rh-immunoglobulin to mother soon after first childbirth. These antibodies will destroy the Rh +ve RBCs of the fetus which have gained access to maternal circulation. In this way active antibodies will not be formed by the mother.

Treatment of hemolytic disease of newborn: Treatment of hemolytic disease of the newborn is replacement of baby's Rh +ve blood with Rh –ve blood exchange transfusion.

NURSING IMPLICATIONS AND APPLICATIONS

Clinical Applications of Blood Grouping

In blood transfusion: Before blood transfusion always cross matching is done.

In preventing hemolytic disease in newborn due to Rh incompatibility (as discussed above).

In paternity disputes: The ABO, Rh and MNS blood grouping is helpful in settling cases of disputed paternity.

In medicolegal cases: Any red stain on a clothing may be claimed to be blood by a supposed victim. Therefore, it is first confirmed that it really is blood by preparing hemin crystals from the stain extract.

In knowing susceptibility to diseases: The incidence of certain diseases is related to blood groups, e.g.

- Individuals with blood group O (non-secretors) are said to be more susceptible to duodenal ulcer (peptic ulcer) than the individuals with blood group A and B (secretors).
- Individuals with blood group A are more susceptible to carcinoma of stomach, pancreas and salivary glands.
- To some extent incidence of diabetes mellitus is more in individuals with blood group A.

BLOOD TRANSFUSION

INDICATIONS

Blood transfusion is a life-saving measure and should be carried out when it is absolutely essential. Common situations in which blood transfusion is indicated are:

Blood loss. Severe blood loss is the most important indication for blood transfusion.

For quick restoration of hemoglobin in patients with severe anemia is required in situations like pregnancy and emergency surgery.

Exchange transfusion is required in hemolytic disease of newborn.

Blood diseases like aplastic anemia, agranulocytosis, leukemias, hemophilia, purpura and clotting defects may require blood transfusion.

Acute poisoning, e.g. carbon monoxide poisoning.

DONOR AND RECIPIENT

Donor refers to a person who donates the blood and the person who receives blood is a recipient.

Universal donor. Blood of the individuals with blood group O does not contain any agglutinogen. So when this blood is transfused to a person with any blood group (A, B, AB or O), theoretically its RBCs will not be agglutinated. Because of this fact an individual with blood group O is called universal donor. However, practically this term is no longer valid, as it ignores the complications produced by existence of Rh factor and other blood group systems.

Universal recipient. Blood of an individual with blood group AB does not contain any agglutinins. So, theoretically when such an individual receives blood from the individual with any blood group (A, B, AB or O), there should be no transfusion reaction. Because of this fact an individual with AB blood group is called universal recipient. However, practically this term is no more valid because it ignores the complications produced by the existence of Rh factor and other blood group systems.

NURSING IMPLICATIONS AND APPLICATIONS

Precautions to be Observed During Blood Transfusion

Absolute indication should always be there for the transfusion of blood.

Cross matching should always be done before the blood transfusion. For it blood is collected from donor as well as recipient. Plasma and RBCs are separated in each. The cross matching involves two steps: major and minor cross matching.

- *Major cross matching involves mixing of donor's cells with recipient's plasma.* This is called major cross matching because of the fact that when mismatched blood is transfused in a recipient, the donor's cells get agglutinated as against their agglutinogen there is sufficiently high concentration of agglutinins in the recipient's plasma.
- *Minor cross matching involves mixing of recipient's cells with donor's plasma.* This is called minor crossmatch due of the fact that reaction of donor's plasma and recipient's cells usually does not occur or is very mild on giving mismatched blood transfusion.

Rh +ve blood should never be transfused to Rh –ve person. It is particularly must for females at any age before menopause, because once she is sensitized by the Rh antigen, the anti-D antibodies are formed and she will not be able to bear a Rh +ve fetus. In other words, Rh+ transfusion may make a woman permanently childless.

Donor's blood should always be screened for diseases which are spread through blood such as AIDS, hepatitis-B, malaria and syphilis.

Blood bag/bottle should be checked for the name of recipient and blood group on the label before starting the blood transfusion.

Blood transfusion should be given at slow rate. If rapid transfusion is given, citrate present in stored blood may cause chelation of calcium ions leading to decreased serum calcium level and tetany.

Proper aseptic measures must be taken during transfusion of blood.

Careful watch on recipient's condition is must for the first 10–15 minutes of starting the transfusion, and from time to time later.

ASSESS YOURSELF

Short and Long Answer Questions

1. **Describe briefly:**
   - Different types of plasma proteins and their functions
   - Stages of erythropoiesis
   - Structure and functions of hemoglobin
   - Life span and fate of red blood cells
   - Different types of leucocytes and their functions
   - Properties and functions of platelets
   - Blood grouping system

2. **Write notes on:**
   - Gamma globulins
   - Reticulocytes
   - Erythrocyte sedimentation rate

- Iron deficiency anemia
- Jaundice
- Phagocytosis
- Hemostasis
- Purpura
- Hemophilia
- Bleeding and clotting time
- Landsteiner's law
- Rh incompatibility
- Precautions during blood transfusion

Multiple Choice Questions

1. **The volume of blood in an average adult is:**
   a. 60 Ml/kg body weight
   b. 70 Ml/kg body weight
   c. 80 Ml/kg body weight
   d. 90 Ml/kg body weight
2. **The normal range of plasma albumin is:**
   a. 2–2.5 gm%
   b. 3–5 gm%
   c. >5 gm%
   d. <2.5 gm%
3. **The osmotic pressure exerted by plasma proteins is:**
   a. 10 mm Hg   b. 20 mm Hg
   c. 25 mm Hg   d. 30 mm Hg
4. **In an adult male, the normal range of red blood cell count is:**
   a. 6–7 million/mm³   b. 5–6.5 million/mm³
   c. 4.5–5.5 million/mm³ d. 3.0–4.5 million/mm³
5. **During formation of RBCs, hemoglobin appears at which stage:**
   a. Pro-normoblast   b. Intermediate normoblast
   c. Late normoblast   d. Reticulocyte

6. **The statement not true for erythropoietin:**
   a. It is a hormone
   b. Secreted from juxta-glomerular apparatus
   c. Hypoxia the main stimulus for its secretion
   d. Secreted by hepatocytes
7. **In differential leucocyte count the normal range of neutrophils is:**
   a. 20–40%
   b. 35–40%
   c. 40–75%
   d. <10%
8. **The antibodies are formed from:**
   a. B Lymphocytes
   b. T Lymphocytes
   c. Helper T cells
   d. Natural killer cells
9. **In which condition the number of eosinophils increases:**
   a. Bacterial infection
   b. Viral infection
   c. Allergic conditions
   d. Leukemia
10. **The statement not true for platelets:**
    a. Also called thrombocytes
    b. Contain contractile proteins
    c. Produce antibodies
    d. Number decreases in purpura
11. **Deficiency of coagulation factor causes:**
    a. Purpura
    b. Hemophilia
    c. Prolonged bleeding time
    d. Decrease on clotting time
12. **The plasma of blood group A person contains:**
    a. Agglutinin α   b. Agglutinin α and β (both)
    c. Agglutinin β   d. None of the above

ANSWER KEY

| 1. c | 2. b | 3. c | 4. b | 5. b | 6. d | 7. c | 8. a |
| 9. c | 10. c | 11. b | 12. c | | | | |

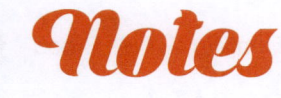
Notes

Chapter

4.2

Anatomy and Physiology of Cardiovascular System

ORGANIZATION AND FUNCTIONS OF CARDIOVASCULAR SYSTEM

ORGANIZATION OF CARDIOVASCULAR SYSTEM

The cardiovascular system (CVS) consists of the heart and the blood vessels. The *heart* acts as a system of two pumps working in series and forms the driving force for blood flow. The blood vessels that take blood from the heart to various tissues are called *arteries*. The smallest arteries are called *arterioles*. Arterioles open into a network of *capillaries* which constitute the microcirculation. The most important function of blood vessels, i.e., the rapid exchange of materials between the blood and extracellular fluid bathing the tissue cells is served by the capillaries. In other words, capillaries serve as the *exchange region*. In some situations, capillaries are replaced by slightly different vessels called *sinusoids*. Blood from capillaries (or from sinusoids) is collected by small *venules* which join to form *veins*. Veins serve as the blood reservoir and return the collected blood to the heart. Functionally the cardiovascular system consists of two main divisions (Fig. 4.2-1):

1. *Systemic circulation*
2. *Pulmonary circulation*.

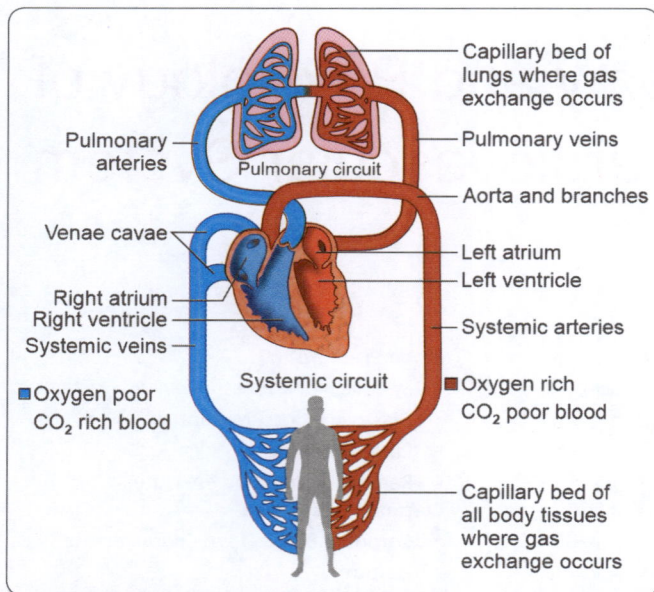

Fig. 4.2-1: General pattern of cardiovascular system comprising systemic and pulmonary circulation

FUNCTIONS OF CARDIOVASCULAR SYSTEM

Primary functions of the cardiovascular system are:
- Distribution of nutrients and oxygen (O_2) to all body cells
- Collection of waste products and CO_2 from different body cells and to carry them to excretory organs for excretion.

Secondary functions that are subserved by the cardiovascular system are:
- Thermoregulation
- Distribution of hormones to the target tissues
- Delivery of antibodies, platelets and leucocytes to aid body defense mechanism.

ANATOMY OF THE HEART

GROSS APPEARANCE, SIZE AND LOCATION

The heart is a cone-shaped, hollow muscular pump designed to ensure the circulation of blood through the tissues of the body. In an adult, the heart is as large as a clenched fist, being approximately 14 cm (5.5 inches) long and 9 cm (3.5 inches) wide. It weighs about 300 g.

Location

The heart lies in the mediastinal area of thoracic cavity between the lungs. It is situated obliquely behind the sternum, a little more to the left than the right (Fig. 4.2-2).

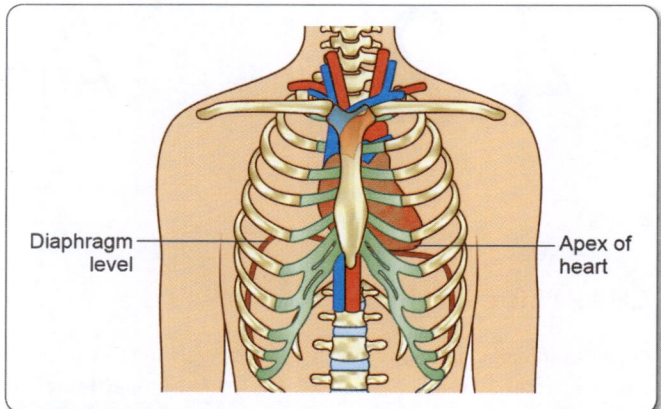

Fig. 4.2-2: Location of heart in the thorax

Gross Appearance and Immediate Relations

Being conical in shape, it is described as having base, apex, sternocostal surface and diaphragmatic surface (Figs 4.2-3A to D).

Sternocostal surface of the heart is facing anteriorly and is related to the body of sternum and costal cartilages.

Diaphragmatic surface is facing inferiorly and is in contact with the diaphragm.

Apex refers to the bluntly pointed terminal part of the heart which is directed downward and to the left. The apex is about 9 cm to the left of the midline at the level of the 5th intercostal space, i.e., a little below and medial to the left nipple. Apex of the heart is formed by the left ventricle.

Base, i.e., posterior aspect of the heart is related to the structures in posterior mediastinum, i.e., descending aorta, inferior vena cava, esophagus and trachea. Base is directed upward and to the right (e.g. apex which is directed downward and to the left).

Laterally the heart is enclosed by lungs.

Superiorly the heart is associated with aorta, superior vena cava, pulmonary artery and pulmonary veins.

CHAMBERS OF HEART

Each half of heart consists of an inflow chamber called the *atrium* and an outflow chamber called the *ventricle* (Fig. 4.2-4). Thus, there are four chambers in the heart.

Atria. Interatrial septum separates the right and leftatria which are thin-walled chambers.

Right atrium receives deoxygenated blood from tissues of the entire body through the *superior* and *inferior venae cavae.* This blood passes into the right ventricle through the right

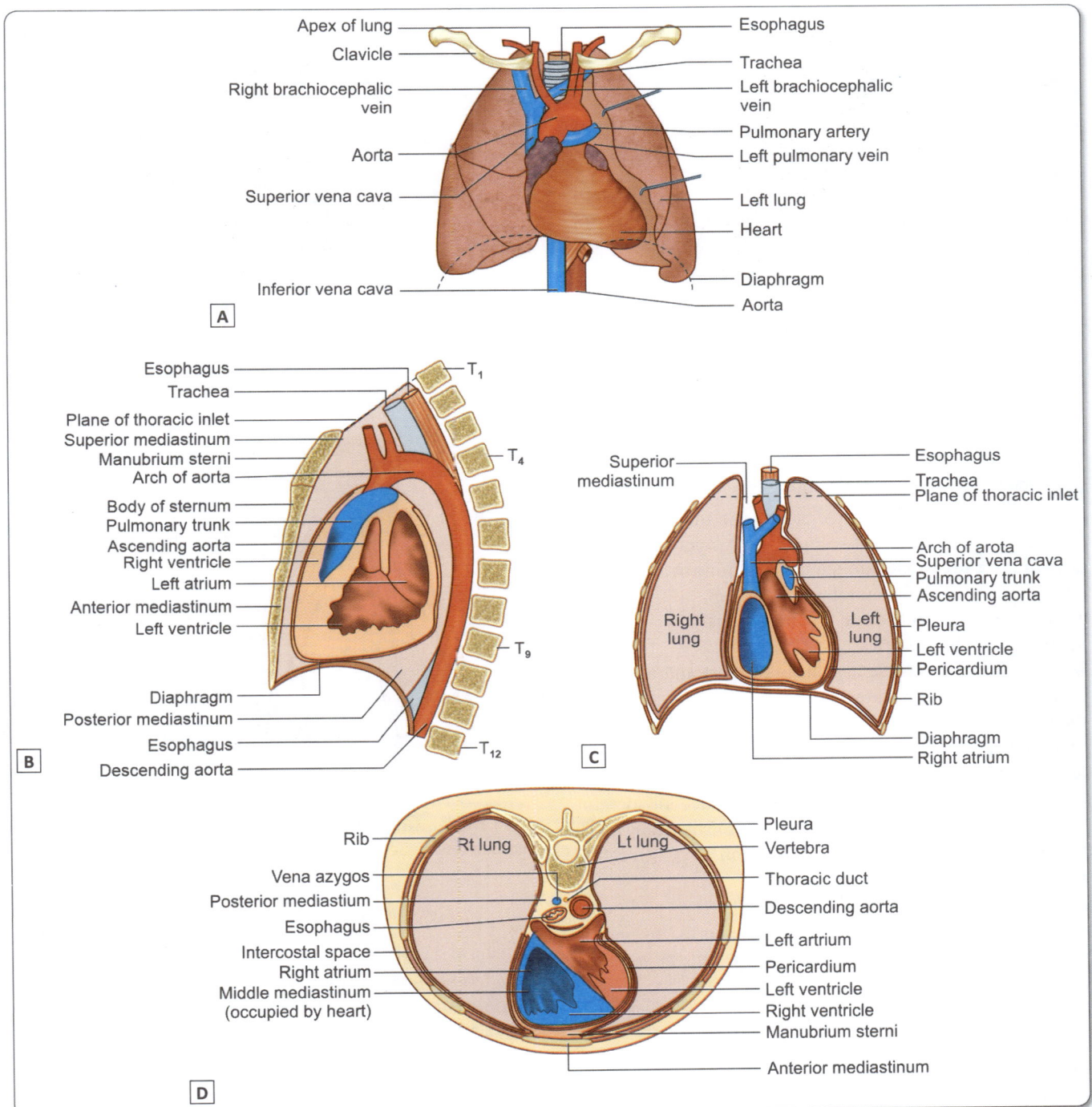

Figs 4.2-3A to D: Gross appearance and structures related to heart: A. Front view; B. Coronal section through heart and lungs; C. Sagittal section of thorax in the area of heart; and D. Transverse section of thorax through heart

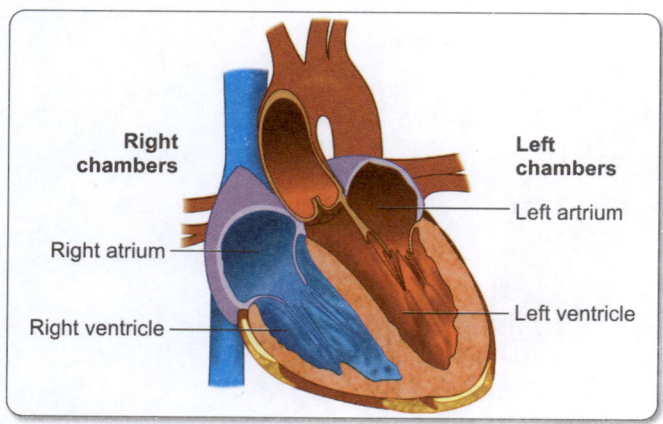

Fig. 4.2-4: Schematic diagram of heart to show the chambers

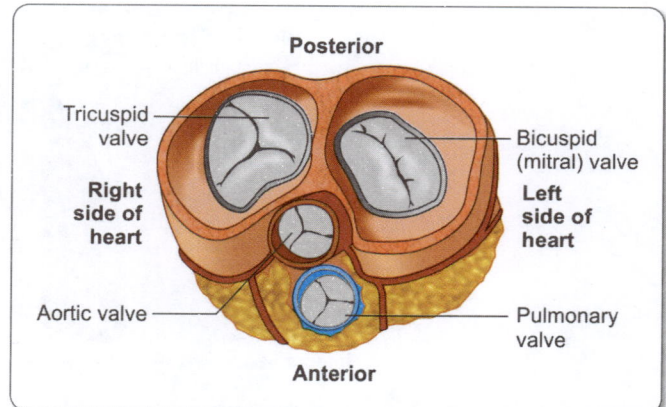

Fig. 4.2-5: Valves of the heart

atrioventricular orifice, which is guarded by *tricuspid valve*. The right atrium has got the pacemaker known as *sinoatrial (SA) node* that produces cardiac impulses and *atrioventricular (AV) node* that conducts these impulses to the ventricles.

Left atrium receives oxygenated blood from the lungs through the four *pulmonary veins* (two right and two left). This blood passes into left ventricle through the *left atrioventricular orifice*, which is guarded by the mitral valve.

Ventricles. Interventricular septum separates the right ventricle from left ventricle.

Interior of each ventricle has an inflow part and an outflow part. *Papillary muscles* are finger-like processes attached to the ventricular wall at one end, but free at the other. They are functionally related to the atrioventricular valves.

Right ventricle receives blood from the right atrium and pumps through the pulmonary trunk (which divides into right and left pulmonary arteries) into the lungs. The *pulmonary valve* is present at the junction of right ventricle and pulmonary trunk.

Left ventricle receives blood from the left atrium and pumps out into systemic circulation through the aorta. *Aortic* valve is present at the junction of left ventricle and the *ascending aorta*.

VALVES OF HEART

There are four valves in human heart, two atrioventri-cular valves and two semilunar valves. Valves allow unidirectional flow of blood.

Atrioventricular Valves

The atrioventricular valves open toward the ventricles and close toward the atria. They allow blood to flow from atria to ventricles. But when ventricles contract, they are closed and thus prevent backflow of blood from ventricles to atria.

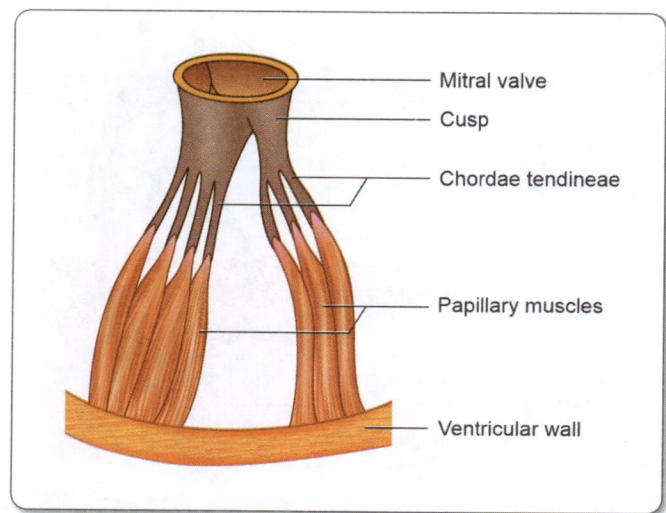

Fig. 4.2-6: Bicuspid valve attached with papillary muscle and chordae tendineae

Right atrioventricular valve is known as *tricuspid valve* and is made of 3 cusps: anterior, posterior and septal (Fig. 4.2-5).

The left atrioventricular valve is called *mitral valve* or *bicuspid valve* and is made of 2 cusps: anterior and posterior (Fig. 4.2-6).

- At the periphery, the cusps (flaps) of the atrioventri-cular valves are attached to the *atrioventricular ring*, which is the fibrous connection between the atria and ventricles. The free edges of the cusps are attached to *papillary muscles* through the cord-like structures called the *chordae tendineae* (Fig. 4.2-6).

- *Papillary muscles* arise from the inner surface of ventricles and contract when the ventricular walls contract. They do not help the valves to close but prevent the bulging of the valves into the atria when ventricles contract.

Semilunar Valves

Aortic valve is the semilunar valve present at the opening of aorta in left ventricle. It is made of three semilunar cusps: one anterior and two posterior (Fig. 4.2-5).

Pulmonary valve is the semilunar valve present at the opening of pulmonary trunk into the right ventricle. It is also made of three semilunar cusps: one posterior and two anterior (Fig. 4.2-5).

- *Semilunar valves open* away from ventricles and close toward the ventricles. These valves open when ventricles contract allowing the blood to flow from left ventricle to aorta and from right ventricle to pulmonary trunk.
- *Semilunar valves close* when ventricles relax, thus preventing backflow of blood from aorta or pulmonary trunk into the ventricles.

CLINICAL ASPECTS

Narrowing of the valve orifice due to fusion of the cusps is known as 'stenosis', viz. mitral stenosis, aortic stenosis, etc.
Dilatation of the valve orifice, or stiffening of the cusps causes imperfect closure of the valve leading to back flow of blood. This is known as incompetence or regurgitation, e.g. aortic incompetence or aortic regurgitation.

STRUCTURE OF THE WALLS OF HEART

Walls of the heart are composed of thick layer of cardiac muscle, the *myocardium*, covered externally by the epicardium, and lined internally by the *endocardium*. Histology plate 4.2-1.

- Walls of the atrial portion of the heart are thin.
- Walls of the ventricular portion of the heart are thick.

Skeleton of the heart consists of fibrous rings that surround the atrioventricular, pulmonary, and aortic orifices and are continuous with the membranous part of the ventricular septum.

Pericardium

The heart and roots of the great vessels are enclosed by a fibroserous sac called pericardium. Its function is to restrict excessive movements of the heart as a whole and to serve as a lubricated container in which different parts of the heart can contract. Pericardium consists of two layers: outer fibrous and inner serous (Fig. 4.2-7).

Fibrous pericardium surrounds the heart like a bag and is attached with the surrounding structures.

Serous pericardium has parietal and visceral layers. The *parietal layer* of serous pericardium lines the fibrous pericardium and is reflected around the roots of the great vessels to become continuous with the *visceral layer of serous*

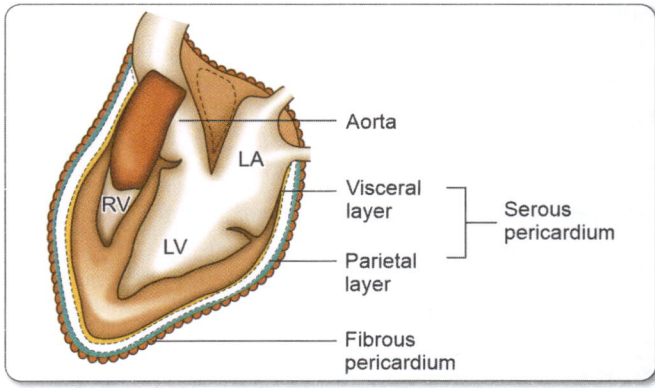

Fig. 4.2-7: Schematic sagittal section of heart showing fibrous and serous pericardium

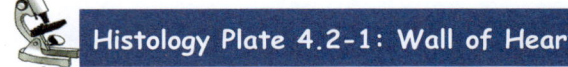

Histology Plate 4.2-1: Wall of Heart

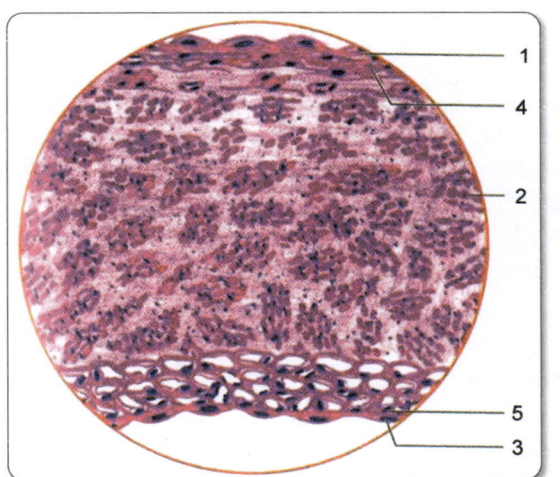

The wall of the heart consists of the following layers from inner to outer side.
- Endocardium—(1)
- Subendocardial layer between endocardium and myocardium—(4)
- Myocardium—(2)
- Subepicardial layer between myocardium and epicardium—(5)
- Epicardium—(3)

pericardium that closely covers the heart and is often called the *epicardium*. The slit-like space between the parietal and visceral layers of the serous pericardium is called *pericardial cavity* which contains small amount of *pericardial fluid* that acts as a lubricant to facilitate movement of the heart.

Myocardium

The myocardium (muscular tissue of the heart) is the main tissue constituting the walls of the heart. It consists of three types of muscle fibers:

1. *Cardiac muscles* forming the walls of the atria and ventricles
2. Muscle fibers forming the *pacemaker* which is the site of origin of cardiac impulse
3. Muscle fibers forming the *conducting system*, which transmits the impulse to the various parts of the heart.

Endocardium

Endocardium is thin smooth and glistening membrane lining the myocardium internally. It consists of a single layer of endothelial cells. The endocardium continues as the endothelium of great vessels opening in the heart.

CLINICAL ASPECTS

Collection of fluid in the pericardial cavity is referred to as *pericardial effusion* or cardiac tamponade. The fluid compresses the heart and restricts venous filling during diastole. It also reduces cardiac output.

Inflammation of the heart can involve more than one layer of the heart. Inflammation of the pericardium is called *pericarditis;* the inflammations of myocardium is *myocarditis;* and of the endocardium is *endocarditis.*

BLOOD SUPPLY TO THE HEART

The blood is supplied to the heart by coronary arteries.

Coronary Arteries

Two coronary arteries (right and left) arise from the root of ascending aorta and supply blood to the myocardium (Figs 4.2-8A and B).

Right coronary artery (RCA) supplies blood to the right ventricle, right atrium, the posterior part of left ventricle, posterior part of interventricular septum and major portion of the conducting system of heart including SA node.

Left coronary artery (LCA) thus supplies mainly to the anterior part of left ventricle, left atrium, anterior part of the interventricular septum and a part of the left branch of bundle of His.

Coronary Veins

Coronary sinus is a wide vein about two centimeters long which drains most of the venous blood from the myocardium (mainly left ventricle) into the right atrium. Its tributaries are the *great cardiac vein*, the *small cardiac vein*, the *posterior vein*

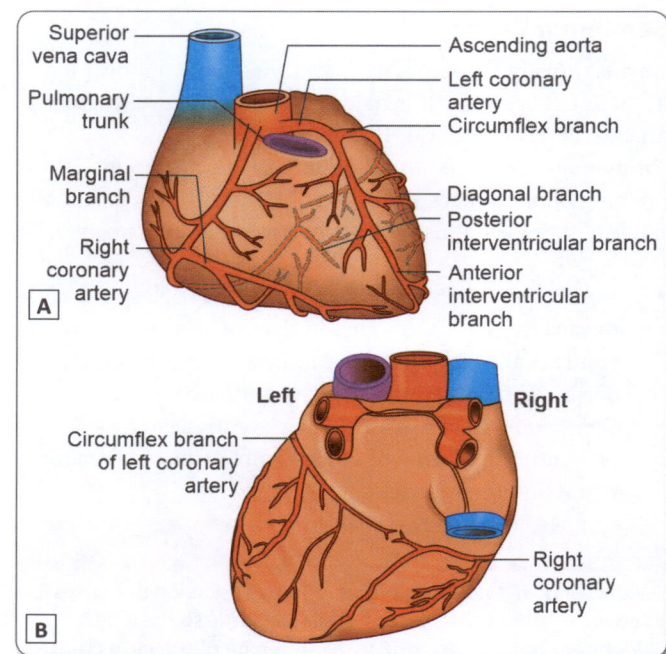

Figs 4.2-8A and B: Major coronary arteries and their branches

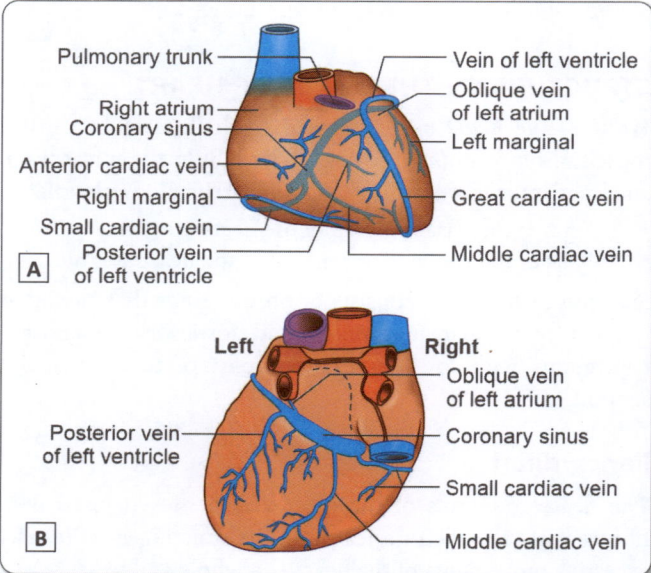

Figs 4.2-9A and B: Veins of the heart; A. Anterior view; B. Posterior view

of left ventricle, and the *oblique vein of left ventricle* (Figs 4.2-9A and B).

Anterior cardiac vein draining venous blood mainly from the right ventricle opens directly into the right atrium.

Thebesian veins and *coronary-luminal vessels* (connections between the coronary vessels and the lumen of heart) constitute the deep venous system. These vessels drain only less than 10% of the venous blood from myocardium directly into the various cardiac chambers, contributing to an *anatomic shunt effect*. The coronary luminal connections carry a larger proportion of the flow in the right ventricle than in the left ventricle.

INNERVATION OF THE HEART

Heart is innervated by both divisions (sympathetic and parasympathetic) of the autonomic nervous system.

BLOOD VESSELS

The blood vessels that comprise the vascular system can be grouped into two systems:

1. Arterial system
2. Venous system

The arterial and venous trees of the body functionally constitute two different systems of circulation—the pulmonary circulation and systemic circulation. The blood vessels described in this section belong to systemic circulation.

ARTERIAL SYSTEM

The arterial tree of systemic circulation includes the aorta and its branches that lead to all body tissues.

Aorta

Aorta is the largest artery of the body. It arises from the left ventricle, arches over the heart to the left, and descends just in front of the vertebral column through the thorax and abdomen up to 4th lumbar vertebra, where it ends by dividing into the left and right common iliac arteries (Figs 4.2-10 and 4.2-11).

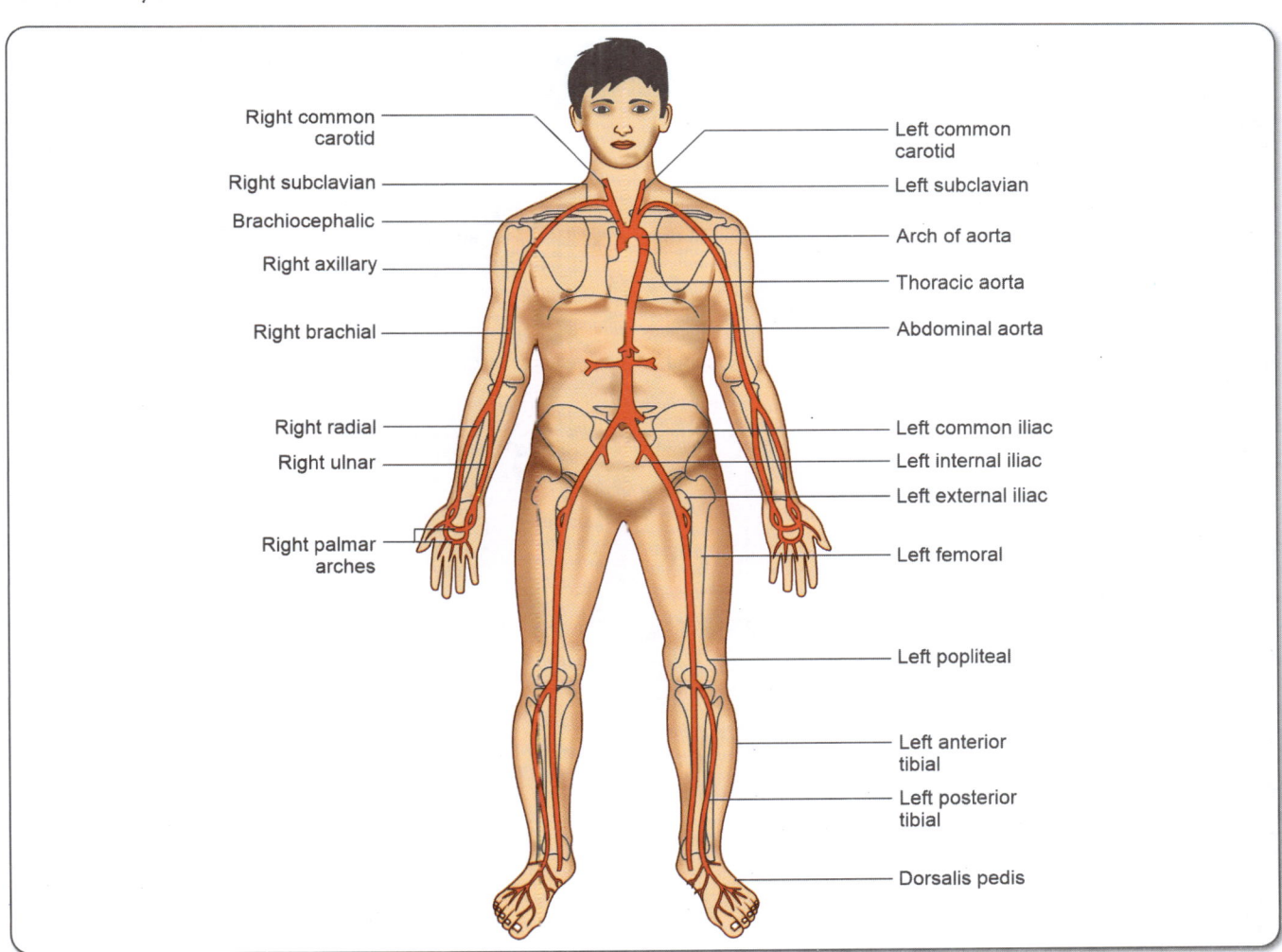

Fig. 4.2-10: The aorta and its main branches

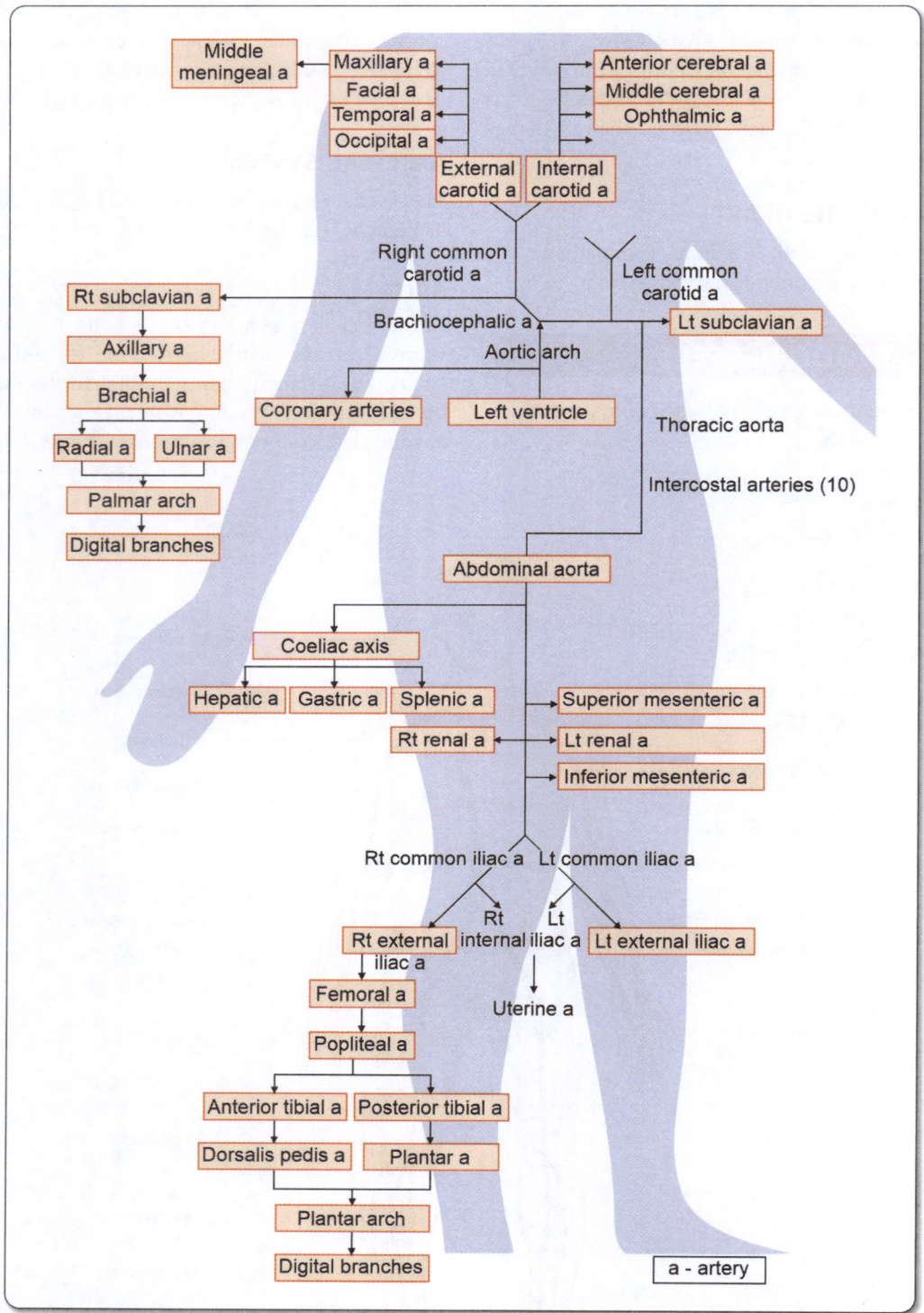

Fig. 4.2-11: Plan of the arterial system

Parts and main branches of aorta are:

- Ascending aorta
- Arch of aorta
- Descending aorta.

Ascending Aorta

Course. The ascending aorta, about 5 cm (2.1 inches) long, after leaving the left ventricle, passes upward and to the right. It then becomes continuous with arch of aorta (Fig. 4.2-12).

Branches. The only branches that arise from the ascending aorta are:

- Right coronary artery
- Left coronary artery.

Coronary arteries. The coronary arteries arise from the aorta just above the level of the aortic valve and supply blood to the heart. The right and left coronary arteries and their main branches travel in the epicardium of heart and subdivide sending penetrating branches through the myocardium.

CLINICAL ASPECTS

The coronary arteries supply the myocardium with oxygen and nourishment. They are, therefore, of great practical importance because disease of their walls may result either in narrowing of the artery or complete blockage of one of the branches:
Angina pectoris. Incomplete obstruction, usually due to spasm of the coronary artery causes angina pectoris, which is associated with agonizing pain in the precordial region and down the medial side of the left arm and forearm.
Myocardial infarction if the block is complete, as in coronary artery thrombosis is called myocardial infarction.

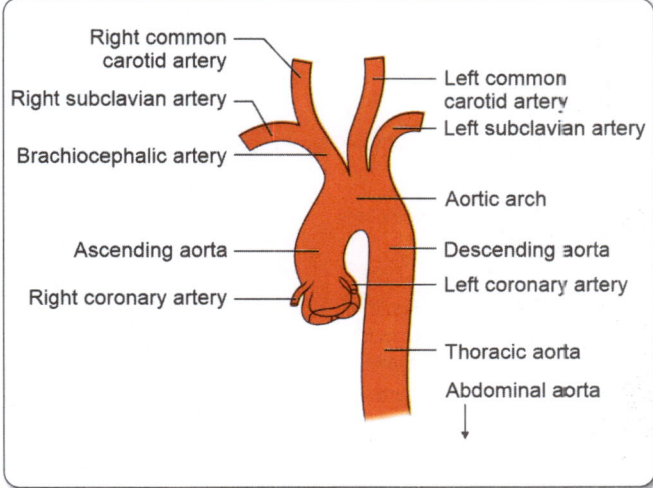

Fig. 4.2-12: The ascending aorta, arch of aorta and descending aorta

Arch of Aorta

Course. The ascending aorta turns backward and to the left to form the arch of aorta which is convex upward. The arch of aorta lies behind the manubrium sterni and becomes continuous with descending thoracic aorta (Fig. 4.2-12).

Branches. Three large branches arise from the arch of aorta (Fig. 4.2-12).

1. Brachiocephalic artery (innominate) artery after arising from the arch of aorta runs upward and to the right for about 5 cm. At the level of sternoclavicular joint, it ends by dividing into two branches:

   a. *The right common carotid artery*, which supplies blood to the right half of the head and neck.
   b. *The right subclavian artery* carries blood to the right upper arm.

2. Left common carotid artery, the second branch from arch of aorta, supplies blood to the left side of neck and head.

3. Left subclavian artery, the third branch from the arch of aorta, supplies blood to the left upper limb.

Descending Aorta

The descending aorta can be divided into two parts:

1. Descending thoracic aorta
2. Descending abdominal aorta.

Descending thoracic aorta

Course. The arch of aorta becomes continuous with descending aorta at the level of 4th thoracic vertebra. The portion of the descending aorta above the diaphragm is called thoracic aorta. The thoracic aorta continues downward in the thorax in front of the remaining thoracic vertebrae and passes through an opening in the diaphragm at the level of 12th thoracic vertebra to become the abdominal aorta (Fig. 4.2-12).

Branches. Along its course, the thoracic aorta gives off numerous visceral and parietal branches, which supply the chest wall and viscera.

Descending abdominal aorta

Course

The portion of descending aorta below the diaphragm is called abdominal aorta, which is related to the lumbar vertebrae and ends at the level of 4th by dividing into right and left common iliac arteries (Fig. 4.2-13).

Branches of abdominal aorta include (Fig. 4.2-13):

Celiac trunk (artery). It arises from the front aspect of abdominal aorta immediately after it has passed through the diaphragm. It is a short trunk which divides into three branches:

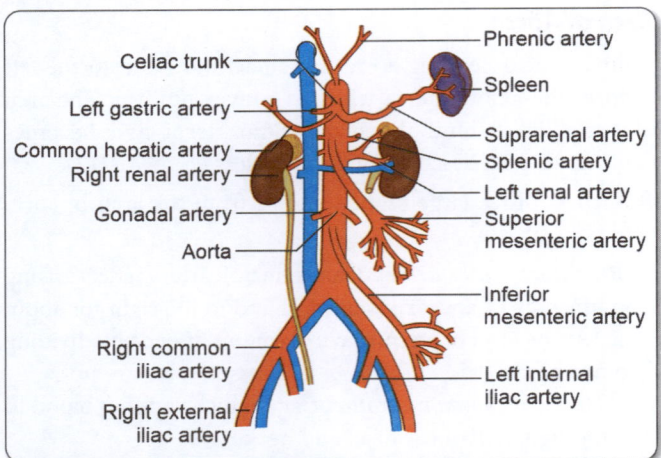

Fig. 4.2-13: Abdominal aorta and its branches

1. *Gastric artery*, which helps to supply the stomach.
2. *Hepatic artery*, which supplies the liver.
3. *Splenic artery*, which supplies the spleen and gives branches to pancreas, stomach and omentum.

Phrenic arteries, supply blood to the diaphragm.

Superior mesenteric artery arises from the anterior surface of abdominal aorta about 1 cm below the celiac trunk. It supplies blood to the small intestine and first portion of large intestine.

Suprarenal artery, supplies the adrenal gland.

Renal arteries. The right and left renal arteries arise from the side of aorta at the level of superior mesenteric artery. These supply the kidney.

Inferior mesenteric artery. It arises lower down from the anterior surface of aorta and sends branches to the lower parts of the colon and to the rectum.

Gonadal arteries. Ovarian arteries in females and spermatic arteries in males supply the ovaries or testis.

Lumbar arteries (3–4 pairs). These arise from the posterior surface of aorta in the region of lumbar vertebrae. These arteries supply the posterior abdominal wall.

Middle sacral artery. This small, single vessel supplies the sacrum and coccyx.

Common iliac arteries. These are terminal branches of abdominal aorta. These vessels supply blood to the lower regions of the abdominal wall, the pelvic organs and the lower extremities.

Regional Arterial Supply

After studying the different parts and branches of aorta, it will be useful to study the regional arterial supply as below:

- Arteries of head and neck
- Arteries of shoulders and upper limbs
- Arteries of the chest
- Arteries of the abdomen
- Arteries of the pelvis
- Arteries of the lower limbs.

Arteries of Head and Neck

Arteries supplying the head and neck area are branches of (Fig. 4.2-14):

- Subclavian arteries
- Common carotid arteries.

Branches of subclavian artery to head and neck area

Branches of subclavian artery supplying the head and neck area are:

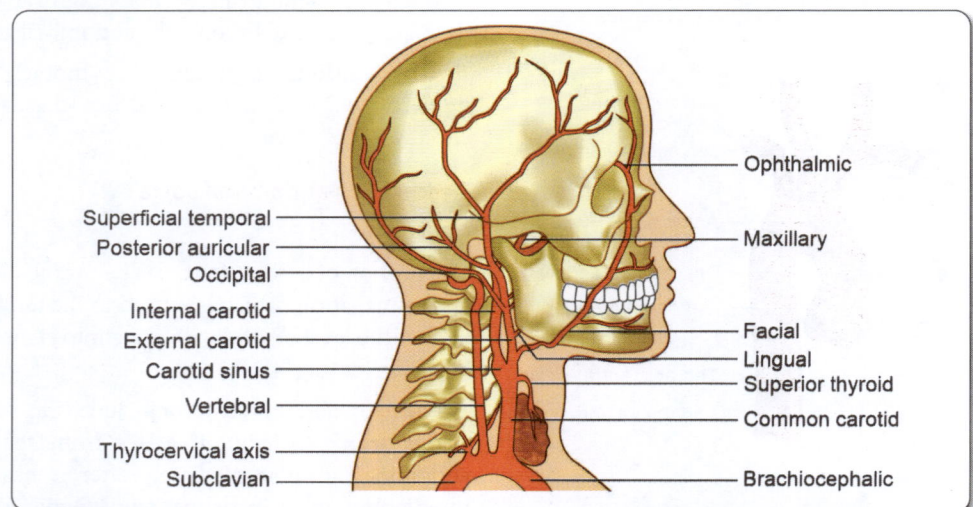

Fig. 4.2-14: Main arteries of head and neck

- Vertebral arteries
- Thyrocervical arteries
- Costocervical arteries.

Vertebral arteries

The vertebral arteries (one each, right and left), after arising from the subclavian arteries, pass upward through the special foramina in the transverse processes of upper six cervical vertebrae. Then, they wind behind the atlas, enter the skull through the foramen magnum, and unite to form a single basilar artery (Figs 4.2-14 and 4.2-15).

Basilar artery

The basilar artery runs along the ventral brain stem and gives branches that supply pons and cerebellum. It terminates by dividing into two posterior cerebral arteries which take part in formation of circle of Willis along with the anterior cerebral arteries (branches of internal carotid arteries) (Fig. 4.2-15).

Thyrocervical arteries

Thyrocervical arteries (Fig. 4.2-14) are short branches of subclavian artery which gives off branches to the thyroid gland, parathyroid gland, larynx, trachea, esophagus, and pharynx, as well as to various muscles in the neck, shoulder and back.

Costocervical arteries

Costocervical arteries are the third vessels to branch from the subclavian. These give off branches which supply to muscles in the neck, back and thoracic wall.

Common carotid arteries

The right common carotid artery is a branch of brachiocephalic artery, while left common carotid artery arises directly from the arch of aorta. Thereafter, the right and left common carotid arteries ascend deeply within the neck ensheathed in the *carotid sheath* along with the internal jugular vein and vagus nerve. At the level of thyroid cartilage of larynx, they divide to form the external and internal carotid arteries (Fig. 4.2-14).

External carotid artery

External carotid artery, as its name suggests, supplies the structure of outer surface of the head and neck.

The branches are shown in Figure 4.2-14:

Superior thyroid artery, supplies to the hyoid bone, larynx and thyroid gland.

Lingual artery, supplies to the tongue, and salivary glands beneath the tongue.

Facial artery passes up over the outer surface of the lower jaw just in front of the angle and supplies the lower part of face, i.e., chin, lips, nose, pharynx and palate.

Occipital artery passes behind the ear and supplies the occipital part of scalp, mastoid process, and various muscles in the neck.

Superficial temporal artery, the terminal branch of external carotid artery, passes in front of the ear to supply the parotid salivary gland and frontal, temporal and parietal portions of the scalp.

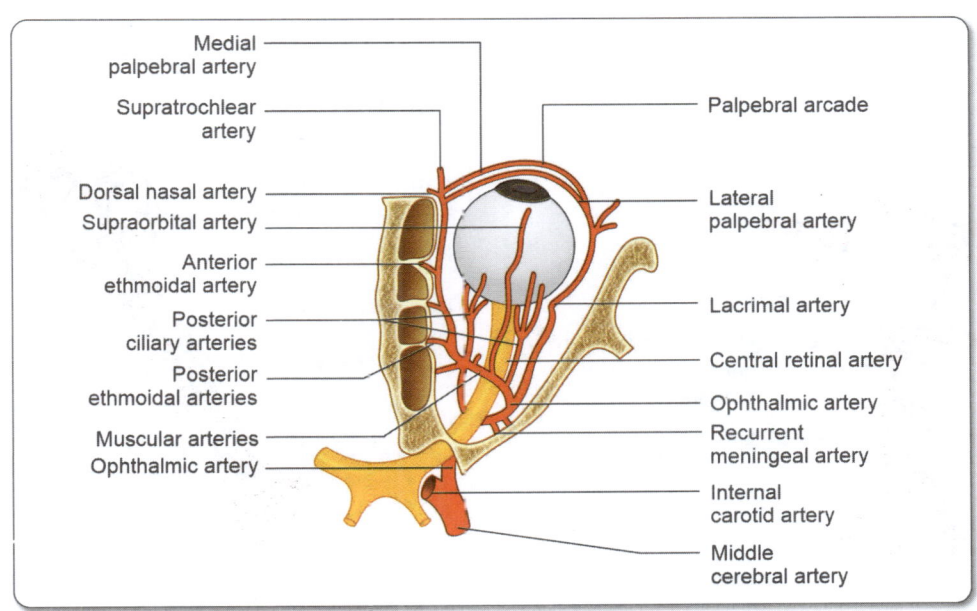

Fig. 4.2-15: Ophthalmic artery and its branches

Maxillary artery, the other terminal branch of the external carotid artery, supplies the structures around the jaws (teeth, gums, cheeks, nasal cavities), and gives off the important *middle meningeal artery* to the interior of the skull.

CLINICAL ASPECTS

The pulse can be felt both in the facial artery, as it crosses the lower jaw and in the temporal artery, where it is placed immediately in front of the external auditory meatus.

Internal carotid artery

Internal carotid artery, a terminal branch of common carotid artery, lies deep in the muscles in the neck. It extends upward to enter the interior of the skull through the carotid foramen in the petrous portion of the temporal bone. In the middle cranial fossa of the skull it ends by dividing into anterior and middle cerebral arteries. It provides major blood supply to the brain.

Branches include:

Ophthalmic artery arises from the internal carotid artery at the level of anterior clenoid process. It enters the orbit through the optic canal and constitutes the main source of blood supply to eyeball and other orbital structures (Fig. 4.2-15).

Posterior communicating artery is a small branch which joins the posterior cerebral artery to form circle of Willis (Fig. 4.2-16).

Choroidal artery is also a small branch which gives off branches to chiasma, optic tract and lateral geniculate body.

Anterior cerebral artery is the smaller terminal branch of internal carotid artery.

Middle cerebral artery is the largest branch of internal carotid artery.

The anterior and middle cerebral arteries communicate with each other and also with basilar artery to form *circle of Willis* (Fig. 4.2-16) which ensures the even distribution of blood to the brain.

Arteries of Shoulder and Upper Limb

Arteries of axilla and upper arm

The axillary artery. The *subclavian artery*, after giving off branches to the neck, continues as axillary artery into the upper arm (Fig. 4.2-17). The axillary artery supplies branches to structures in the axilla, chest wall and shoulder. At the lower boundary of axilla it continues as brachial artery.

Brachial artery. Brachial artery extends along the humerus from the lower border of axilla to the bend of elbow. It supplies to the upper arm structures through its branch (*deep brachial artery*) and shorter branches.

In the cubital fossa (bend of elbow) it ends by dividing into radial and ulnar arteries.

Arteries of forearm

Radial artery. It extends from the elbow to wrist along the radial (lateral) side of the forearm. Near the wrist, it becomes superficial and can be felt lying in front of the bone and thus provides a convenient site for taking pulse (*radial pulse*) (Fig. 4.2-17).

Ulnar artery. It runs from the elbow to the wrist along the ulnar (medial) side of the forearm (Fig. 4.2-17).

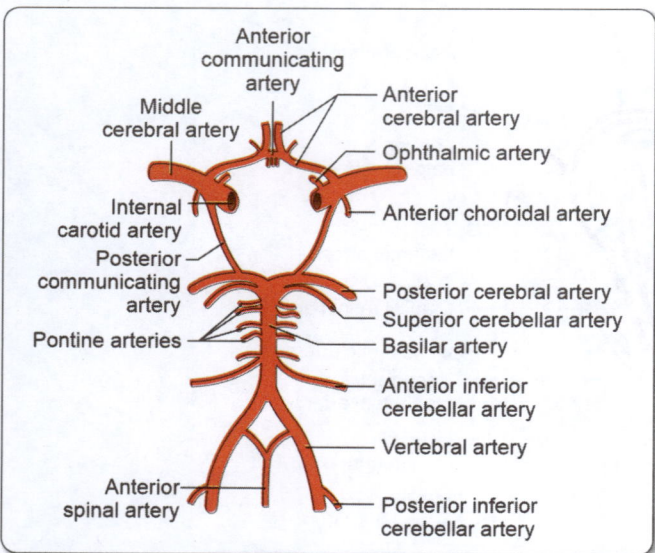

Fig. 4.2-16: Circle of Willis

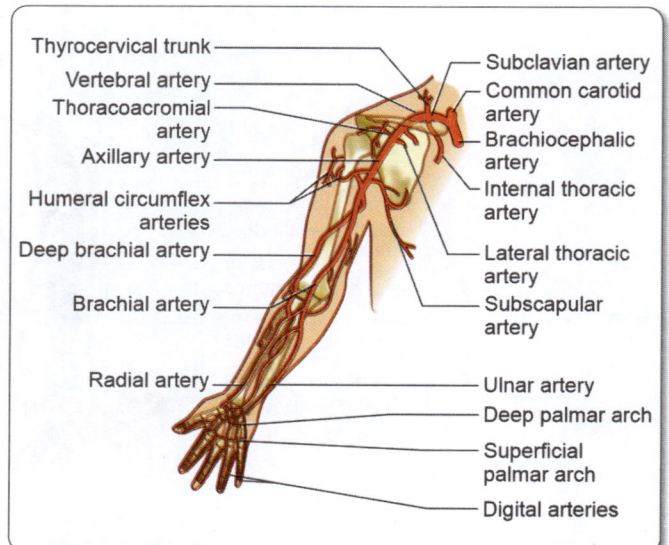

Fig. 4.2-17: Main arteries of shoulder and upper limb

Arteries of hands
Palmar arches

Just in front of the wrist, in the palm, the ends of radial and ulnar arteries anastomose to form two transverse arches: (Fig. 4.2-17)
1. Superficial palmar arch
2. Deep palmar arch.

Branches from the palmar arches supply the structures in hands and fingers.

Arteries of Chest

The walls and viscera of thorax are supplied by branches of subclavian artery and thoracic aorta (Fig. 4.2-18).

Branches of subclavian artery for chest

Internal thoracic artery, a branch of subclavian artery, supplies the chest wall through its branches:
- *Anterior intercostal branches* are six paired arteries (right and left), which supply to the muscles and other structures of six upper intercostal spaces. They also supply the mammary glands.

Branches of descending thoracic aorta to chest
Visceral branches

- *Pericardial arteries* (2–3 in number) supply the pericardium.
- *Bronchial arteries* (3 in number) supply the bronchial tree.
- *Esophageal arteries* (4–5 in number) supply the eosophagus.
- *Mediastinal arteries* (numerous) supply structures in mediastinum.

Parietal branches

Parietal branches of thoracic aorta include:
- *Posterior intercostal arteries*, supply thoracic wall.
- *Subcostal arteries*, supply thoracic wall.
- *Superior phrenic arteries*, supply the superior and posterior surface of diaphragm.

Arteries of Abdomen

Arteries to abdominal wall

Anterior abdominal wall is primarily supplied by branches of:
- Internal thoracic artery, and
- External iliac arteries.

Posterior abdominal wall is supplied by the following paired branches from abdominal aorta (Fig. 4.2-13):
- Inferior pherenic arteries
- Lumbar arteries
- Middle sacral arteries.

Arteries to abdominal viscera

The abdominal viscera is supplied by the following branches of abdominal aorta (Fig. 4.2-13):
- Celiac artery (trunk)
- Superior mesenteric artery
- Suprarenal arteries
- Renal arteries
- Inferior mesenteric artery.

Arteries of Pelvis

Internal iliac artery, a branch of common iliac artery, supplies the various structures of pelvis and gluteal region through its the following branches (Fig. 4.2-19):

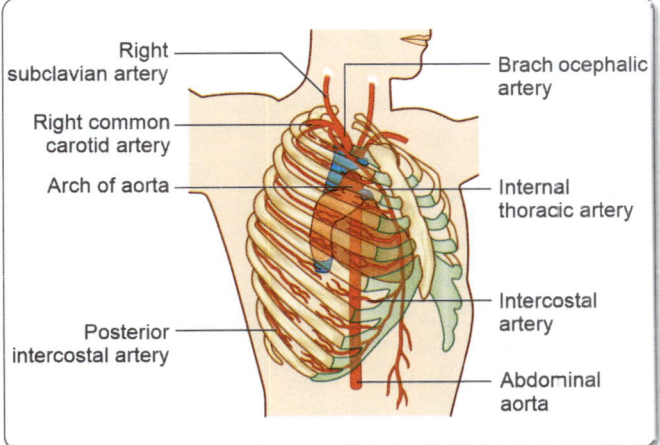

Fig. 4.2-18: Schematic drawing to show arteries supplying to chest wall

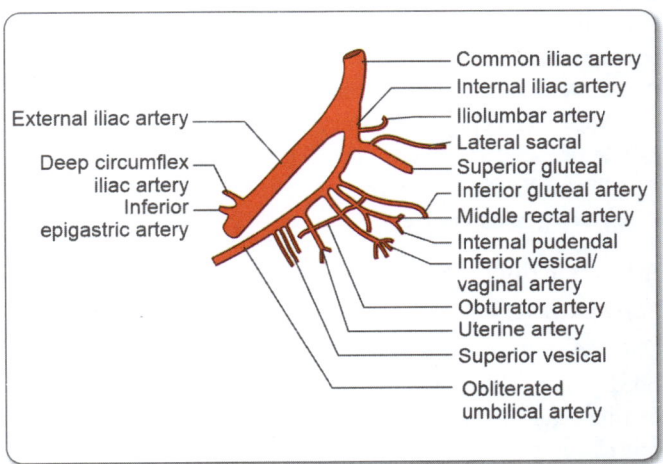

Fig. 4.2-19: Main branches of internal iliac artery

Iliolumbar artery, supplies to the ilium and muscles of the back.

Superior and inferior gluteal arteries, supply to the gluteal muscles, pelvic muscles and skin of the buttocks.

Internal pudendal artery, supplies to distal portion of alimentary canal, the external genitalia and the hip joint.

Superior and inferior vesical arteries, supply to the bladder. In the males these vessels also supply to seminal vesicles and the prostate gland.

Middle rectal artery, supplies to the rectum.

Uterine artery, supplies to uterus and vagina in females.

Arteries of Lower Limb

External iliac artery, the direct continuation of the abdominal aorta, mainly supplies the structures of lower limb. It extends downward from the pelvis in the lower limb and is named, in successive part of its course, the femoral, the popliteal and the posterior tibial artery (Figs 4.2-20A and B).

Arteries in the thigh

Femoral artery

The external iliac artery after passing below the inguinal (Poupart's) ligament becomes the femoral artery.

Course. In the upper half of thigh the femoral artery is comparatively superficial and lies in the space known as *femoral triangle* where pulsations can be felt. The lower part lies more deeply among muscles in a special tunnel called the *adductor (Hunter's) canal.* After passing out of the canal it becomes popliteal artery at the opening in the adductor magnus muscle.

Surface anatomy. Its direction is indicated by a line drawn from a point midway between the anterosuperior iliac spine and the symphysis pubis to a point just above the medial condyle of the femur (adductor tubercle).

Branches. The femoral artery supplies the structures of abdominal wall, external genitalia, thigh and knee joint through its the following branches:

- Superficial circumflex iliac artery
- Superficial epigastric artery
- Superficial and deep external pudendal arteries
- Profunda femoris artery
- Deep genicular artery.

Arteries in popliteal fossa and leg

Popliteal artery

The femoral artery becomes popliteal artery at the proximal border of popliteal fossa (space behind the knee). Branches of this artery supply blood to the knee joint and to certain muscles in the thigh and calf. Its branches also participate in an anastomosis around the knee joint. At the lower border of popliteal fossa, the popliteal artery ends by dividing into anterior and posterior tibial arteries (Fig. 4.2-20).

Anterior tibial artery

It passes downward between the tibia and fibula to supply the front of the leg and is continued downward on the dorsum of foot as the *dorsalis pedis artery.*

Posterior tibial artery

It is the larger branch of popliteal artery, is in fact the direct continuation of the popliteal artery in the back of leg where it lies deep in the calf muscle and gives off the following branches:

Small branches to skin, muscles and other tissues of the lower leg along the way.

Peroneal artery is a large branch of the posterior tibial artery which supplies structures of the medial side of fibula and contributes to the anastomosis of the ankle.

Terminal branches. The posterior tibial artery divides into medial and lateral plantar arteries.

Arteries to the ankle and foot

The dorsalis pedis artery (continuation of anterior tibial artery) anastomoses with the medial and lateral plantar arteries to form the *plantar arch,* similar to the palmar arch of hand. Digital branches from the plantar arch supply blood to the toes.

NURSING IMPLICATIONS AND APPLICATIONS

Pressure Points

Pressure points are the areas where the arteries are near the surface and can be felt and/or compressed against some firm underlying structure. By compressing the arteries at pressure points, it is sometimes possible to arrest severe hemorrhage. Some examples of pressure points in the body are mentioned as follows.

Pressure Points in Head and Neck Area

Facial artery: Against the lower jaw.

Temporal artery: In front of the external auditory meatus.

Occipital artery: Against the occipital bone 6.5 cm behind the ear.

Common carotid: Against the cervical vertebrae to the side of larynx.

Pressure Points in Upper Limb Area

Subclavian artery: Against the first rib in the hollow above the clavicle.

Brachial artery: Against the medial aspect of humerus in the middle of arm.

Radial artery: At the lower end of radius just above the wrist on its anterior surface

Ulnar artery: Against the anterior surface of ulna.

Pressure Points in Lower Limb Area

Femoral artery: Against the pubic bone under the inguinal (Poupart's) ligament.

Posterior tibial artery: Against the posterior surface of medial malleolus.

Dorsalis pedis artery: Against the upper surface of the navicular bone.

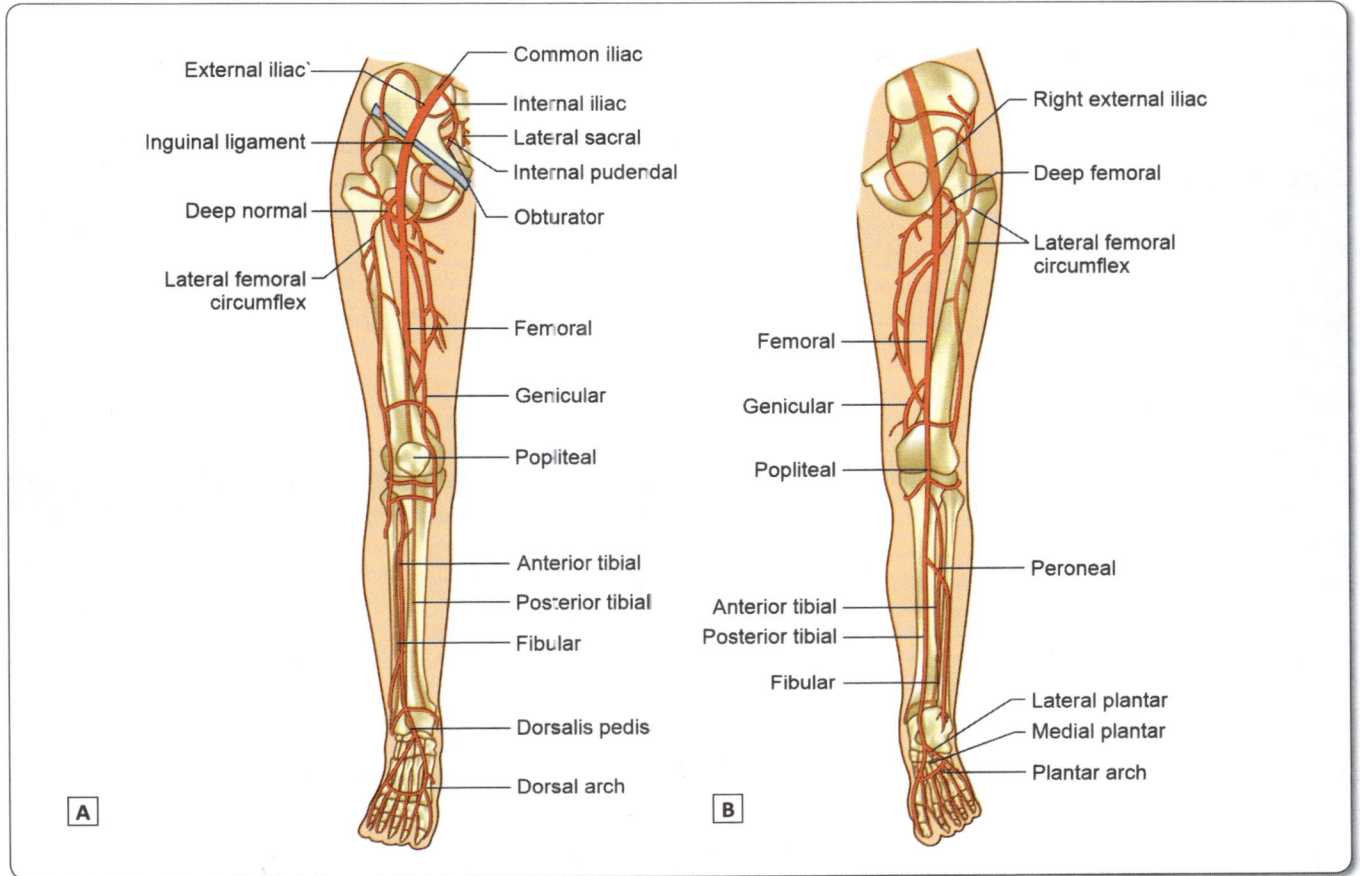

Figs 4.2-20A and B: Main arteries of lower limb

VENOUS SYSTEM

The venous system is concerned with collection of deoxygenated blood from the various tissues of the body and returning it to heart. We have seen that the arteries begin as large vessels which gradually become smaller and they end in arterioles which merge into capillaries. In contrast to it, the veins begin as very small vessels, the *venules*, which unite to form progressive large veins.

Divisions of Venous System

The venous system can be considered to consist of three sets of veins: the pulmonary, the coronary, and the systemic.
Pulmonary veins carry oxygenated blood from the lungs to the left atrium. These form part of pulmonary circulation which is discussed separately.
Coronary veins collect the deoxygenated blood from the myocardium. These veins unite to form the *coronary sinus* which opens into the right atrium directly.

Systemic veins. The systemic veins can be divided into two main groups:
1. *Superficial veins.* These are situated on the surface of the body, just under the skin. These are commonly interconnected in irregular networks, so that many unnamed tributaries may join to form a relatively large vein. Some superficial veins can be easily seen through the skin.
2. *Deep veins.* These are situated deep in the tissue.
    Mainly large veins typically follow the course of main arteries, and often have the same names as their companion in the arterial system. For example, renal veins follow the renal arteries.

Major Venous Trunks

The veins of systemic circulation unite to form larger and larger vessels until two major venous trunks are formed which drain the blood into the right atrium of the heart. These venous trunks are:

1. Superior vena cava
2. Inferior vena cava.

Figure 4.2-21 shows the main veins constituting the venous systems.

Superior Vena Cava

The superior vena cava is formed at the level of lower border of first right costal cartilage by the union of right and left brachiocephalic veins (Fig. 4.2-22). It is about 7 cm long and ends by opening in the right atrium at the level of third right costal cartilage.

Tributaries of superior vena cava

The superior vena cava drains blood from the head, neck, chest and upper limb through the following tributaries (Fig. 4.2-22):

Right brachiocephalic vein. It is only 2.5 cm long. It is formed by the union of right internal jugular and subclavian veins.

The various tributaries which drain into right brachiocephalic vein are (Fig. 4.2-22):

- *Right subclavian veins* bringing deoxygenated blood from the right upper limb.
- *Right internal jugular vein* bringing blood from the right half of head and neck area.
- *Right vertibral vein* draining blood from the structures supplied by vertebral artery.
- *Right internal thoracic vein* draining blood from the area supplied of internal thoracic artery.
- *Right inferior thyroid vein* draining the area supplied by the artery of same name.
- *Right first intercostal vein* draining blood from the structures of first intercostal space.

IMPORTANT TO KNOW

In addition to the above veins the right brachiocephalic vein, the thoracic or right lymphatic duct also drains into it.

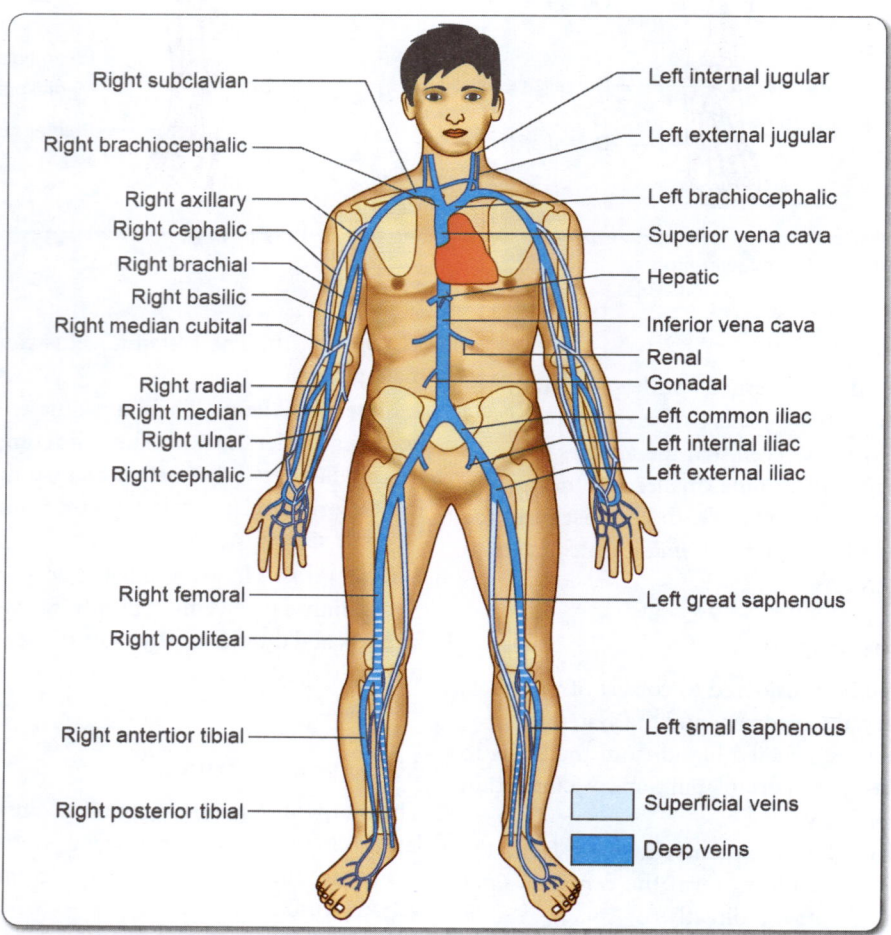

Fig. 4.2-21: Main veins constituting venous system of the body

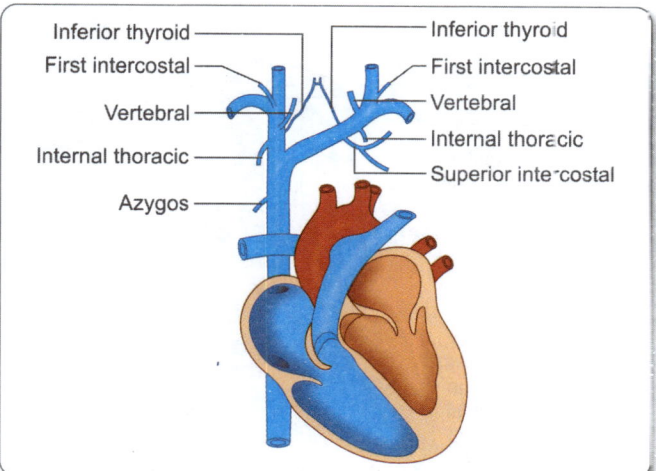

Fig. 4.2-22: Superior vena cava and brachiocephalic veins with their tributaries

Left brachiocephalic vein. It is formed by the left internal jugular and subclavian veins. Its *tributaries* are similar to right brachiocephalic vein, except that it also receives blood from the left superior intercostal vein (Fig. 4.2-22).

Azygos vein opens into the superior vena cava on the right side about its middle (Fig. 4.2-22). It is a large vein which drains blood from the thorax and abdominal wall. The *azygos system* of veins may also serve as a bypass for the inferior vena cava in case of obstruction (for details see veins of thorax).

Inferior vena cava

This is the largest vein in the body. It is formed by the union of the right and left common iliac veins at the body of the 5th lumbar vertebra (Fig. 4.2-21). It ascends upward along the posterior abdominal wall lying to the right of the abdominal aorta. It ends by piercing the diaphragm to open into the right atrium of heart.

Tributaries

It drains the blood from the following structures through various tributaries from:
- *From the lower limbs* the blood is drained into inferior vena cava.
- *From the abdomen* the blood is brought into the inferior vena cava through the tributaries which have the names of the parietal and visceral branches of abdominal aorta. These veins are the lumbar, renal, suprarenal, inferior phrenic, hepatic, and right spermatic or ovarian (Fig. 4.2-21).

Regional Venous Drainage

Till now we have studied the plan of venous system and two major venous trunks which ultimately pour the deoxygenated blood collected from various parts of the body into the right atrium. At this juncture, it will be useful to study the venous drainage from the different regions of the body as below:
- Venous drainage from head and neck.
- Venous drainage from the upper limbs.
- Venous drainage from the thorax and abdominal wall.
- Venous drainage from the abdominal viscera.
- Venous drainage from the pelvis.
- Venous drainage from the lower limbs.

Venous Drainage from the Head and Neck

Venous blood drained from the head and neck area reaches the superior vena cava through two main veins:
1. External jugular vein
2. Internal jugular vein

External jugular vein

External jugular vein is formed in the neck at the level of angle of jaw by the union of *superficial veins* of the scalp. This vein passes downward in front of the sternomastoid muscle and ends by entering the subclavian vein (Fig. 4.2-23).

Tributaries of external jugular vein which return venous blood from the superficial structures of face scalp are the superficial veins of the same name as the branches of external carotid artery.

Internal jugular veins

Internal jugular veins begin at the jugular foramen in the base of skull as direct continuation of the sigmoid portion of the

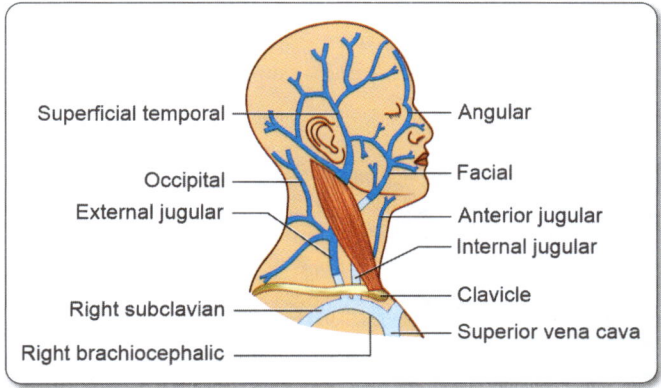

Fig. 4.2-23: Veins of head and neck

transverse (lateral) sinus. They run downward in the neck, deep to the sternomastoid muscle, in close association with the carotid artery with which it is included in the carotid sheath. Finally, the internal jugular veins join with the subclavian veins, carrying blood from the upper limbs, to form the *brachiocephalic veins* which open in the superior vena cava.

Tributaries of internal jugular vein are:

Facial veins. Facial vein is downward continuation of the angular vein which collects blood from the upper part of face through various small veins (Fig. 4.2-23). There is also a communication between the angular vein and the veins inside the skull which pass through the orbit. It is for this reason that boils and carbuncles on the face may be particularly dangerous, for infection may spread through this connection and cause cavernous sinus thrombosis.

Intracranial venous sinuses. The venous blood from the deep area of brain is collected into channels called the dural venous sinuses. These sinuses, lined by endothelium, are formed by layer of dura mater. The main venous sinuses are as shown in Figure 4.2-24.

Superior sagittal sinus. It begins in the frontal region of the skull, carries the blood from the superior part of brain, and runs directly backward in the midline to the occipital region in a fold of dura mater called the *falx cerebri.* Then it turns to the right side and continues as *right transverse sinus.*

Inferior sagittal sinus collects blood from the deeper parts of brain and passes backward to continue as *straight sinus.*

Straight sinus runs backward and downward and continues as *left transverse sinus.*

Transversus sinuses run forward and medially from the occipital region on each side to continue with the sigmoid sinus.

Sigmoid sinuses continue inferiorly as internal jugular veins.

Venous Drainage from the Upper Limb

The veins draining blood from different structures of upper limb are arranged in two groups: superficial and deep veins (Fig. 4.2-25).

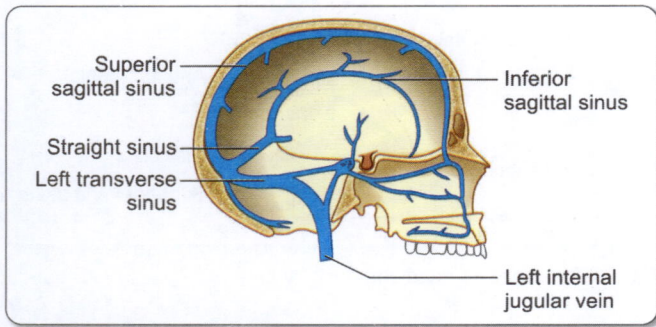

Fig. 4.2-24: Venous system of brain viewed from the right

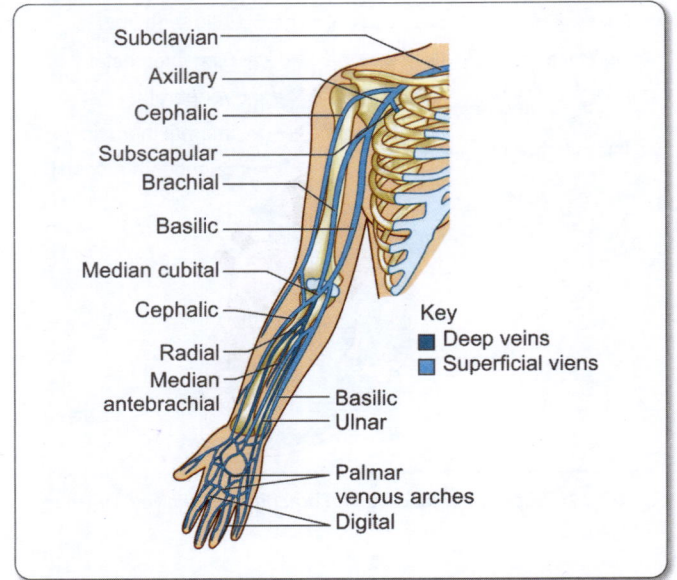

Fig. 4.2-25: Superficial and deep veins of right upper limb

Superficial veins of upper limb

These lie below the skin and are interconnected in complex networks. The superficial veins begin mainly on the back of hand, and some of them converge in cubital space in fornt of elbow joint. The main superficial veins are:

Cephalic vein runs upward from the hand to shoulder on the lateral side of the arm. In the shoulder it pierces the tissues and opens into the *axillary veins.*

Basilic vein runs upward from the back of hand on ulnar side for a distance and then curves forward to the anterior surface. It continues ascending in the medial side until it reaches the middle of upper arm. There, it penetrates deep and joins the axillary vein.

Median vein is a small vein that is not always present. It commences at the palmar surface of the hand, runs upward on the front of forearm and ends in the basilic vein.

Median cubital vein is a small but prominent vein which in the cubital fossa ascends from the cephalic vein on lateral side to join the basilic vein on the medial side. This vein is often used as a site for *venipuncture* for the collection of blood sample and for the injection of fluids or drugs into the blood stream.

Deep veins of upper limb

The deep veins generally parallel the arteries in each region of the upper limb and are given similar names as below:

In the hands blood is collected by *palmar metacarpal veins and deep palmar venous arches* and emptied in the ulnar and radial vein.

In the forearm

Ulnar veins run upward on the medial side
Radial vein runs upward on the lateral side.

In the upper arm

Brachial vein in formed by the union of ulnar and radial veins just above the elbow. The brachial vein continues upward along with the brachial artery.

Axillary vein is the continuation upward of brachial vein. As mentioned above, the superficial basilic and cephalic veins open into the axillary vein in the upper part of upper arm.

Subclavian vein is a continuation of the axillary vein and unites with the internal jugular vein to form the brachiocephalic vein. At the junction with internal jugular vein and left subclavian vein it receives thoracic duct and the right subclavian vein receives the right lymphatic duct.

Brachiocephalic veins of the two sides join to form the superior vena cava which opens in the right atrium of the heart.

Venous Drainage from Thorax and Abdominal Wall

The veins draining blood from the thorax include (Fig. 4.2-26):

Internal thoracic veins receive blood from the tributaries corresponding to branches of internal thoracic artery. These veins open into *brachiocephalic veins.*

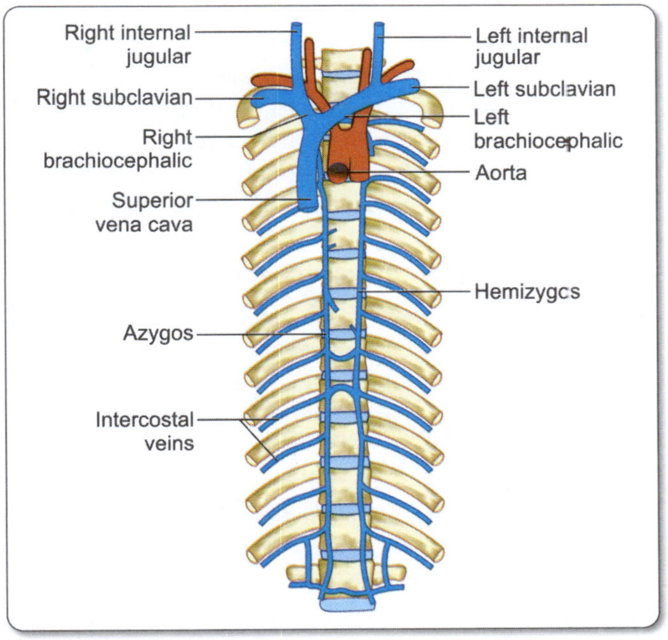

Fig. 4.2-26: Superior vena cava and main veins of the thorax

Intercostal veins. Some of the intercostal veins directly open into the brachiocephalic veins. However, most of the intercostal veins open into the internal thoracic veins.

Lumbar veins drain blood from the thoracic and abdominal wall and open into the inferior vena cava.

Azygos vein. Most of the blood from right side of thoracic cavity and abdominal wall is drained by azygos vein, which ascends on the right side of vertebral column, from the level of 2nd lumbar to 4th thoracic vertebrae, where it empties in the superior vena cava. Tributaries of azygos vein include:

Posterior intercostal veins, which drain the intercostal spaces on the right side.

Ascending lumbar veins, both right and left, open in azygos vein. These drain blood from the thoracic wall and abdominal wall.

Hemiazygos vein. Most of the blood from the left side of thoracic cavity and abdominal wall is drained by hemiazygos vein, which ascends on the left side of vertebral column from the left side of lumbar region to the level of left brachiocephalic vein in which it empties. The hemiazygos vein also sends tributaries to the right azygos vein.

IMPORTANT TO KNOW

Azygos System

The azygos vein (on right side) and hemiazygos vein (or left side) communicate with each other and also with many veins which drain into inferior vena cava. Thus, the azygos system bypasses the blood from inferior vena cava to superior vena cava in case the former is blocked.

Venous Drainage from Abdominal Viscera

As described above the inferior vena cava is the major venous trunk collecting the deoxygenated blood from the abdominal and pelvic viscera. In the abdomen, some veins open directly into the inferior vena cava, while the veins collecting blood from the organs of digestion pour their blood through portal vein into the liver and form the *hepatic portal circulation*, as described as follows.

Veins from abdominal viscera which directly open into inferior vena cava

The lumbar, gonadal, renal, suprarenal, phrenic and hepatic veins open into the inferior vena cava (Fig. 4.2-21). Generally, these veins drain the blood from the structures supplied by arteries with corresponding names. Some differences which exist between the right and left side veins, in the mode of emptying in inferior vena cava, are as follows:

Suprarenal veins. Right suprarenal vein empties into inferior vena cava; the left empties into the left renal or left inferior phrenic.

Inferior phrenic veins. Right inferior phrenic vein empties into the inferior vena cava, one of which empties into the left renal, suprarenal vein and other into the inferior vena cava.

Gonadal veins. The right gonadal (spermatic or ovarian) empties into the inferior vena cava, but the left empties into the left renal vein.

IMPORTANT TO KNOW

Hepatic Portal Circulation

The veins collecting blood from the spleen and abdominal organs of digestion are unique and differ from rest of the veins. These veins originate from the capillary network of the organs of digestion and carry blood from these organs through the portal vein to the liver. In the liver, this blood passes through a second capillary bed, the hepatic sinusoids. This unique venous pathway constitutes the hepatic portal circulation. The importance of this is that the digested foodstuffs absorbed from the alimentary canal go to the liver first. Passage of the blood containing absorbed foodstuffs from the hepatic sinusoids allows the liver cells to absorbs, modify and store them.

Portal vein

Portal vein itself is quite small (about 8 cm long), and is formed behind the pancreas by the union of splenic vein and superior mesenteric vein and opens into the liver (Fig. 4.2-27).

Tributaries of portal vein include the following veins, each of which drains blood from the area supplied by the corresponding artery:

Superior mesenteric vein drains blood from the small intestine, ascending colon, and transverse colon. It unites with the splenic vein to form the portal vein.

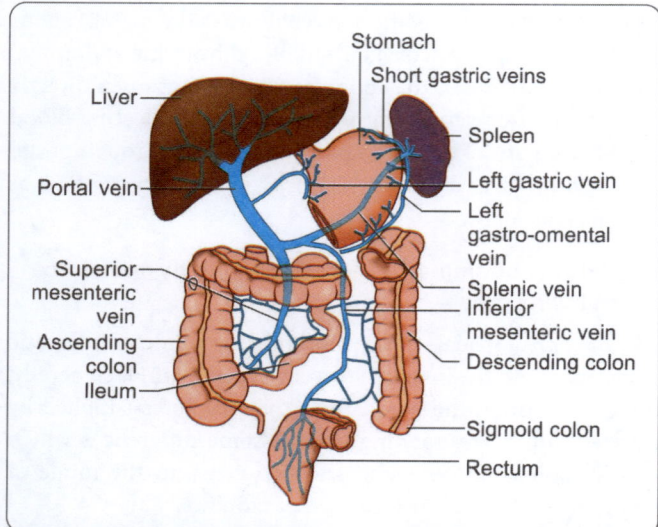

Fig. 4.2-27: Portal vein, its tributaries and termination

Splenic vein. It drains the blood from the spleen, the pancreas and part of stomach. It unites with superior mesenteric vein to form the portal vein.

Inferior mesenteric vein. It drains blood from the descending colon, sigmoid colon and rectum. It opens into the splenic vein.

Gastric veins (right and left) drain blood from the stomach and distal end of esophagus. They drain into the portal vein.

Cystic vein drains blood from the gallbladder, and joins the portal vein.

IMPORTANT TO KNOW

It is important to note that:
- *Blood supplied by hepatic artery* to the liver does not take part in portal circulation. This blood supplies oxygen and nutrients to the liver cells.
- *Obstruction of the portal vein* or its branches causes a rise in blood pressure in the portal venous system, a condition known as *portal hypertension.* This results in enlargement of the spleen, esophageal varices and hemorrhoids.

Venous Drainage from Pelvis

Internal iliac veins

Most of the blood from the pelvis is drained by internal iliac veins through their tributaries. The internal iliac veins begin deep within the pelvis and ascend to the pelvis brim where they unite with external iliac veins to form the *common iliac veins.* The right and left common iliac veins unite to form the inferior vena cava (Fig. 4.2-21).

Tributaries that drain blood from the organs of reproductive, urinary and digestive systems in the pelvic region are the veins corresponding to the branches of internal iliac artery such as the gluteal, pudendal, vesical, rectal, uterine and vaginal. Typically these veins have many interconnections and form plexuses in the region of rectum, urinary bladder, and prostate gland (in the male) or uterus and vagina (in the female).

Venous Drainage from Lower Limbs

The veins draining blood from different structures of the lower limbs (as in the case of upper limbs) are arranged in two groups: (i) Superficial; (ii) deep (Fig. 4.2-21).

Superficial veins of lower limb

The superficial veins of the foot and leg lie below the skin and are interconnected to form complex network. These vessels drain into two major trunks:

1. *Small saphenous vein (Fig. 4.2-28).* It begins on the lateral side of the foot, receives many small tributaries and passes

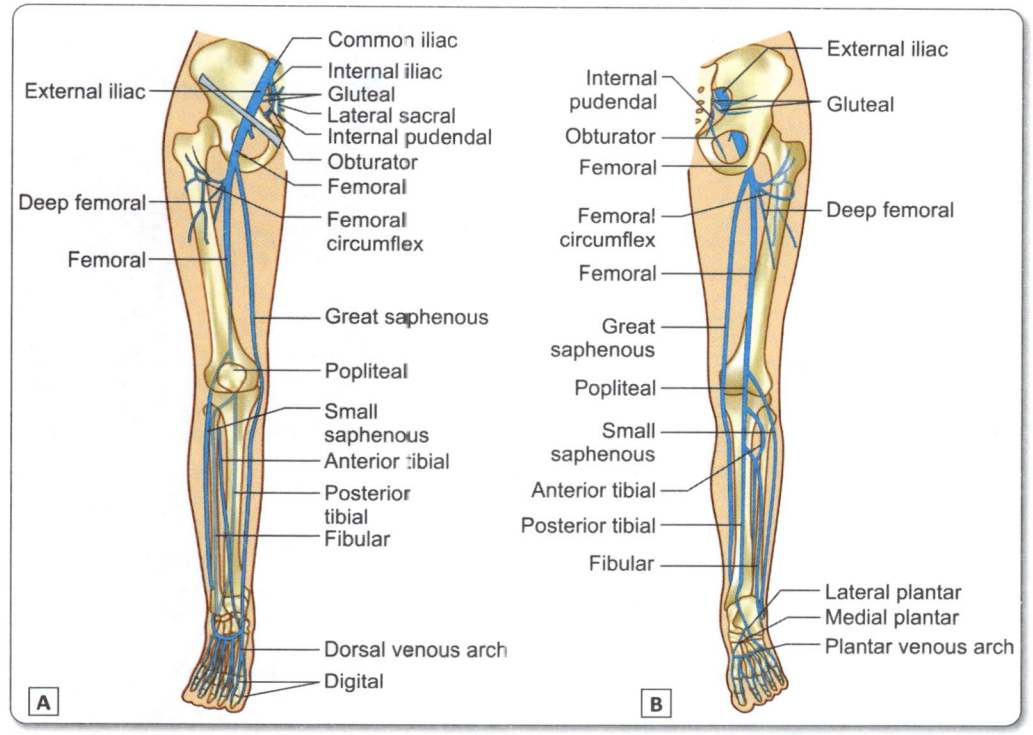

Figs 4.2-28A and B: Superficial and deep veins of lower limb

upward along the center of the back of calf and pierces the deep fascia of the limb over the popliteal space at the back of knee joint to empty into the popliteal vein.

2. Great saphenous vein (Fig. 4.2-28). It begins in the marginal vein of the dorsum of foot, extends along the medial side of leg and thigh, receiving many tributaries on the way. Just below the medial end of the inguinal ligament it passes deeper to enter the *femoral vein.*

The point where it pierces the deep fascia of the limb is called the *saphenous opening.*

Deep veins of the lower limb

The deep veins generally parallel the arteries in each region of the lower limb and are given similar names as discussed here (Fig. 4.2-21).

Anterior and posterior tibial veins begin at the lower end of the leg and ascend upward up to the popliteal fossa accompanied by the corresponding arteries.

Popliteal vein is formed by the union of anterior and posterior tibial veins at the level of knees and pass upward in company with the popliteal artery.

Femoral vein. The popliteal vein enters the Hunter's canal and continues upward through the thigh as the femoral vein. In the femoral triangle, the femoral vein lies along with femoral artery in a sheath of fibrous tissue, called the femoral sheath. Here it receives the long saphenous vein and passes under the inguinal ligament to become the *external iliac vein.*

IMPORTANT TO KNOW

It is important to note that:
- Both superficial and deep veins of the lower limb are provided with valves which are more numerous in the deep veins.
- The saphenous veins communicate extensively with the deep veins of the legs. As a result, there are many pathways by which blood can be returned to the heart from the lower extremities.
- Saphenous veins are subjected to increased blood pressure in standing posture because of gravitational force. Therefore, in persons with prolonged period of standing (e.g. traffic police), these veins are prone to develop abnormal dilatations or varicosities (varicose veins).

PHYSIOLOGICAL ACTIVITIES OF THE HEART

PHYSIOLOGY OF CARDIAC MUSCLE

Structural Organization of Cardiac Muscle

- The cardiac muscle fibers are *striated*. However, unlike the skeletal muscles, the cardiac muscles are *involuntary* (like smooth muscles). Thus cardiac muscles share some characteristics with skeletal muscles and others with smooth muscles.
- The cardiac muscle fibers are *ribbon-like*, *branched* and interdigitate freely with each other. The branches from the neighboring fibers join together. At the point of contact of two muscle fibers, the membranes of both the muscle fibers are fused together and thrown into extensive infolding forming the so called *intercalated disc* (Fig. 4.2-29 and Histology plate 4.2-2).
- Along the sides near the outer border of intercalated disc the two adjacent muscle fibers are connected with each other through the *gap junctions*. The action potential passes from one cardiac muscle cell to the other through gap junctions, which provide *low resistance bridges* and thus the cardiac muscle acts as a *functional syncytium* of many cardiac cells. In this way, the cardiac impulse spreads throughout the muscle mass quickly resulting in a coordinated contraction of the whole tissue.

Structure of a Cardiac Muscle Fiber

Each muscle fiber is about 80 µm long and about 15 µm broad. Its cell membrane is called *sarcolemma* and the cytoplasm is called *sarcoplasm*. Each muscle fiber is made up of number of *myofibrils*, which lie parallel to each other. Each myofibril is 2 µm is diameter, and consists of thick and thin filaments. Essentially, the structure and striations are similar to that of a skeletal muscle.

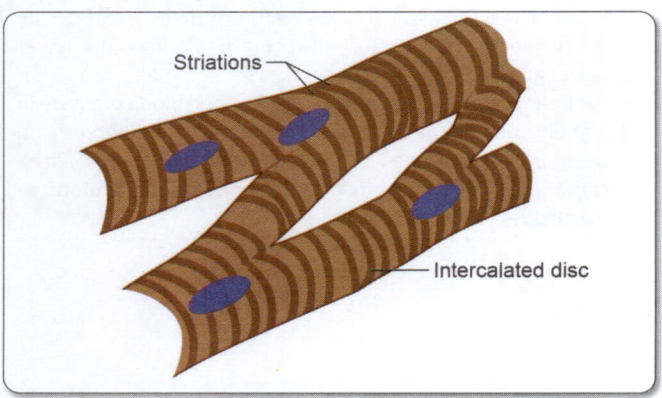

Fig. 4.2-29: Structure of cardiac muscle

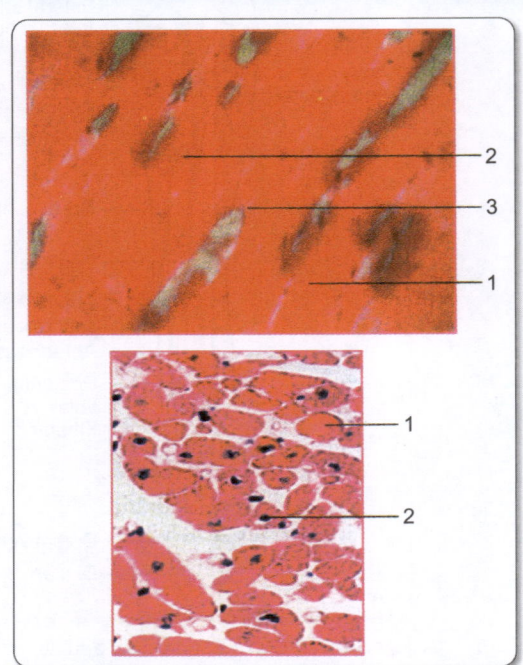

Histology Plate 4.2-2: Cardiac Muscle

Photomicrographs of transverse and longitudinal sections of cardiac muscle fibers (1) and shown. These exhibit single central nucleus (2), branching of the muscle fibers (3) and intercalated disc (4).

Sarcotubular System

The sarcotubular system in cardiac muscles is well developed like that of skeletal muscle. However, the tubules of the T-system penetrate the sarcomere at Z-line. Therefore, in cardiac muscles, there is only one triad per sarcomere as compared to two in skeletal muscle.

Process of Excitability and Contractility: An Electro-mechanical Phenomenon

The cardiac muscle being an excitable tissue produces an action potential (*electrical phenomenon*) when stimulated and responds by contracting (*mechanical phenomenon*). The events which link the electrical phenomenon with mechanical phenomenon constitute the *excitation-contraction coupling phenomenon*.

Electrical Potentials in Cardiac Muscle

Resting membrane potential

The resting membrane potential (RMP) of a normal cardiac muscle fiber is –85 mV to –95 mV (negative interior with reference to exterior).

Action potential

When stimulated, each cardiac muscle fiber shows an electrical activity known as propagated action potential. The action potential recorded from a single cardiac muscle fiber is unusually long and can be divided into five distinct phases (Fig. 4.2-30).

Phases of action potential

Phase 0: Rapid depolarization. The phase 0 (upstroke) is characterized by the depolarization which proceeds rapidly, as in skeletal muscle and nerve. The rapid depolarization and the overshoot are due to rapid influx of Na^+ ions similar to that occurring in nerve and skeletal muscle.

Phase 1: Initial rapid repolarization. Rapid depolarization is followed by a very short-lived slight rapid repolarization. The membrane potential reaches from +30 mV to –10 mV during this phase. The initial rapid repolarization is due to closure of Na^+ channels and opening of K^+ channels resulting in transient outward current.

Phase 2: Plateau. During plateau phase, the cardiac muscle fiber remains in the depolarized state. The membrane potential falls very slowly. The plateau phase lasts for about 100–200 msec. This phase occurs due to slow influx of Ca^{2+}.

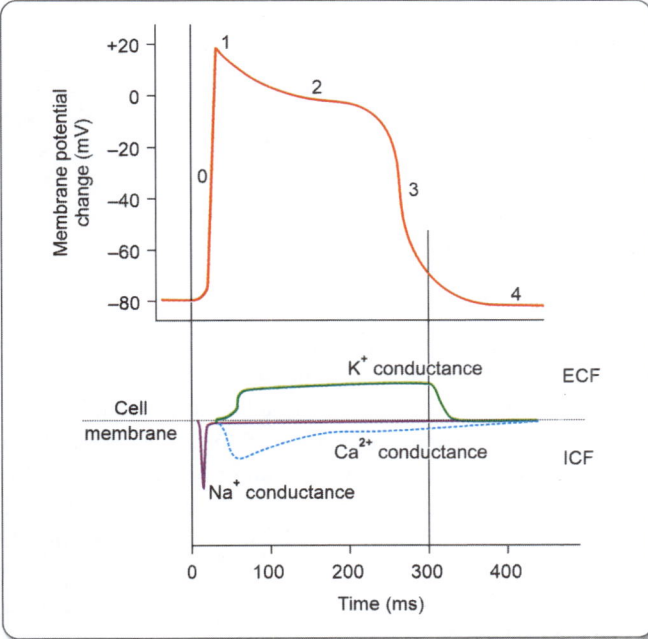

Fig. 4.2-30: Various phases of action potential and ion conductance: Phase 0 = depolarization; Phase 1 = rapid repolarization; Phase 2 = plateau phase; Phase 3 = late rapid repolarization; and Phase 4 = resting potential

Phase 3: Repolarization. During this phase complete repolarization occurs and the membrane potential falls to the approximate resting value.
- *Ionic basis:* The slow repolarization results from closing of Ca^{2+} channels and opening of K^+ channels.

Phase 4: resting potential. In this phase of resting membrane potential (also called polarized state) the potential is maintained at –90 mV.

Duration of action potential

The duration of action potential is about 250 msec at a heart rate 75 beats/minute. The duration of action potential decreases with increased heart rate (150 msec at a heart rate of 200 beats/min).

Spread of action potential through cardiac muscle

The cardiac muscle acts as physiological syncytium due to presence of gap junctions amongst the cardiac muscle fibers. Because of this the action potential spreads through the cardiac muscles very rapidly. Further, as there are two syncytia (the atrial and the ventricular) in the heart, so the action potential is transmitted from atria to ventricles only through the fibers of specialized conductive system.

Excitation-contraction Coupling Phenomenon in Cardiac Muscles

The sequence of events during excitation-contraction coupling in the cardiac muscle are similar to those observed in a skeletal muscle, with the following exception:

In cardiac muscle (as against that in skeletal muscle) extra calcium ions diffuse into the sarcoplasm from T-tubules without which the contraction strength would be considerably reduced, whereas skeletal muscle contraction is hardly affected by calcium concentration in ECF.

Process of Cardiac Muscle Contraction

The molecular mechanism of cardiac muscle contraction by cross-bridge cycling and sliding of filaments is primarily similar to that of skeletal muscles and smooth muscles. However, in cardiac muscle:
- Troponin-tropomyosin complex controls the onset and offset of cross-bridge cycling, similar to that in skeletal muscles, and
- Like smooth muscles, the contractility of cardiac muscle is sensitive to *phosphorylation*.

Relaxation of Cardiac Muscle

Relaxation of cardiac muscle (diastole) occurs when levels of Ca^{2+} ions fall in the cardiac muscle fibers. During diastole the

Ca^{2+} ions are extruded out of the cardiac muscle fiber by a carrier system operating at the sarcolemma, in which two Na^+ ions are exchanged for each Ca^{2+} ion extruded. Thus, the rate of Ca^{2+} ion extrusion depends on the gradient of Na^+ created by Na^+-K^+ ATPase.

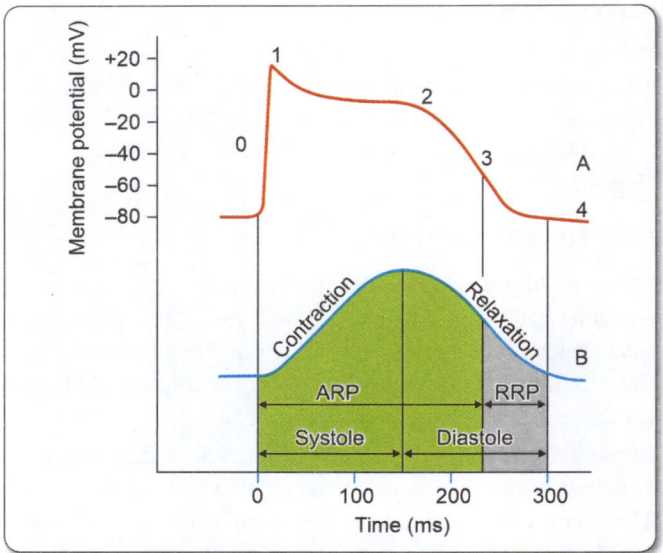

Fig. 4.2-31: Record of action potential (A) and mechanical response (B) from the cardiac muscle fiber shown on same time scale depicting the significance of long refractory period.
Abbreviations: ARP, absolute refractory period; RRP, relative refractory period

CLINICAL ASPECTS

Inhibition of this secondary active transport of Ca^{2+} ions, e.g. by digitalis or other cardiac glycosides raises the intracellular Ca^{2+} concentration and thereby increases myocardial contractility. This effect is utilized in patients with congestive heart failure.

Properties of Cardiac Muscle

The basic properties of cardiac muscle include:
- Excitability (bathmotropism)
- Contractility (inotropism)
- Autorhythmicity
- Conductivity.

Excitability

Excitability (bathmotropism) is the property by which tissues respond to stimuli. The cardiac muscle responds by development of action potential.

The characteristics of cardiac muscle is excitability, which needs a special emphasis in its refractory period.

Refractory period

Refractory period refers to the period the following action potential during which the cardiac muscle does not respond to a stimulus. Cardiac muscle has a long refractory period (250–300 msec in ventricles and about 150 msec in atria). It is of two types:

1. *Absolute refractory period (ARP).* During this period the cardiac muscle does not show any response at all. It extends from phase 0 to half of phase three of action potential, i.e., until the membrane potential reaches approximately –50 mV during repolarization (Fig. 4.2-31). Normal duration of absolute refractory period (ARP) in ventricles is about 180–200 msec.

2. *Relative refractory period.* During this period, the muscle shows response if the strength of stimulus is increased to maximum. It extends from second half of the phase three to phase four of the action potential. Normal duration of relative refractory period in ventricles is about 50 msec.

Significance of long refractory period in cardiac muscle

As shown in Fig. 4.2-31, the cardiac muscle is refractory to any stimulus during the contraction phase (systole), therefore, the complete summation of contractions and thus tetanus cannot be produced in cardiac muscle. This property is very useful.

Since the heart has to function as a pump, it must relax, get filled up with blood and then contract to pump out the blood. A tetanized heart would be useless as a pump.

Contractility

Contractility is the ability of the cardiac muscle to actively generate force to shorten and thicken to do work when sufficient stimulus is applied. Characteristic features of myocardial contractility are:
- All or None Law
- Starling Law of Heart.

All or none law

The response of cardiac muscle to a stimulus is all or none in character, i.e., when a stimulus of subthreshold intensity is applied, the heart does not contract at all (none response), when stimulus of threshold or suprathreshold intensity is applied, it contracts to its maximum ability (all response). This is because of the syncytial arrangement of the cardiac muscle fibers. Therefore, the 'all or none' law in heart is applicable to whole of functional syncytial unit, i.e., the entire atria or entire ventricle, while in skeletal muscle it is applicable only to a single muscle fiber.

Starling's law of heart

According to Starling's law, the force of contraction is the function of the initial length of the muscle fibers; and up to physiological limits the greater the initial length, greater is the force of contraction. In the case of heart muscle, the end diastolic volume forms the preload. The effect of changing end diastolic volume on force of cardiac contraction has been studied by Frank and Starling in 1910. *The Frank-Starling Law of Heart* states that within physiological limits the force of cardiac contraction is proportional to its end diastolic volume (venous return).

Origin and Spread of Cardiac Impulse Conductivity
Conducting system of the heart

Autorhythmicity refers to the property of cardiac muscle which enables the heart to initiate its own impulse at constant rhythmical intervals. Because of this property the heart continues to beat even after all nerves to it are sectioned. This is because of the presence of specialized *pacemaker tissue* in the heart that can initiate repetitive action potentials. The pacemaker tissue makes a *conduction system* that normally spreads impulses through the heart.

The conducting system of the heart consists of specialized fibers of the heart muscle. These include (Fig. 4.2-32):

Sinoatrial node. Sinoatrial (SA) node is located in the wall of right atrium just to the right of opening of superior vena cava. Spontaneous rhythmical electrical impulses arise from the SA node and spread in all directions.

Interatrial tract (Bachman's bundle). It is a band of specialized muscle fibers that run from SA node to left atrium. It causes simultaneous depolarization of the left atrium.

Internodal conduction pathway. Three internodal conduction paths which connect SA node to atrioventricular (AV) node include (Fig. 4.2-32):

- Anterior internodal pathway of Bachman,
- Middle internodal pathway of Wenckebach, and
- Posterior internodal pathway of Thorel.

Atrioventricular node. The atrioventricular (AV) node is located just beneath the endocardium on the right side of lower part of atrial septum, near the tricuspid valve. It is stimulated by the excitation wave that travels through internodal tracts and atrial myocardium.

Atrioventricular bundle of His. The atrioventricular bundle arises from the AV node, descends through the fibrous skeleton of the heart and divides into right bundle branch (RBB) for right ventricle and left bundle branch (LBB) for the left ventricle. The branches break up and become continuous with the plexus of Purkinje fibers.

Purkinje fibers. These are spread out deep to the endocardium and reach all parts of the ventricles, including the bases of papillary muscles.

IMPORTANT TO KNOW

Innervational Characteristics of Heart
- Both SA node and AV node are richly supplied by the sympathetic as well as parasympathetic nerves. Parasympathetic fibers come from the vagus nerve and most sympathetic fibers come from the stellate ganglion.
- SA node is supplied by right vagus nerve and right-sided sympathetics.
- AV node is supplied by left vagus and left-sided sympathetic nerves.

Autorhythmicity
Mechanism of Origin of Rhythmic Cardiac Impulse
Pacemaker

The part of the heart from which rhythmic impulses for heart beat are produced, is called *pacemaker*. In mammalian heart, *SA node acts as a pacemaker* because the rate of impulse generation by SA node is highest. However, when there occurs blockage of transmission of impulse from SA node to AV node, the pacemaker activity may shift from SA node to other sites, e.g. AV node. When pacemaker is other than SA node it is called *ectopic pacemaker*. Ectopic pacemaker causes abnormal sequence of contraction of different parts of the heart.

IMPORTANT TO KNOW

Rate of production of rhythmic impulses by different parts of the heart is:

SA node: 70–80 per minute
AV node: 40–60 per minute
Atrial muscle: 40–60 per minute
Ventricular muscles: 20–40 per minute.

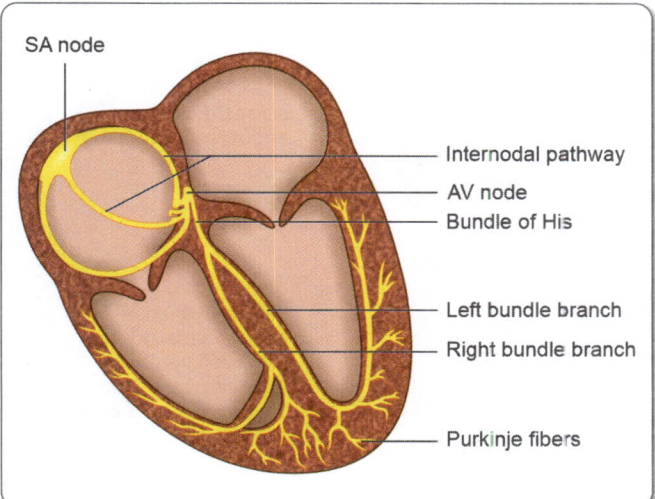

Fig. 4.2-32: Specialized conducting tissues of the heart

Electrical potential in pacemaker tissue. In pacemaker (SA node) fibers, the resting membrane potential is only of –55 mV to –60 mV; and this is not steady, due to slow depolarization which is due to slow diffusion of Na^+ followed by Ca^{2+} influx because of leakage channels (Fig. 4.2-33). Due to this slow depolarization the threshold level –40 mV is reached very slowly. Once the threshold level of –40 mV is reached there occurs a rapid depolarization up to +5 mV followed by rapid repolarization, i.e., there occurs action potential and generation of an impulse. After rapid repolarization, once again the resting membrane potential is reached which is not stable and starts rising slowly to again reach the threshold level to produce the second impulse. This slow rising resting membrane potential inbetween the action potentials is called *prepotential* or *pacemaker potential* (Fig. 4.2-33). Presence of this unique feature in the cells of pacemaker tissue is the underlying mechanism responsible for self-generation of rhythmic impulses (autorhythmicity).

Spread of cardiac impulse

The cardiac impulse which originates in the SA node in the form of action potential spreads throughout the heart through the conduction system (property of conductivity).

SA node and atria. The impulse travels over the muscle fibers of atria from SA nodal fibers, and through the interatrial tract to the left atrium. Conduction through these fibers causes simultaneous depolarization of both the atria. Atrial depolarization is completed in about 0.1 sec. The impulse reaches the AV node from SA node within 0.03 sec after its origin.

AV node. Conduction through AV node is slow, there is a delay of about 0.1 sec. This AV nodal delay is useful, for it provides time for completion of atrial contraction and their emptying (i.e., ventricular filling) before the ventricles contract.

Ventricular conduction. The impulses conducted through the AV node are distributed to ventricles through bundle of His, its branches, and Purkinje fibers in 0.08 – 0.15 sec. In humans, depolarization of the ventricular muscle proceeds as follows (Figs 4.2-34A to E):

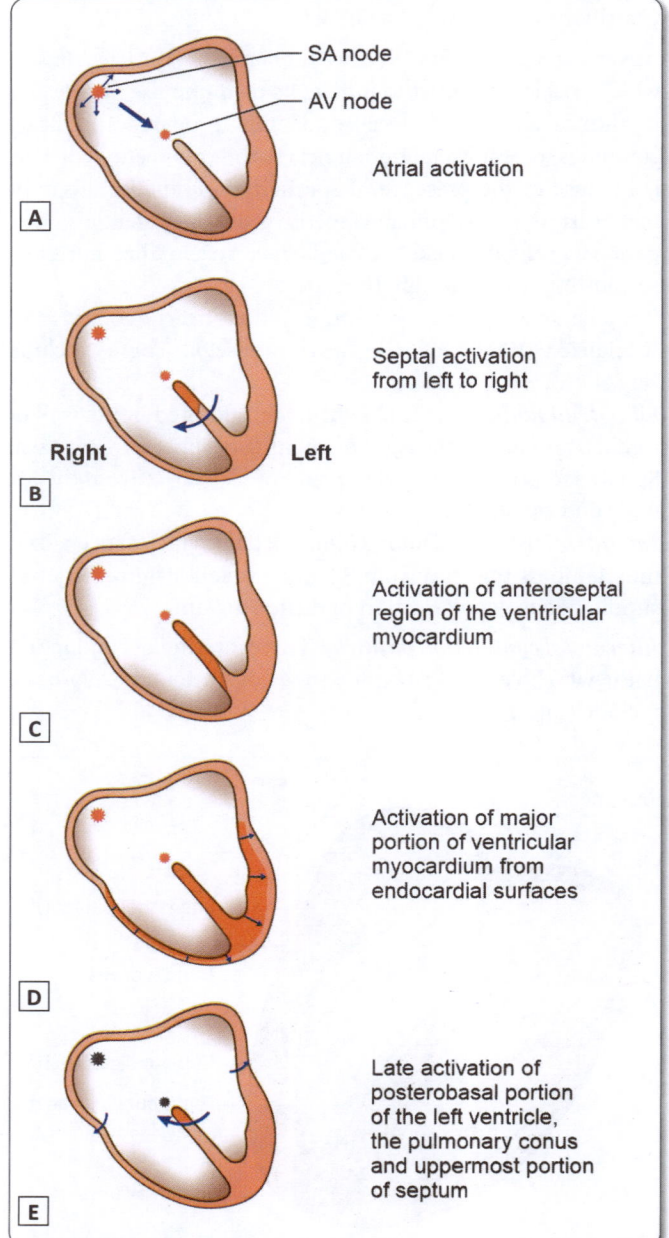

Figs 4.2-34A to E: Spread of cardiac impulse

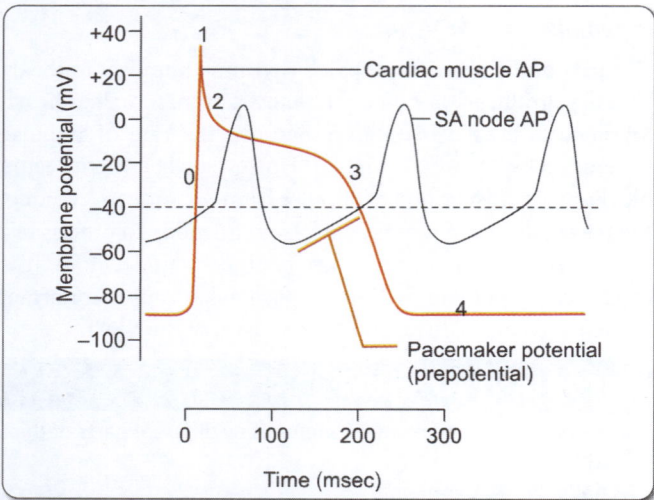

Fig. 4.2-33: Phases of action potential in cardiac muscle fiber (0, 1, 2, 3, 4) and sinoatrial node showing pacemaker potential. AP = action potential

- Starts at the left side of interventricular septum.
- Moves first to the right across the mid portion of the septum.
- The wave of depolarization then spreads down the septum to apex of heart.
- It, then, returns along the ventricular walls to the AV groove, proceeding from the endocardial to the epicardial surface.
- The last parts of the heart to be depolarized are the posterobasal portion of the left ventricle, the pulmonary conus, and the uppermost portion of the septum.

Thus, total time required for conduction from SA node to endocardial surface is 0.22 sec.

ELECTROCARDIOGRAPHY

William Einthoven, a Dutch physiologist, originally developed the technique of electrocardiography. He was awarded Nobel Prize in 1924 for his contribution and is called the father of modern electrocardiography.

Electrocardiography refers to extracellular recording of the summed-up electrical events of all the cardiac muscle fibers generated with each heart beat. Electrically heart behaves as a *dipole*, i.e., two-terminal battery in which the excited part (depolarized segment) forms a negative pole and the non-excited part forms the positive pole. Thus, ECG is nothing but the surface recording of the potential difference between the two poles of the heart dipole at a given time. The record of the potential fluctuations during the cardiac cycle is called the *electrocardiography* (ECG). The machine used to record these potential fluctuations is called *electrocardiograph*.

Electrocardiograph

The electrocardiograph (ECG machine) is essentially a sophisticated string galvanometer. A modern electro-cardiograph amplifies and records the potential fluctuations on a moving strip of paper. Special paper is used which turns black on exposure to heat. The stylus (recording pen) is made hot by electrical current flowing through its tip.

Normal Electrocardiogram

Electrocardiogram (ECG) refers to the record of the potential fluctuations during the cardiac cycle. As a result of sequential spread of the excitation in the atria, the interventricular septum and the ventricular walls (Fig. 4.2-35) and finally repolarization of the myocardium, a series of positive and negative waves designated as P, Q, R, S and T are recorded during each cardiac cycle.

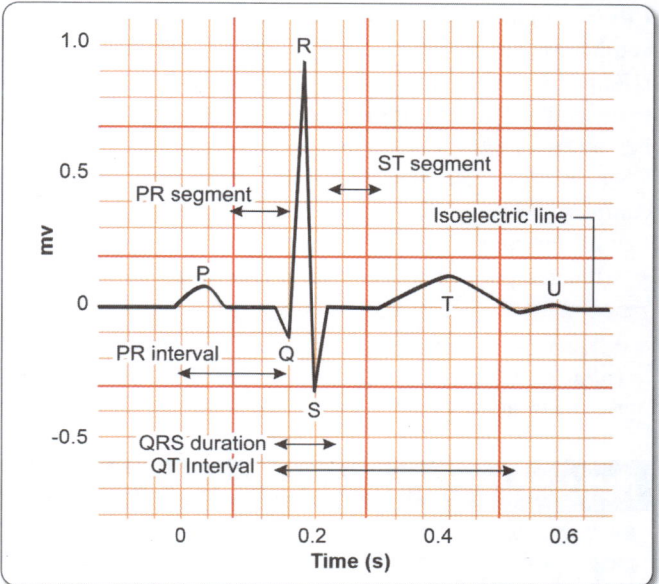

Fig. 4.2-35: Normal electrocardiogram showing various waves

Waves of ECG

P wave. P wave is the positive (upright rounded) deflection. It is produced by the depolarization of atrial musculature so also called atrial complex.

QRS complex. QRS complex consists of three consecutive waves. Q wave is a small negative wave which may be absent normally quite often. It is continued as a tall positive R wave which is followed by a small negative S wave. The QRS complex is caused by ventricular depolarization.

T Wave. T wave is the last, positive, dome-shaped deflection. T wave represents ventricular repolarization.

U wave. It is a small round positive wave. It occurs due to slow repolarization of papillary muscle. It is rarely seen normally. It becomes prominent in hypokalemia.

IMPORTANT TO KNOW

Since atrial repolarization coincides with ventricular depolarization, so it is merged with QRS complex and thus not recorded as a separate wave.

Intervals and Segments of ECG

P-R interval. It is measured from the onset of P wave to the onset of the QRS complex. It measures the *AV conduction time*, including the AV nodal delay. Its *duration* varies from 0.12 sec to 0.21 sec depending on the heart rate.

Clinical significance. Prolonged PR interval indicates AV conduction block.

QT interval. It is the time from the start of the QRS complex to the end of T wave. It indicates total *systolic time of ventricles*, i.e., ventricular depolarization and repolarization.

ST segment. It is an isoelectric period between the end of QRS complex and beginning of T wave.

- Its *duration* is about 0.32 sec.
- It corresponds with *ventricular repolarization.*

CLINICAL ASPECTS

Clinical significance: ST segment is elevated in patients with myocardial infarction.

NURSING IMPLICATIONS AND APPLICATIONS

Electrocardiography is an indispensable tool in the diagnosis, prognosis and planning treatment of the cardiac disorders such as:
- Cardiac arrhythmias
- Myocardial infarction
- Hypertrophy of various cardiac chambers
- Effects on ECG of changes in the ionic composition of blood.

HEART RATE

The normal heart rate in an adult male is 70-80 beats/min.

Factors Affecting Heart Rate

The factors that affect heart rate arc given as follows:

Age. Heart rate varies with age, i.e., it decreases as the age increases due to increase in the degree of vagal tone. The normal range o art rate with different age groups is shown in Table 4.2-1.

Sex. In females the resting heart rate is comparatively higher than in males of same age group.

Temperature. Heart rate increases with rise in body temperature. For each 1°F rise in body temperature, the heart rate increases by 10 beats/min.

TABLE 4.2-1: Heart rate values in relation to age	
Age	**Heart rate (beats/min)**
Birth	140–150
1 month	130–140
1 year	110–115
5 years	105–110
10 years	95–100
15 years	80–85
Adults	70–80
Old age	Up to 100

Blood pressure. Heart rate is inversely related to the arterial pressure; this is referred as *Marey's law.*

Emotions. Tachycardia occurs in emotions such as anxiety, anger and fear. Bradycardia is associated with sudden shock and grief. The emotional effects on heart rate are mediated through corticohypothalamic pathways.

Exercise. During muscular exercise heart rate increases. For details see page 232

Painful stimuli:
- *Superficial pain* causes tachycardia and hypertension (rise in blood pressure).
- *Deep pain* (visceral pain) is associated with bradycardia and hypotension (fall in blood pressure).

Respiration. Heart rate varies with phases of respiration; it increases with inspiration and decreases during expiration. This phenomenon is referred as sinus arrhythmia. It is quite common in infants and children during normal breathing but in adults it is observed only during deep breathing.

Regulation of Heart Rate

Heart rate is mainly controlled by two mechanisms: cardiac innervations. It consists of two divisions of autonomic nervou system, such as parasympathetic and sympathetic, as described I on page 223

HEART AS A PUMP AND CARDIAC CYCLE

The heart as a pump can be considered actually comprising two separate pumps in the series: a *right heart* that pumps the blood through the lungs and a *left heart* that pumps the blood through the peripheral organs. Further, each sided pump consists of an atrium and a ventricle. The atria act as *primary pumps* for the ventricles. The ventricles in turn provide the major force that propels the blood through pulmonary and systemic circulations. To act as a pump, the heart contracts and relaxes rhythmically. The terms *systole* (contractile phase) and *diastole* (relaxation phase) are used for different phases. The electrocardiogram records the *electrical events* that precede and initiate the corresponding *mechanical events* as:

P wave is followed by *atrial contraction.*

QRS complex is are caused by depolarization of the ventricles which initiates *contraction of the ventricles.*

T wave occurs slightly before the end of ventricular contraction.

Cardiac Cycle

The cardiac cycle thus includes both electrical and mechanical events that occur from the beginning of one heart beat to the beginning of the next.

Phases of Cardiac Cycle

Duration of each cardiac cycle at a normal heart rate of 75 beats/min is 60/75 = 0.8 sec. During each cardiac cycle both atria contract (*atrial systole*) and relax (*atrial diastole*), and both ventricles contract (*ventricular systole*) and relax (*ventricular diastole*).

Therefore, each cardiac cycle can be considered to consist of simultaneously occurring atrial and ventricular cycles with the following phases (Figs 4.2-36 and 4.10-37):

Atrial cycle comprises of:

- *Atrial systole* or atrial contraction phase (0.1 sec)
- *Atrial diastole* (0.7 sec).

Ventricular cycle comprises of:

Ventricular systole (0.3 sec) consists of:

- Isovolumic (isometric) contraction phase (0.05 sec)
- Phase of ventricular ejection, which can be further divided into rapid ejection phase (0.1 sec) and slow ejection phase (0.15 sec).

Ventricular diastole (0.5 sec) consists of:

- Protodiastole (0.04 sec)
- Isovolumic (isometric) relaxation phase (0.06 sec)
- Rapid passive filling phase (0.11 sec)
- Reduced filling phase or diastasis (0.19 sec)
- Last rapid filling phase, which coincides with the atrial systole (0.1 sec).

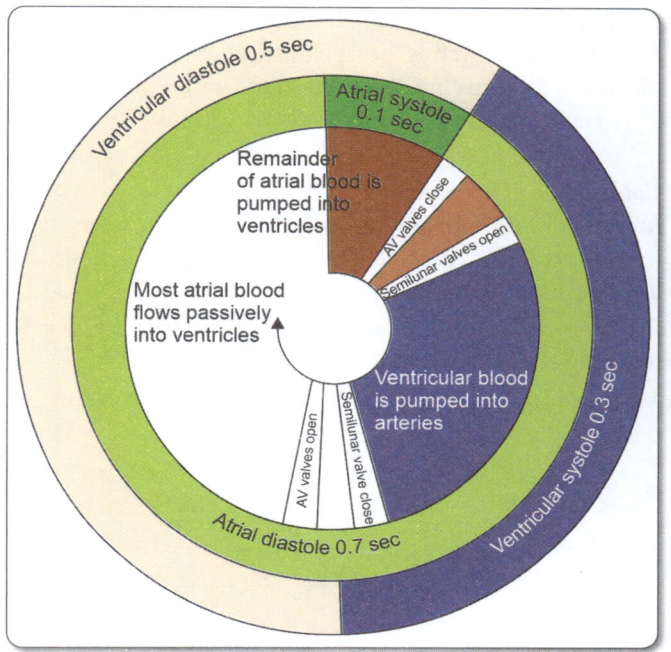

Fig. 4.2-36: Duration of phases of cardiac cycle

Atrial Cycle

Atrial systole

- Atrial systole or the atrial contraction phase lasts for 0.1 sec and coincides with the last rapid filling phase of ventricular diastole (Figs 4.10-36 and 4.10-37).

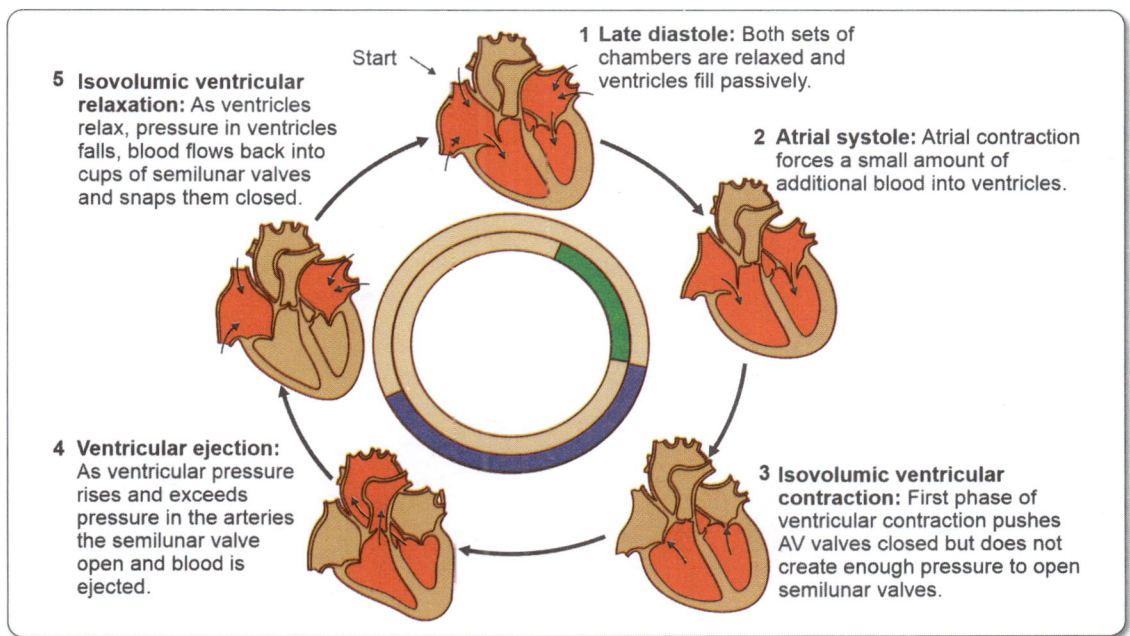

Fig. 4.2-37: Phases of cardiac cycle

- Before the beginning of atrial systole, the ventricles are relaxing, AV valves are open and blood is flowing from the great veins into the atria and from the atria into the ventricles. Thus, the atria and ventricles are forming a continuous cavity.

Contraction of atria causes:

Increase in intra-atrial pressure by 4–6 mm Hg pressure rise in right atrium is reflected into the veins and is recorded as *a-wave* from the jugular vein.

Increase in the ventricular pressure occurs slightly due to pumping of blood in the ventricles.

Narrowing of origin of great veins and decreasing venous return to the heart.

Atrial diastole

After the atrial systole, there occurs atrial diastole (0.7 sec). This period coincides with the ventricular systole and most of the ventricular diastole (Fig. 4.2-36).

During atrial diastole, atrial muscles relax and there occurs gradual filling of the atria due to continuous venous return and the pressure gradually increases in the atria (Fig. 4.2-38).

Ventricular Cycle

Ventricular systole

After the atrial contraction phase is over, the ventricles start contracting. The ventricular systole lasts for 0.3 sec, and has the following phases:

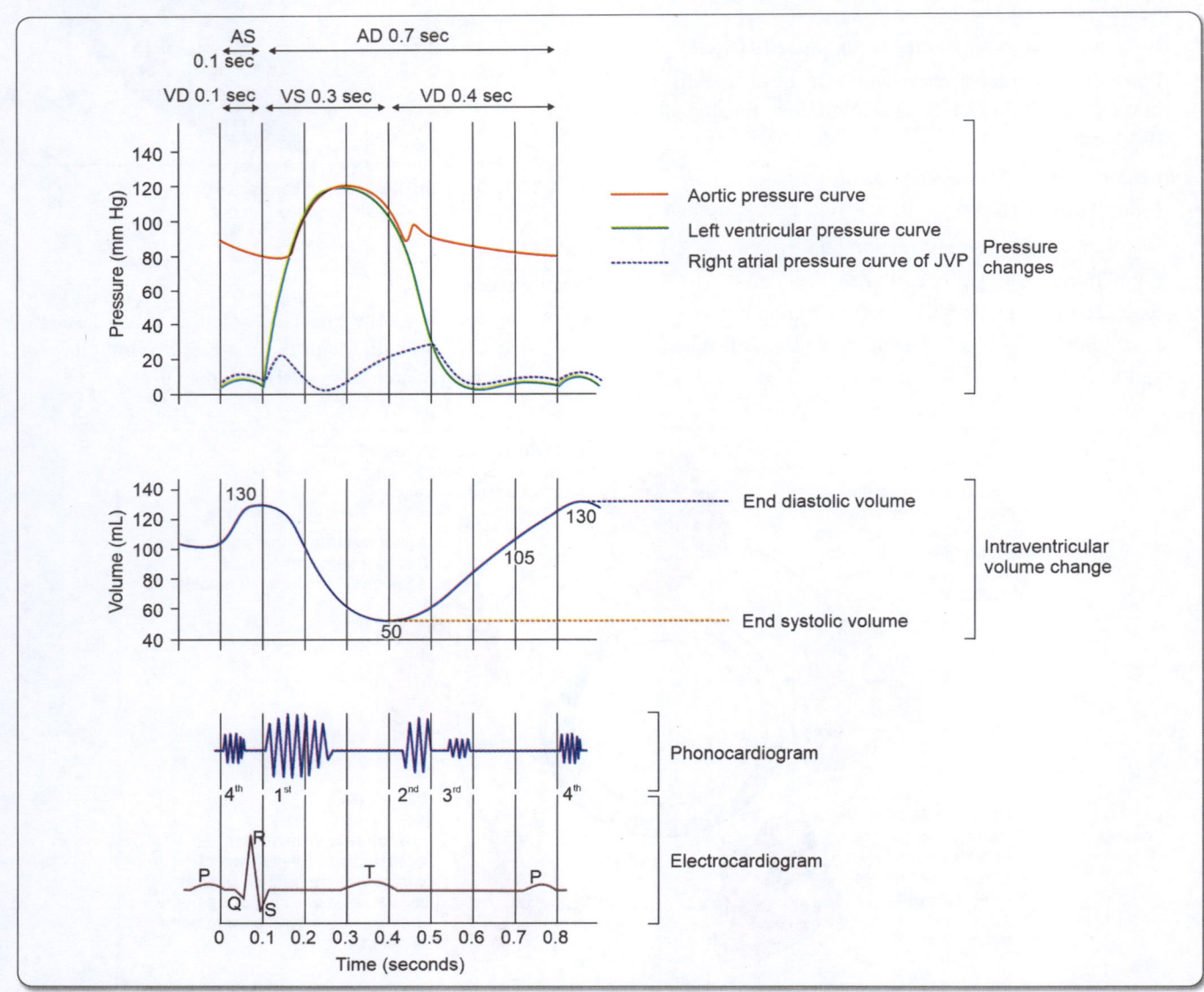

Fig. 4.2-38: Phases and events during cardiac cycle

Phase of isovolumic (isometric) contraction

- With the beginning of ventricular contraction, the ventricular pressure exceeds atrial pressure very rapidly causing closure of AV valves (this event is responsible for production of first heart sound).
- Since the AV valves have closed and semilunar valves have not opened, pressure inside the ventricles rises rapidly to a high level, but the volume of blood in the ventricles does not change, so this phase is called *isovolumic contraction phase.*
- During this phase, due to sharp rise in ventricular pressure, there occurs bulging of AV valves into the atria producing a small but sharp rise in intra-atrial pressure called *c-wave.*
- This phase lasts for 0.05 sec, until the pressure in the left and right ventricles exceeds the pressure in the aorta (80 mm Hg) and pulmonary artery (10 mm Hg) and the aortic and pulmonary valves open.

Phase of ventricular ejection

The ventricular ejection phase begins with the opening of semilunar valves and lasts for about 0.25 sec. It can be further divided into two phases:

1. *Rapid ejection phase*
2. *Slow ejection phase.*

Ventricular diastole

Protodiastole. When the ventricular systole ends, the ventricles start relaxing and intraventricular pressure falls rapidly. This phase lasts for 0.04 sec. During this phase the elevated pressure in the distended arteries (aorta and pulmonary artery) immediately pushes the blood back toward ventricles which snaps the semilunar valves to close. Closure of semilunar (i.e., aortic and pulmonary) valves prevents the movement of blood back into the ventricles and produces the *second heart sound* (S_2). It also causes *dicrotic notch* in the down slope of aortic pressure called the *incisura.*

Isovolumic or isometric relaxation phase

- This phase begins with the closure of semilunar valves and lasts for about 0.06 sec.
- Since semilunar valves have closed and the AV valves have not yet opened, so the ventricles continue to relax as closed chambers in this phase.
- But the ventricular volume remains constant, so this phase is called isvolumic or isometric relaxation phase.
- This phase ends when the AV valves open, as indicated by the peak of *v-wave* on the atrial pressure tracing (Figs 4.2-37 and 4.10-38).

Rapid passive filling phase (0.11 sec)

- During ventricular systole, the atria are in diastole and venous return continues so that the atrial pressure is high. When the AV valves open, the high atrial pressure causes a rapid, initial flow of blood into the ventricles. The rapid passive filling phase produces the *third heart sound* (S_3).
- Once the AV valves open, the atria and ventricles are a common chamber and pressure in both cavities falls as ventricular relaxation continues.

Reduced filling and diastasis (0.19 sec)

In this phase, pressure in atria and ventricles reduces slowly and remains little above zero. This decreases the rate of blood flow from atria to ventricle causing a very slow filling called *diastasis.*

Last rapid filling phase (0.1 sec)

The last rapid filling phase of ventricular diastole coincides with the atrial systole. During this phase additional 25% of the blood enters the ventricles. With this phase, the ventricular cycle is completed.

Events During Cardiac Cycle

The events associated with contraction and relaxation of the heart during a cardiac cycle include pressure changes in the ventricles, atria and aorta; volume changes in the ventricles and valvular events. Most of these have been described during various phases of cardiac cycle.

Pressure Changes in the Aorta

Pressure in the aorta varies between 80 mm Hg and 120 mm Hg during the cardiac cycle. Aortic pressure changes during various phases of cardiac cycle (Fig. 4.2-38) are:

During atrial systole. During atrial systole the pressure in the aorta is about 80 mm Hg.

During ventricular systole. During ventricular systole the aortic pressure starts rising along with the intraventricular pressure and during rapid ejection phase and reaches maximum (120 mm Hg) at the end of rapid ejection phase.

During ventricular diastole. Due to sudden closure of semilunar valve the backflowing blood collides against the closed aortic valve. This collision causes a small but sharp rise in aortic pressure. This small rise produces a notch called *incisura.* This sharp pressure rise is recordable even from peripheral arteries and is called *dicrotic notch.*

During rest of the diastole, the aortic pressure smoothly declines to about 80 mm Hg.

Pressure Changes in Pulmonary Artery

Pressure curve in the pulmonary artery is similar to that of aorta but pressures are low. Pulmonary artery systolic pressure averages 15–18 mm Hg and its pressure during diastole is 8–10 mm Hg.

Volume Changes in the Ventricles During Cardiac Cycle

During atrial systole. Atrial systole coincides with the last rapid filling phase of ventricular diastole. When the atrial contraction begins about 105 mL (75%) of the blood has already flown into the ventricles. The atrial contraction causes additional 25 mL (25%) filling of the ventricles. Thus at the end of atrial systole, i.e., at the end of ventricular diastole the ventricular volume is about 130 mL. This is called end-diastolic volume.

During ventricular systole the volume changes occur as:

During isovolumic contraction phase, as the name suggests, there occurs no change in the ventricular volume.

During ventricular ejection phase about 80 mL of the blood is ejected out by each ventricle. This is called *stroke volume.* The percentage of the end-diastolic volume that is ejected out with each stroke during systole (about 65%) is called *ejection fraction.* Thus, about 50 mL of the blood in each ventricle at the end of ventricular systole is called *end-systolic volume.*

Valvular Events (Heart Sounds)

A total four heart sounds (1st, 2nd, 3rd and 4th) are produced by certain mechanical activities during each cardiac cycle. The heart sounds can be heard with stethoscope (auscultation) and can be recorded (phono- cardiography).

First heart sound (HS$_1$). First heart sound is produced by vibrations set up by the sudden closure of AV valves at the start of ventricular systole (Fig. 4.2-38). It sounds like the spoken word 'LUBB'.

Second heart sound (HS$_2$). It is caused by vibrations associated with closure of the semilunar valves just at the onset of ventricular diastole. It sounds like the spoken word 'DUBB'.

Third heart sound (HS$_3$). Third heart sound is caused by vibrations set up in the cardiac wall by inrush of blood during *rapid filling phase* of ventricular diastole. It cannot be heard by auscultation with stethoscope.

Fourth heart sound (HS$_4$). It is caused by vibrations set up during atrial systole. It is normally not audible.

Arterial Pulse

Arterial pulse is also an event related to cardiac cycle. The blood forced into the aorta during systole not only moves the blood in the vessels forward but also sets up a pressure wave that is transmitted along the *arteries to the periphery.* The pressure wave expands the arterial walls as it travels, and expansion is palpable as the *pulse.*

Examination of arterial pulse is an essential feature of clinical examination. Arterial pulse can be palpated from any superficial artery, e.g. radial, femoral, dorsalis pedis and carotid, etc. Most frequently, pulse is examined from the radial artery because it is conveniently approached without exposing the body, and can be easily palpated as it is placed superficially against the bone.

Examination of the pulse should include the following aspects:

Pulse rate refers to number of pulses per minute.

- *Normal pulse rate* varies with age being 150–180/min in fetus, 130–140/min at birth, about 90/min at the age of 10 years and about 72/min in adults.
- *Increased pulse rate* represents tachycardia and occurs during exercise, in anxiety, in fever, in hyperthyroidism and in atrial and ventricular tachycardias.
- *Decreased pulse rate* represents bradycardia and is seen in hypothyroidism and incomplete heart blocks.

Volume of pulse also known as strength of arterial pulse or amplitude or impact that can be felt. It represents stroke volume or the pulse pressure (i.e., systolic-diastolic pressure).

- *Rapid and thready pulse* occurs in hypovolemia as in severe hemorrhage.
- *Increased volume pulse* is seen during exercise and in ventricular hypertrophy.

Rhythm of pulse is noted as regular or irregular. Under normal conditions and during sinus bradycardia or sinus tachycardia pulse appears at regular intervals.

- *Irregular pulse rhythm* is a feature of extra systole, atrial fibrillation and other cardiac arrhythmias.

Character of pulse is felt on palpation. It denotes the tension and waves in the pulse.

CARDIAC OUTPUT AND VENOUS RETURN

The main function of the heart is to pump blood to meet the metabolic needs of the body. The measure of the heart's ability to pump blood is cardiac output. The *cardiac output* refers to the amount of blood ejected by each ventricle per minute. The *stroke volume* is the amount of blood pumped out by each ventricle per beat or per contraction. Therefore, cardiac output (CO) can be calculated by multiplying the stroke volume (SV) by the heart rate (HR):

$$CO = SV \times HR$$

Under normal conditions, the average heart rate is about 70 beats/min and stroke volume is about 80 mL and thus cardiac output is $80 \times 70 = 5.6$ L.

The cardiac output is expressed in L/min and normally varies from 5 L/min to 6 L/min. In health, the right and left ventricular outputs are nearly equal. Thus, each ventricle pumps about 5–6 L of blood into the circulation per minute. This is made possible because of the fact that the right and left side pumps act in series.

Cardiac index is the cardiac output expressed in relation to the body surface area. The normal cardiac index is about 3.2 L/min/m².

Distribution of the Cardiac Output

Of the total cardiac output, about 75% is distributed to the vital organs of the body and rest of 25% to the skeletal muscles, other organs of the body and skin. The distribution of the cardiac output to various organs of the body is shown in Table 4.2-2.

Regulation of Cardiac Output

The cardiac output increases or decreases in various physiological and pathological conditions as described above. The variations in the cardiac output are brought about by certain factors operating through certain mechanisms by an integrated role.

The cardiac output (CO), as we know, is the product of stroke volume (SV) and heart rate (HR), i.e., CO = SV × HR. Therefore, variations in the cardiac output can be produced by the factors which change stroke volume or heart rate, or both (Fig. 4.2-39).

Cardiac Output Control Mechanisms

The stroke output is regulated by two mechanisms: intrinsic and extrinsic.

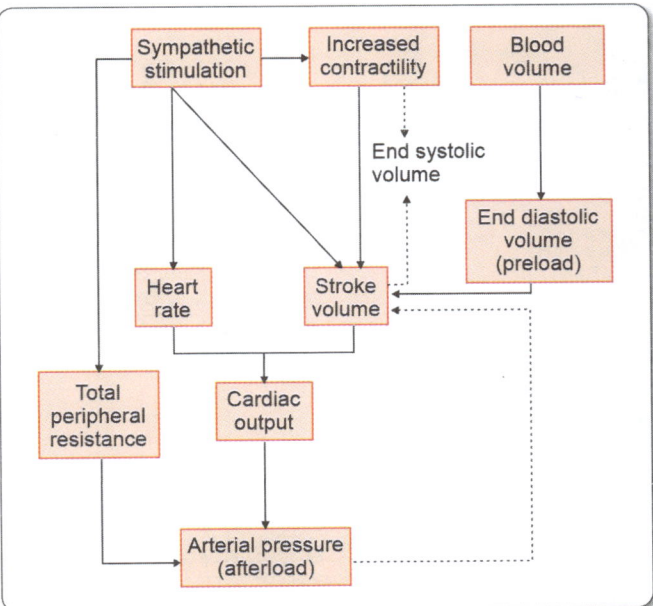

Fig. 4.2-39: Interaction between the factors that regulate cardiac output and arterial pressure. Solid lines indicate increase and dotted lines indicate a decrease

Intrinsic autoregulation (frank-starling mechanism)

According to *Frank-Starling Law* of *Heart*, 'within physiological limits' the force of contraction of *cardiac muscle* is proportionate to the initial length of muscle fibers. In the heart, end-diastolic volume forms the preload. Therefore, precisely the Frank-Starling law of heart can be stated as, within physiological limits, the force of cardiac contraction is proportional to its end-diastolic volume (EDV). Since, in this intrinsic regulation mechanism, cardiac muscle fibers are stretched to increase their initial length, it is also termed *heterometric mechanism*.

Factors Affecting end-diastolic volume (venous return)

The end-diastolic volume refers to the *venous return* to the heart during diastole. For individual at rest, the cardiac output and venous return are approximately 5 L/min. Factors affecting venous return (Figs 4.2-40A and B) are:

Respiratory pump. During inspiration the intrathoracic pressure becomes more negative and there occurs descent of diaphragm which increases the intra-abdominal pressure. The decreased pressure inside the inferior vena cava coupled with increased intra-abdominal pressure during inspiration results in increased flow of blood into the right atrium. This mechanism of increased blood flow during inspiration is called *respiratory pump*. This respiratory pump operates strongly in forced respiration and in severe muscular exercise increasing the venous return.

TABLE 4.2-2: Distribution of cardiac output to various organs		
Body organ	**Amount of blood flow (mL/min)**	**Percentage of total cardiac output**
Liver	1500	about 25 ⎤
Kidney	1300	25 ⎦ 75
Brain	750 ⎤	
Heart	250 ⎥ 1500	25
Lungs	500 ⎦	
Skeletal muscles and other body organs	1000 ⎤	
	1500	25
Skin	500 ⎦	

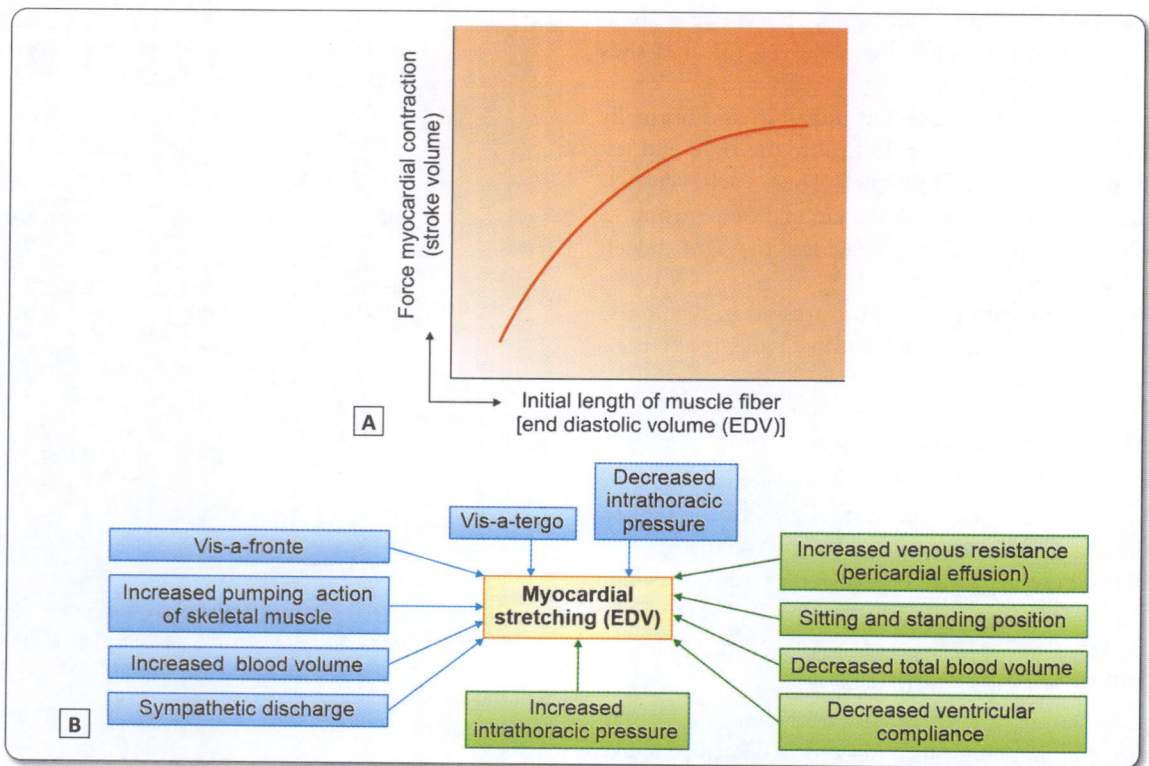

Figs 4.2-40A and B: Frank-Starling curve. A. Factors affecting end-diastolic volume; B. Blue arrows indicate increase and green arrows indicate decrease

Cardiac pump. The cardiac pump influences the venous return by two kinds of forces the 'vis-a-tergo' and 'vis-a-fronte'.

1. *Vis-a-tergo* refers to the forward push from behind, i.e., the propelling force. Vis-a-tergo results from the myocardial contraction during systole and is supplemented by the elastic recoil of the arterial wall (Windkessel effect).

2. *Vis-a-fronte* refers to the suction force acting from the front which basically pulls the blood from the great veins into the right atrium. This suction force is created by ventricular contraction.

Muscle pump. The muscle pump mechanism is responsible for flow of blood from the veins of the limbs to the heart.

Working of muscle pump. Two types of veins are present in the limbs: superficial and deep veins. Blood flows from the superficial veins into deep veins through communicating veins. Due to the presence of valves in the limb veins the blood flows in one direction, i.e., from periphery toward heart and not in reverse direction.

- *When the skeletal muscles contract*, the deep veins present in between the muscles are compressed and due to increased pressure the valve present proximal to the

contracting muscle is opened up while the valve present on distal end is tightly closed and in this way the blood is propelled up toward the heart (Figs 4.2-41A and B).

- *When the skeletal muscle relaxes* a negative pressure is created in the segment of veins. So due to back flow the proximal valve is closed and the distal valve is opened and blood is sucked up (Fig. 4.2-41).

- *With rhythmic contractions of skeletal muscles* in this way, the blood is squeezed out of the limbs toward the heart.

NURSING IMPLICATIONS AND APPLICATIONS

In certain professions (e.g. nurses, traffic police, etc.) the individuals have to keep standing for a long time of a day. In such persons, veins of lower limbs become large, tortuous and bulbous. This condition is called *varicose veins*.

Blood volume. The increased blood volume increases the venous return and a decreased blood volume decreases the venous return.

Sympathetic discharge. On sympathetic stimulation, there occurs increase in the venous tone which decreases the capacity of the venous system (veins are capacitance vessels).

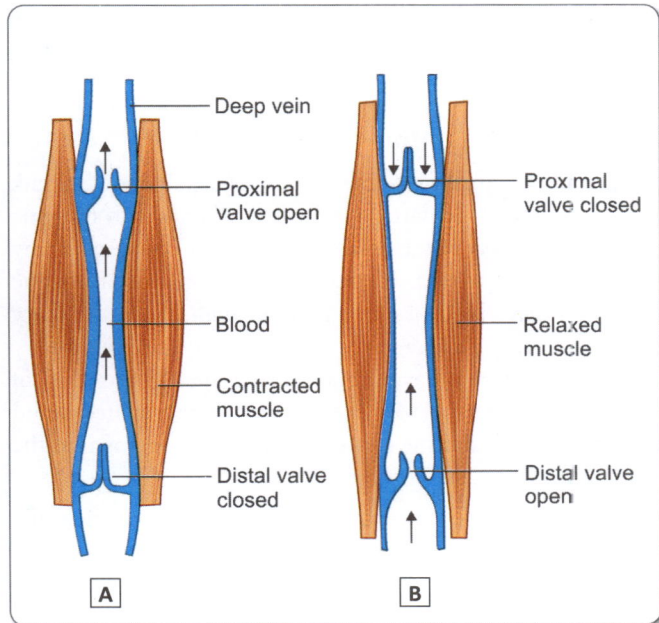

Figs 4.2-41A and B: Mechanism of muscle pump: A. During contraction of muscles; B. During relaxation of muscles

Standing body position is associated with a decreased venous return due to peripheral pooling of the blood.

Extrinsic regulation (autonomic neural mechanism)

In this mechanism stroke volume increases due to *increased myocardial contractility* without any increase in the initial muscle length. Therefore, it is also called *homometric mechanism.* The homometric regulation is governed by autonomic neural mechanism as described below.

Stimulation of the sympathetic nerves to the heart results in increased myocardial contractility and is known as *positive inotropic effect.* The positive inotropic effect of the norepinephrine liberated at the sympathetic nerve endings is augmented by circulating norepinephrine.

Inhibition of sympathetic system has opposite effects.

IMPORTANT TO KNOW

Characteristics of increased myocardial contractility
- The ventricles contract more forcefully and more rapidly. As a result the ventricles are able to do more work per stroke, i.e., ejection fraction increases at the same end-diastolic volume (without increase in venous return).
- Due to more complete emptying of ventricles during each systole the *end-systolic volume is decreased.*
- Due to increased stroke output, *arterial pressure is increased.*

Parasympathetic activity. There is a negative inotropic effect of parasympathetic (vagal) stimulation. This effect, however, is not much because vagal fibers are mainly distributed to the atria and not much to the ventricles.

Role of Heart Rate in Control of Cardiac Output

Since, cardiac output is the product of stroke volume and heart rate, it is tempting to attribute the increase in cardiac output to increase in the heart rate. However, in fact it is not so. It has been seen that when heart rate alone is increased, the cardiac output does not increase at all. The progressive increase in the heart rate is associated with a proportionate decrease in stroke volume because of reduced diastole time and thus reduced end-diastolic volume. Conversely, when the heart rate is reduced the ventricular diastole is prolonged leading to more ventricular filling and thus an increased stroke volume.

During exercise, the sympathetic stimulation produces a marked increase in the heart rate (200–300%) due to positive chronotropism and moderate increase (50–60%) in the stroke volume due to positive inotropism leading to manifold increase in cardiac output.

PHYSIOLOGY OF CIRCULATION

INTRODUCTION

Physiology of circulation is concerned with flow of blood and the pressure in the various segments of the vascular system of the body. It can be discussed under the following headings:
- Functional organization and structure of vascular system
- Hemodynamics

- Blood flow and pressure in different segments of circulatory system
- Blood pressure.

Functional Organization Vascular System

The vascular system is organized into two separate circulations (systemic and pulmonary), arranged in series.

Systemic Circulation

Systemic circulation supplies blood to various systemic organs through parallel distribution channels (Fig. 4.2-42). This parallel arrangement of vessels ensures the supply of blood of the same arterial composition (i.e., same O_2 and CO_2 tension, pH, glucose level and essentially the same arterial pressure) to various body organs. In systemic circulation, from the left ventricle, blood is pumped through the arteries and arterioles

to the capillaries, where it equilibrates with the interstitial fluid. The capillaries drain through the venules into the veins and ultimately to the right atrium.

Pulmonary Circulation

Pulmonary circulation is meant for oxygenation of blood. Since pulmonary circulation is arranged in series with systemic circulation, it receives the same amount of blood over any significant time period. In pulmonary circulation, from the right ventricle, blood is pumped through the pulmonary arteries to the pulmonary capillaries. In the pulmonary capillaries, the blood equilibrates with the O_2 and CO_2 of alveolar air. The capillaries then drain the oxygenated blood through venules and then through pulmonary veins into the left atrium.

Systemic vascular tree. From functional point of view the systemic vascular tree can be divided into the following types of blood vessels:

Large elastic arteries (Windkessel vessels) include aorta and its main branches such as carotid, iliac and axillary arteries

Large muscular arteries (distribution vessels) which include most of the arteries of the body, e.g. arteries like radial, ulnar, popliteal

Arterioles and precapillary sphincters (resistance vessels)

Meta-arterioles and capillaries (exchange vessels)

Venules (postcapillary resistance vessels)

Veins (capacitance vessels)

Arteriovenous anastomoses (shunt or thoroughfare vessels).

Structure of Blood Vessels

General Structural Characteristics

Histologically, walls of most of the blood vessels except the capillaries consist of three coats (Fig. 4.2-43 and Histology plate 4.2-3):

1. *Tunica intima.* It is the innermost coat of the vessel wall. In large arteries, from inside-out, it consists of:

Endothelial lining, which is very smooth and silky, and consists of single layer of cells. It lies in contact with blood.

Basal lamina is a thin layer of glycoprotein which lines the external aspect of the endothelium.

Subendothelial connective tissue is a delicate layer of connective tissue which lies outside the basal lamina.

Internal elastic lamina is a thin membrane formed by elastic fibers.

2. *Tunica media.* It is the middle, thickest coat of the vessel wall. It consists of smooth muscles and elastic tissue. The ratio of these two tissues varies from vessel to vessel. On the

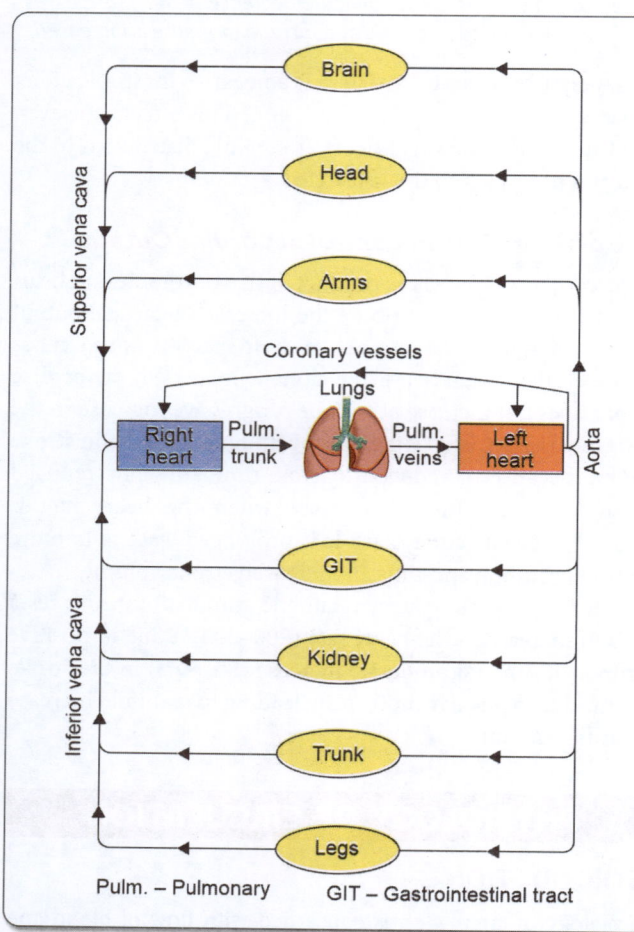

Fig. 4.2-42: A schematic illustration of the organization of cardiovascular system depicting in series arrangement of pulmonary and systemic circulation and parallel arrangement of vessels supplying blood to organs

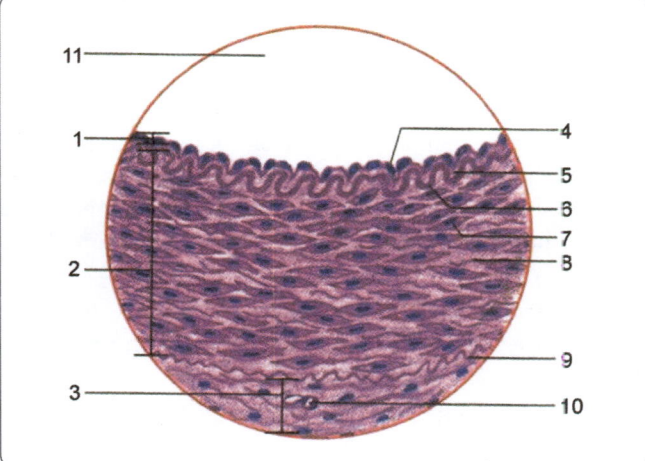

Fig. 4.2-43: Histological structure of an artery. 1. Tunica; 2. Tunica media; 3. Tunica adventitia; 4. Endothelial cells; 5. Subendothelial connective tissue; 6. Internal elastic lamina; 7. Smooth muscle fibers; 8. Elastic fibers; 9. External elastic lamina; 10. Vasa vasorum

Histology Plate 4.2-3: Muscular Artery

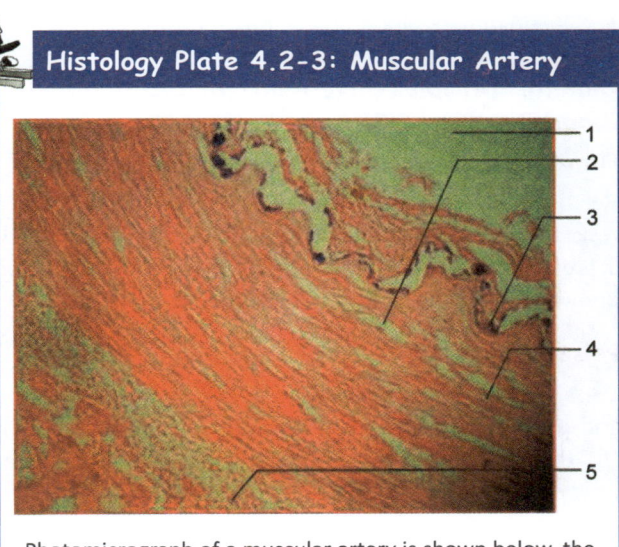

Photomicrograph of a muscular artery is shown below. the following layers are identified:
1. Lumen of the artery
2. Smooth muscle fibers
3. Tunica intima
4. Tunica media
5. Tunica adventitia

outside, tunica media is limited by a membrane formed by elastic fibers called the *external elastic lamina*.

3. *Tunica adventitia.* It is the outermost coat of the vessel wall. It is made of connective tissue in which collagen fibers are prominent. This layer prevents undue stretching or distension of the blood vessel.

Essential Characteristics

Essential characteristics of blood vessels like lumen diameter, wall thickness, approximate total cross-sectional area and percentage of blood volume contained are shown in Table 4.2-3.

Hemodynamics

Hemodynamics, which refers to study of blood flow in various segments of the vascular system, can be discussed under the following headings:
- General principles governing (factors affecting) blood flow

TABLE 4.2-3: Essential characteristics of various types of blood vessels

Vessel	Lumen diameter	Wall thickness	Approximate cross-sectional area (cm²)	Percentage of total blood volume contained in all vessels of each type
Aorta	2.5 cm	2 mm	45	2
Artery	0.4 cm	1 mm	20	8
Arteriole	30 µm	20 µm	400	1
Capillary	5 µm	1 µm	4500	5
Venule	20 µm	2 µm	4000	54
Vein	0.5 cm	0.5 mm	40	
Vena cava	3 cm	1.5 mm	18	
Heart				12
Pulmonary circulation				18

- Types of blood flow
- Regulation of blood flow in different situations.

General Principles Governing (Factors affecting) Blood Flow

Flow-pressure-resistance relationship

Relationship between flow of a fluid with the pressure and resistance offered to it through a rigid tube was studied by a French physiologist Poiseuille in 1842 and Hagen, and is known as Poiseuille's Law or Poiseuille-Hagen law.

Poiseuille's law

Poiseuille's Law expressing the relation between the flow (Q) and pressure gradient (ΔP) in a long narrow tube of length (L), the viscosity of fluid (η), and the radius (r) of the tube is as:

$$Q = \frac{\Delta P \, \pi r^4}{8 \, \eta L}$$

Thus, according to Poiseuille's Law the flow (Q) of a Newtonian fluid through a rigid tube is determined by:

Pressure gradient (ΔP), i.e., difference in the pressure between the two ends of the tube. In other words, fluid always flows from an area of high pressure (P_1) to one of lower pressure (P_2), i.e., $Q \propto \Delta P$ or ($P_1 - P_2$).

Radius of tube (r). The flow of fluid varies directly as the fourth power of radius (r^4). Thus if the radius is halved the flow will decrease by 16 times and vice versa. Thus this factor is very important for flow of blood through the blood vessels.

Viscosity of fluid (η). The flow of fluid varies inversely with the viscosity of fluid, i.e., greater the viscosity, lesser the flow and vice versa.

Length of the tube (L). The flow is inversely proportional to the length of the tube. Longer the length greater will be the total resistance offered.

Resistance (R). According to mathematical calculation in principles of physics, resistance (R) is represented by $8 \, L\eta/\pi r^4$. By replacing $8 \, L\eta/\pi r^4$ with R in Poiseuille's Law, it becomes:

$$Q = \frac{\Delta P}{R}$$

Thus, Poiseuille's Law can be considered analogous to Ohm's Law of current.

The Poiseuille's Law is valid for straight rigid tubes with Newtonian fluid flowing through them. Since, blood vessels are not rigid and the blood is not a Newtonian fluid, therefore, strictly speaking the Poiseuille's Law does not apply to flow of blood through the vascular system. Nevertheless, the important principles relating flow, pressure gradient and resistance remain applicable, so they are discussed in relation to blood flow.

Blood flow: types and distribution

Types of blood flow. Blood flow in the vascular system is of two types:

1. *Laminar blood flow.* Blood flow in the blood vessels is normally streamline, like the flow of liquids in narrow rigid tubes. Such a blood flow is called laminar blood flow and is considered to consist of a series of thin laminae slipping over one another (Fig. 4.2-44A). The laminar blood flow being streamlined is noiseless.

2. *Turbulent blood flow.* In turbulent blood flow, the blood moves in irregular varying paths continuously mixing within the vessel and colliding with the vessel wall. This causes a greater energy loss as compared to laminar flow. The turbulent blood flow is noisy.

NURSING IMPLICATIONS AND APPLICATIONS

Conditions associated with turbulent blood flow are:
- Constriction of the artery by an atherosclerotic plaque (Fig. 4.2-44B) or by any other cause, e.g. application of external pressure while measuring the blood pressure with sphygmomanometer. The turbulent flow generates vibrations (sounds) which can be heard over the artery by a stethoscope, e.g. *Korotkoff sounds* heard while recording the blood pressure or the *murmur* heard over a constricted artery.
- Anemia

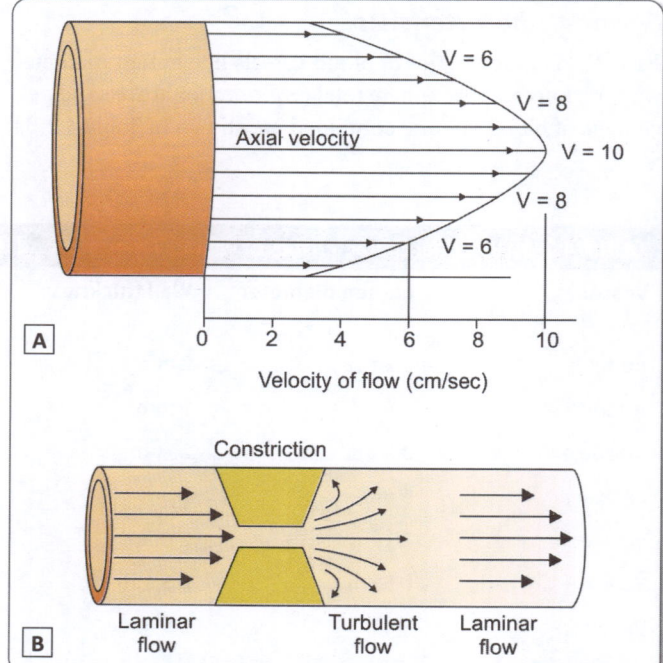

Figs 4.2-44A and B: A. Laminar blood flow; B. Turbulent blood flow caused by constriction of the lumen of blood vessel

Distribution of blood flow to various regions of the body

At rest about 5 L of blood enters aorta per minute. In terms of tissue weight, blood flow to liver, brain and heart is very high. Kidney has high blood flow because it is related to excretory function rather than metabolic requirement. The distribution of blood flow to various organs and regions of the body during resting conditions and during maximum activity conditions is shown in Table 4.2-4.

Pressure and flow in different segments of circulatory system

Pressure and flow functions of elastic arteries

The large elastic arteries (Windkessel vessels) include aorta and its main branches such as carotid, iliac and axillary arteries. These vessels contain elastic tissue in their walls in abundance which provides them two properties of distensibility and elastic recoil. The effect of these two properties of the elastic arteries on pressure and flow of blood is as follows:

Distensibility. The distensibility (compliance) of the elastic arteries allows them to accommodate the stroke volume of heart during systole with only a moderate increase in pressure (from 80 mm Hg to 120 mm Hg) (Fig. 4.2-45A). Due to distension of these vessels a part of energy released from the heart is stored as potential energy in the wall of aorta.

Elastic recoil. During diastole, the stretched elastic wall of the aorta recoils and the potential energy stored in the wall is released onto the blood. This causes the blood to flow during diastole also; in this way the pressure in the aorta does not fall below 80 mm Hg (Fig. 4.2-45B).

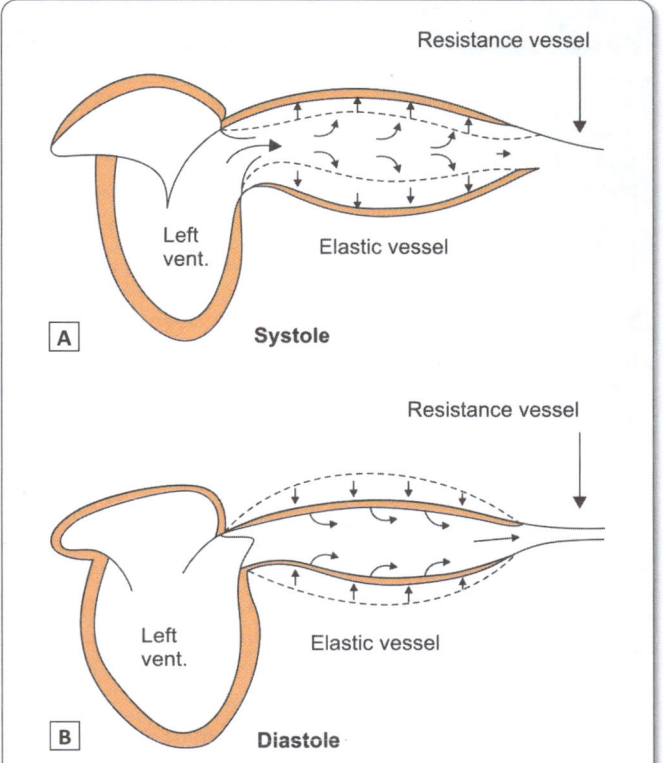

Figs 4.2-45A and B: A. Distensibility; B. Elastic recoil; seen in aorta and its main branches maintain arterial pressure and flow during diastole

Functions of elastic vessels reduce velocity of blood flow to some extent during ventricular contraction (systole) due to property of distensibility.

- They cause increase in velocity of blood flow to some extent during ventricular diastole by elastic recoil. Thus, the Windkessel effect reduces the energy expenditure of heart.
- Pumping actions of the heart along with elastic recoil of aorta together constituten a driving force for blood to move forward (toward periphery). This force is called *vis-a-tergo force*, and is an important determinant for venous return.
- Conversion of pulsatile blood flows from heart to a steady continuous flow. The elastic vessels act together with arterioles (resistance vessels) to convert this pulsatile flow into a steady continuous flow in the tissue capillaries, which allows maximum exchange between the blood and tissues.

TABLE 4.2-4: Distribution of blood flow to various organs of the body during resting and maximum activity conditions

Organs	Blood flow per organ (mL/min)		Blood flow (mL/100 g/min)	
	At rest	During maximum activity	At rest	During maximum activity
Heart	250	1200	80	400
Brain	750	2100	55	150
Liver	1500	3000	58	120
Skeletal muscles	150	1800	4	70
Kidney	1200	1400	400	450
Skin	200	3500	8	150

NURSING IMPLICATIONS AND APPLICATIONS

Due to age-related degenerative changes, the elasticity of large vessels is decreased and so is the Windkessel effect. Therefore, in old age systolic blood pressure increases and diastolic blood pressure decreases. Thus, in normal healthy individual aged about 70 years, typical blood pressure is 160/70 mm Hg. That is, there occurs *systolic hypertension* with *increased pulse pressure* (SBP–DBP).

Pressure and Flow Functions of Arterioles

Structural characteristics. Each arteriole is only a few millimeter long and branches many a time to supply about 10–100 capillaries.

Functions of arterioles are:

Control of blood flow to the organs. The arterioles play a major role in the control of blood flow to organs or tissues. So, they are considered *stopcocks (valves) of circulation.* The constriction of arterioles increases the resistance and decreases the blood flow while dilation of arterioles decreases the resistance and increases the blood flow. The arterioles control blood flow to organs by autoregulation.

Autoregulation. It is the ability of an organ or tissue to adjust its vascular resistance and maintain a relatively constant blood flow over a wide range of arterial pressure (Fig. 4.2-46). Autoregulation is well developed in the kidney, brain, heart, skeletal muscle, and mesentery.

Conversion of pulsatile flow from heart to a steady continuous flow. As described in functions of the elastic vessels, the arterioles along with the elastic vessels convert the pulsatile flow in the arteries to a steady flow in capillaries.

Microcirculation

Architecture of Microcirculation

The microcirculation involves a meshwork of vessels less than 100 μm in diameter. These include small arterioles, meta-arterioles, capillaries, postcapillary venules and arteriovenous shunts (Fig. 4.2-47):

Meta-arterioles. The arterioles divide into smaller muscle-walled vessels, sometimes called meta-arterioles and these in turn feed into capillaries.

Precapillary sphincters refer to a cuff of smooth muscle cells that surround the origin of capillaries. These determine the size of capillary exchange area at one particular moment in the tissue. For example, increase in the sphincter patency increases the number of open capillaries. Precapillary sphincters respond to local or circulating vasoconstrictor substances.

Capillaries arise directly from arterioles or meta-arterioles. These vessels allow easy exchange of gases and nutritive substances across them and so are also called *exchange vessels.* Capillaries constitute the most important segment of the circulatory system. Their structure and functions will be discussed in detail.

Postcapillary venules, which measure 20–60 μm in diameter, are the *most permeable part* of the micro-circulation.

Arteriovenous anastomosis (shunt or thoroughfare vessels). These are short, low-resistance connections between the arterioles and veins, bypassing the capillaries. These are abundantly innervated by vasomotor sympathetic fibers. These vessels are especially found in the skin of fingers, toes and earlobes where they are involved in the regulation of body temperature.

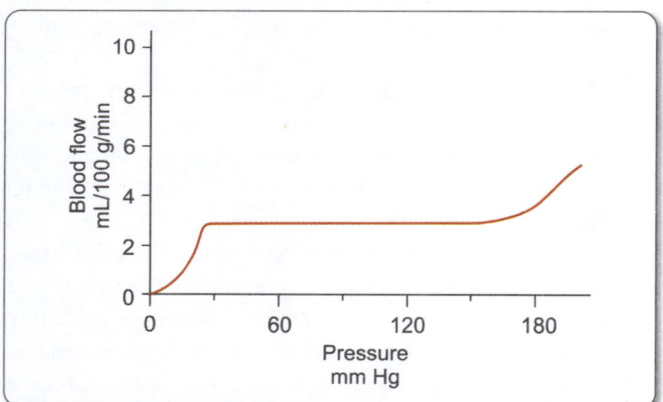

Fig. 4.2-46: Autoregulation of blood flow. Note the blood flow remains relatively constant over a wide range of arterial pressure. This is accomplished by change in resistance proportionate to change in arterial pressure

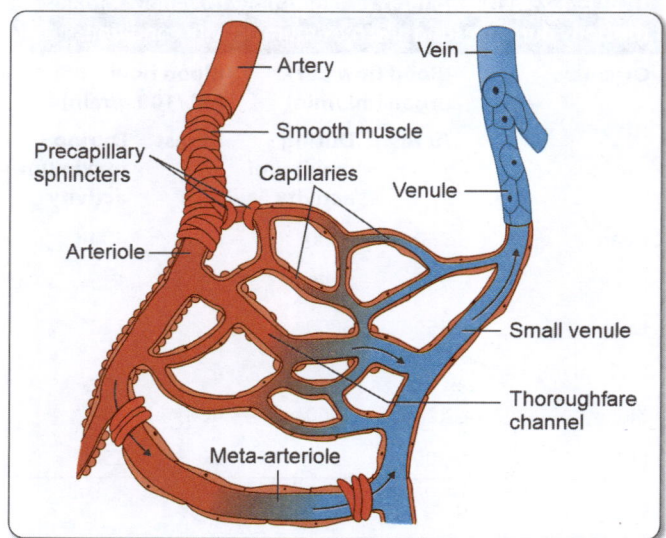

Fig. 4.2-47: Architecture of microcirculation

Structural Characteristics of Capillaries

Each capillary has an average diameter of 5 μm, length of 50 μm, wall thickness of 1 μm and cross-sectional area of 40 μm².

The capillary wall essentially consists of a single layer of endothelial cells which are lined on the outside by a basal lamina (glycoprotein), overlying the basal lamina there may be isolated branching perivascular cells called *pericytes*.

The endothelial structure of capillaries varies in different organs depending on the function of the particular tissue. Under electron microscope, three types of capillaries have been identified:

1. *Continuous capillaries* are characterized by a single layer of endothelial cells which are almost continuous, except for small clefts of 6–7 nm in size in between the cells (Fig. 4.2-48A). These are the most common types of capillaries and are found in most of the body tissues viz. skeletal muscle, adipose tissue, connective tissue, pulmonary circulation and so on.

2. *Fenestrated capillaries* consist of thin endothelial cells with large fenestrations (20–100 nm in diameter) (Fig. 4.2-48B) which make the capillaries porous. Fenestrated capillaries are found in renal glomeruli, intestinal villi, most endocrinal glands.

3. *Discontinuous capillaries* are characterized by large gaps (600–3000 nm in diameter) between endothelial cells (Fig. 4.2-48C). Through these gaps even-formed elements of blood can pass freely. Such capillaries are also called sinusoids and are found in bone marrow, liver and spleen.

Transcapillary Exchange

The capillary blood brings oxygen, electrolytes and nutrients to the tissues and removes the waste products of cellular metabolism. The exchange of these substances occurs across the thin membrane formed by the endothelial cells.

Filtration and reabsorption across microvascular endothelium. The rate of filtration and absorption at any point along the capillary wall depends on the balance of forces known as *Starling forces*. According to Starling hypothesis, the filtration absorption is expressed as:

$$K (P_c + \pi_i) - (P_i + \pi_c)$$

K = The permeability-surface area coefficient
P_c = The hydrostatic capillary pressure,
P_i = The hydrostatic interstitial pressure,
π_c = Oncotic pressure of blood
π_i = Oncotic pressure of the interstitium.

Thus, P_c–P_i, represents the hydrostatic pressure gradient, and

$\pi_c - \pi_i$, represents the oncotic pressure gradient.

Hydrostatic capillary pressure (P_c) tends to force the fluid out through the capillary membrane. The values of hydrostatic capillary pressure in most of the tissues are:

- At the arterial end = 30–40 mm Hg
- At the venous end = 10–15 mm Hg
- In the middle = 25 mm Hg.

Hydrostatic interstitial pressure (P_i) tends to force fluid inward through the capillary membrane. It is about –2 mm Hg in subcutaneous tissue.

Oncotic pressure of blood or plasma colloid osmotic pressure (π_c) results from the osmotic pressure of plasma proteins. It tends to pull fluid inward through the capillary membrane. It is about 25–27 mm Hg.

Oncotic pressure of the interstitium (π_i) is due to the presence of proteins in the interstitial space. It tends to pull fluid out of the capillary membrane. The effective oncotic pressure in the interstitium is estimated to range between 5 mm Hg and 10 mm Hg (average 8 mm Hg).

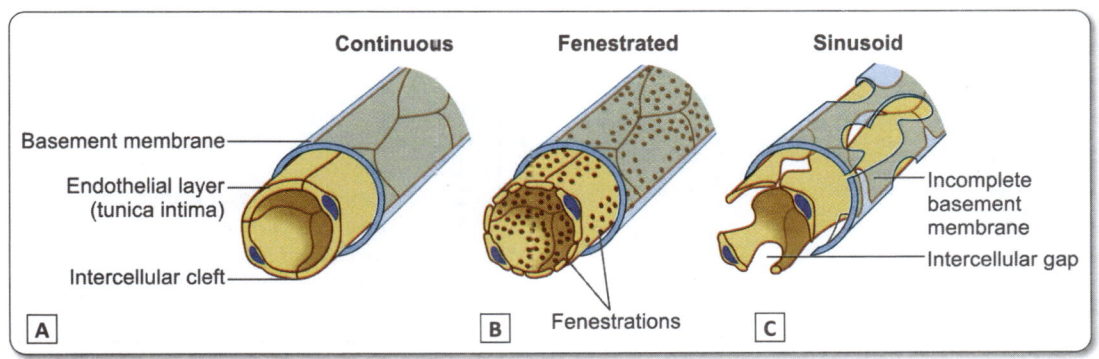

Figs 4.2-48A to C: Structure of different types of capillaries. A. Continuous; B. Fenestrated; C. Sinusoidal

TABLE 4.2-5: Calculation of net filtration force at the capillaries	At the arteriolar end (mm Hg)	At the venous end (mm Hg)
• **Forces tending to move fluid outward**		
■ Capillary hydrostatic pressure (P_c)	35	10
■ Interstitial oncotic pressure (π_i)	3	3
Total outward force ($P_c + \pi_i$)	**38**	**13**
• **Forces tending to move fluid inward**		
■ Oncotic pressure of blood (π_c)	25	25
■ Interstitial hydrostatic pressure (P_i)	−2	−2
Total inward force ($\pi_c + P_i$)	**23**	**23**
• **Filtering force**	38 − 23	13 − 23
	15	− 10
• **Net filtering force of the whole capillary**	(15 − 10) = 5	

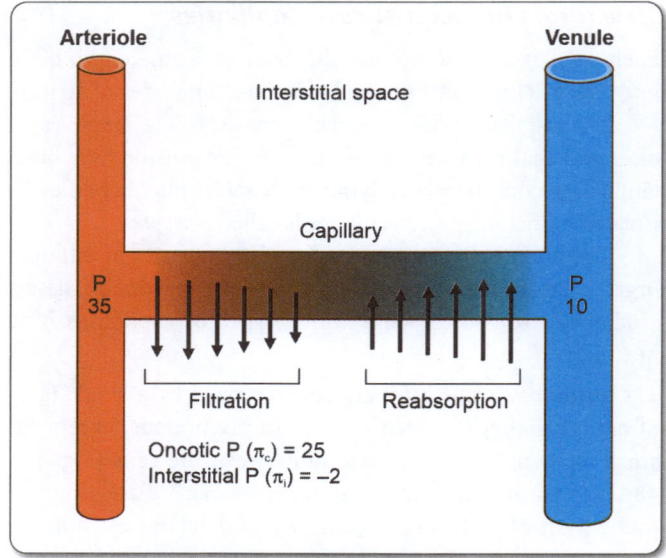

Fig. 4.2-49: Filtration and reabsorption in a capillary due to balance of starling forces

NURSING IMPLICATIONS AND APPLICATIONS

Calculation of Net Filtration at the Capillaries
- From the above description, the net forces acting on the fluid at the arteriolar and venous end of a typical muscle *capillary* can be calculated (Table 4.2-5):

In the example given above we have studied the balance of Starling forces at the arteriolar and venous end of the capillary only. However, over the length of the capillary the hydrostatic pressure gradually declines to zero near the middle of capillary. From here the inward forces become dominant and reabsorption process starts to reach its maximum at the venular end (Fig. 4.2-49).

Venous Circulation

Structural Characteristics of Veins (Histology Plate 4.2-4)

Walls of veins, as compared to arteries, at equivalent levels in the vascular tree are thin-walled and contain small amount of elastic tissue and smooth muscle, and have larger lumen. Because of their structural characteristics they are more distensible and collapsible.

Lumen of the veins is larger than the equivalent arteries.

Valves are present in the veins of the dependent parts of the body that prevent the backflow of venous blood.

Histology Plate 4.2-4: Large Vein

Photomicrograph of a large vein in shown below. the following layers are identified:
1. Tunica intima
2. Tunica media (this layer in thin)
3. Tunica adventitia (thick layer)
4. Endothelial cells
5. Longitudinally oriented smooth muscle fibers
6. Lumen

Functions of the Veins

Blood reservoirs. Because of their feature of *distensibility and collapsibility* the veins serve as blood reservoirs. About 60–70% of the circulating blood is present in the venous system. Due to this property veins are also called the *capacitance vessels.*

Conduits. The systemic veins carry blood from the tissues to the right atrium, and the pulmonary veins collect blood from the lungs and return it to the left atrium.

Maintenance of cardiac output. Veins help to maintain the cardiac output whenever there is loss of blood. After blood loss from an external or internal injury reflex increase in sympathetic discharge produces contraction of the smooth muscles in the walls of the veins. As a result of venular contraction, there occurs a decrease in their capacity leading to increased venous return to heart. In this way veins help to maintain cardiac output by maintaining normal venous return in spite of blood loss.

BLOOD PRESSURE

Blood pressure is the lateral pressure exerted by the flowing blood on the walls of the vessels. It is usually measured in mm Hg. Without any further qualification the term blood pressure denotes the *arterial pressure.* While describing the pressure exerted by the blood column in other types of blood vessels, the type of vessel is also mentioned, e.g. *capillary pressure* and *venous pressure.*

Systolic Blood Pressure

- The maximum arterial pressure during systole is called *systolic blood pressure*, and occurs during ventricular ejection.
- Normal systolic blood pressure in a young adult is 120 mm Hg (range: 105–135 mm Hg).
- Systolic blood pressure undergoes considerable fluctuations, e.g. it is increased during excitement, exercise and meals, and is decreased during sleep and rest.

Diastolic Blood Pressure

- Diastolic blood pressure refers to the minimum arterial pressure during diastole and occurs just before the onset of ventricular ejection.
- Normal diastolic blood pressure in a young adult is 80 mm Hg (range 60–90 mm Hg).

Conventional Expression of Blood Pressure

Conventionally, systolic and diastolic blood pressures are denoted as numerator and denominator, respectively. For example, blood pressure of a normal person is written as 120/80 mm Hg.

Pulse Pressure

- Pulse pressure is the arithmetic difference between systolic and diastolic blood pressures
- Normally, average pulse pressure is 40 mm Hg.

Mean Arterial Pressure

- Mean arterial pressure (MAP) is the average of all pressures measured millisecond by millisecond throughout the cardiac cycle.
- Practically, MAP is roughly equal to diastolic pressure (DP) plus one-third of pulse pressure (PP), i.e.,

$$DP + \frac{1}{3}PP$$

- Normal value of MAP is 93 mm Hg (range: 90–100 mm Hg).

Determinants of (Factors affecting) Arterial Blood Pressure

The arterial blood pressure (BP) is a function of the product of cardiac output (CO) and total peripheral resistance (PR), i.e.

   Arterial BP = cardiac output (CO) × peripheral resistance (PR)

Therefore, arterial blood pressure is affected by conditions that affect either cardiac output or peripheral resistance.

Changes in cardiac output affect the systolic pressure more than diastolic pressure while changes in peripheral resistance affect diastolic pressure more than the systolic pressure. As discussed in the section on cardiac output, the cardiac output is a function of *heart rate* and *stroke volume*, so these two are important determinants of the blood pressure.

- The peripheral resistance depends upon the viscosity of blood, elasticity of the vessel wall, and velocity of the blood flow. Thus, these factors are also important determinants of the blood pressure.

Effect of some of the important determinants of the blood pressure described here briefly.

Regulation of Blood Pressure

Arterial blood pressure is controlled by several mechanisms which under physiological conditions maintain the normal mean arterial pressure (MAP) within a narrow range of 95–100 mm Hg. Various mechanisms controlling arterial pressure can be grouped as:
- Rapid blood pressure control mechanisms
- Intermediate blood pressure control mechanisms
- Long-term blood pressure control mechanisms

Rapid Blood Pressure Control Mechanism (Nervous Regulating Mechanism)

Rapid blood pressure control mechanism or the so called short-term control mechanism primarily includes the following three nervous reflexes:

1. Baroreceptor reflexes (see page 226)
2. Central nervous system ischemic response (see page 226)
3. Chemoreceptor reflexes (see page 228).

Salient features of rapid control mechanisms are:

- These *act very rapidly*, i.e., within seconds to few minutes of alterations in the blood pressure.
- These are *short-term mechanisms*, i.e., these act for few hours to few days and are thus insignificant in long-term regulation of blood pressure.
- These are useful in preventing *acute decreases in blood pressure* (e.g. during severe hemorrhage) as well as in preventing *excessive increases in blood pressure* (e.g. as might occur in response to excessive blood transfusion).

Intermediate Blood Pressure Control Mechanisms

The intermediate blood pressure control mechanisms that are important in blood pressure control after several minutes of acute pressure changes are:

- Renin-angiotensin vasoconstrictor mechanism (see page 229)
- Stress relaxation and reverse stress relaxation mechanism, and
- Capillary fluid shift mechanism.

Salient features of intermediate blood pressure control mechanisms are:

- These mechanisms come into play after several minutes of acute pressure changes and reach full function within a few hours.
- These mechanisms play their role from few days to few weeks.
- All these mechanisms basically try to control the alterations in blood pressure by altering the blood volume.

Stress relaxation and reverse stress relaxation mechanisms

Stress relaxation mechanism refers to vasodilatation occurring due to stress on the vascular smooth muscles. When pressure in the vessels becomes too high (e.g. the following massive slow intravenous transfusion), the vessels become stretched and continue to stretch for minutes or hours. This causes relaxation of blood vessels simply by vascular tone adjustment.

This leads to an increase in the capacity of the arterial system with a concomitant fall in blood pressure.

Reverse stress relaxation mechanism operates when the blood pressure is low due to less stress on the vessel walls and tries to restore it back to normal. For example, when blood pressure falls due to prolonged slow bleeding, there occurs tightening of blood vessel walls by vascular tone adjustment secondary to less stress on the vessel wall (reverse stress relaxation mechanism). This mechanism tries to restore the blood pressure back to normal. This mechanism can correct up to 15% change in blood volume below normal.

Capillary fluid shift mechanism

Capillary fluid shift mechanism helps in restoring both low and high blood pressure back to normal:

When blood pressure is raised, the mean capillary pressure is also high resulting in shift of fluid from circulation to the interstitial fluid compartments. This reduces the blood volume to restore the arterial pressure.

When blood pressure is lowered, the mean capillary pressure is also low, resulting in absorption of fluid from the interstitial compartments to circulation. Thus the blood volume is increased which helps to return the blood pressure back to normal.

The capillary fluid shift mechanism is about two times more effective than baroreceptor reflex mechanism in controlling the blood pressure, but it acts much more slowly (intermediate acting mechanism) than baroreceptor mechanism (rapid acting mechanism).

Long-term Blood Pressure Control Mechanisms

Kidneys play main role in the long-term control of blood pressure by the following mechanisms:

Direct mechanism, i.e., 'renal-body fluid feedback mechanism'.

Indirect mechanisms control kidney functions indirectly via the following hormonal mechanisms:

- Aldosterone system
- Renin-angiotensin system.

Renal-body fluid system for arterial pressure control

The most important mechanism for the long-term control of blood pressure is linked to control of circulatory volume by the kidney. In fact, it is similar to the capillary fluid shift mechanism except that only the renal glomerular capillaries are involved in the process. The renal-body fluid system corrects blood pressure by causing appropriate changes in blood volume through *diuresis* and *natriuresis*.

CLINICAL ASPECTS

VARIATIONS IN BLOOD PRESSURE

Physiological Factors Affecting Blood Pressure

Age: In healthy humans, both systolic and diastolic pressures rise with age.

- *At birth* systolic blood pressure is 40 mm Hg (range: 20–60 mm Hg). It then rises rapidly up to one month of age.
- *At one month* of age the systolic blood pressure becomes about 80 mm Hg and then rises slowly.
- *At about 17 years* of age normal adult level of blood pressure is 120/80 mm Hg.
- *At about 70 years of age* the normal value of blood pressure is 160/90 mm Hg. The increase in blood pressure associated with advancing age is due to increase in rigidity of vessel wall.

Sex: Before menopause, females have little lower (4–6 mm Hg) systolic blood pressure than males of corresponding age. *After menopause,* systolic blood pressure in females is little higher (4–6 mm Hg) than males of same age group.

Effect of meals: Systolic blood pressure increases by 4–6 mm Hg after meals and this effect lasts for about one hour. *Diastolic blood pressure* either remains unchanged or decreases slightly due to vasodilatation in splanchnic vessels.

Emotions: Increased sympathetic activity during emotional situations leads to increase in systolic blood pressure.

Climatic temperature: Exposure to cold produces rise in the blood pressure, while *exposure to hot temperature* lowers the blood pressure.

Diurnal variation: Systolic blood pressure shows a diurnal variation of about 6–10 mm Hg; the values being lower in the morning and higher in the afternoon. In night workers, however, a reverse rhythm is observed.

Exercise: In muscular exercise, generally systolic blood pressure rises and diastolic blood pressure falls.

Effect of gravity: In standing position, due to hydrostatic (gravitational) effect of the blood column, the pressure in the vessels below heart level is increased and in the vessels above heart level it is decreased.

Effect of change in posture: Immediately on standing, there occurs peripheral pooling of blood in dependant parts leading to decreased venous return and decreased cardiac output and momentary fall in systolic blood pressure.

Sleep: In complete relaxed state during early hours of sleep there occurs fall in blood pressure up to 15–20 mm Hg. However, in disturbed sleep blood pressure increases due to increased sympathetic discharge.

Body build: Systolic blood pressure is slightly higher in obese individuals as compared to thin-built individuals.

Pathological Variations in Blood Pressure

Hypertension

Hypertension (HT) refers to a condition in which value of systolic blood pressure is persistently >140 mm Hg and/or that of diastolic blood pressure is above 90 mm Hg. If there is increase only in systolic blood pressure, it is called *systolic hypertension* in which pulse pressure is raised. It is of two types:

i. *Primary hypertension* also known as *essential hypertension* is characterized by a raised blood pressure without any underlying disease. Risk factors for primary HT include: heredity, obesity, mental tension and smoking.

ii. *Secondary hypertension* refers to a condition in which blood pressure is raised due to some other underlying disease. Common causes of secondary hypertension are:

- *Cardiovascular diseases*, e.g. atherosclerosis.
- *Renal diseases*, e.g. glomerulonephritis.
- *Endocrinal disorders* like hyperaldosteronism (excessive secretion of aldosterone from adrenal cortex).
- *Neurologic disorders* which may produce hypertension include raised intracranial pressure.
- *Pregnancy-induced hypertension* (PIH) is noticed in some of the pregnant women. Its exact cause is not known.

Hypotension

Hypotension refers to a condition in which values of blood pressure are below the normal range. Clinically, when the systolic blood pressure is < 90 mm Hg, it is considered hypotension. It is of the following types:

Primary hypotension also known as essential hypotension is a disorder of unknown etiology.

Secondary hypotension, occurs secondary to some other underlying diseases such as myocardial infarction, neurogenic shock, hemorrhagic shock, hypoactivity of pituitary gland and hypoactivity of adrenal glands.

Postural hypotension refers to sudden fall in blood pressure when patients stand up from lying down posture. It occurs due to some dysfunction of autonomic nervous system.

CORONARY CIRCULATION

The blood supply to the heart is by coronary arteries (for anatomical details of coronary vessels see page 182)

Coronary Blood Flow: Characteristic Features

A continuous flow of blood to the heart is essential to maintain an adequate supply of O_2 and nutrients.

Normal coronary blood flow at rest is about 250 mL (70 mL/100 g tissue/min), i.e., about 5% of the resting cardiac output (5 L). 3- to 6-fold increase in the coronary blood flow may occur during exercise.

Phasic Changes in Coronary Blood Flow

The coronary blood flow shows changes during phases of cardiac cycle. The blood flow is determined by the balance between *pressure head* (i.e., aortic pressure) and the resistance (i.e., extravascular pressure exerted by the myocardium on the coronary vessels) offered to blood flow during various phases of cardiac cycle as shown in Figure 4.10–50 as described here:

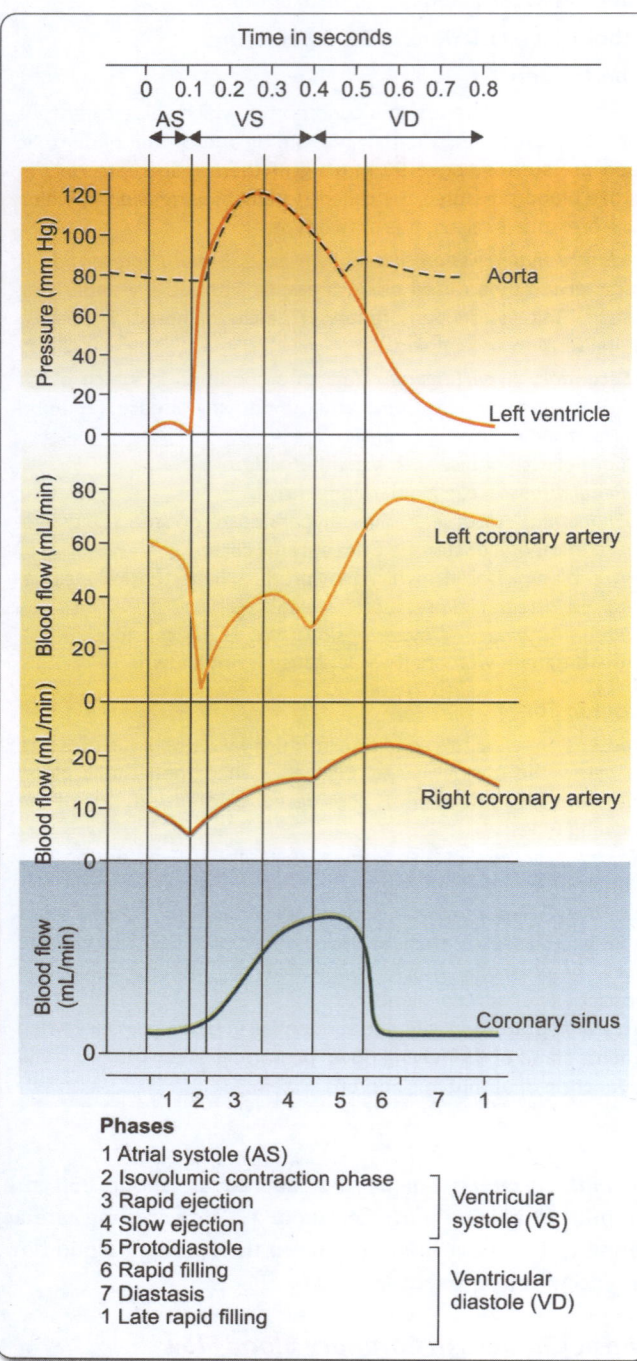

Fig. 4.2-50: Blood flow in right and left coronary arteries and coronary sinus during different phases of cardiac cycle

Blood flow to left ventricle

During systole, the tension developed in the left ventricle is so high that it has throttling effect on the branches of coronary arteries. As a result, the average blood flow through the capillaries of left ventricles falls.

During diastole the cardiac muscles relax and blood flow increases. Thus, most of the coronary blood flow (over 70%) occurs during diastole.

Blood flow to right ventricle and atria

Blood passing through coronary capillaries of right ventricle also shows phasic changes similar to left ventricle. However, the changes in right ventricular flow are far less because force of contraction of the right ventricle is much less. Thus, the blood flow to the right ventricle and atria occurs both during systole and diastole.

CARDIOVASCULAR REGULATION

Cardiovascular regulation. Cardiovascular control makes *circulatory adjustments* which are essential to cope up with the timely needs of each and every organ of the body and is thus of fundamental importance for survival.

Circulatory adjustments which ensure that all of the organs receive sufficient blood flow are: Control of blood volume, and control of arterial pressure. These circulatory adjustments are made by the cardiovascular control mechanisms primarily by regulating the following parameters.

Regulation of cardiac performance, i.e. alterations in the activities of heart which include:

Chronotropic action, i.e., effect on heart rate which may be in the form of:

- Increased heart rate (tachycardia) or positive chronotropic effect
- Decreased heart rate (bradycardia) or negative chronotropic effect.

Inotropic action, i.e., effect on force of contraction which may be in the form of:

- Increase in the force of contraction (positive inotropic effect)
- Decrease in the force of contraction (negative inotropic effect.

Dromotropic action, i.e., effect on conduction of impulse through the heart, which may be in the form of:

- Increase in the velocity of impulse conduction (positive dromotropic effect)
- Decrease in the velocity of impulse conduction (negative dromotropic effect).

Bathmotropic action, i.e., effect on the excitability of the cardiac muscle, which may be in the form of:

- Increased excitability of cardiac muscle (positive bathmotropic effect)
- Decreased excitability of cardiac muscle (negative bathmotropic effect).

Regulation of performance of blood vessels which primarily includes:

Alterations in diameter of arterioles which change the peripheral resistance and also the hydrostatic pressure in the capillaries

Alteration in diameter of veins which changes the venous pressure and thus venous return and the cardiac output.

CARDIOVASCULAR CONTROL MECHANISM

The cardiovascular control mechanism which plays its role in making circulatory adjustments during the routine and emergency cardiovascular stresses can be grouped as:

- Neural control mechanism
- Humoral control mechanism
- Local control mechanism

Neural Control Mechanism

Neural regulation of circulation is of fundamental importance since it responds within seconds.

The neural cardiovascular regulating mechanism consists of:

- Medullary cardiovascular control centers.
- Autonomic nervous system supplying the heart and blood vessels.
- Afferent impulses to medullary centers.
- Role of skeletal nerves and muscles in controlling blood pressure.

Medullary Cardiovascular Control Centers

1. Vasomotor center

It is the primary cardiovascular regulatory center located in the medulla oblongata of brain stem. It consists of groups of neurons situated bilaterally in the reticular substance of medulla at the floor of fourth ventricle. The medullary cardiovascular center is constituted by the following different areas (Fig. 4.2-51):

Pressor area. Stimulation of pressor area produces:

- *Arteriolar constriction* which increases the systemic blood pressure
- *Venoconstriction* which decreases blood stored in the venous reservoir and increases venous return,
- *Increase in heart rate* or positive chronotropic effect
- *Increase in force of contraction* or positive inotropic effect.

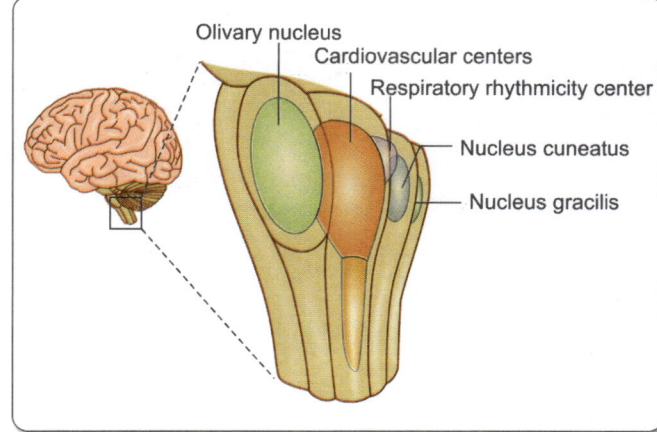

Fig. 4.2-51: Medullary cardiovascular control centers

Depressor area. Stimulation of neurons forming depressor area produces decrease in the sympathetic activity due to inhibition of the tonically discharging impulses of the pressor area causing:

- *Arteriolar dilation* which decreases systemic blood pressure
- *Venodilatation* which increases storage of blood in venous reservoir and decreases venous return and cardiac output
- *Decrease in heart rate* or negative chronotropic effect
- *Decrease in force of contraction* or negative inotropic effect.

2. Medullary parasympathetic center

Medullary parasympathetic center or *cardiac vagal center* earlier also called cardioinhibitory center (CIC) is now called by its specific name, i.e., the *nucleus ambiguus* (NAm). Nucleus ambiguus receives afferents via nucleus tractus solitarius (NTS) and in turn sends inhibitory pathway in the form of vagal fibers to *heart* to decrease heart rate and force of cardiac contraction.

Medullary relay station for cardiorespiratory afferents

Nucleus tractus solitarius (NTS) of the vagus nerve forms the so called medullary relay station. It receives afferents from most of the baroreceptors and chemoreceptors. Cells of the NTS, in turn, relay the information to vasomotor center and cardiac vagal center (nucleus ambiguus) that control sympathetic and parasympathetic outputs, respectively.

Autonomic Nerve Supply to Heart and Blood Vessels

1. Autonomic nerve supply to heart

Sympathetic supply. Spinal sympathetic center is formed by neurons located in the intermediolateral horns of the

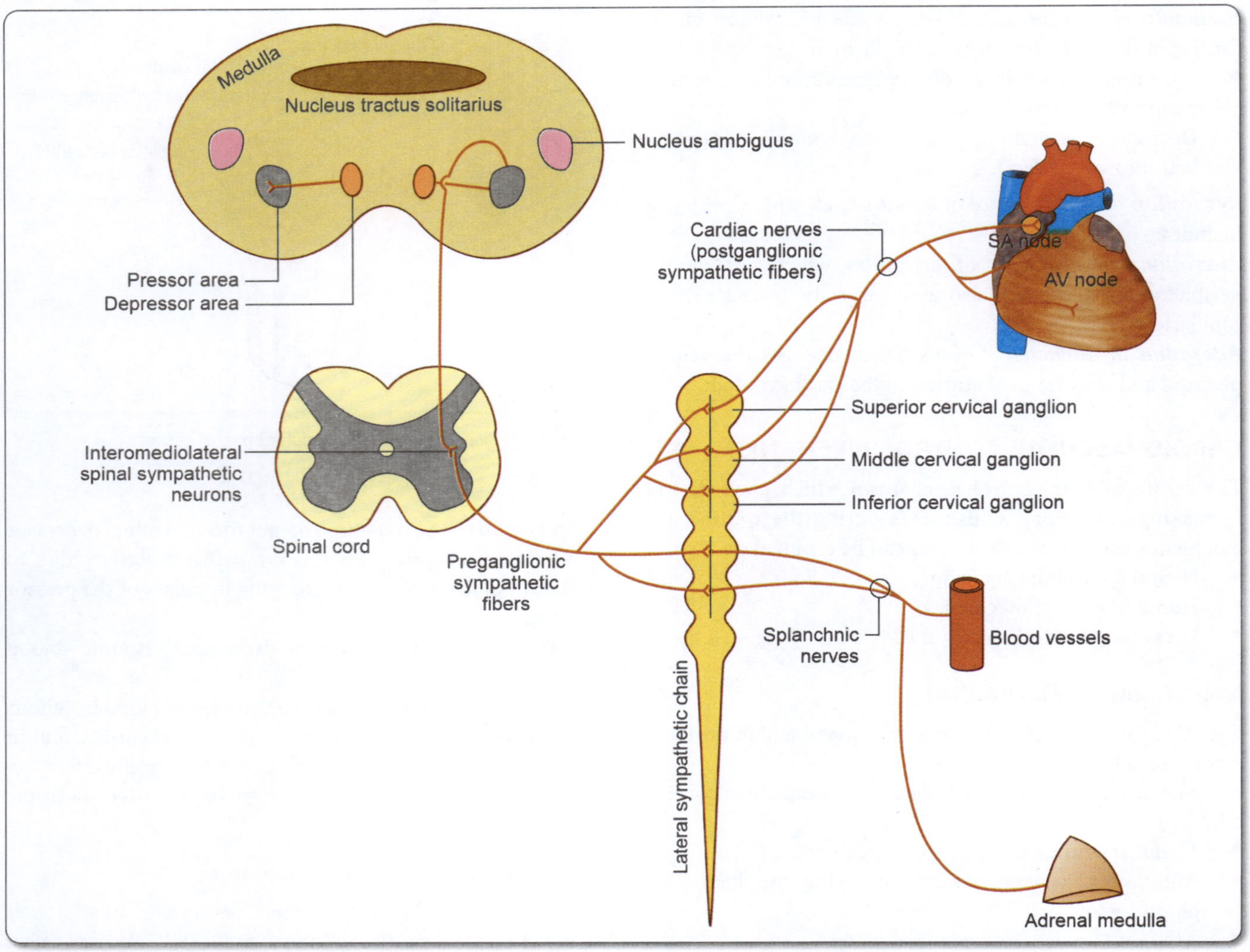

Fig. 4.2-52: Sympathetic innervation of the heart

spinal cord extending from T_1 to L_2 spinal segments. (Fig. 4.2-52).

Parasympathetic supply. Parasympathetic fibers to the heart are carried through two vagii (Fig. 4.2-53).

Vagal tone. There is a good deal of tonic vagal discharge, called the *vagal tone*, in humans and other large animals. In adult humans the resting heart rate which is about 72 beats/min rises to 150–180 beats/min after the administration of vagolytic drugs such as atropine, because of the unopposed sympathetic tone.

2. Autonomic nerve supply to blood vessels

The autonomic efferents supplying the blood vessels produce two types of effects.

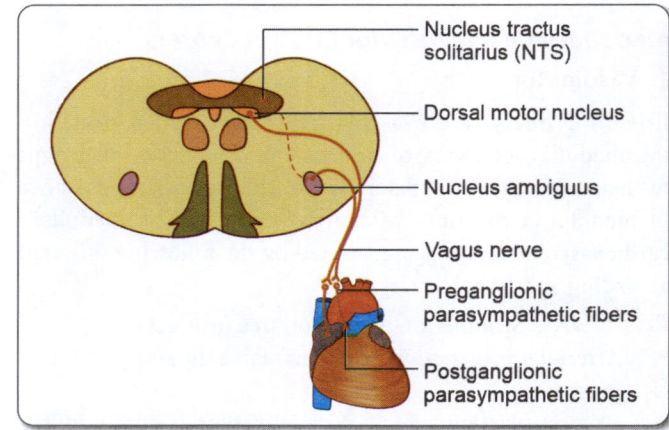

Fig. 4.2-53: Parasympathetic innervation to heart and blood vessels

1. *Vasoconstriction effect.* Sympathetic vasoconstrictor fibers show tonic (i.e., continuous) discharge at the rate of about 1 impulse/sec. Therefore, when the sympathetic nerves are cut (*sympathectomy*), there occurs:

- *Vasodilatation*
- *Venodilatation* (increased venous capacity)
  Stimulation of sympathetic fibers produces:
- *Constriction of arterioles*
- *Venoconstriction* (decreased venous capacity)

2. *Vasodilatation effect.* Neural vasodilatation effect on blood vessels is produced by the following mechanisms:

- *Decrease in discharge of noradrenergic vasoconstrictor nerves.*
- *Sympathetic cholinergic vasodilator nerves:* Some of the organs of the body such as skeletal muscles, heart, lungs, liver, kidney and uterus in addition to adrenergic vasoconstrictor sympathetic fibers also receive innervation by *cholinergic vasodilator sympathetic* fibers having acetylcholine and vasoinhibitory peptide (VIP) as neurotransmitter.

- *Parasympathetic vasodilator nerves:* Blood vessels, in general, do not have parasympathetic innervation with the following exceptions:
- *Sacral outflow parasympathetic fibers* represented by *nervi erigentes* which supplies sexual erectile tissue.
- *Cranial outflow of parasympathetic fibers* along chorda tympani is branch of facial nerve to salivary glands.

Vasodilation by axon reflex. Conduction of normal sensory afferent impulses from the skin to spinal cord is called *orthodromic conduction.* However, in certain situations the antidromic conduction of impulses cause release of substance P from the nerve endings which produces vasodilation.

3. Afferent impulses to medullary cardiovascular control centers

The medullary control centers are influenced by afferent control impulses from the higher centers and a large number of other areas (Fig. 4.2-54). These include:

Afferent impulses from higher centers controlling vasomotor center

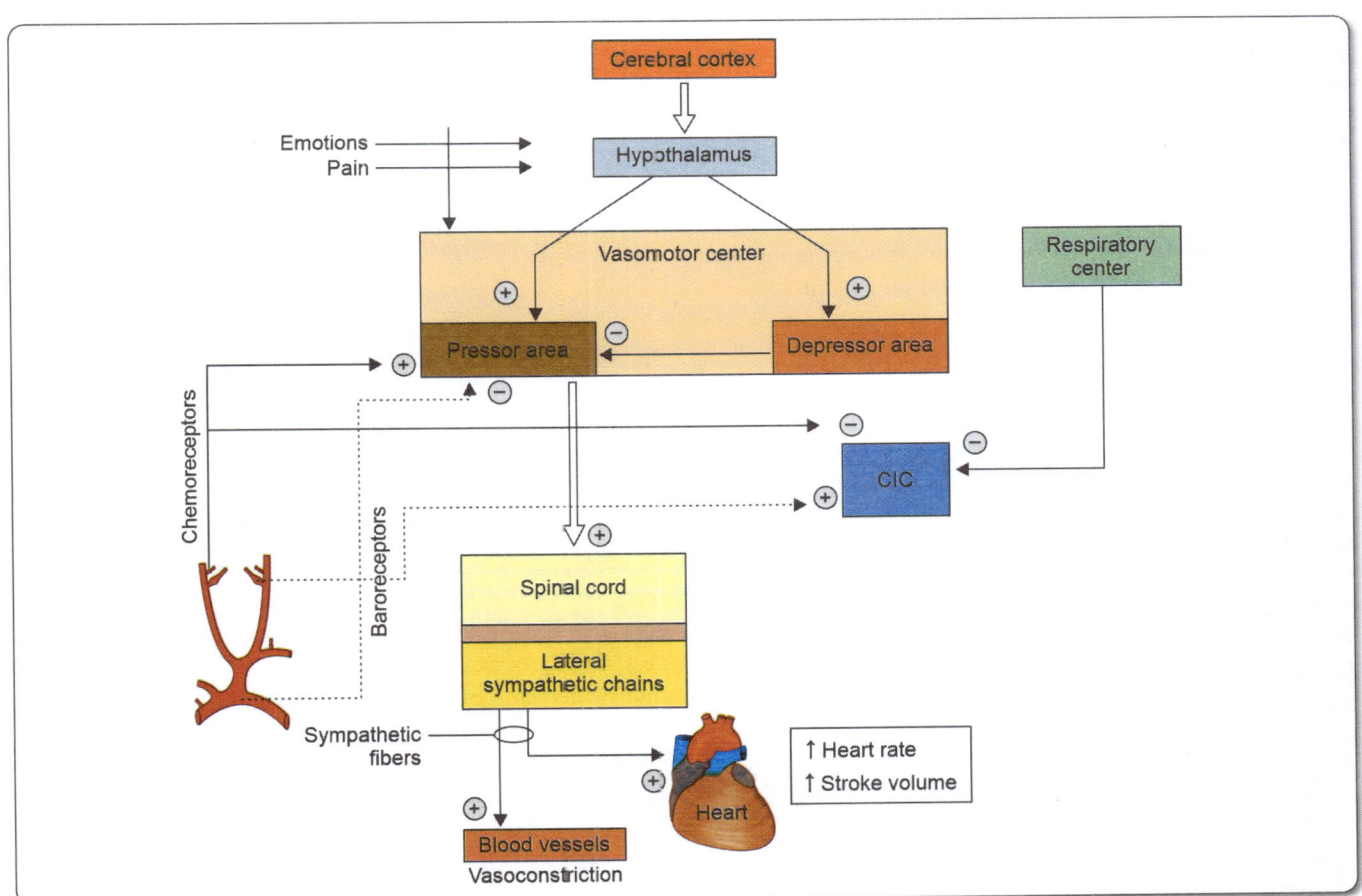

Fig. 4.2-54: Scheme to show afferent impulses affecting medullary cardiovascular control centers

Afferent impulses from respiratory centers

Cardiovascular reflex mechanisms operating through medullary control centers are:

- *Baroreceptor reflex*
- *Chemoreceptor reflexes*

Direct effects on vasomotor area

- Central nervous system ischemic response
- Cushing reflex

Afferents from nociceptive stimuli.

a. Afferent impulses from higher centers controlling vasomotor center and cardiac vagal center

Cerebral cortex. There are descending tracts to the vasomotor area from cerebral cortex (particularly the limbic cortex) that relay in the hypothalamus. Some examples of the influence of limbic system on the VMC are:

- *Tachycardia and hypertension* produced by emotions
- *Bradycardia and fainting* occurring during sudden emotional shock.
- *Fight or flight response* is a complex set of responses which increases cardiac output and raises blood pressure in anticipation of flight or physical defence.

Hypothalamus. The hypothalamus serves to integrate many somatic and autonomic responses. Examples are:

- *Temperature regulation.*
- *Emotional stresses.*

Reticular formation of pons, mesencephalon and diencephalon also influences the vasomotor area. For example: *Pain* usually causes rise in blood pressure via afferent impulses in the reticular formation converging on the vasomotor area. However, prolonged severe pain may cause vasodilation and fainting.

b. Afferent Impulses from respiratory centers

Impulses arising from the respiratory centers affect the heart rate by changing the vagal tone and the alterations produced are known as *sinus arrhythmia*, which occurs during forced breathing.

During inspiration, the impulses arising from the respiratory centers inhibit the cardiac vagal center causing reduced vagal tone and *sinus tachycardia.*

During expiration, the respiratory centers stop sending inhibitory impulses to the cardiac vagal center causing increased vagal tone and sinus bradycardia.

c. Cardiovascular reflex mechanisms affecting medullary control centers

Cardiovascular reflex mechanisms are multiple sub-conscious special nervous control mechanisms that operate through medullary control centers all the time to maintain the arterial pressure within normal range. These include:

- Baroreceptor reflex mechanisms
- Chemoreceptor reflex mechanism. (For details see page 228)

d. Direct effects on vasomotor area

The vasomotor center is directly affected by locally produced hypoxia and hypercapnia. Examples of direct effects are central nervous system ischemic response and cushing reflex.

Central nervous system ischemic response. When blood pressure falls below 60 mm Hg, the blood flow to the vasomotor area is decreased enough to cause CNS ischemia. As a result of CNS ischemia, the CO_2/lactic acid accumulates locally and excites the neurons of VMC which causes strong sympathetic stimulation leading to vasoconstriction. There occurs immediate increase in the blood pressure. This is called *CNS ischemic response.* This acts as an emergency arterial pressure control system.

Cushing reflex. When intracranial pressure is increased it compresses the arteries in the brain and blood supply to the vasomotor area is compromised. The hypoxia and hypercapnia produced locally increase the discharge from VMC. The resultant rise in systemic pressure tends to restore the blood supply to medulla. This effect is called *cushing reflex.* The resultant increase in blood pressure also causes reflex bradycardia via baroreceptor response. Thus, bradycardia is an important feature of raised intracranial pressure.

e. Afferents from nociceptive stimuli

Afferents carrying pain sensations also affect VMC and evoke either pressor or depressor reflex effect as:

- Increase in the blood pressure and tachycardia is caused due to somatic pain afferents
- Hypotension and bradycardia are produced by *visceral pain afferents.*

Baroreceptor Reflex Mechanisms

Baroreceptors also known as mechanoreceptors or pressure receptors are the stretch receptors located in the walls of heart and large blood vessels. These are spray type nerve endings, i.e., they are extensively branched, knobby, coiled, and intertwined ends of myelinated nerve fibers.

Location of Carotid and Aortic Arch Baroreceptors

Carotid baroreceptors are located in carotid sinus which is a small dilatation of the internal carotid artery just above the bifurcation of the common carotid artery into external and internal carotid branches (Fig. 4.2-55).

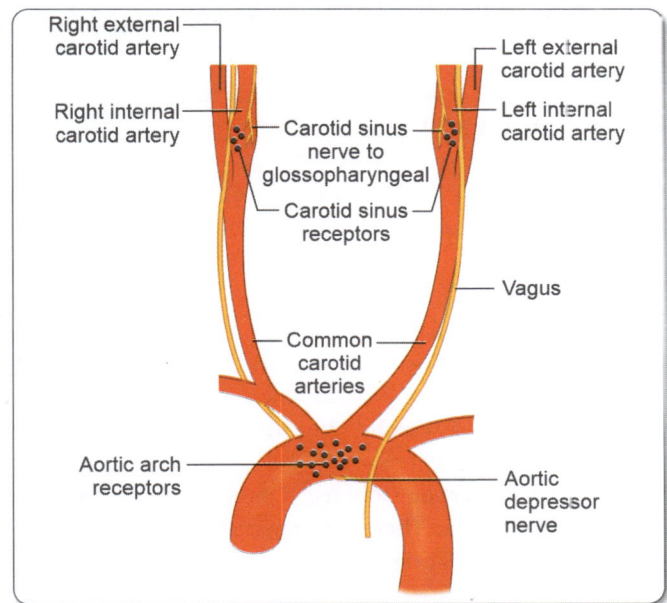

Fig. 4.2-55: Location of baroreceptors (carotid sinus and aortic arch) and chemoreceptors (carotid bodies and aortic bodies)

Aortic arch baroreceptors are located in the wall of arch of aorta (Fig. 4.2-55).

Other systemic arterial baroreceptors (similar to carotid and aortic baroreceptors) are also found at the root of right subclavian artery and junction of thyroid artery and in the common carotid artery.

Innervation of baroreceptors (Fig. 4.2-56)

Carotid sinus baroreceptors are innervated by carotid sinus nerve (Hering's nerve) which is a branch of glossopharyngeal nerve, and ***all other baroreceptors*** are supplied by the vagus nerve.

Afferent fibers from the baroreceptors pass via the glossopharyngeal and vagus nerves to the medulla. Most of them end in the nucleus of the tractus solitarius (NTS), where they secrete an excitatory transmitter, presumably glutamate.

Buffer nerves. The carotid sinus nerve and vagal fibers from the carotid sinus and aortic arch baroreceptors respectively are commonly called buffer nerves, as these are involved in buffering the blood pressure, i.e., preventing sudden rise and fall in blood pressure.

Projections from NTS terminate on to the:
- *Depressor area of VMC*
- *Cardiac vagal center* (nucleus ambiguus),

Response of carotid and aortic baroreceptors to pressure

Response from carotid baroreceptors have been studied in detail. Salient features of these receptor responses to pressure are:

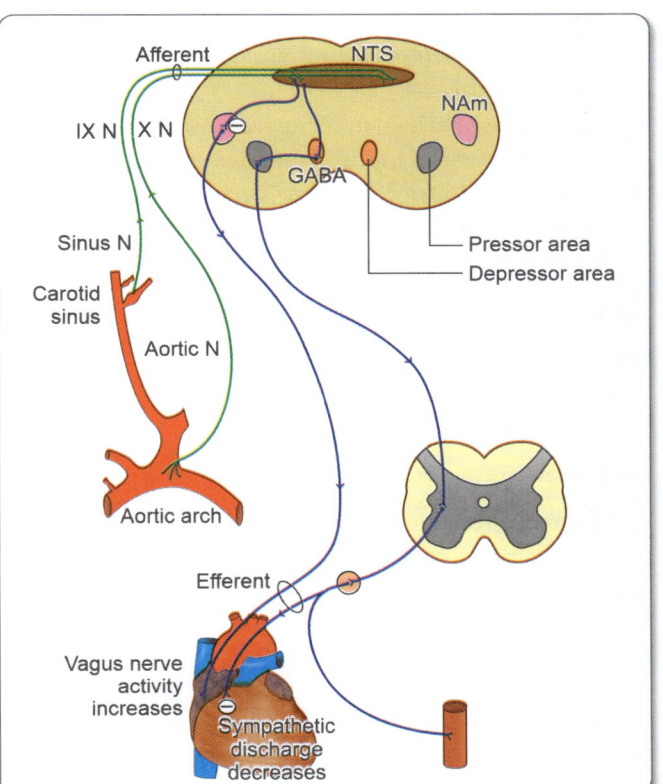

Fig. 4.2-56: Neural pathway of baroreceptor reflex
Abbreviations: GABA, gamma aminobutyric acid; NTS, nucleus tractus solitarius; NAm, nucleus ambiguus

Baroreceptor response. At normal blood pressure levels, the fibers of the buffer nerves discharge at a low rate which increases when the pressure in the carotid sinus and aortic arch rises, and declines when the pressure falls (Fig. 4.2-57).

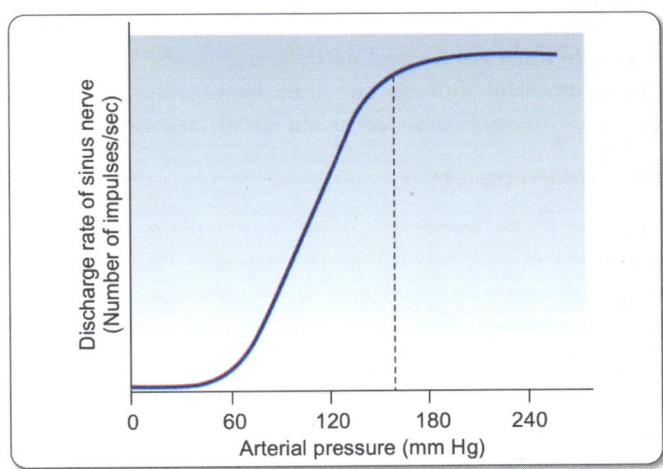

Fig. 4.2-57: Response of carotid sinus baroreceptors at different levels of arterial pressure

- The minimum pressure, about 60 mm Hg, at which carotid baroreceptors are stimulated is called *threshold of baroreceptor reflex.*
- Above threshold level the baroreceptors respond progressively more rapidly till the discharge rate reaches a *plateau*, at 150–160 mm Hg. Thus, the carotid baroreceptors exhibit a great sensitivity as they respond to pressure that varies approximately 50–160 mm Hg.

Cardiac baroreceptors

Cardiac baroreceptors are located in the walls of heart subendocardially. All cardiac receptors are innervated by vagus nerve. These include:

Atrial stretch receptors

Atrial stretch receptors are present in the walls of atria. Atrial stretch receptors have been studied in detail by Prof. A.S. Paintal (an Indian scientist) in 1953. The atrial stretch receptors have been associated with the following roles in the cardiovascular control:

As low-pressure receptors, the atrial stretch receptors along with pulmonary receptors play an important role to minimize arterial pressure changes in response to change in blood volume.

Atrial reflex control of heart rate (Bainbridge reflex). Bainbridge noted that sudden rise in atrial pressure after rapid infusion of saline or blood in anesthetized animals produced tachycardia, if the initial heart rate was low. Thus, this reflex helps to prevent damming of blood in the veins, atria and pulmonary circulation.

Atrial reflex control of blood volume (volume reflex) when there is volume overload the atrial stretch receptors help to return the blood volume back toward normal by decreasing the secretion of antidiuretic hormone (ADH), which diminishes the reabsorption of water from tubules, and by release of a chemical *atrial natriuretic peptide* (ANP) which causes powerful diuresis and thus blood volume back to normal. This combined mechanism constitutes volume reflex.

Ventricular receptors

The ventricular baroreceptors are scattered throughout the left ventricle and interventricular septum. They discharge irregularly and no physiological significance can be attached to these receptors.

Pulmonary baroreceptors. Pulmonary baroreceptors are located in the walls of pulmonary trunk and its divisions— the right and left pulmonary artery play an important role to minimize arterial pressure changes in response to change in blood volume as discussed above.

Role of Chemoreceptor Reflexes in Cardiovascular Control

Chemoreceptors are chemosensitive cells that respond to the following changes in blood:

- Oxygen lack (decreased pO_2)
- Carbon dioxide excess (increased pCO_2)
- Hydrogen ion excess (decreased pH).

Location of chemoreceptors

The chemoreceptors are present in (Fig. 4.2-55):

- *Carotid bodies.* These are 1–2 mm in size and are located in the bifurcation of each common carotid artery. These are innervated by carotid sinus nerve which is a branch of glossopharyngeal nerve.
- *Aortic bodies* are one to three in number located adjacent to arch of aorta. These are innervated by aortic nerve (branch of vagus nerve).

Functions of chemoreceptors

The chemoreceptors exert their role in cardiovascular regulation. In hypoxia, there occurs increased chemoreceptor discharge, which not only produces hyperventilation but also excites the vasomotor center (VMC) leading to peripheral vasoconstriction and increase in arterial blood pressure. Thus, unlike the inhibitory action of arterial baroreceptors, the chemoreceptors have an excitatory effect on the VMC.

> **IMPORTANT TO KNOW**
>
> It is important to note that the chemoreceptors are not stimulated strongly until the arterial pressure falls below 60 mm Hg. Therefore, it is at lower pressures that this reflex becomes important and helps to prevent still further fall in pressure.

Role of Skeletal Nerves and Muscles in Controlling Blood Pressure

Abdominal compression reflex. Whenever VMC is stimulated, e.g. by baroreceptor reflex or chemoreceptor reflex, other areas of reticular formation of brain stem are also stimulated along with. They send simultaneous impulses through skeletal nerves to skeletal muscles of the body, especially abdominal muscles. The contraction of abdominal muscles compresses the abdominal venous reservoirs increasing the venous return to heart and thereby the cardiac output. This response is called *abdominal compression reflex.*

Role of skeletal muscles during exercise. During exercise, the skeletal muscles, especially that of limbs contract and compress the venous reservoirs. This causes translocation of large quantities of blood from the peripheral vessels into heart and lungs. This increases the cardiac output.

Humoral Control Mechanisms

Humoral regulation of circulation refers to the regulation by substances secreted into or absorbed into body fluids, e.g hormones, ions, etc. Most important humoral factors affecting circulation are:

Circulating Vasodilators

The circulating vasodilators include kinins and atrial natriuretic peptide (ANP).

Kinins are peptides (bradykinin and lysylbradykinins) found in the plasma, and body tissues. They cause *vasodilation* by relaxing vascular smooth muscle (VSM) via NO and increase *capillary permeability.*

Atrial natriuretic peptide. For details see page 290

Circulating vasoconstrictor. The circulating vasoconstrictors include catecholamines, angiotensin II and vasopressin.

Catecholamines are released on sympathetic stimulation and include epinephrine and norepinephrine. Catecholamines stimulate both α and β adrenergic receptors. The catecholamines increase peripheral resistance and raise the diastolic blood pressure.

The renin-angiotensin system has important roles in the regulation of blood pressure and in the regulation of extracellular fluid volume. Renin, a protease enzyme, is secreted by *juxtaglomerular cells* of the kidney into the blood.

- *Renin* catalyzes the conversion of *angiotensinogen* (α_2– globulin substrate present in the plasma) to angiotensin I. Angiotensin I is converted into angiotensin II by the action of *angiotensin converting enzyme* (ACE) present in the endothelium of blood vessels throughout the body, especially in the lungs and kidneys.

$$\underset{\text{Angiotensinogen}}{} \xrightarrow{\text{Renin}} \underset{\text{Angiotensin I}}{} \xrightarrow{\text{ACE}} \text{Angiotensin II}$$

- *Angiotensin II* has three principal effects by which it can elevate the arterial pressure:
  1. Vasoconstriction
  2. Decrease in salt and water excretion by kidney
  3. Stimulation of thirst.

Vasopressin or antidiuretic hormone (ADH) is secreted in minute quantities and therefore mainly affects water reabsorption in renal tubules. However, after a severe hemorrhage its concentration rises to a high level and then it has vasoconstrictor effect.

Ions and Other Chemical Factors

The increased concentration of many different ions and chemical factors can also alter local blood flow by causing vasodilation or vasoconstriction.

- Calcium ions cause vasoconstriction
- Potassium ions cause vasodilatation
- Hydrogen ions (decreased pH) cause vasodilation
- Carbon dioxide causes vasodilation in most tissues and marked vasodilation in the brain.
- Glucose or other vasoactive substances, when increased in quantities, raise the osmolarity of blood and cause vasodilation.

Local Control Mechanisms

Local cardiovascular control mechanisms are primarily concerned with the control of blood flow to the tissues locally. These include:

- Mechanisms involved in acute control of blood flow
- Mechanisms involved in long-term blood flow regulation.

A. Mechanisms Involved in Acute Control of Blood Flow

The mechanisms that are involved in most tissues of the body are:

Autoregulation (control of flow during changes in arterial pressure). Autoregulation is the ability of an organ or tissue to adjust its vascular resistance and maintain a relatively constant blood flow over a wide range of arterial pressure.

Role of local vasodilator metabolites. The accumulation of local vasodilator metabolites increase local blood flow. The greater the rate of metabolism in the tissue greater is the rate of production of metabolites. These include:

- Decrease in O_2 tension and pH
- Increase in pCO_2 and osmolality
- Rise in temperature
- Potassium (K^+) and lactate ions
- Histamine
- Adenosine.

CLINICAL ASPECTS

Local vasodilator metabolites increase blood flow during the following conditions:

Active hyperemia It refers to the vasodilation which occurs when the tissue metabolic rate increases.

Reactive hyperemia It is a phenomenon by which the local blood flow to the organ is controlled after a period of ischemia

---

Role of local vasoconstrictors. Serotonin released from platelets in the injured tissue is responsible in part for the vasoconstriction which occurs in hemostasis.

Role of substances secreted by endothelial cells. The vasoactive substances secreted by endothelial cells play important role in control of local blood flow. These include:

- Prostaglandins and thromboxane A_2
- Endothelium-derived relaxing factor (EDRF)
- Endothelins.

B. Mechanisms Involved in Long-Term Blood Flow Regulation

The long-term blood flow regulation develops over a period of days to months to match the metabolic needs of the tissues. Long-term blood flow regulation is required by:

- Ischemic tissues
- Tissues that are growing rapidly
- Tissues that become chronically hyperactive.

The long-term blood flow regulation is brought about by an increase in the physiological size of the vessels in a tissue, and by an increase in the number of blood vessels. One of the major factors that stimulate the increased vascularity of the tissues is a low oxygen concentration.

Angiogenesis. The growth of the new vessels is called angiogenesis. *Angiogenic factors* such as vascular endothelial growth factor (VEGF), fibroblast growth factor (FGF), and angiogenin are the substances which are responsible for angiogenesis.

Development of collateral blood vessels. Collateral blood vessels refer to those new vessels which develop around a blocked artery or vein and allow the affected tissue to be at least partially resupplied with blood. An important example is the development of collateral blood vessels after thrombosis of one of the coronary arteries in old people.

CARDIOVASCULAR HOMEOSTASIS IN HEALTH

Cardiovascular homeostasis in health refers to the compensatory adjustments of the cardiovascular system to challenges faced by the circulation in everyday life. The common situations during which cardiovascular adjustments are required in day-to-day life include:

- Gravitational changes
- Intrathoracic pressure changes
- Exercise.

CARDIOVASCULAR ADJUSTMENTS DURING GRAVITATIONAL CHANGES

Gravitational changes occur under the following conditions in life:

- Posture change from lying to standing
- Prolonged quiet standing,

Adjustments during Posture Change from Lying to Standing

When posture is changed from lying (recumbent) to standing (erect) the hemodynamic changes occur as a result of the effect of gravity on the blood column which tends to reduce the cardiac output and blood pressure. However, since in humans the compensatory mechanisms are so well developed that in normal persons no effect is felt on posture changes in day-to-day life. The sequence of events which occur during change in posture from lying to standing are (Fig. 4.2-58).

In standing position, due to *hydrostatic (gravitational) effect of blood column*, the blood pressure at the level of feet in both the arteries and veins is increased approximately by 80 mm Hg.

Increased intraluminal pressure has no effect on thick-walled arteries, but the thin-walled veins distend and accommodate more blood (venous pooling).

Venous pooling (300–500 mL) results in decreased venous return and so the cardiac output and thence the blood pressure is also reduced.

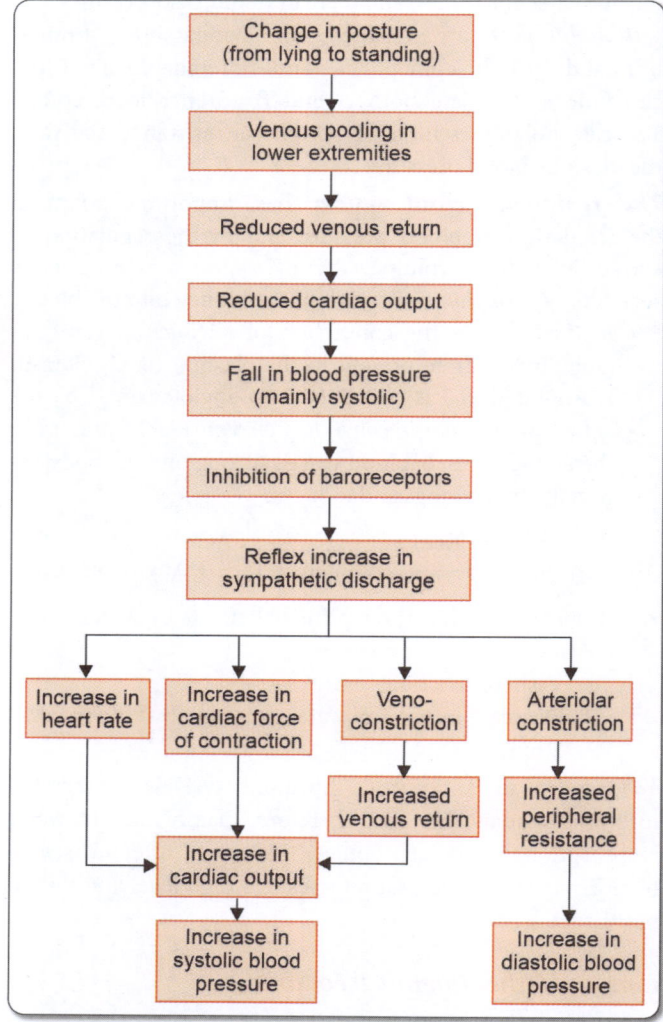

Fig. 4.2-58: Summary of events maintaining normal blood pressure during change of posture from lying to standing

A drop in the blood pressure in carotid sinus and aortic arch within seconds triggers the *baroreceptor-mediated compensatory mechanism* which causes the following changes:

- *Heart rate* is increased by 5–10 beats/min.
- *Force of cardiac contraction* is increased leading to increase in stroke volume and cardiac output.
- *Peripheral resistance* is increased due to arteriolar constriction in the cutaneous, renal and splanchnic circulation. Increase in peripheral resistance increases the diastolic pressure.
- *Venoconstriction* in the body transfers blood from the capacitance vessels toward the heart increasing the venous return.
- *Increased secretion of renin and aldosterone* which also help in normalization of blood pressure.

In spite of the above-mentioned compensatory changes the stroke volume and cardiac output in standing posture are about 25% less than in supine position.

However, due to a 25% increase in the total peripheral resistance the blood pressure becomes almost normal.

The above events are summarized in Figure 4.2-58.

Changes during Prolonged Quiet Standing

During prolonged quiet standing (a situation particularly met with military or police personnel, i.e., standing in attention for long periods), along with the venous pooling the fluid begins to accumulate in the interstitial spaces because of increased hydrostatic pressure in the capillaries. The cardiac output is decreased due to decreased venous return. A stage may come when cerebral blood flow decreases to less than about 60% and symptoms of cerebral ischemia develop. The individual may faint and fall down.

The fainting, in a sense, is also a homeostatic mechanism, because falling to horizontal position promptly restores venous return, cardiac output and cerebral blood flow to adequate levels.

CLINICAL ASPECTS

POSTURAL HYPOTENSION

Postural hypotension or orthostatic hypotension in which there occurs a sudden fall in blood pressue on changing posture from lying to erect, which causes symptoms of cerebral ischemia. The individual experiences transient blurring of vision, dizziness or even fainting. It is diagnosed by recording blood pressure in lying and standing postures. A decrease in systolic blood pressure by 30 mm Hg or more on standing from supine position is diagnostic. Postural hypotension develops in individuals in whom the cardiovascular compensatory mechanisms (described above) are very slow to develop.

CARDIOVASCULAR ADJUSTMENTS DURING MUSCULAR EXERCISE

Severe muscular exercise is the most stressful physiological condition that the cardiovascular homeostasis mechanisms face in everyday life, since, in addition to cardiovascular adjustments, respiratory and other adjustments also occur in the body.

Cardiovascular Responses to Exercise

To meet the increased energy demand of muscles during exercise the primary cardiovascular response is in the form of:

- Increase in the skeletal muscle blood flow
- Redistribution of blood flow in the body
- Increase in the cardiac output
- Blood pressure changes
- Changes in blood volume.

1. *Skeletal muscle blood flow:* At rest the blood flow to the skeletal muscle is about 2–4 mL/100 g/min of muscle tissue. During strenuous exercise muscle blood flow can increase up to 20 times, i.e., about 50–80 mL/100 g/min muscle tissue. This is called *exercise hyperemia*. This tremendous increase in muscle blood flow during exercise is made possible by:

- Arteriolar dilatation
- Opening up of closed capillaries which greatly increase the surface area and the rate of blood flow.

2. *Redistribution of blood flow:* As mentioned earlier the tremendous increase in skeletal muscle blood flow is possible due to increased cardiac output and redistribution of cardiac output in the following manner (Table 4.2-6).

TABLE 4.2-6: Redistribution of cardiac output in standing posture during exercise

	At rest	During heavy exercise	Change
Cardiac output	5 L/min	24 L/min	Increased 5–6 times
Blood flow to:			
• Skeletal muscles	750–800 mL/min	20 L/min mL/min	25 times
• Heart	250 mL/min	1 L/min	4 times
• Brain	750 mL/min	750 mL/min	No change
• Viscera	2600 mL/min	500 mL/min	Decreased by 80%
• Skin	500 mL/min	400 mL/min	Initially decreased
		1000 mL/min	Later increased

Coronary blood flow. During exercise coronary blood flow is increased by 4–5 times with 100% O_2 utilization. This occurs due to:

- *Increased coronary blood flow* due to sympathetic stimulation
- *Coronary vasodilatation.*

Visceral blood flow is temporarily curtailed in coordination with increase in muscle blood flow. It is brought about by the increased sympathoadrenal discharge.

Splanchnic blood flow is decreased by 80% in severe exercise.

Renal blood flow is also decreased by 50–80% in severe exercise.

Cutaneous blood flow at rest is about 500 mL/min.

- *Decrease* in cutaneous blood flow occurs initially in the beginning of exercise due to reflex vasoconstriction.
- When body temperature rises, to dissipate the heat generated during exercise, the blood flow through the skin increases.

Cerebral blood flow remains unchanged.

Adipose tissue blood flow is increased by 4 times during exercise. This helps to deliver fatty acids mobilized from triglyceride stores to the working muscles.

3. *Increase in cardiac output:* Normal cardiac output is about 5–6 L/min. In maximum exercise it may increase by 5–6 times. Since, cardiac output is the product of heart rate and stroke volume, an increase in both contributes to the increase in cardiac output during exercise.

4. *Blood pressure changes during exercise:*

a. *In systemic circulation:*

- *Systolic blood pressure* is always raised by exercise since it depends upon the cardiac output which is increased in exercise.
- *Diastolic blood pressure* which primarily depends upon the peripheral resistance may mildly increase or decrease or remain unchanged. Mostly the vaso-dilatation in the skeletal muscles balances the vasoconstriction in other tissues; so diastolic blood pressure is usually not changed much.
- *Mean blood pressure* is usually increased.

b. *In pulmonary circulation:*

- *Systolic blood pressure* in pulmonary artery may rise during heavy exercise to 25 mm Hg to 30 mm Hg from 15 mm Hg to 20 mm Hg at rest
- *Diastolic blood pressure* may rise from 5 mm Hg to 8 mm Hg at rest to 8 mm Hg to 10 mm Hg
- *Mean blood pressure* may reach 15 mm Hg from 8 mm Hg to 12 mm Hg at rest.

5. *Changes in blood volume during exercise:* Blood volume during exercise is decreased by 15% resulting in hemoconcentration. Blood volume is decreased due to more plasma loss at the capillary level due to:

- Increased hydrostatic pressure in capillaries
- Increased tissue fluid osmotic pressure due to accumulation of osmotically active metabolites in tissue spaces.

The cardiovascular responses to exercise are summarized in Figure 4.2-59.

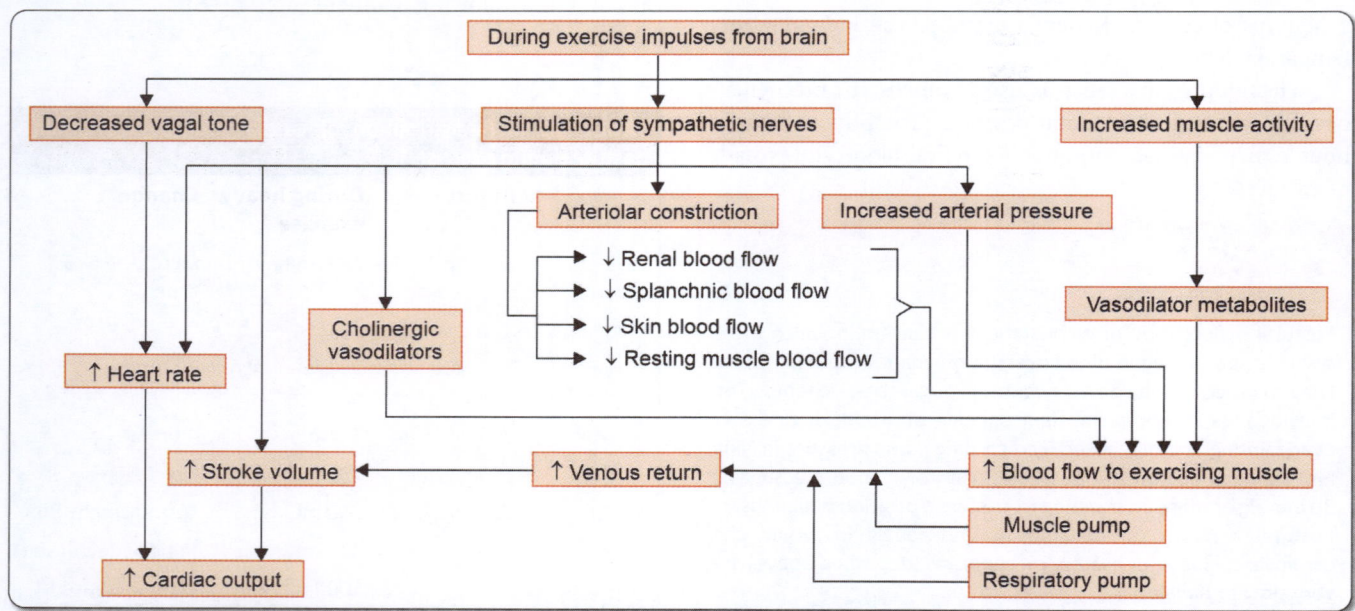

Fig. 4.2-59: Summary of cardiovascular responses to exercise

NURSING IMPLICATIONS AND APPLICATIONS

Cardiovascular homeostasis mechanism operates in almost all cardiorespiratory and many other multiorgan diseases. The most important condition which needs special description is circulatory shock.

CIRCULATORY SHOCK

Circulatory shock or simply called shock is a syndrome characterized by inadequate delivery of oxygen and nutrients to critical organs such as heart, brain, liver, kidneys and gastrointestinal tract.

Types and Causes of Shock

Depending upon the cause of inadequacy of cardiac output (relative or absolute) the circulatory shock may be of the following types:

- Hypovolemic shock
- Low-resistance or distributive or vasogenic shock
- Cardiogenic shock
- Obstructive shock.

i. Hypovolemic Shock

Hypovolemic shock also known as cold shock is caused by a low blood volume resulting in decreased cardiac output.

Depending on the causes the hypovolemic shock may be of the following types:

Hemorrhagic shock: It occurs as a result of external or internal blood loss caused by ruptured vessels.

Dehydration shock: Fluid loss when insufficient amount can dehydrate the body and reduce the circulating blood volume. Fluid loss can occur from:

- *GIT* in diarrhea or vomiting
- *Kidney* in diabetes mellitus, diabetes insipidus, or excessive use of diuretics
- *Skin* in burns.

Traumatic shock: It is a special type of hypovolemic shock in which there is associated neurogenic shock caused by severe pain which inhibits the vasomotor center.

ii. Low-resistance or Distributive or Vasogenic Shock

Low-resistance or distributive or vasogenic shock occurs when neural reflexes or toxic substances cause excessive vasodilation within the vascular system. Low-resistance shock is also called *warm shock* because skin is warm and not cold and moist as it is in hypovolemic shock. Depending upon the causes, the low-resistance shock is of the following types:

Neurogenic shock: It occurs due to:

- *Marked reduction in sympathetic vasomotor tone*
- *Pronounced increase in the vagal tone* as in vasovagal syncope or emotional fainting.

Anaphylactic shock: Anaphylaxis refers to an acute allergic reaction. Large quantities of histamine and histamine-like substances released in allergic reaction cause widespread and marked *vasodilation* reducing peripheral resistance. Also, there is marked *increase in capillary permeability* leading to fluid loss and adding hypovoltemic element to the low-resistance shock.

Septicemic shock: Septicemia is a condition in which bacteria circulate and multiply in the blood and form toxic products and cause high fever and marked vasodilatation due to peripheral arteriolar paralysis.

iii. Cardiogenic Shock

Cardiogenic shock occurs due to decreased pumping ability of the heart because of some cardiac abnormality.

Causes of cardiogenic shock are:

- Myocardial infarction
- Cardiac arrhythmias
- Congestive heart failure
- Severe valvular dysfunctions.

iv. Obstructive Shock

Obstructive shock or, to be more precise, the extracardiac obstructive shock occurs due to impairment of ventricular filling during diastole due to some external pressure on the heart. Due to decreased ventricular filling the stroke volume and hence the cardiac output is decreased causing circulatory shock.

Causes of obstructive effusion shock are:

- Pericardial cardiac tamponade, i.e., bleeding into the pericardium with external pressure on the heart
- Tension pneumothorax
- Constrictive pericarditis
- Pulmonary embolism.

Symptoms and Signs

Symptoms and signs observed in patients with shock are:

- *Pale, cold and moist skin* occurs due to decreased blood flow to skin and increased sweating (due to increased sympathetic discharge).
- *Cyanotic tinge of skin* may sometimes occur because of increased O_2 extraction from the blood.
- *Tachycardia* and *fall in pulse pressure* produce *thin and thready pulse*, the characteristic feature of hypovolemic shock.
- *Increased rate and force of respiration* is due to greater sino-aortic chemoreceptors discharge.
- *Oliguria*, another important feature of hypovolemic shock, is due to renal arteriolar constriction.
- *Restlessness and apprehension* may occur due to stimulation of brain stem reticular formation by circulating catecholamines, since hemorrhage is a potent stimulator of secretion of these hormones from the adrenal medulla.

IMPORTANT TO KNOW

Under normal circumstances the circulatory compensatory mechanisms eventually cause full recovery without help of outside therapy during the stage of non-progressive shock. However, a timely outside therapy may hasten the recovery.

Treatment of Shock with Physiological Basis

The treatment of shock is aimed at correcting the cause and helping physiological compensatory mechanisms.

Contd...

(i) General measures for shock treatment are:
- *Room temperature:* Where the patients of shock are kept should be cold. If exposed to warmth there will be sweating which will cause further hypovolemia and aggravate the shock.
- *Raising the foot end of the patient's bed* by 6" – 12" (*Trendelenburg position*) helps in promoting the venous return and thereby increasing the cardiac output. It is especially useful in hemorrhagic and neurogenic shock when the blood pressure is too low.

(ii) Replacement therapy is very useful in hypovolaemic shock.
- *In hemorrhagic shock*, the best therapy is transfusion of whole *blood*. When whole blood is not available the *plasma* may be used. Plasma maintains the colloid osmotic pressure of the blood, but the hematocrit decreases with this therapy. If neither whole blood nor plasma is available, a plasma substitute such as *dextran* may be used.

(iii) Sympathomimetic drugs are useful as:
- *Dopamine* should be the sympathomimetic drug of choice.
- Epinephrine or norepinephrine drug may also be used when dopamine is not available.

(iv) Oxygen therapy: Oxygen therapy may have some beneficial effects.

(v) Glucocorticoids: Glucocorticoids are particularly useful in anaphylactic shock.

ASSESS YOURSELF

Short and Long Answer Questions

1. **Draw a labeled diagram to show:**
   a. Phases of action potential of the cardiac muscle fiber
   b. Relation of the following events during different phases of cardiac cycle
   - Pressure changes in the left ventricle
   - Pressure changes in aorta
   - Pressure changes in right atrium
   - Volume changes in the ventricles
   - Heart sounds
2. **Describe briefly:**
   - Property of refectory period
   - All or None Law
   - Staring Law of Heart
   - Heart Rate
   - Conducting system of heart
   - Pace maker potential
3. **Define cardiac output, its determinants and regulation**
4. **Write notes on:**
   - End diastolic volume
   - Blood pressure
   - Renin-angiotensin system
   - Coronary circulation
   - Cardiovascular changes during exercise
   - Postural hypotension
   - Hemodynamics

Multiple Choice Questions

1. **The apex of the heart normally lies in which intercostal space:**
   a. 2nd
   b. 3rd
   c. 4th
   d. 5th

2. **The tricuspid valve is present between:**
   a. Superior vena cava and right atrium
   b. Pulmonary vein and left atrium
   c. Right atrium and right ventricle
   d. Left atrium and left ventricle

3. **The true statement for mitral valve is:**
   a. Is a bicuspid valve
   b. Is a tricuspid valve
   c. Is a semilunar valve
   d. Lies between right atrium and right ventricle

4. **The pericardial fluid is present between which pericardial layers:**
   a. Fibrous and serous
   b. Fibrous and visceral
   c. Serous and visceral
   d. Pericardium and epicardium

5. **Right coronary artery supplies blood to:**
   a. Anterior part of left ventricle
   b. Sinu-Atrial node
   c. Bundle of His
   d. Anterior part of inter ventricular septum

6. **Brachiocephalic artery originates from:**
   a. Ascending aorta   b. Arch of aorta
   c. Descending aorta   d. Common carotid artery

7. **Which of the following is a branch of iliac trunk:**
   a. Superior mesenteric artery
   b. Suprarenal artery
   c. Splenic artery
   d. Renal artery

8. **The true statement for basilar artery:**
   a. Is a branch of vertebral artery
   b. Supplies blood to medulla oblongata
   c. Arises directly from subclavian artery
   d. Participates in formation of circle of Willis

9. **Which is not the branch of femoral artery:**
   a. Superficial circumflex iliac artery
   b. Superficial epigastric artery
   c. Profunda femoris
   d. External iliac artery

10. **Azygos vein drains blood from:**
    a. Left side of thoracic cavity
    b. Right side of thoracic cavity
    c. Left side of abdominal wall
    d. Left side of vertebral column

11. **In cardiac muscle fiber the 0 phase of action potential occurs due to:**
    a. Efflux of Na^+
    b. Influx of Na^+
    c. Influx of K^+
    d. Efflux of Ca^{2+}

12. **The property of autoryhthmicity of cardiac muscle is because of:**
    a. Resting membrane potential
    b. Pacemaker potential
    c. Action potential
    d. All or none property

13. **QRS Complex of electrocardiogram is caused by:**
    a. Atrial depolarization
    b. Ventricular depolarization
    c. Conduction of impulse through AV node
    d. Conduction of impulse through Bundle of His

14. **The true statement for PR interval of ECG is:**
    a. Normal duration is above 0.32 sec
    b. Measured from the beginning of P wave to the end of QRS complex
    c. Measures AV conduction time
    d. Shortened in AV conduction block

15. **In normal cardiac cycle the duration of atrial systole is:**
    a. 0.1 Sec
    b. 0.3Sec
    c. 0.5 Sec
    d. 0.7 Sec

16. **In isovolumic contraction phase of ventricular systole pressure in the left ventricle increases to:**
    a. 10 mm Hg
    b. 20 mm Hg
    c. 80 mm Hg
    d. 120 mm Hg

17. **The first heart sound is produced due to:**
    a. Closure of AV valves
    b. Opening of AV valves
    c. Closure of semilunar valves
    d. Opening of semilunar valves

18. **The statement not true for Venous return:**
    a. Increased by cardiac pump
    b. Increased by muscle pump
    c. Increased by sympathetic stimulation
    d. Increased during pregnancy

19. **The condition that increases peripheral resistance is:**
    a. Increase in velocity of blood flow
    b. Increase in blood volume
    c. Increases in the viscosity of blood
    d. Turbulence in blood flow

20. **Which component of microcirculation is not innervated by sympathetic:**
    a. Arterioles
    b. Meta-arterioles
    c. Pre-capillary sphincters
    d. Capillaries

21. **For tissue fluid formation the hydrostatic pressure at arterial end of capillary is:**
    a. 0 mm Hg
    b. 10 mm Hg
    c. 25 mm Hg
    d. 32 mm Hg

22. **In which phase of cardiac cycle coronary blood supply to heart increases:**
    a. Isovolumic phase of ventricular systole
    b. Rapid ejection phase of ventricular systole
    c. Isovolumic relaxation phase of ventricular diastole
    d. Proto-diastole

23. **The statement not true for vasodilation effect is:**
    a. Decreased discharge of sympathetics
    b. Increased discharge of parasympathetics
    c. Axon reflex
    d. Administration of Ach

24. **Which of the following causes vasoconstriction:**
    a. Atrial natriuretic peptide
    b. Acetyl choline
    c. Histamine
    d. Dopamine

ANSWER KEY

1.	d	2.	b	3.	a	4.	c	5.	b	6.	b	7.	c	8.	d
9.	d	10.	b	11.	b	12.	b	13.	b	14.	c	15.	a	16.	c
17.	a	18.	d	19.	c	20.	d	21.	d	22.	c	23.	a	24.	d

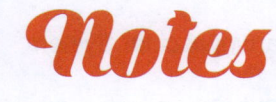

Notes

Anatomy and Physiology of Lymphatic System and Immunity

LYMPHATIC SYSTEM

GENERAL CONSIDERATIONS

The lymphatic system has been called the 'middle man' between blood and the body tissues. The whole of the tissues, however, are bathed in fluid called tissue fluid. All interchanges of nourishment and waste products between the blood and the body tissues take place through the medium of tissue fluid. Colloid material from the tissue fluid cannot re-enter the blood capillaries; hence lymph capillaries are ever present to receive colloids, as well as, electrolytes, water, and other substances and return them to the blood stream. The lymphatic system is, therefore, a subsidiary or second circulatory system, which drains the tissue fluids.

Constituents of Lymphatic System

Lymph is, thus, the interstitial fluid that flows into the lymphatic capillaries. From the lymphatic capillaries, the lymph passes through vessels of successively increasing size and a large number of lymph nodes before entering the blood. The lymphatic system, thus, comprises:
- The lymph
- Lymphatic vessels
- Lymph nodes, and other lymph organs.

Functions of Lymphatic System

Returns proteins from tissue spaces to blood. The lymphatic system recovers approximately 200 g of protein daily that has been lost from the microcirculation.

Absorption of nutrients, especially fats, from the gastrointestinal tract.

Acts as transport mechanism to remove red blood cells that have lost into the tissues as a result of hemorrhage.

Supplies nutrients and oxygen to those parts where blood cannot reach.

Role in defence mechanism. Lymph nodes associated with lymphatic system act as efficient filters. They have sinuses lined with phagocytic cells that engulf bacteria, red cells and other particulate material.

LYMPH

Lymph is essentially the name given to the tissue fluid when it has entered the lymphatics.

Formation and Composition
Formation

The formation of lymph is closely associated with the formation of tissue fluid.

As discussed in capillary exchange, most (90%) of the fluid filtered at arterial end of the capillary is reabsorbed at its venous end; and the remaining 10% enters the circulation through lymphatics and is called lymph. Thus, the lymph is a transudate formed from blood in the tissue spaces, i.e., it is derived from the interstitial fluid.

Composition

Composition is similar to plasma except that:

Protein content is usually lower than that of plasma (2–5 g%). Protein content of the lymph usually varies with the region it drains.

Fat content. Since, the lymphatic system also provides a route of absorption of long-chained fatty acids and cholesterol from the intestine (in the form of *chylomicrons*), therefore, after a fatty meal these fat globules may be so numerous that lymph becomes milky and is then called *chyle*.

Cellular content. Suspended in the lymph are cells that are chiefly lymphocytes. Most of these lymphocytes are added to the lymph as it passes through lymph nodes.

Lymph Flow

Lymph enters the lymphatic capillaries under the influence of osmotic pressure of tissue fluid. The flow of lymph in the lymph vessels, like venous blood, is under low pressure and is controlled largely by the outside forces which include:

- Contraction of smooth muslces in the walls of large lymph vessels
- Contraction of skeletal muscles
- Movements of different body parts
- Arterial pulsations
- Compression of tissue by objects outside the body
- Negative intrathorcic pressure and action of respiratory muscles.

IMPORTANT TO KNOW

Normal lymph flow is 2–4 L/day (80–150 mL/hour) for the entire body.

Rate of lymph flow varies in different organs and is highest in the gastrointestinal tract and the liver.

In lymphatics rate of lymph flow is 100 mL/hour through thoracic duct and about 20 mL/hour through other lymphatic channels.

LYMPH VESSELS

The lymphatic system constitutes an accessory route for the removal of interstitial fluid. The small lymph vessels are called lymph capillaries and the large lymph vessels are called lymphatic trunks and the largest lymph vessel is thoracic duct.

Lymph Capillaries

The lymph capillaries originate as closed endothelial tubes that are permeable to fluid and high-molecular weight compounds.

Structure of lymph capillaries (Fig. 4.3-1) is basically similar to that of blood capillaries with the following differences:

- The basal lamina around the endothelial cells is absent or poorly developed
- Pericytes or connective tissue are not present around the lymph capillaries
- There are no visible fenestrations in the endothelium
- The junctions between endothelial cells are open. In fact, the edges of the endothelial cells overlap in such a way that they form minute flap valves.

Lymphatic Vessels

The lymphatic capillaries are present in most tissues of the body except brain, cartilage, splenic pulp, bone marrow and avascular structures (e.g. cornea, crystalline lens, nail and hairs). The lymphatic capillaries join to form the lymphatic

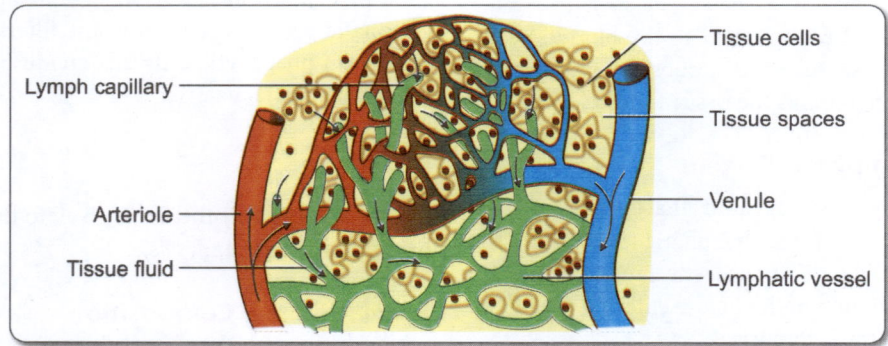

Fig. 4.3-1: Structure of lymph capillary

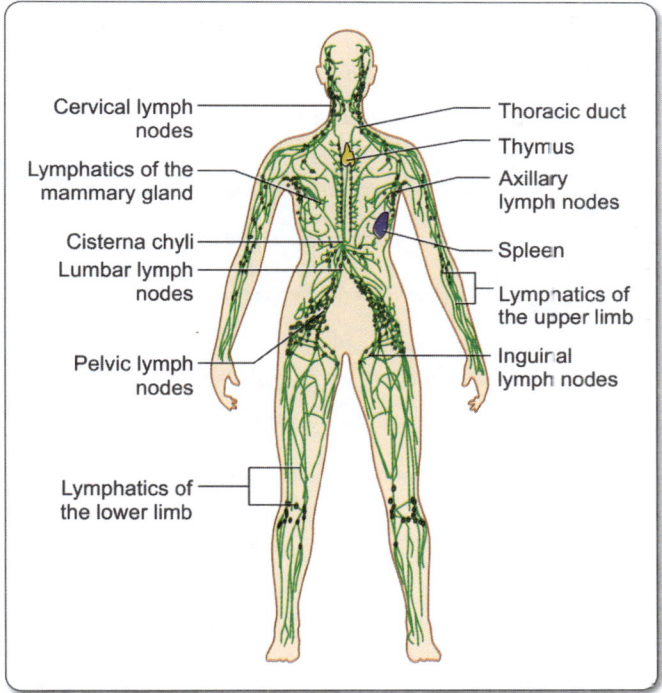

Fig. 4.3-2: Distribution of lymph vessels and lymph nodes in the human body

vessels. The lymphatic vessels are distributed throughout the body like the veins (Fig. 4.3-2). The lymphatics continue to unite and form larger and larger vessels until finally they converge to form the lymphatic trunks and collecting ducts.

Lymphatic Trunks and Collecting Ducts
Lymphatic Trunks

The lymphatic trunks are larger lymph vessels which drain lymph from relatively large regions of the body, and they are named for the region with which they are associated. Examples of lymphatic trunks include (Fig. 4.3-2):

Lumbar trunk. It drains lymph from the lower limbs, lower abdominal wall, and the pelvic organs.

Intestinal trunk. It drains lymph from the various viscera of abdomen.

Intercostal trunk. It drains from portions of thorax.

Bronchomediastinal trunk. It also receives lymph from the portion of thorax.

Subclavian trunk. It drains lymph from the upper limb.

Jugular trunk. It drains lymph from portions of the neck and head.

Collecting Ducts

The lymphatic trunks then join to form two collecting ducts—the thoracic duct and right lymphatic duct (Figs 4.3-2 and 4.3-3).

Thoracic Duct

It is the largest lymph vessel in the body. It carries lymph from both sides of the body below the diaphragm and from the left side above the diaphragm. Near its termination, it receives the *left subclavian lymphatic trunks* carrying lymph from left upper limb, the *left jugular lymphatic trunk* carrying lymph from left half of head and neck, and sometimes the *left bronchomediastinal lymphatic trunk* carrying lymph from left half of thorax (usually this trunk enters the subclavian vein independently).

The thoracic duct ends by opening into the junction of the left subclavian vein and the internal jugular vein (Fig. 4.3-3).

Right Lymphatic Duct

Right lymphatic duct drains lymph from the right half of the body above the diaphragm. It is formed by the *right bronchomediastinal trunk* carrying lymph from the right half of thorax, *right jugular trunk* draining lymph from the right half of head and neck, and *right subclavian trunk* carrying lymph from the right upper limb. The right lymphatic duct ends by opening into the right subclavian vein (Fig. 4.3-3).

Structure of Larger Lymph Vessels

Structure of larger lymph vessels is similar to that of veins:

- *Three coats,* i.e., tunica intima, tunica media and tunica adventitia can be distinguished.
- *Valves* similar to those in veins are present in abundance in small as well as large lymphatic vessels. The valves often give lymph vessels a beaded appearance.

LYMPHATIC ORGANS AND TISSUES

The lymphoid component of the immune system consists of a network of lymphoid organs, tissues and cells and the product of these cells. Lymphoid organs can be classified into:

Central or primary lymphoid organs, which include:
- Thymus
- Bursa equivalent (fetal liver and bone marrow)

Peripheral lymphoid organs which include:
- Lymph nodes
- Spleen
- Mucosa associated lymphoid tissues (MALT).

Primary (Central) Lymphoid Tissues
Thymus

The thymus gland is located in mediastinum just above the heart. It consists of many lobules. Histologically, each lobule consists of outer *cortex* and inner *medulla*. Both cortex and medulla contain *epithelial cells* and *thymocytes*. The main function of the thymus is development of cell-mediated immunity.

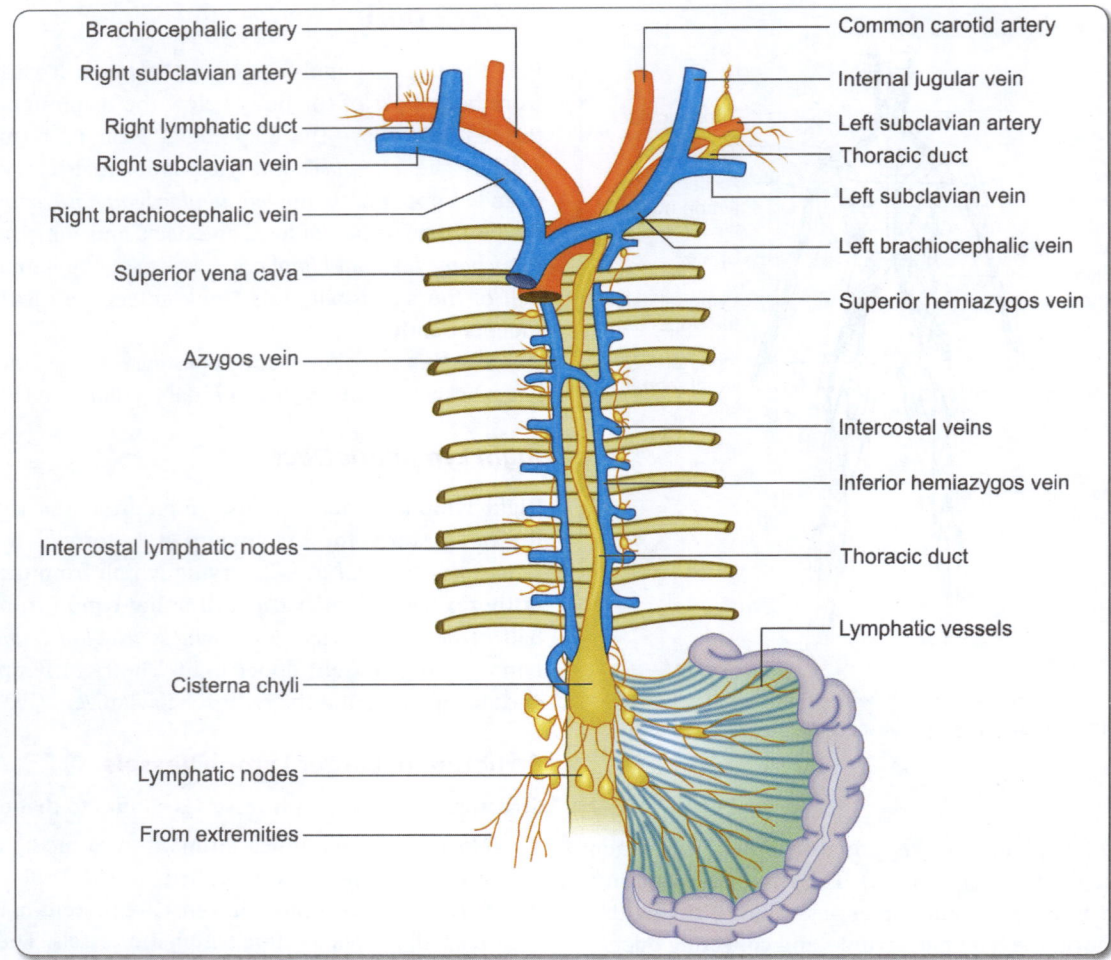

Fig. 4.3-3: The thoracic duct and right lymphatic duct

Bursa Equivalent

In the human being the fetal liver and bone marrow appear to be the equivalent of avian bursa of Fabricius. *Bursa of Fabricius* in birds is also a site of lymphocytic proliferation and differentiation. Immunocompetent lymphocytes produced in the bursa are called bursa lymphocytes or B lymphocytes or B cells. The mature B cells migrate from the bursa into outer or superficial cortex of the germinal follicles and medullary cords of lymph nodes and lymphoid follicles of spleen. These sites are known as *bursa-dependent* or *thymus-independent* areas.

Peripheral Lymphoid Organs

Lymph Nodes

The lymph nodes are small bean-shaped or oval structures which form part of lymphatic network distributed throughout the body.

Structural characteristics of lymph node (Fig. 4.3-4)

Capsule of connective tissue covers each lymph node. From the capsule, trabeculae penetrate into the lymph node.

Afferent lymphatics enter into each lymph node at its convex surface and drain into the peripheral subcapsular sinus.

Efferent lymphatics leave the lymph node at the concavity (hilum) as a single large lymph vessel.

Microscopic structure

Microscopically, the lymph node consists of two parts—peripheral cortex and central medulla.

Cortex of the lymph node consists of several rounded aggregates of lymphocytes called *lymphoid follicles*, representing B cell area of the node.

Paracortex is deeper part of cortex, i.e., the zone between the peripheral cortex and the inner medulla and represents the T-cell area (the *bursa-independent area*).

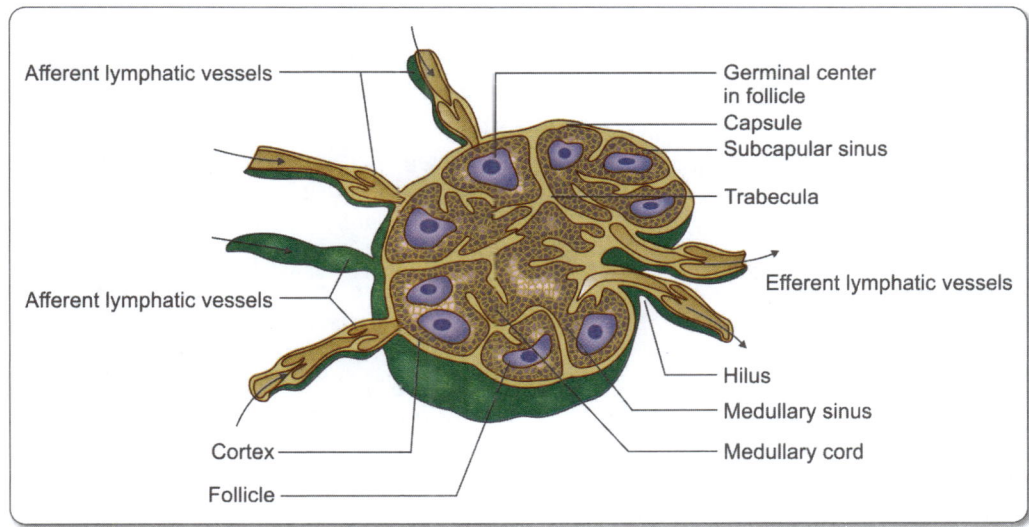

Fig. 4.3-4: Structure of a lymph node

Medulla is predominantly composed of cords of plasma cells and some lymphocytes (*medullary cords*).

Location of lymph nodes

There are many groups of lymph nodes in the body, arranged in superficial and deep sets (just as there are superficial and deep sets of lymphatics). Occasionally, a lymph node exists alone; mostly they are found in groups or chains. Superficial nodes are arranged along the veins and deep nodes along the arteries. Location of some of the important lymph node groups is as follows:

Head and neck region lymph nodes are:

Superficial lymph nodes, draining the superficial tissues of the head and neck, are (Fig. 4.3-5):

- Occipital lymph nodes
- Retroauricular lymph nodes
- Parotid lymph nodes
- Submandibular lymph nodes
- Submental lymph nodes
- Superficial cervical lymph nodes.

Deep cervical lymph nodes. Lymph from all the superficial lymph nodes mentioned above drains into deep cervical lymph nodes which are located along the internal juguar vein (Fig. 4.3-2).

Shoulder girdle and upper limb region lymph nodes includes

Axillary lymph nodes, located in the axilla, are the chief lymph nodes draining the upper limbs, skin and muscle of chest, back and upper half of abdomen. Axillary lymph nodes are superficial nodes arranged in many groups (Fig. 4.3-2).

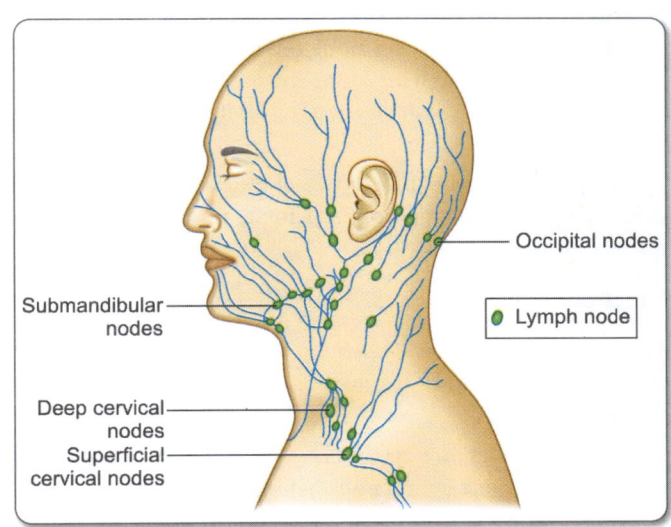

Fig. 4.3-5: Lymph nodes of head and neck region

Other lymph nodes of upper limb not of much significance are:
- *Supratrochlear lymph nodes* (one or two nodes) lying just above the medial epicondyle of humerus.
- *Infraclavicular lymph nodes* (one or two nodes) lie just below the clavicle.

Thorax region. The lymph nodes of the thorax region are divided into:

Parietal nodes of thoracic region, which drain the thoracic wall, include parasternal lymph nodes, intercostal lymph nodes and diaphragmatic lymph nodes.

Visceral sets of thoracic lymph nodes include brachiocephalic lymph nodes, posterior mediastinal lymph nodes and tracheobronchial lymph nodes which drain lymph from the thoracic viscera.

Abdominal and pelvic region ymph nodes. The lymph nodes draining the abdominal and pelvic viscera are arranged along the aorta and its major branches, and are named accordingly, e.g.:

- *Aortic lymph nodes (lateral, retro, and preaortic)*
- *Coeliac lymph nodes*
- *Superior mesenteric lymph nodes*
- *Inferior mesenteric lymph nodes*
- *Common iliac lymph nodes*
- *External iliac lymph nodes*
- *Internal iliac lymph nodes.*

Lower limb region lymph nodes include:

Inguinal lymph nodes, located in the groin region, are the chief lymph nodes draining the lower limbs. They are arranged in the following group (Fig. 4.3-2):

- *Superficial inguinal lymph nodes*
    - Upper group lying along the inguinal ligament
    - Lower group lying along the great saphenous vein.
- *Deep inguinal lymph nodes*, lying along the medial side of femoral vein.

Popliteal lymph nodes, one or two in number, of insignificant existence present in the popliteal fossa are the other lymph nodes of lower limb.

Functions of lymph nodes

To mount immune response in the body. Processing of antigens and antibody production occurs in the lymphoid follicles.

The lymph nodes act as inline filters. Lymph must pass through at least one lymph node before mixing with the blood stream. Over 99% of the lymph passes through the lymph sinuses and only 1% penetrates the lymphoid follicles.

NURSING IMPLICATIONS AND APPLICATIONS

- The cancer cells are also carried by the lymph vessels. Therefore, for metastatic point of view knowledge about lymphatic drainage is important.
- During examination palpation of lymph nodes (in the neck, axilla and inguinal region) must be done. If there is enlargement of the lymph nodes is noted then fine needle aspiration cytology (FNAC)to be done for proper diagnosis and treatment.

Spleen

The spleen is the largest lymphoid organ of the body. The average weight of the spleen is about 150 g.

Structural characteristics of spleen are shown in (Figure 4.3-6)

Capsule of connective tissue surrounds the spleen. From the capsule connective tissue *trabeculae* extend into the pulp of the organ and serve as supportive network. The spleen consists of homogeneous, soft, dark red mass called *red pulp*. In the red pulp are seen scattered white nodules called *white pulp* (Malpighian bodies).

Microscopically, the structural characteristics are:

- *Red pulp* consists of the thin-walled *blood sinuses* with *splenic cords* between them.
- *White pulp* consists of lymphocytes surrounding an eccentrically placed central artery.

Functions of spleen

Role in immune response. The spleen is an active site for production of T and B lymphocytes and antibodies.

Role in removal of old RBCs, *WBCs and platelets.* Tissue macrophages present in the spleen play important role in removal of old RBCs, WBCs and platelets.

Role in hematopoiesis. During 4th and 5th month of fetal life, erythropoiesis occurs in spleen.

Role in iron metabolism. Spleen macrophages recycle the iron liberated from the phagocytozed RBCs, for synthesis of fresh hemoglobin in the bone marrow.

Role as a reservoir. Spleen serves as a reservoir for mobilization of RBCs in some animals like cat and dog. In human being spleen serves as reservoir for *platelets*.

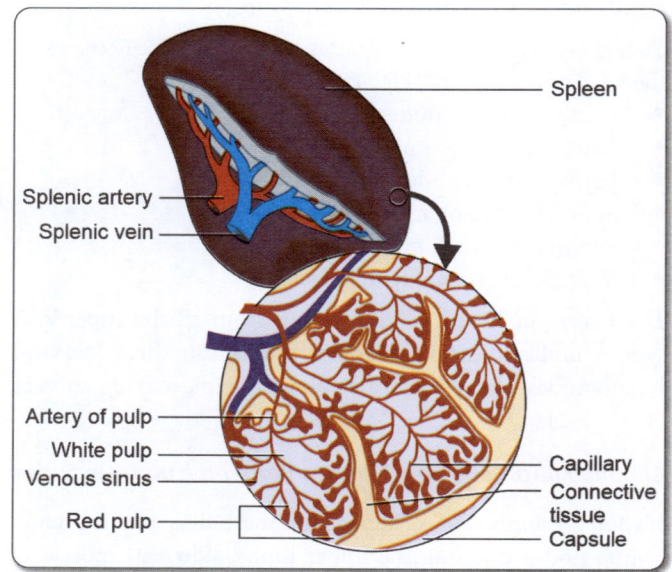

Fig. 4.3-6: Structural characteristics of spleen

Mucosa-Associated Lymphoid Tissue

Mucosa associated lymphoid tissue (MALT) includes: Tonsils, adenoids and Peyer's patches of small intestine also known as gut-associated lymphoid tissue (GALT). GALT plays a primary role in defence against infectious organisms entering via the gastrointestinal tract (GIT).

ARCHITECTURE OF IMMUNE SYSTEM

The immune system consists of immunological cells distributed in two main components:

1. Mononuclear-phagocytic system
2. Lymphoid component.

MONONUCLEAR-PHAGOCYTIC SYSTEM

Mononuclear-phagocytic system (MPS) also known as *tissue-macrophage system* is the new name given to the system previously called *reticuloendothelial system (RES)*.

Constituent Cells of Mononuclear-phagocytic System

The mononuclear-phagocytic system includes the following constituents:

- Precursor cells of the monocyte series
- Promonocytes
- Monocytes from the bone marrow and blood.

Functions of Mononuclear-phagocytic System

The mononuclear-phagocytic system (MPS) plays the following roles in the body:

- Role in inflammation and healing
- Role in defence against the bacteria invading the body tissues
- Role in the immune response
- Role in removal of old RBCs, WBCs and platelets.

IMMUNITY

Immunity refers to resistance of the body to pathogens and their toxic products. It can be classified as:

Innate immunity

- Nonspecific
- Specific innate immunity

Acquired immunity

- Active acquired immunity
- Passive acquired immunity.

Innate Immunity

Innate or natural immunity is the inborn capacity of the body to offer resistance to pathogens and their toxic products. It is due to genetic and constitutional make up of an individual. It may be *specific* (against a particular organism) or *nonspecific*.

Mechanisms of Innate Immunity

Mechanical barrier. The intact skin and mucosa in the body act as barrier against invading microorganism.

Surface secretions constitute one of the important mechanisms of innate immunity. These include:

- *Secretions* from the sebacious glands of skin kill many bacteria and fungi
- *Saliva*
- *Gastric juice*
- *Tears.*

Humoral defence mechanisms provide innate immunity by the nonspecific microbicidal substances present in the body fluids, e.g. *lysozyme*, *basic polypeptides*, *complements* and *interferons* (antiviral substances).

Cellular mechanisms of defence which provide non-specific innate immunity are:

- *Phagocytes*, i.e., neutrophils and the monocyte-macrophage system cells constitute the most important nonspecific cellular defence against the invading microorganisms.
- *Natural killer (NK) cells* refer to a subpopulation of lymphocytes which provide nonspecific cellular defence against viruses, tumor cells and other infected cells.
- *Eosinophil* granules contain enzymes and toxic molecules that act against larvae of helminths.

Acquired Immunity

The resistance that an individual acquires during his lifetime is known as acquired immunity. It is antigen-specific and may be antibody-mediated or cell-mediated. It is of two types: Active and passive.

Active Immunity

Active immunity is acquired by the synthesis of antibodies (humoral immunity) and production of immunocompetent cells (cell-mediated immunity) by the individual's own immune system in response to antigenic stimulation. Active immunity can be induced naturally or artificially.

Natural active immunity. Natural active immunity results either from a subclinical or clinical infection. For example, natural active immunity to poliomyelitis.

Artificial active immunity. Artificially, the active immunity is induced by introducing antigens in the body in the form of vaccines and this process is called *active immunization*. The vaccines are preparations of live or killed microorganisms or their products. Examples of vaccines are:

Bacterial vaccines:
- *Live:* BCG vaccine for tuberculosis
- *Killed:* TAB vaccine for typhoid

Bacterial product vaccines:
- Tetanus toxoid
- Diphtheria toxoid

Viral vaccines:
- *Live:* Sabin vaccine for poliomyelitis, mumps measles and rubella (MMR) vaccine for measles, mumps and rubella, and
- *Killed:* Salk vaccine for poliomyelitis, neural and non-neural vaccines for rabies.

Passive Immunity

Passive immunity refers to the immunity that is transferred to a recipient in a ready-made form. Here the individual's immune system does not play active role.

Natural passive immunity is transfer of ready-made antibodies from the mother as:
- *In fetus* the IgG antibodies are transferred from the mother through the placenta.
- *After birth*, immunoglobulins are passed to the newborn through the breast milk. Human colostrum is rich in IgA antibodies which are resistant to digestion in stomach and small intestine.

Immunization of pregnant women with tetanus toxoid is recommended in countries where neonatal tetanus is common.

Artificial passive immunity. Artificially, passive immunity can be transferred to the recipients by injecting readymade antibodies. This is done by administration of hyperimmune sera. Examples of artificial passive immunity include injection of:
- *Antitetanus serum (ATS)*
- *Antidiphtheric serum (ADS)*
- *Antigas gangrene serum (AGS).*

The passively administered antibodies are removed by metabolism. Therefore, immunity conferred is short-lived.

ANTIGENS

Antigens are substances that can stimulate an immune response in the body. Most antigens are proteins, but some are carbohydrates, lipids and nucleic acids. The specificity of an antigen is due to specific areas of its molecule called *determinant sites* or *epitopes*.

Some Facts about Antigenicity

Immunogenicity, i.e., ability of an antigen to stimulate an immune response.

Antigen specificity is determined by chemical grouping and acid radicals.

Species specificity. Tissues of all individuals in a species contain species-specific antigens. However, some degree of cross-reactivity is seen between antigens from related species.

Isoantigens are the antigens which are found in some but not all members of a species. On the basis of isoantigens a species may be divided into different groups. The best example of isoantigens is human blood group antigens on the basis of which all humans can be divided into blood groups A, B, AB and O.

Histocompatibility Antigens

Histocompatibility antigens refer to the antigens present on the plasma membrane of cells of each individual of a species. These antigens are encoded by genes known as histocompatibility genes which collectively constitute major histocompatibility complex (MHC). These are present on the surface of leucocytes known as human leucocyte associated antigens (HLA). No two persons except identical twins have the same MHC proteins.

There are two subclasses of MHC genes:
1. **MHC class I** molecules are found on the surface of virtually all the cells of the body excluding red blood cells.
2. **MHC class II.** In man, MHC class II antigens are only found on immunologically reactive cells such as B lymphocytes, macrophages, monocytes and activated T lymphocytes.

ANTIBODIES

Antibodies or immunoglobulins (Igs) are gamma globulins, which are produced in response to antigenic stimulation. These react specifically with the antigens, which stimulated their production. All antibodies are immunoglobulins but all immunoglobulins are not antibodies. Immunoglobulins have been divided into five distinct classes or isotypes namely IgG, IgA, IgM, IgD and IgE.

Structure of Antibody

IgG has been studied extensively. It serves as a model of basic structural unit of all immunoglobulins. An immunoglobulin is a Y-shaped molecule made of four polypeptide chains: 2 heavy

(H) and 2 light (L). These are held together by disulphide bonds (Fig. 4.3-7).

Functions

The specific functions of various immunoglobulins appear as

- *IgG* protects the body fluids
- *IgA* protects the body surfaces
- *IgM* protects the blood stream
- *IgE* mediates type I hypersensitivity
- *IgD's* role is not clearly known.

DEVELOPMENT OF IMMUNE RESPONSE

Development of immune response implies *development of acquired active immunity* in the body. The immune system of the body responds to an antigen by two ways:

1. Humoral or antibody-mediated immunity (AMI)
2. Cell-mediated immunity (CMI).

Development of Humoral Immunity

The humoral immunity is mediated by antibodies and so is also called antibody-mediated immunity (AMI). The antibodies are produced by plasma cells which in turn are produced by B lymphocytes.

Role of Humoral Immunity

- The humoral immunity provides defence against most extracellular bacterial pathogens and viruses that infect through the respiratory and intestinal tract.
- It participates in immediate hypersensitivity reactions of type I, II and III.
- Humoral immunity is also associated with certain autoimmune diseases.

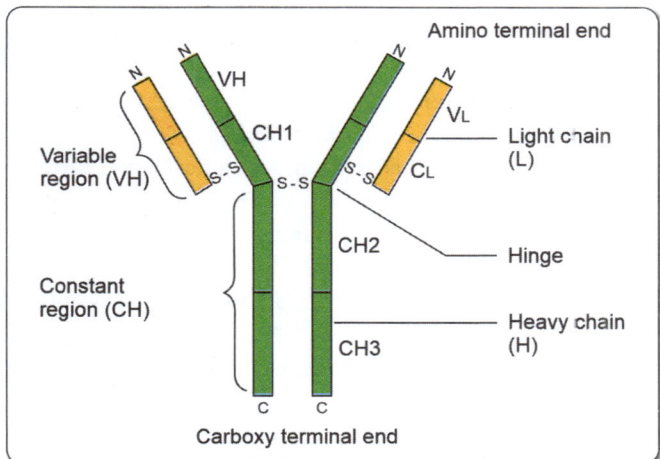

Fig. 4.3-7: Basic structure of an antibody showing the arrangement of heavy and light chains and its variable and constant domains

Types of Humoral Immune Responses

The antibody response to stimulation by antigen is of two types (Fig. 4.3-8):

1. *Primary response* refers to the response of the body's immune system to an antigen which is introduced into the body for the first time. Always there is a latent period varying from 4 days to 4 weeks before the primary response in the form of a rise in the serum antibodies titer can be detected.

2. *Secondary response* refers to the response of the body's immune system to an antigen which is introduced into the body on a second occasion. Such a response occurs more quickly and more abundantly. This is because of the fact that the immune system is liable to retain the memory of a prior antigenic exposure for long periods (immunological memory) and produce enhanced response when encountered with the same antigen for the second time.

Stages of Humoral Immune Response (Fig. 4.3-9)

1. *Antigen processing and presentation.* Once the antigen enters the body, it is phagocytosed by the macrophages (nonspecific response), broken down into polypeptide fragments. The fragments of the processed antigen are then presented to immunocompetent lymphocytes by the macrophages. So, the macrophages are also called *antigen presenting cells.*

2. *Recognition of antigen by lymphocytes.* Processed antigen then bind to specific receptors that present on the surface of lymphocytes is called *recognition of antigen by lymphocytes.* Thus many million different T and B lymphocytes, each with the ability to respond to particular antigen, are present in the body.

3. *Lymphocyte activation.* The lymphocytes that have combined with antigen are activated, i.e., the lymphocytes become larger and look like a lymphoblast. This is known as *blast transformation.* Activated B lymphocytes and helper T

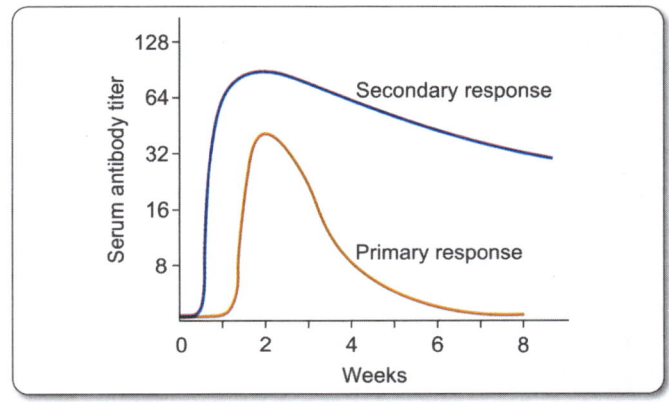

Fig. 4.3-8: Response of body immune system to an antigen

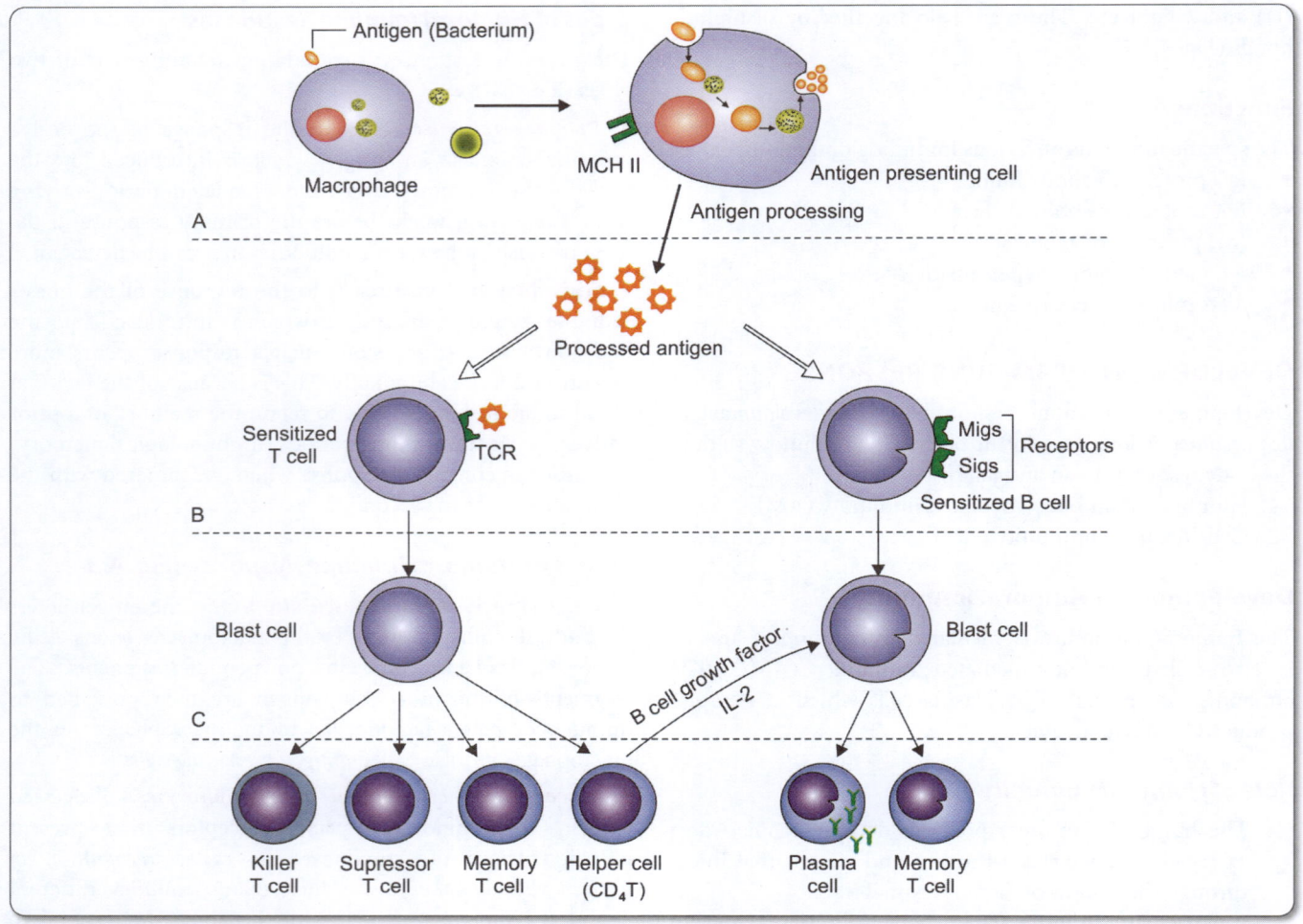

Figs 4.3-9A to C: Broad outline of development of humoral immune response: A. Antigen processing and presentation to immunocompetent cell; B. Recognition of antigen by the lymphocytes; C. Activation of lymphocytes (blast transformation)

cells (CD4 cells) play major role in humoral immunity. The B lymphocytes proliferate and transform into:

- Plasma cells
- Memory B cells.

> **IMPORTANT TO KNOW**
>
> - *Role of plasma cells*: The plasma cells secrete antibodies.
> - *Role of memory B cells*: Memory B cells have a long lifespan and remain inactive. When the body is exposed to the same antigen for the second time, they are able to recognize it, become active, i.e., they are responsible for secondary response of antibodies.

4. *Production of antibodies.* The plasma cells so formed secrete antibodies which are also called immunoglobulins (IGS). Each plasma cell produces about 2000 molecules of antibodies per second. A plasma cell secretes an antibody of a single specificity.

5. *Inactivation of antigen or attack phase or effector phase of immune response.* Antibodies act on the invading antigen in two ways:

a. *Direct attack on the invading agents.* Antibodies can inactivate the invading agent by the following reactions:

- *Agglutination:* By this reaction, a large number of particles (bacteria or red cells) with antigens on their surface are bound together to form a clump. Clumping increases the susceptibility to phagocytosis.
- *Precipitation:* In this reaction antigen-antibody complex forms insoluble precipitate.
- *Neutralization:* Antibodies cover the toxic sites of antigen and neutralize them.
- *Cytolysis:* Antibodies attack the membranes of cellular agents thereby causing rupture of cells.

b. *Attack on the antigen through complement system.* The complement system includes 11 enzymatic proteins which are named as C1 to C9, B and D. All these are present in the blood as plasma proteins. These are also present in the tissue fluid.

Development of Cellular Immune Response

The cellular immunity refers to specific acquired immunity which is accomplished by effector T cells and macrophages (Fig. 4.3-10). It is also called cell-mediated immunity (CMI).

Role of Cellular Immunity

- Cellular immunity protects the host against fungi, most of the viruses and intracellular bacterial pathogens, like *Mycobacterium tuberculosis*, *M. leprae* and *Brucella*.
- It participates in allograft rejection and graft versus host reaction.
- CMI participates in delayed hypersensitivity reaction.
- CMI is also associated with certain autoimmune diseases.
- It provides immunological surveillance and immunity against cancer (tumor immunity).

Types of Cellular Immune Response

Like humoral immune response, the cellular immune response is also of two types:

1. *Primary cellular response* which is produced by initial contact with a foreign antigen.

2. *Secondary cellular response* which is produced when the host is subsequently exposed to the same antigen. The secondary cell-mediated immune response is usually more pronounced and occurs more rapidly.

Stages of Cellular Immune Response

Antigen processing and presentation

Antigen entering the host body is phagocytosed and degraded into polypeptide fragments by the antigen processing cells (APCs) which include macrophages and dendritic cells present in the peripheral lymphoid tissue. The antigen polypeptide fragments then become associated with MHC antigen and are expressed on the surface of APC.

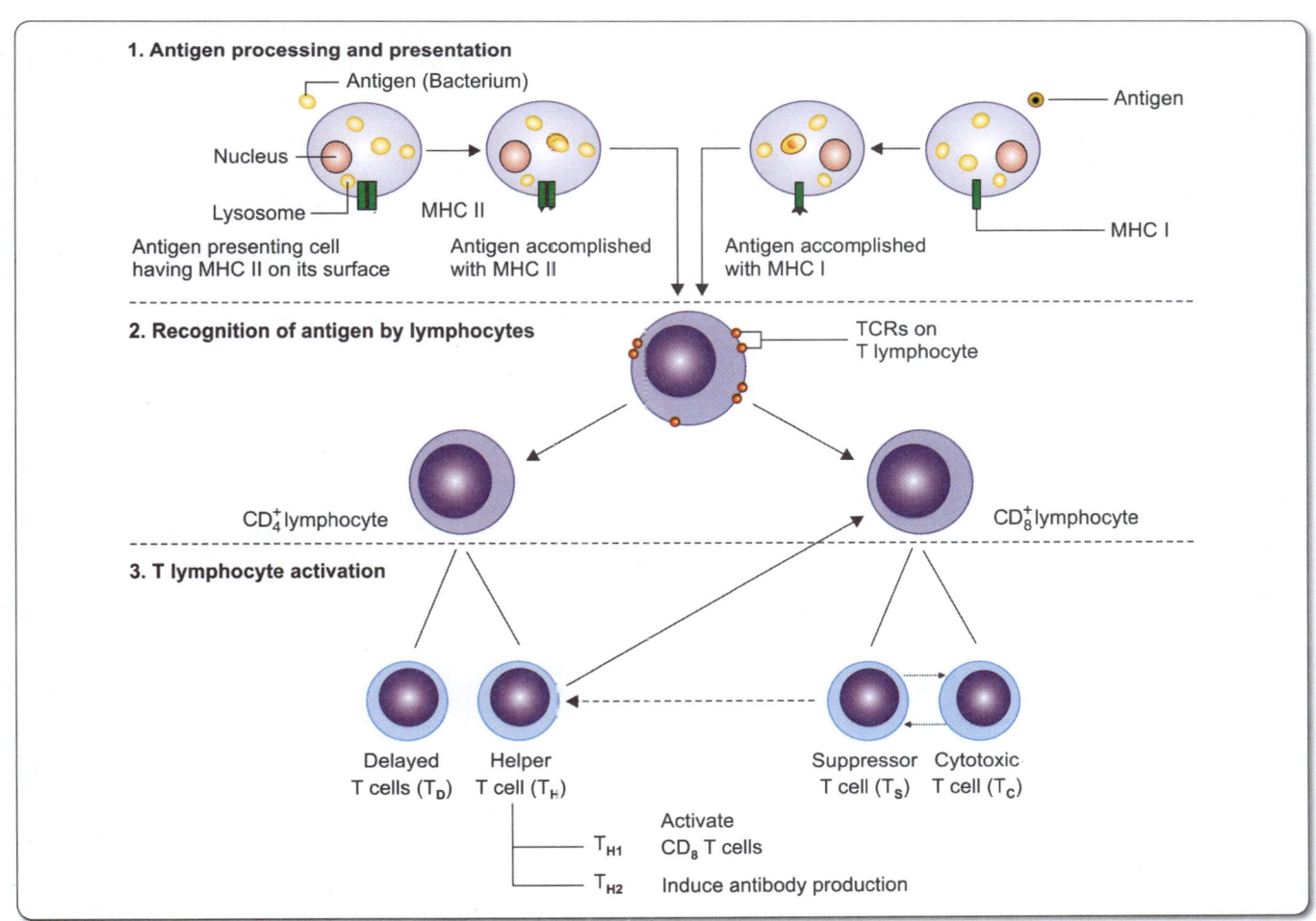

Fig. 4.3-10: Broad outline of development of cellular immune response

Recognition of antigen by lymphocytes

The T lymphocytes possess the antigenic recognition receptors known as *T cell receptors* (TCRs). Further, the mature T lymphocytes can be differentiated into two antigenic subtypes CD_4^+ cells and CD_8^+ cells.

1. CD_8^+ cells recognize the combination of foreign antigen and class I MHC antigen
2. CD_4^+ cells recognize the combination of foreign antigen and class II MHC antigen.

T lymphocyte differentiation (activation)

The CD_8^+ type of T lymphocytes after combining with foreign antigen MHC I complex are activated and differentiated into:
- Cytotoxic T cells (Tc cells)
- Suppressor T cells (Ts cells).

CD_4^+ type of T lymphocytes after combining with foreign antigen MHC-II complex are activated and differentiated into:
- Helper T cells (T_H cells)
- Delayed type hypersensitivity T cells (TD cells).

T-T cooperation. The differentiation of T lymphocytes into T_H, T_C, T_S and T_D cells is interdependent. This interdependence is called T-T cooperation.

Release of differentiated T cells. The differentiated T lymphocytes so formed are released into the lymph and then enter the blood and are distributed throughout the body.

The T lymphocytes circulate again and again throughout the body sometimes lasting for months or years.

T lymphocyte memory cells are also formed. These spread throughout the lymphoid tissues of entire body of T cells occurs far more rapidly and much more powerfully than in first response (secondary response).

Attack phase of cell-mediated immunity is as under.

Role of cytotoxic T cells. (Tc cells) and natural killer cells (NK cells) are responsible for the attack phase of cell-mediated immunity.

Role of helper T cells (T_H cells). Helper T cells are of two types: T_H^1 and T_H^2.

1. *Helper T_1 (T_H^1) cells* play their roles by secreting three cytokines:
   a. *Interleukin 2 (IL-2)*
   b. *γ interferon (IFN-γ)* has the direct ability to kill antigen bearing cells.
   c. *Tumor necrosis factor-B (TNF-B)* can induce apoptosis in antigen-bearing cells.
2. *Helper T_2 (T_H^2) cells* secrete interleukins 4, 5, 6, 10 and 13 and are primarily with activation of B lymphocytes to produce antibodies (T-B cooperation) (Fig. 4.3-11).

Role of suppressor T lymphocytes (T_S cells)
- Suppressor T cells regulate the activity of cytotoxic T cells; also suppress the activities of helper T cells.

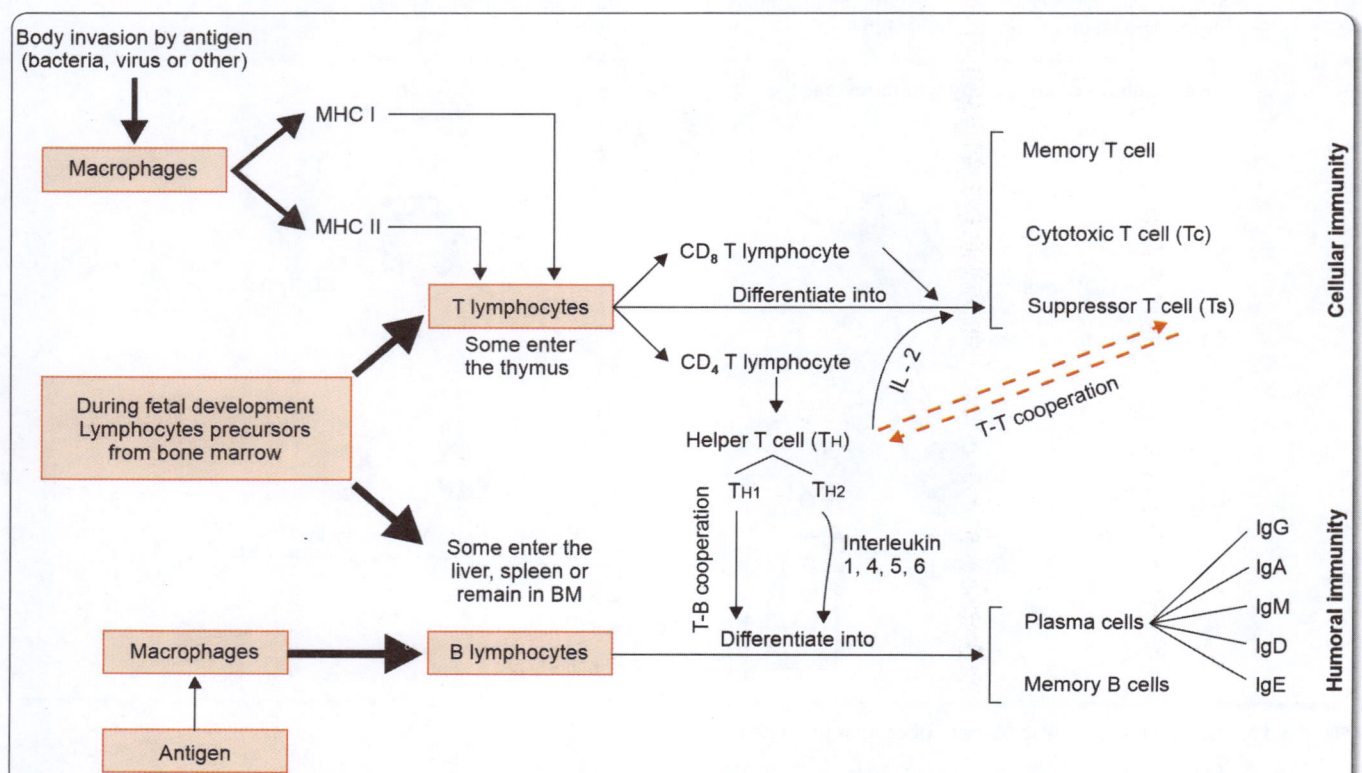

Fig. 4.3-11: Summary of immune response

IMPORTANT TO KNOW

Cytokines

Cytokines are small protein molecules which act like hormones to regulate immune response.

The cytokines are secreted not only by lymphocytes and macrophages but also by endothelial cells, neuroglia cells, and other types of cells. Broadly, cytokines can be grouped as:

Interleukins (IL). These are the principal cytokines and include IL-1 to IL-13.

Other cytokines include:
- Chemokines
- Growth factors
- Colony stimulating factors
- Tumor necrotic factors (TNF α and TNF β)
- Interferons (IFN).

CLINICAL ASPECTS

IMMUNE TOLERANCE

Immune tolerance may be defined as a state of unresponsiveness to an antigen. It occurs in two forms:

1. *Natural tolerance* refers to nonresponsiveness to a self-antigen. During embryonic development, when immune system is immature, any antigen which comes in contact with immature immune system is recognized as self-antigen. Therefore, it does not evoke any response in later life when body is exposed to the same antigen.
2. *Acquired tolerance* means unresponsiveness to a potential antigen. It results due to impairment of immune system; hence there is lack of responsiveness to potential antigens.

AUTOIMMUNITY

During fetal life, when many antigens are presented to immune system, they are recognized as self-antigens and antibodies and cytotoxic T cells are not produced.

Therefore, tolerance to self-antigen is produced. However, sometimes body starts producing antibodies or T cells against self-antigen (own cells or tissue) leading to an autoimmune disease. Therefore, autoimmunity may be defined as immune response to self-antigen.

Autoimmune Diseases

Common autoimmune diseases include:

Autoimmune anemia: For example:
- *Hemolytic anemia:* Antibodies react with own RBCs.
- *Pernicious anemia:* Antibodies react against gastric mucosa.

Thrombocytopenic purpura: Autoantibodies react with self-platelets.

Graves' disease: Autoantibodies bind to thyroid cells and stimulate them.

Hashimoto's disease: T cells react against with antigen on the thyroid cells.

Insulin-dependent diabetes mellitus: Antibodies damage the β cells (insulin-producing cells) of the pancreas.

Rheumatoid arthritis: Antibodies damage the joints.

Rheumatic fever: Antibodies cross-react with valves of the heart.

HYPERSENSITIVITY

Hypersensitivity is an abnormal response which produces physiological or histopathological damage in the host. There are the following types of hypersensitivity reactions:
- Type I (Anaphylaxis or IgE-mediated)
- Type II (Antibody-mediated cytotoxicity)
- Type III (Immune complex-mediated disorders)
- Type IV (Delayed type or T cell-mediated hypersensitivity).

IMMUNODEFICIENCY DISEASES

Immunodeficiency diseases occur when body defence mechanisms are impaired.

Immunodeficiency diseases may be classified as primary or secondary.

Primary Immunodeficiency

Primary immunodeficiency occurs due to defect in the development of the immune system.

Secondary Immunodeficiency Disease

Acquired deficiencies of immunological response mechanisms can occur secondarily to number of diseases. Secondary immunodeficiency is more common than the primary immunodeficiency. Acquired immunodeficiency syndrome (AIDS) is the most important.

NURSING IMPLICATIONS AND APPLICATIONS

Acquired Immunodeficiency Syndrome

AIDS, i.e., is characterized by reduction in the number of helper T cells because of infection by human immunodeficiency virus (HIV). AIDS was first of all detected in USA in 1981.

Spread of Disease

AIDS is a major worldwide life-threatening disease spreading rapidly. Daily about 8500 persons get infected with HIV. The high-risk groups include sex workers, drug addicts, homosexual males, persons with extramarital relations and recipients of unscreened blood transfusion.

Transmission

There are mainly three routes of transmission:

1. *Parenteral route* is through blood contact involving:
   - Unscreened blood transfusion
   - Tattooing
   - Use of infected razors, syringes and needles
   - Use of poorly sterilized dental instruments
   - Organ transplants.

2. *Sexual route* accounts for about 85% of HIV infection due to multiple sex partners, sex workers, homosexuality and artificial insemination. The virus is present in sufficient concentration in the semen and vaginal secretions of the infected person.

3. *Transplacental route:* Infection can be transmitted from infected mother to her fetus (vertical transmission) across the placenta and also to infant through breast milk (perinatal transmission).

AIDS does not spread through mosquito bites, hugging, kissing and sharing meals.

Prevention

Preventive measures against HIV infection include:

Education: National AIDS control organization (NACO) has been set up under Ministry of Health and Family Welfare. Awareness is being imparted through all means of publicity and by non-government organization (NGO)s in schools, colleges, factories, farms, etc.

Screening is compulsarily carried out in case of blood donors, organ donors, semen donors, foreigners, and sex workers.

AIDS-positive persons are advised to prevent sexual contacts and pregnancy.

Ban on prostitution.

Safer sex with single partner, use of condoms and barrier creams.

Use of disposable syringes, needles, blood bags and I/V sets.

Proper sterilization of razors, blades and dental equipment by using 70% alcohol, 35% sodium hypochloride, 5% formaldehyde, boiling for 15 minutes or autoclaving.

ASSESS YOURSELF

Short and Long Answer Questions

1. **Describe briefly:**
   a. Lymphatic system and its functions
   b. Peripheral lymph organs and their functions

2. **Discuss the classification of immunity and write a note on stages of immunological response.**

3. **Differentiate between:**
   - Active and passive immunity
   - Primary and secondary immune response
   - Humoral and cell mediated immunity

4. **Write notes on:**
   - Histocompatibility antigens
   - Cytokines
   - Hypersensitivity
   - Acquired immunodeficiency syndrome

Multiple Choice Questions

1. **Thoracic duct receives lymph from:**
   a. Right half of body above the diaphragm
   b. Right thorax
   c. Left subclavian lymphatic trunk
   d. Right lymphatic duct

2. **The statement not true for spleen:**
   a. It is a main primary lymphoid organ
   b. Removes old RBCs, WBCs and Platelets
   c. Plays role in immune response
   d. White pulp consists of lymphocytes

3. **Which of the following is not included in mononuclear phagocyte system:**
   a. Monocytes
   b. Promonocytes
   c. Reticulocytes
   d. Precursor cells of monocyte series

4. **Which of the following participates in humoral defence mechanism:**
   a. Phagocytes
   b. Natural killer cells
   c. Granules of eosinophils
   d. Plasma cells

5. **Which of the following is an example of viral vaccine:**
   a. BCG vaccine
   b. Tetanus toxoid
   c. Sabin vaccine
   d. TAB vaccine

6. **The function of IgA immunoglobulins is:**
   a. Body fluid protection
   b. Protection of body surfaces
   c. Protection of blood stream
   d. Role in hypersensitivity

7. **The antibodies are produced by:**
   a. T lymphocytes   b. Helper T cells
   c. Cytotoxic Tcells   d. Plasma cells

8. **Which is not an autoimmune disease:**
   a. Hemolytic anemia
   b. Thrombocytopenic purpura
   c. Diabetes
   d. Hypertension

9. **Which is an example of passive artificial immunity:**
   a. Anti-gangrene serum
   b. Immunization of pregnant female by tetanus toxoid
   c. Breast milk feeding to newborn baby
   d. Killed vaccine for typhoid

10. **Histocompatibility MHC Class–I antigen is present in which immunologically reactive cells:**
   a. B lymphocyte
   b. Macrophages
   c. Monocytes
   d. Surfaces of all cells except RBCs

ANSWER KEY

| 1. | c | 2. | a | 3. | c | 4. | d | 5. | c | 6. | b | 7. | d | 8. | d |
| 9. | a | 10. | d | | | | | | | | | | | | |

Notes

Section

V

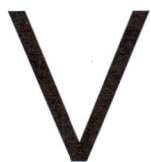

Endocrine System

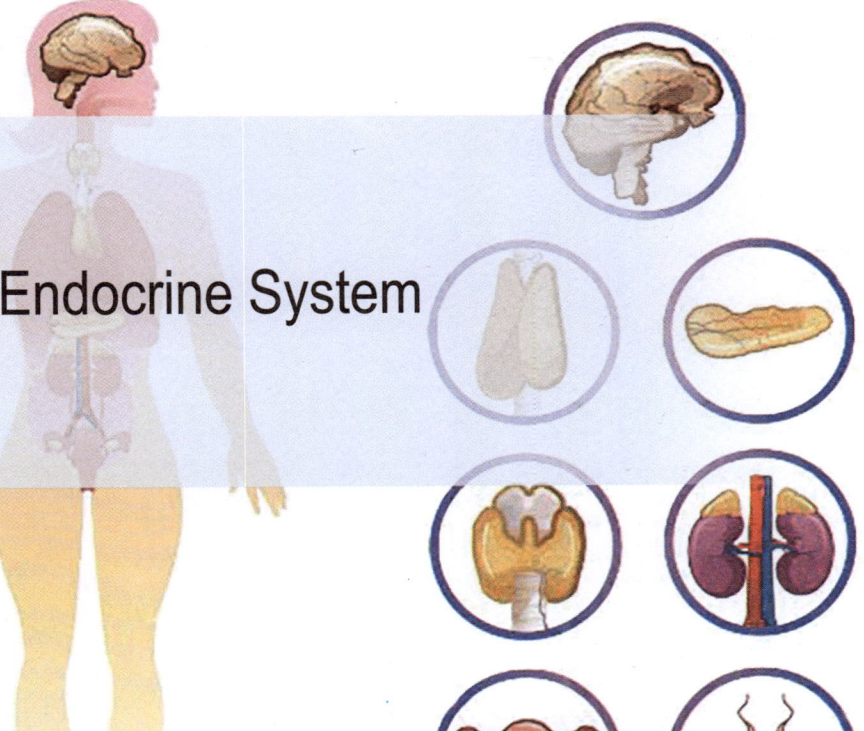

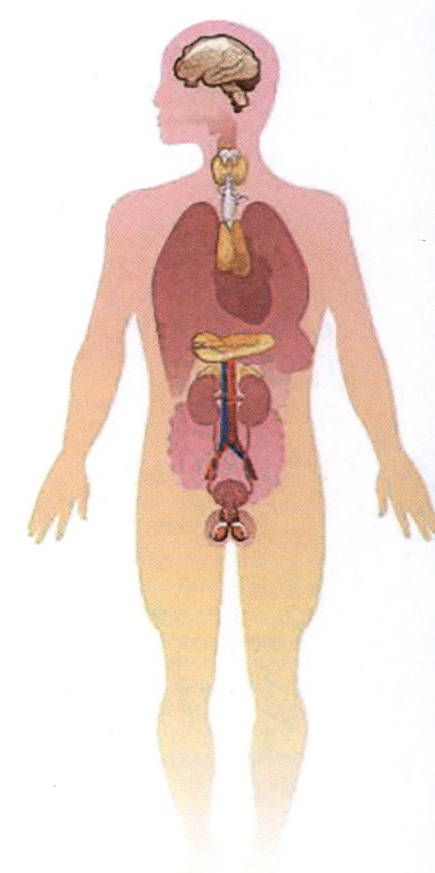

Section Outline

Anatomy and Physiology of Endocrine Organs

ORGANIZATION AND GENERAL PRINCIPLES OF ENDOCRINE SYSTEM

ORGANIZATION OF ENDOCRINE SYSTEM

The biological functions of the multicellular living organisms are very well-coordinated. This coordination is achieved by two main control systems—nervous system and the endocrine system. Nervous system is principally related with functions of the body in external and internal environment. The nervous system coordinates the body functions through transmission of impulses via nerve fibers. Endocrine system is mainly concerned with different metabolic functions of the body especially the chemical reactions and transport of various substances. The endocrine functions are accomplished through a wide range of chemical messengers, the hormones.

The endocrine system consists of various endocrine glands and neurosecretory cells located in the hypothalamus. The various endocrine glands present in the body (Fig. 5.1-1) are:

Pituitary gland (hypophysis). Pituitary gland is also known as hypophysis which in Greek means 'lying under' of the brain. It has two main parts: adenohypophysis and neurohypophysis. *Adenohypophysis* secretes growth hormone (GH) or somatotropins, follicle-stimulating hormone (FSH), luteinizing hormone (LH), prolactin, thyrotropin or

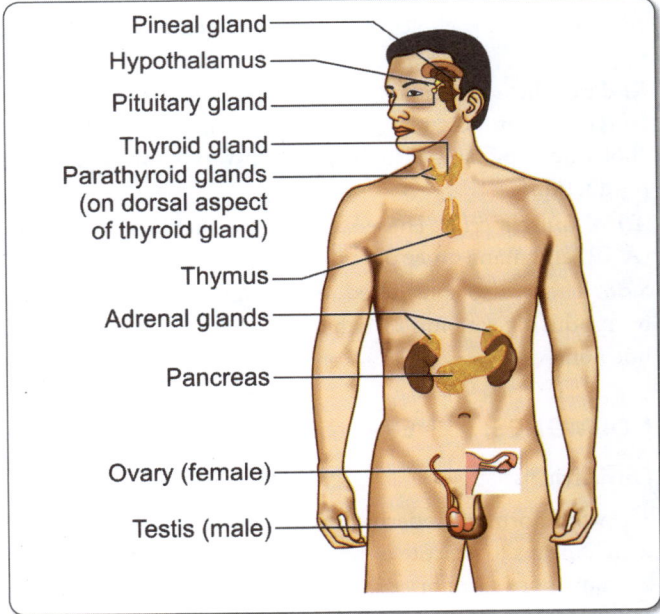

Fig. 5.1-1: Positions of the endocrine glands in the body

thyroid-stimulating hormone (TSH), and corticotropin or adrenocorticotropic hormone (ACTH). The *neurohypophysis* stores the antidiuretic hormone (ADH) or vasopressin and oxytocin synthesized by the hypothalamus.

Thyroid gland. The thyroid gland is present in the neck in front of trachea. It secretes thyroxine (T_4) and triiodothyronine (T_3). The C cells or parafollicular cells secrete calcitonin.

Parathyroid glands. These are four in number, very small glands situated behind the lobes of the thyroid gland and secrete parathormone.

Adrenal glands. These are situated on the upper poles of the two kidneys, hence also called suprarenal glands. The outer cortex region of the adrenal glands secretes cortisol, aldosterone and sex steroids and the inner medullary region secretes catecholamines (adrenaline and norad-renaline).

Pancreatic islets (islets of Langerhans). These are small groups of cells, which secrete insulin, glucagon and somatostatin.

Gonads. These include ovaries in females and testes in males. Ovaries secrete estrogens and progesterone (female sex steroids) and testes secrete (testosterone male sex hormone).

Pineal gland. It is a small gland present in the roof of third ventricle in the brain. It secretes melatonin and other biogenic amines.

Placenta. During pregnancy, placenta secretes various hormones like human chorionic gonadotropin (hCG), estrogen, progesterone, somatotropins and relaxin.

Gastrointestinal mucosa. It also secretes various hormones collectively known as gastrointestinal (GIT) hormones, e.g., gastrin, secretin, cholecystokinin-pancreozymin (CCK-PZ), etc.

Kidneys. In addition to their renal functions, the kidneys secrete erythropoietin, prostaglandins and 1,25-dihydroxy-cholecalciferol, and also help in activation of angiotensin production.

Atrial muscle cells. These secrete atrial natriuretic peptides (ANP) and many other peptides.

Skin. This is also considered to act as an endocrine structure by producing vitamin D, which is now considered to be a hormone.

HORMONES: GENERAL CONSIDERATIONS

Definition

The word hormone is derived from the Greek word, "*hormon*", which means to execute or to arouse. In the classic definition, hormones are secretory products of the ductless glands which are released in catalytic amounts into blood stream and transported to specific target cells (or organs), where they elicit physiologic, morphologic and biochemical responses.

Hormone Transport, Plasma Concentration and Half-life

Hormone Transport

After secretion into blood stream, hormones may circulate in two forms:

1. Unbound form. Some hormones circulate as free molecule, e.g., catecholamines and most peptide and protein hormones circulate unbound.

2. Bound form. Some hormones, such as steroids, thyroid hormones, and vitamin D, bound to specific globulins that are synthesized in the liver. The binding of hormones to proteins is advantageous as it:

- Protects the hormone against clearance by the kidney
- Slows down the rate of degradation by the liver
- Provides circulating reserve of the hormone.

Plasma Concentration

Hormones are usually secreted into the circulation in extremely low concentrations.

Half-life

Most hormones are metabolized rapidly after secretion. In general:

- Peptide hormones have short half-life
- Steroids and thyroid hormones have significantly longer half-life because they are bound to plasma proteins.

Functions of Hormones

Hormones regulate existing fundamental processes but do not initiate reactions de novo.

Regulation of Biochemical Reactions

Hormones regulate the metabolic functions in a variety of ways:

- They stimulate or inhibit the rate and magnitude of biochemical reactions by controlling enzymes and thereby cause morphologic, biochemical, and functional changes in target tissues.
- They modulate energy producing processes and regulate the circulating levels of energy-yielding substances (e.g., glucose, fatty acids). However, they are not used as energy sources in biochemical reactions.

Regulation of Bodily Processes

Hormones regulate different bodily processes such as growth, maturation, differentiation, regeneration, reproduction and behavior.

Thus, main function of endocrine glands is to maintain homeostasis in internal environment.

Regulation of Hormone Secretion

The quantity of hormones secreted is regulated in accordance with their requirement. General mechanisms that govern the secretion of hormones include:

- Feedback control
- Neural control
- Chronotropic control.

Feedback control

Feedback control is of two types:

1. Negative feedback control
2. Positive feedback control.

Negative feedback control. Generally, the influence of blood concentration of the hormone concerned or its effect is to inhibit further secretion of the hormone and is called negative feedback control (Fig. 5.1-2A).

Positive feedback control. It is less common, acts to amplify the initial biological effects of the hormone (Fig. 5.1-2B).

Neural control

Neural control acts to evoke or suppress hormone secretion in response to both external and internal stimuli.

External stimuli which can modulate hormone release through neural mechanisms may be visual, auditory, olfactory, gustatory and tactile.

Internal stimuli which influence hormonal release through neural mechanism include pain, emotion, sexual excitement, fright, stress and changes in blood volume.

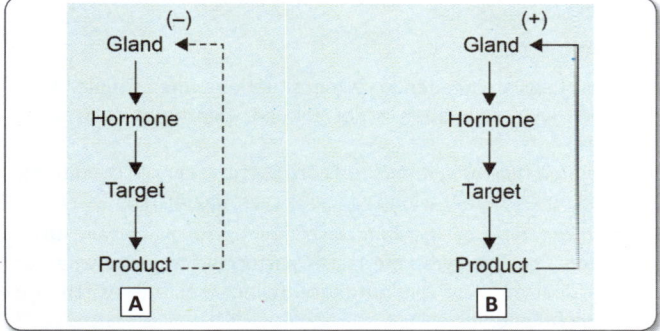

Figs 5.1-2A and B: Hormonal regulation by feedback control mechanism. A. Negative feedback; B. Positive feedback

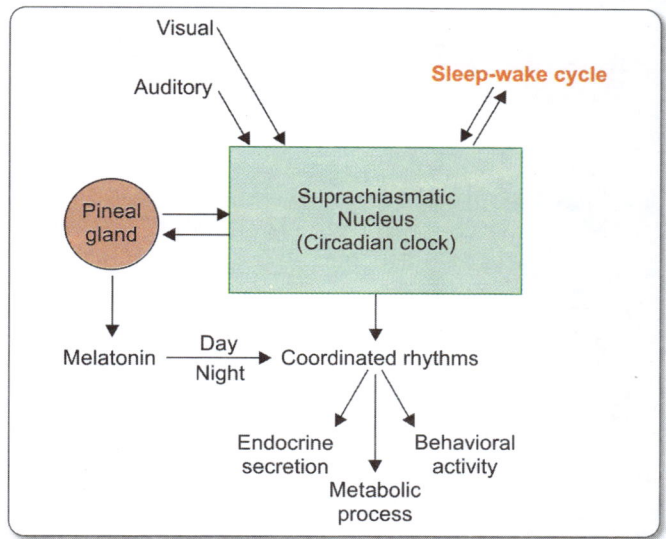

Fig. 5.1-3: The origin of circadian rhythms in endocrine gland secretion, metabolic process and behavioral activity

Chronotropic control

Chronotropic control of hormone secretion accounts for:

- Oscillating and pulsatile release of certain hormones
- Diurnal variation in hormonal levels
- Menstrual rhythm
- Seasonal rhythm
- Developmental rhythm.

The source of regular oscillatory cycles is a pulse generator located in the suprachiasmatic nucleus (SCN) of the hypothalamus (Fig. 5.1-3).

The intrinsic circadian clock is also located in the SCN, which is responsible for endocrine, metabolic and behavioral coordinated rhythms.

HORMONE RECEPTORS AND MECHANISM OF ACTION

Characteristics of Hormone Receptors

All hormones act through specific receptors. Almost all hormone receptors are large proteins present in hormone sensitive target cells.

Receptor specificity. There are specific receptors for each hormone. This is the reason that all hormones circulate to all parts of the body, yet each hormone has specific target tissue for its action (Fig. 5.1-4).

Mechanism of Action of Hormones

The main mechanisms of hormone actions are:

- Action through change in membrane permeability

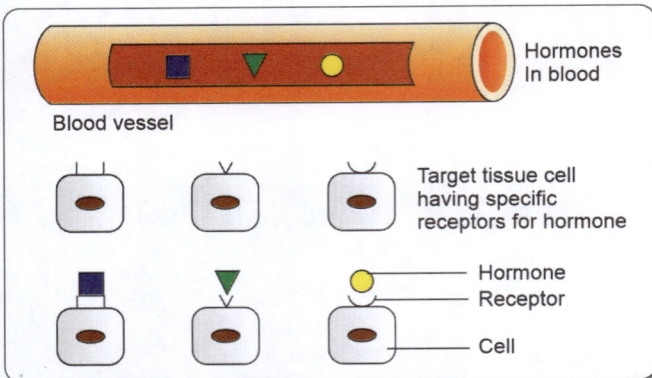

Fig. 5.1-4: Specificity of hormone action is because of specific receptors

- Action through effect on gene expression by binding of hormones with intracellular receptors
- Action through secondary messengers which activate intracellular enzymes when hormones combine with membrane receptors
- Action through tyrosin kinase activation.

TABLE 5.1-1: Modes of action of steroid and peptide hormones	
Steroid hormones	**Peptide hormones**
Lipid-soluble—can freely pass through cell membrane	Water soluble—unable to diffuse through cell membrane
Bind to receptors in the cytoplasm	React with receptors on the surface of the cell membrane
Form a hormone-receptor complex, enter the nucleus and have a direct effect on specific genes within DNA	Hormones do not enter the cell. Require a second messenger system to transmit signal to effector molecules inside cells of activation
Method of action is relatively slow	Method of action is fast
Include sex hormones synthesized by the ovary (oestrogen/progesterone), testis (testosterone) and the adrenal cortex	Include hormones synthesized by the hypothalamus (oxytocin and antidiuretic hormone(and hormones secreted by glands in the gastrointestinal tract

CLINICAL ASPECTS

MEASUREMENT OF HORMONES

Measurement of blood level of hormones is essential to confirm the endocrine disorders associated with either deficiency or excess of a hormone. Since the hormones exist in the blood in very low concentration, the conventional methods of estimation such as colorimetry are not of much use. Therefore, they are measured by hormone assays and some special techniques which include:

Bioassay

In this method, hormone levels were assessed by injecting the unknown sample of plasma in experimental animals and observing quantitatively the specific biological effect. The effect chosen was a characteristic action of the hormone for which a clear dose-response relationship existed.

Immunoassay

The immunoassay methods, frequently employed for estimation of hormone levels, include:
- Radioimmunoassay (RIA)
- Enzyme-linked immunosorbent assay (ELISA).

Radioimmunoassay

The radioimmunoassay is performed as:
- An unknown sample of plasma in which the concentration of a particular hormone (H) to be estimated is mixed with commercially available purified specific antibody (anti-H) and an appropriate amount of the purified hormone tagged with radioactive isotope (H+). The mixture is incubated in the cold.
- The antibodies have high affinity for the hormone. There occurs a competition between the free hormone (H) present in the unknown sample of plasma and the tagged hormone (H+) for binding to the specific antibody (anti-H).

Enzyme-linked immunosorbent method

Enzyme-linked immunosorbent assay (ELISA) method is principally similar to RIA, i.e., it is also based on the principle of antigen-antibody reaction. Any antigen that is protein can be measured by this technique. In this method, radioactivity is not measured, instead specific antibody hormone (antigen) complex is stained with suitable dye, and the intensity of color is measured by spectrophotometer. This technique is useful in estimating peptide and steroid hormones.

Cytochemical Assay

This test is much more sensitive than the immunoassay, but is cumbersome and time-consuming and so rarely used. In this technique, genesis of hormone can be detected in slices or cut out of the endocrine gland by incubating them in culture medium. This test is very useful in measuring the minute basal levels of hormone secretion.

Dynamic Tests

Dynamic tests are needed in certain situations when simple blood hormone level estimation is not enough. Two types of dynamic tests are:

Suppression type of dynamic tests are useful in certain conditions, e.g., to know whether a lung cancer is secreting ACTH.

Stimulation type of dynamic tests are useful in certain other conditions, e.g., metyrapone test is performed to know whether the corticotrophs of the pituitary (which secrete ACTH) are normally functioning or not.

PITUITARY GLAND AND HYPOTHALAMUS

INTRODUCTION AND FUNCTIONAL ANATOMY

Introduction

The hypothalamic-pituitary unit forms a unique component of the entire endocrine system that regulates growth, lactation, fluid homeostasis, and the functions of thyroid gland, adrenal glands, and gonads.

Functional Anatomy

Gross Anatomy of Pituitary Gland

Pituitary gland, also called hypophysis cerebri, is a small gland, weighs about 0.5 g and is approximately 1 cm in diameter. It is situated in the hypophyseal fossa (sella turcica) of the sphenoid bone.

Physiologically, the pituitary gland consists of three distinct parts or lobes (Fig. 5.1-5):
1. Anterior lobe or adenohypophysis
2. Posterior lobe or neurohypophysis
3. Intermediate lobe or pars intermedia.

Development of Pituitary Gland

Anterior pituitary is ectodermal in origin. It develops from *Rathke's pouch*, which is an embryonic upward outpouching from the roof of the primitive oral cavity.

Posterior pituitary or neurohypophysis develops from a lowered outpouching of neuroectodermal tissue from the central areas of hypothalamus (tuber cinereum and median eminence).

From the above, it is quite clear that the anterior and posterior pituitary develop independently from widely different origins, and it is only a coincidence that when fully formed, they happen to lie so close together that they are considered parts of the same organ.

Parts of Pituitary Gland

Adenohypophysis. The glandular anterior lobe of pituitary gland is called adenohypophysis. It constitutes about 80% of the pituitary gland. It can be further divided into three parts (Fig. 5.1-5):
1. *Pars distalis*
2. *Pars intermedia*
3. *Pars tuberalis*

Neurohypophysis. The posterior lobe of pituitary is a neural structure and hence called neurohypophysis. It consists of three parts (Fig. 5.1-5):
1. *Pars posterior.*
2. *Infundibular stem.*
3. *Median eminence.*

Pituitary stalk. The median eminence and infundibulum constitute the neural stalk. The posterior pituitary maintains its neural connection with hypothalamus by this neural stalk. The neural stalk surrounded by pars tuberalis of adenohypophysis constitutes the pituitary stalk.

Intermediate lobe of pituitary gland is rudimentary in humans as well as in a few other mammalian species. In certain lower animals, this lobe secretes melanocyte-stimulating hormone (MSH) in response to changes in exposure to light and other environmental factors.

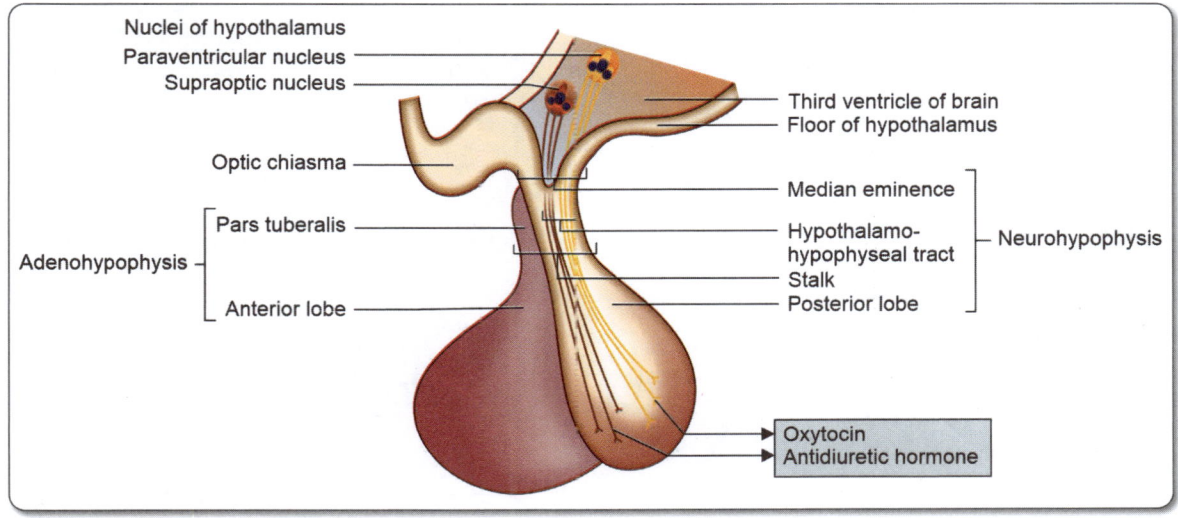

Fig. 5.1-5: Anatomical subdivisions of pituitary gland

Histological Structure of Pituitary Gland

The histology of pituitary gland is shown in histology plate 5.1-1.

Adenohypophysis

Pars Distalis consists of cords of cells separated by fenestrated sinusoids. The cells can be divided into two main types: The chromophobes and chromophils.

Chromophobes. These are agranular cells and it is considered that the chromophils are derived from the chromophobes.

Chromophils. These are granular cells, constitute 50% of the cells of anterior pituitary. Chromophils are further classified as: acidophils (35%), and basophils (15%).

- *Acidophilic cells (α cells):* The granules of these cells are acidophilic.
- *Basophilic cells (β cells):* The granules of these cells are basophilic.

Folliculostellate cells. These cells send processes between the secretory cells. Recently it has been demonstrated that these contain and secrete the cytokine 1L-6, but their physiological role is still not clear.

Pars Tuberalis. It mainly consists of undifferentiated cells with few acidophils and basophils.

Pars Intermedia. It contains β cells, few secretory cells and chromophobe cells.

Neurohypophysis

Histologically posterior pituitary contains following structures:

Unmyelinated nerve fibers. These are the axons of the neurons located in the supraoptic and paraventricular nuclei

Histology Plate 5.1-1: Pituitary gland

A photomicrograph of pituitary gland is shown. Pars distalis (1) is the largest part of the gland. Pars intermedia (2) consists of colloid filled cysts. Neurohypophysis (4) is composed of unmyelinated nerve fibers (3) and pituicytes.

of hypothalamus. These carry precursor of posterior pituitary hormones and end as close terminals near the blood capillaries (Fig. 5.1-6).

Pituicytes are the special type of supporting cells, having long dendritic processes. These are present in between the axons.

Glial cells like astrocytes and oligodendrocytes are also seen.

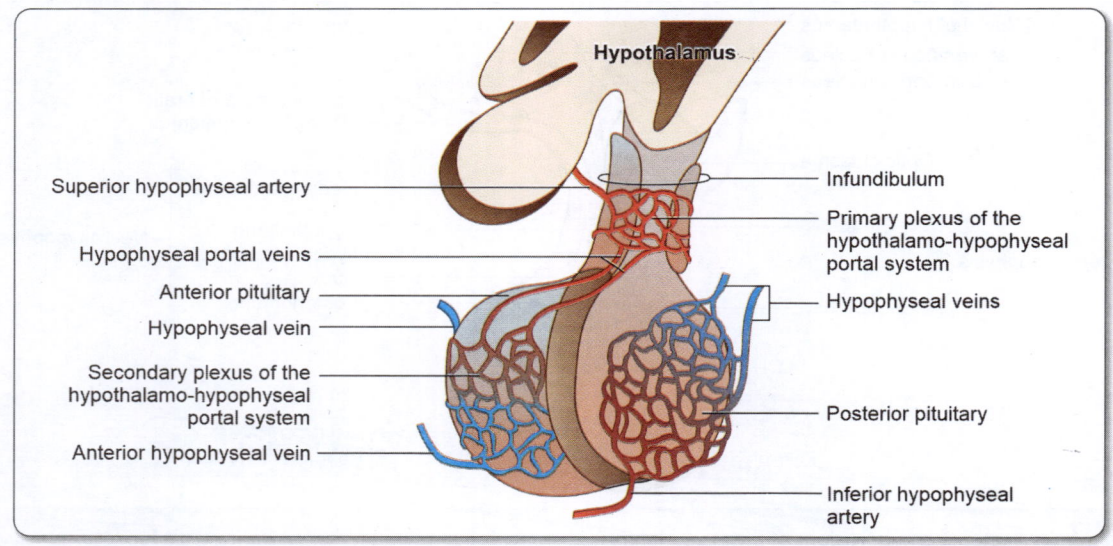

Fig. 5.1-6: Hypothalamo-hypophyseal portal system

Blood Supply of Pituitary Gland

Arterial Supply

The arterial blood to the pituitary gland is supplied by the branches of:
- Internal carotid arteries (superior and inferior hypophyseal branches)
- Anterior cerebral artery
- Posterior cerebral artery.

Hypothalamo-hypophyseal portal system (Figs 5.1-6 and 5.1-7)

- The branches from superior hypophyseal artery form a ring around the upper part of the pituitary stalk and further branch to form a *capillary network*.
- The blood from this capillary network is drained by *long portal veins* in the infundibulum.
- Then in the anterior lobe, these long portal veins break up into another set of capillary network and represent as *sinusoids of pars anterior*. This arrangement is called *hypothalamo-hypophyseal portal system*.
- The inferior hypophyseal (branch of internal carotid artery) branches to form a capillary network at the lower end of infundibulum stem.

- The short portal vessels arise from this capillary network and supply blood mainly to posterior pituitary and some parts of anterior pituitary.
- The short portal vessels provide link between the anterior and posterior pituitary.

Venous Drainage

The blood from anterior pituitary is drained to cavernous sinus and then into jugular vein.

> **IMPORTANT TO KNOW**
>
> The anterior pituitary lies outside the blood-brain barrier, hence, it is accessible to influences from general circulation (hormones and neurotransmitter by the brain and hormones secreted in the general circulation).

ENDOCRINE ASPECTS OF HYPOTHALAMUS

Functional Anatomy

Hypothalamus is a specialized center in the brain that functions as a master coordinator of hormonal action. It is a part of the brain situated below the thalamus and is very

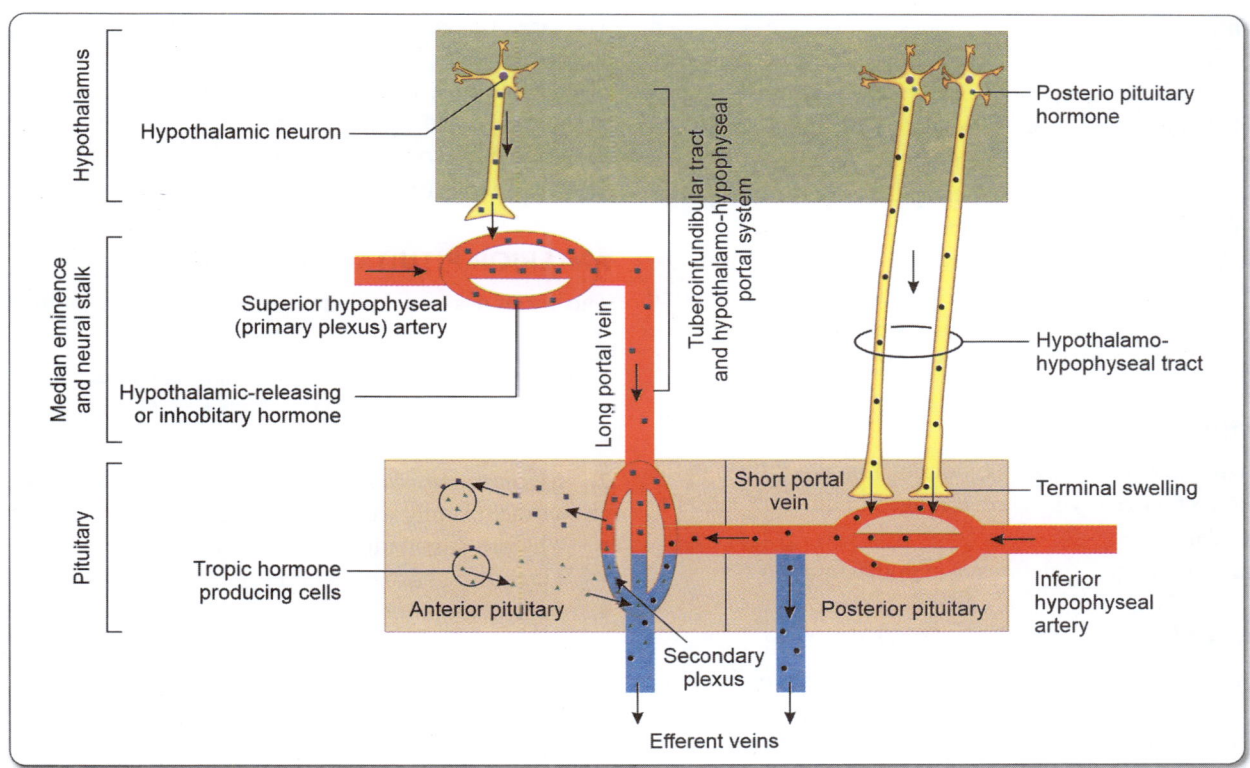

Fig. 5.1-7: Schematic diagram to explain anatomical and functional relationship between hypothalamus and pituitary gland

closely connected to pituitary gland. Thus hypothalamus provides an important link between the endocrine system and the nervous system. Further details of functional anatomy of hypothalamus is given in Chapter 10.2, page 502.

Hypothalamic-Pituitary Relationship

The influences from the hypothalamus are conveyed to pituitary gland by two different tracts:

Hypothalamohypophyseal tract. It is composed of axons of the large neurosecretory cells of the supraoptic and paraventricular nuclei of hypothalamus. These fibers pass to neurohypophysis through the infundibular stem and form a series of dilated terminals known as Herring bodies (Fig. 5.1-6). The neurosecretory cells of supraoptic and paraventricular nuclei secrete peptide hormones (vasopressin and oxytocin), which travel down their axons in neurosecretory granules to be stored in the nerve terminals lying the neurohypophysis. Upon stimulation of the cell bodies, the granules are released from the axonal terminals by exocytosis.

Tuberoinfundibular tract and hypothalamohypophyseal portal system. It consists of fibers arising from the arcuate nuclei of the tuberal region of the hypothalamus, and extend to the median eminence (Fig. 5.1-6). The cell bodies of these hypothalamic neurons synthesize certain releasing and inhibiting hormones which are conveyed by the tuberoinfundibular tract to the median eminence region where they are stored in the nerve terminals. When hypothalamic neurons are stimulated by nerve impulses, the releasing or inhibiting hormones are discharged into the median eminence and enter the capillary plexus of superior hypophyseal artery. From here they are transported down the portal vessels (long portal veins) and then exited from the secondary capillary plexus to reach the specific endocrine target cells in the adenohypophysis where they regulate the secretion of tropic hormones of anterior pituitary (Fig. 5.1-7).

Functions of Hypothalamus

The hypothalamus serves its endocrine functions through the neurosecretory cells which are arranged in different nuclei of hypothalamus.
The main endocrine functions of hypothalamus are:

Control of Anterior Pituitary Function

Hypothalamus controls the functioning of anterior pituitary through various hypothalamic-hypophysiotropic hormones, i.e., various hypothalamic-releasing and -inhibiting hormones. The hypothalamic-releasing and -inhibiting hormones are released in response to neural stimuli.

Various hypothalamic-releasing and -inhibiting hormones include:

- Growth hormone releasing hormone (GHRH)
- Growth hormone inhibiting hormone (GRIH) also called somatostatin
- Corticotropin-releasing hormone (CRH)
- Thyrotropin-releasing hormone (TRH)
- Gonadotropin-releasing hormone (GnRH)
- Prolactin-releasing hormone (PRH)
- Prolactin-inhibiting hormone (PIH).

Functions of hypothalamic-releasing and -inhibiting hormones. In general, they control the release of various tropic hormones from anterior pituitary. However, now it has known that besides regulating the secretion of specific tropic hormone, a hypothalamic hormone may also influence the secretion of another anterior pituitary hormone. For example:

- TRH, besides promoting secretion of TSH, also stimulates the secretion of prolactin.
- Somatostatin, discovered as a growth hormone inhibiting hormone (GHIH), also inhibits the secretion of TSH.
- Growth hormone releasing hormone (GHRH) also stimulates the secretion of ACTH and prolactin.
- GnRH promotes the release of both LH and FSH.

Control of Posterior Pituitary Function

The large (magnocellular) neurosecretory cells forming the supraoptic and paraventricular nuclei of hypothalamus are responsible for synthesis of the two posterior pituitary peptide hormones (oxytocin and ADH). These hormones reach the posterior pituitary through hypothalamic-hypophyseal tract described above (Figs 5.1-6 and 5.1-7).

ANTERIOR PITUITARY HORMONES

The hormones of adenohypophysis are broadly classified into three categories:

1. *Hormones of growth hormone family* include:
- Growth hormone (GH)
- Prolactin (PRL)

2. *Glycoprotein hormone family.* The hormones of glycoprotein family secreted by anterior pituitary include:
- Thyroid-stimulating hormone (TSH)
- Luteinizing hormone (LH)
- Follicular-stimulating hormone (FSH).

3. *Pro-opiomelanocortin peptides (POMC).* The hormones of this group are:
- Adrenocorticotropic hormone (ACTH)
- Melanocyte-stimulating hormone (MSH), α-MSH and β-MSH are produced in the intermediary lobe (which is rudimentary in humans)

- β-lipotropin
- β-endorphin.

Physiological aspects of growth hormone are discussed in detail in this chapter. Other hormones are discussed under their respective headings, e.g., TSH with thyroid hormone, and ACTH with adrenal gland and prolactin in reproductive system.

Growth Hormone

Growth hormone (GH), also called *somatotropin*, is the most important hormone for postnatal growth and development to adult size. It also helps to maintain lean body mass and bone mass in adults.

Structure

Growth hormone consists of a single unbranched chain containing 191 amino acids. Its molecular weight is 2000.

Synthesis

Growth hormone is synthesized by acidophilic cells called *somatotrophs* of anterior pituitary.

Plasma Levels

The basal plasma GH level varies from 2–4 ng/mL.

Secretion

Growth hormone is released in *pulsatile* fashion.
- *Secretion is increased* by sleep, stress, hormones related to puberty, starvation, exercise, and hypoglycemia.
- *Secretion of GH is decreased* by somatostatin, somatomedins, obesity, hyperglycemia, and pregnancy.

Circulation

Circulating GH is bound to a plasma protein (GH binding protein).

Metabolism

Growth hormone is rapidly metabolized, probably at least in part, in the liver. Metabolic clearance and daily urinary GH excretion correlates well with the integrated 24-hour plasma GH profile.

Regulation of GH secretion

Hypothalamus controls GH secretion by releasing two hormones, growth hormone releasing hormone (GHRH) and growth hormone release inhibiting hormone (GRIH) (Fig. 5.1-8).

Growth hormone releasing hormone (GHRH). It stimulates the secretion of GH from the anterior pituitary.

Growth hormone release inhibiting hormone (GRIH). It is also called somatostatin and is a polypeptide. It inhibits the release of GH from the anterior pituitary.

The negative feedback control mechanism for GH involves the role of somatomedins, GH and GHRH (Fig. 5.1-8).
- *Negative feedback control by somatomedins:* Somatomedins are insulin-like growth factors (IGF) that are produced when growth hormone acts on target tissues. Somatomedins inhibit the secretion of GH directly or by stimulating the secretion of somatostatin from the hypothalamus.
- *Negative feedback control by GH:* Growth hormone also inhibits its own secretion by stimulating the secretion of somatostatin from the hypothalamus.
- *Negative feedback control by GHRH:* GHRH inhibits its own secretion from the hypothalamus. This mechanism is called *ultrashort feedback loop.*

Actions of growth hormone

Growth hormone promotes growth and also influences the normal metabolism, therefore, besides acting on one specific organ, its actions are generalized.

Growth promoting actions of GH

Growth hormone promotes linear growth of an individual by its effects on the bone, cartilage and other connective tissues.

Effects on cartilage. GH stimulates the proliferation of chondrocytes (cartilage cells) present in the epiphyseal end plates of long bones.

Effects on bone. GH stimulates osteoblastic activity which converts cartilage into bone. This process continues up to adolescence till there is fusion of epiphyseal end plate with shaft of the bone. The bone mass also increases during this period.

Metabolic actions of GH

Effects on protein metabolism. Growth hormone has an anabolic effect on protein metabolism. It promotes the protein deposition in the tissues by following effects:
- Increases the rate of amino acid uptake into the cells.
- Increases protein synthesis in ribosomes.
- Stimulates transcription (RNA synthesis from DNA).

Effects on fat metabolism. GH promotes lipolysis in adipose tissue (catabolic effect) and then increases fat utilization for energy.

Effects on carbohydrate metabolism. GH is antagonistic to insulin and produces hyperglycemia by following effects:
- Decreases the uptake as well as utilization of glucose by the tissues for energy production, and
- Inhibits glycolysis and thus glycogen stores tend to increase.

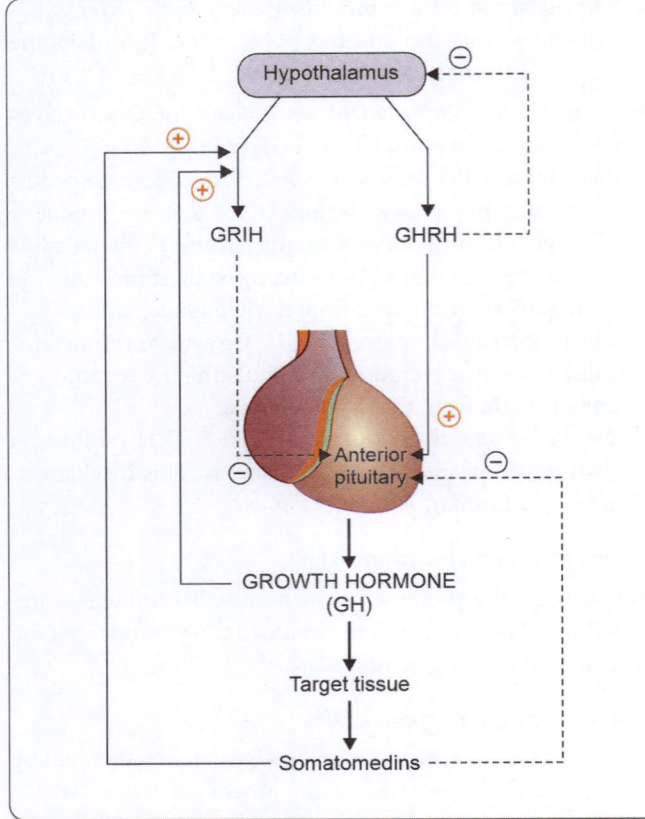

Fig. 5.1-8: Control of growth hormone secretion; GRIH, growth hormone inhibiting hormone; GHRH, growth hormone releasing hormone

Effects on mineral metabolism. Growth hormone promotes bone mineralization in growing children.

Thyroid-Stimulating Hormone

Thyroid-stimulating hormone (TSH), as its name suggests, is a tropic hormone responsible for the stimulation of the thyroid gland *(for details see page 270).*

Prolactin

Prolactin (PRL) has many effects on the body, chief of which is that it stimulates the mammary glands of the breast to produce milk *(for details see page 466).*

Glycoprotein Hormone Family

Adrenocorticotropic hormone

Adrenocorticotropic hormone (ACTH) stimulates the adrenal cortex, the outer part of the adrenal gland, to produce its hormones *(for details see page 280).*

Follicle-stimulating hormone

Follicle-stimulating hormone (FSH) stimulates the follicle cells of the gonads to produce gametes—ova in females and sperm in males.

Luteinizing hormone

Luteinizing hormone (LH) stimulates the gonads to produce the sex hormones—estrogens in females and testosterone in males.

NURSING IMPLICATIONS AND APPLICATIONS

ABNORMALITIES OF ANTERIOR PITUITARY HORMONES

The abnormalities related to pituitary hormones occur either due to excess or deficiency of the hormones secreted. The most common causes of pituitary hormone disturbances are pituitary tumors which may cause symptoms of excess of one or more hormones and simultaneous deficiency of other hormones, hence a mixed picture may evolve. The various hormones of pituitary, their site of action and diseases produced by them are given in Table 5.1-2.

Pituitary disorders seen in clinical practice are:
- Hypopituitarism
- Abnormalities of growth hormone,
- Prolactin deficiency
- Cushing's syndrome

Hypopituitarism

Hypopituitarism is a clinical condition of hyposecretion of one or more pituitary hormones. Hypopituitarism can be due to hypothalamic causes or pituitary causes. Since anterior pituitary has a large reserve, the endocrine abnormalities are produced only when large part of pituitary is destroyed.

Abnormalities of Growth Hormone Secretion

The abnormalities of growth hormone secretion include:
- Hypersecretion of GH
- Hyposecretion of GH.

Hypersecretion of GH

Hypersecretion of GH occurs in tumors of acidophilic cells of anterior pituitary. Depending upon the age of an individual, excess of GH may cause:
- Gigantism
- Acromegaly.

Gigantism: It is a clinical condition resulting from hypersecretion of GH in growing children before the closure of epiphysis of long bones. The main feature of gigantism is *abnormal height* (7–8 feet due to excessive growth of long bones) with huge status and the person becomes "giant" (Fig. 5.1-9).

Contd...

TABLE 5.1-2: Pituitary hormones: Site of action and diseases associated with their deficiency and excess

Hormone	Site of action	Diseases	
		Excess	Deficiency
Anterior pituitary			
Growth hormone (GH)	All somatic cells	Gigantism in adolescents	Dwarfism
Adrenocorticotropic hormone (ACTH)	Adrenal cortex	ACTH-dependent Cushing's syndrome	Hypoadrenalism (rare)
Thyroid-stimulating hormone (TSH)	Thyroid	Hyperthyroidism	Hypothyroidism
Prolactin	Breast	Hyperprolactinemia	—
Gonadotropins	Gonads	Hypergonadism	Hypogonadism
Melanocytic-stimulating hormone (MSH)	Skin	Hyperpigmentation	—
Posterior pituitary			
Antidiuretic hormone	Kidneys	—	Diabetes insipidus

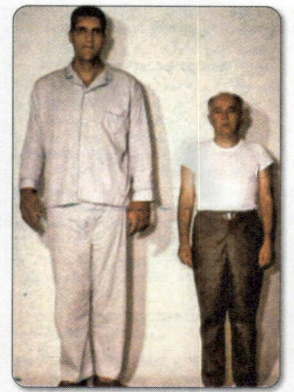
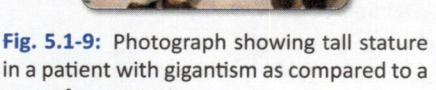
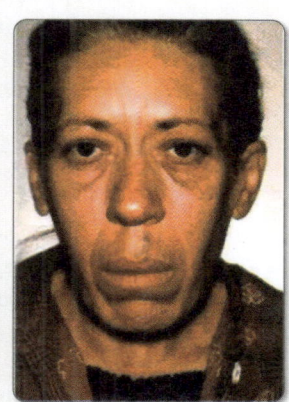
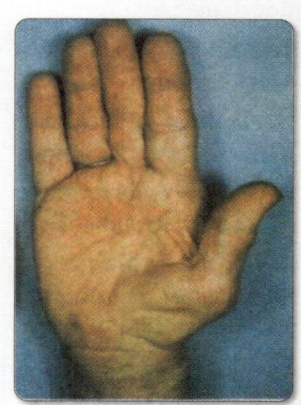

Fig. 5.1-9: Photograph showing tall stature in a patient with gigantism as compared to a man of average size

Fig. 5.1-10: Coarse facial features, broad thick nose, prognathism, prominent eyebrows and thickened skin in acromegaly

Fig. 5.1-11: Large spade-like hand with short thick wide fingers in acromegaly

Acromegaly: It is a clinical condition that occurs due to excess of GH in adults (after epiphyseal closure of long bones has occurred) and causes excessive growth in those areas where cartilage persists.

Clinical features are:
- *Acromegalic face*, which is characterized by thick lips, macroglossia, broad and thick nose, prominent eyebrows, thickened skin, and coarse facial features (Fig. 5.1-10).
- *Prognathism*, i.e., protrusion of the lower jaw due to elongation and widening of mandible associated with increased spacing of the teeth.
- *Acral part abnormalities* include large spade-like hands, thick wide fingers, large feet with increase in size of the shoes. Height is normal, build is stout and stocky (Fig. 5.1-11).
- *Kyphosis* may occur due to improper vertebral growth.
- *Excessive growth of internal organs*, i.e., cardiomegaly, hepatomegaly, splenomegaly and renomegaly may be associated.
- *Increased sympathetic activity* may cause increased sweating and hypertension.

Hyposecretion of GH

Deficiency of GH in childhood leads to stunted growth or *dwarfism*. ***Deficiency of GH in adulthood*** results in *mild anemia* which is refractory to usual treatment with hematinics like iron.
- Reduction in muscle mass, and
- Hypoglycemia may also occur.

Growth hormone related dwarfism (Pituitary dwarfism) occurs due to deficiency of GH in early childhood.

Characteristic features: Deficiency of GH causes retardation of growth in all parts of the body proportionately. Consequently, a pituitary dwarf with a chronological age of 20 years has the body structure like that of a normal child of 7–10 years of age. Thus a pituitary dwarf has following features:
- Shortness of stature (dwarf)
- Normal mental activity
- Plumpness (fatness)
- Immature faces
- Delicate extremities
- Sexual maturity does not occur when associated with gonadotropin deficiency.

POSTERIOR PITUITARY HORMONES

The two important hormones released from posterior pituitary are:

1. Antidiuretic hormone (ADH)
2. Oxytocin (OTC).

Antidiuretic Hormone

Antidiuretic hormone (ADH), as the name indicates, prevents diuresis and is chiefly concerned with conservation of body water. Since it also causes vasoconstriction, it is also called vasopressin or more precisely arginine vasopressin (AVP).

Structure

ADH and OTC both are homologous neurohormones, polypeptide in nature.

Synthesis

Antidiuretic hormone as well as OTC are synthesized in the cell bodies of magnocellular neurons of both paraventricular and supraoptic nuclei of hypothalamus. The secretory granules containing hormone precursors, known as Herring bodies, are transported down the axons by axoplasmic flow to the nerve endings in the posterior pituitary.

Secretion

ADH and OTC are released when a nerve impulse is transmitted from the cell body in the hypothalamus down the axon, where it depolarizes the neurosecretory vesicles.

Transport

The hormone and other secreted products separately enter the closely adjacent capillary. The hormone then reaches the target cells and by circulatory interconnections to the anterior pituitary also.

Metabolism

The circulating vasopressin is rapidly inactivated in the liver and kidney.

Actions of ADH

ADH acts through vasopressin receptors. The vasopressin receptors are of three types:

1. V1-A receptors are involved in vasoconstrictor effect
2. V1-B receptors are involved in ADH action on anterior pituitary
3. V2 receptors are involved in ADH action on kidney

Action on kidney. The main role of ADH is regulation of water balance in the body by acting on the distal convoluted tubules and collecting ducts of the renal nephron. ADH increases the permeability of these cells to water.

Vasoconstrictor effect. ADH in large doses causes vasoconstriction and leads to rise in blood pressure. Hemorrhage is a potent stimulus to ADH secretion.

Action on anterior pituitary. ADH travels to the anterior pituitary via the portal veins and causes increased ACTH secretion.

Regulation of ADH Secretion

The main factors which regulate the ADH secretion are:

Effective osmotic pressure of plasma or plasma osmolality

Plasma osmolality in normal individuals is maintained very close to 285 mOsm/L by ADH. Change in plasma osmolality is a very potent regulator of ADH secretion. Thus, water deprivation (which increases plasma osmolality) stimulates ADH secretion. On the other hand, a water load (which decreases plasma osmolality) decreases ADH secretion.

Mechanism of Action

Changes in plasma osmolality affect the osmoreceptors.

- *Osmoreceptors* refer to group of neurons located in the anterior hypothalamus.
- The rise in plasma osmolality even by 1–2% results in shrinkage of osmoreceptors causing reflex increase of ADH secretion.

CLINICAL ASPECTS

Abnormalities of ADH Secretion

Abnormalities of ADH secretion include:
- Syndrome of inappropriate hypersecretion of ADH, and
- Diabetes insipidus.

Syndrome of Inappropriate Hypersecretion of ADH

Syndrome of inappropriate hypersecretion of antidiuretic hormone (SIADH) refers to a condition in which ADH secretion is increased despite the presence of hypoosmolality. Excessive ADH secretion leads to water intoxication, i.e., overhydration, and because of this, SIADH is also called *dilution syndrome*.

Diabetes Insipidus

Diabetes insipidus refers to a clinical condition of polyuria that occurs either due to deficiency of ADH (vasopressin) release or failure of renal response to ADH.

Characteristic features

The diabetes insipidus is characterized by decreased renal absorption of water leading to following features:

Polyuria, i.e., passage of large amount of urine, up to 3–20 liters, is the most important single feature of diabetes insipidus.
Polyuria is followed by:
Obligatory polydypsia (drinking of large amount of water). It occurs due to stimulation of thirst mechanism.
Dehydration may occur in severe cases. Its signs and symptoms include dry tongue and dry mouth. Fall of blood pressure and loss of consciousness may be seen in acute severe cases.

Changes in blood volume

Changes in circulating blood volume, central blood volume, cardiac output and blood pressure affect the secretion of ADH.

Other factors affecting ADH secretion

Factors, other than the two major stimuli (i.e., hypovolemia and plasma osmolality), which affect ADH secretion are:

- *Stress* of pain, chronic emotional stress, and surgical procedures cause increase in ADH secretion.
- *Adrenaline* decreases the ADH.

Oxytocin

In both sexes, oxytocin is produced by the hypothalamus and stored and secreted into the bloodstream from the posterior pituitary gland.

Oxytocin stimulates contractions of the uterus during labor, to stimulate the ejection of milk during lactation, and to promote maternal nurturing behavior. Oxytocin is thought to influence a number of other physiological and behavioral processes as well, particularly sexual and social behavior in males and females *(for details see page 464).*

THYROID GLAND, PARATHYROID GLANDS AND THYMUS

THYROID GLAND

Anatomy of Thyroid Gland

Thyroid gland is the largest endocrine gland in the body (weighing about 15–25 g in adults). It consists of two lobes joined together by a narrow isthmus and is located on either side of trachea just below the larynx at the level of 5th to 7th cervical and 1st thoracic vertebra. The lobes are conical in shape. Each lobe is about 5 cm long and 3 cm wide (Fig. 5.1-12). Structures in relation to thyroid gland are:

- Two parathyroid glands are present on the posterior surface of each lobe.
- Recurrent laryngeal nerve lies close to the lobes.

Blood Supply

Arterial blood supply. Superior thyroid artery (a branch of external carotid artery), and inferior thyroid artery (a branch of subclavian artery) supply the blood to the thyroid gland. It receives high blood supply (400–600 mL/100 g/min).

Venous drainage. It occurs through thyroid veins which ultimately drain the blood into internal jugular vein.

Histological Structure

Histologically, each *lobe* of thyroid gland is divided into various *lobules* by fibrous tissue septa. Each lobule is made up of an aggregation of several *follicles.* (Histology Plate 5.1-2) (Fig. 5.1-13A). Each follicle is lined by *follicular cells.*

Follicular cells. These vary in shape with the degree of glandular activity. Normally (at an average level of activity) the cells are *cuboidal* and the colloid in the follicles is moderate in amount. During high degree of activity, the cells become columnar and flat when inactive (Fig. 5.1-13B). These cells secrete thyroid hormones.

Parafollicular cells or *C cells* are scattered between follicular cells and basement membrane (Fig. 5.1-13). and secrete calcitonin.

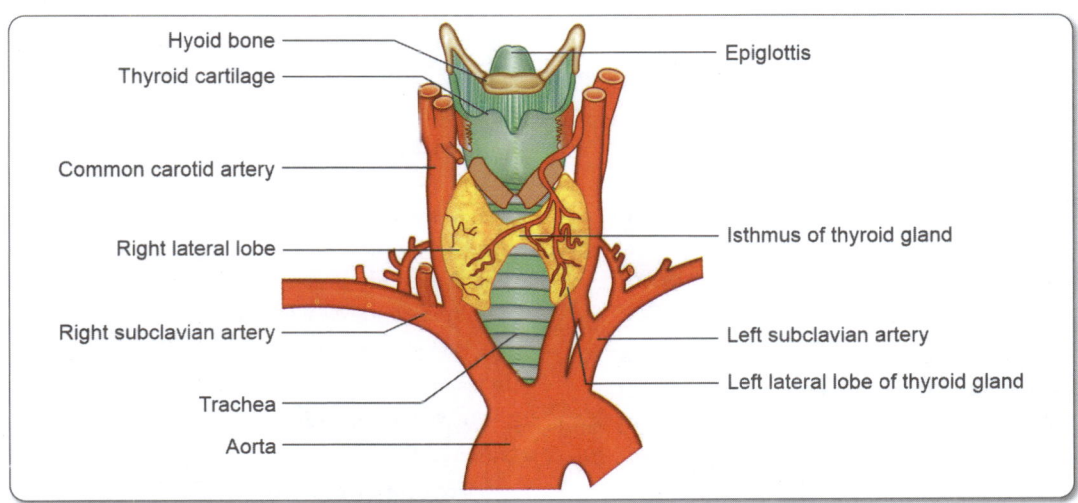

Fig. 5.1-12: Location of thyroid gland and its relations

Histology Plate 5.1-2: Thyroid Gland

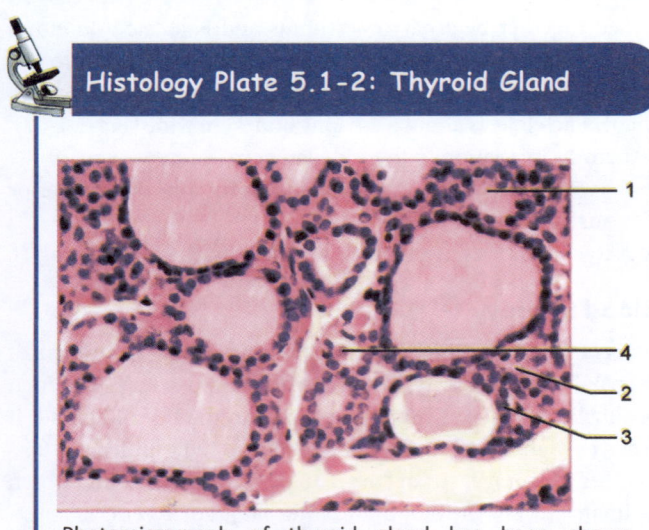

Photomicrograph of thyroid gland has been shown illustrating rounded colloid filled follicles (1) separated by interfollicular connective tissue (2). Follicles are lined by simple cuboidal epithelium (3). Groups of parafollicular cells (4) are present in connective tissue.

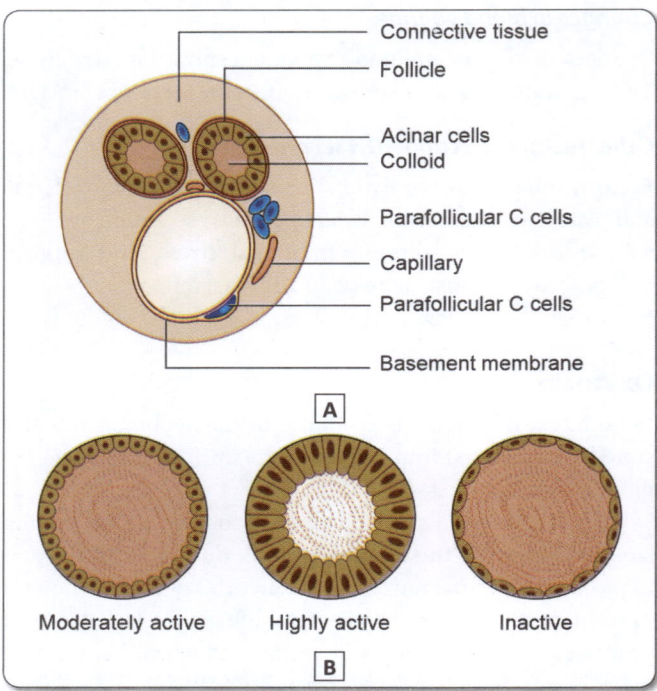

Figs 5.1-13A and B: A. Histological structure of thyroid gland; B. Variations in follicular cell size with activity

Colloid. This is a homogeneous material that fills the cavity of each follicle. The major constituent of the colloid is thyroglobulin, a glycoprotein with a molecular weight of 660,000. During active state, the follicles are depleted of colloid; and in resting state when unstimulated, the follicles accumulate colloid.

Thyroid Hormones

The two principal thyroid hormones include thyroxine (T_4) and triiodothyronine (T_3).

Thyroxine or T_4 (tetraiodothyronine) constitutes 90% of thyroid output.

Triiodothyronine or T_3 (triiodothyronine) constitutes 10% of thyroid output; however, it is responsible for most of the tissue actions of thyroid hormone.

Calcitonin is a hormone secreted by parafollicular cells of thyroid gland. It is concerned with calcium homeostasis.

Biosynthesis and Storage of Thyroid Hormones

Iodine metabolism

Iodine is essential for the synthesis of thyroid hormones. It is ***ingested in the form of iodides hormone.***

Sources of iodine are sea fish (richest), bread, milk and vegetables. Iodine is added ***to the table salt to prevent iodine deficiency.***

- Daily average intake of iodine is 500 µg.
- Daily requirement of iodine is 100–200 µg.

Mostly 80% (i.e., 400 µg/day) of the iodides absorbed from gastrointestinal tract into the circulation are selectively removed from circulation by cells of thyroid gland. Plasma iodide level is 0.15–0.3 µg%.

Synthesis of thyroid hormones

Thyroxine (T_4) and triiodothyronine (T_3) are synthesized from tyrosine and iodide by the enzyme complex peroxidase. The steps involved in the synthesis of thyroid hormones are (Fig. 5.1-14):

1. ***Iodine trapping.*** The first step in the synthesis of thyroid hormones is *uptake of iodide* by the thyroid gland and is called iodine trapping.

2. ***Synthesis and secretion of thyroglobulin.*** Thyroglobulin is a large glycoprotein that is synthesized in the thyroid epithelial cells as peptide units. These units move to the apical plasma membrane and release into the lumen of follicle (Fig. 5.1-14).

It is also the storage site of the two hormones within the thyroid gland.

3. ***Oxidation of iodide.*** Then iodine is transported into the lumen of the follicles.

Thyroid is the only tissue that can oxidize iodide to iodine. TSH promotes this reaction while antithyroid drugs (thiourea, thiouracil, methimazole) inhibit.

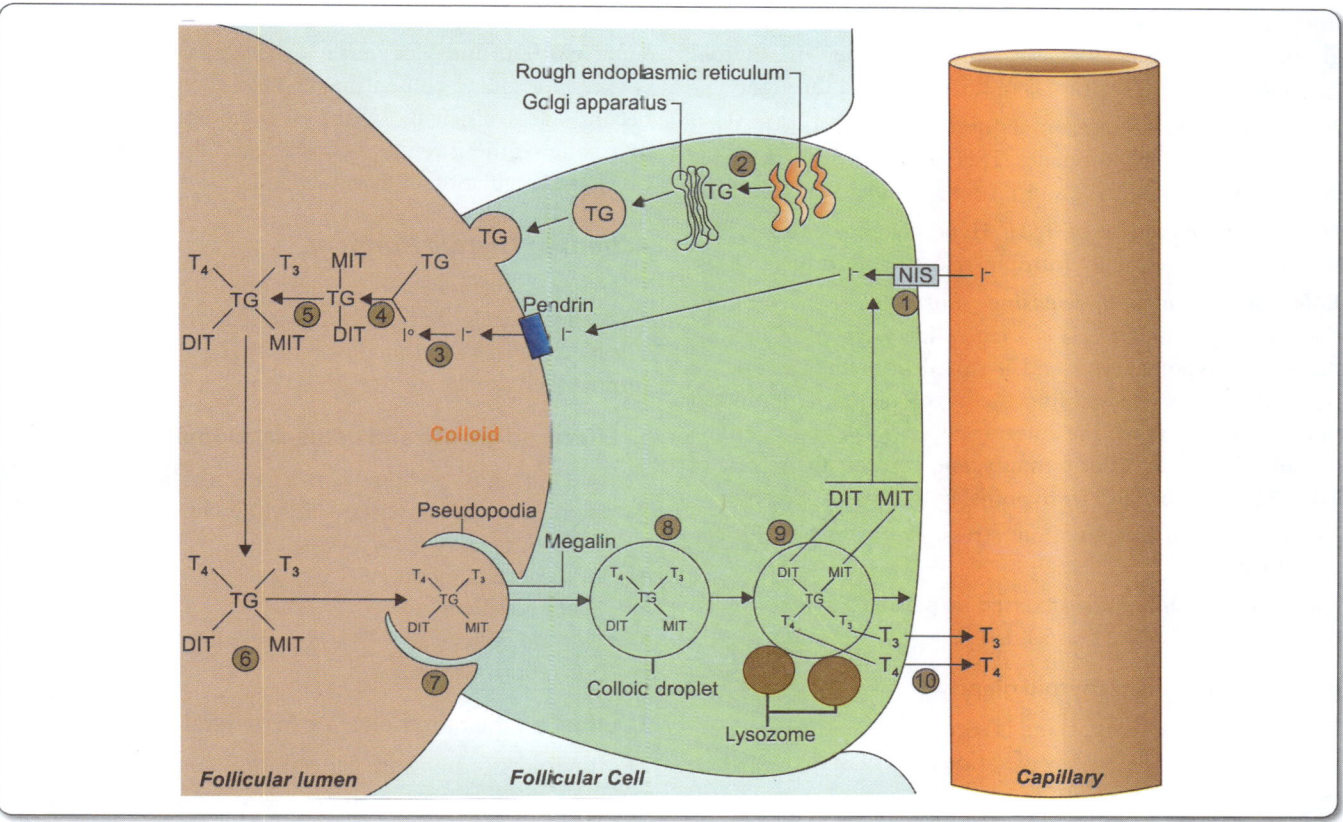

Fig. 5.1-14: Steps in synthesis and release of thyroid hormones: 1, iodine trapping; 2, synthesis of thyroglobulin; 3, oxidation of iodine; 4, organification of thyroglobulin; 5, coupling reaction; 6, storage of thyroid hormone in colloid; 7, take up of colloid by epithelial cell by endocytosis; 8, colloid vesicle; 9, release of T_3 and T_4 after proteolysis; and 10, diffusion of T_3 and T_4 into the capillary

Abbreviations: DIT, diiodotyrosine; MIT, monoiodotyrosine; TG, thyroglobulin

4. *Organification of thyroglobulin* refers to iodination of tyrosine residues present in the thyroglobulin molecule to form monoiodotyrosine (MIT) and diiodotyrosine (DIT).

5. *Coupling reaction.* Two molecules of DIT couple to form thyroxine (T_4). One molecule of MIT, when coupled with one molecule of DIT, produces triioidothyronine (T_3). The enzyme peroxidase is required during coupling.

Storage

Once thyroglobulin has been iodinated, it is stored in the lumen of the follicle as colloid for several months. It is estimated that the stored thyroid hormones can meet the body requirement for 1–3 months.

Transport and Metabolism of Thyroid Hormones

Transport of T_4 and T_3. Secreted T_4 and T_3 circulate in the blood stream in two forms: bound and free.

1. *Bound form:* Most of the circulating T_4 (99.95%) and T_3 is bound to specific binding protein.

2. *Free form:* These free, unbound hormones, represent the biologically active hormone.

Metabolism and excretion of thyroid hormones. The major pathways of peripheral metabolism of circulating thyroid hormone include deiodination, deamination (decarboxylation), and conjugation with glucuronic acid.

Regulation of Thyroid Hormone Secretion

The secretion of thyroid hormones is regulated by:
- Negative feedback mechanism (through hypothalamus-anterior pituitary-thyroid gland axis)
- Autoregulation of thyroid gland.

A. Regulation through negative feedback mechanism

The negative feedback mechanism operating through hypothalamus-anterior pituitary-thyroid gland axis (Fig. 5.1-15) plays an essential role in controlling secretion of thyroid hormones by:

Role of thyroid-stimulating hormone (TSH). It is a glycoprotein which increases the secretion of thyroid hormones. TSH production is in turn regulated through:

Feedback control by plasma T_4 and T_3. (Fig. 5.1-15). A fall in T_4 and T_3 levels stimulates TSH secretion from anterior pituitary, while a rise in T_4 and T_3 levels inhibits TSH secretion.

Hypothalamic control of TSH. Hypothalamus adjusts TSH secretion by secreting thyrotropin-releasing hormone (TRH).

Role of thyrotropin-releasing hormone. Thyrotropin-releasing hormone (TRH) is a tripeptide secreted by arcuate nucleus of hypothalamus and is stored in median eminence from where it is released into the hypothalamo-hypophyseal portal vessels to reach the anterior pituitary. TRH acts on the basophils in the anterior pituitary, and controls the release of TSH. Secretion of TRH by hypothalamus is controlled by:

Nervous stimuli like emotion, stress, exposure to cold, etc. and also by

Negative feedback control exerted by plasma T_3 and T_4 levels on the hypothalamus (Fig. 5.1-15).

B. Autoregulation of thyroid gland

The secretion of thyroid gland is regulated by iodine contents in food. If there is deficiency of iodine content in the diet, then the *iodine trapping* mechanism of the follicular cells becomes super-efficient and vice versa is also true, i.e., when there is excess of iodine content in the food then iodine trapping becomes less efficient. In this way, iodine availability for thyroxine synthesis remains constant and this phenomenon is called autoregulation of thyroid gland.

Actions of Thyroid Hormone

The thyroid hormones do not have any discrete target organ. They affect cellular activity of almost all the tissues of the body. The biochemical functions attributed to thyroid hormones are summarized as follows:

1. Effects on growth and tissue development

Thyroid hormones are important for normal body growth and development. Some important effects are on:

- Development of nervous tissue
- Bone development
- Teeth development
- Normal cycle of growth and maturation
- Subcutaneous tissues.

2. Effect on the metabolic rate in general

The thyroid hormone in general stimulates the metabolic activities and increases the basal rate of oxygen consumption and heat production in most tissues of the body except the brain, retina, gonads, lungs and spleen.

3. Effects on metabolism

Effect on carbohydrate metabolism. T_4 and T_3 lead to increase of almost all aspects of glucose metabolism, i.e., rapid uptake of glucose by the cells, enhanced glycolysis, enhanced gluconeogenesis, and increased insulin secretion and its effects on carbohydrate metabolism.

Effect on fat metabolism. Thyroid hormones cause increase in the levels of fatty acids and a decrease in the quantity of cholesterol, phospholipids and triglycerides in plasma.

Effect on protein metabolism. In physiological amounts, the thyroid hormones function as anabolic hormone leading to positive nitrogen balance, and

Metabolic effects through other hormones. T_4 and T_3 potentiate the respective stimulatory effects of epinephrine, norepinephrine, glucagon, cortisol and growth hormone on gluconeogenesis, lipolysis, ketogenesis, and proteolysis of the labile protein pool.

Effect on vitamin metabolism. Thyroid hormones cause increased need for vitamins leading to relative vitamin deficiency in hyperthyroidism.

Effect on water and electrolyte balance. Thyroid hormones play role in regulation of water and electrolyte balance.

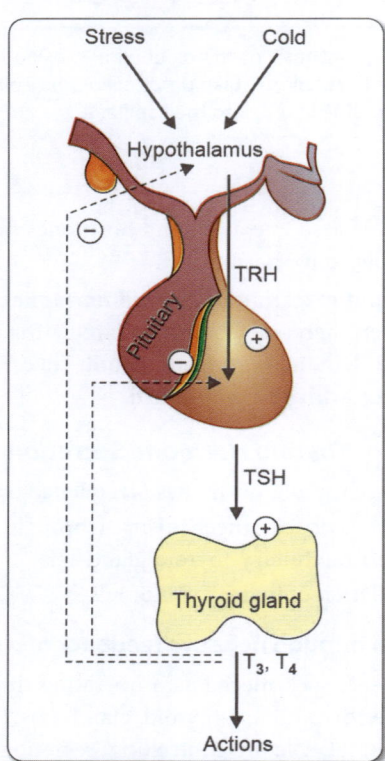

Fig. 5.1-15: Regulation of thyroid hormone secretion by negative feedback control mechanism through hypothalamus-anterior pituitary-thyroid gland axis

4. Respiratory effects

Thyroid hormones stimulate O_2 utilization, which is accomplished by following effects:

Increase in the resting respiratory rate, minute ventilation, and ventilatory responses to hypercapnia and hypoxia.

Increase in oxygen carrying capacity of blood by slightly increasing the red blood cell mass.

5. Cardiovascular effects

In general, the thyroid hormones have the following effects on cardiovascular system:

Tachycardia, i.e., increased heart rate (at rest, even during sleep) is an important physical sign.

Force of cardiac contraction is increased by inotropic effects via adrenergic stimulation.

Cardiac output is increased as a result of increased blood volume, increased heart rate and increased force of contraction

6. Effects on nervous system

a. *Effect on development of nervous system*

T_3 seems to be necessary for proper axonal and dendritic development as well as normal myelination in the nervous system. Critical period for development of nervous system is up to 1 year of life.

b. *Effect on functioning of nervous tissue in adults*

T_4 enhances wakefulness, alertness, responsiveness to various stimuli, auditory sense, awareness of hunger, memory, and learning capacity.

7. Effects on gastrointestinal tract

Effects of thyroid hormones on gastrointestinal tract (GIT) include:

- Increase in appetite and, therefore, increase in food intake, and
- Increase in motility of gastrointestinal tract.
- Excess of thyroid hormone often causes diarrhea.

8. Effects on reproductive system

In males, lack of thyroid hormones causes complete loss of libido, and excess of hormones causes impotence.

In females, lack of thyroid hormones has varying effects:

- Menorrhagia and polymenorrhagia
- Irregular periods or even amenorrhea occur in some women.

CLINICAL ASPECTS

ABNORMALITIES OF THYROID GLAND

Hyperthyroidism

Hyperthyroidism refers to increased secretion of thyroid hormones. Its common causes are:
- Graves' disease (described below), and
- Toxic nodular goiter.

Graves' Disease

Graves' disease is an autoimmune disease characterized by development of thyroid-stimulating antibodies (TSAb) against the TSH receptors, also called long-acting thyroid stimulator (LATS). These antibodies bind to TSH receptors and mimic TSH action on thyroid growth and hormone synthesis.

Symptoms and Signs (Fig. 5.1-16)

General features include marked increase in basal metabolic rate (BMR), weight loss despite an increased intake of food, and increased heat production causing discomfort in warm environments, excessive sweating and a greater intake of water.

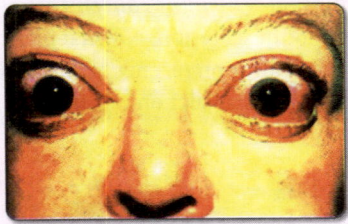

Fig. 5.1-16: Graves' disease

Cardiovascular features are:
- Increased pulse rate or sinus tachycardia
- Arrhythmias (atrial fibrillation is the most common).

Neuromuscular features are nervousness, irritability, restlessness, psychosis, tremors of hand, muscular weakness, and exaggerated tendon reflexes.

Gastrointestinal features are diarrhea or steatorrhea and vomiting.

Dermatological features are perspiration (increased sweating or hyperhidrosis), loss of hair, redness of palm.

Reproductive features are impotence in males and oligomenorrhea or amenorrhea, abortions and infertility in females.

Ophthalmological signs are lid retraction producing staring look and lid lag, and exophthalmos, i.e., bulging out of eyeball.

Hypothyroidism

Hypothyroidism is a clinical syndrome caused by low levels of circulating thyroid hormones. Depending upon the etiology, hypothyroidism can be primary or secondary.

Primary hypothyroidism is caused by disorder of thyroid gland.

Secondary hypothyroidism is caused by diseases of anterior pituitary and hypothalamus.

Clinical Features

Clinical features depend upon the age at which deficiency manifests and duration and severity of the disease. Two different clinical entities are:
- Infantile hypothyroidism (cretinism)
- Adult hypothyroidism (myxedema).

Contd...

Infantile hypothyroidism (cretinism): It occurs when thyroid deficiency occurs during first year of life and is characterized by (Fig. 5.1-17) mental retardation, marked retardation of growth (dwarf), delayed milestones of development, potbelly, protruding tongue, flat nose, dry skin and sparse hairs.

   Treatment should be prompt otherwise mental deficiency will persist.

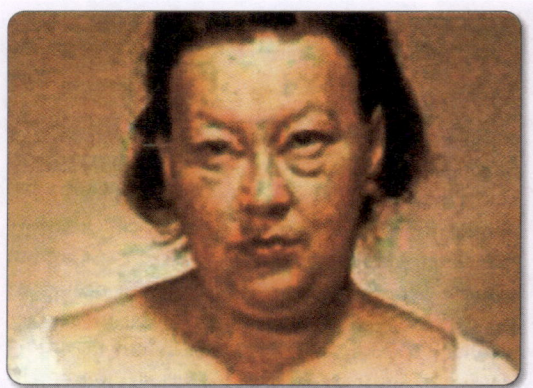

Fig. 5.1-18: Patient with myxedema showing puffy face, thick lips and periorbital edema

Dermatological features: Dry thick skin (toad skin), sparse hair, non-pitting edema due to infiltration by myxedematous tissue (myxedema).

Reproductive features: Menorrhagia and infertility (common), galactorrhea and impotence (less common).

Gastrointestinal features: Constipation (common) and adynamic ileus (less common).

Hematological features include anemia.

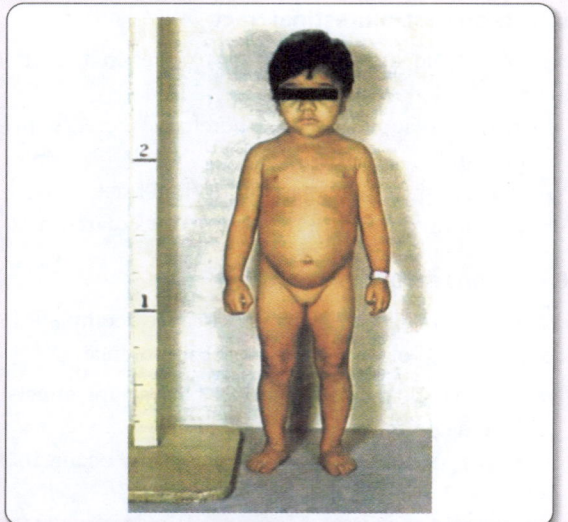

Fig. 5.1-17: Clinical features of cretinism. Note short stature and potbelly

Adult hypothyroidism is also called myxedema because of characteristic infiltration of skin by myxedematous tissue (Fig. 5.1-18). Symptoms and signs include:

General features: Tiredness and weight gain without an appreciable increase in caloric intake (due to lower than normal metabolic rate). Decreased heat production lower body temperature causing intolerance to cold, and decreased sweating.

Cardiovascular features: Adrenergic activity is decreased causing bradycardia. Other features include pericardial effusion and precipitation of angina.

Neuromuscular features: Movement, speech and thought are all slowed, and lethargy, sleepiness, delayed relaxation of ankle jerks, aches and pain are common.

Goiter

Goiter refers to any abnormal increase in the size of the thyroid gland. The term goiter does not denote the functional status of thyroid gland, because it may be associated with:

Euthyroid, i.e., normal thyroid hormone level

Hypothyroidism, i.e., low thyroid hormone level

Hyperthyroidism, i.e., high thyroid hormone levels as seen in Graves' disease and toxic nodular goiter.

Iodine deficiency goiter or endemic goiter occurs when the daily dietary intake of iodine falls below 10 µg (normal requirement 100–200 µg/day). It decreases the synthesis and secretion of thyroid hormone leading to increased TSH levels and proliferation of thyroid gland tissue (goiter). It is mostly found in the geographic regions away from the sea coast where the water and soil are low in iodine content. Consumption of iodized salt is advocated to overcome the problem of endemic goiter. In certain cases, administration of thyroid hormone is also indicated.

Calcitonin

Synthesis and Structure

Calcitonin is synthesized in the C-cells or parafollicular cells of the thyroid gland. These cells are of neural crest origin which during development migrate to the developing thyroid gland.

Regulation of Secretion

The secretion of calcitonin is regulated by following factors:

Increase in plasma calcium concentration is the major regulator of calcitonin secretion. Normal plasma calcium level is 9–11 mg%. Concentration reaches to 9.5 mg% and that above this calcium level, plasma calcitonin is directly proportional to plasma calcium.

Gastrointestinal hormones such as gastrin, cholecystokinin, glucagon, and secretin have all been reported to stimulate calcitonin secretion, with gastrin being the most potent stimulus. *Other factors* like β-adrenergic agonist, dopamine, and estrogen also stimulate calcitonin secretion.

Plasma Levels, Half-life and Degradation

- *Plasma levels* of circulating calcitonin range from 10–20 pg/mL.
- *Degradation.* Circulating calcitonin is heterogeneous, and it is largely degraded and cleared by the kidney.

Actions and Physiological Role of Calcitonin

The major effect of calcitonin is to rapidly lower the plasma calcium level and it also decreases the plasma phosphate. These effects of calcitonin are due to its following actions:

Action on the bone. The main action of calcitonin on the bone is to oppose the bone resorptive action of PTH.

Action on kidney. Calcitonin increases loss of calcium and phosphate in the urine. This effect also contributes in producing hypocalcemia and hypophosphatemia.

PARATHYROID GLANDS

Anatomy of Parathyroid Glands

The parathyroid glands are two pairs of small endocrine glands closely located or the back of the thyroid gland (Fig. 5.1-19). Each gland is about the size of a split pea, measuring $6 \times 4 \times 2$ mm. The total weight of four normal glands is about 140 mg.

Histological Structure

The parenchyma of the parathyroid gland is made up of cells that are arranged in cords. The cells of the parathyroid glands are of two main types: chief cells and oxyphil cells.

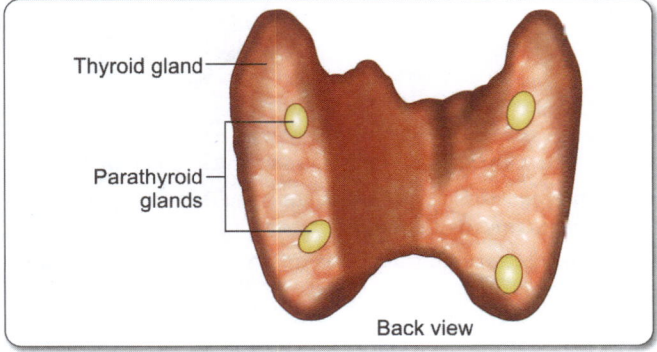

Fig. 5.1-19: Location of parathyroid glands (viewed from behind)

Chief cells, also called principal cells, are much more numerous. Chief cells secrete the parathyroid hormone (PTH) or parathormone.

Oxyphil cells. First appear at puberty and their function is still not clear.

Parathyroid Hormone (PTH)
Structure

Parathyroid hormone is a single chain polypeptide, containing 84 amino acids and has molecular weight 9500.

Synthesis

Parathyroid hormone is synthesized from a precursor molecule called prepro-PTH. PTH is released from chief cells by exocytosis in response to decrease in plasma ionized calcium concentration.

Regulation of PTH Secretion

Role of plasma ionized calcium. The secretion of PTH is mainly regulated by circulating levels of ionized calcium. The secretion of PTH is inversely related to the plasma calcium concentration. Maximum secretion occurs when plasma ionized calcium levels fall below 3.5 mg%.

Role of serum magnesium concentration.
- *Mild decrease* in serum Mg^{2+} concentration stimulates PTH secretion, while
- *Severe decrease* in serum Mg^{2+} concentration inhibits PTH secretion and produces symptoms of hypoparathyroidism (e.g., hypocalcemia).

Role of plasma phosphate concentration. A rise in plasma concentration of phosphate causes an immediate fall in ionized calcium concentration, which in turn stimulates PTH secretion.

Role of vitamin 1,25-(OH)$_2$D$_3$. It decreases PTH secretion.

Plasma Levels and Degradation of PTH

Plasma level of PTH is about 130 pg/mL.
Degradation of PTH occurs rapidly in the peripheral tissues. PTH is predominantly split in the liver.

Actions of PTH

The prime function of PTH is to maintain plasma calcium level by acting on three major target organs: directly on bone and kidney, and indirectly on the gastrointestinal tract (Fig. 5.1-20).

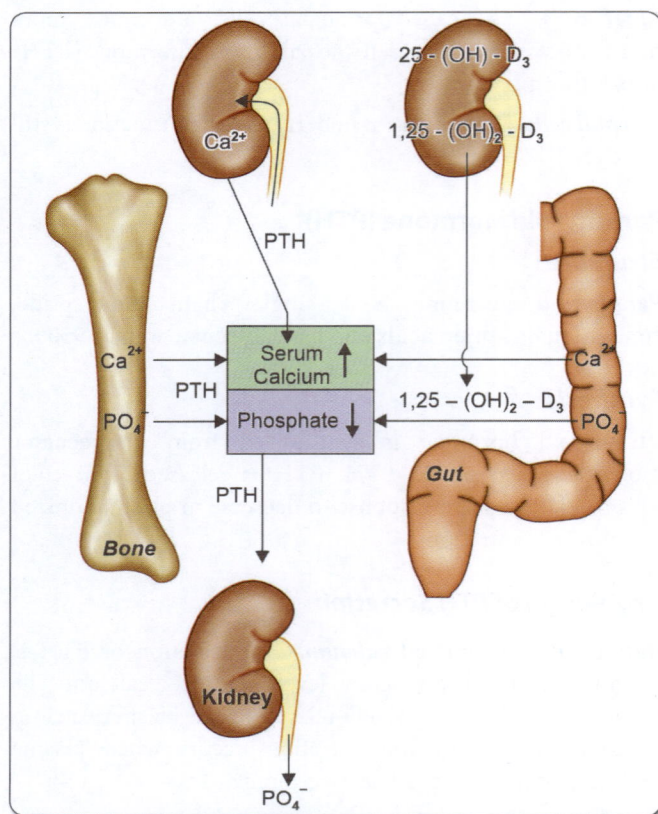

Fig. 5.1-20: Action of parathyroid hormone (PTH) on bone, kidney and intestine

Actions on the bone. PTH stimulates calcium and phosphate resorption from bones, i.e., causes decalcifi-cation or demineralization of bone.

Actions on kidney. The actions of PTH on kidney are:

Increase in calcium reabsorption. PTH increases the reabsorption of calcium from the ascending limb of loop of Henle and the distal tubules of kidney and helps to prevent hypocalcemia.

Inhibition of phosphate reabsorption in the proximal tubule. It is the most dramatic effect of PTH on the kidney. This effect produces phosphaturia and hypophosphatemia.

Stimulation of reabsorption of Mg^{2+} by the renal tubules.

Stimulation of synthesis of 1,25-dihydroxy-cholecalciferol. It is a very important action of PTH in the kidney.

Actions on intestines. Parathormone greatly enhances both calcium and phosphate absorption from intestine indirectly by increasing synthesis of 1,25-dihydroxy-cholecalciferol in the kidney.

CLINICAL ASPECTS

ABNORMALITIES OF PARATHYROID GLANDS

Hyperparathyroidism and Hypercalcemia

Hyperparathyroidism is a clinical condition characterized by excessive secretion of parathyroid hormone (PTH).

Clinicobiochemical features: The main characteristic feature of hyperparathyroidism is involvement of bones which may present as hypercalcemia, hypercalciuria or renal calculi (renal stones). Hypercalcemia may produce muscle weakness, lethargy, constipation and peptic ulceration. Hypercalcemia is also responsible for hypertension and cardiac arrhythmia.

Hypoparathyroidism and Hypocalcemia

Hypoparathyroidism refers to a clinical condition characterized by low level of plasma calcium either due to deficient production of PTH or its unresponsiveness.

Characteristic Features of Hypoparathyroidism

Characteristic features of hypoparathyroidism are:

Hypocalcemia: Total serum calcium may be decreased to 4–8 mg% and the ionized calcium to 3 mg%. Fall in the levels of ionized calcium leads to a clinical condition called *tetany* (described below):

Hyperphosphatemia: It is an increase in serum inorganic phosphate levels to 6–16 mg%.

Tetany

Tetany refers to a clinical condition resulting from increased neuromuscular excitability.

Clinical features: The following symptoms may be seen:

- *Trousseau's sign (carpal spasm):* The hands in carpal spasm adapt a peculiar posture in which there occurs flexion at metacarpophalangeal joints, extension at interphalangeal joints and there is apposition of thumb (Fig. 5.1-21). This peculiar posture of hand is called *obstetric hand*.

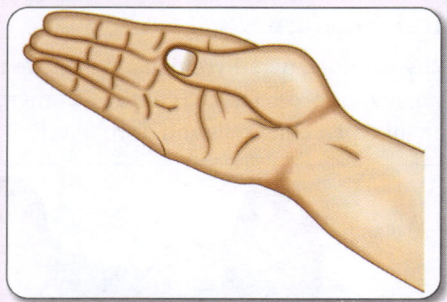

Fig. 5.1-21: Carpal spasm (Trousseau's sign) in a patient with tetany

- *Laryngeal stridor* (loud sound) results from spasm of laryngeal muscles. It may produce asphyxia.

Management of tetany includes treatment of hypocalcemia— an intravenous injection of 20 mL of 10% calcium gluconate is given to correct hypocalcemia and relieve tetany.

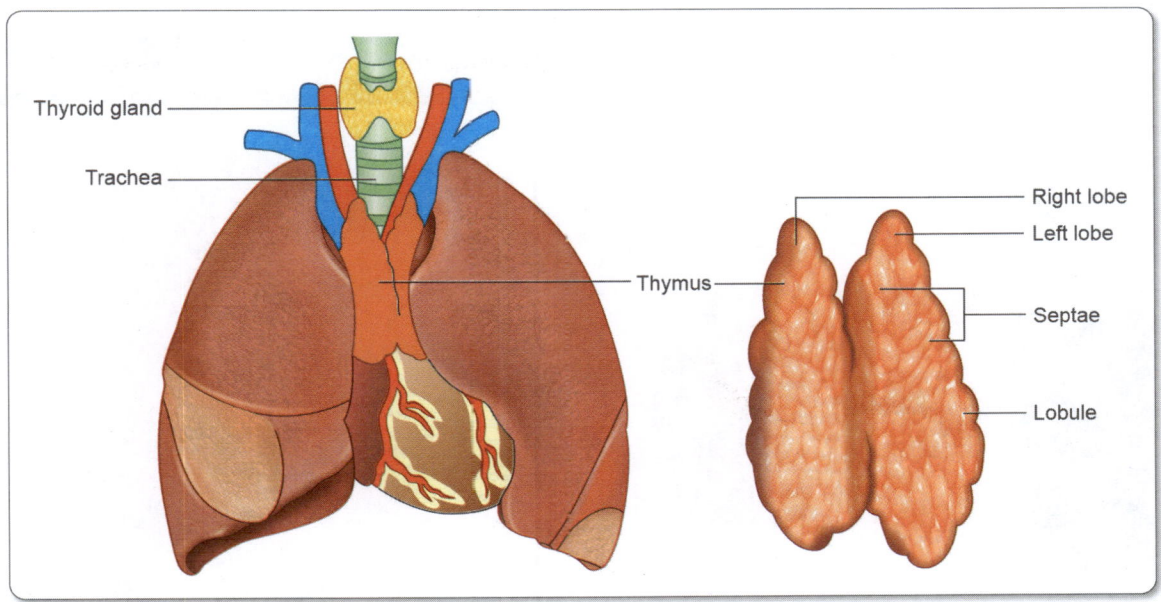

Fig. 5.1-22: Location of thymus gland in an adult

THYMUS

Anatomy

Thymus is a small lymphoid structure located in the lower part of neck in front of the trachea, below the thyroid gland (Fig. 5.1-22). The thymus consists of two lobes connected by areolar tissue. The lobes are covered by a fibrous capsule which sends septa. At birth, it is small (weighing 10–12 g), gradually enlarges till puberty when it weighs 20–30 g, and then it starts decreasing in size and in old age weighs about 3–6 g. The sex glands exert a depressant effect on the thymus, therefore, castration (removal of gonads) prolongs the period of persistence of the thymus.

Histological Structure

Histologically, thymus consists of the inner medulla and outer cortex.

Medulla. It comprises reticular epithelial cells, a few lymphocytes and concentric corpuscles of Hassall.

Cortex. It includes actively multiplying, closely packed lymphocytes and contains no Hassall's corpuscles.

Functions

Thymus has two functions:

1. Immunological functions (For details see Chapter 4.3, page 239)
2. Endocrine functions.

Endocrine function of thymus. Thymus tissue secretes two hormones, thymosin and thymin.

Thymosin. It is a peptide which promotes proliferation of T-lymphocytes in the thymus and peripheral lymphoid tissue.

Thymin. It is also called thymopoietin, inhibits acetylcholine release at motor nerve endings and thus suppresses neuromuscular activity and is one of the cause of Myasthenia Gravis (*for detail see page 388*).

ADRENAL GLANDS

ANATOMY OF ADRENAL GLAND

There are two adrenal glands, situated one on either side, at the upper pole of kidney, hence also called "suprarenal gland" (Figs 5.1-23A and B). Normally, each gland weighs about 5 g and consists of two parts, the adrenal cortex and the medulla.

Histological Structure

Adrenal Cortex

The adrenal gland is covered by a connective tissue capsule from which septa extends into the gland substance. The mature human adrenal cortex consists of three distinct layers or zones of cells (Fig. 5.1-24 and Histology Plate 5.1-3).

1. *Zona glomerulosa,* constituting outer one-fifth of cortex, is a small zone present under the capsule. It consists of cells that secrete *aldosterone* and *corticosterone.*

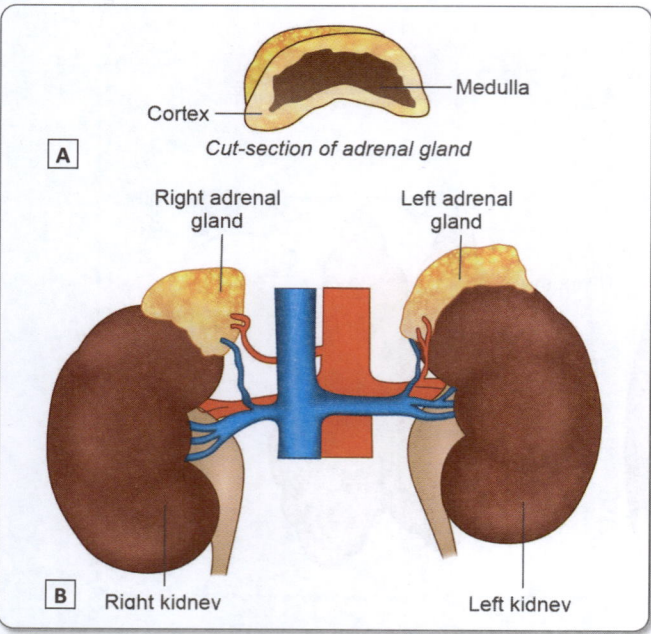

Figs 5.1-23A and B: Adrenal gland. **A.** Division; **B.** Location

2. *Zona fasciculata* is the widest zone forming middle three-fifths of the cortex. It is made up of cells that are arranged in two cell thick straight columns. Sinusoids intervene between the columns.

3. *Zona reticularis* forms the inner one-fifth of the cortex. It is made up of a network of compactly arranged cords of cells (hence the name zona reticularis).

Adrenal Medulla

Histologically, it is made up of chromaffin cells, innervated by preganglionic sympathetic neurons.

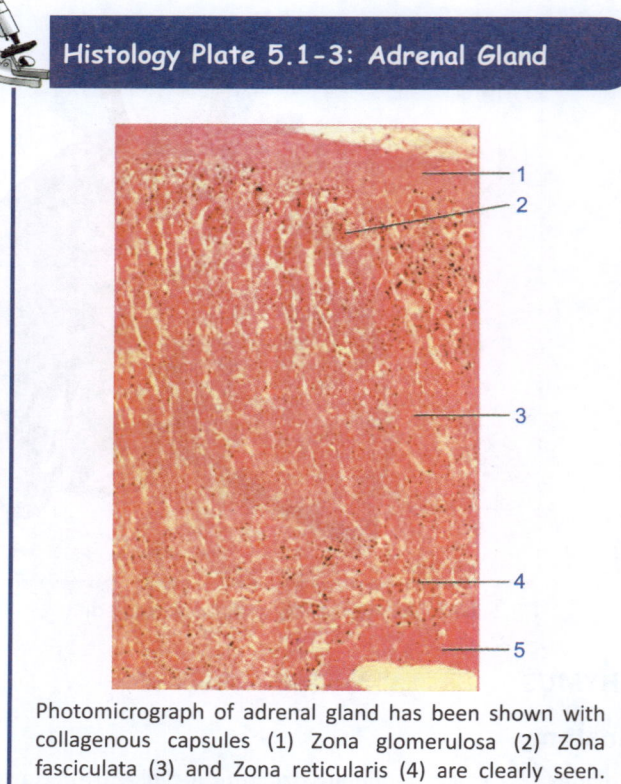

Histology Plate 5.1-3: Adrenal Gland

Photomicrograph of adrenal gland has been shown with collagenous capsules (1) Zona glomerulosa (2) Zona fasciculata (3) and Zona reticularis (4) are clearly seen. Medulla (5) is present in lower part.

Functionally, these cells are considered to be modified postganglionic neurons which do not have axons. Catecholamines are stored in the chromaffin granules. In addition to the catecholamines, the chromaffin granules also contain proteins, lipids, and adenine nucleotides (mainly ATP).

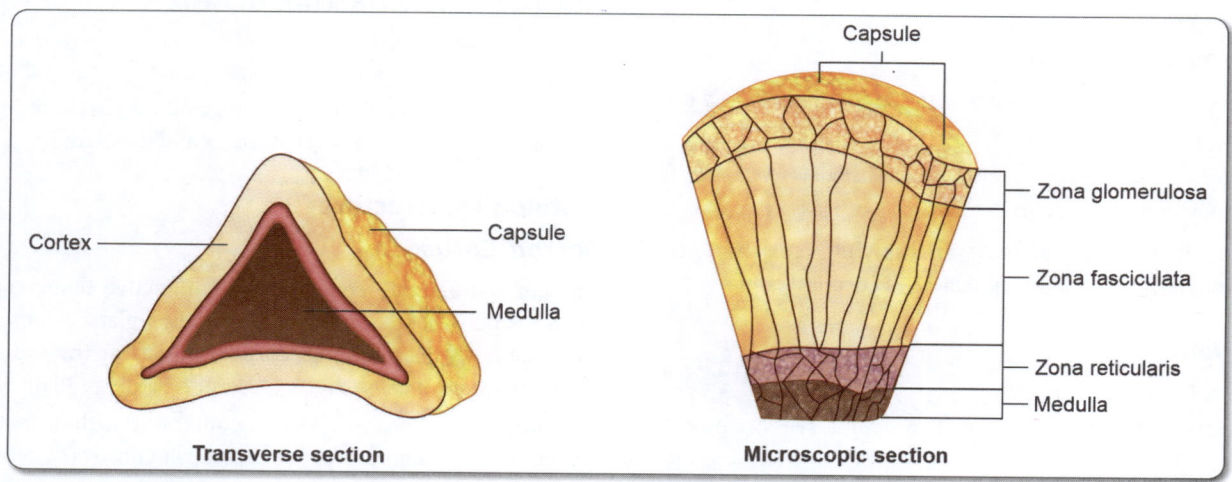

Fig. 5.1-24: Histological structure of adrenal gland

Nerve endings, present in the adrenal medulla, are the *cholinergic preganglionic* sympathetic fibers that synapse directly on chromaffin cells. These fibers traverse the splanchnic nerve and are myelinated emanating mainly from the lower thoracic segments (T_5 and T_9) of the ipsilateral intermediolateral grey column of the spinal cord (Fig. 5.1-25).

Blood Supply (Fig. 5.1-26)

Arterial blood supply. The arterial blood reaches the adrenal gland to the outer capsule from superior suprarenal artery (a branch of the inferior phrenic artery), middle suprarenal artery (a branch of the abdominal aorta), and inferior suprarenal artery (a branch of the renal artery). The arterial blood enters sinusoidal capillaries in the cortex and then drains into medullary veins which supply blood to medulla and thus form a *portal system.* This arrangement of portal circulation exposes the medulla to relatively high concentrations of corticosteroids from the cortex.

Venous drainage. The venous blood drains via single central vein. The right suprarenal vein drains into the inferior vena cava and left suprarenal vein into the left renal vein.

HORMONES OF ADRENAL CORTEX

Hormones secreted by adrenal cortex, called *corticosteroids,* can be grouped as:

Glucocorticoids. These include *cortisol* and *corticosterone,* that have widespread effect on glucose and protein metabolism.

Mineralocorticoids. Aldosterone is the chief mineralo-corticoid. It regulates sodium balance and ECF volume in the body.

Adrenal sex steroids. These include dehydroepian-drosterone (DHEA) and its sulphate ester.

Glucocorticoids

Synthesis

The glucocorticoids are synthesized largely by the cells forming zona fasciculata with a small contribution by the cells of zona reticularis of adrenal cortex.

Plasma Levels, Transport, Metabolism, and Excretion of Glucocorticoids

Plasma levels

Plasma levels of glucocorticoids and other corticosteroids are shown in Table 5.1-3. The plasma levels of total cortisol show diurnal fluctuation and range from 10–25 µg% with an average of 14 µg%. The rate of secretion of cortisol, which is about 15 mg/day under normal condition, may increase to 300–400 mg/day under conditions of severe stress.

Transport

In the plasma, cortisol circulates in two forms:

1. *Bound form.* Most of the plasma cortisol (5%) is bound to specific corticosteroid, binding α_2-globulin (CBG), which is

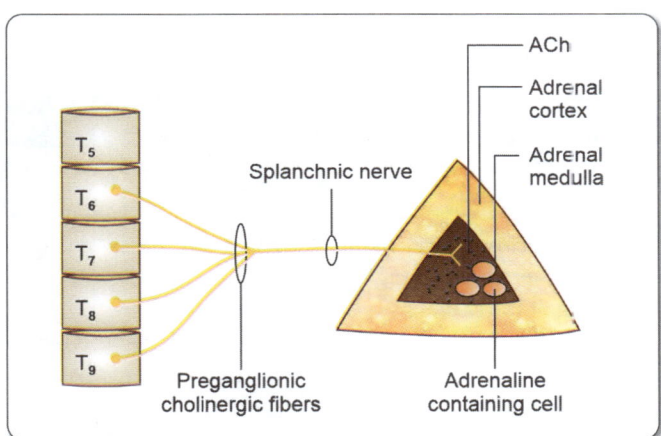

Fig. 5.1-25: Preganglionic sympathetic fibers synapsing directly on chromaffin cells in the adrenal medulla

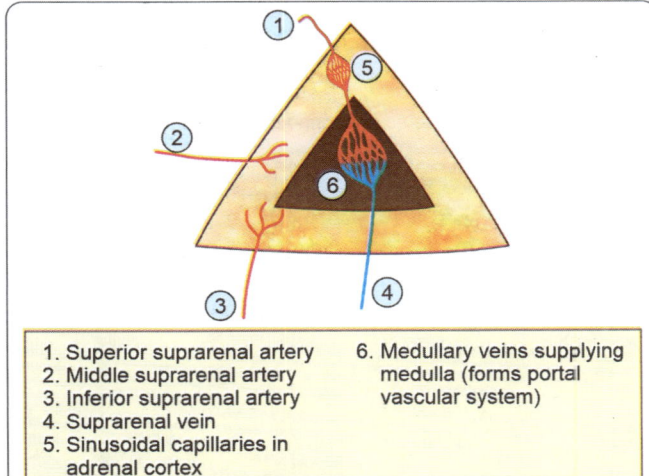

1. Superior suprarenal artery
2. Middle suprarenal artery
3. Inferior suprarenal artery
4. Suprarenal vein
5. Sinusoidal capillaries in adrenal cortex
6. Medullary veins supplying medulla (forms portal vascular system)

Fig. 5.1-26: Schematic diagram to show arterial supply and venous drainage of adrenal gland

TABLE 5.1-3: Average 8 am plasma levels and secretion rate of corticosteroids in adult humans		
Corticosteroid	**Plasma concentration (µg/dL)**	**Secretion rate (mg/day)**
Cortisol	14.0	15
Corticosterone	1.0	03
Aldosterone	0.009	0.15
Dehydroepiandrosterone (DHEA) sulphate	115	15

a glycoprotein and is also called *transcortin*. A small amount (15%) is bound to albumin.

2. Free form. The free form of cortisol constitutes only 5–10% of the total plasma cortisol.

Metabolism and excretion

Corticosteroids are degraded in the liver and excreted in the urine and feces.

Actions of Glucocorticoids

Glucocorticoids are essential for survival. The actions of glucocorticoids are grouped as:

I. Metabolic effects of glucocorticoids

The different metabolic effects of glucocorticoids are:

Effects on carbohydrate metabolism. Glucocorticoids exert an anti-insulin effect, which leads to hyperglycemia by following actions:

Increased gluconeogenesis. Glucocorticoids increase the rate of glucose production from non-carbohydrate sources by as much as 6–10 folds.

Decreased utilization of glucose in peripheral tissues.

Effects on protein metabolism. The effects exerted by glucocorticoids are:

Catabolic effect. Cortisol enhances the release of amino acids by proteolysis in skeletal muscle and other extrahepatic tissues.

Antianabolic effect. It is the ability of the glucocorticoids to inhibit the synthesis of protein.

Effects on fat metabolism. They are complex and include:

Lipolytic effects. Although cortisol itself has only a slight lipolytic activity, its presence is necessary for epinephrine, growth hormone, and other lipolytic substances to stimulate hydrolysis of stored triglycerides at maximal rates.

- Fatty acid synthesis is inhibited in the liver by cortisol.

Lipogenic role. Glucocorticoids stimulate lipogenesis.

Effects on electrolyte and water metabolism. Glucocorticoids control distribution of body water and electrolytes by following actions:

Retention of sodium and water.
Promotion of diuresis.

II. Physiological actions on various organs and systems

In addition to the metabolic effects, the glucocorticoids affect various organs and systems throughout the body (Fig. 5.1-27):

Effects on muscle:
Contractility and work performance of skeletal and cardiac muscles are maintained by the cortisol.

Decrease in muscle mass and strength is caused by an excess of cortisol. This occurs due to decrease in muscle protein synthesis and increase in muscle catabolism.

Effects on bone. The glucocorticoids cause:
- *Increased bone resorption.*
- *Inhibition of bone formation.*

IMPORTANT TO KNOW

Because of the above effects on bone, *osteoporosis* results in skeletal deformity.

Effects on connective tissue. Cortisol decreases collagen synthesis thereby resulting into:
Thinning of the skin
Thinning of walls of capillaries, which leads to their easy rupture and to intracutaneous hemorrhage.

Effects on vascular system. Cortisol is essential for maintaining normal blood pressure by:
- Sustaining myocardial performance
- Enhancing the vasopressure effect of catecholamines (especially norepinephrine) and angiotensin II, and maintaining normal blood volume.

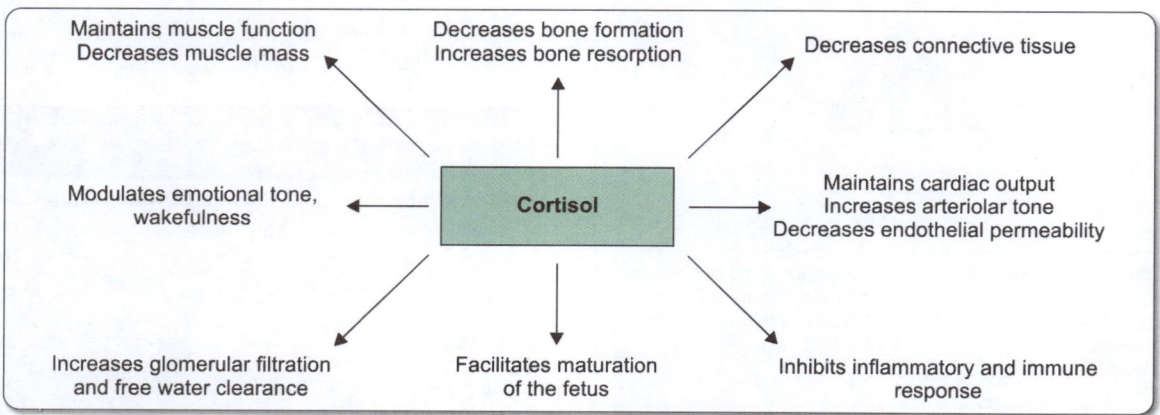

Fig. 5.1-27: Effects of glucocorticoids on various tissues, organs and systems of the body

Effects on kidney:

- Increase in glomerular filtration rate (GFR) by increasing glomerular plasma flow
- Rapid excretion of water load
- Increase in calcium and phosphate excretion by decreasing their reabsorption in the proximal tubules.

Effects on central nervous system. Glucocorticoid receptors (GR) are present in various parts of the brain, especially in the limbic system. Through these receptors, the glucocorticoids modulate excitability behavior and mood.

Effects on gastrointestinal tract. The glucocorticoids increase gastric acid secretion and can lead to peptic ulceration following long-term use of cortisol.

Effects on blood cells and lymphatic organs. The excess of glucocorticoids leads to:

- Eosinopenia and basopenia
- Lymphopenia
- Neutrophilia
- Polycythemia
- Thrombocytosis.

III. Anti-inflammatory, anti-immunity and anti-allergic effects

These effects are not produced by the glucocorticoids which are normally secreted physiologically, but are produced by their large doses when administered therapeutically and are thus called the pharmacological actions of glucocorticoids.

IV. Role of glucocorticoids in fetal life

Maturation of CNS, retina, skin and lungs is facilitated by the cortisol in utero.

V. Role of glucocorticoids in stress

Various stresses, e.g., trauma, cold, illness, starvation are associated with activation of the hypothalamic-hypophyseal-adrenal axis. Increased secretion of glucocorticoids is one of the various mechanisms involved in adaptation to various stresses.

Regulation of Glucocorticoid Secretion

The glucocorticoid secretion is regulated by hypothalamic-anterior pituitary-adrenal cortex axis which exerts its effect through (Fig. 5.1-28):

- Corticotropin releasing hormone (CRH)
- Adrenocorticotropic hormone (ACTH)
- Glucocorticoid negative feedback effect.

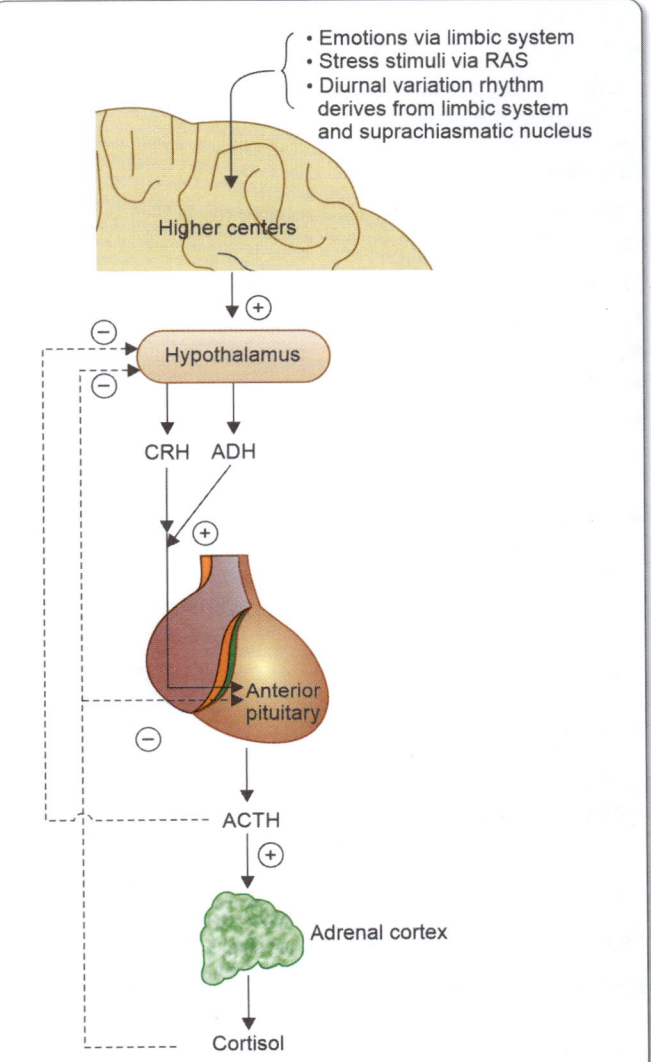

Fig. 5.1-28: Hypothalamic-anterior pituitary-adrenal axis and negative feedback mechanism
Abbreviations: ACTH, adrenocorticotropic hormone; ADH, antidiuretic hormone; CRH, corticotropin-releasing hormone

IMPORTANT TO KNOW

Since CRH and ACTH are related to regulation of glucocorticoid release, they are described in detail here rather than along with other hormones of hypothalamus and anterior pituitary, respectively.

1. Role of corticotropin-releasing hormone

Corticotropin-releasing hormone (CRH) is secreted by the small cells of paraventricular nucleus of hypothalamus. CRH is a polypeptide with 41 amino acids.

Actions of CRH

Stimulation of synthesis and release of ACTH by acting on the *corticotrophs.*

Other actions of CRH related to or independent of ACTH include:

- Central arousal
- Increase in blood pressure
- Diminution of reproductive function by decreasing synthesis of gonadotropin-releasing hormone (GnRH) and gonadotropins
- Decrease in feeding activity and growth
    - Stimulation of release of cytokines in immune cells.

2. Role of adrenocorticotropic hormone

Adrenocorticotropic hormone (ACTH) is secreted by *corticotrophs.*

Actions of ACTH

Actions on adrenal cortex. ACTH is primarily concerned with growth and functions of adrenal cortex.

Extra adrenal actions of ACTH. They occur only with very high levels which are seen in abnormal conditions.

Regulation of ACTH secretion

Hypothalamic control on ACTH secretion is mainly exerted through CRH (see above). The hypothalamic control is responsible for following characteristics of ACTH secretion:

Diurnal variation in the levels of ACTH (and thus of cortisol) is due to variation in CRH release. A large peak in the levels of ACTH and cortisol occurs in the morning (6–8 AM) during awakening (plasma level of ACTH range between 20 and 100 pg/mL with an average of 50 pg/mL). Thereafter, the average level decreases markedly (5 pg/mL), just before or after the subject falls asleep. In night workers, the rhythm is reversed.

Pulsatile release of ACTH is also due to pulsatile release of CRH—up to three pulses per hour, and each pulse lasts about 20 minutes. Cortisol pulses follow the ACTH pulses (Figs 5.1-29A to C).

Negative feedback inhibition of ACTH is caused by (Fig. 5.1-28):

- Plasma cortisol levels (long-loop negative feedback), and
- Plasma ACTH levels (short-loop negative feedback).

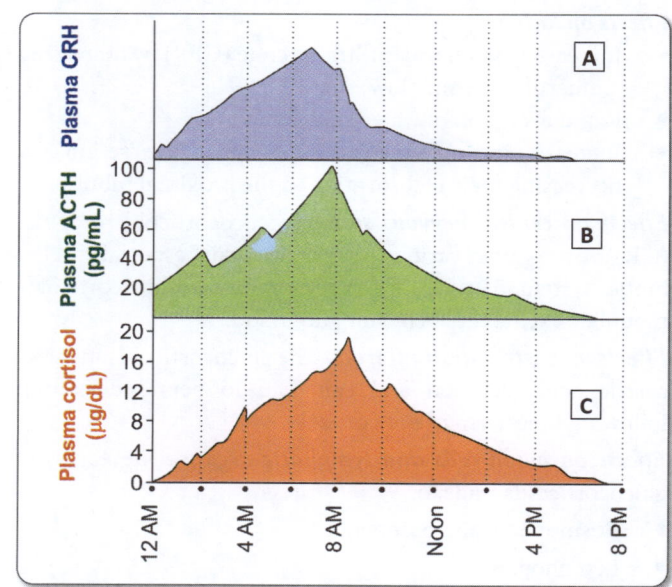

Figs 5.1-29A to C: Diurnal variations and pulsatility in secretion of CRH (A), ACTH (B) and cortisol (C). Note the ACTH peak follows CRH peak and cortisol peak follows ACTH peak by 10 minutes

3. Negative feedback control of glucocorticoid secretion

Chronically elevated plasma levels of free cortisol exert a direct negative feedback action on its own secretion. This effect is exerted at two levels (Fig. 5.1-28):

1. On hypothalamus to decrease formation of CRH
2. On anterior pituitary to decrease formation of ACTH.

Mineralocorticoids

The mineralocorticoids include:

- Aldosterone. It is the chief mineralocorticoid,
- Deoxycorticosterone (DOC), and 18-hydroxy-deoxycorticosterone (18-OH-DOC) are secreted in small amount and have some mineralocorticoid activity.

Since aldosterone is the major mineralocorticoid, so discussion in this section is limited to it.

Synthesis

Aldosterone, the chief mineralocorticoid, is synthesized exclusively by the *zona glomerulosa cells.*

Plasma Levels, Transport, Metabolism and Excretion

Plasma levels

Depending upon the dietary intake of sodium, the aldosterone secretion ranges from 50 µg/day (with dietary sodium intake of 150 mEq) to 250 µg/day (with dietary sodium intake of 10 mEq).

Actions of Aldosterone

A. Primary actions of aldosterone

1. *Effects on renal tubules*

Aldosterone acts on late distal tubules and collecting ducts of kidney and causes following effects:

1. **Sodium reabsorption** from the tubular fluid into renal tubular epithelial cells, and
2. **Potassium excretion**

2. *Effects on sweat glands, salivary glands and colon*

Sweat glands and salivary glands. They produce primary secretions which contain large amount of sodium chloride. The sodium chloride is absorbed as the secretion passes through the ducts, and in turn K^+ and HCO_3^- are excreted. Thus aldosterone decreases the loss of Na^+ and Cl^- in sweat and salivary secretion.

Colon. The aldosterone stimulates sodium reabsorption from the colon while enhancing potassium excretion in the feces.

B. Secondary effects of aldosterone

The secondary effects include:

1. Hypokalemia, i.e., decrease in plasma K^+ levels may occur in aldosterone excess due to increased urinary excretion of K^+.

2. Hypernatremia.

Regulation of Aldosterone Secretion

Aldosterone secretion is controlled by following factors (Fig. 5.1-30):

1. Renin-angiotensin system

The secretion of aldosterone is influenced by changes in the circulating fluid volume which are sensed in the kidney. The signals arising from the kidney increase aldosterone secretion when ECF volume is decreased and vice versa.

Conditions associated with decreased ECF are:

- Sodium deprivation (e.g., dietary restriction)
- Hemorrhage
- Upright posture for several hours
- Acute diuresis.

Steps involved in the secretion of aldosterone by renin-angiotensin system are:

Decrease in ECF volume leads to decrease in renal arterial blood flow and pressure.

Decrease in renal perfusion pressure causes the juxtaglomerular cells of the afferent arterioles to secrete renin. **Renin** catalyzes the conversion of angiotensinogen (alpha 2-globulin substrate present in the plasma) to angiotensin I.

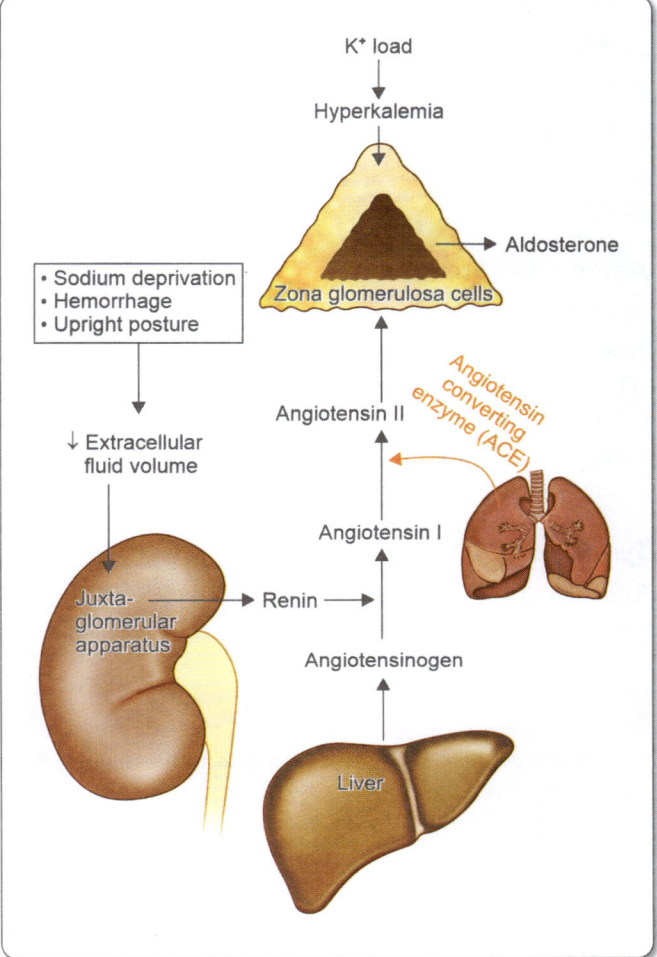

Fig. 5.1-30: Regulation of aldosterone secretion

Angiotensin I is converted into angiotensin II by the action of angiotensin converting enzyme (ACE) present in the endothelium of blood vessels, especially in the lungs.

Angiotensin II binds to specific plasma membrane receptors present on adrenal zona glomerulosa cells and increases the secretion of aldosterone.

Aldosterone secretion may be increased to 4–8-fold by renin-angiotensin system.

2. Plasma potassium concentration

There exists a vital negative feedback relationship between plasma potassium concentration and aldosterone secretion, i.e., *an increase in plasma concentration* by only 0.5 mEq/L immediately raises plasma aldosterone levels 3-fold.

3. Role of ACTH

ACTH also plays role in mineralocorticoid secretion by direct stimulating effect.

4. Role of atrial natriuretic peptide (ANP)

ANP inhibits renin secretion, leading to decrease the effect of angiotensin II.

Adrenal Sex Steroids

Adrenal sex steroids include:

Dehydroepiandrosterone (DHEA), its sulphate ester (DHEA-S) and *androstenedione* are the major androgenic precursor products of adrenal cortex.

Estrogen and progesterone are produced in very small amounts.

Synthesis

The adrenal sex steroid precursors are synthesized in the *zona reticularis*. The 17-hydroxylated derivatives of pregnenolone and progesterone are the starting points for synthesis of androgen precursors.

Plasma Levels

Normal plasma level of DHEA is 150–200 µg% at 25 years of age in both sexes.

Contribution of Adrenal Glands Toward Sex Steroids

During fetal life, adrenal cortex is hyperplastic and secretes large amount of DHEA which acts as the main precursor for synthesis of estrogen by placenta.

In adult woman, the adrenal glands supply 50–60% of the androgenic hormone requirement. DHEA-S contributes to increased muscle mass, growth of pubic and axillary hair and libido.

In adult man, since testes produce a large quantity of testosterone, the adrenal androgen precursors are of little biological importance. However, they may be partly responsible for development of male sex organs in childhood.

CLINICAL ASPECTS

The important applied aspects in relation to the adrenal cortex which need mention include:
- Hyperactivity of adrenal cortex
- Hypoactivity of adrenal cortex

Hyperactivity of Adrenal Cortex

Disorders of hyperactivity of adrenal cortex include:
- Cushing's syndrome (hypercortisol state)
- Conn's syndrome (hyperaldosteronism).

Cushing's Syndrome

Cushing's syndrome refers to the group of clinical conditions occurring due to prolonged excessive levels of glucocorticoids.

Characteristic features of Cushing's syndrome are (Figs 5.1-31A and B):
- *Truncal or centripetal obesity* occurs due to redistribution of body fat (which is in the abdominal wall, back and face) from extremities producing characteristic features of:
  - Buffalo hump
  - Moon face
  - Purple striae or cutaneous abdominal striae or livid stretch marks. Causes rupture of subdermal tissues producing reddish purple striae.
- *Muscle weakness* and backache due to protein catabolism.
- *Sodium and water retention* may cause weight gain, edema and hypertension.
- *Hyperglycemia* occurs due to gluconeogenesis and inhibition of peripheral utilization of glucose. It may lead to glycosuria and adrenal diabetes.
- *Hirsutism and menstrual irregularity* may occur due to increased adrenal androgens.

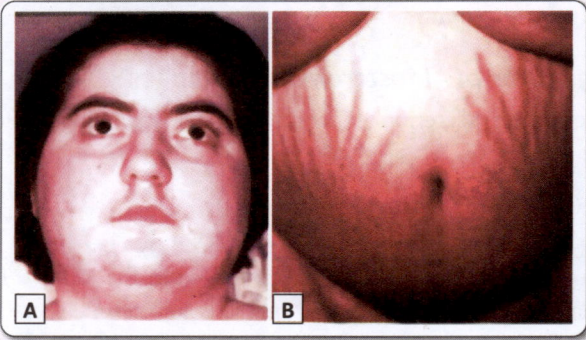

Figs 5.1-31A and B: Photograph of a patient with Cushing's syndrome. A. Moon face; B. Truncal obesity and purple striae on the abdomen

- *Susceptibility to osteoporosis and bone fracture* is increased due to protein depletion and bone resorption.
- *Susceptibility to infections* is increased due to immunosuppression.
- *Psychological, emotional and personality changes* may occur due to CNS effects of glucocorticoids.
- *Blackening of skin* may occur due to pigmentation caused by melanocyte-stimulating hormone (MSH)-like effects of excessive adrenocorticotropic hormone (ACTH).
- *Susceptibility to peptic ulceration* is increased.

Hyperaldosteronism

Hyperaldosteronism (Conn's syndrome) refers to over-production of the hormone aldosterone, a major sodium-retaining hormone.

Contd...

Characteristic features of hyperaldosteronism are:
- *Sodium and water retention* leading to hypertension and edema.
- *Hypokalemia* may occur due to increased potassium excretion producing muscle weakness.
- *Metabolic alkalosis* may occur due to secretion of more amount of H$^+$ into renal tubules. Metabolic alkalosis may produce hypocalcemia causing tetany.

Hypoactivity of Adrenal Cortex

Adrenocortical deficiency, depending upon the site of lesion, can be divided into two types:
1. *Primary adrenocortical deficiency* occurs due to involvement of adrenal cortex and is associated with high ACTH levels due to feedback mechanism. The conditions producing primary adrenocortical deficiency include:
   - Addison's disease
   - Congenital adrenal hyperplasia.
2. *Secondary adrenocortical deficiency* occurs due to involvement of either hypothalamus or pituitary or due to exogenous glucocorticoid administration and is associated with *low ACTH level* due to less production.

Addison's Disease

Characteristic features occur due to chronic deficiency of hormones secreted by all the three zones of adrenal cortex:
1. *Glucocorticoid insufficiency* produces weight loss, malaise, anorexia, nausea, vomiting, weakness and diarrhea. Since glucocorticoids are essential for adaptation to stress, therefore, in Addison's disease exposure to any type of stress, e.g., even mild infection may be fatal.
2. *Mineralocorticoid deficiency* produces hyponatremia, hyperkalemia, acidosis and decreased ECF volume with hypotension.
3. *Loss of androgens* causes sparse hair in females.
4. *Increased ACTH secretion* occurs due to feedback mechanism and causes diffuse pigmentation of the skin and mucous membranes (because of its MSH- like actions).

Addisonian Crisis or Adrenal Crisis

It refers to acute adrenal insufficiency characterized by sudden collapse. The condition becomes fatal if not treated in time.

Congenital Adrenal Hyperplasia

Congenital adrenal hyperplasia is caused by congenital deficiency of one of the enzymes involved in the biosynthesis of glucocorticoids, particularly *21-hydroxylase deficiency* and deficiency of *11-hydroxylase*.

Characteristic features: Features occurring because of above pathophysiological changes are virilism and excessive body growth.
- *In boys*, adrenal hyperplasia leads to:
  - Precocious body growth leading to stocky appearance called *infant hercules*.
  - Precocious sexual development with enlarged penis even at age of 4 years.
- *In female fetus*, high plasma androgen levels cause *masculinized pattern* of development (*virilism*). Sometimes the female fetus may be born with male type external genitalia. This condition is called *pseudohermaphroditism*.

HORMONES OF ADRENAL MEDULLA

The adrenal medulla secretes *catecholamines* which include epinephrine, norepinephrine and dopamine. About 80% of adrenal medullary catecholamine is epinephrine and rest is norepinephrine.

Synthesis and Storage of Catecholamine Hormones

Synthesis of Catecholamines

Epinephrine and norepinephrine are synthesized in different cells from L-tyrosin.

Storage of Catecholamines in Storage Granules

The epinephrine formed in the cytoplasm is then taken back up by the chromaffin granules, in which it is stored as the predominant adrenomedullary hormone.

Factors regulating catecholamine synthesis are:
- Acute sympathetic stimulation
- Chronic stimulation of preganglionic fibers
- ACTH
- Cortisol
- Epinephrine.

Regulation

Nervous Control of Secretion

The catecholamine secretion is entirely controlled by the splanchnic nerves supplying the medulla. These fibers, when stimulated, act by releasing acetylcholine close to the adrenal medullary chromaffin cells.

Physiological and psychological stimuli for release

The adrenal medullary activation occurs as a part of generalized sympathetic response to any emergency situation. Therefore, this has also been called *sympathetic alarm* reaction. The various sensory stimuli associated with rapid release of epinephrine (and probably norepinephrine) from adrenal medulla include:
- Perception or even anticipation of danger or harm (anxiety)
- Pain
- Trauma
- Hypovolemia from hemorrhage or fluid loss

Circulation, Metabolism and Excretion

- *Secreted epinephrine* and norepinephrine from the adrenal medulla is in the ratio of 4:1.
- *Basal plasma levels* (in recumbent humans) of free epinephrine are 30 pg/mL and that of free norepinephrine are 300 pg/mL.
- *Variation in plasma levels* of catecholamines according to physiological or pathological states are quite common.
- Catecholamines are metabolites in liver and kidney. The metabolites are excreted in urine and bile.

Adrenergic Receptors and Actions of Catecholamines

Adrenergic Receptors

The adrenergic receptors are of two types:

1. **Alpha (α) receptors.** These are further of two types (α$_1$ and α$_2$). The alpha-adrenergic receptors are sensitive to both epinephrine and norepinephrine. These receptors are associated with most of the excitatory functions of the body but have one major inhibitory function (i.e., inhibition of intestinal motility).

2. **Beta (β) receptors.** These are further of three types β$_1$, β$_2$ and β$_3$. Beta-adrenergic receptors respond to epinephrine and in general are relatively insensitive to norepinephrine. These receptors are associated with most of the inhibitory functions of the body but have an important excitatory function (i.e., excitation of myocardium).

Actions of Catecholamines

The catecholamines exert their effects by binding with adrenergic receptors as described above.

- Actions of catecholamines on individual organs and systems are similar to those resulting from stimulation of sympathetic nervous system.
- In general, the effects produced by adrenomedullary stimulation last longer (about 10 times) than those produced by sympathetic stimulation.

I. Metabolic actions of catecholamines

General metabolic effects of epinephrine

- Increased O$_2$ consumption (by 20–40%) and increased CO$_2$ output.
- Raised basal metabolic rate (BMR) and respiratory quotient (RQ).
- Increased heat production due to stimulation of cellular oxidative processes.

Effect on carbohydrate metabolism. Epinephrine produces hyperglycemia and makes the glucose available for the brain and other tissues to meet the emergency.

Effects on fat metabolism. Catecholamines cause increase in lipolysis by stimulating hormone-sensitive lipase in adipose tissue and muscles.

II. Physiological actions of catecholamines

Effects on cardiovascular system. The net effects of epinephrine and norepinephrine are shown in Table 5.1-4:

Effects on other systems include:

On CNS, catecholamines activate reticular activating system (RAS) thus leading to arousal and alerting responses producing anxiety, apprehension, and coarse tremors of extremities.

On GIT, epinephrine causes contraction of sphincters of gut; the net result is production of constipation.

On urinary bladder, epinephrine produces retention of urine.

On skin, catecholamines act on pilomotor muscle producing piloerection of hair.

On skeletal muscle, during exercise epinephrine increases blood supply (by causing vasodilation).

On eyes, epinephrine causes dilation of the pupil (mydriasis).

On respiration, epinephrine via β$_2$ receptors relaxes smooth muscles of bronchioles producing bronchodilation. It also increases rate and force of respiration.

- **On blood,** epinephrine produces following effects:
- Increases RBC count, and
- Increases plasma protein concentration

CLINICAL ASPECTS

DISEASES OF ADRENAL MEDULLA

Pheochromocytoma

Pheochromocytoma is a rare benign tumor arising from the epinephrine- and norepinephrine-secreting chromaffin cells of adrenal medulla.

Clinical features, produced by the excess of epinephrine and norepinephrine, include:

- Episodic or non-episodic hypertension with postural drop.
- Attacks of tachycardia, palpitation, sweating, pallor, headache and chest discomfort.
- Abdominal pain, vomiting, constipation and glucose intolerance.
- Weight loss and weakness.

TABLE 5.1-4: Cardiovascular effects of catecholamine

Parameter	Epinephrine	Norepinephrine
Heart rate	↑	↓
Cardiac output	↑	↓
Peripheral resistance	↓	↑
Systolic blood pressure	↑	↑
Diastolic blood pressure	↓	↑
Mean arterial pressure	↓ or N	↑

An Integrated Response to Stress

Stress, may it be emotional, physical or biological, evokes an integrated response of sympathoadrenal medullary system and hypothalamic-pituitary-adrenal cortex axis.

Steps involved in stress adaptation by an integrated response of the above system are:

Perception of stress signals. Stress is perceived by many areas of the brain, from the cortex down to brain stem including limbic system and reticular activating system (RAS).

Stimulation of hypothalamus. Major stresses activate the CRH and ADH neurons in the paraventricular nucleus and adrenergic neurons.

Activation of hypothalamic-pituitary-adrenal axis: CRH and ADH release stimulates ACTH release and ultimately elevates plasma cortisol levels.

Activation of sympathoadrenal medullary system. Sudden exposure to any type of stress initially produces the sympathetic alarm reaction. Stimulation of adrenergic neurons of hypothalamus ultimately leads to release of epinephrine from adrenal medulla and norepinephrine from the sympathetic ganglia.

Integrated role of hormones released by hypothalamic-pituitary-adrenal axis and sympathoadrenal medullary system in stress adaptation. Together these hormones help in adaptation to stress by their following actions (Fight and Flight):

- *Increase in glucose production* and shift glucose utilization toward the central nervous system away from peripheral tissues.
- *Free fatty acid supply* to heart and to the muscles.
- *Cardiovascular adjustments*: Catecholamines and cortisol raise blood pressure and cardiac output, and they improve the delivery of substrates to tissues.
- *Arousal, defensively useful behavioral activation* and *focused attention* result from the adrenergic stimuli to the pertinent brain centers.
- *Inhibition of activities that are not useful during stress and divert individuals, and their resources, from defensive responses to danger* is an important part of adaptation to stress. For example, inhibition of growth hormone, gonadotropin release, and sexual activity.
- *Interaction with immune system.*

PANCREATIC HORMONES

Functional Anatomy

The endocrine part of the pancreas comprises numerous rounded collections of cells known as *pancreatic islets* or the *islets of Langerhans*. These are embedded within the exocrine part, and they constitute 1–1.5% of the human pancreatic mass (Histology Plate 5.1-4).

Islets of Langerhans

Each islet contains four types of cells (Fig. 5.1-32):

1. *Beta (β) cells* make up 60–70% of the total cells and constitute the central core of the islet. These cells secrete insulin.

2. *Alpha (α) cells* form about 20% of the total cells and constitute the outer rim of the islet. These cells secrete glucagon.

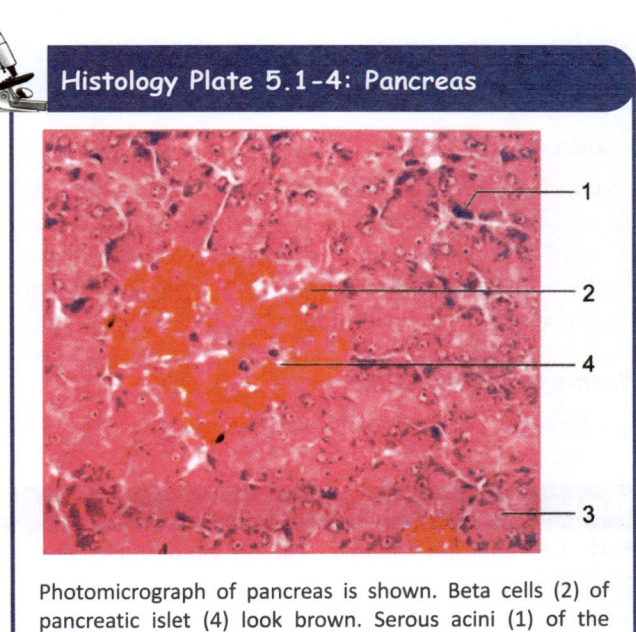

Histology Plate 5.1-4: Pancreas

Photomicrograph of pancreas is shown. Beta cells (2) of pancreatic islet (4) look brown. Serous acini (1) of the pancreas are stained. Centroacinar cells (3) can also be seen.

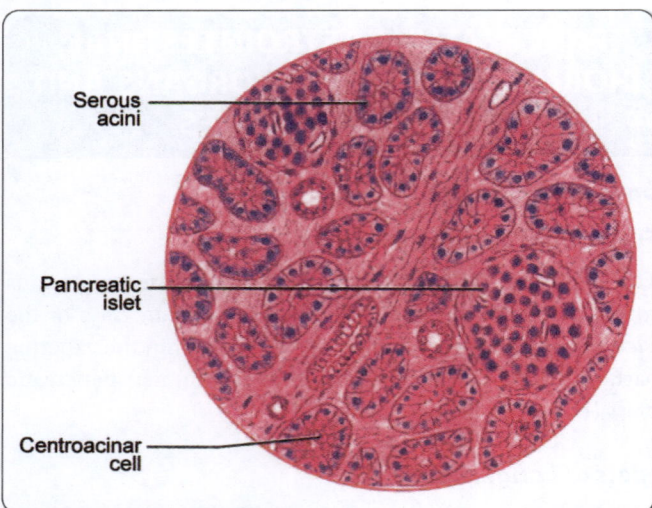

Fig. 5.1-32: Schematic histological structure of pancreas

3. Delta (δ) cells form about 10% of total cells and are intermixed. These are source of somatostatin.

4. PP cells are also peripherally placed scattered amongst the α cells. These are source of pancreatic peptide.

Gap junctions link beta cells to each other, alpha cells to each other, and beta cells to alpha cells for rapid communication.

Insulin

Insulin is a polypeptide hormone secreted by the β cells of islets of Langerhans of pancreas. Historically, insulin is the first hormone to be isolated, purified, crystallized and synthesized.

Some of the important factors stimulating and inhibiting insulin secretion are depicted in Table 5.1-5.

Plasma Levels of Insulin

- Average basal peripheral plasma insulin level is 10 µU/mL.

TABLE 5.1-5: Factors stimulating and inhibiting insulin secretion	
Factors stimulating insulin secretion	**Factors inhibiting insulin secretion**
• ↑ Blood glucose • ↑ Amino acids • ↑ Fatty acids • Glucagon • GIP • ACh • Growth hormones, cortisol	• ↓ Blood glucose • Somatostatin • Norepinephrine, epinephrine

- Three to ten fold increase in plasma insulin level is noted after a typical meal. The peak occurs after 30 to 60 minutes of initiating the meal.

Actions of Insulin

A. Metabolic effects
B. Effects on ion transport
C. Role in cell growth and development.

A. Metabolic effects of insulin

The insulin plays a key role in the metabolism of carbohydrates, lipids and proteins. The major targets for insulin actions are the muscle mass, the liver and adipose tissue.

Effects on carbohydrate metabolism. Insulin decreases blood glucose concentration by following mechanisms:

Insulin increases uptake of glucose in target cells.

Insulin promotes glucose utilization by:

- *Glycolysis* (oxidation of glucose) is increased in muscle and liver by insulin.
- *Glycogen* formation (glycogenesis) from glucose in muscle and liver is promoted by insulin.

Insulin decreases glucose production by inhibiting:

- Gluconeogenesis
- Glycogenolysis.

Effects on lipid metabolism. The metabolism of both endogenous and exogenous fat is profoundly influenced by insulin in target tissues—liver, adipose tissue and muscle.

- Insulin increases lipogenesis
- Insulin decreases lipolysis
- Insulin reduces ketogenesis
- Effect of insulin on lipoprotein metabolism. It appears that insulin is required for the utilization of VLDL and LDL.

From the effects of insulin on carbohydrate and fat metabolism described above, it is obvious that insulin regulates use of glucose and FFA for energy production.

Effects of insulin on protein metabolism. Insulin is an anabolic hormone; it stimulates protein synthesis and inhibits protein degradation.

B. Effects of insulin on ion transport

Insulin increases K^+, PO_4^{3-} and Mg^{2+} uptake into the skeletal muscle cells and of K^+ and PO_4^{3-} into hepatic cells from ECF by increasing membrane permeability.

Another effect of insulin on electrolytic balance is to increase reabsorption of K^+, PO_4^{3-} and Na^+ by the tubules of the kidney.

C. Role of insulin in cell growth and development

Insulin is an important factor for growth and development with following roles:

Anabolic action of insulin is as important as growth hormone for promotion of normal growth.

Direct stimulatory effect on macromolecules. Insulin also stimulates the synthesis of macromolecules in tissues such as cartilage and bone; and thereby directly contributes to body growth.

Stimulation of other growth factors such as somatomedins (insulin-like growth factors 1 and 2, i.e., IGF-1 and IGF-2), epidermal growth factor (EGF), nerve growth factor (NGF), and relaxin.

Glucagon

Glucagon is secreted by α-cells of islets of Langerhans. Basal levels of glucagon in a normal fasting individual are 100–150 pg/mL.

Actions of Glucagon

The actions of glucagon, in almost all respects, are exactly opposite to those of insulin. It promotes mobilization of stored nutrients such as glucose, fatty acids, and ketoacids and thus is a hormone of energy release. Its metabolic effects are as follows:

Effects on carbohydrate metabolism. Glucagon predominantly acts on the liver and increases the blood sugar level by following actions:
- *It increases glycogenolysis.*
- *It increases gluconeogenesis.*

Effects on lipid metabolism. Glucagon is a powerful *lipolytic agent*. It activates lipase in adipose tissue which releases FFA and glycerol into the circulation. In the liver, excess of FFAs are oxidized resulting in energy production and ketone body synthesis (ketogenesis). Thus glucagon is a ketogenic as well as a hyperglycemic hormone.

Effects on protein metabolism. Glucagon increases the amino acid uptake of liver, which in turn promotes gluconeogeneis. Thus, glucagon *lowers plasma amino acids.*

Calorigenic effect. Glucagon also has a calorigenic effect. This effect is probably related to increased hepatic deamination of amino acids.

Other actions of glucagon. Other miscellaneous actions of glucagon include:
- Inhibition of renal tubular sodium reabsorption, resulting in natriuresis.
- Modest increase in force of contraction of the heart.

- Stimulation of secretion of growth hormone, insulin and pancreatic somatostatin.
- Glucagon may act locally in the regulation of appetite.

Regulation of Glucagon Secretion

I. Role of blood levels of nutrients

There exists a feedback relationship between blood levels of glucagon and nutrients (Fig. 5.1-33).

Blood glucose level. Hypoglycemia causes to 4-fold increase in plasma levels of glucagon and high blood glucose concentration inhibits glucagon secretion (Fig. 5.1-33).

Plasma amino acids. Secretion of glucagon is increased by a protein-rich meal.

Free fatty acids and ketoacids. Glucagon stimulates production and release of free fatty acids (FFA) and ketoacids, which in turn suppress glucagon secretion, i.e., there is a feedback relationship (Fig. 5.1-33).

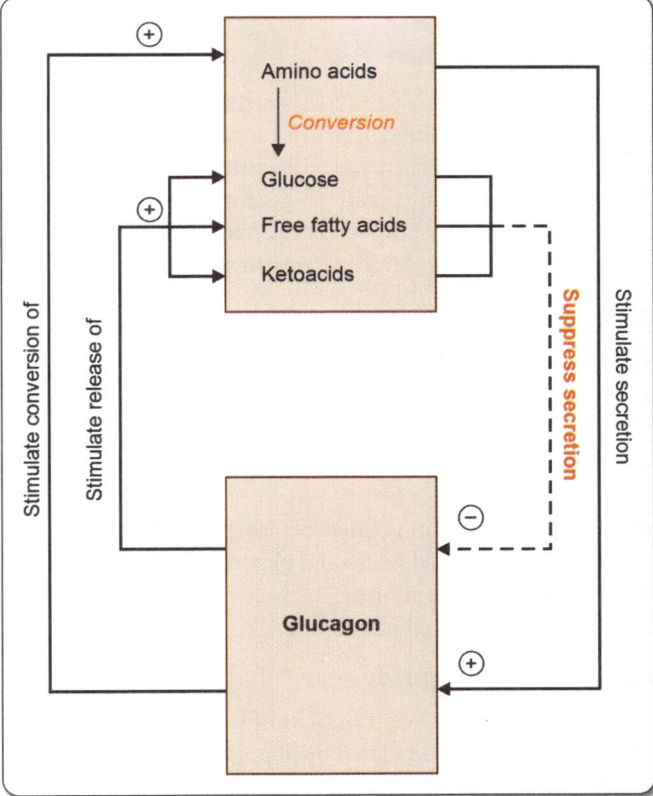

Fig. 5.1-33: Feedback relationship between glucagon and nutrients. Glucagon stimulates production and release of glucose, free fatty acids and ketoacids, which in turn suppress glucagon secretion, and glucagon in turn stimulates the conversion of amino acids to glucose

II. Role of gastrointestinal hormones

Gastrointestinal (GT) hormones such as CCK-PZ, gastrin and GIP increase glucagon secretion.

III. Role of nervous system

Sympathetic nerve stimulation to pancreas increases glucagon secretion. Various stresses, fasting, exercise and infection increase the glucagon secretion in part by their stimulatory effect on sympathetic nervous system and partly by release of glucocorticoids.

Vagal stimulation and acetylcholine also acutely increase glucagon secretion.

The neurohormone, somatostatin, inhibits the secretion of glucagon.

Somatostatin and Pancreatic Polypeptide

Somatostatin

Structure and synthesis

Pancreatic somatostatin is a neuropeptide, synthesized by δ cells.

Regulation of secretion

Somatostatin secretion is increased after ingestion of food, because increased blood glucose, amino acids, fatty acids and gastrointestinal tract hormones stimulate its secretion. Glucagon, β-adrenergic and cholinergic neurotransmitters also stimulate somatostatin secretion. Insulin and α-adrenergic neurotransmitters inhibit somatostatin secretion.

Actions

Somatostatin has following effects:
- Acts on the islets of Langerhans and inhibits secretion of insulin and glucagon.
- Increases the motility of stomach, duodenum and gallbladder.
- Decreases secretion of hydrochloric acid, pepsin, gastrin, secretin, intestinal juices and panceatic juice.
- Inhibits the absorption of glucose, xylose, and triglycerides across the mucosal membrane.

Pancreatic Polypeptide

It is synthesized by PP cells of islets of Langerhans.
Its secretion is also stimulated by hypoglycemia and inhibited by glucose administration.

Actions and physiological importance

Its best known action is to inhibit exocrine pancreatic secretion. Its true physiological importance is not known.

Hormonal Regulation of Blood Glucose Level

A healthy individual is capable of maintaining the blood glucose level within a narrow range.
- Fasting blood glucose level in a postabsorptive state varies between 70 and 110 mg%.
- Postprandial blood glucose level, i.e., after a large carbohydrate meal or following oral administration of glucose in the dose of 1 g/kg body weight, the blood glucose level increases to about 140 mg% (less than 150 mg%) in a period of less than 1 hour. However, this response to oral administration of carbohydrate, when plotted on a time scale, is called *glucose tolerance curve* (Fig. 5.1-34) and is used clinically as a test to study the maintenance of blood glucose levels.

Role of Hormones in Regulation of Blood Glucose

Under normal circumstances, the various hormones play a significant role in maintaining the blood glucose levels within normal physiological range. This is accomplished by preventing the occurrence of hyperglycemia and hypoglycemia.

Prevention of occurrence of hyperglycemia

The occurrence of hyperglycemia after a pure carbohydrate load or a mixed meal in a healthy individual is prevented by a manifold (4–5 times) increase in insulin secretion (for details see actions of insulin).

Prevention of occurrence of hypoglycemia

Hypoglycemia, which may occur due to fasting or prolonged exercise, is prevented in a healthy individual by a number

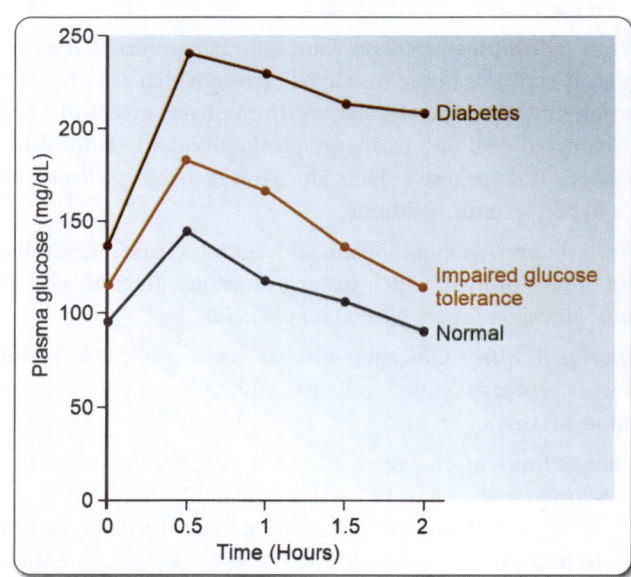

Fig. 5.1-34: Glucose tolerance curve

of hormones, which include glucagon, epinephrine, growth hormone and glucocorticoids. It is obvious that there is only one hormone, insulin, which prevents hyperglycemia, whereas at least four hormones are available for prevention of hypoglycemia.

Important applied aspects of endocrine pancreas which need mention are:
- Diabetes mellitus
- Hypoglycemia.

DIABETES MELLITUS (HYPERGLYCEMIA)

Diabetes mellitus is a clinical syndrome of hyperglycemia occurring due to deficiency of insulin.

Types and Stages of Diabetes Mellitus

Diabetes mellitus can be classified into following types:

Primary diabetes mellitus in which cause is not known. It is of further two types:
- Insulin-dependent diabetes mellitus (IDDM)
- Non-insulin-dependent diabetes mellitus (NIDDM).

Secondary diabetes mellitus: It is associated with certain pathological conditions such as pancreatitis, cystic fibrosis, acromegaly, Cushing's syndrome, etc.

Insulin-dependent Diabetes Mellitus (IDDM)

Insulin-dependent diabetes mellitus (IDDM), or type I diabetes, is considered an autoimmune disorder in which antibodies destroy the β cells of islets causing an absolute deficiency of insulin.

Characteristic features of IDDM are:
- It manifests before 40 years of age (usually between 12–15 years) and is also called juvenile onset diabetes. It accounts for 10–20%.
- Patients are usually lean.
- Classical triad of presenting symptoms consisting of polyuria, polydipsia and polyphagia is associated with weight loss.
- Ketosis and acidosis are common complications of this diabetes mellitus.
- Plasma insulin levels are very low or undetectable.

Non–insulin-dependent Diabetes Mellitus (NIDDM)

Non–insulin-dependent diabetes mellitus (NIDDM) or type II diabetes is also a genetic disorder. It is supposed to occur due to decrease in insulin receptors on the insulin responsive (target) cells.

Characteristic features of NIDDM are:
- It manifests after 40 years of age and so is also called *adult onset diabetes*.
- It is most common and accounts for 80–90% of diabetic population.
- Most of the patients are obese.
- Symptoms begin gradually and may be ignored and many a time diagnosis is made on urine examination which shows glycosuria.
- Plasma insulin levels are often normal or even elevated.
- Ketoacidosis is not very common.

Hyperglycemia and its Consequences

Hyperglycemia (elevation of blood glucose concentration) is the characteristic feature of uncontrolled diabetes mellitus. It occurs due to lack of insulin. The consequences of hyperglycemia are:
- *Glycosuria*, i.e., excretion of glucose into the urine.
- *Polyuria*, i.e., passage of large amount of urine frequently.
- *Loss of electrolytes* (sodium, potassium and phosphate) in urine.
- *Cellular dehydration*, high glucose concentration increases osmotic pressure of extracellular fluid and osmotic transfer of water from cells to extracellular fluid leading to dehydration of cells.
- *Polydipsia*, i.e., excessive drinking of water, results from activation of thirst.
- *Increased caloric loss* is the result of loss of glucose in urine.
- *Polyphagia*, i.e., excessive eating, occurs due to stimulation of satiety center.
- *Loss of body weight* occurs because of loss of calories in the urine and mobilization of fats and proteins for energy production.

HYPOGLYCEMIA

Hypoglycemia refers to a clinical condition caused by blood glucose levels below 45 mg% (2.5 mmol/L).

Symptoms and Signs of Hypoglycemia

Symptoms and signs of hypoglycemia occur due to effects of low levels of glucose per se (mainly on nervous system especially brain) and because of sympathetic stimulation (mainly on CVS, GIT and skin).

CNS *symptoms* are called *neuroglycopenic symptoms*. Since metabolism of brain mainly depends on blood glucose level, it is depressed when glucose level falls below 50–70 mg%. CNS becomes quite excitable which results in hallucinations, extreme nervousness, tremors, confusion, difficulty in concentration, incoordination, convulsions, and drowsiness. When blood glucose levels fall further, (<30 mg%) hypoglycemic coma may develop, which needs to be differentiated from hyperglycemic coma in diabetics, and needs an emergency treatment by immediate administration of large quantity of glucose intravenously.

CVS symptoms in hypoglycemia are palpitation, tachycardia, and cardiac arrhythmias.

GIT symptoms include nausea and vomiting.

Skin symptoms are sweating and hypothermia.

GASTROINTESTINAL HORMONES

General Consideration

Gastrointestinal hormones are secreted by the glandular cells scattered in the epithelium of the gastrointestinal tract, mainly stomach and small intestines. These hormones are released into the blood capillaries in response to stimulation by various chemicals (present in the chyme) or mechanically. Through portal circulation the hormone reaches its target region situated nearby in GIT. The gastrointestinal hormones are characterized by two main features.

1. Each hormone may affect more than one target tissue, and
2. Each target tissue responds to more than one hormone at a time. (For details see page 102).

HORMONES OF OTHER ORGANS

In addition to main endocrine glands, other organs also have endocrine functions, e.g., atrial natriuretic peptide (ANP) is secreted by heart, renin by kidney, melatonin by pineal gland and so on.

Hormones of the Heart

The hormones of the heart include:
- *Atrial natriuretic peptide (ANP).* It is the first natriuretic hormone isolated from the heart.
- *Brain natriuretic peptide (BNP).* It is the second natriuretic hormone first isolated from the porcine brain and hence named as BNP. In human, it is isolated from the heart.

Actions of ANP include:
- It increases sodium excretion by increasing glomerular filtration rate, and inhibiting Na^+ reabsorption at the level of renal tubules.
- It lowers the blood pressure by:
  - Relaxing vascular smooth muscles of arterioles and venules, and
  - Increasing capillary permeability.

Hormones of the Kidney

The main function of the kidney is excretion of waste products but it also secretes three hormones:
1. Renin
2. 1,25 dihydroxycholecalciferol
3. Erythropoietin.

Renin

Renin is a glycoprotein. In humans, renin is secreted by granular cells of *juxtaglomerular apparatus* of kidney into the blood stream. The only action of active renin is to convert angiotensinogen into angiotensin-1. (*For details see page 281*).

1,25-dihydroxycholecalciferol

1,25-dihydroxycholecalciferol or vitamin D, also called calcitriol, is now considered a hormone. 1,25-dihydroxycholecalciferol, the active form of vitamin D_3, is synthesized from its precursor called vitamin D_3. It reaches the blood from two different sources:

1. *Dietary sources* include fish, fish liver oil, egg's yolk. Its daily requirement is 400 IU or 10 μg.

2. *Cutaneous source.* The keratinocytes located in the inner layer of epidermis synthesize vitamin D_3 by action of ultraviolet rays (from sunlight) on 7-dehydroxycholesterol.

The synthesis of 1,25-dihydroxycholecalciferol from vitamin D_3 occurs in the liver and in the kidney.

Functions

1,25-dihydroxycholecalciferol (calcitriol) are:
- The main function is to maintain plasma calcium and phosphate levels by acting at three different sites: intestine, bone and kidney.
  1. It helps in calcium absorption from gut,
  2. It helps in reabsorption of calcium from renal tubular fluid, and
  3. On bones it increases bone resorption.
- It also plays an important role in regulation of growth and development by production of growth factors.

Erythropoietin

Erythropoietin is a glycoprotein. In adults, it is mainly (85%) secreted by juxtaglomerular cells of the kidney with some contribution (15%) from hepatocytes in the liver. The main role of erythropoietin is to stimulate bone marrow for erythropoiesis. (*For details see Chapter 4.1, page 153*).

Pineal Gland

Gross Anatomy and Location

The pineal gland, also known as epiphysis, is a small structure (5 mm × 7 mm) shaped like a pine cone. It is situated in the groove between two superior colliculi in the diencephalic area of brain above the hypothalamus (Fig. 5.1-35). It forms the posterior boundary of the third ventricle.

Structure

The stroma of pineal gland has two types of cells: neuroglial cells and parenchymal cells. The parenchymal cells possess the secretory function.

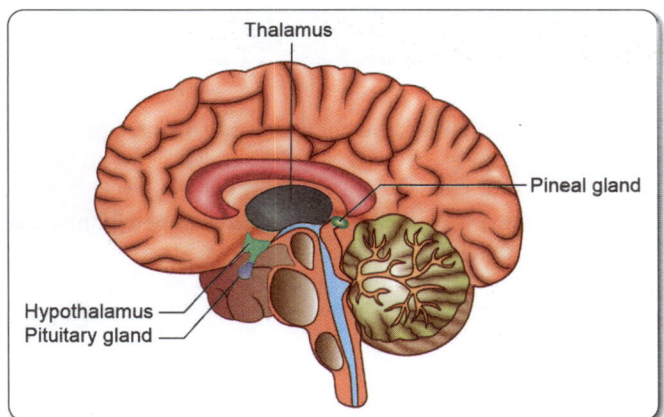

Fig. 5.1-35: Location of pineal gland in the groove between two superior colliculia

In infants, the pineal gland is quite large and the cells are arranged in alveoli, but

In adults, the size of pineal gland decreases and gets calcified, i.e., small concretions of calcium phosphate and carbonate (pineal sand) appear in the tissues.

Melatonin

The hormone melatonin is synthesized by parenchymal cells of the pineal gland from tryptophan.

Functions of melatonin are:

Role in circadian rhythm of the body. The melatonin secretion shows diurnal variations, i.e., it is secreted more in the dark period than in the light period of the day-night cycle. This correlates with various internal activities in different periods of the day, i.e., *circadian rhythm.*

Effect on the gonads. Melatonin exerts both inhibitory and facilitatory effects on the gonads due to diurnal change in melatonin secretion. It inhibits onset of puberty.

Effect on MSH and ACTH secretion. Melatonin decreases the secretion of these hormones.

Sleep. Melatonin has role in induction of sleep.

LOCAL HORMONES

Local hormones are the substances which are produced in many tissues, and execute their actions in the same area or in immediate neighborhood. Commonly produced local hormones are:

Prostaglandins and Related Substances

Prostaglandins and related substances such as thromboxanes, prostacyclins, leukotrienes are lipid in nature and are synthesized from *arachidonic acid.* Prostaglandins are named so because first of all these were isolated from prostatic fluid of semen. However, now they are known to be synthesized in almost all the tissues of the body. Prostaglandins have multitudinous physiological effects in:

- Inflammatory response
- Regulation of blood pressure
- Initiates labor by stimulating uterine contractions
- Role in blood coagulation; prostaglandins inhibit platelet aggregation
- Regulation of blood flow to kidneys
- Potentiate pain during inflammation
- Inhibit secretion of gastric HCl.

Thromboxane A$_2$ is synthesized by platelets. It promotes:
- Vasoconstriction
- Platelet aggregation.

Prostacyclin is produced in vascular endothelium. It produces vasodilatation.

Leukotrienes are mediators of allergic responses and inflammation. These are released when specific allergens combine with antibodies on the surface of mast cells. They produce bronchoconstriction, arteriolar constriction and increase vascular permeability.

Histamine

This hormone is synthesized by basophils in the blood and mast cells in the tissues. It is released during inflammatory response and is responsible for increasing capillary permeability. Histamine also causes:
- Contraction of smooth muscles of bronchi
- Stimulation of gastric HCl secretion and gut motility.

Serotonin (5-HT)

Serotonin (5-Hydroxytryptamin, 5-HT) is present in blood platelets, in brain tissue and in intestinal wall. It plays important role in hemostasis in GIT secretions and motility.

Other Local Hormones

These include acetylcholine, ADP, AMP, plasma polypeptides (angiotensin, plasma kinins, e.g., bradykinin).

ASSESS YOURSELF

Short and Long Answer Questions

1. **Describe briefly:**
   - Functions of growth hormone and its regulation
   - Biosynthesis of thyroid hormone
   - Role of calcitropic hormones in maintenance of calcium balance
   - Functions of glucocorticoids and their regulation
   - Functions of mineralocorticoids and their regulation

2. **Differentiate between:**
   - Acromegaly and gigantism
   - Pituitary and thyroid dwarf
   - Type I and Type II diabetes mellitus

3. **Write notes on:**
   - Hypothalamo –hypophyseal portal system
   - Diabetes insipidus
   - Myxedema
   - Bone cells
   - Cholecalciferol
   - Tetany
   - Cushing syndrome
   - Blood supply of adrenal glands
   - ACTH
   - Glucose tolerance test
   - Islets of Langerhans
   - Somatostatin
   - Pineal gland
   - Melatonin

Multiple Choice Questions

1. **The hypothalamic nucleus responsible for pulsatile secretion of a hormone is:**
   a. Supra-optic   b. Para-ventricular
   c. Supra-chiasmatic   d. Anterior nucleus

2. **Which is the best method of measurement of a hormone**
   a. Bioassay
   b. Cytochemical assay
   c. Dynamic Tests
   d. Enzyme linked immunosorbent method

3. **Anterior pituitary develops from:**
   a. Median eminence   b. Rathke's pouch
   c. Tuber cinereum   d. Hypothalamus

4. **Which is not the part of neurohypophysis?**
   a. Pars intermedia   b. Pars posterior
   c. Median eminence   d. Infundibular stem

5. **In lower animals, melanocyte stimulating hormone is secreted by:**
   a. Adenohypophysis
   b. Neurohypophysis
   c. Pituitary stalk
   d. Intermediate lobe of pituitary

6. **In adenohypophysis, the alpha cells are mainly present in:**
   a. Pars distalis   b. Pars tuberalis
   c. Pars dintermedia   d. Pituitary stalk

7. **The statement not true for hypothalamo–hypophyseal portal system is:**
   a. Present in the upper part of pituitary stalk
   b. Blood from capillary network is drained by long portal veins
   c. Transmits neurotransmitter from supraoptic nucleus of hypothalamus
   d. Short portal vessels provide link between anterior and posterior pituitary

8. **Secretion of growth hormone is increased by:**
   a. Hyperglycemia   b. Sleep
   c. Pregnancy   d. Somatostatin

9. **Secretion of growth hormone is decreased during:**
   a. Pregnancy   b. Puberty
   c. Starvation   d. Stress

10. **Prolactin mainly has effect on:**
    a. Metabolism   b. General growth
    c. Mammary glands   d. Gonad

11. **Gigantism occurs due to hypersecretion of:**
    a. Corticotropin   b. Growth hormone
    c. Somatostatin   d. Antidiuretic hormone

12. **Diabetes insipidus occurs due to:**
    a. Hypersecretion of ADH
    b. Hyposecretion of ADH
    c. Hypersecretion of insulin
    d. Hyposecretion of insulin

13. **Follicles of thyroid glands are lined by:**
    a. Cuboidal cells   b. Para follicular cells
    c. Folliculo stellate cells d. Chromophobes

14. **For biosynthesis of thyroid hormone, daily requirement of iodine is:**
    a. 100–200 µg   b. 250–300 µg
    c. 300–400 µg   d. 500 µg

15. **The statement not true for thyroid hormone:**
    a. Stored in epithelial cells of thyroid
    b. Mainly present in colloid form
    c. Formed from iodine and tyrosine
    d. Thyroid stimulating hormone increases the synthesis

16. **Thyroxin causes:**
    a. Hyperglycemia   b. Increase in cardiac output
    c. Constipation   d. Bradycardia

17. **Increased secretion of thyroid hormone leads to:**
    a. Cretinism   b. Myxedema
    c. Dwarfism   d. Exophthalmos

18. **Parathyroid hormone is secreted from:**
    a. Chief cells   b. Oxyphil cells
    c. Para follicular cells   d. Stellate cells

19. **Parathormone maintains calcium balance by:**
    a. Increasing synthesis of vitamin D
    b. Bone resorption
    c. Stimulating phosphate reabsorption from kidney
    d. Decreasing serum Mg^{2+} level

20. **The true statement for adrenal cortex:**
    a. Zona glomerulosa forms middle three fifth of cortex
    b. Zona glomerulosa secretes corticosteroids
    c. Zona fasciculata is present just beneath the capsule
    d. Zona reticularis forms one fifth of the cortex

21. **Adrenal medullary chromaffin cells are innervated by:**
    a. Preganglionic cholinergic neurons
    b. Preganglionic adrenergic neurons
    c. Postganglionic sympathetic neurons
    d. Postganglionic parasympathetic neurons

22. **Chromaffin cells of adrenal medulla secrete:**
    a. ACTH   b. Cortisol
    c. Epinephrine   d. Acetylcholine

23. **Main metabolic effect of glucocorticoids is**
    a. Increase of glucogenolysis
    b. Anabolic effect
    c. Increase in glucose utilization by peripheral tissues
    d. Lipolytic effect

24. **Which is not the action of glucocorticoids is:**
    a. Bone resorption
    b. Bone formation
    c. Increases cardiac muscle contractility
    d. Increases glomerular filtration rate

25. **The primary action of aldosterone is:**
    a. Sodium reabsorption from kidney
    b. Potassium reabsorption from kidney
    c. Hyperkalemia
    d. Increase in Glomerular filtration rate

26. **Which of the following increases aldosterone secretion?**
    a. Decrease in ECF   b. Hypernatremia
    c. Hypokalemia   d. Hypertension

27. **Hypersecretion of glucocorticoids occurs in:**
    a. Cushing syndrome   b. Conn's syndrome
    c. Addison's disease   d. Diabetes mellitus

28. **Which is not the feature of Cushing syndrome?**
    a. Moon face   b. Buffalo hump
    c. Purple stria   d. Hyperpigmentation of skin

29. **Which pancreatic islets cell secretes insulin?**
    a. Alpha   b. Beta
    c. Delta   d. PP cells

30. **Which of the following stimulates insulin secretion:**
    a. Somatostatin   b. Norepinephrine
    c. Hypoglycemia   d. Hyperglycemia

31. **The main stimulatory effect of insulin is:**
    a. Body growth   b. Gluconeogenesis
    c. Lipolysis   d. Protein degradation

32. **Glucagon is secreted from which pancreatic islets cell?**
    a. Alpha   b. Beta
    c. Delta   d. PP cells

33. **Glucagon secretion is inhibited by:**
    a. Hyperglycemia   b. Hypoglycemia
    c. Protein rich meal   d. Gastrin

34. **The characteristic feature of non-insulin dependent diabetes mellitus is:**
    a. Manifestation at age 10 to 15 years
    b. Weight loss
    c. Obesity
    d. Low level of insulin

ANSWER KEY

1. c	2. d	3. b	4. a	5. d	6. a	7. c	8. b
9. a	10. c	11. b	12. b	13. a	14. a	15. a	16. b
17. d	18. a	19. b	20. b	21. a	22. c	23. d	24. b
25. a	26. a	27. a	28. d	29. b	30. d	31. a	32. a
33. a	34. c						

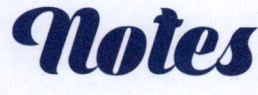
Notes

Section

VI

Sensory Organs

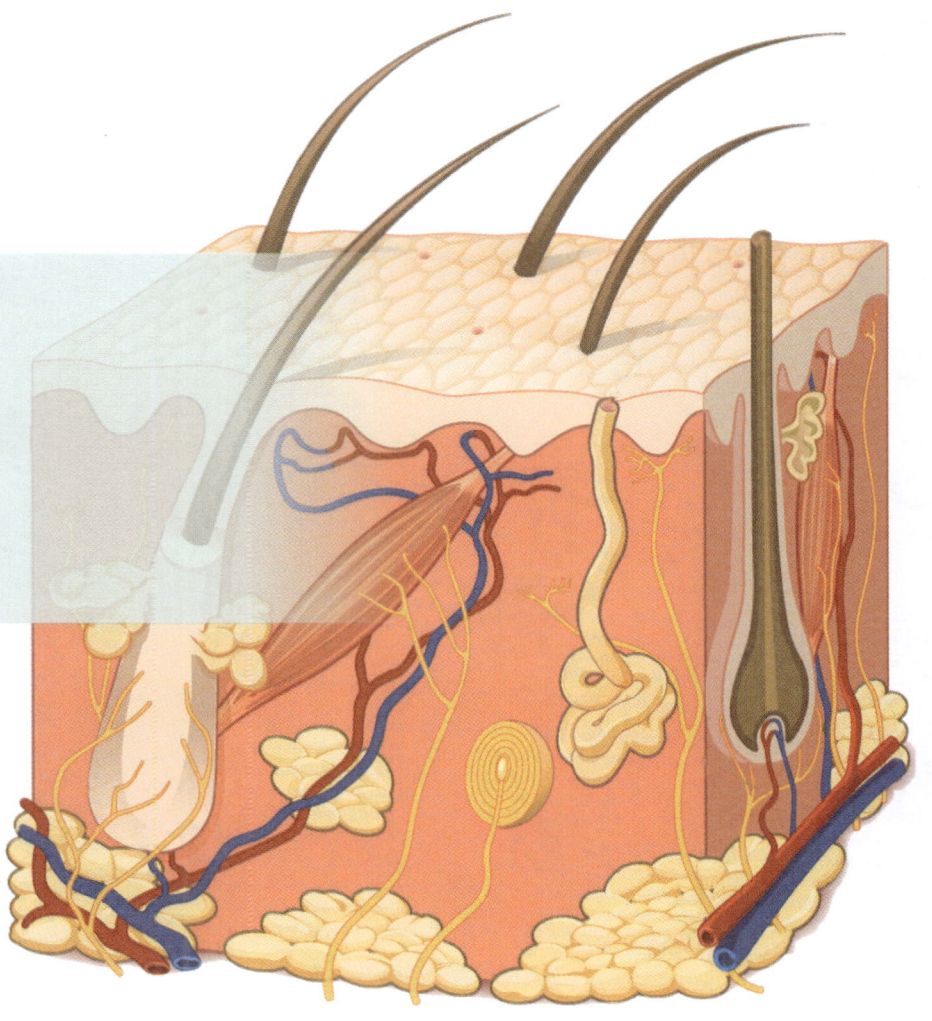

Section Outline

Integumentary System: Skin and Fascia

SKIN

GENERAL CONSIDERATIONS

Skin refers to the outer or external covering of the body. In addition to providing complete covering to the body, the skin performs many other important functions, and therefore, it is regarded as an important organ of the body. At the orifices, the skin is continuous with the mucous membranes of the body.

Thickness and Surface Area of Skin

Thickness

Skin accounts for 7% of the body weight. Its thickness varies from about 0.5–3 mm. The surface area of skin is about 1.5–2 (1.7) m² in an adult.

Distribution of Surface Area

For distribution of the surface area of the skin, rule of nine can be followed. It is particularly used to assess the area of skin involved in burns. The rule of nines is as given in (Fig. 6.1-1):
Head and neck: 9%
Each upper limb: 9% (two limbs 18%)
Front of trunk: 18%

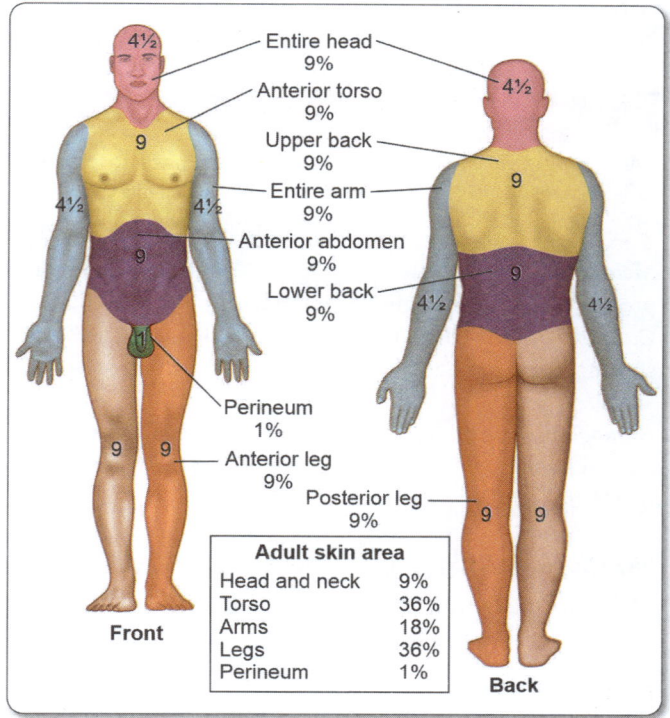

Fig. 6.1-1: Distribution of surface area as per rule of nines

Back of trunk including buttocks: 18%
Each lower limb: 18% (two limbs 36%)
Perineum: 1%

IMPORTANT TO KNOW

Calculation of Surface Area

The surface area of an individual can be calculated by *Du Bois formula,* which is:

$$a = w \times h \times 71.84$$

where:
    a = Surface area in square centimeters
    w = Weight in kilograms
    h = Height in centimeters

Color of Skin

The color of skin varies with the race, age, part of the body and exposure to sunlight. The determinants of skin color are the pigments present at different levels and places in the skin. These include:

Melanin. The pigment melanin is brown in color and present in the germinative zone of the epidermis. It is synthesized in cells called *melanocytes* located in the deep germinative layer.

The melanocytes synthesize melanin from the amino acid tyrosine in the presence of an enzyme called tyrosinase. On exposure to sunlight (ultraviolet radiations), both the amount and darkness of melanin produced is increased.

CLINICAL ASPECTS

An inherited inability of an individual in any race to produce melanin results in the condition called albinism. In this condition, the pigment is absent in skin, hairs and uveal tissue of the eyes.

Melanoid. It is a pigment which resembles melanin. It is present diffusely throughout the epidermis.

Carotene. It is yellow to orange in color; is found in the stratum corneum and the fat cells of dermis and superficial fascia.

Hemoglobin (purple) and *oxyhemoglobin* (red) present in the blood circulating in the capillaries of the dermis give pinkish hue to the skin.

Skin Surface Ridges and Grooves

The outer surface of skin is marked by certain ridges and grooves (surface irregularities). These include the following:

Epidermal ridges

Also known as papillary ridges or friction ridges, these are seen on the skin of the palms and soles and their digits. They form narrow ridges separated by fine parallel grooves, arranged in curved arrays. They conform to the contours of the underlying dermal papillae and develop during the third and fourth month of gestation. The function of the ridges is to increase the grip of the hand or foot by increasing friction.

NURSING IMPLICATIONS AND APPLICATIONS

The study of ridge pattern constitutes a branch of science, called *dermatographics.* The ridge pattern, which is determined genetically by multifactorial inheritance, is unique for each individual. It does not change throughout life, except to enlarge and this can serve as the basis for identification through fingerprints or footprints. The major patterns in the human fingerprints include loops, whorls and arches.

Tension lines

These are the epidermal grooves, which form a network of linear furrows which divide the surface into polygonal or diamond-shaped area. These lines to some extent correspond to variations in the pattern of fibers in the dermis. These can be seen conspicuously on the dorsum of hand as an example.

Flexor lines

Also known as *skin creases* or *skin joints,* these are certain permanent epidermal grooves along which the skin folds during habitual movements (chiefly flexion) of the joints. The skin along these lines is thin and firmly bound to the deep fascia. The lines are prominent, opposite the flexure of the joints, particularly on the palms, soles and digits.

STRUCTURE OF SKIN

The skin consists of two distinct layers (Fig. 6.1-2):
1. Epidermis
2. Dermis.

Epidermis

Epidermis is the most superficial avascular part of skin. It is composed of keratinized stratified squamous epithelium. It is ectodermal in origin and gives rise to appendages of the skin.

Thickness of Epidermis

Thickness of epidermis varies in different parts of the body. It is thickest in the palms of hands and soles of the feet.

Layers of Epidermis

The keratinized stratified squamous epithelium forming the epidermis is organized in four (in thin skin) or five (in thick skin) layers of cells. From the deepest to the most superficial these layer are (Fig. 6.1-3):

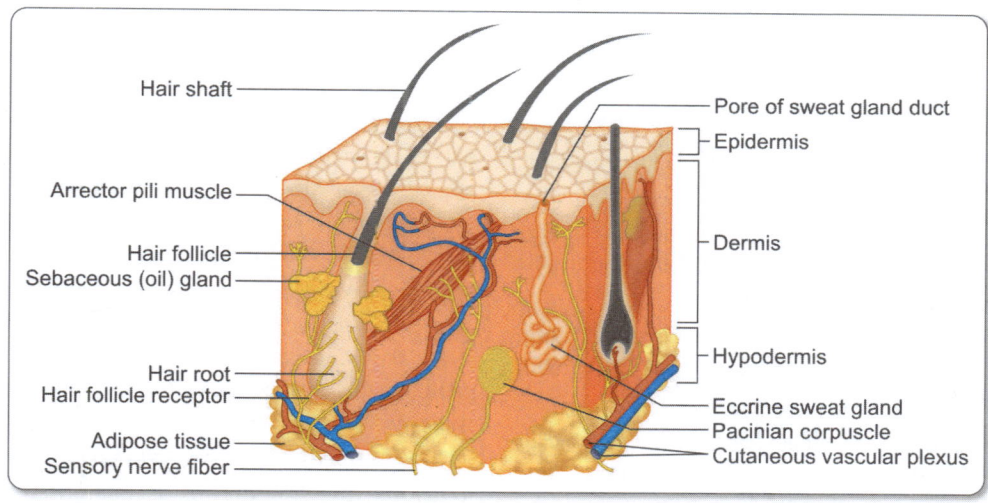

Fig. 6.1-2: Structure of skin

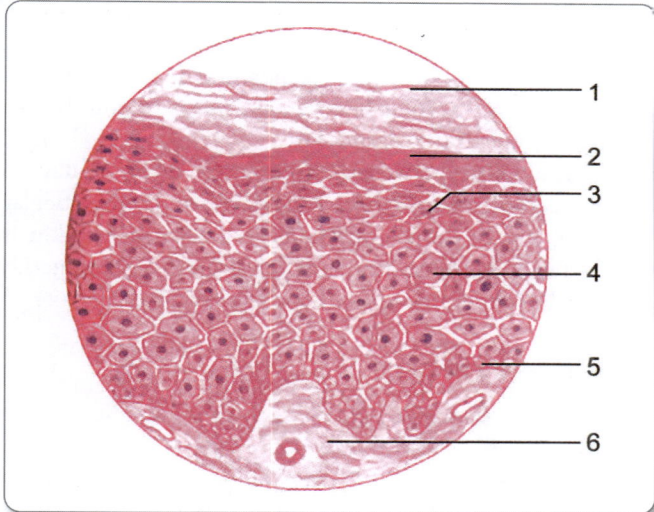

Fig. 6.1-3: Layers of epidermis: 1. Stratum corneum; 2. Stratum lucidum; 3. Stratum granulosum; 4. Stratum spinosum; 5. Stratum basale; 6. Dermis

1. *Stratum basale.* Stratum basale or basal layer, also called stratum germinativum or germinal layer or malpighian layer is the deepest layer formed of single layer of cuboidal to columnar cells. These cells are capable of continued cell division. Thus, these cells proliferate and pass toward the surface to replace cornified cells lost due to wear and tear. As the cells migrate superficially, they become more and more flattened, and lose their nuclei.

The stratum basale also contains *melanocytes* which synthesize melanin.

2. *Stratum spinosum.* This layer is formed of 4–8 layers of polyhedral cells (*keratinocytes*) with rounded central nucleus. Cells of this layer are connected to those of neighboring cells by spine-like processes which are actually desmosomes, linking the adjacent cells tightly.

The stratum spinosum and stratum basale collective form the so-called *germinative zone* (the zone where new cells are germinated).

3. *Stratum granulosum.* This is the granular cell layer consisting of 2–4 layers of flattened, diamond-shaped cells with flat nuclei. The cytoplasm of these cells contains darkly stained keratohyalin granules, which give an overall darker appearance to this cell layer.

4. *Stratum lucidum.* This layer is well formed in thick nonhairy skin of palms and soles and is usually absent in thin hairy skin. When well formed, it appears as a thin, clear, homogenous band between the stratum granulosum and stratum corneum. It consists of several rows of clear or flat, dead cells that contain droplets of a substance called eleidin. This layer is named because eleidin is translucent (lucidum = clear). Eleidin is formed from keratohyalin and is eventually transformed to keratin.

5. *Stratum corneum.* If also known as horny layer and is made up of several non-nucleated dead cells called squames in which the cytoplasm has been replaced by the fibrous protein keratin. The squames are held together by a material containing lipids and carbohydrates. These cells are continuously shed and replaced. The stratum corneum is waterproof and serves as an effective barrier against light and heat waves, bacteria, and many chemicals.

Cells in the Epidermis

The cells present in the epidermis are:

Keratinocytes form about 85% of the cells and are responsible for regeneration of epidermal cells.

Melanocytes are present in the stratum basale and stratum spinosum of the epidermis. They produce melanin pigment which gives color to the skin (Fig. 6.1-4).

Langerhan's cells. These are phagocytic macrophage cells present in the stratum spinosum layer of the epidermis. These play important role in protecting the skin against viral and other infections.

Merkel's cells. These are modified sensory receptor cells present mainly in the stratum basale.

Maintenance of Epidermis

The healthy epidermis is maintained as a result of three synchronized processes:

1. *Desquamation* (shedding) of the keratinized cells from the surface.

2. *Effective keratinization* of the cells approaching the surface.

3. *Continual cell division* in the germinative zone with newly formed cells being pushed to the surface.

Source of Nutrition

There are no blood vessels or nerve endings in the epidermis. The deeper layers of epidermis are bathed in interstitial fluid from the dermis which provides oxygen and nutrients, and is drained away as lymph.

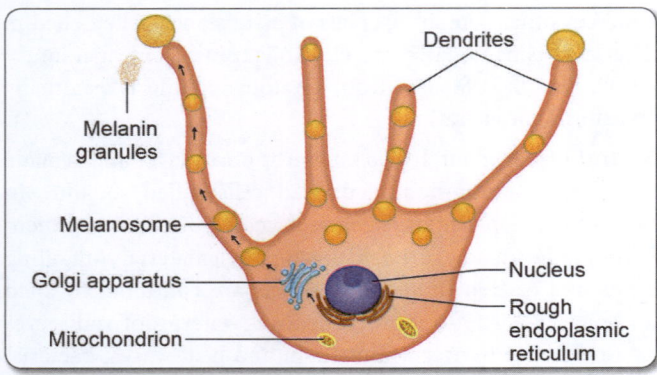

Fig. 6.1-4: Melanocytes

Dermis

Dermis or corium is the deep vascular layer of the skin. It is made up of connective tissue containing collagenous and elastic fibers mixed with blood vessels, lymphatics and nerves. It varies in thickness in different parts of the body, but is generally thicker than epidermis. The connective tissue forming dermis is arranged into a superficial papillary layer and a deep reticular layer:

Papillary layer of dermis is formed of loose areolar connective tissue containing fine collagenous, reticular and elastic tissue. This layer of connective tissue projects as dermal papillae which fit into the concavities on the undersurface of epidermis. Some dermal papillae contain *Meissner's tactile corpuscles* which are touch receptors.

Reticular layer of dermis is composed chiefly of dense connective tissue containing bundles of collagen and elastic fibers which form a network. Fibroblasts, macrophages and mast cells are the main cells found in dermis. Spaces between the fibers are occupied by a small quantity of adipose tissue, hair follicles, nerves, sebaceous glands, and ducts of the sweat glands. Varying thickness of reticular layer is responsible for differences in the thickness of skin.

The toughness and elasticity of the skin is due to combination of collagenous and elastic fibers in the reticular layer. Rupture of the elastic fibers occurs when the skin is overstretched, resulting in permanent *striae* or stretch marks, that may be found in pregnancy and obesity.

FUNCTIONS OF SKIN

Protective function. Skin performs protective function for the body structures by following mechanisms:

Mechanical protection. The skin provides mechanical protection to underlying tissues. For this function, skin is thickest over area, exposed to greatest friction.

Physical barrier. Due to keratinized stratum corneum, the skin forms a relatively waterproof layer and acts as barrier against microbial invasion, chemicals (acids and alkalies), wet and draught, hot and cold and mechanical injuries.

Immune mechanism. Specialized immune cells called Langerhans cells are present in the dermis. These cells phagocytose the antigen entering the skin and present it to the T-lymphocytes in the lymphoid tissue. In this way, an immune response is stimulated.

Reflex action. The sensory nerve endings present in the skin initiate the reflex action against any unpleasant or painful stimuli. As a result, the body protects itself from further damage.

Absorption of ultraviolet rays. The melanin and thick first layer of epidermis absorb ultraviolet rays of the sun and thus, prevent the skin from getting ultraviolet radiation injury.

Regulation of body temperature is an important function performed by the skin. Heat is lost through evaporation of sweat; and heat is conserved by the fat and hair. For details see page 305.

Sensory function. Skin contains nerve endings and receptors sensitive to touch, pain and temperature, which play an important role in the sensory perception. For details see page 524.

Absorptive function. Though skin forms a relatively waterproof barrier, the oily substances are freely absorbed by the skin. Some drugs are administered as transdermal patches, e.g., hormones used as replacement therapy in postmenopausal women, anti-inflammatory drugs such as diclophenac sodium patch, and nicotine patch as an aid to stop smoking.

Secretory functions. Skin secretes sweat and sebum.

Excretory function. Skin also acts as an excretory organ or it helps in eliminating excess of water, salts and waste products like urea (especially when kidney function is impaired) through sweat.

Synthesis. In the skin vitamin D is synthesized from ergosterol by the action of ultraviolet rays of sun.

Regulation of pH. Skin plays a role in the regulation of body pH. A good amount of acid is excreted through the sweat.

Role in maintaining water balance. The epidermis is such a membrane that it does not allow water to pass in and out. The importance of this function is seen in persons who have lost extensive areas of skin through burns. An important cause of death in such cases is water loss from the body.

CLINICAL ASPECTS

WOUND HEALING

The most frequently injured tissue of the body is skin. The skin wounds heal well, as it has got an excellent power of regeneration.

Types of Wound Healing

Depending upon the type of wound and prevailing local and systemic factors wound healing is of two types:

1. Primary wound healing
2. Secondary wound healing.

Primary Wound Healing

Factors Favoring Primary Wound Healing

The primary wound healing, also known as healing by first intention, occurs under following circumstances:

- When cut edges are sharp and clean and can be brought together
- Wound is not contaminated by foreign bodies or toxic materials
- Wound is not infected
- Immunity is not impaired
- Blood supply to the area is good.

Secondary Wound Healing

Factors Responsible for Secondary Wound Healing

The secondary wound healing or healing by second intention occurs under following situations:

- When destruction is much and some tissue is lost.
- When the cut surfaces cannot be brought together.
- When the wound is infected.

SKIN BURNS

Burns refer to the injury caused to skin and other body tissue by heat, electricity, ionizing radiations, strong chemicals. Thus, skin burns may be:

- Thermal burns
- Electric burns
- Radiational burns
- Chemical burns (caused by acids and alkalies).

Scalds refer to the burns caused by hot fluids.

Types of Burns

Depending upon the depth of burnt area, the burns may be:

- *First-degree burns or partial thickness or superficial burns,* when only the epidermis is involved.
- *Second-degree burns,* when epidermis and upper region of dermis is also involved.
- *Third-degree or full thickness (deep) burns* involve entire thickness of skin.

Estimation of extent of burns in adults is made following the 'rule-of-nines' as described earlier.

Estimation of severity of burns: Burns are *considered critical* if:

- Over 25% of the body has second-degree burns
- Over 10% of the body has third-degree burns
- Third-degree burns involve face, hands and feet.

PRESSURE SORES

Pressure sores or bed sores, also known as decubitus ulcer, refer to the area of sloughing of skin, which occur over the pressure areas where the skin is compressed for long periods between the bony prominences and a hard surface.

Predisposing Factors for Pressure Sores

Pressure sores occur when the patient lies over the bed for a prolonged period without moving the body parts as occurs is:

Contd...

- Paralyzed patients
- Patients having multiple limb fractures
- Old debilitated patients
- Comatosed patients.

Occurrence of bed sores in such patients is precipitated by moisture, infection, poor nutritional status, sensory impairment and poor circulation.

SKIN INFECTIONS

Common skin infections are:

Viral infections. These include:

- *Warts and verrucas* are caused by human papillomavirus (HPV). These present as small firm growths on the hands, face and soles of the feet.
- *Chickenpox and shingles* are caused by zoster virus.
- *Cold sores (herpes labialis) and genital herpes* are caused by herpes simplex virus type I and type II, respectively.

Bacterial infections of skin of common occurrence are:

- *Impetigo* is a highly infectious condition manifesting as superficial skin pustules usually around the nose and mouth. Common causative bacteria are *Staphylococcus aureus* and *Streptococcus pyogenes*.
- *Cellulitis* is a diffuse infection of the skin and subcutaneous tissue. The causative bacteria enter the body through a break in the skin and these include *Streptococcus pyogenes* or *Clostridium perfringens*. If untreated, it may be complicated by necrotizing fasciitis or even septicemia.
- *Acne vulgaris* is characterized by pustule formation on the face in adolescents. Basically it occurs due to infection in the blocked sebaceous glands in hair follicle. Increased level of male sex hormones during puberty are implicated in the etiology.

Fungal infections of skin are:

- *Candidiasis* is an intertriginous infection affecting submammary folds, axillae and digital clefts. It is a common cause of vulvovaginitis in females.
- *Pityriasis versicolor.* It is characterized by small confluent scaly depigmented patches.
- *Dermatophytosis* (Ringworm infection). The lesions are red, scaly and itchy. The groin and feet (tinea pedis) are common sites.

MALIGNANT TUMORS OF SKIN

Common malignant tumors of the skin are:

Basal cell carcinoma: It is the most common malignant tumor of skin. It most commonly involves skin of face and head and neck area, i.e., the most sun-exposed sites.

Squamous cell carcinoma: It commonly arises from the mucocutaneous junctions in the body such as lid margin, lips, penis, etc.

Malignant melanoma: It is a rare tumor that may arise from a pre-existing nevus, or de novo from the melanocytes present in the skin.

SKIN GRAFTING

Skin grafting is a surgical procedure involving transfer of normal skin to the damage area of the skin. It is required when a large area of the skin has *been lost during burns or due to injury.*

NURSING IMPLICATIONS AND APPLICATIONS

Prevention and Treatment of Bed Sores

Nursing care is very important for prevention of bed sores in bed ridden patients. Bed sores can be prevented by opting following five tips.

1. *Proper hydration and nutrition* is crucial for preventing bed sores. When the internal body is well taken care of, the skin will be less prone to sores and any resulting infection. Therefore, nourishing the patient with good healthy protein rich diet and hydration can help.
2. *Exercise.* It is very important for bed ridden patients to perform movements, so that air flow can occur to every part of the body. The attending nurse should help in doing movements of the body in such patients and preventing bed sores.
3. *Repositioning* Frequent repositioning the patient (once in every two hours) and checking of pressure points for development of bed sore is also important point for nursing care to bedridden patients.
4. *Extra-cushioning* by putting extra pillows under high pressure points such as tail-bone and shoulders can improve air flow.

5. *Cleanliness and dryness:* Keeping everything clean, dry and disinfected of the patient (skin and linen, etc.) can prevent the bed sores.

Treatment of Bed Sores

The treatment of bed sores include:

- Clean and wash the wound gently with saline during every change of dressing
- Remove the dead tissue prior to dressing using high pressure water jet or surgical instrument.
- Apply dressing using antimicrobial ointments to protect the wound, and to facilitate the healing.
- Use of dynamic type of mattresses, which are made of static foam help to release the pressure.
- Oral or systemic use of antibiotics is to treat infection.
- Proper diet rich in protein or protein supplements to boost healing process is also being recommended.

APPENDAGES OF SKIN

Appendages of the skin refer to the structures developed from the embryonic epidermis. These include:

- Nails
- Hairs
- Sebaceous glands
- Sweat glands.

Nails

Nails are hardened keratin plates (cornified zone) which make solid covering over the dorsal surfaces of the terminal portions of the fingers and toes.

Parts

Each nail has following parts (Figs 6.1-5A and B):

Nail root is the proximal hidden part which is buried into the nail groove and is overlapped by the nail fold of skin.

Free edge is the part of the nail that projects beyond the distal end of digit.

Nail body is the visible part of nail which is adherent to the underlying skin. The whitish crescentric area at the proximal end of the nail body is called *lunule*.

Skin surrounding the nail is named as below:

Nail fold or nail wall refers to the fold of skin overlapping the proximal and lateral borders of the nail.

Nail bed refers to the epidermis lying beneath the nail root and nail body. The germinative zone of the nail bed beneath the root and lunula is thick and proliferative (germinal matrix), and is responsible for the growth of the nail. The rest of nail bed is thin (sterile matrix) over which the growing nail glides.

Nail groove refers to the furrow between the nail fold and nail bed.

IMPORTANT TO KNOW

Important facts about nails are:

- *Pinkish color* of the nails is due to very vascular corium below the translucent nail bed. In anemia, the nails are pale and white.
- *Nail growth* is faster in summer than in winter, in the fingers than in toes, and in the longer fingers than in the shorter ones. It takes about 90–120 days for the whole nail (body) to grow.

Hairs

Distribution and Development of Hair

Distribution

Hairs are keratinous filaments distributed all over the body except for the palms, soles, dorsal surface of distal phalanges, umbilicus, glans penis, inner surface of prepuce, the labia minora and inner surface of labia majora. The length, thickness and color of the hairs vary in different parts of the body and in different individuals.

Development

The invaginations of the germinative layer of epidermis into the dermis occur by 3rd and 4th month of fetal life to form the *hair follicles* from which the hairs are derived.

Lanugo (primary hairs) refer to the delicate hairs which cover the fetal skin by the 5th and 6th month. The lanugo are mostly shed by birth.

Vellus (secondary hairs) are fine hairs, which replace the lanugo during infancy. These are retained in most parts of the body except in non hairy areas.

Terminal hair are thick and dark hair, which replace the vellus in the area of scalp, eyebrows and other hairy areas of adult skin.

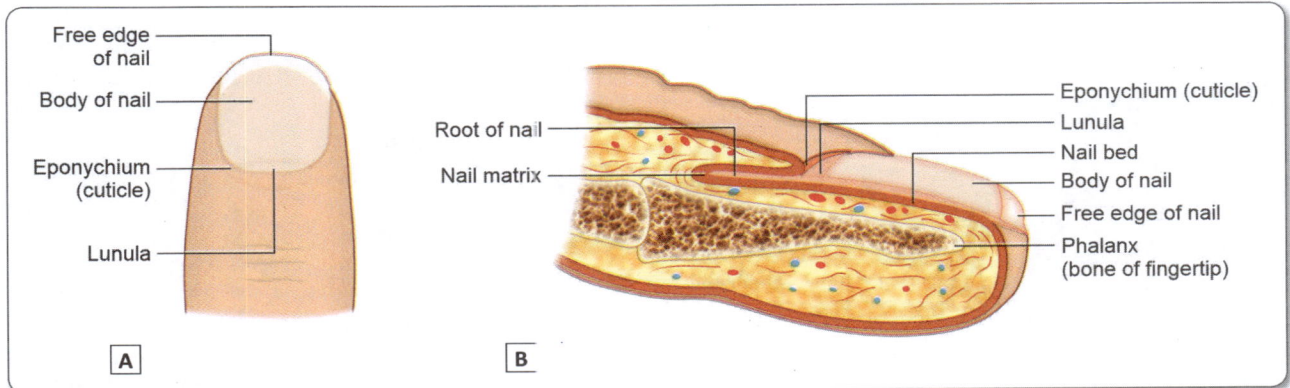

| A | B |

Figs 6.1-5A and B: Structure of a nail: A. Finger nail viewed from above; B. Cross-section of the finger nail and nail bed

Parts and Structure of the Hair Proper (Fig. 6.1-6)

Parts of hair

Each hair consists of following parts:

Shaft refers to the superficial portion, most of which projects above the surface of skin.

Root is the embedded part of the hair that penetrates into the dermis and even into the subcutaneous tissue.

Microscopic structure of hair

Microscopically each hair consists of three layers:

1. *Medulla* is the innermost part composed of rows of polyhedral cells containing granules of eleidin and air spaces.

2. *Cortex* is the middle part which forms the major part of hair and consists of elongated cells that contain pigment granules in dark hairs, but mostly air in white hair.

3. *Cuticle* is the outermost part which consists of a single layer of thin flat scale-like cells that are the most heavily keratinized.

Structures Surrounding the Hair

Hair follicle is the downgrowth of the epidermal cells into the dermis which surrounds the hair. The wall of hair follicle consists of three layers, the inner root sheath, outer root sheath and connective tissue sheath. The hair follicle is expanded at its proximal end to form the *hair bulb*. Each hair bulb is invaginated at its end by the *hair papilla* (vascular connective tissue) which forms the neurovascular hilum of hair and its sheath. Hair grows at the hair bulb by proliferation of its cells capping the papilla.

Arrector pili is a smooth muscle supplied by sympathetic nerves that connects the undersurface of the follicles to the superficial papillary layer of the dermis. Contraction of this muscle erects the hair, depresses the adjacent skin forming goose skin and compresses the sebaceous glands, so as to expel its secretion.

Sebaceous Glands

Distribution

Sebaceous glands are widely distributed all over the dermis of skin except for the palms and soles. They are especially abundant in the scalp and face and are also very numerous around the apertures of nose, ear, mouth, and anus.

Locations

Sebaceous glands associated with hair are situated in the angle between the hair follicle and the arrector pili muscle.

Structure

The sebaceous glands are simple or branched *alveolar glands* formed of secretory parts and excretory ducts.

Secretory part of each gland is made up of a cluster of about 2–5 piriform alveoli.

Ducts of the sebaceous glands open into the hair follicles, with the exception of lips, glans penis, inner surface of prepuce, labia minora, nipple and areola of the breast and tarsal glands of eyelids, where the ducts open on surface of skin.

> **IMPORTANT TO KNOW**
>
> *Secretion* of sebaceous glands, known as sebum, is oily in nature. It keeps the hair soft and pliable and gives it a shiny appearance. On the skin it provides some waterproofing and acts as a bactericidal and fungicidal agent preventing the successful invasion of microbes. It also prevents drying and cracking of the skin. The secretion is under hormonal control especially the androgens.

Sweat Glands

Sudoriferous or sweat glands are distinguished into two principal types on the basis of structure and location. These are:

1. Eccrine sweat glands
2. Apocrine sweat glands.

Eccrine Sweat Glands

Distribution

Eccrine sweat glands are more abundant and distributed in almost every part of the skin except for the margins of lips, nail beds of fingers and toes, glans penis, glans clitoris, and ear drums. These glands are most numerous in the skin of palms and soles.

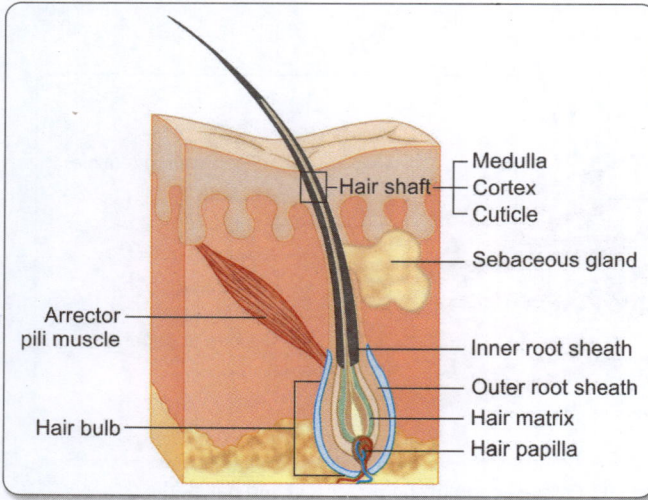

Fig. 6.1-6: Structure of hair

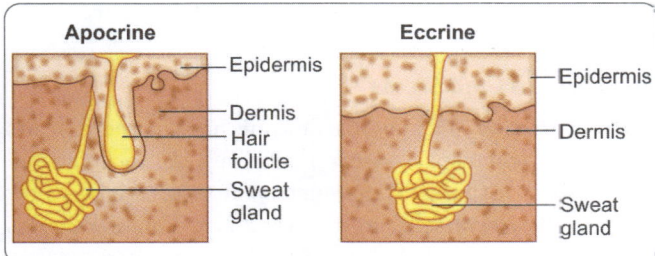

Fig. 6.1-7: Types of sweat glands

Structure (Fig. 6.1-7)

Each gland is a single tube having two parts:

1. *Body* of the gland is highly coiled secretory part which lies in the deeper part of corium or in the subcutaneous tissue.

2. *Duct* is the straight part of the gland which traverses the dermis and epidermis and opens on the surface of skin.

Nervous control

The eccrine sweat glands are supplied and controlled by cholinergic sympathetic nerves.

Secretion

The eccrine sweat glands are *merocrine* in nature, i.e., they produce their thin watery secretion without any disintegration of epithelial cells.

Function

The glands help in regulation of the body temperature by evaporation of sweat and also help in excreting the body salt.

Apocrine Glands

Distribution

Apocrine glands are distributed primarily to the skin of the axilla, eyelids (Moll's glands), pubic region, and areola of the breasts. Ceruminous glands of the external auditory meatus are modified apocrine sweat glands.

Structure (Fig. 6.1-7)

These are simple branched tubular glands. The secretory portion of the glands is located in the dermis and excretory duct opens into the hair follicle.

Secretion

Apocrine glands begin to function at puberty and produce a more viscous secretion having a characteristic odor.

Nervous control

The apocrine glands are also merocrine in nature, but are regulated by a dual autonomic control.

Function

They do not respond sufficiently to temperature changes as do eccrine glands. Therefore, some workers are not inclined to call them sweat glands. In animals, they produce chemical signals pheromones, which are important in courtship and social behavior.

REGULATION OF TEMPERATURE

The human body has the remarkable capacity of maintaining the core temperature at 37°C. This process is called thermoregulation. It is an important mechanism as the extremes of temperature can affect the ability of the body to function properly. Hypothalamus plays the major role in thermoregulation.

FACTORS AFFECTING BODY TEMPERATURE

Following are few factors that can increase or decrease the internal body temperature:

Factors that increase internal body temperature are:
- Fever
- Exercise
- Digestion

Factors that decrease internal body temperature are:
- Use of drugs
- Alcohol use
- Metabolic conditions, such as hypothyroidism.

MECHANISM OF THERMOREGULATION

Role of Hypothalamus

The temperature of the body is regulated by neural feedback mechanisms which operate primarily through the hypothalamus. The hypothalamus acts as the principal integrating center for heat regulation. By adjusting a balance between heat production and heat loss, it helps to maintain body temperature at 37°C. Hypothalamus accomplishes this function by two centers: heat loss center and heat gain center.

Role of Skin

The skin helps in regulating body temperature through vasodilatation and vasoconstriction of blood vessels in the skin, sweating and insulating fat layer of hypodermis.

Mechanisms for Decreasing the Internal Temperature

Exposure to Heat Stress

The tonic sympathetic discharge is reflexly abolished by hypothalamic mechanism. Thus, the blood flow to skin is increased by the following responses in a chronological sequence:

- First of all, A–V anastomoses of hands, feet and ear lobules dilate due to reduction in the sympathetic tonic discharge.
- Secondly, rest of the cutaneous vessels dilate due to progressive withdrawal of sympathetic vasoconstrictor activity.
- Thirdly, sweat glands get activated due to the cholinergic sympathetic discharge. The bradykinin produced by the secretory activity of the sweat glands acts locally as a powerful vasodilator and increases blood flow to skin.

All the above mechanisms collectively may increase the cutaneous blood flow. The increased blood flow carries heat to the surface of the body, where it is dissipated by radiation, evaporation and conduction to the environment.

Mechanisms that Increase Body Temperature During

Exposure to Cold Stress

Vasoconstriction. Via hypothalamic mechanism, there occurs widespread cutaneous vasoconstriction due to increased sympathetic discharge. Consequently, cutaneous blood flow is markedly decreased. In this way, heat conservation is accomplished by markedly diminishing the rate of blood flow to skin.

Thermogenesis (Generation of heart):

Shivering is one of the prime examples of thermogenesis or generating heat in the body.

Hormonal thermogenesis. Secretion of nore-pinephrine, epinephrine and thyroxine increase the metabolism and hence, results in an increase in body temperature.

CLINICAL ASPECTS

FEVER

Fever, also known as pyrexia, refers to an increase in the body temperature above the normal range. It is the most common symptom/sign of the ill health.

Causes: Common causes of fever are:
- *Infections* caused by bacteria, viruses, protozoa (e.g., malaria) and other infecting agents are usually associated with fever.
- *Tissue destruction*, as in myocardial infarction, uninfected neoplasms, serum sickness and rheumatism, etc. is also associated with fever.
- *Pyrexia of unknown origin*. This term is used when cause of fever cannot be ascertained.

Pathogenesis: Fever develops when the hypothalamic set point is reset at a higher temperature by the pyrogens.

Role of pyrogens: Toxins liberated from the infecting organism and tissue destruction act on the phagocytic cells (monocytes, macrophages and Kupffer cells) to produce cytokines that act as endogenous pyrogens, which act on the anterior hypothalamus to increase the production of prostaglandin E2. Prostaglandin E2 acts on the hypothalamus to increase the thermostat 'set point'.

HEAT EXHAUSTION AND HEAT STROKE

Heat exhaustion refers to a condition of circulatory failure caused by excessive sweating following prolonged exposure to heat. It is characterized by dehydration, salt loss, decreased blood volume, decreased arterial pressure and syncope (fainting).

Heat stroke usually occurs when heavy physical work is performed in hot and humid environment. In this condition, normal response to increased temperature (sweating) is impaired and core temperature increases to the point of tissue damage. It is characterized by convulsion, loss of consciousness and even death may occur when body temperature exceeds 41°C.

HYPOTHERMIA

If the body temperature falls to 95°F (35°C) or lower, hypothermia develops. Hypothermia results when the ambient temperature is so low that the body's heat generating mechanisms (e.g., shivering and metabolism) cannot adequately maintain core temperature near the set point. Infants and old people develop hypothermia more easily than the adults. It has been observed that:
- At rectal temperature of 28°C, the body's ability to spontaneously return to normal temperature.
- Humans can tolerate body temperature of 21–24°C without permanent ill effects, i.e., if rewarmed with external heat, returns to a normal state.

Effects of hypothermia on body include:
- Slowing of metabolic and physiologic processes,
- Retardation of glucose metabolism,
- Slowing of respiration and heart rate,
- Lowering of blood pressure,
- Slowing of reflexes and occurrence of muscular rigidity,
- Loss of consciousness and
- Death may occur when temperature remains below 25°C for some time.

NURSING IMPLICATIONS AND APPLICATIONS

Nursing care of patients with high temperature include:
- Removal of excessive clothing, blankets and linen.
- Adjustment of the room temperature to make the environmental temperature comfortable for the patient.
- Administration of prescribed medication (antibiotics and antipyretics)
- Tepid sponge bath to facilitate the body in cooling down to provide comfort to the patient
- Raising of head end of patient's bed to improve expansion of lung enabling the patient to breathe more effectively.

FASCIA

INTRODUCTION

Fascia has been described along with skin in this chapter, because like skin it also forms a covering around the body structures. Fascia is a sheet/band of fibrofatty tissue that lies deep to the skin and invests muscles and other deep structures. In reality, it is a packing material; a connective tissue that remains between areas of more specialized tissue. It varies widely in structure and thickness according to the functional requirements. The fascia is classified into:
- Superficial fascia
- Deep fascia

SUPERFICIAL FASCIA

Superficial fascia is also known as hypodermis or subcutaneous tissue or tela subcutanea. It is a general coating of the body beneath the skin, comprising loose areolar tissue with varying amount of fat.

Distribution and Special Features

Superficial fascia is widely distributed below the skin in the body (Fig. 6.1-8). It has some special features in different regions of the body.

Most distinct areas. Superficial fascia is most distinct in the lower part of the anterior abdominal wall, perineum, and the limbs.
- *Very thin* superficial fascia is seen over dorsal aspect of hands and feet, sides of neck and around the anus.
- *Very dense* superficial fascia is seen in the scalp, palms and soles.
- *Stratification* of superficial fascia (into two layers) occurs in the lower part of anterior abdominal wall, perineum and uppermost small part of the thighs.

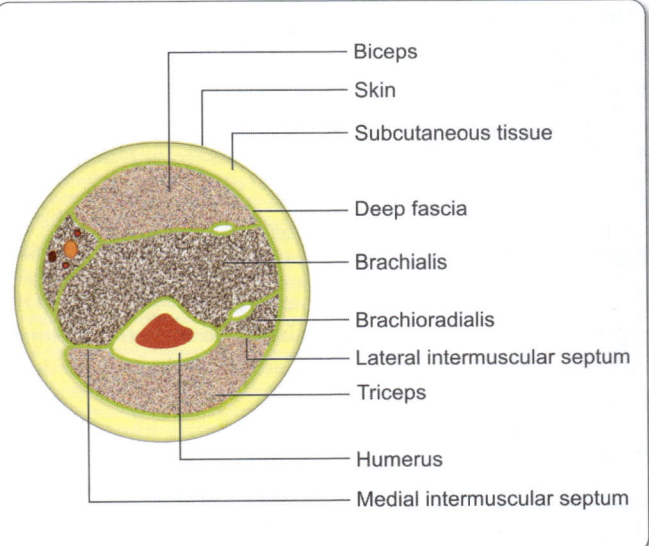

Fig. 6.1-8: Cross-section of an arm showing the arrangement of superficial and deep fascia

Labels: Biceps, Skin, Subcutaneous tissue, Deep fascia, Brachialis, Brachioradialis, Lateral intermuscular septum, Triceps, Humerus, Medial intermuscular septum

Fat of Superficial Fascia

Fat is most important constituent of the superficial fascia. The subcutaneous layer of fat is called *panniculus adiposus.* This acts as a barrier to the heat loss from the body and is responsible for the shape and contours of the body. Some features of the distribution of fat in the body are as below:

Males versus females. In females, fat is more abundant, more evenly distributed and forms a thicker layer than in males. In females, fat is in the superficial fascia of lower abdomen and upper thighs, whereas in males it is inside the abdominal cavity.

Areas of the body with excessive fat. Fat is abundant in the gluteal region (buttocks), lumbar region (flanks), front of thighs, anterior abdominal wall below the umbilicus, mammary gland, postdeltoid region, and the cervicothoracic region.

Area of the body with no fat. Fat is absent from the eyelids, external ear, penis, scrotum, labia minora, clitoris and nipples.

Contents of Superficial Fascia

In addition to fibrofatty tissue, the superficial fascia also contains. Small blood vessels, lymphatics and lymph nodes.

Various Modifications of superficial fascia, such as:
- Mammary gland
- Subcutaneous muscles of fascia, which include dartos, platysma, palmaris brevis and corrugator cutis ani

Functions of Superficial Fascia

- Facilitates movements of skin
- Conserves body heat, as the fat present in it is bad conductor of heat
- Serves as a soft medium for the passage of blood vessels and nerves to the skin.

DEEP FASCIA

Deep fascia is a fibrous sheet which invests the body beneath the superficial fascia. In other words, it is dense, inelastic and tough membrane which separates superficial fascia from the underlying deeper structures. It is devoid of fat.

Distribution and Arrangement

Deep fascia is widely distributed in the body. Some features about distribution and arrangement of deep fascia in the body are as below:

Best versus ill-defined areas of deep fascia:
- It is *best defined* in the limbs where it forms tough and tight sleeves. In the iliotibial tract of fascia lata, it is specially well developed.
- In the neck, the deep fascia is *well developed* and forms a collar.
- Over rectus sheath and external oblique aponeurosis of abdominal wall it is *quite thin* and barely demonstrable.
- It is *absent* in the area of face and ischiorectal region.

Extensions (prolongations) from deep fascia run along various body structures such as muscles, nerves, vessels. These are described in detail under modifications of deep fascia.

Arrangement of deep fascia vis-a-vis superficial fascia in the body is depicted in a cross-section of an arm.

Modification of Deep Fascia

Deep fascia is modified in different areas to serve special functions. Some of the important modifications of deep fascia are summarized below:

Modifications of deep fascia in relation to muscles are:

Intermuscular septa are the extensions from the deep fascia which envelop the functionally different group of muscles into separate compartments.

Epimysium refers to the extension of deep fascia which arises from the intermuscular septum and surrounds the single muscle belly.

Perimysium refers to sheath of connective tissue which extends from the epimysium which encloses each muscle fasciculus. Fasciculi are bundles of muscle fibers which form a muscle.

Endomysium is the extension from the perimysium which surrounds each muscle fibers (Fig. 6.1-9).

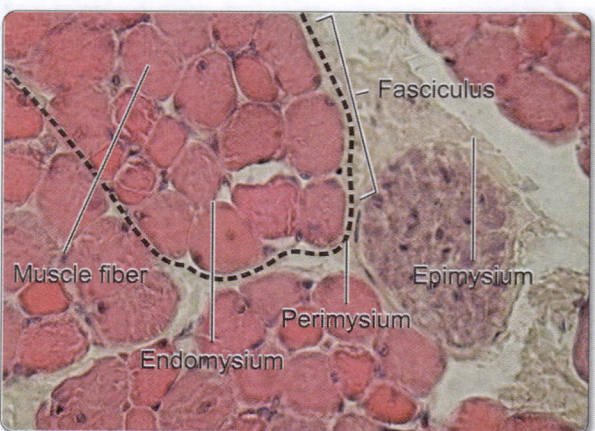

Fig. 6.1-9: Transverse section of skeletal muscle showing arrangement of perimysium and endomysium

Modification of Deep Fascia in Relation to Blood Vessels

Deep fascia forms *perivascular sheaths* around large arteries and veins. Examples include carotid sheath, axillary sheath and femoral sheath. The perivascular sheath around the arteries is dense and rather loose around the veins to give an allowance for the vein to distend.

Modifications of Deep Fascia in Relation to Nerves

Epineurium refers to deep fascia covering around each nerve.

Perineurium is the covering around each nerve fasciculus.

Endoneurium refers to the fascial covering around each nerve fiber.

These connective tissue coverings support the nerve fibers and carry capillaries and lymphatics.

Modifications in Deep Fascia in Relation to Joints

Synovial membrane, capsule and bursa are modified forms of deep fascia in relation to most of the joints.

Tendon sheaths and associated bursae are the modifications of deep fascia which prevent wear and tear of the tendons and minimize friction.

Retinaculae refer to thickened bands of deep fascia in relation to some joints, e.g., wrist and ankle (Fig. 6.1-10). The retinacula act as pulley during the movements of joints and also keep tendons in position.

Modification in Relation to Palms and Soles

In the region of palm and sole, deep fascia is modified to form *aponeurosis*, e.g., palmar and plantar aponeurosis which protect the underlying structures, e.g., nerves, blood vessels and delicate tendons.

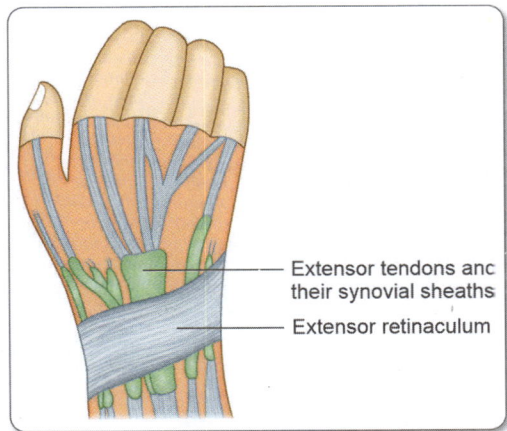

Fig. 6.1-10: Extensor retinaculum of wrist

Extensor tendons anc their synovial sheaths

Extensor retinaculum

Modifications in Relation to Bones

- Deep fascia becomes continuous with the *periosteum in bare bones.*
- Interosseous membrane refers to the modified deep fascia present in between the two bones of forearms and legs. This membrane keeps the two bones at optimum distance and increases surface area for attachment of muscles.

Modification in Relation to Neck

In the neck area the deep fascia is very well developed and forms an investing layer called collar which gives the neck a proper shape.

Functions of Deep Fascia

Keeps in position the underlying structures.

Preserves the characteristic surface contour of the limbs.

Provides extra surface for attachment of muscles.

Helps in venous and lymphatic return. The contraction of calf muscles in the tight sleeve of deep fascia helps in pushing the venous blood and lymph toward heart.

Assists muscles in their action by the degree of tension and pressure it exerts upon their surfaces.

Prevents the loss of power. Modification of deep fascia in the form of retinacula (as mentioned earlier) act as pulley and serves to prevent the loss of power. In such situations, the friction is minimized by the synovial sheaths of the tendons.

CLINICAL ASPECTS

Surgical plane to drain pus from the deeper tissues is helped by knowledge of applied anatomy. A deeply accumulated pus often tends to track down from its primary site to a more dependent part of the body. The course taken by the pus is determined by the fascial planes and neurovascular bundles.

Edema or collection of fluid in the legs can develop following damage to fascia of leg, as it can affect the venous return leading to accumulation of blood and fluid.

Dupuytren's contracture refers to the contraction of palmar fascia leading to flexion deformity of fingers.

ASSESS YOURSELF

Short and Long Answer Questions

1. **Draw a diagram to show various layers of skin.**
2. **Describe the functions of skin.**
3. **Mechanism of thermoregulation.**
4. **Write notes on:**
   - Appendages of skin
   - Sebaceous gland
   - Arrector pilorum
   - Hypothermia
   - Fever

Multiple Choice Questions

1. **The surface area of skin of lower limb is:**
   a. 1%   b. 9%
   c. 18%   d. 36%
2. **In which layer of skin melanin pigment present:**
   a. Stratum basale   b. Stratum granulosum
   c. Stratum lucidum   d. Papillary layer of dermis

3. **The Merkel cells are present in which layer of the skin:**
   a. Reticular layer of dermis
   b. Papillary layer of dermis
   c. Stratum basale of epidermis
   d. Stratum corneum of epidermis
4. **True about epidermal ridges of the skin:**
   a. Form linear furrows
   b. Present on the dorsum of hand
   c. Firmly bound to underlying fascia
   d. Seen on skin of palm and sole
5. **Stratum spinosum layer of epidermis consists of:**
   a. Single layer of cuboidal to columnar cells
   b. 4 to 8 layers of keratinocytes
   c. 2 to 4 layers of granular cells
   d. Thick non hairy skin layer
6. **Which of the following cells not belong to epidermis?**
   a. Keratinocyte   b. Langerhans cells
   c. Merkel's cells   d. Fat cells

7. **Which type of hair cover the fetal skin?**
    a. Vellus   b. Lanugo
    c. Terminal   d. None of these
8. **Sebaceous glands:**
    a. Consist of 2–5 alveoli
    b. Ducts open into hair follicles
    c. Arrector pili muscle expel the secretions
    d. Mainly present on lips
9. **Statement not true for arrector pili muscle:**
    a. Supplied by parasympathetic nerves
    b. Contraction causes erection of hair
    c. Supplied by sympathetic nerve
    d. Goose skin on contraction

10. **Statement not true for eccrine sweat gland:**
    a. Its body present in subcutaneous tissue
    b. Innervated by cholinergic sympathetic fibers
    c. Help in regulation of body temperature
    d. Secretes pheromones
11. **Which area of body has no fat?**
    a. Gluteal region
    b. Lumbar region
    c. Eyelids
    d. Abdominal wall

ANSWER KEY

1.	d	2.	a	3.	c	4.	d	5.	d	6.	d	7.	b	8.	d
9.	a	10.	d	11.	c										

SENSE OF VISION

Sense of vision is a complex function of the visual apparatus consisting of two eyeballs, visual pathway and their central connections. In addition to these essential organs, there are accessory organs which are necessary for the protection and functioning of the eyeball.

ACCESSORY ORGANS OF THE EYE AND ORBIT

Accessory organs of the eye include eyebrows, eyelids, conjunctiva, lacrimal apparatus and extraocular muscles.

Eyebrows

The two eyebrows are arched structures placed horizontally over the superciliary ridge of the frontal bone, separated from each other by a smooth hairless prominent area known as glabella. The surface of the eyebrows is covered by hairs which project obliquely from the skin and form an important part of the eyebrows. They protect the eyeball from sweat, dust and other foreign bodies.

Eyelids

The eyelids are mobile tissue curtains placed in front of the eyeballs. These act as shutters protecting the eyes from injuries and excessive light. These also perform an important function of spreading the tear film over the cornea and conjunctiva.

Eyelashes are short curved hair present on the lid margins (free edges of the eyelids).

Structure. From anterior to posterior the eyelid consists of following layers (Fig. 6.2-1)

Skin. It is elastic and very thin.

Subcutaneous loose areolar tissue.

Layer of striated muscles. It consists of orbicularis oculi muscle which closes the lids. In addition, the upper eyelid also contains levator palpebrae superioris muscle which raises the upper eyelids.

Submuscular areolar tissue. The nerves and vessels of the eyelids lie in this layer.

Fibrous layer. It is the framework of the lids and consists of two parts: the central *tarsal plate* and the peripheral *septum orbitale*.

Layer of nonstriated muscle fibers is formed by palpebral muscle of Müller.

Conjunctiva. The lids on their inner surface are lined by a thin mucous membrane called the palpebral conjunctiva.

Conjunctiva

The conjunctiva is a translucent mucous membrane which lines the posterior surface of the eyelids and anterior aspect of the eyeball up to limbus.

Parts: Conjunctiva consists of following parts (Fig. 6.2-2):

Palpebral conjunctiva lines the posterior surface of the eyelids.

Bulbar conjunctiva covers the anterior part of eyeball up to the limbus.

Fornices. Superior and inferior conjunctival fornices are the cul-de-sacs formed at the junction of bulbar conjunctiva with the palpebral conjunctiva.

Plica semilunaris is a pinkish crescentric fold of conjunctiva present in the medial canthus.

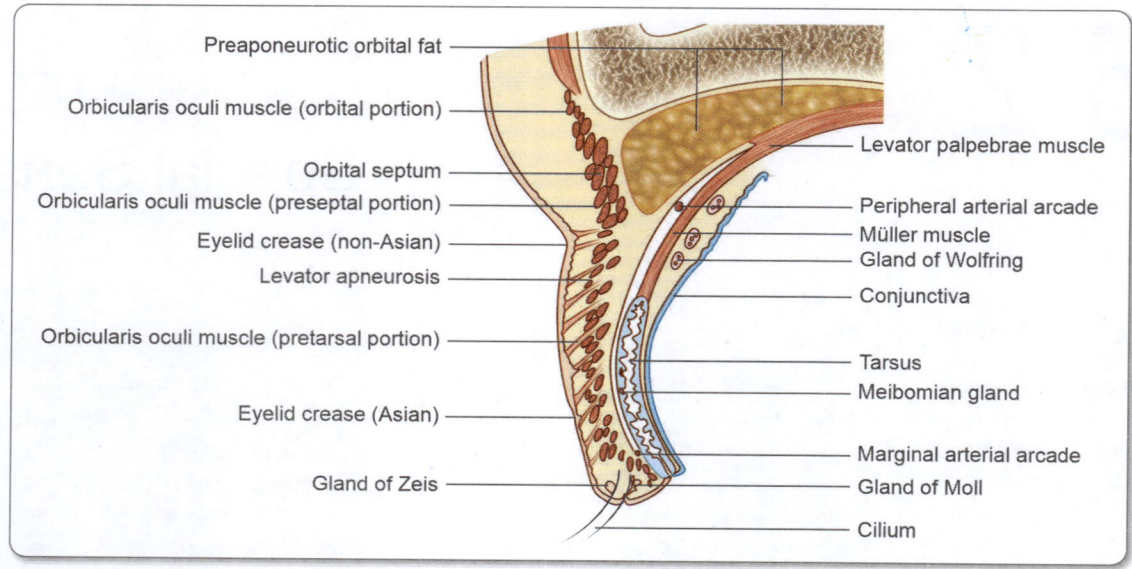

Fig. 6.2-1: Structure of upper eyelid

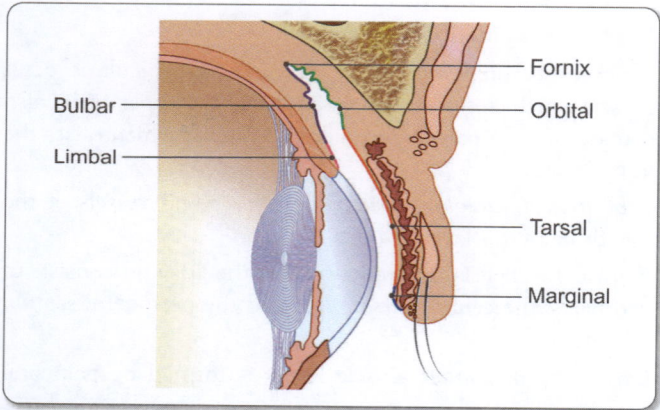

Fig. 6.2-2: Parts of conjunctiva

Lacrimal Apparatus

The lacrimal apparatus (Fig. 6.2-3) comprises the structures concerned with the formation (main lacrimal gland and accessory lacrimal glands) and drainage (lacrimal passages: puncta, canaliculi, lacrimal sac and nasolacrimal duct) of tears.

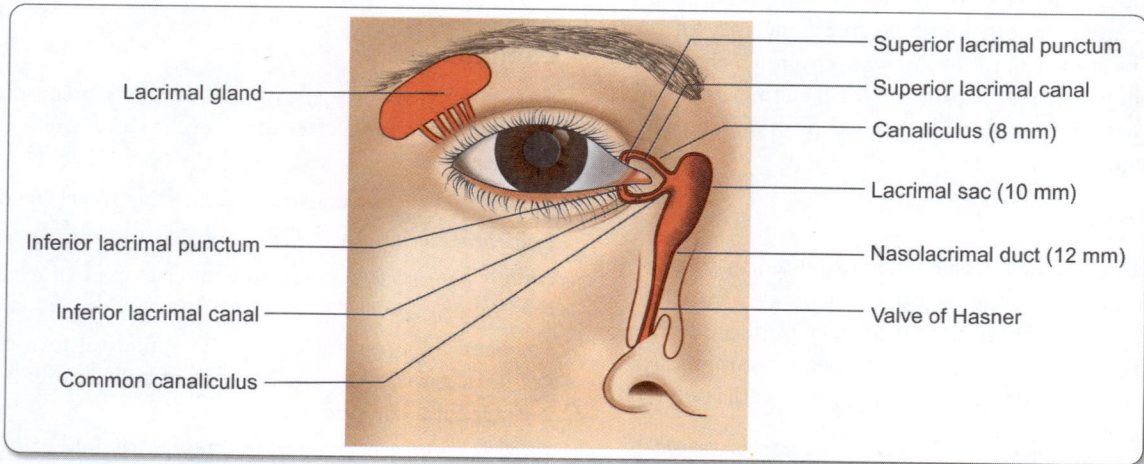

Fig. 6.2-3: The lacrimal apparatus

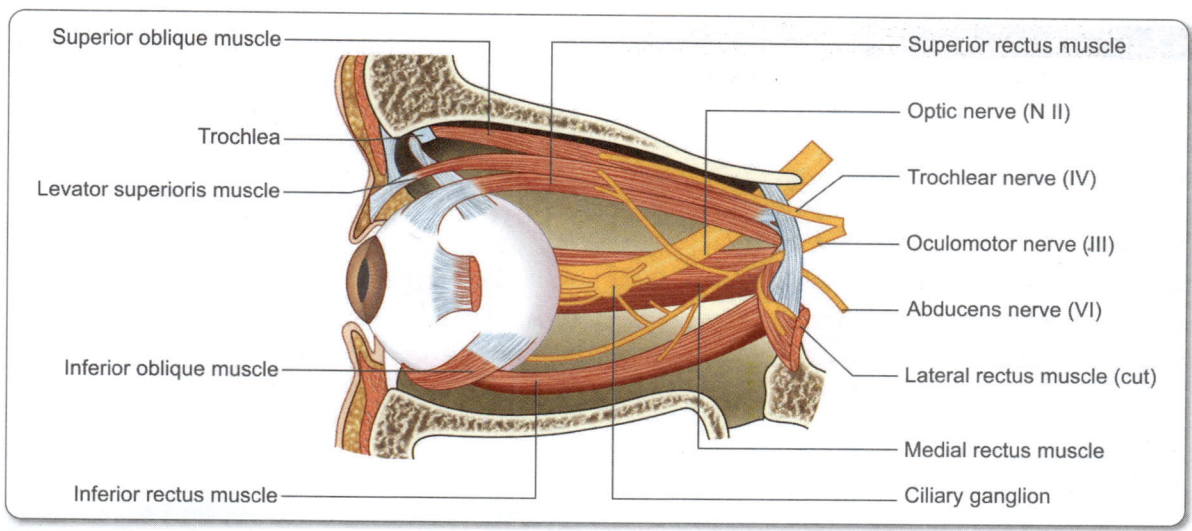

Fig. 6.2-4: Extraocular muscles

Main Lacrimal Gland

The main lacrimal gland is situated at the upper and outer angle of the orbit, in a depression known as the fossa for the lacrimal gland. It consists of an upper orbital and a lower palpebral part. Each gland is about the size and shape of an almond. It is composed of secretory epithelial cells. The ducts of lacrimal gland which are about 12 in number open in the superior fornix. The gland secretes tears composed of water, salt and lysozyme (a bactericidal enzyme).

Accessory Lacrimal Glands

These are microscopic glands situated beneath the palpebral conjunctiva between fornix and edge of the tarsal plate.

Lacrimal Passages

Lacrimal puncta. These are two small rounded or oval openings situated on a small elevation called *lacrimal papilla*, about 6 mm from the inner canthus on each eyelid margin.

Lacrimal canaliculi. These are narrow tubular passages which join the puncta to lacrimal sac.

Lacrimal sac. It lies in the lacrimal fossa located in the anterior part of medial orbital wall. The sac continues with the nasolacrimal duct inferiorly.

Nasolacrimal duct (NLD). It is a membranous canal about 15–18 mm long. It extends from the lower part of lacrimal sac to inferior meatus of the nose. Direction of NLD is downward, backward and laterally. Hasner's valve, which prevents reflux from the nose is present at the lower end of NLD.

CLINICAL ASPECTS

Overflow of tears from the conjunctival sac may be either:
- **Hyperlacrimation:** Excessive secretion of tears due to ocular inflammation or surface ocular disease, emotional and psychiatric causes and lacrimal gland diseases.
- **Epiphora:** Watering due to obstruction to outflow of tears (lacrimal canaliculi or NLD) or lacrimal pump failure or punctual malposition.

Extraocular Muscles (Fig. 6.2-4)

A set of six extraocular muscles (4 recti and 2 obliques) controls the movements of each eye. These muscles are attached to the outer coat of the eyeball at one end and to the walls of the orbital cavity at the other end.

Actions of Extraocular Muscles

The extraocular muscles rotate the eyeball around vertical, horizontal and antero-posterior axes. The action of each muscle is shown in Figure 6.2-5 and depicted in Table 6.2-1.

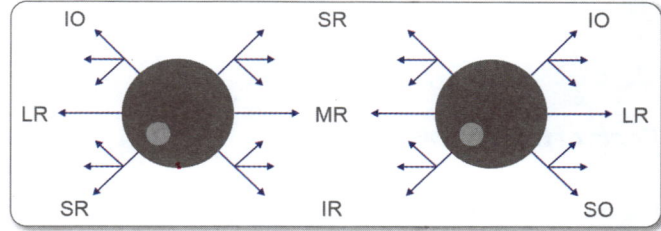

Fig. 6.2-5: Action of extraocular muscles. (SR: superior oblique; LR: lateral rectus; IO: inferior oblique; MR: medial rectus; IR: inferior rectus and SO: superior oblique).

TABLE 6.2-1: Actions of extraocular muscles

Muscle	Primary action	Secondary action
Medial rectus	Adduction	–
Lateral rectus	Abduction	–
Superior rectus	Elevation	Intorsion
Inferior rectus	Depression	Extorsion
Superior oblique	Intorsion	Depression
Inferior oblique	Extorsion	Elevation

CLINICAL ASPECTS

Squint

Weakness or paralysis of a muscle causes squint or strabismus, which may be concomitant or paralytic.

Concomitant squint is congenital; there is no limitation or movement, and no diplopia.

In paralytic squint, movements are limited, diplopia and vertigo are present.

Nystagmus is characterized by involuntary, rhythmical oscillatory movements of the eyes. This is due to incoordination of the ocular muscles.

Orbit

The bony orbits are quadrangular truncated pyramids situated between the anterior cranial fossa above and the maxillary sinuses below. Seven bones take part in its formation. It has four walls (medial, lateral, superior and inferior), a base and an apex. For detail see page 342.

Eyeball

Each eyeball is a cystic structure kept distended by the pressure inside it.

IMPORTANT TO KNOW

Dimensions of an Adult Eyeball

Anteroposterior diameter	:	24 mm
Horizontal (transverse) diameter	:	23.5 mm
Vertical diameter	:	23 mm
Circumference	:	75 mm
Volume	:	6.5 mL
Weight	:	7 g

Coats of the Eyeball

The eyeball comprises three coats: outer (fibrous coat), middle (vascular coat) and inner (nervous coat) (Fig. 6.2-5).

Outer fibrous coat

It is a dense strong wall which protects the intraocular contents. Anterior one-sixth of the fibrous coat is transparent and is called cornea. The posterior 5/6th opaque part is called sclera. Junction of the cornea and sclera is called limbus.

Cornea. The cornea is a transparent, avascular, watchglass-like structure with a smooth shining surface. The average diameter of the cornea is 11–12 mm. Its thickness in the central part is 0.52 mm and in the peripheral part 0.67 mm.

Nerve supply of cornea is purely sensory, derived from the ophthalmic division of the 5th cranial nerve.

Sclera. The sclera is a strong, opaque, white fibrous layer. It is a relatively avascular structure about 1 mm in thickness. It is pierced by nerves and vessels entering the eyeball.

Histologically, sclera consists of three layers-episcleral tissue, sclera proper and lamina fusca.

IMPORTANT TO KNOW

The cornea was the first tissue organ transplanted due to its avascularity. Surgical removal of damaged cornea and replacement with donor's healthy cornea is now common medical procedure. Under 'National Programme for Control of Blindness and Visual Impairment (NPCBI), every year from 25th August to 8th September 'National Eye Donation Fortnight' is observed to create mass public awareness about importance of eye donation and to motivate people to pledge their eyes for donation after death.

CLINICAL ASPECTS

Injury to cornea may cause opacities. These opacities may interfere with vision and result in blindness.

Middle vascular coat (Fig. 6.2-6)

The middle vascular coat, also known as uveal tract, from anterior to posterior, can be divided into three parts—iris, ciliary body and choroid. The blood supply of uveal tract is derived from the short posterior ciliary arteries, long posterior ciliary arteries and anterior ciliary arteries.

Iris. It is a colored, circular diaphragm with a central aperture of 3–4 mm in size known as pupil. The pupil regulates the light reaching the retina. The pupil constricts and dilates by the contraction of *sphincter pupillae* and *dilator pupillae* muscle of the iris, respectively. The sphincter pupillae is supplied by the parasympathetic nerves while the dilator pupillae is supplied by the sympathetic nerves.

Ciliary body. The ciliary body is middle part of the uveal tract. In cut section it is triangular in shape with base forward. Anteriorly, the iris is attached to about the middle of the base of ciliary body. Posteriorly, the ciliary body becomes continuous with the choroid.

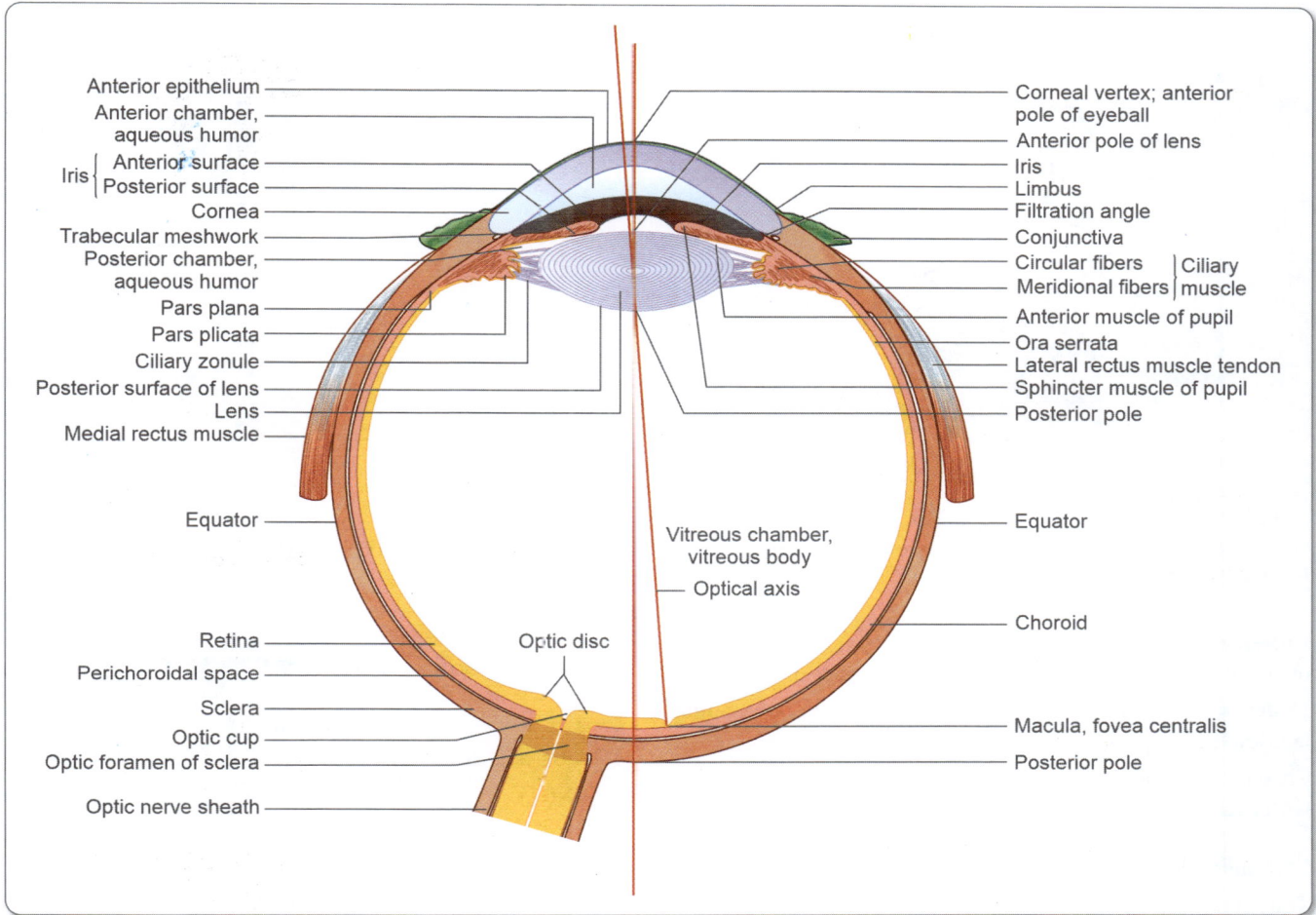

Fig. 6.2-6: Gross anatomy of eyeball

- The ciliary body contains a nonstriated muscle called the *ciliary muscle* which is supplied by parasympathetic fibers and takes part in the process of accommodation of the eye.
- There are about 70–80 finger-like projections from the ciliary body. These are called *ciliary processes* and are the site of aqueous humor production—a watery fluid which maintains the intraocular pressure of the eyeball.

Choroid. It is a dark brown highly vascular layer situated in between sclera and retina. It supplies nutrition to the outer layers of retina.

Inner nervous coat (retina) (Figs 6.2-7A and B)

Retina, the innermost tunic of the eyeball, is a thin, delicate, transparent membrane. It is the most highly developed tissue of the eye. It is concerned with the visual functions.

Gross anatomy: Grossly, retina can be divided into optic disc, macula lutea and the peripheral retina.

Ora serrata is the anterior serrated termination of the retina.

Macula lutea (yellow spot) is a comparatively dark area situated at the posterior pole temporal to the optic disc. Its central depressed area of 1.5 mm in diameter is called *fovea centralis*, which is the most sensitive part of the retina. Visual acuity is maximum in this part of retina.

Optic disc. It is a well-defined circular, pink-colored disc of 1.5 mm diameter. It has only nerve fiber layer, so it does not excite any visual response. It produces *blind spot* in the field of vision.

Interior of the Eyeball

Interior of the eyeball contains, from anterior to posterior—the aqueous humor, lens and vitreous.

Aqueous humor

It is a watery fluid present in the anterior and posterior chambers of the eyeball.

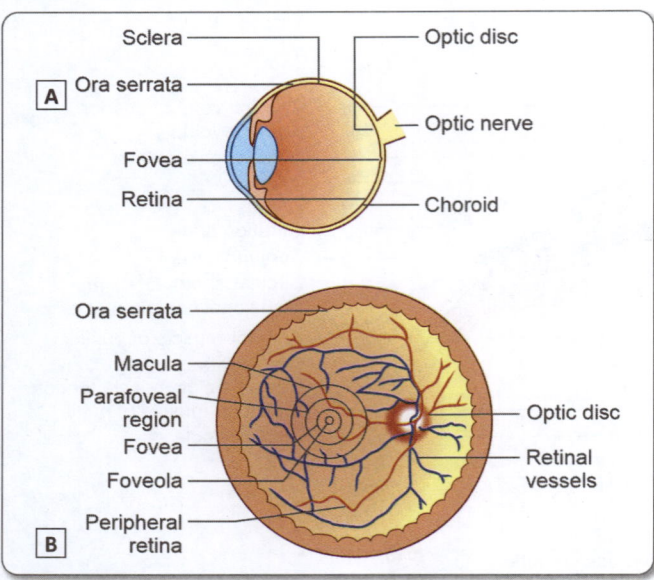

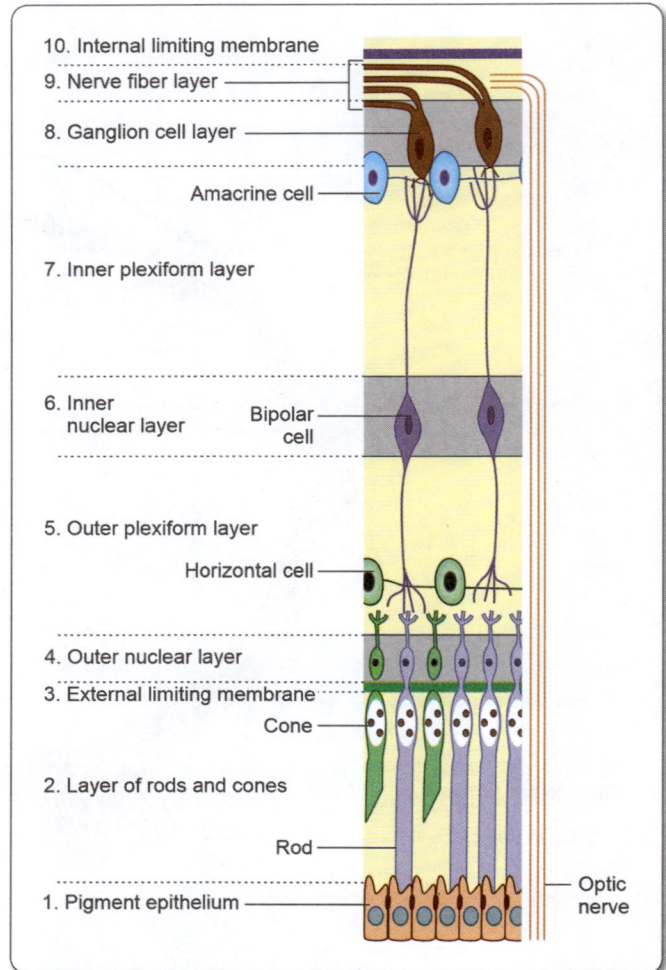

Figs 6.2-7A and B: Gross anatomy of retina

Fig. 6.2-8: Microscopic structure of retina

Anterior chamber is the space bounded anteriorly by the back of cornea and posteriorly by the anterior surface of iris.

Posterior chamber is the space between the front of crystalline lens and back of iris.

Through pupil, anterior and posterior chambers communicate with each other. For details see page 318.

Crystalline lens

The lens is a transparent, biconvex, crystalline structure placed between the iris and the vitreous. It is suspended from the ciliary body by the suspensory ligament or zonules of Zinn. Refractive power of the lens is about 15–16 Diopter. Lens is elastic in nature and its power changes with accommodation. Elasticity of the lens gradually decreases with the age. It is a vascular structure and derives its nutrition from the aqueous humor.

Vitreous humor

Vitreous humor is an inert, transparent, jelly-like structure that fills the posterior four-fifths of the cavity of eyeball. It serves the optical function. It consists of 90% water, some salts and mucoproteins.

RETINA AND VISUAL PATHWAY

Structure of Retina

Retina consists of ten layers, which from without inwards, are as follows (Fig. 6.2-8):

1. *Layer of pigment epithelium.* It is a single layer of hexagonal cells containing melanin pigments.

2. *Layer of rods and cones.* Rods and cones are end organs of vision and are also known as photoreceptors.

3. *External limiting membrane.* It is a thin fenestrated membrane.

4. *Outer nuclear layer.* It consists of nuclei of the rods and cones.

5. *Outer plexiform layer.* It consists of connections of axons of rods and cones with the dendrites of the bipolar cells.

6. *Inner nuclear layer.* It consists of nuclei of bipolar cells, which constitute first order neurons of vision.

7. *Inner plexiform layer.* It consists of synapses of the axons of the bipolar cells with the dendrites of the ganglion cells.

8. *Ganglion cell layer.* It consists of ganglion cells.

9. *Nerve fiber layer.* It consists of axons of the ganglion cells which pass through lamina cribrosa to form the optic nerve.

10. *Internal limiting membrane.* It separates the retina from the vitreous.

CLINICAL ASPECTS

Retinal detachment occurs between outer single pigmented layer and inner nine nervous layers. Actually, it is an inter-retinal detachment.

Visual Pathway

Each eyeball acts as a camera; it perceives the images and relays the sensations to the brain (occipital cortex) via visual pathway which comprises optic nerve, optic chiasma, optic tract, geniculate body and optic radiations (Fig. 6.2-9).

Optic nerve. Each optic nerve (second cranial nerve) starts from the optic disc and extends up to the optic chiasma. It is the continuation backward of the nerve fiber layer of retina, which consists of the axons of the ganglion cells. The optic nerve is about 47–50 mm in length.

Optic chiasma. It is a flattened structure lying above the pituitary fossa. Fibers originating from the nasal halves of the retina decussate at the chiasma.

Optic tracts. These are cylindrical bundles of nerve fibers which originate from the posterolateral angle of the chiasma

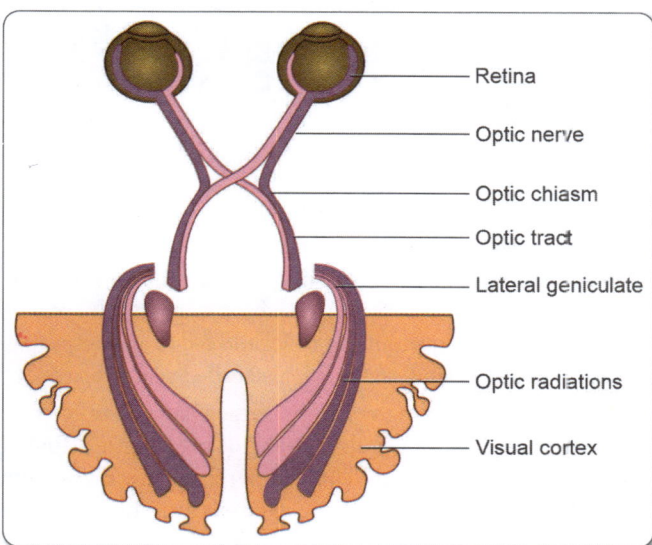

Fig. 6.2-9: Components of visual pathway

and outward and backward to end in the lateral geniculate bodies. They consist of the temporal fibers of the same side and the nasal fibers of the opposite side.

Lateral geniculate bodies. These are oval structures situated at the posterior termination of the optic tracts. The fibers of the optic tracts end in the lateral geniculate bodies and nerve fibers of the optic radiations originate from them.

Optic radiations. These extend from the lateral geniculate bodies to the visual cortex.

Visual cortex. It is located on the medial aspect of the occipital lobe, above and below the calcarine fissure. It is subdivided into the visuosensory area (striate area 17) that receives the fibers of the radiations, and the surrounding visuopsychic area (peristriate area 18 and parastriate area 19).

PHYSIOLOGY OF EYE AND VISION

Function of the eyes is to provide sense of sight (vision), which is the choicest gift from the Almighty to humans and other animals. The eyeballs are able to perform their function with the help of the following physiological activities.

- Maintenance of clear media of the eye
- Maintenance of normal intraocular pressure
- Neurophysiology of vision
- Mechanism of sight
- Physiology of binocular vision.

Maintenance of Clear Media of the Eye

The main factor responsible for transparency of the refractive media of the eye is their avascularity. The structures forming refractive media of the eye from anterior to posterior are as follows:

Tear film. It keeps the cornea moist and provides oxygen and nutrients.

Cornea. It forms the main refracting medium of the eye.

Aqueous humor. It is a clear watery fluid filling the anterior chamber and posterior chamber of the eye.

Crystalline lens. It is a biconvex lens which has been provided with a unique mechanism of changing its power (*accommodation*). Due to this characteristic, it helps in sharp focussing of the images of the objects present at varying distances from the eye.

Vitreous humor. It is clear jelly-like material which in addition to being a refractive medium also helps in maintaining the shape of the eyeball.

Maintenance of Normal Intraocular Pressure

Aqueous Humor

The aqueous humor is a clear watery fluid filling the anterior chamber (0.25 mL) and posterior chamber (0.06 mL) of the eyeball. In addition to its role in maintaining a proper intraocular pressure, it also plays an important metabolic role by providing substrates and removing metabolites from the avascular cornea and the lens.

Aqueous humor is derived from plasma within the capillary network of ciliary processes. It flows from the posterior chamber into the anterior chamber through the pupil. From the anterior chamber the aqueous is drained out by two routes:

1. Trabecular (conventional outflow)
2. Uveoscleral (unconventional outflow).

Maintenance of Intraocular Pressure

The intraocular pressure (IOP) refers to the pressure exerted by intraocular fluids on the coats of the eyeball. The normal IOP varies between 10 mm Hg and 21 mm Hg (mean 16 ± 2.5 mm Hg). The normal level of IOP is essentially maintained by a dynamic equilibrium between the formation and outflow of the aqueous humor.

CLINICAL ASPECTS

Glaucoma is a disease process in which IOP is raised above the tolerance limit of the affected eye, resulting in damage to the optic nerve head and irreversible visual field defects.

Over production of aqueous humor or lack of its drainage or combination of both raise the intraocular pressure. The condition is called glaucoma. It must be treated urgently.

NEUROPHYSIOLOGY OF VISION

Neurophysiology of vision is a complex phenomenon which is still poorly understood. The main mechanisms concerned with vision are as follows:

Initiation and Transmission of Visual Sensation

Light falling upon the retina initiates photochemical changes in the visual pigments of rod and cone cells. The photochemical reaction initiates the visual sensation in the form of changes in electrical potential, which are transmitted through the bipolar cells to the ganglion cells and along the fibers of the optic nerve to the brain.

Photoreceptors (Fig. 6.2-10)

- Rods and cones (*photoreceptors*) are the end organs of vision which transform light energy into visual (nerve) impluse.

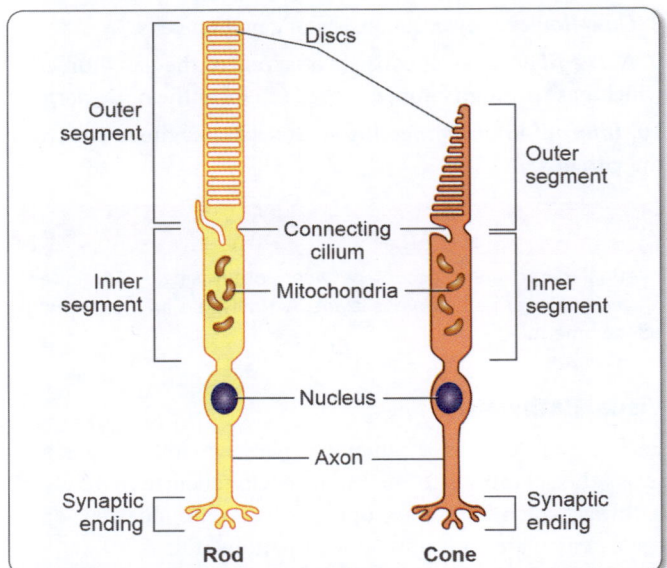

Fig. 6.2-10: Structure of rods and cones

- Rods contain a photosensitive substance, visual purple (*rhodopsin*), and subserve the peripheral vision and vision of low illumination (scotopic vision).
- Cones also contain a photosensitive substance and are primarily responsible for highly discriminatory central vision (photopic vision) and color vision.
- There are about 120 million rods and 6.5 million cones.

Structure of photoreceptor. Each photoreceptor consists of a cell body and nucleus (which lie in the outer nuclear layer) (Fig. 6.2-10).

Visual Pigments

Rhodopsin (visual purple). Rhodopsin is the photosensitive visual pigment present in the discs of the rod's outer segments. It consists of a protein opsin (called scotopsin) and a carotenoid called retinal (the aldehyde of vitamin A).

The absorption spectrum of rhodopsin lies within the narrow limits of 493–505 nm. It absorbs primarily yellow wavelength of light, transmitting violet and red to appear purple by transmitted light; it is, therefore, also called visual purple.

Cone pigments. Cone pigments are somewhat different from the rhodopsin, they respond to specific wavelength of light, giving rise to color vision. These differences are present in the opsin portion of the molecule, whereas the chromophore 11-cis-retinal remains the same.

Light-induced Changes

Light falling upon the retina is absorbed by the visual pigments and initiates *photochemical changes* which in turn trigger a sequence of events that cause phototransduction.

Visual Perception

It is a complex integration of light sense, form sense, sense of contrast, and color sense.

Light Sense

It is awareness of the light. The minimum brightness required to evoke a sensation of light is called the *light minimum*. It should be measured when the eye is dark adapted for at least 20–30 minutes.

The human eye in its ordinary use throughout the day is capable of functioning normally over an exceedingly wide range of illumination by a highly complex phenomenon termed the *visual adaptation*. The process of visual adaptation primarily involves:

- *Dark adaptation* (adjustment in dim illumination)
- *Light adaptation* (adjustment to bright illumination).

Dark Adaptation

It is the ability of the eye to adapt itself to decreasing illumination. When one goes from bright sunshine into a dimly-lit room, one cannot perceive the objects in the room until some time has elapsed. During this period, eye is adapting to low illumination. The time taken to see in dim illumination is called *dark adaptation time*. The rods are much more sensitive to low illumination than cones. Therefore, rods are used more in dim light (*scotopic vision*) and cones in bright light (*photopic vision*).

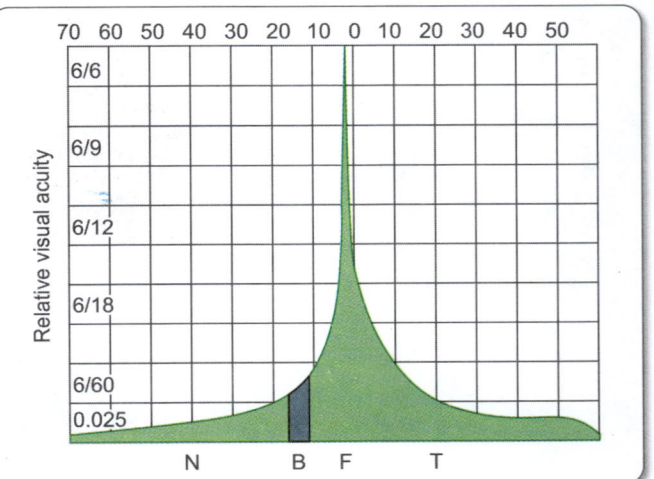

Fig. 6.2-12: Visual acuity (form sense) in relation to regions of retina: N (Nasal retina); B, Blind spot; F, Fovea region and T, Temporal retina

Light Adaptation

When one passes suddenly from dim to brightly lighted environment, the light seems intense and uncomfortably bright until eyes adapt to increased illumination. Unlike dark adaptation the process of light adaptation is very quick and occurs over a period of 5 minutes.

Form Sense

It is the ability to discriminate between the shapes of the objects. Cones play a major role in this faculty. Therefore, form sense is most acute at the fovea, where there are maximum number of cones, and decreases very rapidly toward the periphery (Fig. 6.2-12). Visual acuity recorded by Snellen's Test Chart is a measure of the form sense.

Color Sense

Color sense is the ability of the eye to discriminate between colors excited by light of different wavelengths. Some broad facts about color vision are:

- Color vision is a function of cones and thus better appreciated in photopic vision.
- There are three different types of cones, viz. red sensitive, green sensitive and blue sensitive, which combinedly perform the function of color vision.
- All colors are a result of admixture in different proportion of three primary colors: the red (723–647 nm), green (575–492 nm), and blue (492–450 nm) (Young-Helmholtz theory).

Contrast Sensitivity

Contrast sensitivity is the ability to perceive slight changes in luminance between regions, which are not separated

---

IMPORTANT TO KNOW

Dark adaptation curve plotted with illumination of test object in vertical axis and duration of dark adaptation along the horizontal axis shows that visual threshold falls progressively in the darkened room for about half an hour until a relative constant value is reached (Fig. 6.2-11).

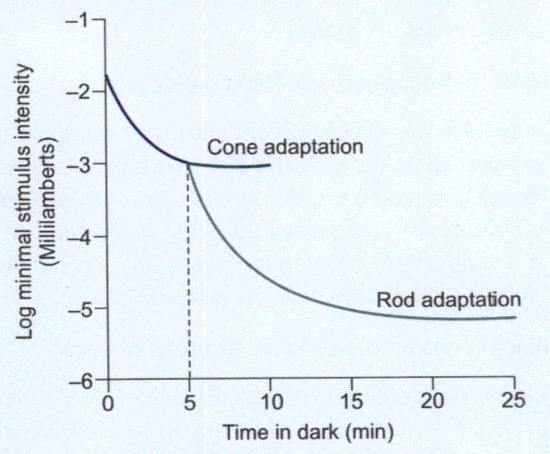

Fig. 6.2-11: Dark adaptation curve

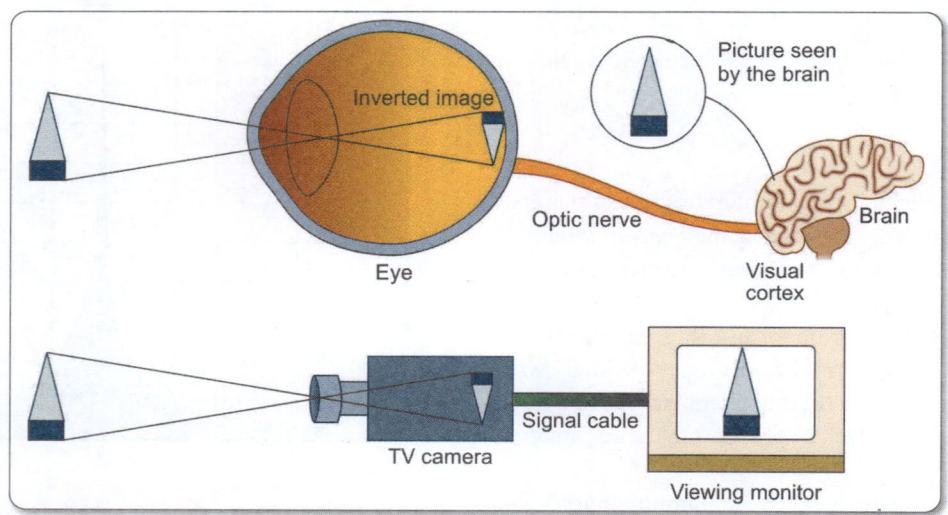

Fig. 6.2-13: Sense of sight in many ways similar to close circuit color TV system

by definite borders and is just as important as the ability to perceive sharp outlines of relatively small objects.

Mechanism of Sight

The functioining of the eye as an optical instrument can be compared with a camera (Fig. 6.2-13) as follows:

- *Eyelids* act as shutter of the camera.
- *Cornea and crystalline lens* act as focussing system of the camera.
- *Iris* acts as diaphragm, which regulates the size of the aperture (*pupil*) and therefore the amount of light entering the eye.
- *Choroid* helps in forming the darkened interior of the camera.
- *Retina* acts as light-sensitive plate or film on which image is formed.

The optic nerve and its connections convey the details of the image to the occipital region of the cerebral cortex where they are processed before reaching consciousness.

Optics of Eye: Image Formation

The optics of eye is very complex. However, for understanding, it has been simplified. The focussing structures of eye (cornea and crystalline lens) form a convex lens of +60 D which focus

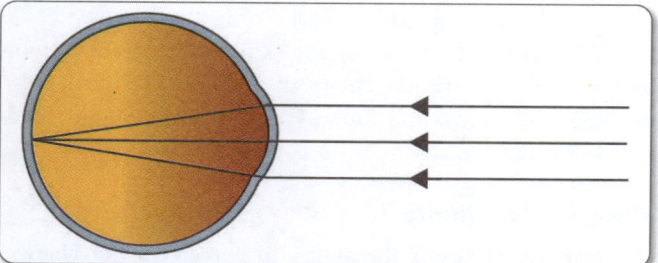

Fig. 6.2-14: Refraction in an emmetropic eye

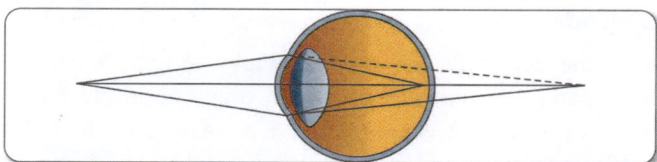

Fig. 6.2-15: Effect of accommodation on divergent rays entering the eye

the light rays on the sensitive layer of retina (Fig. 6.2-14). Optically normal eye is called *emmetropic accommodation*.

Accommodation

Our eyes have been provided with a unique mechanism by which we can even focus the diverging rays coming from a near object on the retina in a bid to see clearly (Fig. 6.2-15). This mechanism is called accommodation. In it, there occurs:

- Increase in the power of the crystalline lens
- Constriction of pupil
- Convergence of eyeballs.

Changes in the curvature of lens surface

The principal change in the lens during accommodation is seen in the anterior surface of the lens as compared to posterior surface. As the refractive index of lens (1.39) is more than the refractive index of aqueous and vitreous, increase in convexity of the lens increases its dioptric power and thus allows the near objects to be focussed clearly on the retina.

Pupillary constriction and convergence of eyes

In addition to the changes in the lens and zonular system the pupil constricts and the eyes converge, almost simultaneously. These changes occur in a bid to achieve clear vision for near objects.

CLINICAL ASPECTS

COMMON DEFECTS OF THE IMAGE-FORMING MECHANISM

Emmetropia

Emmetropia (optically normal eye) can be defined as a state of refraction, when the parallel rays of light coming from infinity are focused at the sensitive layer of retina with the accommodation being at rest (Fig. 6.2-14).

Ametropia

Ametropia (a condition of refractive error) is defined as a state of refraction, when the parallel rays of light coming from infinity (with accommodation at rest) are focussed either in front or behind the sensitive layer of retina, in one or both the meridia. The ametropia includes myopia, hypermetropia and astigmatism.

Hypermetropia

Hypermetropia (hyperopia) or long-sightedness is the refractive state of the eye wherein parallel rays of light coming from infinity are focussed behind the retina with accommodation being at rest (Fig. 6.2-16).

Optical correction: Basic principle of treatment of hypermetropia is optical correction with convex (plus) lenses, so that the light rays are brought to focus on the retina (Fig. 6.2-17).

Myopia

Myopia or short-sightedness is a type of refractive error in which parallel rays of light coming from infinity are focussed in front of the retina when accommodation is at rest (Fig. 6.2-18).

Optical Correction: Basic principles of treatment of myopia is optical correction with concave (minus) lenses, so that clear image is formed on the retina (Fig. 6.2-19).

Astigmatism

Astigmatism is a type of refractive error wherein the refraction varies in the different meridian. Consequently, the rays of light entering the eye cannot converge to a point focus but form focal lines.

Presbyopia

Presbyopia (eyesight of old age) is not an error of refraction but condition of physiological insufficiency of accommodation, leading to failing vision for near.

- Since, we usually keep the book at about 25 cm, so we can read comfortably up to the age of 40 years. After the age of 40 years, the near point of accommodation recedes beyond the normal reading or working range. This condition of failing near vision is due to age-related decrease in the amplitude of accommodation.
- *Treatment* of presbyopia is the prescription of appropriate convex glasses for near work.

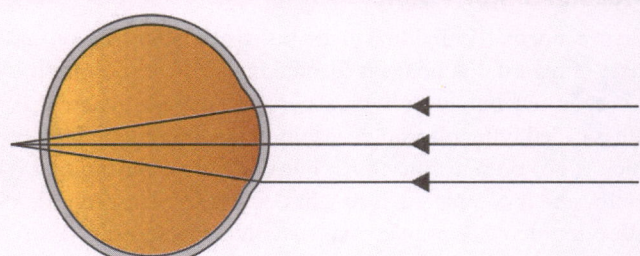

Fig. 6.2-16: Refraction in hypermetropic eye

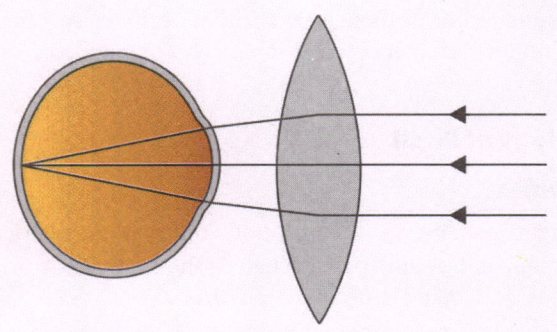

Fig. 6.2-17: Refraction in hypermetropic eye corrected with convex lens

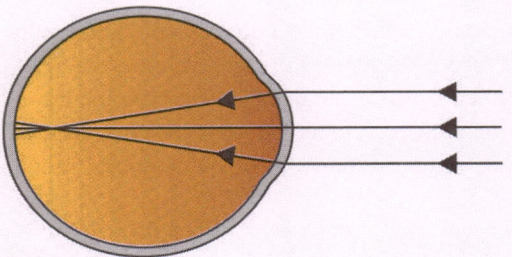

Fig. 6.2-18: Refraction in myopic eye

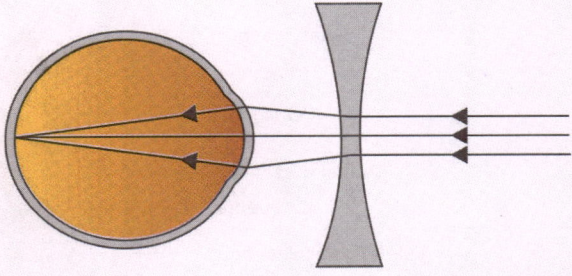

Fig. 6.2-19: Refraction in myopic eye corrected with concave lens

Binocular Single Vision and Field of Vision

Binocular Single Vision

When a normal individual fixes his visual attention on an object of regard, the image is formed on the fovea of both the eyes separately, but the individual perceives a single image. This state is called binocular single vision. It is a conditioned reflex which is not present since birth but is acquired during first 6 months and is completed during first few years. The process of its development is complex and partially understood.

Field of Vision

The visual field is a three-dimensional area that can be seen around an object of fixation. The extent of normal visual field with a 5 mm white color object is superiorly 60°, inferiorly 70°, nasally 60° and temporally 90° (Fig. 6.2-20).

Physiology of Pupil

Light Reflex

When light is shone in one eye, both the pupils constrict. Constriction of the pupil to which light is shone is called *direct light reflex* and that of the other pupil is called *consensual (indirect) light reflex*. Light reflex is initiated by rods and cones.

Pathway of light reflex (Fig. 6.2-21)

Afferent fibers extend from retina to the pretectal nucleus in the midbrain. These travel along the optic nerve to the optic chiasma where fibers from the nasal retina decussate and travel along the opposite optic tract to terminate in the contralateral pretectal nucleus, while the fibers from the temporal retina remain uncrossed and travel along the optic tract of the same side to terminate in the ipsilateral pretectal nucleus.

Internuncial fibers connect each pretectal nucleus with Edinger-Westphal nuclei of both sides. This connection forms the basis of consensual light reflex.

Efferent pathway consists of the parasympathetic fibers which arise from the Edinger-Westphal nucleus in the midbrain and travel along the third (oculomotor) cranial nerve. The preganglionic fibers enter the inferior division of the third nerve and via the nerve to the inferior oblique reach the ciliary ganglion to relay. Postganglionic fibers travel along the short ciliary nerves to innervate the sphincter pupillae.

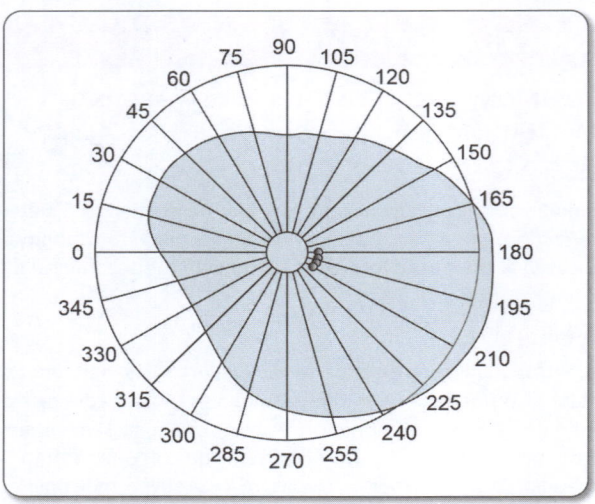

Fig. 6.2-20: Extent of normal visual field

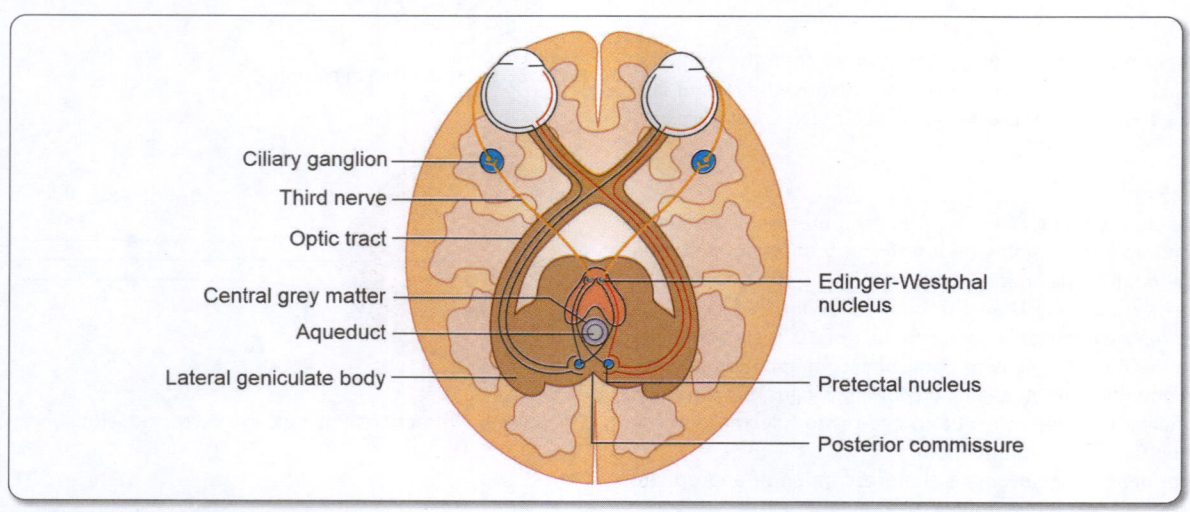

Fig. 6.2-21: Pathway of light reflex

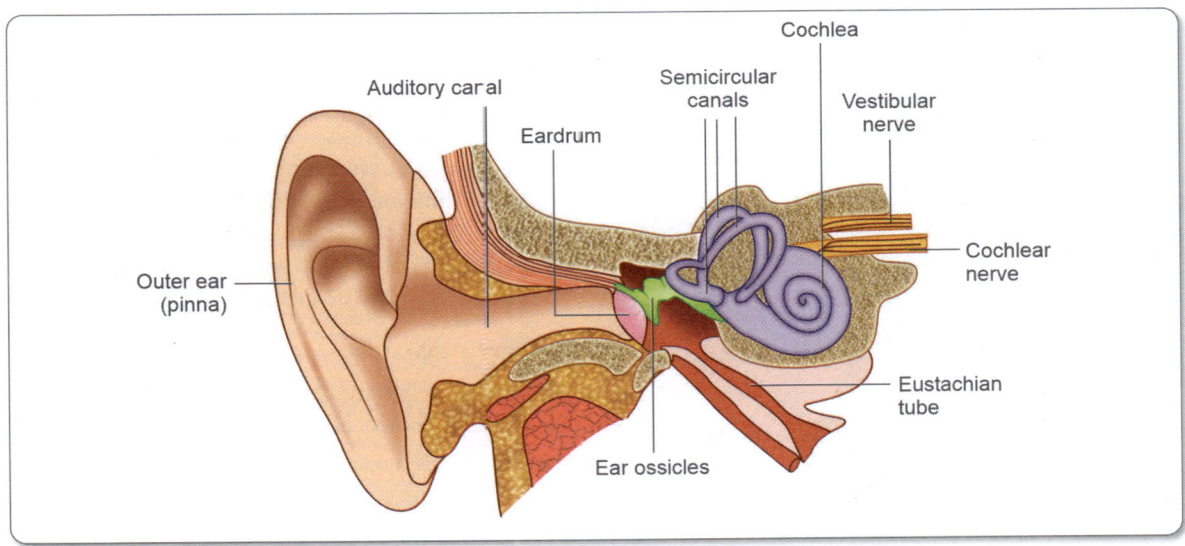

Fig. 6.2-22: Structure of three subdivisions of the ear

SENSE OF HEARING

EAR

Functional Anatomy

The mechanism of hearing is closely associated with the mechanism of equilibrium, therefore, the inner ear acts as an organ of hearing and equilibrium. For hearing, the sound waves have to pass through the three subdivisions of the ear, which are (Fig. 6.2-22):

1. External ear
2. Middle ear
3. Internal ear

External Ear

The external ear consists of the pinna (auricle) and the external auditory meatus.

Pinna or auricle consists of a single convoluted plate of elastic cartilage covered by skin. In humans, the pinna is not moveable.

Functions: The pinna collects and reflects the sound waves into the external auditory canal.

External auditory meatus extends from the pinna to the tympanic membrane. It is lined with skin, which secretes wax (from the ceruminous glands) and oil (from the sebacious glands).

CLINICAL ASPECTS

- Accumulation of wax in the external acoustic meatus is often a source of excessive itching.
- Impaction of large foreign bodies like seeds, grains and insects is common syringing is done to remove these.

Middle Ear

The middle ear or the tympanic cavity is an air-filled rectangular space in the petrous part of temporal bone. It consists of following structures.

Tympanic membrane. It is a cave-shaped structure with concavity directed toward the external auditory meatus. Point of maximum convexity is called umbo. It consists of connective tissue covered with skin on the outside and mucous membrane on the inside (Fig. 6.2-23).

Eustachian tube. The pharyngotympanic tube connects the middle ear cavity with pharynx. Air can pass through this tube into the middle ear. Therefore, it serves the function of equalization of pressure on two sides of tympanic membrane.

Ear ossicles. The three ear ossicles (auditory ossicles) include malleus, incus and stapes. They are attached to each other by ligaments and form a chain (Fig. 6.2-24).

Malleus. It resembles hammer and consists of a head, neck and three processes. *Manubrium* (handle) of the malleus is

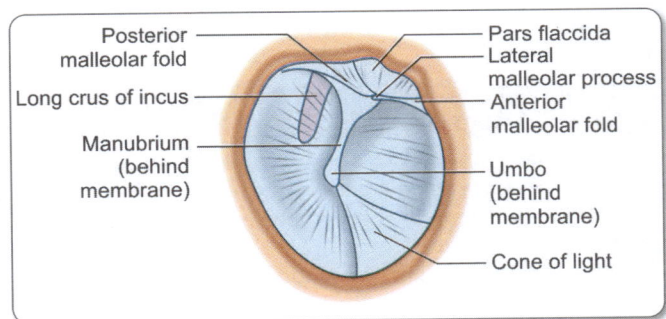

Fig. 6.2-23: Tympanic membrane

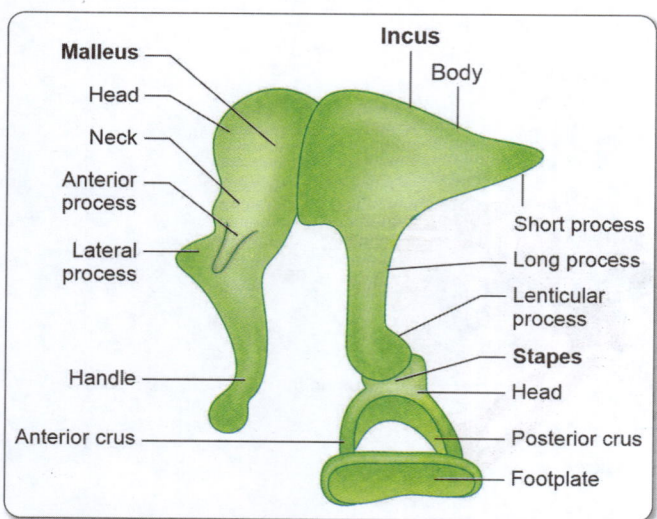

Fig. 6.2-24: Ear ossicles and their parts

connected to inner surface of the tympanic membrane, and *head* articulates with incus posteriorly.

Incus. It is the middle ossicle that resembles an anvil in shape. It consists of a body and two processes. The body of incus articulates with the head of malleus.

Stapes. It resembles a stirrup. Its head articulates with the incus, and the oval footplate contacts the membrane of the oval window of the cochlea.

Windows. Medial wall (labyrinthine wall) of the middle ear contains two windows:

1. *Oval window* (fenestra vestibuli) is present above, in which footplate (face plate or stapes) is attached. It leads to the vestibule of the internal ear and transmits the sound vibrations of the ossicles to the perilymph of scala vestibuli.

2. *Round window* (fenestra cochlea) is present in the lower part, and is closed by a thin membrane called *secondary tympanic membrane*. It accommodates the pressure waves transmitted to the perilymph of the scala tympani.

Muscles. The middle ear contains two muscles: the tensor tympani and stapedius. Both muscles of the middle ear act simultaneously and reflexly in response to loud sound and attenuate the sound.

CLINICAL ASPECTS

- Inflammation of the auditory tube (eustachian catarrh) is often secondary to an attack of common cold. This causes pain in the ear which is aggravated by swallowing, due to blockage of the tube.
- *Otosclerosis*: Sometimes bony fusion takes place between the foot plate of the stapes and the margins of the fenestra vestibuli. This leads to deafness.

Internal Ear

The internal ear or labyrinth is situated in the petrous part of the temporal bone. It consists of bony labyrinth and membranous labyrinth (Figs 6.2-25A to C). *Bony labyrinth* consists of three parts: vestibule, semicircular canals and the cochlea. *Membranous labyrinth* is lodged within the bony labyrinth. The inner ear can be divided into two main parts—vestibular apparatus, and auditory receptor apparatus. The vestibular apparatus is concerned with equilibrium.

Auditory apparatus

The auditory apparatus is formed by the *duct of cochlea* which lies within the bony cochlea.

Bony cochlea is a spiral tube which in humans has a two and three-fourths turns around a central bone called the *modiolus*. Around the modiolus and winding spirally like the thread of a screw, is a thin plate of bone called *osseous spiral lamina*. It divides the bony cochlea incompletely, and gives attachment to the basilar membrane. Two membranes (basilar membrane and Reissner's membrane) divide the bony cochlea into three compartments (Fig. 6.2-26):

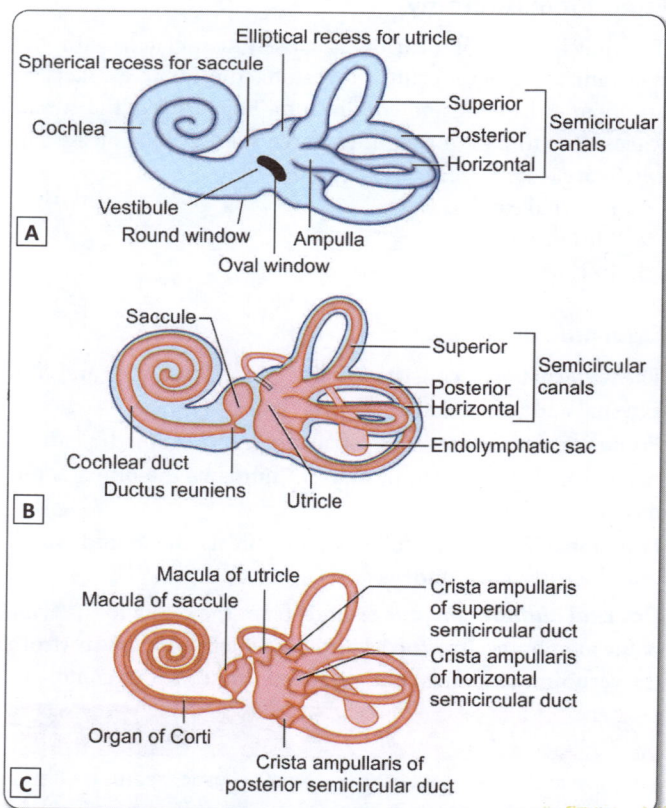

Figs 6.2-25A to C: Structure of inner ear: A. Left bony labyrinth; B. Cut section of bony labyrinth; C. Left membranous labyrinth

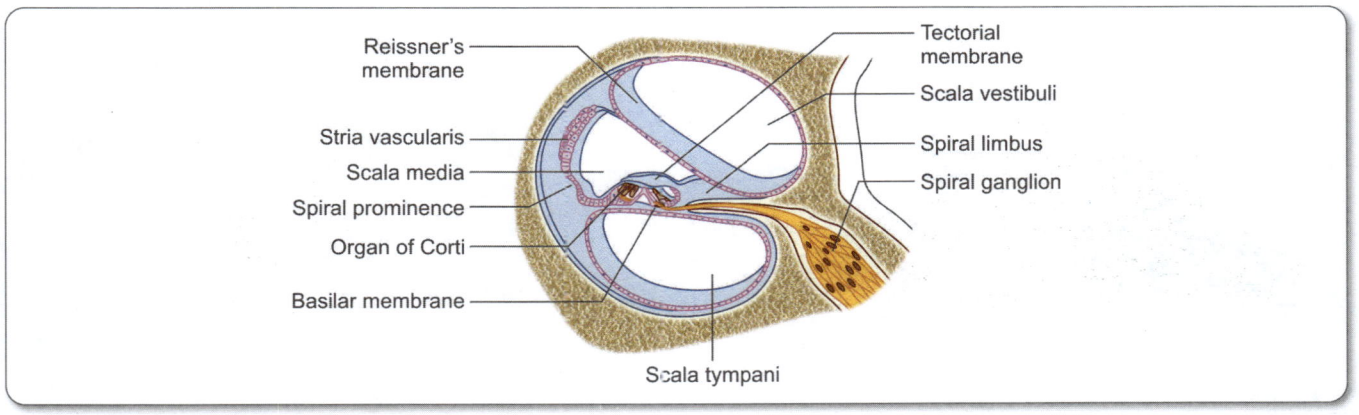

Fig. 6.2-26: Vertical section through cochlea showing scala vestibuli, scala media (cochlear duct) and scala tympani. Note the location of organ of Corti over the basilar membrane in the cavity of cochlear duct

- Scala vestibuli
- Scala media (membranous chochlear duct)
- Scala tympani.

Scala vestibuli is separated from the scala media by *Reissner's membrane* and is closed by the footplate of stapes which separates it from the air-filled middle ear (Figs 6.2-26 and 6.2-27).

Scala tympani is separated from the scala media by the *basilar membrane* and is closed by *secondary tympanic membrane*. It is also connected with subarachnoid space through the aqueduct of cochlea (Figs 6.2-26 and 6.2-27).

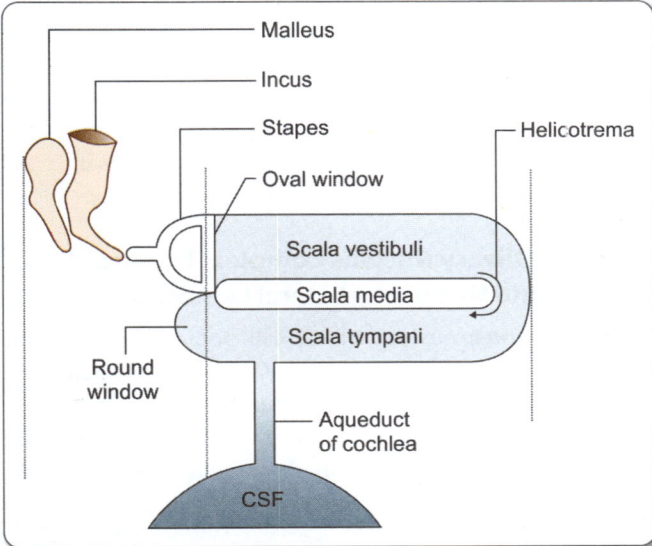

Fig. 6.2-27: Diagrammatic depiction of arrangement of perilymphatic system, three compartments of cochlea (scala vestibuli, scala media, and scala tympani), and ear ossicles of the middle ear. Note the CSF passes into scala tympani through aqueduct of cochlea

Scala vestibuli and scala tympani are filled with perilymph and communicate with each other at the apex of cochlea through an opening called *helicotrema*.

Scala media or *cochlear duct* or *membranous cochlea* appear triangular on cross-section. Its three walls are formed by (Fig. 6.2-26):
- Basilar membrane
- Reissner's membrane
- Stria vascularis.

Perilymph and endolymph

Perilymph is the fluid present in the scala tympani and scala vestibuli compartments of the cochlea. Its composition is similar to extracellular fluid (ECF) in that it is high in Na^+ and low in K^+.

Endolymph is the fluid present within the scala media or the membranous cochlea. Its composition is similar to intracellular fluid (ICF) in that it is high in K^+ and low in Na^+. It is secreted by the stria vascularis which forms the lateral wall of scala media.

Organ of corti

The organ of Corti, the sense organ of hearing, is situated on the top of the basilar membrane in the scala media (Fig. 6.2-28). It contains the auditory receptors or the peripheral receptors of sense of hearing. Important components of the organ of Corti are:

Rods of Corti. These are two projections (inner and outer rods) from the basilar membrane into the scala media. In between the two rods is the *tunnel of Corti* which contains a fluid called *cortilymph*. The exact function of the rods and cortilymph is not known.

Hair cells. Hair cells are receptor cells that transduce sound energy into electrical energy. Two groups of hair cells lie on

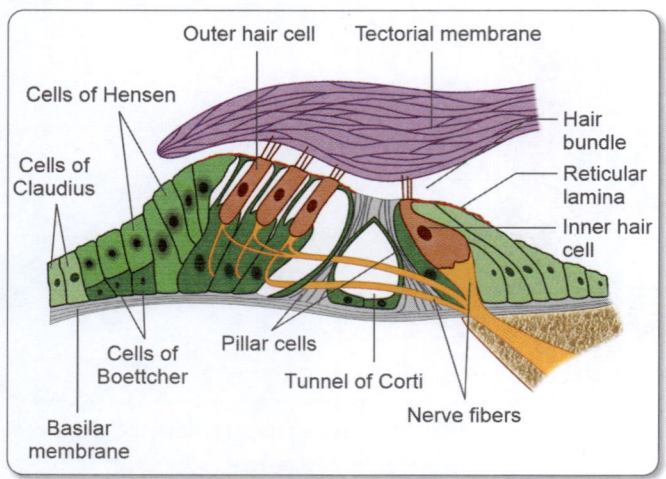

Fig. 6.2-28: Structure of organ of Corti. Note the connections between tectorial membrane and cilia of hair cells

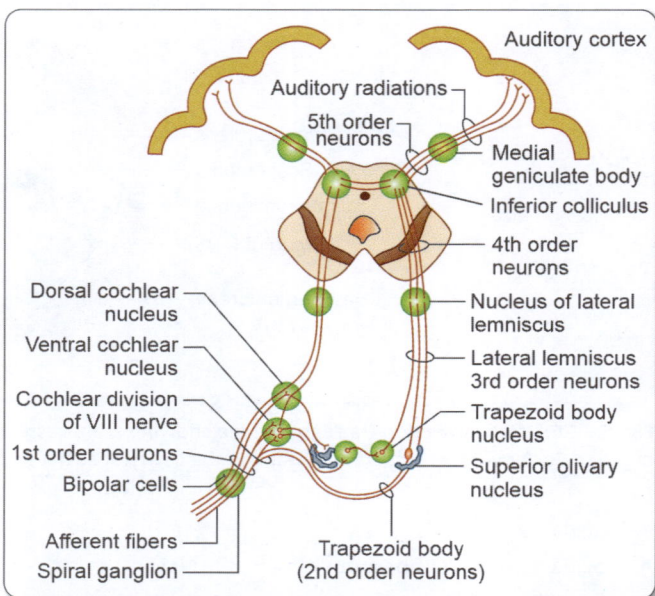

Fig. 6.2-29: Central auditory pathways

the basilar membrane—inner hair cells and outer hair cells these are responsible for *detecting the presence of sound*.

Supporting cells (Fig. 6.2-28): These support the hair cells.

Tectorial membrane. It consists of gelatinous matrix with delicate fibers. This membrane is attached to the upper surface of spiral lamina, and its free edge extends just beyond the outermost neuroepithelial cells.

- The shearing force between the hair cells and tectorial membrane produces the stimulus to hair cells.

Nerve supply of hair cells

Afferent fibers supplying the hair cells constitute the cochlear division of VIII cranial nerve. Cell bodies of these fibers are located in the spiral ganglion.

Efferent fibers to the hair cells come from both the ipsilateral and contralateral sides.

CLINICAL ASPECTS

Acoustic neuroma is a tumor of Schwann cells of VIII nerve. If neuroma extends into internal auditory meatus, VII nerve will get pressed. There will be VIII nerve paralysis and VII nerve paralysis as well.

AUDITORY PATHWAYS

Auditory pathways comprise following relay stations (Fig. 6.2-29):

Spiral Ganglion

First order neurons are the bipolar cells of the *spiral ganglion*.

Dendrites of these bipolar cells constitute the afferent fibers innervating the hair cells.

Axons of these bipolar cells form the cochlear division of VIII cranial nerve. The cochlear nerve ends in the cochlear nuclei in medulla.

Cochlear Nuclei

Second order neurons have their cell bodies in the cochlear nuclei which are situated in the medulla. There are two cochlear nuclei: dorsal and ventral. The axons of second order neurons from cochlear nuclei pass medially in the dorsal part of pons.

- The crossing fibers of two sides form a conspicuous mass of fibers called the *trapezoid body*.
- Some crossing fibers run separately in the dorsal part of pons and do not form part of the trapezoid body.

Superior Olivary Nucleus Complex, Trapezoid Nucleus and Nucleus of Lateral Lemniscus

Third order neurons have their cell bodies mainly in the *superior olivary complex* (made up of a number of nuclei) and also in trapezoid nucleus, and nucleus of lateral lemniscus.

The fibers from these collections ascend through *lateral lemniscus* and ascend to the midbrain and terminate in the inferior colliculus.

Inferior Colliculus

Fourth order neurons have their cell bodies in *inferior colliculus* where the fibers of lateral lemniscus terminate. Fibers arising in the inferior colliculus enter the inferior brachium to reach the medial geniculate body.

Medial Geniculate Body

Fifth order neurons have their cell bodies in the medial geniculate body where most of the fibers arising in inferior colliculus terminate. Fibers arising in the medial geniculate body form the *acoustic radiation*, which ends in the acoustic area of the cerebral cortex.

Auditory Cortex

Major areas constituting auditory cortex present in the temporal lobe are:
- Primary auditory cortex (areas 41 and 42)
- Auditory association areas (areas 22, 21 and 20).

PHYSIOLOGY OF HEARING

Hearing, i.e., detection of sound waves, may serve to warn of impending danger or localize friends. But most importantly, audition allows social communication. Physiology of audition can be discussed under the following headings:
- Stimuli or sound waves
- Conduction of sound waves
- Transduction of sound waves
- Neural transmission of signals
- Encoding of signals.

Stimuli or Sound Waves

Stimuli for the receptors of hearing are sound waves. Sound is a form of energy produced by a vibrating object. A sound wave consists of alternating phases of compression and rarefaction of molecules of the medium (air, liquid, or solid) in which it travels.

Physical Properties of Sound

Physical properties of sound and certain terms which are frequently used in audiology and acoustics are (Figs 6.2-30A to E).

Speed or velocity of sound waves is different in different media. *In the air*, at 0° C, at sea level, sound travels at a rate of approximately 330 m/sec (1100 ft/sec).

Frequency of sound refers to number of waves per second.
- The *unit* of frequency is hertz (Hz).
- Range of human hearing is approximately 20–20,000 Hz.
- Range of average speaking voice is approximately 2000–5000 Hz.

Amplitude (intensity) of sound is the strength which determines its loudness. The intensity of sound is measured in terms of maximum pressure change at the tympanic membrane which is more commonly expressed as *sound pressure level* (SPL). The unit of SPL is decibel (dB).

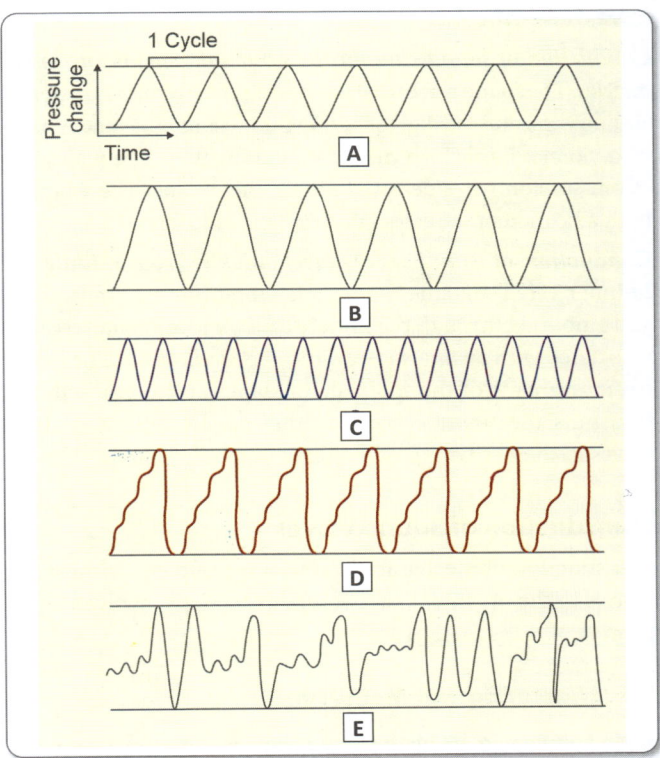

Figs 6.2-30A to E: Characteristics of sound wave: A. Pure tones; B. Increase in amplitude (intensity) of sound wave thus the sound is louder; C. Increase in frequency (pitch); D. Complex waveform due to mixture of pure tones and overtones; determines the quality of sound (timber); and E. aperiodic irregular waveform (noise)

Pure tone refers to A single frequency sound, e.g., a sound of 25–50 or 100 Hz

Complex sound refers to that with more than one frequency. For example, human voice is a complex sound.

Pitch is the subjective sensation produced by frequency of sound. Higher the frequency greater is the pitch.

Overtones. A complex sound is a mixture of pure tones. The lowest frequency at which a source vibrates is called *fundamental (or primary) frequency.* All other frequencies which are multiples of the fundamental frequency are called *overtones* or *harmonics*.

Conduction of Sound Waves

Role of External Ear

External ear captures the sound waves.

Pinna collects and reflects the sound waves into the external auditory meatus.

External auditory meatus conducts the sound waves to tympanic membrane. Its S-shaped course helps in amplifying the sound waves.

Role of Middle Ear

Conduction of sound stimulus by tympanic membrane to ear ossicles. The sound waves that pass through the pinna and external auditory meatus strike the tympanic membrane and enable it to vibrate. Eustachian tube does the function of equalization of pressure on two sides of tympanic membrane. The vibrating tympanic membrane causes the ear ossicles to vibrate.

Conduction of sound waves mechanically from middle ear to inner ear. Tympanic membrane vibrations are transmitted and amplified through the middle ear by movement of ossicles associated with an *impedance matching mechanism*. The to and fro movements of the footplate of stapes at the oval window transmits the sound waves to inner ear by setting up fluid waves in the perilymph of the scala vestibuli (Fig. 6.2-31).

Transduction of Sound Waves

Transduction of mechanical sound wave into electrical signal occurs in the organ of Corti of inner ear. Steps involved in the process of transduction are:

Vibration of Basilar Membrane

Sound waves entering the inner ear from the oval window spread along the scala vestibuli as a traveling wave. As the sound energy passes from scala vestibuli to scala tympani, it causes the basilar membrane to vibrate.

Stimulation of the Hair Cells

The up-and-down movements of the basilar membrane in turn cause the organ of Corti to vibrate up and down. The bending of stereocilia stimulates (excites) the hair cells.

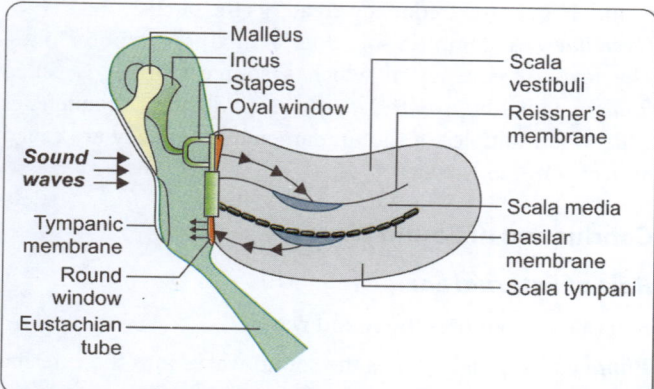

Fig. 6.2-31: Diagrammatic depiction of the mechanism of vibrations of basilar membrane produced by in and out motion of stapes (for details see text)

Membrane Potential Changes in the Hair Cells

The movements of hair cells of organs of Corti cause their depolarization and development of receptor potential leading to generation of action potential in the neuron. In this way sound wave is transduced into electrical signal.

Neural Transmission of Signals

The electrical signals from hair cells are transmitted through a complex auditory pathway to the auditory cortex.

Neural Processing of Auditory Information Encoding of Signals

In the auditory cortex the sound wave in the form of nerve impulse is processed and perceived. Neural processing of auditory information involves:

- Encoding of frequency (pitch determination)
- Encoding of intensity (determination of loudness)
- Feature detection
- Localization of sound in space.

CLINICAL ASPECTS

Noise and Masking

Noise is defined as an aperiodic complex sound. There are three types of noise:
1. **White noise:** In this all frequencies are in audible spectrum. It is used for masking
2. **Narrow-band noise**
3. **Speech noise:** It is a noise having all frequencies in the speech range (300–3000 Hz).

Masking refers to a phenomenon in which the presence of one type of sound decreases the ability of the ear to hear another type of sound.

Hearing Loss, Deafness and Tinnitus

Hearing Loss

Hearing loss refers to impairment of hearing and its severity may vary from mild to profound.
Deafness is labelled when there is little or no hearing at all.
Types of hearing loss. Hearing loss can be of two types:
1. Conductive hearing loss
2. Sensorineural hearing loss.

Tinnitus:

Tinnitus refers to ringing sensation in the ear. It is caused by irritative stimulation of either the inner ear or the vestibulocochlear nerve.

SENSE OF SMELL

The sense of smell or olfaction is well-developed in animals like dog and rabbit to give warning of the environmental dangers.

Such animals are called *macrosomatics*. In humans, apes and monkeys (primates) the sense of smell is comparatively less developed, but still it is important for pleasure and for enjoying the taste of food. Therefore, the humans and primates are called *microsomatics*.

SITE OF OLFACTION NOSE

The olfactory stimuli are detected by specialized receptors located on the free nerve endings of the olfactory nerves which are located in the olfactory mucosa of nose in human beings.

Olfactory Mucosa

In humans, the olfactory mucosa is confined to upper one-third of nasal cavity (Figs 6.2-32A and B).

Histologically, the olfactory mucosa consists of three types of cells—receptor cells, supporting cells and basal cells. Receptor cells are bipolar neurons which lie between the supporting (sustentacular) cells.

Nerve Supply of Olfactory Mucosa

Special sensory nerves innervating the olfactory mucosa are 15–20 bundles of olfactory nerve fibers (1st cranial nerve) which convey sense of smell.

General sensory nerves supplying the olfactory mucosa are branches of trigeminal nerve (V cranial nerve). The irritative character of some odorants results from stimulation of free nerve endings of the trigeminal nerve.

OLFACTORY PATHWAYS

Olfactory pathways comprise:

Olfactory Nerves

About 15–20 olfactory nerve filaments which consist of the axons of the bipolar olfactory neurons which pierce the cribriform plate on either side to reach olfactory bulb.

Olfactory Bulb (Fig. 6.2-33)

It is an oval flattened strip of grey matter lying on the cribriform plate, which receives the olfactory nerve filaments. The olfactory bulb contains three types of cells: mitral cells, tufted cells, and interneurons (granule cells and periglomerular cells). The mitral and tufted cells constitute 2nd order neurons. *Axons of the mitral and tufted cells* leave the olfactory bulb and run in the olfactory tract.

Olfactory Tract

It lies in the olfactory sulcus on the orbital surface of the frontal lobe and proceeds backward from each olfactory bulb to the region of anterior perforated substance on the base of brain where it divides into lateral, intermediate and medial olfactory striae.

Olfactory Cortex

It includes the anterior olfactory nucleus, prepiriform cortex, olfactory tubercle and amygdala. All these are parts of limbic system.

PHYSIOLOGY OF OLFACTION

Odoriferous Stimuli

The odoriferous (smell-producing molecules) stimuli enter the nasal cavity while breathing. The odorant molecules must

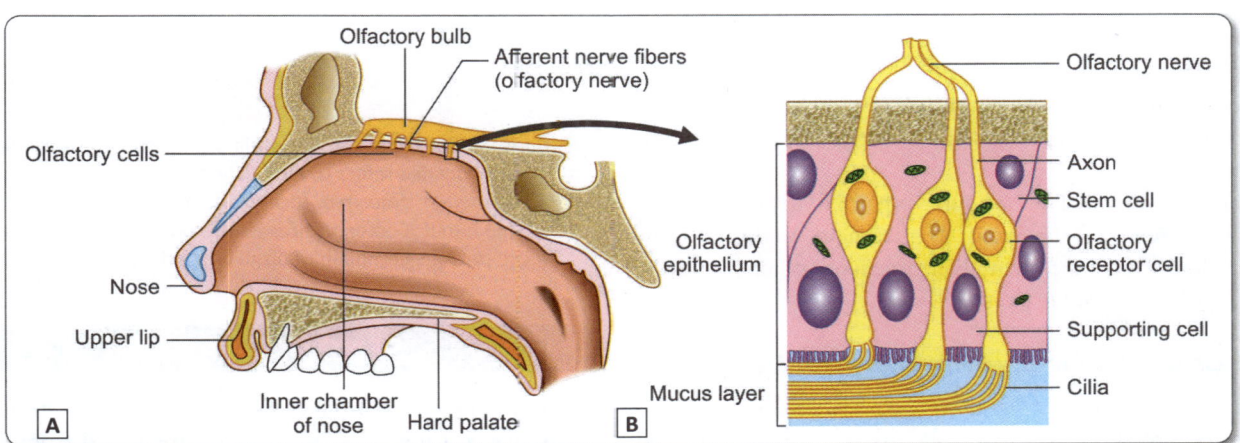

Figs 6.2-32A and B: Location of olfactory mucosa (A) and histological features of olfactory mucosa (B)

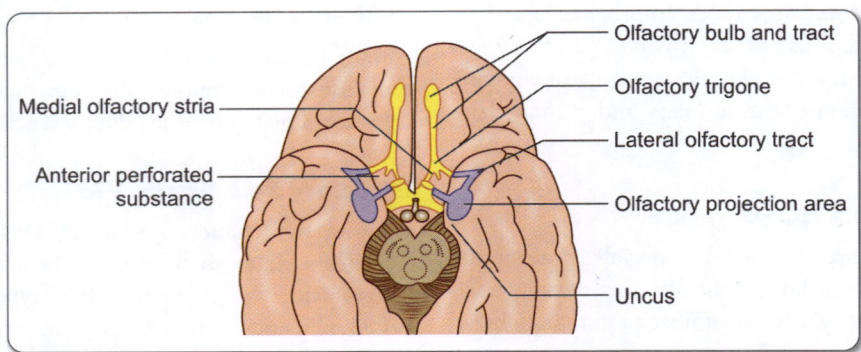

Fig. 6.2-33: Olfactory bulb and olfactory tract

dissolve in the mucous layer (lining the olfactory mucosa) before they can come in contact with olfactory receptors.

Types of Odorant Stimuli

There seems to be over 50 *primary smell sensations*. Although the olfactory capability of humans is somewhat limited compared with that of macrosomatic animals, nevertheless humans are able to perceive more than 10,000 different odorous molecules.

Olfactory Receptors

The cilia of the olfactory neurons are specialized for odor detection. They have specific receptors for odorants.

Steps of Transduction in the Olfactory Receptor Neurons

Binding of odorant molecule to receptors. It has been suggested that the mucous layer covering the olfactory mucosa contains one or more odorant-binding proteins (OBP) that concentrate and transfer the odorant molecules to the receptors present on the cilia of olfactory neurons.

Depolarization receptor potential. The interaction of an odorant with its receptor produces a depolarizing receptor potential.

Action potentials. The receptor potential depolarizes the initial segment of the axon to threshold leading to the generation of action potentials in the sensory axon and the *transmission of signal to olfactory bulb.*

Processing of Olfactory Sensation in the Olfactory Bulb

The odorant information is extensively processed, and perhaps refined in the olfactory bulb before it is sent to the olfactory cortex.

Transmission of Odorant Information to the Olfactory Cortex and Neocortex

- From the olfactory bulb the odorant information is first transmitted to *olfactory cortex*, which includes piriform cortex, parts of amygdala, the olfactory tubercle and parts of entorhinal cortex.
- From the olfactory cortex, information is relayed to the frontal cortex (directly) and orbitofrontal cortex (via thalamus).

Factors influencing Olfactory Function

Threshold of olfactory receptors. The threshold of olfactory receptors varies from substance to substance. For example, methyl mercaptan, a substance which gives garlic its characteristic odor, has extremely low threshold.

Intensity/concentration of the odor. The concentration of an odoriferous substance must be changed by about 30% before a difference can be detected.

Adaptation. Olfactory sensation adapts very rapidly with continued exposure to an odor.

CLINICAL ASPECTS

- *Anosmia and hyposmia:* Anosmia is total loss of sense of smell while hyposmia refers to diminished olfactory sensitivity.
- *Paraosmia or dysosmia:* It refers to distortion or perversion of smell. In it, person interprets the odors incorrectly. Often these persons complain of disgusting odors.

SENSE OF TASTE

Sense of taste (gustation) is a chemical sense that is stimulated by food and drink. Taste must be distinguished from flavor, which includes the olfactory, tactile, and thermal attributes of food in addition to taste.

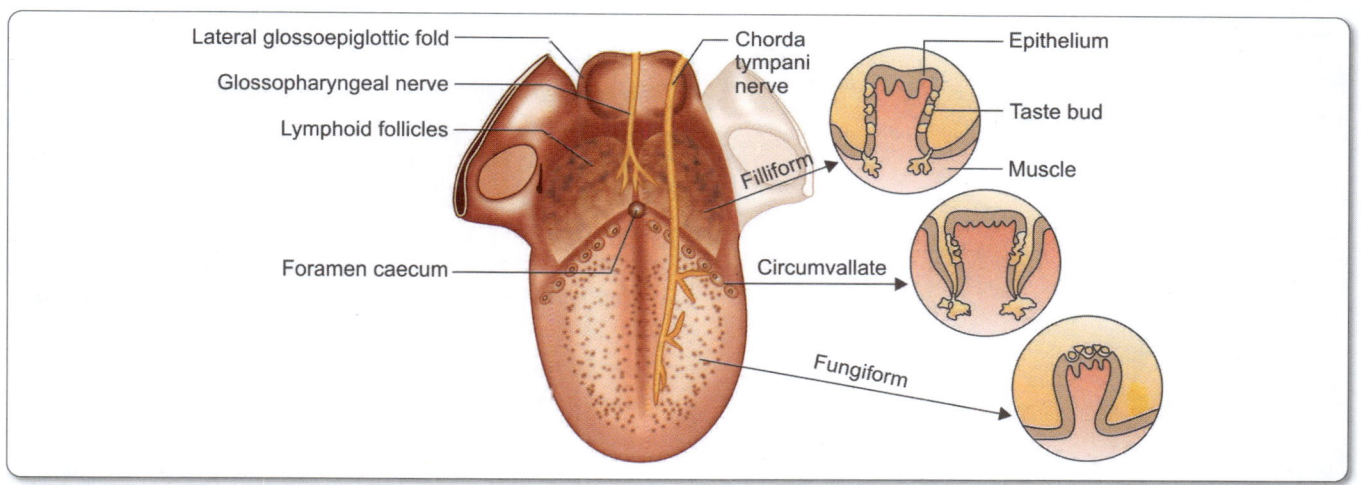

Fig. 6.2-34: Structure and distribution of papillae on the tongue and arrangement of tastebuds in the three types of papillae. Innervation by the cranial nerves is also indicated

SITE OF TASTE

The taste (gustatory) stimuli are detected by specialized chemoreceptors called taste receptors or taste cells. The taste receptors are clustered in the taste buds located on the tongue, palate, pharynx, epiglottis, and upper third of esophagus.

Tongue, the main site of taste detection, contains numerous taste buds on its dorsal surface. The mucous membrane of the dorsal surface of tongue exhibits numerous papillae, which increase the surface area of the mucosa available for taste receptors. The taste buds are located in the walls of these papillae.

Taste Bud

It consists of cluster of cells with a small opening (taste pore) in the surface. It consists of the following cells (Fig. 6.2-34).

Receptor cells. These are modified epithelial cells elongate, bipolar-shaped and extend from the epithelial opening of the taste bud to its base. The taste cells are innervated by sensory neurons (primary gustatory afferent fibers) at its basal pole.

Basal replacement cells. These are small round cells present at the bottom of taste bud (Fig. 6.2-35).

Supporting cells. In addition to taste cells and basal cells, the taste buds contain supporting or sustentacular cells.

Innervation

The special sensory nerve fibers innervating the taste cells come from the branches of the facial, glossopharyngeal and vagus nerve (7th, 9th and 10th cranial nerve, respectively). The tactile and temperature receptors of the mouth, tongue, and pharynx are innervated by the trigeminal nerve (5th cranial nerve).

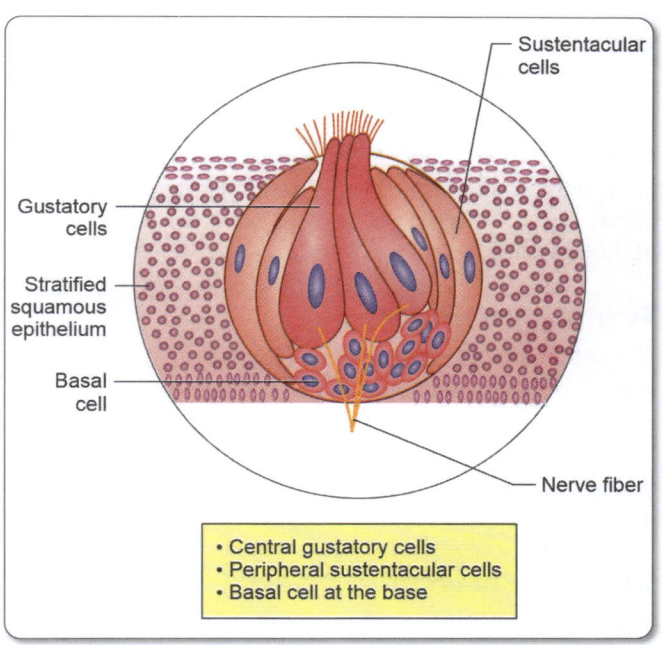

Fig. 6.2-35: Structure of a tastebud

TASTE PATHWAYS

The taste pathways consist of three orders of neurons (Fig. 6.2-36):

First Order Neurons

The cell bodies of the first order neurons innervating the taste cells in taste buds are located in different ganglia of the 7th, 9th and 10th cranial nerves as:

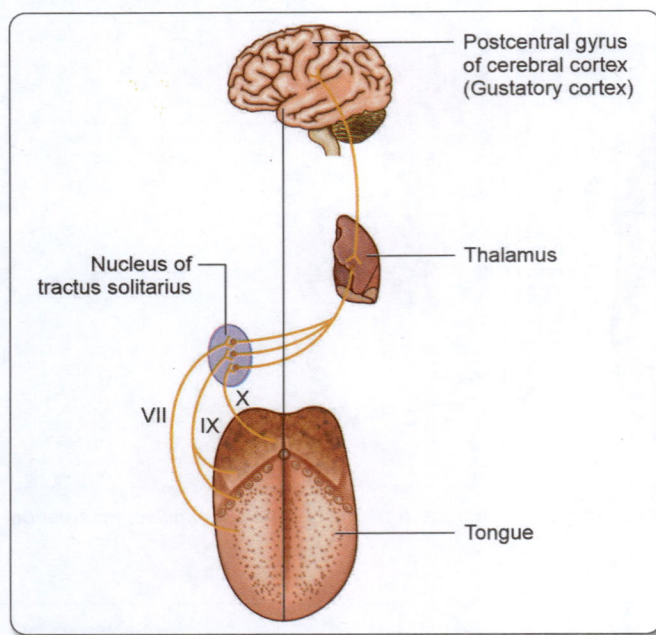

Fig. 6.2-36: The taste pathways

Termination of First Order Neurons

Ultimately all the taste fibers, traveling in different cranial nerves join the tractus solitarius to terminate in the nucleus of tractus solitarius.

Second Order Neurons

The cell bodies of second order neurons are located in the *nucleus of tractus solitarius (NTS)* in the medulla. Axons of second order neurons cross the midline to join the medial lemniscus and terminate with 5th cranial nerve fibers (carrying pain, touch, **and temperature** fibers) in the ventral posterior medial nucleus of thalamus.

Third Order Neurons

The cell bodies are located in the *thalamus*. Axons of third order neurons proceed to terminate in the inferior part of the postcentral gyrus, i.e., the part of sensory cortex.

PHYSIOLOGY OF TASTE

Gustatory Stimuli

Types of Stimuli and Most Sensitive Areas of Tongue

Conventionally four basic types of taste sensations have been described: *sweet*, *salt*, *sour* and *bitter*. All other taste sensations (hundreds in humans) are assumed to result from various combinations of these primary (basic) taste sensations.

Substances Producing Primary (Basic) Taste Sensations

Sweet sensation is produced by a number of organic molecules including sugars, glycols, alcohols, aldehydes, esters, etc. Tip of the tongue was considered the area most sensitive to sweet stimuli.

Salty sensation is produced by the anions of ionizable salts, especially the sodium chloride. The front half of each side of the tongue was thought to be the area most sensitive to salty stimuli.

Sour sensation. It is produced by acids. The posterior half of each side of the tongue was the area considered most sensitive to sour stimuli.

Bitter sensation is produced by alkaloids such as quinine, caffeine, nicotine and strychnine.

Transduction of Gustatory Stimuli

Transduction of gustatory stimuli into electrical signals is initiated at the level of receptors. The taste receptors are chemoreceptors which are stimulated by substances dissolved in the mouth by saliva. The dissolved substances act on the microvilli of taste receptors exposed in the taste pore of taste buds. This interaction typically depolarizes the cell. This causes the development of *receptor potential* in the receptor cell which in turn generates action potential in the sensory nerves.

Transmission of Information about Taste to the Cortex

Each sensory fiber contacts a number of taste cells and each taste cell synapses with numerous sensory fibers. Thus the electrical activity recorded from a single sensory fiber represents the input of many taste cells. As described in the taste pathway (Fig. 6.2-36), the signals carried by sensory fibers travel through several different nerves to the gustatory cortex.

Encoding of Taste Information

The identity of a taste stimulus appears to be encoded in the gustatory cortex by a unique pattern of inputs from many separate fibers that provide components of the patterns for different stimuli.

Sensation of Flavors

The multitude of different sensation of flavors that one experiences results from a combination of gustatory, olfactory and somatosensory inputs.

CLINICAL ASPECTS

Abnormalities of Taste Sensations

Ageusia refers to absence of taste sensation.
Hypogeusia refers to diminished taste sensitivity.
Dysgeusia refers to disturbed sense of taste.

ASSESS YOURSELF

Short and Long Answer Questions

1. **With the help of well-labeled diagram, describe the coats of an eyeball and their functions.**
2. **Describe the process of photo transduction.**
3. **Describe the functions of middle ear.**
4. **Briefly discuss physiology of hearing.**
5. **Describe the pathway of auditory conduction.**
6. **Describe briefly the physiology of olfaction.**
7. **Write notes on:**
   - Accommodation
   - Refractive errors
   - Presbyopia
   - Visual pigments
   - Optical pathway
   - Dark adaptation
   - Visual acuity
   - Intraocular pressure
   - Light reflex
   - Organ of Corti
   - Membranous labyrinth
   - Bony ossicles
   - Taste buds
   - Gustatory stimuli and taste pathway

Multiple Choice Questions

1. **The statement not true for conjunctiva:**
   a. Bulbar conjunctiva covers anterior part of eyeball
   b. Palpebral conjunctiva covers the lids
   c. Bulbar conjunctiva covers anterior surface of cornea
   d. Fornices are covered by conjunctiva
2. **The nasolacrimal duct opens into:**
   a. Inferior meatus of nose
   b. Superior concha
   c. Middle concha
   d. Inferior concha
3. **The primary function of lateral rectus muscle is:**
   a. Abduction   b. Adduction
   c. Elevation   d. Depression
4. **The nerve supply of cornea is by:**
   a. Ophthalmic nerve   b. Optic nerve
   c. Maxillary nerve   d. Facial nerve
5. **The true statement about ciliary body:**
   a. Forms the part of uveal tract
   b. Ciliary muscle is innervated by sympathetic fibers
   c. Highly vascular body
   d. Consists of striated muscle fibers
6. **The anterior chamber of eye lies between:**
   a. Back of cornea and anterior surface of lens
   b. Posterior surface of cornea and anterior surface of Iris
   c. Posterior surface of iris and anterior surface of lens
   d. Posterior surface lens and retina
7. **The refractive power of lens is:**
   a. 13 Diopter
   b. 16 Diopter
   c. 43 Diopter
   d. 60 Diopter
8. **The innermost layer of retina is:**
   a. Layer of rods and cones
   b. Layer of pigmented epithelium
   c. Inner nuclear layer
   d. Internal limiting membrane
9. **The nerve signal starts from which layer of retina:**
   a. Layer of rods and cones
   b. Layer of pigmented epithelium
   c. Inner nuclear layer
   d. Ganglion cell layer
10. **Crossing over of fibers from nasal retina takes place at:**
    a. Optic tracts
    b. Optic chiasma
    c. Lateral geniculate body
    d. Optic radiations
11. **The photosensitive pigment of rods is:**
    a. Rhodopsin   b. Photopsin
    c. Melanin   d. Carotene
12. **Visual acuity is maximum at:**
    a. Optic disc   b. Blind spot
    c. Fovea centralis   d. Nasal retina

13. **The wavelength of absorption spectrum of red cones is:**
    a. 450 – 490 nm
    b. 490 – 575 nm
    c. 645 – 720 nm
    d. < 490 nm

14. **Refractive error when parallel rays of light focused behind the retina is:**
    a. Myopia
    b. Hypermetropia
    c. Astigmatism
    d. Presbyopia

15. **Long sightedness is corrected by using:**
    a. Concave lens
    b. Convex lens
    c. Bifocal lens
    d. Cylindrical lens

16. **Which of the following of olfactory mucosa is responsible for smell sensations:**
    a. Basal cells
    b. Free nerve endings
    c. Supporting cells
    d. Bipolar cells

17. **The mitral cells of olfactory bulb constitute:**
    a. 1st order neurons
    b. 2nd order neurons
    c. 3rd order neurons
    d. 4th order neurons

18. **The statement not true for the taste buds:**
    a. Basal cells are primary gustatory afferent fibers
    b. Innervated by 7th, 9th and 10th cranial nerves
    c. First order neurons are located in the ganglia of 7th, 9th and 10th cranial nerves
    d. Receptor cells are modified basal cells

19. **Which is not the part of olfactory cortex:**
    a. Piriform cortex
    b. Amygdala
    c. Frontal cortex
    d. Inferior part of post central gyrus

20. **Nucleus tractus solitarius is located in the:**
    a. Orbitofrontal cortex
    b. Midbrain
    c. Pons
    d. Medulla

21. **The taste receptors are mainly:**
    a. Mechanoreceptors
    b. Thermo receptors
    c. Irritant receptors
    d. Chemical receptors

22. **Disturbed taste sensation is known as:**
    a. Ageusia
    b. Dysgeusia
    c. Hypogeusia
    d. Paraosmia

ANSWER KEY

1. c	2. a	3. a	4. a	5. a	6. b	7. b	8. d
9. d	10. b	11. a	12. c	13. c	14. a	15. b	16. a
17. b	18. d	19. d	20. d	21. d	22. b		

Section
VII

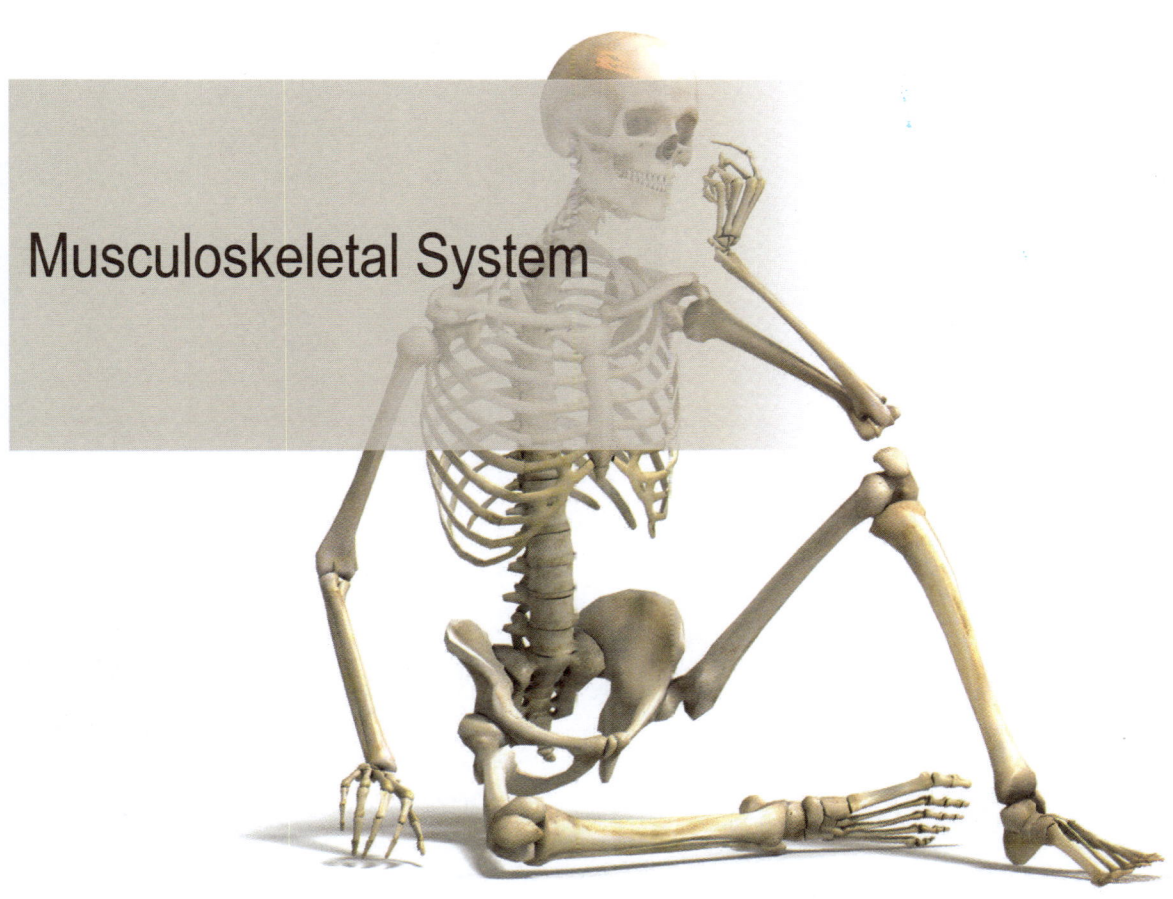

Musculoskeletal System

Section Outline

Human Skeleton

INTRODUCTION

The skeleton forms the main supporting framework of the body, and is primarily designed for a more effective production of movements by the attached muscles. A familiarity with the names, shapes and positions of individual bones will be very useful in understanding the regional anatomy of the body and functioning of the other organ systems.

DIVISIONS OF HUMAN SKELETON

The human skeleton can be grouped into two principal divisions:

1. Axial skeleton, and
2. Appendicular skeleton.

A total of 206 bones constitute the adult human skeleton, of these 80 bones form the axial skeleton and 126 bones form the appendicular skeleton Fig. 7.1-1 and Table 7.1-1.

AXIAL SKELETON

The axial skeleton consists of the bones that lie around the axis of body (a straight line that runs vertically along the body's center of gravity). These include (Fig. 7.1-1):

- Skull
- Hyoid bone
- Vertebral column
- Sternum or breast bone
- Thoracic cage.

SKULL

The skull, including the mandible, is a highly modified region of the axial skeleton. The skull is composed of a large number of separate bones which are united by sutures (fibrous immovable joints). The skull can be divided into two parts: Cranium and facial skeleton.

Cranium

The cranium is the upper bowl-shaped part of the skull which contains the brain. The cranium consists of eight bones (two parietal, two temporal, and one each the occipital, frontal, sphenoid, and ethmoid bone), which are described briefly (Figs 7.1-2 and 7.1-3):

Parietal Bones

The paired parietal bones form the roof and sides of the cranium (Fig. 7.1-2). They articulate with each other at the midline in the sagittal suture, with the occipital bone posteriorly in the lambdoid suture, and with the frontal bone anteriorly at the coronal suture. The parietal bone articulates inferiorly with the temporal bone and the greater wing of the sphenoid bone.

TABLE 7.1-1: Bones forming the axial and appendicular divisions of skeleton system

Axial skeleton				
Skull			**Vertebral column**	26
• Cranium	8		**Thorax**	
• Face	14		• Sternum	1
Hyoid	1		• Ribs	24
Auditory ossicles (3 in each ear)	6			
Appendicular skeleton				
Pectoral (shoulder) girdles			**Pelvic (hip) girdle**	
• Clavicle	2		• Hip bone and pelvis	2
• Scapula	2		**Lower extremities**	
Upper extremities			• Femur	2
• Humerus	2		• Fibula	2
• Ulna	2		• Tibia	2
• Radius	2		• Patella	2
• Carpals	16		• Tarsals	14
• Metacarpals	10		• Metatarsals	10
• Phalanges	28		• Phalanges	28

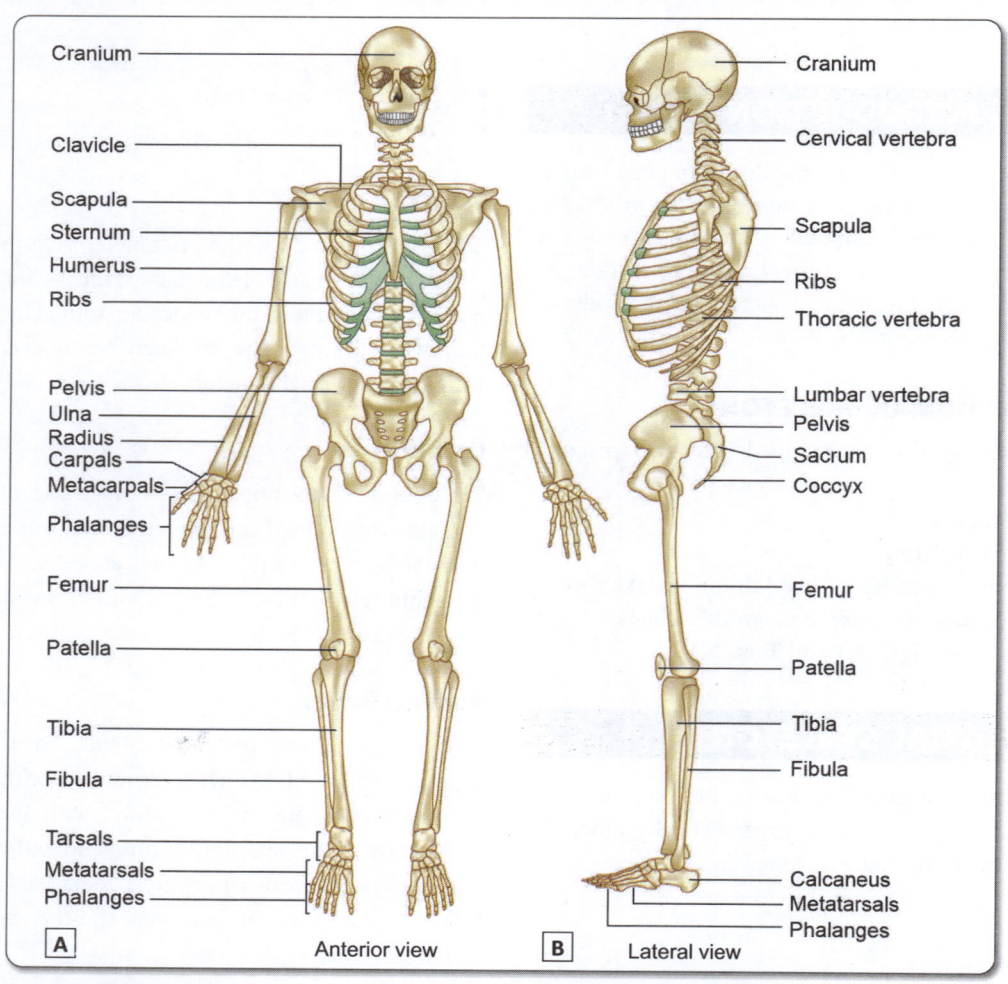

Figs 7.1-1A and B: The human skeleton; A. Anterior view; B. Lateral view

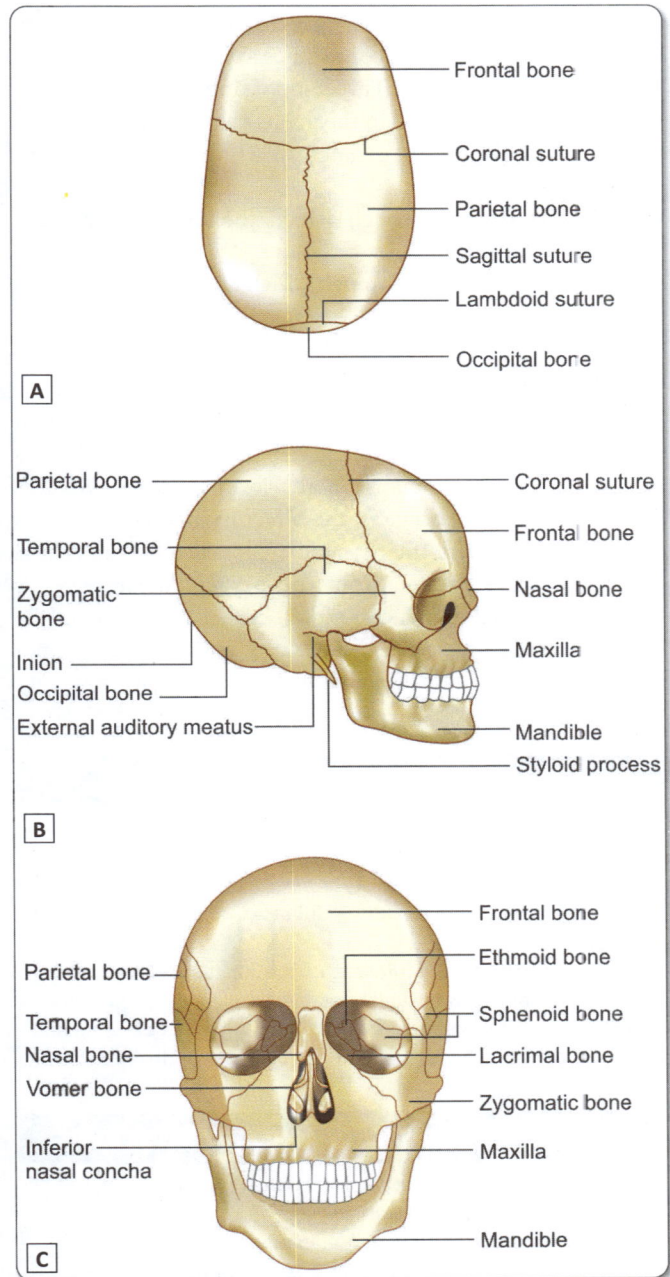

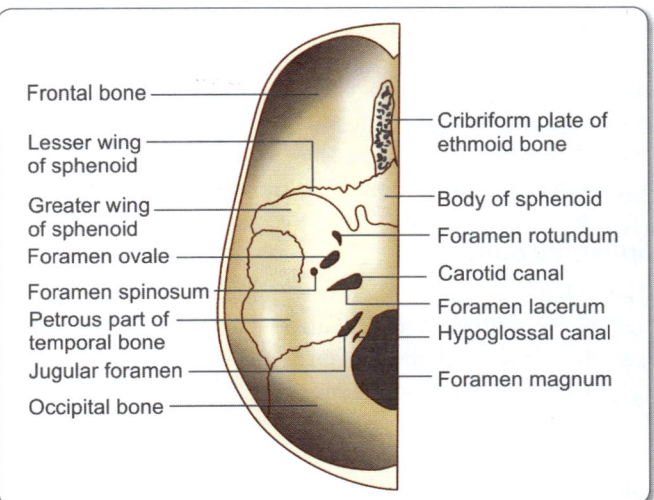

Fig. 7.1-3: View of cranial cavity and inner surface of bones forming base of the skull

Figs 7.1-2A to C: Bones of skull: A. Superior view of cranium; B. Lateral view of skull; C. Anterior view

Occipital Bone

The occipital bone forms the posterior aspect of the skull and the posterior floor of the cranial cavity. A prominence, the external occipital protuberance, or inion, is found on the external surface at the posterior midline (Fig. 7.1-2). The large foramen magnum is found in the inferior aspect of the occipital bone. The inner surface of the bone forms the posterior cranial fossa in which there are depressions in which the cerebellum, pons, and medulla oblongata lie. Fig. 7.1-3 shows the inner aspect of the cranial floor. The occipital bone articulates with the temporal bones, the parietal bones, and the sphenoid bone.

Temporal Bones

Each of the temporal bones is composed of two portions: a large, flat plate, the squamous portion; and a thickened, wedge-shaped area, the petrous portion. The squamous portion forms the side of cranium and articulates with the parietal bone and the sphenoid bone. An anterior projection, the zygomatic process, articulates with the zygomatic bone (Fig. 7.1-2). The petrous portion extends within the cranium and houses the midline and inner ear structures. The mastoid process and styloid process project from the inferior aspect, and between these two is located the stylomastoid foramen, through which the facial nerve exits the skull. The petrous portion articulates with the occipital bone in the floor of the skull. The carotid canal runs superiorly and anteriorly through the petrous portion and provides entrance for the internal carotid artery into the cranial cavity.

Frontal Bone

The single frontal bone forms the anterior portion of the cranium, the anterior floor of the cranial cavity, and the superior part of the face (Fig. 7.1-2). At the top of the skull, this bone articulates with the parietal bones; inferiorly it articulates with the sphenoid bone, ethmoid bone, and lacrimal bones; and inferoanteriorly it articulates with the nasal bones, maxillary bones and zygomatic bones. The inner surface of the cranial cavity portion of the frontal bone forms the anterior cranial fossa, in which the frontal lobes of the cerebral hemispheres lie. The frontal sinuses are located within the anterior portion of the frontal bone.

Sphenoid Bone

The sphenoid bone is a single bone, the body of which lies in the midline and articulates with the occipital bone and the temporal bones to form the base of the cranium (Fig. 7.1-4). The sphenoid bone joins the zygomatic bones to form the lateral walls of the orbits. Anteriorly and inferiorly, the sphenoid bone articulates with the maxillary and the palatine bones, superiorly with the parietal bones, and anteriorly and superiorly with the ethmoid and frontal bones. The depression on the superior cranial surface of the body of the sphenoid bone, the hypophyseal fossa (or the sella turcica), houses the pituitary gland; a portion of the body is hollow, forming the sphenoid sinus cavity.

Two pairs of wings project from the body of the sphenoid bone.

1. *The lesser wings* project from the anterior aspect of the body and are more superior and smaller than the greater wings. They are attached to the body by two small roots, and it is the gap between the two roots that forms the optic foramen or canal through which the optic nerve exits the orbit.

The lesser wings articulate with the frontal and ethmoid bones.

2. *The greater wings* project from the lateral aspects of the body and articulate with the frontal bone, the parietal bones, the squamous portions of the temporal bones, and the zygomatic bones. The pterygoid process projects from the

base of the greater wing and articulates with the vertical stem of the palatine bones; each contributes to a shallow depression, the pterygopalatine fossa. Three important:

- Foramina are located in the greater wing (Fig. 7.1-3)
- Foramen rotundum, through which the maxillary nerve passes
- Foramen ovale, through which the mandibular nerve passes; and
- Foramen spinosum, through which the middle meningeal artery passes.

Ethmoid Bone

The single ethmoid bone resembles a rectangular box that contains a midline perpendicular plate. This plate bisects the top of the box, the horizontal cribriform plate, which is perforated for the passage of the olfactory nerves. The sides of the box parallel to the perpendicular plate are the orbital plates and are separated from the perpendicular plate by the ethmoid air cells. The ethmoid bone articulates with the sphenoid and frontal bones superiorly and with the vomer inferiorly; the orbital plates also articulate with the maxillary and lacrimal bones.

IMPORTANT TO KNOW

Fontanelles. In the newborn the skull bones are not completely joined together but are separated by membranous connective tissue. The gaps or soft spots are known as fontanelles. Six fontanelles are present during infancy, with the two most notables are:

- *Anterior fontanelle* is present at the junction of frontal and parietal bones, and usually closed by the age of 18 months.
- *Posterior fontanelle* is present at the junction of occipital and parietal bones, and usually closed by 2–3 months after birth.

NURSING IMPLICATIONS AND APPLICATIONS

Nurse should adapt a habit to palpate the fontanelles of all babies when brought to the doctor, because it will give an idea whether it is depressed/raised/enlarged.

- The depressed fontanelle indicates dehydration
- Raised fontanelle indicates increase in intracranial pressure.
- In hydrocephalus the fontanelles are raised

Formina and Fissures of Skull

The skull bones possess various foramina and fissures through which nerves blood vessels and ligaments pass that connect the brain with rest of the body structures. The important foramina and fissures and structures passing through them are enlisted in Table 7.1-2.

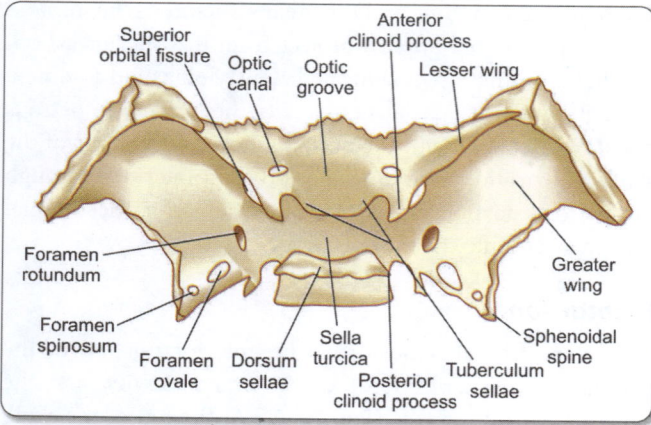

Fig. 7.1-4: Sphenoid bone

TABLE 7.1-2: The important foramina and fissures and structures passing through them	
Foramen magnum	• Lower part of medulla, continuing inferiorly as spinal cord • The meninges • Spinal accessory nerves, Vertebral arteries • Anterior and posterior spinal arteries • Apical ligament of dens
Jugular foramen	• Glossopharyngeal nerve (IX cranial nerve) • Vagus nerve (IX cranial nerve) • Accessory nerve (XI cranial nerve) • Sigmoid sinus continues as internal jugular vein • Inferior petrosal sinus
Foramen ovale	• Mandibular nerve, Accessory meningeal artery, Lesser petrosal nerve, Emissary vein (MALE)
Foramen rotundum	Maxillary nerve
Stylomastoid foramen	Facial nerve, stylomastoid vessels
Carotid canal	Internal carotid artery, sympathetic plexus
Optic canal	Optic nerve, covered by meninges, ophthalmic artery
Internal acoustic meatus	Facial nerve, vestibulocochlear nerve, labyrinthine vessels
Mandibular foramen	Inferior alveolar nerve, inferior alveolar vessels
Superior orbital fissure	• Lacrimal nerve, frontal nerve, trochlear nerve • Upper and lower divisions of oculornotor nerve • Abducent nerve • Superior ophthalmic vein
Inferior orbital fissure	Maxillary nerve, infraorbital vessels, zygornatic nerve
Infraorbital foramen	Infraorbital nerve, infraorbital vessels

Facial Skeleton

The lower part of the skull is described as the facial skeleton or the *viscerocranium*. It consists of 14 bones, of which only two are single.

The single frontal bone forms the forehead and articulates with the nasal bones, the maxillae, and the zygomatic bones in the formation of the face. The sutures joining adjacent bones of the face are generally named according to the names of the two bones that are connected (e.g. the suture between the frontal arches). They also articulate with the maxillary bones and with the greater wings of the sphenoid bone.

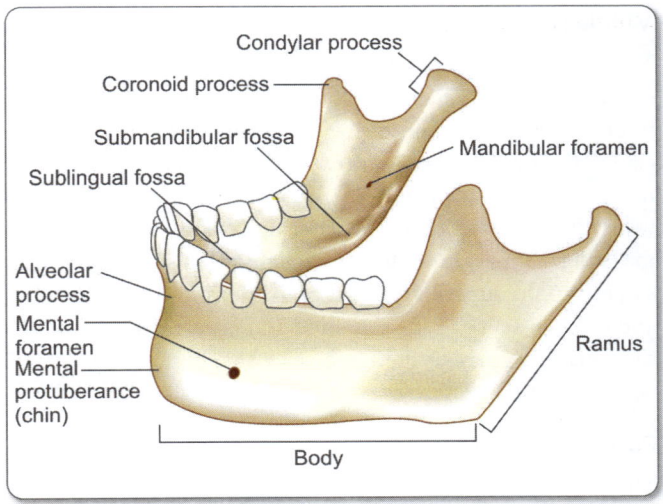

Fig. 7.1-5: Mandible

Mandible (Fig. 7.1-5)

The mandible forms the movable lower jaw. It is a horseshoe-shaped bone consisting of a curved horizontal body and two perpendicular processes, the rami.

Cavities of the Skull

The skull contains multiple cavities which reflect its multiple functions:

Cranial cavity. It houses, supports and protects the brain.

Nasal cavity. It is concerned with respiration and olfaction.

Oral cavity. It is the first part of the gastrointestinal tract responsible for mastication and initial food processing, and houses taste receptors.

Orbits. The orbits contain the eyes and other related structures and are described in detail Chapter 6.2, page 314.

Cranial Cavity

The cranial cavity houses the brain and its meninges and their associated vessels in addition to the intracranial portions of the cranial nerves. The base of the cranial cavity can be subdivided into three fossae: Anterior, middle, and posterior.

Anterior cranial fossa

The anterior cranial fossa is limited in front and laterally by the frontal bone and posteriorly by the lesser wing of the sphenoid. Its floor is formed by the orbital plate of the frontal bone, the cribriform plate of the ethmoid (with a median crest-like ridge, the crista galli which forms the anterior attachment of falx cerebri), and the lesser wings and anterior part of the body (jugum) of the sphenoid (Fig. 7.1-3).

Middle cranial fossa

The middle cranial fossa lies at a lower plane than the anterior cranial fossa but is higher than the posterior cranial fossa. Its floor is shaped like a butterfly, namely it consists of a narrow central or median part and expanded lateral parts (wings). It is bound anteriorly by the posterior free edge of the lesser wing of the sphenoid, the anterior clinoid processes and the anterior margin of the sulcus chiasmatis. Posteriorly, it extends to the superior borders of the petrous temporal bones and dorsum sellae of the sphenoid and laterally it is bound by the squamous part of the temporal bone, part of the parietal bones, and the greater wings of the sphenoid.

Posterior cranial fossa

This is the deepest of the three cranial fossae, its floor lying below the level of the middle fossa. Its roof is formed by the tentorium cerebelli. It lodges the hindbrain, the cerebellum, pons, and medulla oblongata. The fossa is bound anteriorly by the superior border of the petrous temporal bone and the dorsum sellae and surrounds the foramen magnum, the cerebellum being housed in the cerebellar fossae on the squamous part of the occipital bone.

Pituitary fossa

The pituitary fossa (hypophyseal fossa) is an indentation in the roof of the body of the sphenoid bone in the middle cranial fossa. It is bound anteriorly by the tuberculum sellae, in front of which lies the sulcus chiasmatica, and posteriorly by the dorsum sellae, a ridge of the bone at either end of which lie the posterior clinoid processes. The pituitary fossa houses the pituitary gland or hypophysis cerebri.

Orbits

The bony orbits are quadrangular truncated pyramids situated between the anterior cranial fossa above and the maxillary sinuses below (Fig. 7.1-6). Each orbit is formed by portions of seven bones: (1) frontal, (2) maxilla, (3) zygomatic, (4) sphenoid, (5) palatine, (6) ethmoid, and (7) lacrimal. It has four walls (medial, lateral, superior and inferior), base and an apex.

Medial walls of two orbits are parallel to each other and, being thinnest, are frequently fractured during injuries.

Inferior orbital wall (floor) is triangular in shape and is quite thin.

Lateral wall of the orbit is triangular in shape. It covers only posterior half of the eyeball.

Roof is triangular in shape and is formed mainly by the orbital plate of frontal bone.

Base of the orbit is the anterior open end of the orbit. It is bounded by thick orbital margins.

Orbital apex. It is the posterior end of orbit with four orbital walls converge. It has two orifices, the *optic canal* which transmits optic nerve and ophthalmic artery and the *superior orbital fissure* which transmits a number of nerves, arteries and veins.

Contents of the Orbit

The *volume* of each orbit is about 30 cc. Approximately one-fifth of it is occupied by the eyeball. Other contents of the orbit include part of optic nerve, extraocular muscles, lacrimal gland, lacrimal sac, ophthalmic artery and its branches, third, fourth and sixth cranial nerves and ophthalmic and maxillary divisions of the fifth cranial nerve, sympathetic nerve, orbital fat and fascia.

Paranasal Sinuses (Fig. 7.1-7)

Anatomically, the orbital cavity is bounded on three sides by the air-containing cavities—the paranasal sinuses also called paraorbital sinuses. The paranasal sinuses are four on each side. These are:

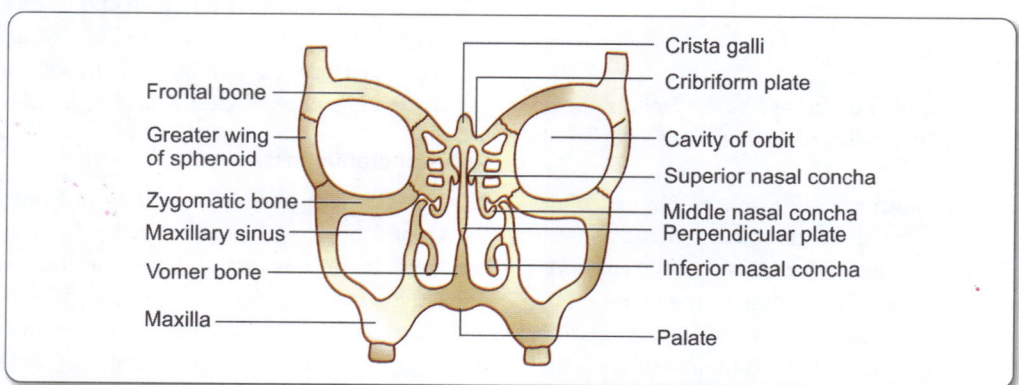

Frontal bone
Greater wing of sphenoid
Zygomatic bone
Maxillary sinus
Vomer bone
Maxilla

Crista galli
Cribriform plate
Cavity of orbit
Superior nasal concha
Middle nasal concha
Perpendicular plate
Inferior nasal concha
Palate

Fig. 7.1-6: Schematic coronal section through orbit and nasal cavity

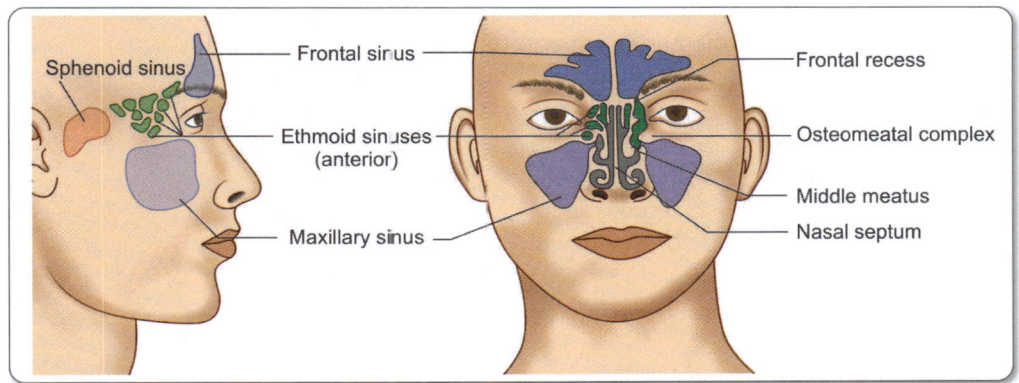

Fig. 7.1-7: Paranasal sinuses

Maxillary Sinus

Maxillary sinus is the largest of paranasal sinuses and occupies the body of maxilla.

On an average, maxillary sinus has a capacity of 15 mL in adults. It is pyramidal in shape with the following features:

Base of the maxillary sinus forms part of the lateral wall of the nose.

Apex of this pyramidal cavity is directed laterally into the zygomatic process.

Anterolateral wall is formed by facial surface of the maxilla and is related to soft tissue of cheek.

Posterior wall is related to infratemporal and pterygopalatine fossae.

Floor is formed by maxillary alveolar process and is situated about 1.25 cm below the floor of the nose. Roots of the molars and premolars are in close relation to the floor separated from it by a thin lamina of bone. With advancing age, the floor undergoes absorption, which may expose the roots, especially of the first molar. Orodental fistulae can result from extraction of teeth.

Roof of the maxillary sinus is formed by the orbital plate of the maxilla, which also forms the floor of the orbit. Growths of the maxillary sinus may push the roof upward causing proptosis with upward displacement of the eyeball.

Osteum of the maxillary sinus is situated high up in its medial wall and opens in the posterior part of ethmoidal infundibulum into the middle meatus. It is unfavorably situated for natural drainage.

Frontal Sinuses

Frontal sinuses are situated between the inner and outer tables of frontal bone and are separated by a thin septum. On an average the height of the frontal sinus is 3 cm, the breadth 2.5 cm and depth 2 cm. Its anatomical features are as follows:

Anterior wall of the sinus is related to the skin over the forehead.

Inferior wall or floor of the sinus is related to the orbit and its contents.

Posterior wall of the sinus is related to meninges and frontal lobe of the brain.

Opening of the frontal sinus is situated in its floor and leads to the middle meatus directly or through a canal called *frontonasal duct*.

Ethmoidal Sinuses

Ethmoidal sinuses are thin-walled air cavities mostly situated in the lateral mass of the ethmoid. These are completed by the adjoining bones, viz., frontal palatine, sphenoid, maxillary and lacrimal. Collectively, they form an *ethmoid labyrinth*.

The ethmoidal sinuses vary from 3–18 in number and occupy the space between upper third of lateral nasal wall and the medial wall of the orbit.

The sinuses are divided by irregular septa into anterior, middle and posterior groups (Fig. 7.1-5). The *anterior and middle sinuses* open into the middle meatus and the posterior sinuses open into the superior meatus. Relations of ethmoid labyrinth are as follows:

Roof of the ethmoidal sinuses is formed by anterior cranial fossa lateral to cribriform plate. Meninges of brain form important relations here.

Lateral wall of these sinuses is related to the orbit.

Sphenoid Sinuses

The sphenoidal sinuses situated in the body of sphenoid bones are separated by a thin bony septum which is often obliquely placed and thus the right and left sinuses are rarely symmetrical. Some important anatomical relations of the sphenoid sinuses are as follows:

Roof of the sinus in anterior part is related to the olfactory tract, optic chiasma and frontal lobe. In the posterior part, roof is related to pituitary gland in the sella turcica.

Lateral wall of the sinus in the anterior part is related to internal carotid artery, maxillary nerve and optic nerve anterosuperiorly (which often ridge each sinus). In the posterior part, each lateral wall is related to cavernous sinus, internal carotid artery and cranial nerves—3rd, 4th, 6th and all the divisions of 5th.

Floor of the sinus lies above the nasal cavity and houses pterygoid canal, which may ridge it.

Anterior wall of the sphenoidal sinus is related to the posterior ethmoidal sinus which may in fact be bulging in it (Fig. 7.1-7).

Osteum of the sphenoid sinus is situated in the upper part of its anterior wall and drains into sphenoethmoidal recess.

HYOID BONE (FIG 7.1-8)

The hyoid bone is a unique component of the axial skeleton because it does not articulate with any other bone.

Location. The hyoid bone is located in the neck between the mandible and larynx. It is suspended from the styloid process of the temporal bone by ligaments and muscles.

Features. The hyoid bone consists of a horizontal body and paired projections called the *lesser cornu* and the *greater cornu* (Fig. 7.1-8). Muscles and ligaments attach to these paired projections.

Functions. It supports the tongue and provides attachment for some of the muscles.

VERTEBRAL COLUMN

The vertebral column, also known as backbone, is a strong, flexible column formed by vertebrae piled one upon another (Figs 7.1-9A and B).

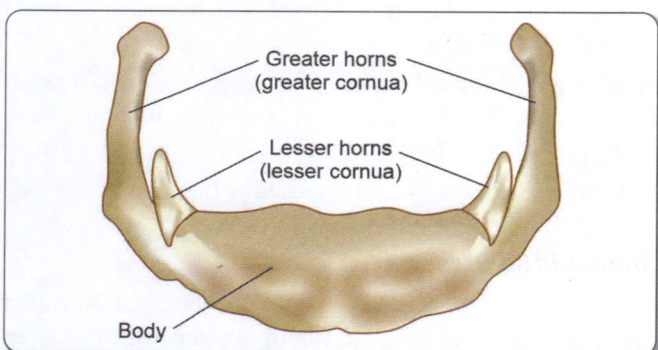

Fig 7.1-8: Hyoid bone

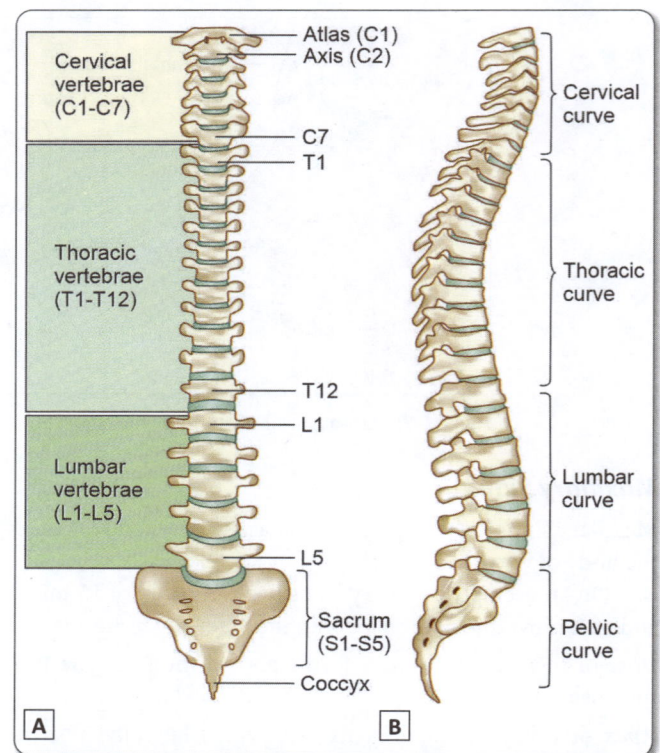

Figs 7.1-9A and B: The vertebral column: A. Anterior view and; B. Right lateral view showing various curves

Curves of Vertebral Column

When viewed from the side, the vertebral column presents four curves (2 primary and 2 secondary) which are alternately convex and concave.

Primary Curves

The two concave curves (*thoracic* and *pelvic*) are called primary curves because they exist in fetal life and are designed for the accommodation of viscera.

Secondary Curves

The two convex curves (*cervical* and *lumbar*) are called secondary or compensatory curves because they are developed after birth.

Structure of Vertebral Column

The vertebral column is made up of:
- Vertebrae (a series of small bones)
- Intervertebral discs
- Ligaments.

Vertebrae

The vertebral column is formed of 33 vertebrae in all. These include:

- Cervical vertebrae (in the neck): 7 (Movable)
- Thoracic or dorsal vertebrae (in the thorax): 12 (Movable)
- Lumbar vertebrae (in the loin): 5 (Movable)
- Sacral vertebrae (in the pelvis): 5 (Fused)
- Coccygeal vertebrae (in the pelvis): 4 (Fused)

From the above it is clear that in terms of separate bones, the vertebral column consists of 26 bones (24 separate movable vertebrae, one sacrum (made of 5 fused vertebrae) and one coccyx (made of 4 fused vertebrae).

General anatomical features of a typical vertebra

The movable vertebrae though differ in size, shape and have some distinguishing features, all have many similar structural characteristics. A typical vertebra has the following parts (Figs 7.1-10A and B):

Body of a vertebra

It forms the anterior, solid cylindrical mass of bone. The size varies with the site. They are smallest in the cervical region and become larger toward the lumbar region. The bodies of adjoining vertebrae are firmly united to one another through intervertebral discs (Fig. 7.1-10B).

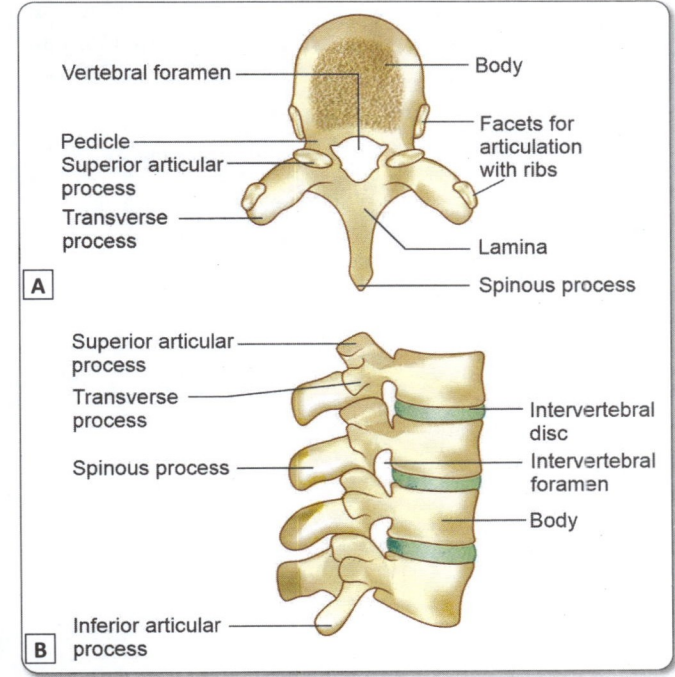

Figs 7.1-10A and B: Structure of a typical vertebra: A. Viewed from above; B. Lateral view of several vertebrae with intervertebral discs

Pedicles and laminae

Pedicles (right and left) are two short, thick processes which project backward from the body, one on each side, to join with the *laminae*. The two laminae (right and left) join posteriorly with each other in the midline. The pedicles and laminae together constitute the *vertebral neural arch*. This arch encloses the *vertebral foramen*. Collectively the vertebral foramina form the *vertebral canal* which houses the spinal cord and its meninges.

Processes

Each vertebra has several processes:

Articular processes are four in number, two to connect with bone above, and two to connect with the bone below.

Transverse processes are two in number, one at each side where the pedicle and lamina join.

Spinous process, one from each vertebra, projects backward from the junction of the laminae in midline.

Special anatomical features of different vertebrae

Typical cervical vertebrae

Typical cervical vertebrae (C_3 to C_7) have the following special features:

Transverse processes have a foramen through which a vertebral artery passes toward brain.

Spinous processes are short.

Bodies of the cervical vertebrae are smaller than the thoracic but the arches are larger.

Atypical cervical vertebrae

First and second cervical vertebrae are atypical and need special description.

First cervical vertebra, also called *atlas*, looks very different from a typical cervical vertebrae, as it has no body and no spine. It simply consists of a ring of bone with two short transverse processes (Fig. 7.1-11).

Second cervical vertebra, also called *axis*, is characterized by the presence of the dens or odontoid process (a thick finger-like projection arising from the upper part of body) (Fig. 7.1-12). The odontoid process fits into the space between the anterior arch of the atlas and its transverse ligament to form the *median atlanto-occipital joint*. The movement at this joint is turning the head from side to side.

Thoracic vertebrae

Thoracic vertebrae have the following distinguishing features (Fig. 7.1-13):

Costal facets for articulation with ribs are present on the sides of the bodies and on the transverse process.

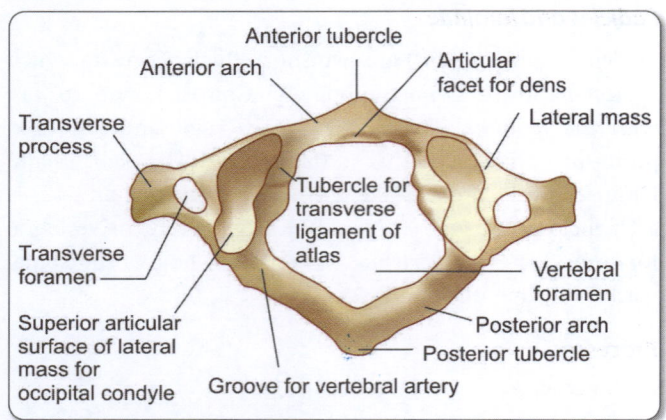

Fig. 7.1-11: The first cervical (atlas) vertebra viewed from above

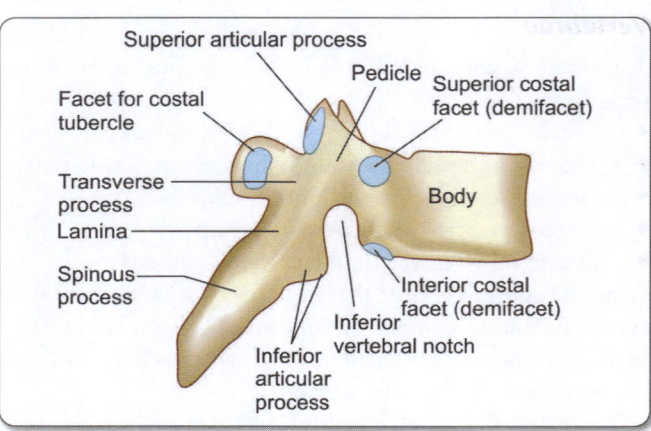

Fig. 7.1-13: Side view of a typical thoracic vertebra

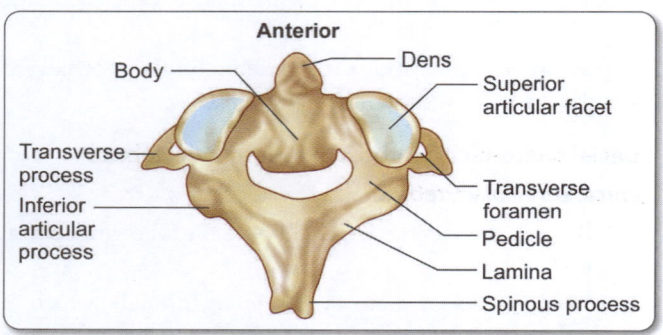

Fig. 7.1-12: The second cervical (axis) vertebra viewed from above

Size of these vertebrae is larger than those of cervical vertebrae.
Spinous processes are long and are directed downward.

Lumbar vertebrae

Lumbar vertebrae can be distinguished from cervical vertebrae by the absence of foramina transversaria and from the thoracic vertebrae by the absence of costal facets for attachment of the ribs. Further, the bodies of these vertebrae are the largest and heaviest in the spine. The processes are short, heavy and thick.

Sacrum

It is a large triangular or wedge-shaped bone formed by the union of five sacral vertebrae. Its features are (Figs 7.1-14A and B):

Pelvic surface is concave, comparatively smooth and marked by four transverse ridges. At the ends of ridges are four pairs of pelvic sacral foramina.

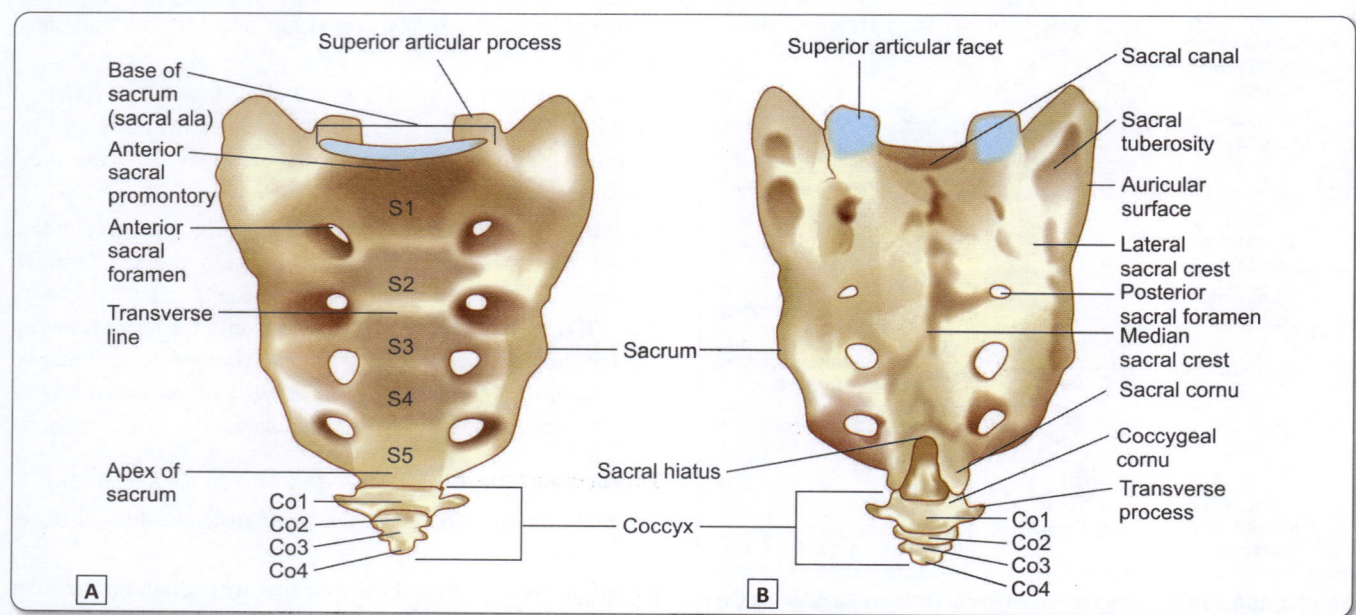

Figs 7.1-14A and B: The sacrum and coccyx bones viewed: A. Anterior view; B. Posterior view

Dorsal surface is convex and irregular.

Base or upper part of the sacrum articulates with the 5th lumbar vertebra.

At sides, this bone articulates with the ilium to form sacroiliac joint and its *inferior tip* articulates with the coccyx.

Coccyx

It is a small triangular bone formed by fusion of coccygeal vertebrae (Fig. 7.1-14). It is the most rudimentary part of the vertebral column. At the base it articulates with the tip of sacrum.

Intervertebral foramina

Intervertebral foramina are formed one on each side between the pedicles of two adjacent vertebrae. Thus half boundary of each foramen is formed by the vertebra above and half by the one below. Through these foramina pass the spinal nerves, blood vessels and lymph vessels on each side between every pair of vertebrae throughout the length of the vertebral column.

Intervertebral Discs

As mentioned above in-between the bodies of adjoining vertebrae from the axis to the sacrum are present fibrocartilaginous plates called the intervertebral discs. These discs are thinnest in the cervical region and become progressively thick toward the lumbar region. They are kept in place by the posterior longitudinal ligament of the vertebral canal.

Parts

The *peripheral part* of the disc, a rim made of fibrocartilage, is called *annulus fibrosus*. The *central part* of the disc is relatively soft and is called the *nucleus pulposus*.

Functions

The intervertebral discs have a shock absorbing function. The cartilaginous joints formed by them throughout the vertebral column also contribute to the flexibility of the vertebral column as a whole.

Ligaments of Vertebral Column

The ligaments of vertebral column which hold the vertebrae together and help to maintain the intervertebral discs in position are:

Transverse ligament. It is attached to the bony ring of atlas (first cervical vertebra). It maintains the odontoid process of the axis in correct position in relation to the atlas.

Anterior longitudinal ligament. It extends along the anterior surfaces of the bodies of vertebrae from axis to the sacrum. It connects the bodies of the vertebrae to each other anteriorly.

Posterior longitudinal ligament. It lies inside the vertebral canal and extends along the posterior surface of the bodies from the axis to sacrum. Thus, it binds the bodies of vertebrae together posteriorly.

Ligamenta flava. These are broad thin ligaments that connect the laminae of adjacent vertebrae.

Ligamentum nuchae. It extends from the protuberance of the occiput to the spinous process of 7th cervical vertebra. It connects apices of the spinous processes of cervical vertebrae.

Supraspinous ligament. It is the downward continuation of ligamentum nuchae. It extends from the 7th cervical vertebra to the sacrum and connects spinous processes of these vertebrae.

Interspinal ligaments. Adjacent spinous processes are connected by interspinal ligaments which extend from the root to the apex of each process and meet the ligamenta flava in front and supraspinal ligament behind.

Intertransverse ligaments. These connect the transverse processes and are placed between them.

Movements of Vertebral Column

The spinal curves confer springiness and strength upon the vertebral column, and the elasticity is further increased by ligamenta flava and the discs of fibrocartilage. As a result the vertebral column as a whole is movable, being capable of:

- *Flexion*, i.e., bending forward freely,
- *Extension*, i.e., bending backward (less freely),
- *Lateral flexion*, i.e., bending from side to side (less freely), and
- *Rotation* of limited amount is possible in cervical and thoracic regions.

Functions of Vertebral Column

Protection to the delicate spinal cord is provided by the bony vertebral canal formed collectively by the vertebral foramina.

Passage for the exit of spinal nerves, blood vessels and lymph vessels is provided by the intervertebral foramina, formed one on each side by the pedicles of adjacent vertebrae.

Movability to the trunk is provided by the elasticity and flexibility of the vertebral column as a whole.

Support to the cranium and trunk is provided by the vertebral column.

Shock absorption is possible due to the pads formed by intervertebral discs. These pads mitigate the effects of contusion arising from falls or blows, protecting the brain.

Axis of the trunk giving attachment to the ribs, shoulder girdle and upper limbs, and the pelvic girdle and lower limbs, is formed by the vertebral column.

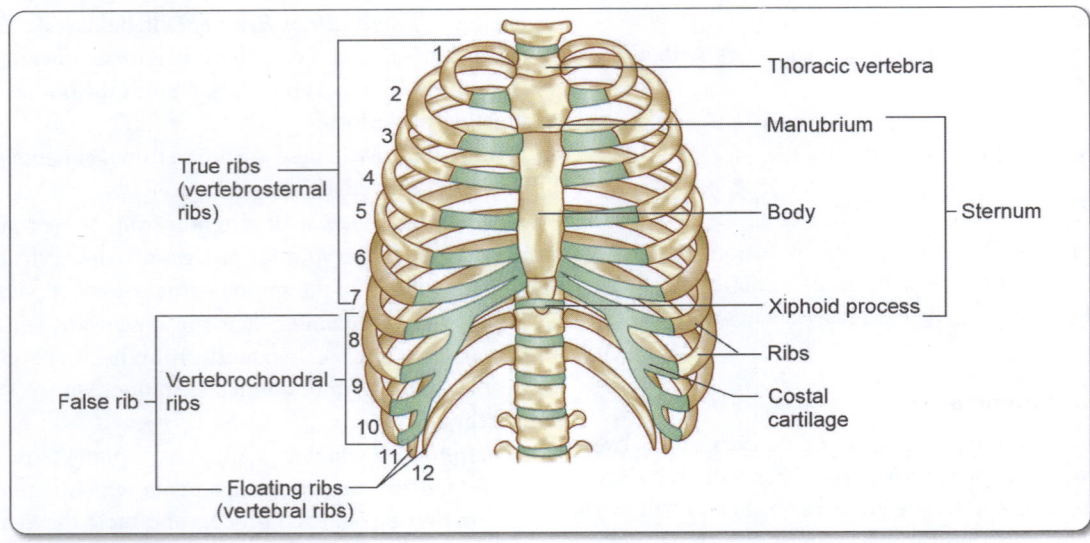

Fig. 7.1-15: Anterior view of thoracic cage

THORACIC CAGE

The skeleton of the thorax or thoracic cage protects the heart, lungs and other thoracic organs. The thoracic cage is formed by (Fig. 7.1-15):

- Sternum (1)
- Ribs (12 pairs), and
- Thoracic vertebrae (12)

Sternum

Sternum is a flat, narrow bone about 6 inches long, situated in the median line in the front of the chest. It consists of three parts (Fig. 7.1-16):

1. *Manubrium*, the uppermost part, bears notches for attachment with the clavicles and costal cartilages of first two pairs of ribs.

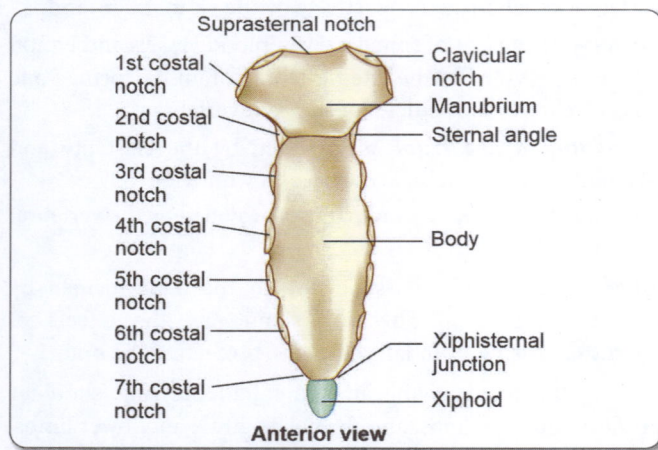

Fig. 7.1-16: The sternum and its attachments

2. *Body*, the middle part, possesses notches for attachment with costal cartilages of ribs.

3. *Xiphoid process*, the lower part, has no ribs attached to it but gives attachment to some of the abdominal muscles.

CLINICAL ASPECTS

- *Sternal puncture.* For bone marrow examination sternum manubrium is the common site for bone marrow aspiration for diagnosis of type of anemia and leukemias
- For cardiothoracic surgery (for example heart surgery) sternum has to be cut open to get access to heart and other thoracic contents.

NURSING IMPLICATIONS AND APPLICATIONS

Sternal angle or angle of Louise. The manubrium makes a slight angle at its junction with body of sternum is called sternal angle or angle of Louise. It is an important landmark for the following:

- The second rib attaches with sternum at this level, therefore srenal angle is an important landmark for counting the lower ribs and intercostal spaces
- For determining the location of apex beat of the heart
- Trachea bifurcates into principal bronchi at this level

Ribs

The twelve pairs of ribs form the side walls of thorax (Fig. 7.1-15). Each rib is a long curved bone having a posterior end and an anterior end (Fig. 7.1-17). Posterior ends of all the twelve ribs are attached to the vertebral column. Depending upon the attachment of anterior end, the ribs have been classified into three groups:

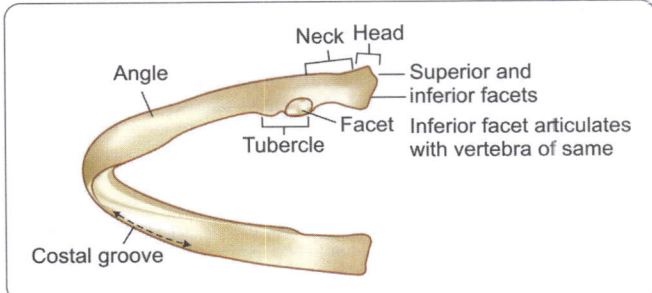

Fig. 7.1-17: A typical rib viewed from below

1. ***True ribs.*** The anterior end of the upper seven pairs of ribs is attached to the sternum through a bar of costal cartilage. These are called true ribs.

2. ***False ribs.*** The costal cartilages of 8th, 9th and 10th ribs are not attached to the sternum directly, but end by getting attached to the next higher cartilage. That is, they are attached indirectly to the sternum and are called false ribs.

3. ***Floating ribs*** refer to 11th and 12th ribs, the anterior ends of which are free (floating).

APPENDICULAR SKELETON

The appendicular skeleton consists of a total of 126 bones. The appendages are:
- Shoulder girdle and upper limbs
- Pelvic girdle and lower limbs

SHOULDER GIRDLE AND UPPER LIMBS

Each shoulder girdle consists of two bones, 1 clavicle and 1 scapula; and each upper limb is formed by 30 bones (1 humerus, 1 radius, 1 ulna, 8 carpal bones, 5 metacarpal bones and 14 phalanges (Fig. 7.1-18).

Clavicle or Collar Bone

The clavicle is a long bone with a double curvature (Fig. 7.1-19). It is placed horizontally at the upper and anterior part of thorax above the first rib. The inner or *sternal end* of the clavicle articulates with the sternum and the outer or *acromial end* articulates with the scapula. The clavicle forms the only bony link between upper limb and axial skeleton.

CLINICAL ASPECTS

Clavicle bone is prone to fracture when there is fall on outstretched arm.

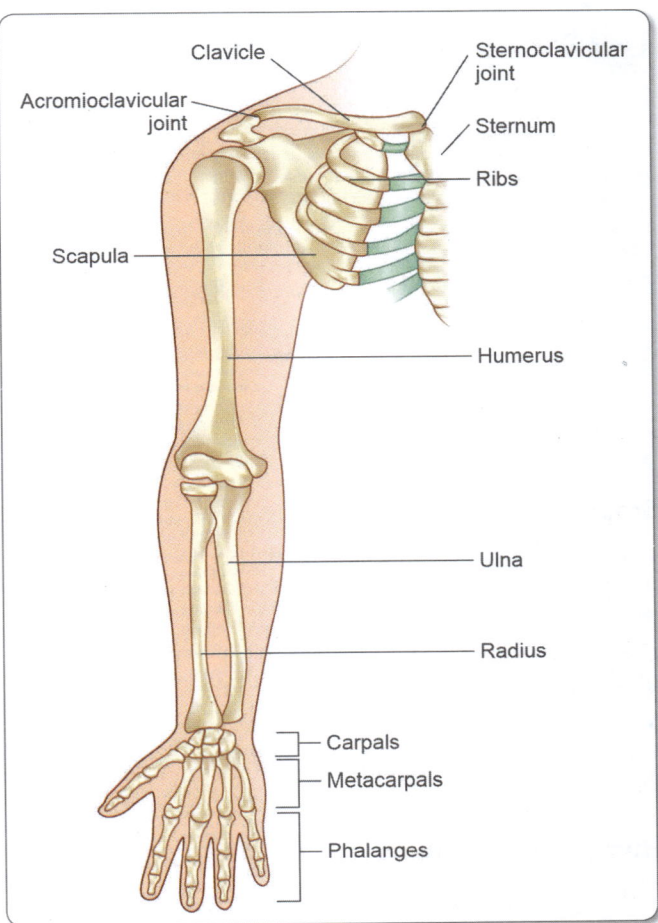

Fig. 7.1-18: Anterior view of skeleton of right shoulder girdle and upper limb

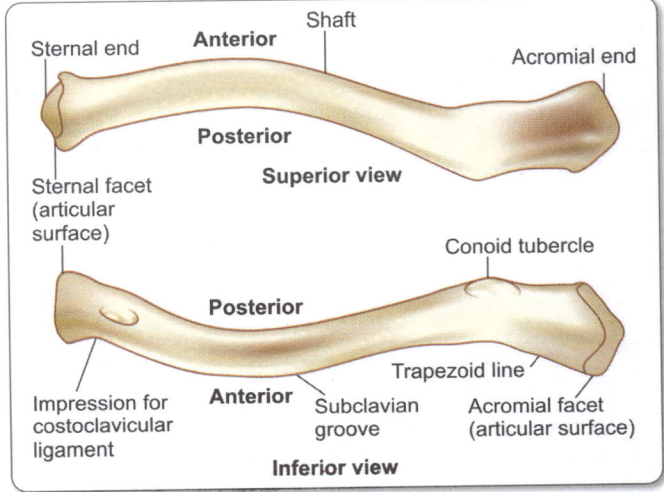

Fig. 7.1-19: The right clavicle seen from above

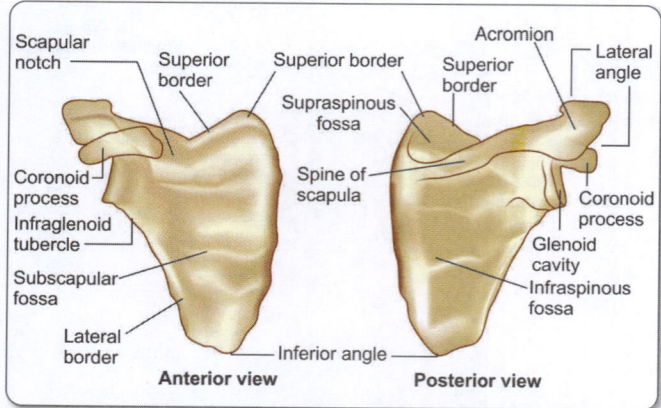

Fig. 7.1-20: The right scapula

Scapula

The scapula, also called shoulder blade, is a flat triangular bone placed behind the upper part of thorax. The scapula presents the following important features (Fig. 7.1-20):

Glenoid cavity is a shallow socket present at the lateral angle. It receives the head of humerus forming the shoulder joint.

Spine forms a prominent ridge on the posterior surface of scapula and terminates in a triangular, the *acromian process*, which articulates with clavicle.

Humerus or Arm Bone

Humerus is the largest and longest bone of the upper limb. It presents the following parts (Fig. 7.1-21):

Rounded head at the upper end which articulates with the glenoid cavity of the scapula to form the shoulder joint.

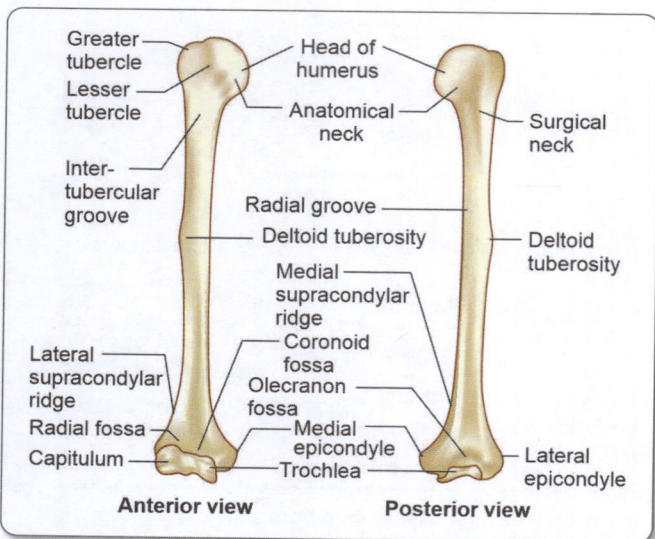

Fig. 7.1-21: Humerus or arm bone

Shaft of the humerus is connected above to the head through a narrow part neck and below to the condyle.

Condyle is the lower end of humerus which presents two surfaces that articulate with the radius and ulna to form the elbow joint.

Radius

The radius along with ulna forms the bones of the forearm. It is located on the thumb side between the elbow and wrist and is somewhat shorter than its companion.

Features of some parts of the radius are (Fig. 7.1-22):

*   *Head* is thick disc-like and articulates with lower end of humerus and upper end of ulna.
*   *Shaft* is connected to the head through a constricted neck. It presents *radial tuberosity* which gives attachment to the biceps muscle.
*   *Lower end* of radius articulates with scaphoid and lunate bones of the wrist and the ulna. The lateral *styloid process* present at the lower end gives attachment to the ligaments of the wrist.

CLINICAL ASPECTS

Colles fracture is the fracture of distal end of the radius and is quite common in elderly people.

Ulna

Ulna, placed on the medial side of radius, is comparatively longer bone of the forearm.

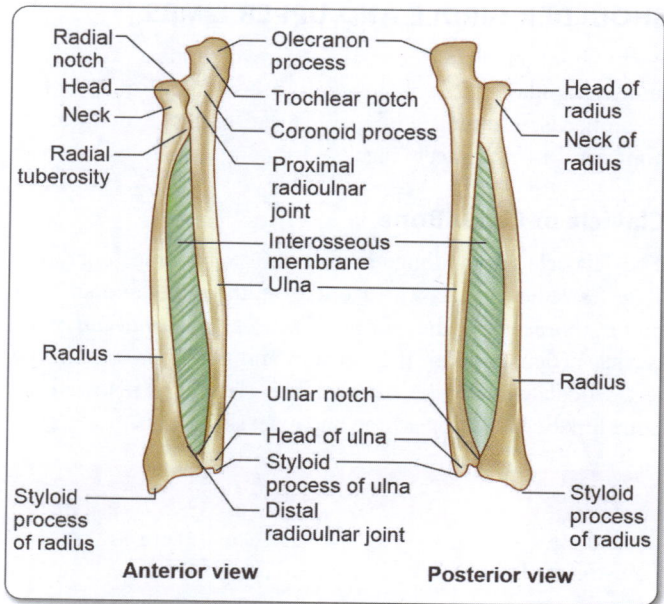

Fig. 7.1-22: Right radius and ulna with interosseous membrane

Features of some parts of ulna are (Fig. 7.1-22):

Upper end of ulna presents two processes—the *olecranon process* and *coronoid process*. In-between these two processes is present the *trochlear notch* which articulates with the trochlea of humerus.

Shaft of ulna is attached to that of radius with interosseous membrane.

Lower end presents knob-like *head* which articulates with a notch of the radius (ulnar notch) laterally and with a disc of fibrocartilage inferiorly which separates it from the wrist. The *medial styloid process* present at the lower end of ulna gives attachment to ligaments of wrist.

Bones of the Hand

Hand is composed of a wrist, a palm and five fingers. Bones of the hand include (Fig. 7.1-23):

Carpal bones, eight in number, bonded together in two rows of four bones each, form the bones of wrist. The compact mass of eight bones is called *carpus*. The carpus at its proximal surface articulates with the lower end of radius and ulna and at its distal surface articulates with the metacarpal bones.

Metacarpal bones, five in number (one in line with each finger) form the skeleton of the palm of hand (Fig. 7.1-23). These bones are cylindrical, with rounded distal ends that make the knuckles on a clenched fist. Proximally the metacarpal bones articulate with the carpus and distally with the phalanges.

Phalanges form the bones of fingers. Each finger consists of three phalanges—a proximal, a middle and a distal. The thumb has two phalanges.

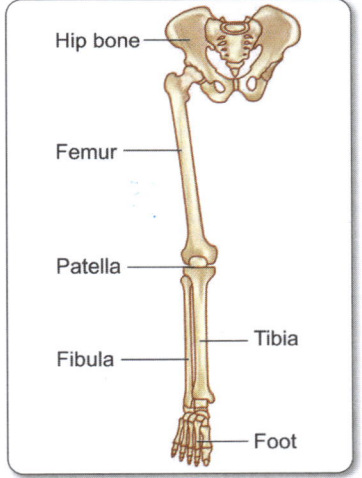

Fig. 7.1-24: Pelvic girdle

PELVIC GIRDLE AND LOWER LIMBS

Pelvic Girdle (Fig. 7.1-24)

Pelvic girdle is formed by two hip bones also known as innominate bones or ossa coxae.

Innominate or Hip Bones (Fig. 7.1-25)

Each hip bone consists of three parts (bones)—the ileum, ischium and pubis—which are fused together in the region of *acetabulum* (a socket into which the head of femur fits and forms the hip joint). Features of three fused bones forming hip bone are (Fig. 7.1-25):

Ileum, the upper expanded part of hip bone forms the prominence of hip. Posteriorly it joins the sacrum at sacroiliac joint. It bears an *iliac crest* and *anterior superior iliac spine*.

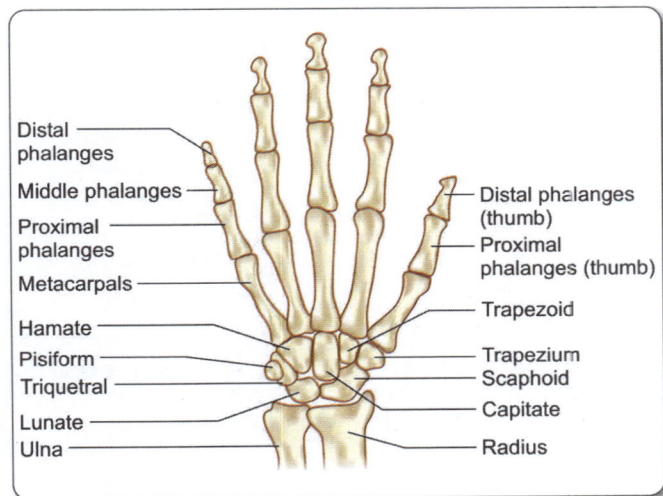

Fig. 7.1-23: Bones of hand

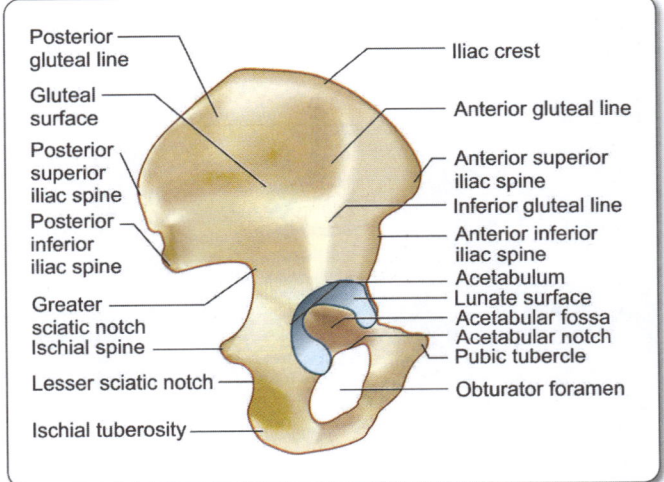

Fig. 7.1-25: The hip bone showing the union of ilium, ischium and pubis in the acetabulum

Ischium forms the inferior and posterior part of hip bone. It bears *ischial tuberosity* and ischial spine. The largest foramen in the skeleton, called the *obturator foramen*, is situated between the ischium and pubis.

Pubis, the anterior part of the hip bone, the two pubis bones are fused anteriorly at *symphysis pubis*.

Pelvis

Pelvic girdle, together with sacrum and coccyx forms the ring-like structure of pelvis which resembles a basin (Fig. 7.1-26).

Parts

The pelvis is divided into two parts by the brim of pelvis:
1. *Greater* or *false pelvis* is above the pelvic brim
2. *Lower* or *true pelvis* is below the pelvic brim.

Sex differences in Pelvises

Female pelvis is wider, pubic arch is broader, distance between the ischial spines and the ischial tuberosities is greater and sacral curvature is shorter. These differences between male and female pelvises are related to the function of the female pelvis as a birth canal.

Functions of Pelvis

- Provides a *stable support* for the trunk of the body and attachments to the legs. Weight of the body is transmitted through the pelvis to the legs and then onto the ground.
- *Protects* the organs such as urinary bladder, distal end of large intestine, and the internal reproductive organs.
- *True pelvis* in females functions as a birth canal.

Skeleton of Lower Limbs

The bones of each free lower limb is formed by the following 30 bones:

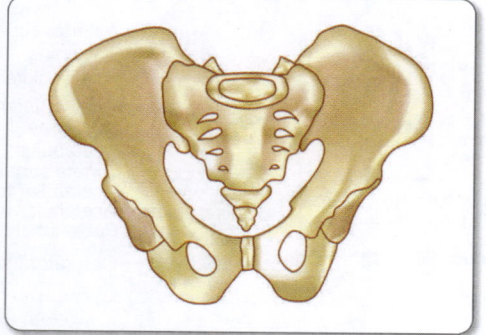

Fig. 7.1-26: The pelvis formed by two hip bones along with sacrum and coccyx

- Femur   1
- Patella   1
- Tibia   1
- Fibula   1
- Tarsal bones   7
- Metatarsals   5
- Phalanges   14

Femur

The femur or thigh bone, the longest and strongest bone of the body, extends from hip to the knee.

Parts of femur bone are (Figs 7.1-27A and B):

Head of femur is almost spherical and fits into the acetabulum of the hip bone to form hip joint. Fovea capitis is a pit on the head which marks the attachment of a ligament that holds the femur into acetabulum.

Neck and two processes (*greater trochanter* and *lower trochanter*) are present just below the head. These processes provide attachment for muscles of the legs and buttocks.

Shaft is long and connects upper end with lower end of the femur.

Lower end of the femur presents two large eminences—the medial and lateral *condyles*—and articulates with tibia and patella.

CLINICAL ASPECTS

Fracture at the neck of the femur is very common in elderly people.

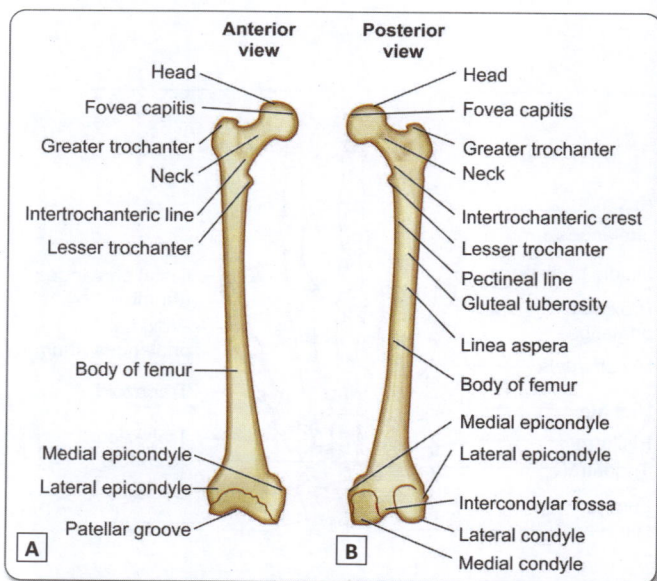

Figs 7.1-27A and B: Skeleton of pelvic girdle and right lower limb

Patella

The patella, also known as knee cap, is a flat sesamoid bone placed in the tendon of quadriceps femoris muscle. Its posterior surface articulates with the patellar surface of lower end of femur.

Tibia

The tibia, or shin bone, is the larger of the two lower leg bones and is located on the medial side. Salient features of tibia are (Fig. 7.1-28):

Upper end is expanded into two condyles, lateral and medial. Superior surfaces of condyles are concave and receive the convex condyles of femur to form the knee joint. Head of fibula articulates with the inferior aspect of lateral condyle.

Shaft of the tibia presents tibial tuberosity on its anterior surface below the condyles. Tibial tuberosity provides an attachment for the patellar ligament.

Lower end of tibia articulates with talus and fibula to form the ankle joint. A downward projection of lower end of tibia medial to the ankle joint is called *medial malleolus.*

Fibula

Fibula is a long, slender bone located on the lateral side of fibula. Its salient features are (Fig. 7.1-28):

Upper end is slightly enlarged to form the irregular head which articulates with tibia but does not enter the knee joint. Thus, fibula does not bear any of the body weight.

Shaft of fibula is attached with shaft of the tibia through an interosseous membrane.

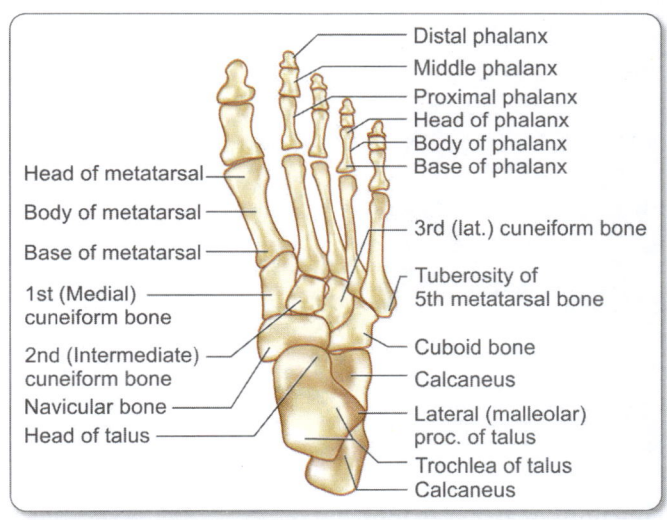

Fig. 7.1-29: Bones of foot (superolateral view)

Lower end is enlarged to form lateral malleolus which articulates with the ankle and can be felt as a prominence on the lateral side.

Bones of Foot

The foot consists of an ankle, instep and five toes. Bones of the foot include (Fig. 7.1-29):

Tarsal bones, seven in number, form the posterior part of the foot. Of these:

Talus articulates with the lower end of tibia and fibula at the ankle joint.

Remaining 6 tarsal bones are bound firmly together, forming a mass on which talus rests.

Calcaneus, or heel bone, is the largest tarsal bone. It is located below the talus where it projects backward to form the base of heel.

Metatarsal bones, five in number (one in line with each toe), form the skeleton of instep (Fig. 7.1-29). These bones are elongated and articulate posteriorly with the tarsus and anteriorly with the phalanges.

Phalanges. There are three phalanges in each toe, except the great toe which has only two.

Arches of Foot

The tarsal and metatarsal bones of the foot are arranged and bound by ligaments in such a way that arches of the foot are formed (Fig. 7.1-30):

* *The longitudinal arch* is highest on the medial side and extends from the heel to the toe.
* *The transverse arches* run across the foot in the metatarsal region.

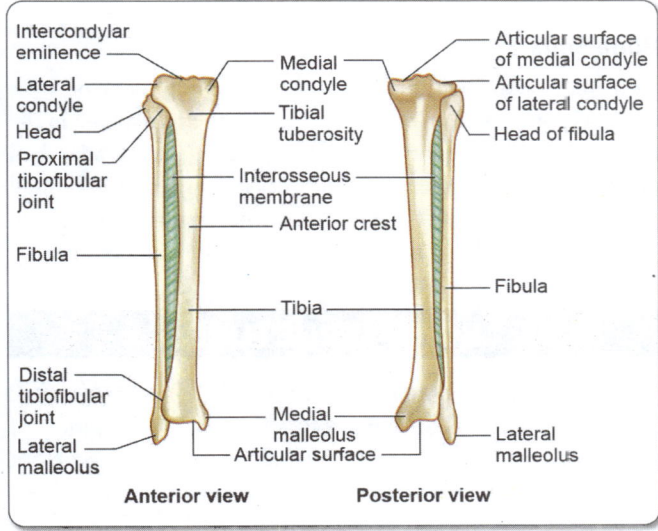

Fig. 7.1-28: Right tibia and fibula with interosseous membrane

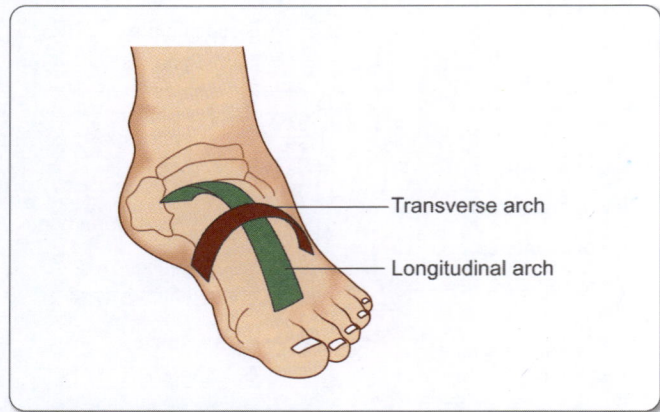

Fig. 7.1-30: Arches of the foot

Functions of arches of foot

The arches of foot provide a stable, springy base for the body. Sometimes, however, the tissues that bind the metatarsals together become weak, producing a condition called *fallen-arches* or flatfoot.

BONE: TYPES, PARTS AND COMPOSITION

Types of Bones

Bone is a specialized tough connective tissue that forms skeleton of the body. Depending upon the size and shape the bones have been classified as:
- Long bones, e.g., limb bones
- Short bones, e.g., wrist and ankle bones
- Flat bones, e.g., scapula, skull bones and mandible
- Irregular bones, e.g., vertebrae
- Sesamoid bones, e.g., patella.

Parts of Long Bone

Parts of a typical long bone are (Fig. 7.1-31):

Diaphysis (shaft) is the mid portion of the long bone.

Epiphysis is the widened part on either end of the bone.

Metaphysis is the portion between the diaphysis and epiphysis.

Epiphyseal cartilage or growth plate refers to a layer of cartilage that is present between the epiphysis and metaphysis during growing age.

Composition of Bone

Bone is composed of a collagenous framework (matrix) impregnated with bone salts. The dry, fat-free bone consists of one-third organic bone matrix, and two-thirds minerals (inorganic).

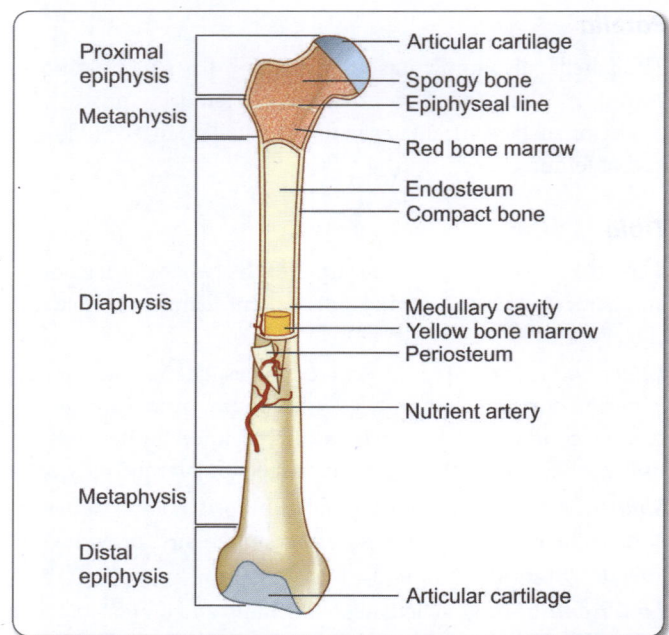

Fig. 7.1-31: Parts and gross structure of long bone as seen in longitudinal cut section

Bone Matrix

Bone matrix, also called osteoid, consists of collagen fibers embedded in the gelatinous ground substance.

Collagen fibers are arranged in lamellae. The fibers of one lamellus run parallel to each other. Over 90% of the organic matrix is type I collagen.

Ground substance is formed by the extracellular fluid and proteoglycans (which include chondroitin sulfate and hyaluronic acid). These substances are concerned with the regulation and deposition of bone salts.

Bone Salts

The bone salts constitute the inorganic component of bone which is comprised primarily of calcium and phosphate in the form of hydroxyapatite crystals $[Ca_{10}(PO_4)_6(OH)_2]$, adsorbed on the surface of hydroxyapatite crystals are present small amounts of other salts such as sodium, potassium, magnesium and carbonate. The bone salts strengthen the bone matrix.

BONE STRUCTURE

Structurally, two types of bones are known: *Compact* or *cortical bone*, and *trabecular* or *spongy* or *cancellous* bone. In most of the bones, both compact and cancellous forms are present, but thickness of each type varies in different regions of the bone.

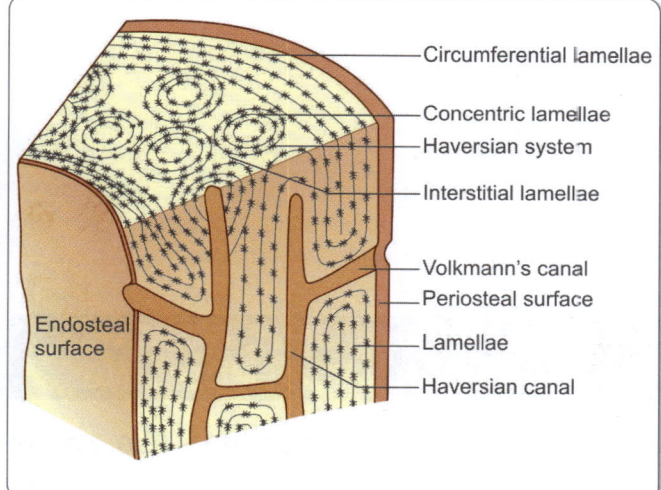

Fig. 7.1-32: Structure of compact bone

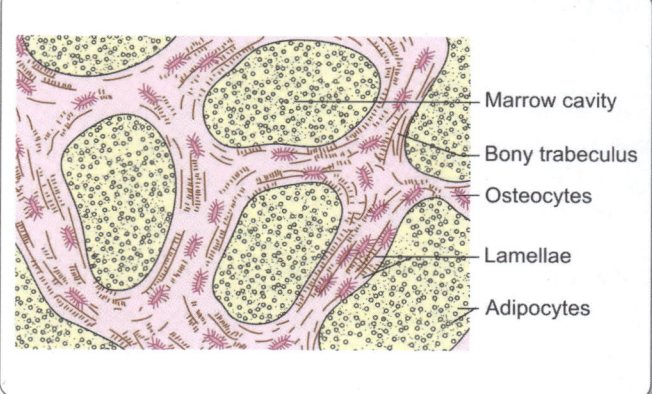

Fig. 7.1-33: Structure of trabecular spongy bone

STRUCTURE OF COMPACT BONE

The compact bone makes the outer layer of most bones and accounts for the 80% of the bone in the body.

Histologically, the compact bony tissue is made up of several minute cylindrical structures called *osteons* or *Haversian system* (Fig. 7.1-32). Each osteon is formed by several layers of collagen lamellae (Haversian lamellae) arranged concentrically around a centrally placed canal called the *Haversian canal* which contains the blood vessels, lymph vessels and nerve fibers. In-between the concentric layers of collagen tissue are present many *lacunae* (small cavities) which contain *osteocytes*. The osteocytes send long process called canaliculi all around.

The compact bone is lined externally by periosteum and internally by endosteum. Both periosteum and endosteum of the long bones contain osteoprogenitor cells which can differentiate into osteoblasts or osteoclasts.

STRUCTURE OF TRABECULAR OR SPONGY BONE

The trabecular or spongy or cancellous bone is present inside the compact bone and makes up the 20% of bone in the body. It is made up of spicules or plates or trabeculae which are separated by wide spaces that are filled in by bone marrow.

The trabeculae are thin and consist of irregular lamellae of bone with lacunae containing osteocytes. The trabeculae are covered by a thin layer of connective tissue called *endosteum* which contains osteoblasts, osteoclasts and osteoprogenitor (stem) cells (Fig. 7.1-33 and Histology Plate 7.1-1).

Histology Plate 7.1-1: Spongy bone

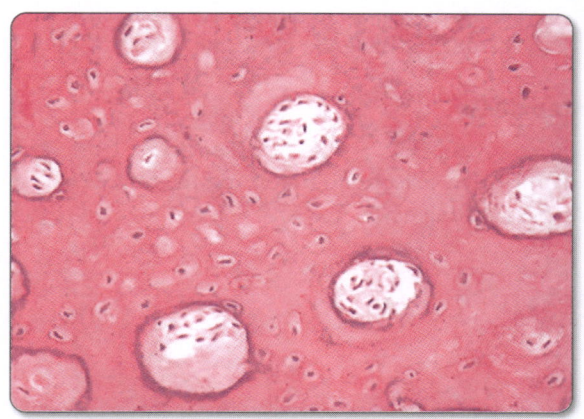

In high magnification, various lacunae are seen in the spongy bone and osteocytes are clearly visible.

CELLS OF BONE

Osteoprogenitor Cells

These are stem cells of mesenchymal origin that can proliferate and convert themselves into osteoblasts whenever there is need for bone formation. They resemble fibroblasts in appearance.

Osteoblasts

Bone forming cells are called osteoblasts. These are situated in the outer surface of bone, the marrow cavity and epiphyseal plate cells.

Functions

Role in laying down of the organic matrix of bone. Osteoblasts are responsible for synthesis of bone matrix by secreting type I collagen and a protein called *matrix gla protein* (MGP).

Role in calcification. Enzyme alkaline phosphatase present in the cell membranes of osteoblasts plays important role in the calcification of bone matrix.

Osteocytes

Cells of mature (or developed) bone are called osteocytes. As mentioned above they represent osteoblasts, which during bone formation are 'imprisoned' in the lacunae between the bone lamellae. The cytoplasmic processes from the osteocytes run into canaliculi and ramify throughout the bone matrix. The processes from neighboring cells have contact with each other forming tight junction.

Functions

Osteocytes play an important role in maintaining the exchange of calcium between the bone and extracellular fluid.

Osteoclasts

Bone removing cells are called osteoclasts. These are giant multinucleated cells found in relation to surfaces where bone removal is taking place.

Function

Osteoclasts are responsible for bone resorption during bone remodeling.

Bone Lining Cells

Bone lining cells are flattened cells which form a continuous epithelium-like layer on bony surfaces. They are present on the periosteal surface as well as endosteal surface.

BONE DEVELOPMENT, GROWTH, FORMATION AND REMODELING

BONE DEVELOPMENT AND GROWTH (FIG. 7.1-34)

All bone is of mesenchymal origin. The process of bone formation is called ossification. Development of bone tissue starts before birth and completed by 21 years of life. There are two mechanisms of bone formation:

1. Endochondral bone formation
2. Intramembranous bone formation.

1. Endochondral bone formation. During fetal development, formation of most of the bones is preceded by the formation of a cartilaginous model which is subsequently replaced by bone. This kind of ossification is called endochondral bone formation.

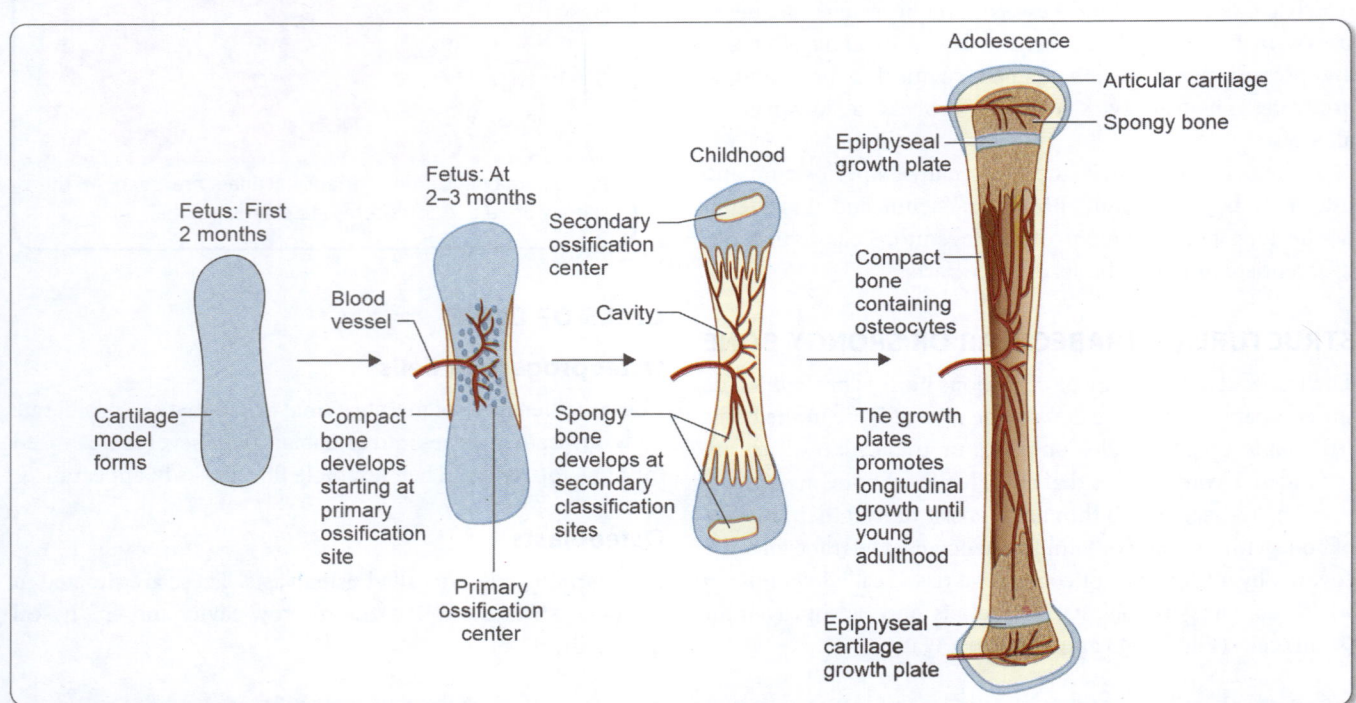

Fig. 7.1-34: Bone development and growth

2. Intramembranous bone formation. Formation of some bones, e.g., clavicle, vault of skull and mandibles is not preceded by formation of a cartilage model, but they are formed directly in a fibrous membrane. This kind of ossification is called intramembranous bone formation.

Development of Long Bones

The steps of formation of long bone are:

Formation of a Cartilage Model

In the region, where a long bone is to be formed, the mesenchyme first lays down a cartilaginous model of bone.

Ossification and Calcification

The ossification is carried out by osteoblasts which enter the central part of the cartilaginous model. This area is called *primary center of ossification* (Fig. 7.1-34). Gradually bone formation extends from the primary center toward the ends of shaft.

Growth in Length and Girth

After birth *secondary centers* of endochondral ossification appear in the cartilages forming the ends of bones. These centers enlarge and convert the cartilaginous ends into bone. The portion of the bone formed from one secondary center is called *epiphysis*. During growth, the bone of diaphysis and the bone of epiphysis are separated by a plate of actively proliferating cartilage, the *epiphyseal plate*. The portion of the diaphysis adjoining the epiphyseal plate is called metaphysis. It is highly vascular and region of active bone formation. The bone increases in length as this plate lays down new bone on the end of shaft. The growth of the bone stops when the epiphysis fuses with the diaphysis (*epiphyseal closure*). The normal age at which the epiphysis closes in different bones of the body is well known.

Even after bone growth has ceased, the calcium turnover function of bone is most active in the metaphysis which acts as a storehouse of calcium.

PROCESS OF BONE FORMATION

During growth bone formation is carried out by active osteoblasts. Bone is continuously deposited by these cells. The process of bone formation includes osteoid formation and mineralization of bone matrix.

Osteoid Formation

The osteoblasts synthesize and lay down the type I procollagen molecules into the adjacent extracellular space. These cells also secrete a gelatinous matrix in which the fibers get embedded.

Bone Matrix Mineralization

Soon after formation of osteoid the process of bone matrix mineralization starts. It occurs in two phases: an initial slow process of mineralizations followed by rapid mineralization process.

The process of mineralization greatly depends upon the *calcium × phosphate* ion product in extracellular fluid. This product must be above 30/dL for this process to occur. Most of the calcium phosphate is deposited within 6–12 hours. After the process of mineralization of bone matrix is completed, the osteoid is converted into a bone lamella (Fig. 7.1-35). After the formation of one bone lamella (as described above) another layer of osteoid is laid down by osteoblast. The osteoblasts move away from the bone lamella to line the new layer of osteoid. However, some osteoblasts are caught between the lamella and the osteoid.

Conversion of Trabecular Bone to Compact Bone

All newly formed bone is cancellous. It is converted into compact bone (Fig. 7.1-36):

- Each space between the trabeculae of cancellous bone comes to be lined by osteoblasts (Figs 7.1-36A and B).
- The osteoblasts lay down lamellae of bone as already described. The first lamella is formed over the inner wall of the original space and is, therefore, shaped like a ring (Fig. 7.1-36C).
- Subsequently, concentric lamellae are laid down inside this ring thus forming an *osteon*. The original space becomes smaller and smaller and persists as a *Haversian canal* (Fig. 7.1-36D).

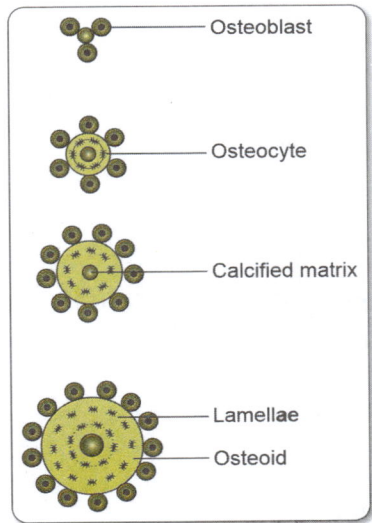

Fig. 7.1-35: Schematic depiction of process of formation of bone lamella

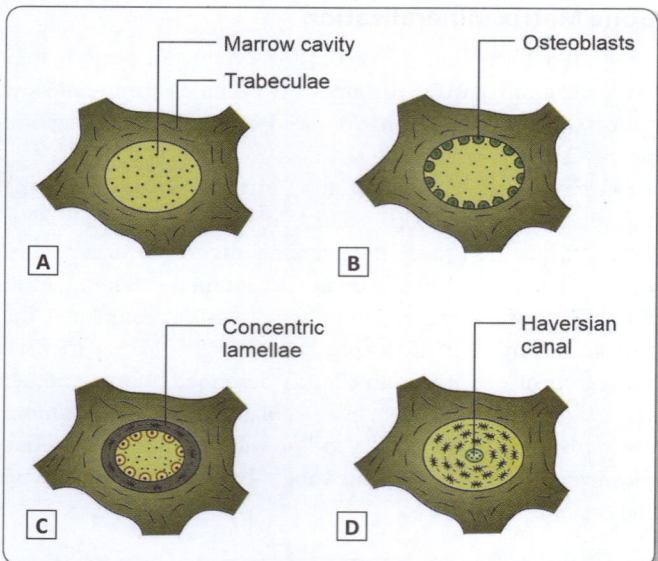

Figs 7.1-36A to D: Steps of conversion of trabecular bone into compact bone

BONE REMODELING AND RESORPTION

Bone Remodeling

Definition

Bone remodeling refers to a process of bone resorption followed by bone formation which keeps on occurring throughout life in a cyclic manner.

Phases of Bone Remodeling Cycle

A bone remodeling cycle takes about 100 days and consists of two phases: the resorption phase and the succeeding formation phase.

1. Resorption phase lasts for initial 10 days. In this phase mineralized bone is reabsorbed by osteoclasts releasing calcium and phosphate.

2. Formation phase lasts for next 90 days and is characterized by reformation of bone by osteoblasts (assimilating calcium and phosphate).

Physiological Significance of Continuous Bone Remodeling

Bone adjusts its strength in proportion to the degree of bone stress. For example, in athletes, soldiers and others in whom the bone stress is more, the bones become heavy and strong.

Shape of bone can be rearranged for proper support of mechanical force in accordance with the stress.

Old bone becomes relatively weak and brittle. The development of new bone matrix maintains the toughness of bone.

Bone Resorption

Bone resorption, like bone formation, is a continuous process. In bone resorption, there occurs destruction of entire matrix of bone resulting in diminished bone mass.

Osteoclasts are the cells responsible for bone resorption.

REGULATION OF BONE GROWTH AND REMODELING

Regulation of bone growth and remodeling include:
- Regulation of osteoid formation
- Regulation of bone resorption
- Regulation of bone remodeling.

Regulation of Osteoid Formation

The factors affecting process of osteoid formation include protein intake and a number of growth factors such as Tissue growth factor beta (TGF-β), Insulin growth factor I and II (IGF-I and IGF-II), Platelet-derived growth factor (PDGF), and fibroblast growth factors, etc. Besides these growth factors, insulin, GH, sex hormones (estrogens, androgen), thyroid hormones, calcitriol and calcitonin also affect the process of osteoid formation.

Regulation of Bone Resorption

The bone resorption is stimulated by PTH, calcitriol, epithelial growth factor (EGF), PDGF and some other growth factors. The response is mediated through release of prostaglandins. Thyroxine and vitamin A also increase bone resorption.

Regulation of Bone Remodeling

The paired activity of osteoclast and osteoblast cells in bone remodeling is well regulated.

FUNCTIONS OF BONES

Bones subserve the following important functions:

Protective function. The framework formed by the bones protects the vital organs and soft tissues of the body, e.g., thoracic cage protects lungs and heart, and skull protects brain.

Mechanical functions served by the bones include:
- *Support* to body
- *Attachment* to muscles and tendons
- *Movements* are performed at the joints by leverage effects of bones.

Metabolic functions of bone include their important role in homeostasis of calcium and phosphate metabolism.

Hemopoietic function includes the formation of blood cells in the red bone marrow.

CLINICAL ASPECTS

OSTEOPOROSIS

Osteoporosis is referred to weak and porous bones that are incapable of maintaining normal bone functions.

Primary risk factors include *female gender*, *history of smoking*, *low body weight*, *advanced age* and *menopause* (or other *hormonal aberrations*). Any factor that interferes with the appropriate mineralization of bone can lead to osteoporosis.

Calcium and *Vitamin D* supplements are generally recommended in addition to healthy or balanced diet and regular physical activity.

OSTEOGENESIS IMPERFECTA

Osteogenesis imperfecta is a disorder of bones with *genetically pattern of inheritance*. This disorder is marked by: Bone fractures that are mostly pathological (which means without any force of impact or injury).

PAGET'S DISEASE OF BONE

Paget disease is another common *musculoskeletal* disease that may also involve the hearing. This disorder is characterized by high growth of bones that primarily affect *long bones of the body*. The bones increase in size but are also weak and vulnerable to injuries, fractures and dislocations.

OSTEOMALACIA

Osteomalacia is an acquired condition caused by *deficiency of vitamin D* in adults *and in children is referred to as rickets*.

FRACTURE

Fracture refers to a breech or break in the continuity of bones. Most commonly bones fractured are long bones of the body (*like humerus, ulna, radius, femur, tibia* and *fibula*). In some susceptible individuals, the spinal and pelvic bones can also get fractured (as a result of accidents, falls or assault).

FIBROUS DYSPLASIA

When fibrous tissue (*a type of scar tissue*) replaces the normal bone, the disorder is referred to as fibrous dysplasia. Most common sites are (*femur*), shinbone (*tibia*), *humerus, pelvic bones, ribs, skull* and *facial bones*. It may also occur as part of pituitary gland (presenting with signs of precocious puberty).

OSTEITIS FIBROSA CYSTIC

Hypersecretion of certain hormones like parathyroid gland leads to excessive resorption of bones leading to osteitis fibrosa cystic *bone lesions*.

CHONDROBLASTOMA

Chondroblastoma is *benign tumors* that usually involve terminal ends of long bones (*like upper limb bones or thigh bones*). It is most common in individuals younger than 25 years.

OSTEOCHONDRITIS DISSECANS

It is a rare bone condition in which the cartilage and bone separate from the edges of the long bones due to interruption in the blood supply. The primary pathophysiological feature of this disorder is an unstable joint. Most commonly involved joints are *knee, elbows, ankles* and *pelvis*. The dislodged pieces of bone are referred to as "joint mice". The primary sign and symptoms are:

- *Clicking or cracking sensation whenever the affected joint is moved.*
- *Limitation of range of motion.*
- *Weakness of muscles.*
- *Pain and stiffness that aggravate after mild to moderate physical activity.*

NURSING IMPLICATIONS AND APPLICATIONS

1. Care of patient with joint replacement (Hip joint/Knee joint). The nursing care in such patients include:
- Assessment of vital signs
- Toileting help
- Measurement of drain output
- Feeding the patient if necessary
- Appropriate positioning is important to minimize the risk of dislocation
- Ambulatory assistance

2. *Orthopedic Rehabilitation.* For orthopedic rehabilitation, nurse has to focus on the prevention and treatment of musculo-skeletal disorders with special skills like:
- Neurovascular status monitoring
- Traction
- Passive movement therapy
- Casting and internal fixation

3. *Bone marrow biopsy* can be done from the following sites;
- Iliac crest
- Manubrium sterni, and
- Upper end of fibula

Applications

Sternal puncture (See page 348)

Epidural anesthesia: For painless delivery anesthetic agent is injected into the epidural space through sacral hiatus.

Paracentesis thoracis: For draining fluid from the pleural cavity recommended site for putting the needle is intercostal space between 8th and 9th rib to avoid injury to diaphragm.

Bone Fracture

Ribs: Fracture of middle ribs is common. The broken rib ends may injure the lung/spleen, fracture of lower ribs may lead to diaphragmatic hernia.

Hip dysplasia is displacement of head of the femur from acetabulum.

Fracture of neck of the humerus causes injury to axillary nerve leading to numbness/weakness of shoulder and upper arm.

Prolapse of intervertebral disc presses on the nerve roots to cause varied symptoms (pain, numbness, hypotension and giddiness) depending on the level of prolapse.

ASSESS YOURSELF

Short and Long Answer Questions

1. **Describe briefly:**
   - Functions of bones
   - Composition of bone
   - Parts of long bone
2. **Differentiate between:**
   - Compact and spongy bone
   - Endochondral and intramembranous bone formation
   - Osteoblast and osteoclasts
   - Axial and appendicular skeleton
3. **Write notes on:**
   - Cavities of skull
   - Thoracic cage
   - Paranasal sinuses

Multiple Choice Questions

1. **Which of the following not included in the axial skeleton:**
   a. Skull   b. Sternum
   c. Scapula   d. Vertebral column
2. **Patella belongs to skeleton of:**
   a. Pectoral girdle   b. Pelvic girdle
   c. Upper extremity   d. Lower extremity
3. **The number of metatarsals is:**
   a. 10   b. 14
   c. 16   d. 28
4. **The parietal bones articulate with each other at:**
   a. Lambdoid suture   b. Sagittal suture
   c. Coronal suture   d. None of these
5. **The true statement for temporal bone:**
   a. Zygomatic process is its anterior projection
   b. Its petrous part is large and flat
   c. Its Squamous part lies in the cranium
   d. Its squamous part articulates with occipital bone
6. **Which of the following facial bone is single:**
   a. Maxilla   b. Zygomatic
   c. Frontal   d. Sphenoid
7. **The statement not true for orbit:**
   a. Formed by parts of seven bones
   b. Medial wall is frequently fractured
   c. Its roof is formed by maxillary bone
   d. It has two orifices
8. **Number of lumbar vertebrae in vertebral column is:**
   a. 4   b. 5
   c. 7   d. 12

9. **Which of the following is an atypical vertebra:**
   a. Thoracic   b. Lumbar
   c. 2nd cervical   d. 5th cervical
10. **True about xiphoid process of sternum:**
    a. Attached with clavicle
    b. Two pairs of ribs are attached to it
    c. Forms the middle part of sternum
    d. No rib attached to it
11. **Which of the following ribs is true rib:**
    a. 7th pair   b. 8th pair
    c. 9th pair   d. 12th pair
12. **The true statement about clavicle:**
    a. Attached to the glenoid cavity
    b. Its inner end is called acromion end
    c. Forms only link with axial skeleton and upper limb
    d. Articulates with spine of scapula
13. **Female pelvis differs from male pelvis having:**
    a. Narrow pelvic arch
    b. Short sacral curvature
    c. Less distance between ischial spine and ischial tubrisity
    d. Narrow pelvis
14. **The head of femur:**
    a. Fits into glenoid cavity
    b. Fits into acetabulum
    c. Articulates with fovea capitis
    d. Attached to hip bone through greater trochanter
15. **Colles fracture is fracture of:**
    a. Neck of femur   b. Clavicle
    c. Lower end of radius d. Lower end of ulna
16. **The statement not true for osteoblasts:**
    a. Formed from osteo progenitor cells
    b. Located on the outer surface of the bone
    c. Secrete collagen I
    d. Maintain calcium exchange between bone and ECF
17. **The bone which is formed by intramembranous bone formation process:**
    a. Humerus   b. Clavicle
    c. Scapula   d. Pelvis
18. **The secondary center of ossification is present at:**
    a. Metaphysis
    b. Epiphyseal plate
    c. Cartilages at the ends of bones
    d. Diaphysis

ANSWER KEY

1.	c	2.	d	3.	c	4.	b	5.	a	6.	c	7.	c	8.	b
9.	c	10.	d	11.	a	12.	c	13.	b	14.	b	15.	b	16.	d
17.	b	18.	a												

DEFINITION AND CLASSIFICATION

Joints or articulations are junctions between two or more bones or cartilages. The joints can be classified according to their structural composition and according to the amount of movement they are capable of.

A. Structural classification. On the basis of intervening tissue:
- Fibrous joints
- Cartilaginous joints
- Synovial joints

B. Functional classification. According to the degree of movement permitted:
- Immovable joints (synarthroses)
- Slightly movable joints (amphiarthroses)
- Freely movable joints (diathroses)

C. Regional classification. (On the basis of location):
- Skull type
- Vertebral type
- Limb type

GENERAL DESCRIPTION OF JOINTS

For the purpose of description of structure and general features of various joints, the following mixed classification is considered (Figs 7.2-1A to J):
- Fibrous (or immovable or skull type) joints.
- Cartilaginous (or slightly movable or vertebral type) joints.
- Synovial (or freely movable or limb type) joints.

FIBROUS JOINTS

Fibrous or immovable joints (synarthroses) are also called skull type joints, since they are generally limited to skull. These joints have fibrous tissues between the two articulating surfaces. These are of the following types:
- Sutures
- Syndesmosis
- Gomphosis
- Schindylesis

Sutures

Sutures refer to the immovable joints found between the bones. For example, between skull bones.

Salient features of sutures or sutural joints are:
- A thin layer of fibrous tissue may be present between the two bones (Fig. 7.2-2A).
- According to the shape of bony margins, the sutures can be plane, serrate, *denticulate* (dentate), squamous or limbus type.
- Periosteum on the outer and inner surfaces of these bones bridge the gaps between them and form the primary bond at the suture.
- No active movement takes place at an immovable joint.

Syndesmosis

Syndesmosis is a type of fibrous joint in which two bones are connected by an interosseous ligament. This usually allows slight but occasionally more extensive movement between them (Fig. 7.2-2B). For example, *inferior tibiofibular joint*.

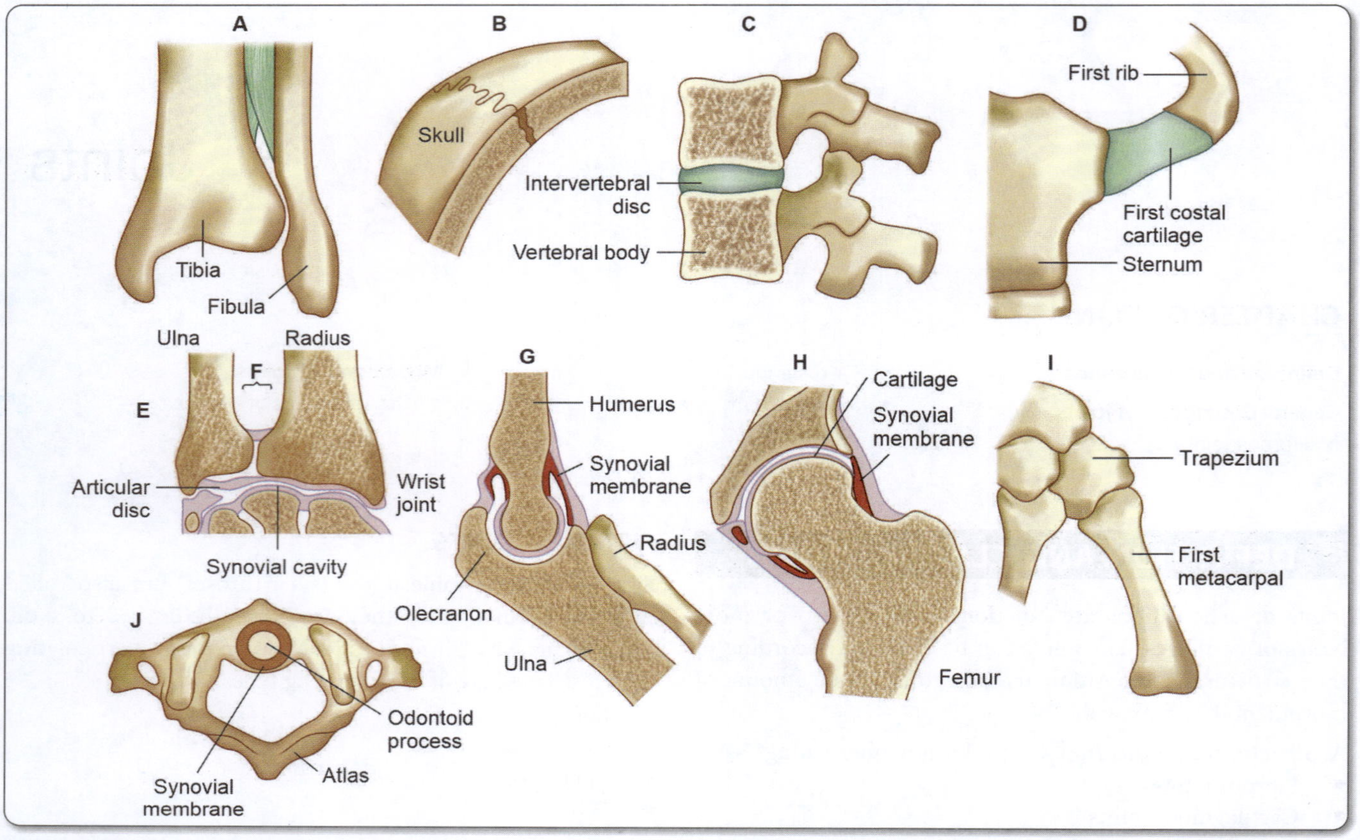

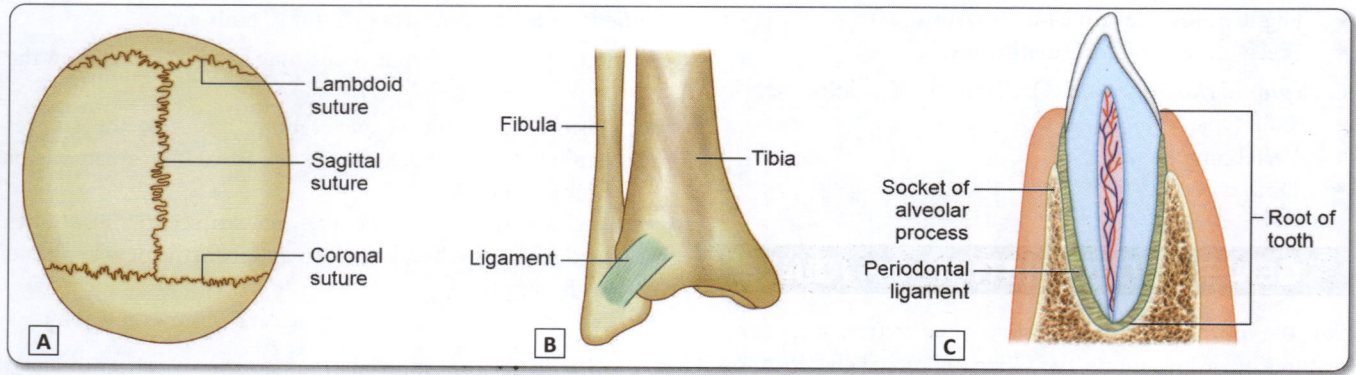

Figs 7.2-1A to J: General description of joints. A. Syndesmosis; B. Suture (skull); C. Symphysis (vertebral bodies); D. Synchondrosis (first rib and sternum); E. Condyloid (wrist); F. gliding (radioulnar); G. Hinge (elbow); H. Ball and socket (hip); I. Saddle (carpometacarpal); and J. Pivot (atlantoaxial)

Figs 7.2-2A to C: The fibrous joints. A. Suture; B. Syndesmosis; C. Gomphosis

Gomphosis

Gomphosis is also known as *'peg and socket joint'*. These joints are typically seen as a joint between tooth and jaw (*articulation dentoalveolus*). The cavity in jaw and root of tooth is connected by some fibrous tissues (Fig. 7.2-2C).

Schindylesis

Schindylesis refers to a wedge and groove type joint between two bones. For example, rostrum of sphenoid and ala of vomer.

CARTILAGINOUS JOINTS

Cartilaginous or slightly movable joints (amphiarthroses) are also called vertebral type of joints. As the name indicates, in such joints, the two bones are joined by cartilage. Cartilaginous joints are of two varieties:

1. Primary cartilaginous joints
2. Secondary cartilaginous joints.

1. *Primary cartilaginous joints (Synchondroses).* These are temporary joints seen in childhood during development of the bones. For example, first rib is joined to manubrium sterni through cartilage (Fig. 7.2-3A).

2. *Secondary cartilaginous joints (Symphyses).* In such joints, the articular surfaces of the two bones are covered by a thin layer of hyaline cartilage, and united by a disc of fibrocartilage (Fig. 7.2-3B).

Salient features of such joints are:
● These joints are permanent and persist throughout life.
● Typically such joints occur in the median plane of the body.
● These permit limited movements due to compressible pad of fibrocartilage.

Examples of secondary cartilaginous joints include:
● Pubic symphysis, and
● Joints between bodies of vertebrae.

SYNOVIAL JOINTS

Synovial or freely movable joints (diarthroses) are also called limb joints.

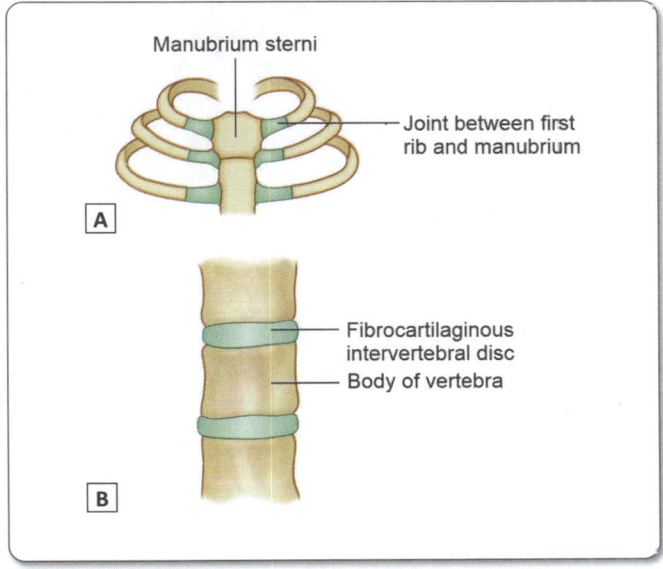

Figs 7.2-3A and B: The cartilaginous joints. A. Primary; B. Secondary

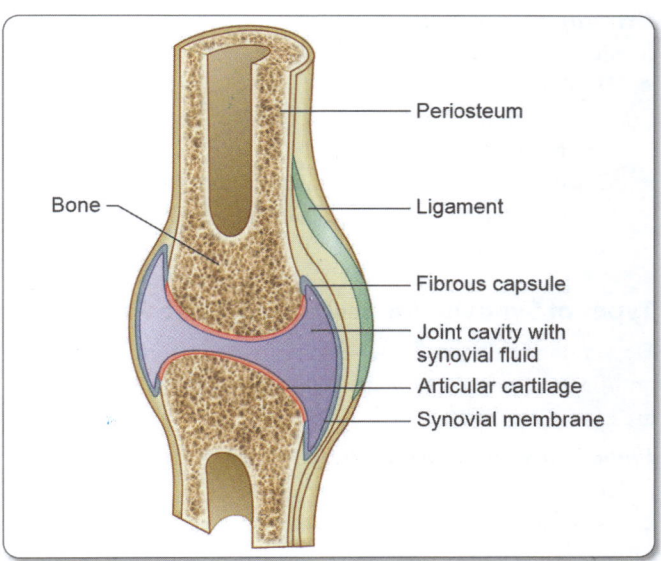

Fig. 7.2-4: The synovial joint

Structural Characteristics

Structural characteristics of synovial joints are (Fig. 7.2-4):

Articular or hyaline cartilage caps the ends of two bones taking part in the joint. This cartilage has neither blood vessels nor lymphatics (nor has it any nerves). It receives nourishment from the synovial fluid.

Articular capsule, made up of fibrous tissue, encloses the ends of two bones making the joint. The fibrous capsule is sufficiently loose to allow free movements at the joint but is strong enough to protect it from injury.

Synovial membrane, a thin sheet of connective tissue and epithelial cells, lines the inside of fibrous capsule. Synovial membrane also covers all intracapsular structures that do not bear weight. It secretes synovial fluid.

Synovial fluid, slippery like egg white, is a dialysate of blood plasma plus a mucin called hyaluronic acid (which provides viscidity and lubricating properties to the synovial fluid). Synovial fluid serves the following *functions:*
● *Lubricates* the intracapsular joint structures.
● *Nourishes* the structures within the joint cavity.
● *Maintains* joint stability.
● *Phagocytes* present in it remove microbes and cellular debris from the joint cavity.

Other intracapsular structures which are present in some joints (not all) include:
● *Fat pads and menisci* (semilunar cartilage) are present in knee joints.
● *Bursae,* the closed fluid filled sacs, are also present in some joints, e.g., knee joint. They act as cushion to prevent friction.

Extracapsular structures which support the joints from outside the capsule include:

- *Ligaments,* made of dense fibrous tissues, blend with the capsule in the form of thick cords and bands and provide additional stability to most synovial joints.
- *Muscles or their tendons* which are attached on the bones forming joints also provide stability to the joints during movements.

Types of Synovial Joints (Figs 7.2-5A to F)

Depending upon the shape of the articulating part of the bone and/or the range of movement permitted, the synovial joints are of various types:

Plane joints or gliding joints. They are characterized by flat articulating surfaces which allow only gliding movement, e.g., carpal joints and joints of small tarsal bones (Fig. 7.2-5A).

Hinge joints. In such joints, one articulating surface is concave and other convex. These are *uniaxial joints* which allow movements in one direction (flexion and extension) like a door on its hinges. Examples of hinge joints include elbow joint, knee joint, and interphalangeal joints of the fingers and toes (Fig. 7.2-5B).

Pivot joints. In such joints one bone end is rod-shaped, that fits into a ring made, partly of bone and partly of ligament. Thus, pivot joints are uniaxial joints in which movement in such joints is limited to rotation about a central axis as with a neck in a collar. Examples of such a joint are joint between first and second cervical vertebrae and the superior radio-ulnar joint (Fig. 7.2-5C).

Condyloid joints. In such joints, an oval-shaped condyle of one bone fits into an eliptical cavity of another bone as in the case of the joints between the metacarpals and phalanges. These joints are *biaxial*, i.e., allow a variety of movements in two planes, e.g., flexion and extension, and adduction and abduction; however, rotational movements are not allowed.

Ellipsoid joints. In such joints, the convex articulating surface is elliptical rather than round and the other is a socket, e.g., the radiocarpal (wrist) joint. Such joints are *biaxial* and allow movements in various planes but no rotations (Fig. 7.2-5D).

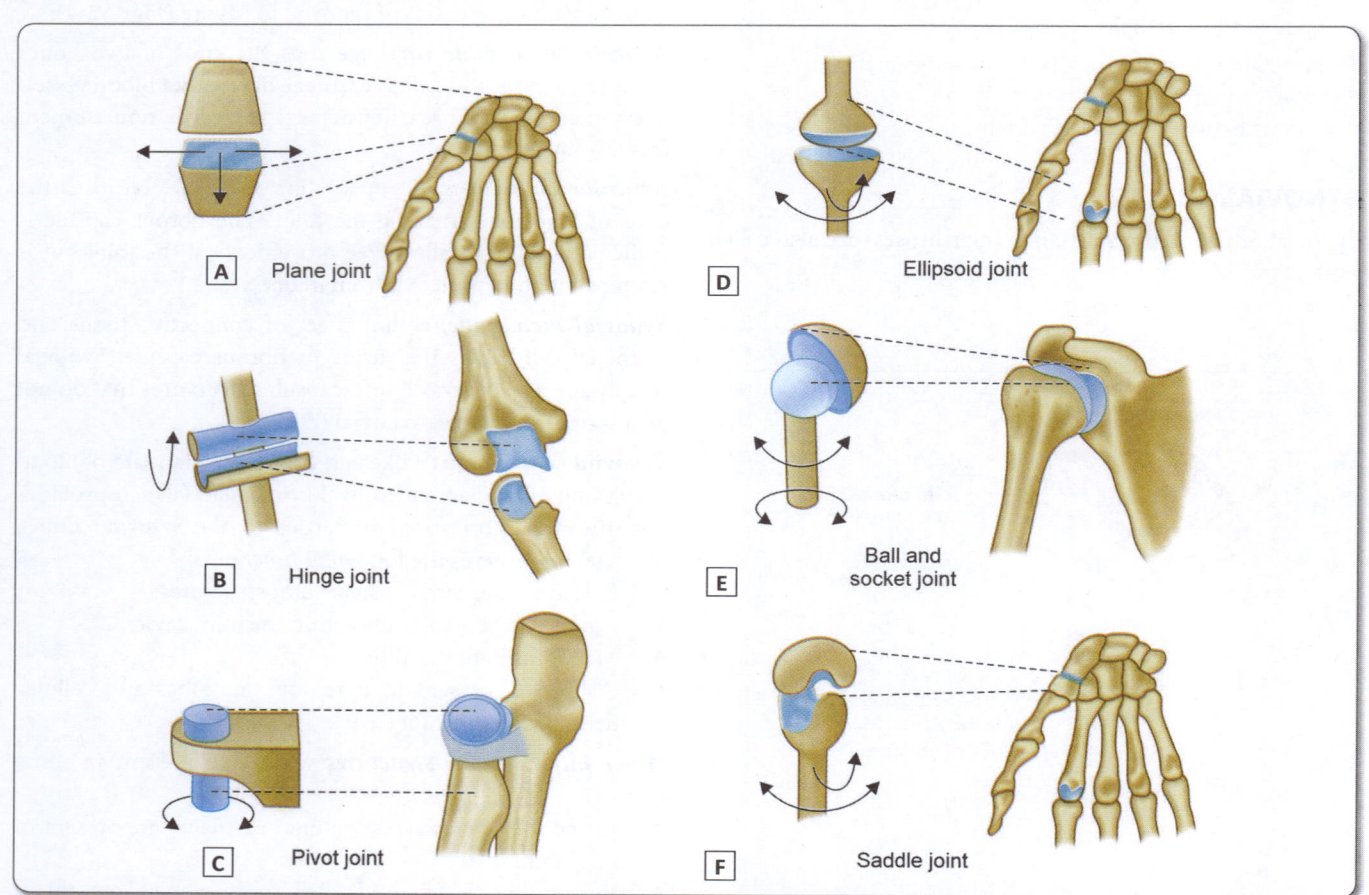

Figs 7.2-5A to F: Types of synovial joints

Ball and socket joint. In such joints, a ball-shaped head of one bone fits into a cup-shaped socket of another bone. These joints are *multiaxial* and thus allow movements in all planes, as well as rotational movement around a central axis. Examples of such joints are shoulder joint and hip joint (Fig. 7.2-5E).

Saddle joints. In such joints, articulating surfaces have both concave and convex regions; surface of one bone fits into complementary surface of another. In other words, the surfaces are reciprocally saddle-shaped. Being *multiaxial* such joints allow a variety of movements. Example includes joint between carpal and metacarpal bones of thumb (Fig. 7.2-5F).

CLINICAL ASPECTS

TRAUMATIC LESIONS OF JOINTS

Joints are subjected to considerable stress and are commonly injured during strenuous physical activity resulting in dislocations and sprain.

DISLOCATION OF JOINT

This is a condition in which the articular surfaces of a joint are separated and displaced in such a way that one surface loses its contact completely from the other. If a partial contact is still retained, it is better called *subluxation.* Dislocation usually occurs from a fall or other form of trauma and is characterized by pain, deformity, and loss of function. X-ray is confirmatory. The joints of shoulders, knee, elbows, fingers and mandible are common sites for dislocation.

SPRAINS

They are the result of stretching or tearing of the ligaments or tendons at a joint, i.e., soft tissue injury without dislocating the bones. They are usually caused by wrenching or twisting of joint excessively.

PENETRATING INJURIES

May be caused by a compound fracture of one of the articulating bones, or trauma caused by gun shot.

ARTHRITIS

Arthritis refers to inflammation of one or more joints. It can be caused by a variety of diseases. The most common types are:

Rheumatoid Arthritis

This is systemic disease with widespread involvement of joints and connective tissue. In this condition, the synovial membrane of the freely movable joints becomes inflamed and grows thicker. This change is usually followed by damage to the articular cartilages on the ends of bones and an invasion of joint by fibrous tissue.

Gouty Arthritis

Gout is a metabolic disorder of purine metabolism. Uric acid crystals may be deposited in the joints. The joint most frequently involved is the metatarsophalangeal of the great toe.

DEGENERATIVE DISORDERS

Osteoarthritis

This is a common degenerative noninflammatory condition which occurs in joints that are subject to a great deal of wear and tear. It usually occurs in individuals after the age of 45 years. The articular cartilage of involved joint shows degenerative change in the center (fibrillation of cartilage) and proliferative change around the edges (osteophages). The spine and joints of the lower extremity are most frequently involved causing pain and restricted movement of affected joints.

MOVEMENTS OF JOINTS

As mentioned above, a variety of movements are possible depending upon the type of joint. These can be grouped as below:

Rotation. It is the movement of a bone around its own axis in a pivot joint; for example, shaking your head to say 'no' (Figs 7.2-6A to C)

Abduction. It is a movement from the midline or axis of the body; for example, moving the arm away from the body or spreading the fingers apart (Fig. 7.2-6D)

Adduction. It is a movement toward midline of the body; for example, closing arms to the chest or bringing together (Fig. 7.2-6D).

Circumduction. It describes a movement in which a long bone circumscribes a conical space by rotation around an imaginary for example, swinging the arms or legs (Fig. 7.2-6E).

Flexion. It means to bend: Flexion brings two bones closer together and decreases the angle between them; for example bending the elbow or the knee (Fig. 7.2-6F)

Extension. It means to straighten, the opposite of flexion. It is extension between the two bones; for example, extending the flexed elbow.

Supination. It is a specialized rotation of the forearm that turns the palm of the hand forward or anteriorly. If the elbow is flexed, supination turns the palm of hand upward or superiorly (Fig. 7.2-6G)

Pronation. It is the opposite of supination. It is a specialized rotation of the forearm that turns the palm of hand backward or posteriorly. If the elbow is flexed, pronation turns the palm of the hand downward or inferiorly (Fig. 7.2-6H)

Dorsiflexion. Flexion of ankle in which the dorsum of the foot is lifted upward, decreasing the angle between the foot and the leg; for example, standing on your heels (Fig. 7.2-6I)

Plantar flexion. It is the movement of the ankle that increases the angle between the foot and leg; for example, standing on your toes (Fig. 7.2-6I).

Inversion. It is the movement of the sole of the foot inward or medially (Fig. 7.2-6J).

Eversion. It is the opposite of inversion. It is the movement of the sole of the foot outward or laterally (Fig. 7.2-6K).

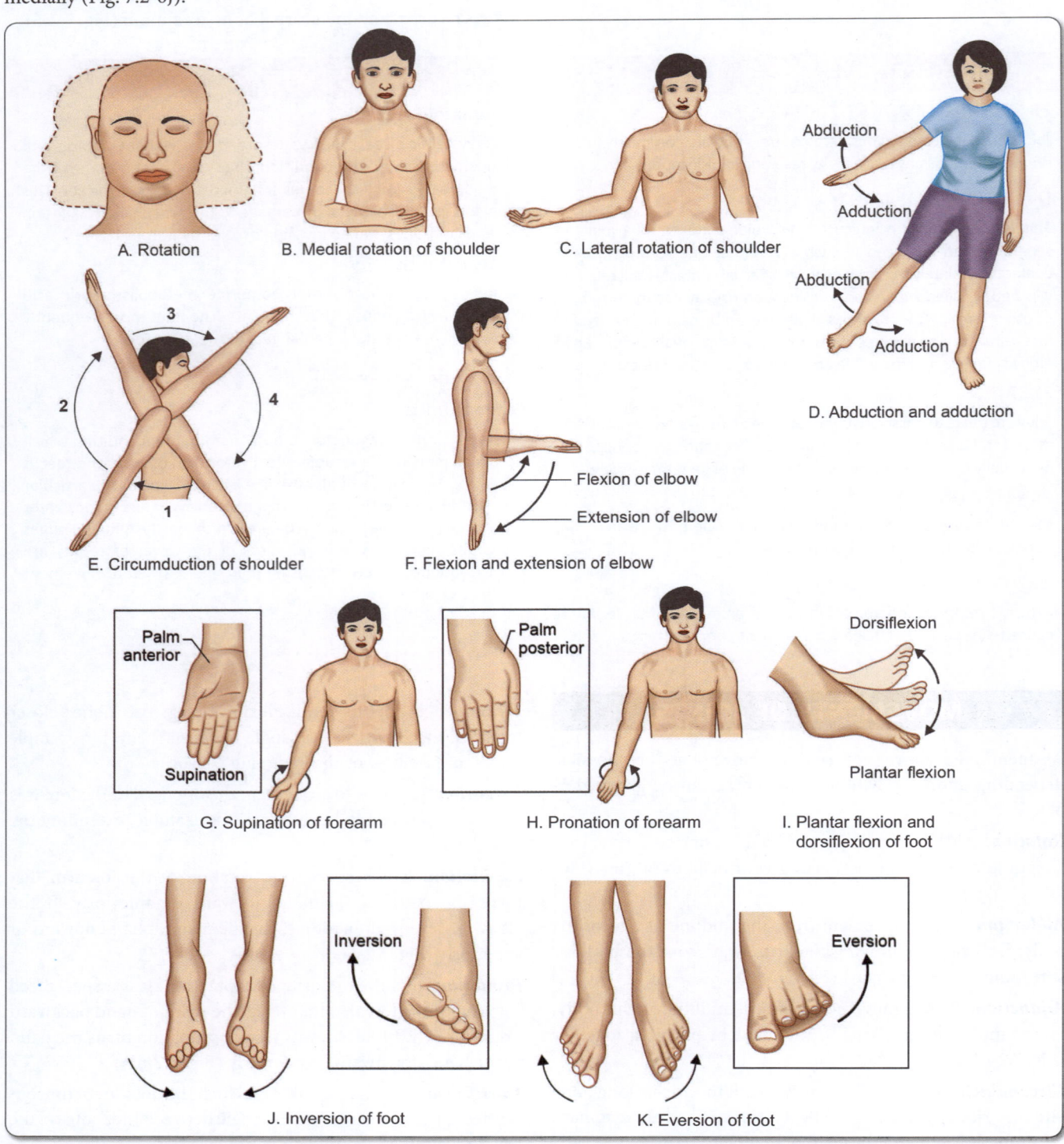

A. Rotation

B. Medial rotation of shoulder

C. Lateral rotation of shoulder

Abduction
Adduction
Abduction
Adduction

D. Abduction and adduction

E. Circumduction of shoulder

Flexion of elbow
Extension of elbow

F. Flexion and extension of elbow

Palm anterior
Supination

G. Supination of forearm

Palm posterior

H. Pronation of forearm

Dorsiflexion
Plantar flexion

I. Plantar flexion and dorsiflexion of foot

Inversion

J. Inversion of foot

Eversion

K. Eversion of foot

Figs 7.2-6A to K: Common types of body movement

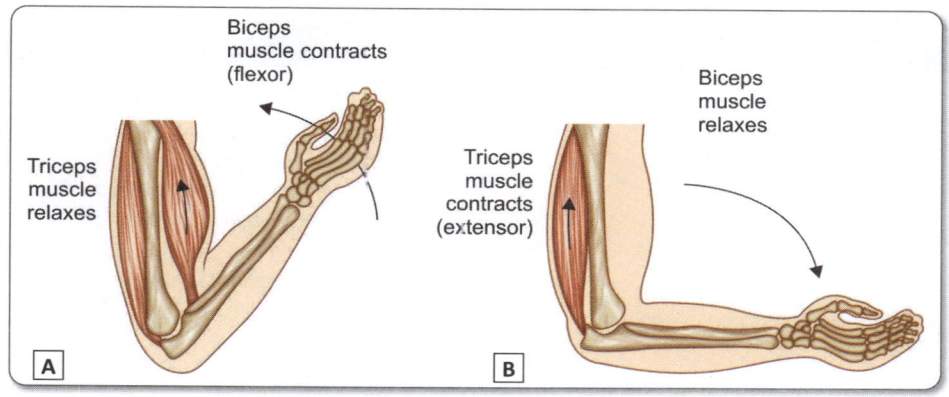

Figs 7.2-7A and B: Muscles: A. Agonist; B. Antagonist

GROUP ACTIONS OF MUSCLES

Each movement at a joint is coordinated by several skeletal muscles acting in group rather than individually. According to their group actions, the muscles are named and classified as below.

Agonist (Prime Mover)

Agonist refers to the muscle, which produces the desired action. For example, biceps brachi agonist; which produces flexion at the elbow joint is considered agonist. Similarly, triceps brachii which produces extension at elbow is considered agonist for this movement (Figs 7.2-7A and B).

Antagonist (Opponent)

The term antagonist is used for a muscle producing opposite movement than the primary mover at the same joint. For example, triceps, which produces extension at elbow joint is antagonist of biceps which produces flexion at the elbow. Similarly, for extension movement, the triceps is agonist and biceps is antagonist (Fig. 7.2-7B).

It is important to note that a particular movement is brought about by coordinated movement of both agonists and antagonists. For example, for producing flexion movement at elbow the agonist (i.e., biceps muscle) contracts and the antagonist (i.e., triceps) relaxes (Fig. 7.2-7A). Thus, in other words, the antagonist having opposite action cooperates for a movement with the agonists by relaxing. This is due to reciprocal innervation of the opposite group of muscles, regulated by the spinal cord through stretch reflex. Reciprocal innervation is goverened by the *Sherrington's law*, which states that when the agonist muscles get full innervation from the brain, simultaneously the antagonist gets zero innervation.

Fixator

Fixator refers to a group of muscles, which stabilize the proximal joints of a limb, so that the desired movement at the distal joint may occur. For example, for flexion at elbow, the deltoid and pectoralis major muscles act as fixator, as they stabilize and fix the arm and shoulder in a suitable position so that flexion at elbow can be produced by contraction of agonist (biceps) and relaxation of antagonist (triceps).

Synergist

Synergist refers to the group of muscles, which while contracting produce same movement at the particular joint. For example, brachialis and brachioradialis muscles also produce flexion at elbow by their contraction. So, they act as synergists to the biceps brachii muscle (Fig. 7.2-8).

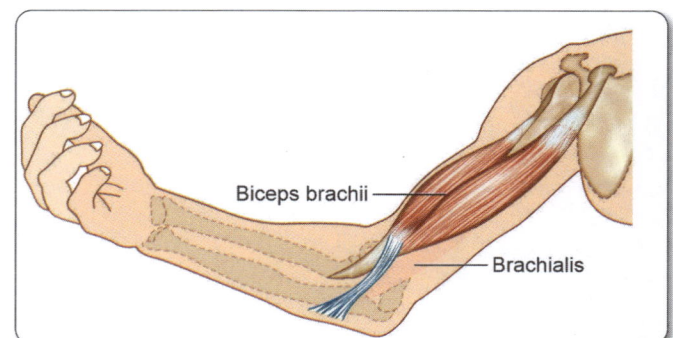

Fig. 7.2-8: Synergist muscles

ASSESS YOURSELF

Short and Long Answer Questions

1. **Describe the following:**
   - Classification of joints
   - Functions of synovial fluid
2. **Write notes on:**
   - Cartilaginous joints
   - Osteoarthritis
   - Sutures

Multiple Choice Questions

1. **Which is the example of syndesmosis?**
   a. Joints between skull bones
   b. Pubic symphysis
   c. Inferior tibio-fibular joint
   d. Carpal joints

2. **Which is the pivot joint?**
   a. Radius- carpal joint
   b. Joint between 1st and 2nd cervical vertebrae
   c. Carpal–metacarpal joint
   d. Elbow joint

3. **Angular movements take place at:**
   a. Knee joint
   b. Wrist joint
   c. Ankle joint
   d. Hip joint

4. **The true statement about synovial membrane:**
   a. It is a closed sac
   b. Acts as cushion to prevent friction
   c. It is a sheet of connective tissue
   d. It is a ligament

ANSWER KEY

1. c   **2.** b   **3.** a   **4.** c

Muscles of Human Body

GENERAL DESCRIPTION OF SKELETAL MUSCLES

Motion is one of the most important aspects of human body. This function is accomplished by the concerted role of bony skeleton, joints and the skeletal muscles of the body. In addition to the motion, the skeletal muscles also serve some other functions.

GROSS ANATOMY

Muscle Belly, Origin and Insertion

The main mass of a skeletal muscle is termed as the muscle belly. The fibrous ends of the muscle taper into tendons. Skeletal muscles produce movements by exerting force on tendons, which in turn pull the bones. For producing a movement at any joint, the muscle has to be attached on both the bones forming the joint. Ordinarily, the attachment of a muscle tendon to the stationary bone is called the *origin* and to the movable bone is called *insertion*. This can be compared to a door spring on a door. The part of spring fixed on the immovable frame can be considered analogous to the origin of muscle, and the part of spring attached on movable door can be considered analogous to the insertion of a muscle.

Tendons

Tendons are the fibrous ends of the muscles by which they are attached to the bones. Tendons vary considerably:
- They may be hardly noticeable, so that muscles appear to be directly attached to bone both at its origin and insertion.
- More usually, the tendons are well developed at the insertion of muscle.
- Frequently, tendons are long, round, or flattened bands, usually surrounded by sheaths of synovial membrane, especially in the neighborhood of joints.
- Sometimes, the tendons form a broad, flat expansion termed as *aponeurosis,* e.g., the lumbar aponeurosis.

NERVE SUPPLY AND MUSCLE MECHANICS

Nerve Supply

The skeletal muscles being voluntary muscles are controlled by somatomotor and somatosensory parts of the central nervous system. The nerve controlling the muscle action is called *motor nerve.* Each muscle gets the motor as well as sensory nerve supply either through a mixed nerve or through two separate nerves—one motor and other sensory.

Mechanics of Muscle

When a muscle contracts, the force of contraction is said to have three components:

1. Swing, which is transaxial. For example, this component is maximum during the contraction of brachialis muscle while flexing the elbow.

2. Shunt, which is transarticular. This component is maximum when the origin of the muscle is close to a joint while insertion is at a distance, e.g., brachio- radialis muscle.

3. Spin, which is rotatory along its axis. For example, the spin component is predominant in the pronator quadratus muscle, wrapped on the anterior surfaces of lower ends of radius and ulna bones.

NOMENCLATURE OF SKELETAL MUSCLES

The human body contains about 700 skeletal muscles, each of which bears a name. The muscles have been named in a number of ways:

According to the shape of the muscle. For example, *Deltoid,* a triangular-shaped muscle, is named after the Greek letter delta which is triangular in shape.

Trapezoid muscle is trapezoid in shape.

According to the number of heads of origin. For example,

Biceps (2 heads of origin)

Triceps (3 heads of origin)

Quadriceps (4 heads of origin) muscles.

According to the function of muscle. For example,

Flexor carpi radialis produces flexion at the wrist.

Extensor carpi radialis produces extension at the wrist joint.

Adductor longus produces adduction.

Abductor hallucis longus produces abduction.

Levator scapulae produces upward movement of scapula.

Based on the region in which muscle is located: For example, *Pectoralis major* and *pectoralis minor* are named because they are located in pectoral region (front of the chest).

Gluteus maximus, gluteus medius and *gluteus minimus* muscles are named so because they are located in the gluteal region (region of buttock) and are large, medium and small in size, respectively.

Temporalis muscle is located in temple region.

Intercostal muscles are located in between the ribs.

According to the direction of muscle fibers. For example, *Rectus abdominis,* because of straight fibers (rectus = straight):

Oblique abdominis, because of oblique fibers.

Transversus, because of transverse fibers.

According to attachment. For example, sternomastoid, stylohyoid, cricothyroid.

According to gross appearance. For example, semitendinosus, semimembranosus, etc.

MUSCLE TISSUE

All muscles comprise elongated cells called myocytes. Myocytes contain myofibrils comprised actin and myosin, two major protein filaments that help in contraction of the muscles.

There are three types of muscle tissue in the body:
1. Skeletal muscles (striated muscles)
2. Smooth muscles (non-striated muscles)
3. Cardiac muscles (discussed in chapter 4.2, page 198)

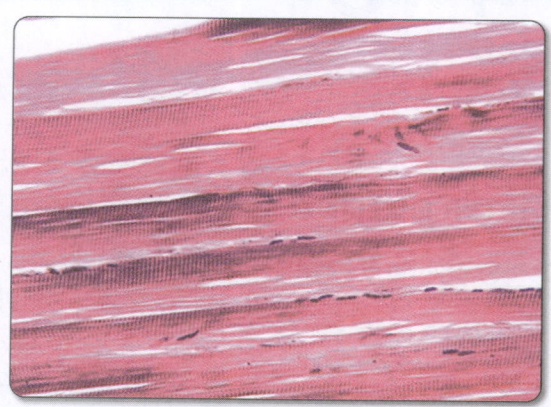

Histology Plate 7.3-1: Skeletal Muscle

Cross-striations of skeletal muscle are more visible with special stains. The darker-staining A bands, lighter-staining I bands and peripherally located nuclei are clearly visible in this photomicrograph.

Skeletal Muscle

Skeletal muscle mainly attaches to the skeletal system *via* tendons to maintain posture and control movement. Skeletal muscle is under voluntary control, although this can be subconscious for example, when maintaining posture or balance. When viewed under the microscope, skeletal muscle cells appear to have a striped, or striated, pattern of light and dark regions. These stripes are caused by the regular arrangement of actin and myosin proteins within the cells into structures known as myofibrils (Histology Plate 7.3-1). Myofibrils are responsible for the skeletal muscles' great strength and ability to pull with incredible force and propel the body.

Smooth Muscle or Visceral Muscle

Smooth muscle tissue is associated with other organs and tissue systems such as the digestive system or respiratory system. It plays an important role in the regulation of flow in such tissues for example, aiding the movement of food through the digestive system *via* peristalsis. These are involuntary muscles. Each visceral muscle cell is long and thin with a single central nucleus and many protein fibers. The protein fibers are arranged into strings called intermediate filaments and masses known as dense bodies. Intermediate filaments contract to pull the dense bodies together and contract the visceral muscle cell. Striations, which reflect the alignment of myofibrils in other muscle types, are not visible in smooth muscle (Histology Plate 7.3-2 for details see page 398).

Histology Plate 7.3-2: Smooth Muscle

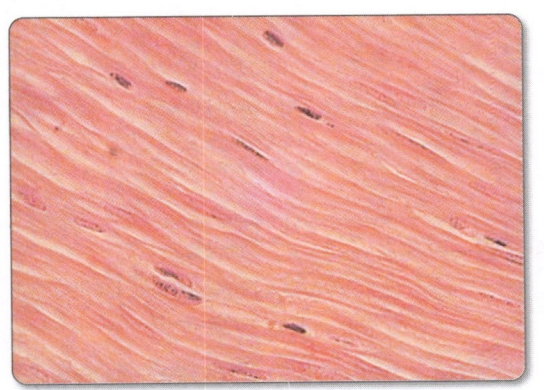

In smooth muscles, the fibers are spindle shaped cells having tapering ends. The nuclei are centrally placed and no striations are seen.

MAIN SKELETAL MUSCLES OF HUMAN BODY

Muscles of the human body are too numerous to be considered in any detail. They can, however, be divided into several main groups and subgroups, and salient features of some of the muscles may be considered as below:

- Muscles of head and neck
- Muscles of pectoral girdle and upper limb
- Muscles of trunk
- Muscles of back
- Muscles of pelvis
- Muscles of pelvic girdle and lower limb.

MUSCLES OF HEAD, FACE AND NECK

These can be divided into the following subgroups:

- Muscles of scalp and facial expression
- Muscles of mastication
- Muscles that move the head
- Muscles of eyes (see Chapter 6.2, page 313)
- Muscles of ears (see Chapter 6.2, page 324)
- Muscles of pharynx (see Chapter 3.1, page 109)
- Muscles of larynx (see Chapter 2.1, page 63)

Muscles of Scalp and Facial Expression

Muscles of facial expression connect the bones of the skull to various regions of the overlying skin. Because of their attachment to skin they enable us to express our feelings as surprise, sadness, anger, fear, pain, happiness, disgust, etc.

Common Muscles of Scalp and Facial Expression

- Epicranius (Occipitofrontalis)
- Orbicularis oculi
- Orbicularis oris
- Buccinator
- Zygomaticus
- Platysma

Nerve Supply

These muscles are supplied by branches of the 7th cranial (facial) nerve.

Origin, Insertion, Nerve Supply and Action

These are summarized in Table 7.3-1.

TABLE 7.3-1: Origin, insertion, nerve supply and actions of muscles of facial expression

Muscle	Origin	Insertion	Nerve supply	Actions
Occipitofrontalis (frontal belly)	Epicranial aponeurosis	Skin superior to supraorbital margin	Facial (CN VII) nerve	Raises eyebrow
Orbicularis oculi	Maxillary and frontal bones	Skin around eye	Facial (CN VII) nerve	Closes eye
Orbicularis oris	Muscles near the mouth	Skin of central lip	Facial (CN VII) nerve	Closes lips, protrudes lips
Buccinator	Outer surfaces of maxilla and mandible	Orbicularis oris	Facial (CN VII) nerve	Compresses cheeks inward
Zygomaticus	Zygomatic bone	Orbicularis oris	Facial (CN VII) nerve	Raises corner of mouth
Platysma	Fascia in upper chest	Lower border of mandible	Facial (CN VII) nerve	Draws angle of mouth downward

Abbreviation: CN—Cranial nerve

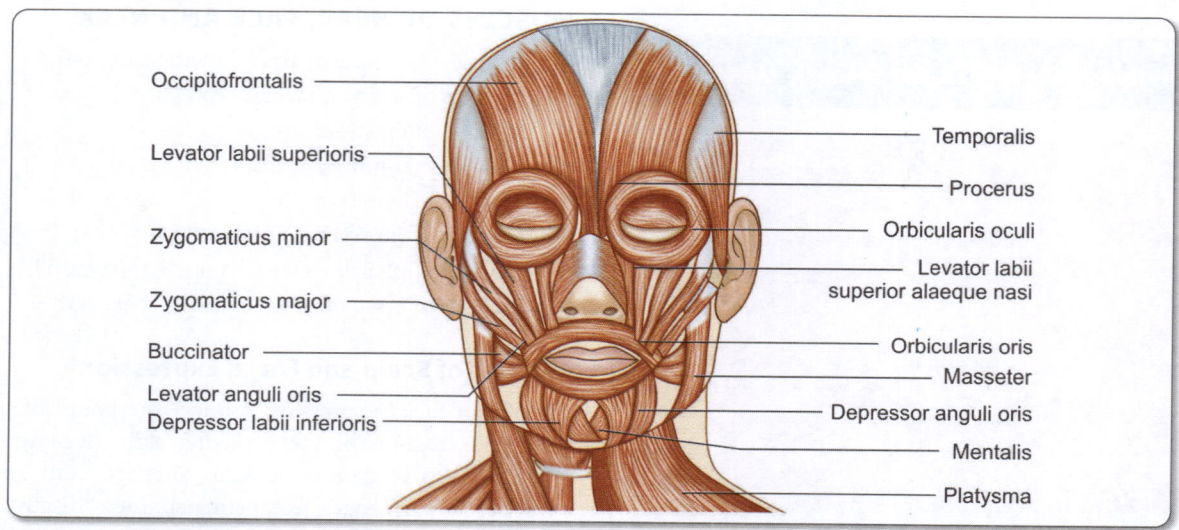

Fig. 7.3-1: The skeletal muscles of facial expression, muscles of mastication and muscles of neck which move the head

Muscles of Mastication

Muscles of mastication produce chewing movements, which include closure of jaw (for biting), side-to-side grinding motions, movements of opening, closing and protruding the jaw. Four pairs of muscles of mastication, that are attached to the mandible, include (Fig. 7.3-1):

1. Masseter (2)
2. Temporalis (2)
3. Internal pterygoid (2)
4. External pterygoid (2)

Nerve Supply

Muscles of mastication are supplied by branches of 5th cranial (trigeminal) nerve.

Origin, Insertion, Nerve Supply and Actions

These are depicted in Table 7.3-2.

Muscles that Move the Head

The muscles in the neck and upper back, which attach the head to the trunk are responsible for movements of the head (flexion, extension, tilt and rotation). These muscles include (Fig. 7.3-2):

- Sternocleidomastoid
- Splenius capitis
- Semispinalis capitis
- Longissimus capitis

Origin, Insertion Nerve Supply and Actions

These are summarized in Table 7.3-3.

MUSCLE OF SHOULDER GIRDLE AND UPPER LIMB

These can be divided into the following subgroups:
- Muscles that move the pectoral girdle
- Muscles that move the upper arm

TABLE 7.3-2: Origin, insertion, nerve supply and actions of muscles of mastication

Muscle	Origin	Insertion	Nerve supply	Actions
Masseter	Lower border of zygomatic arch	Lateral surface of mandible	Mandibular division of trigeminal (CN V) nerve	Raises jaw
Temporalis	Temporal bone	Coronoid process and anterior ramus of mandible	Mandibular division of trigeminal (CN V) nerve	Raises jaw
Internal pterygoid	Sphenoid, palatine, and maxilla bones	Medial surface of mandible	Mandibular division of trigeminal (CN V) nerve	Closes jaw, pulls jaw sideways
External pterygoid	Sphenoid bone	Anterior surface of mandibular condyle	Mandibular division of trigeminal (CN V) nerve	Pulls jaw forward

Abbreviation: CN—Cranial nerve

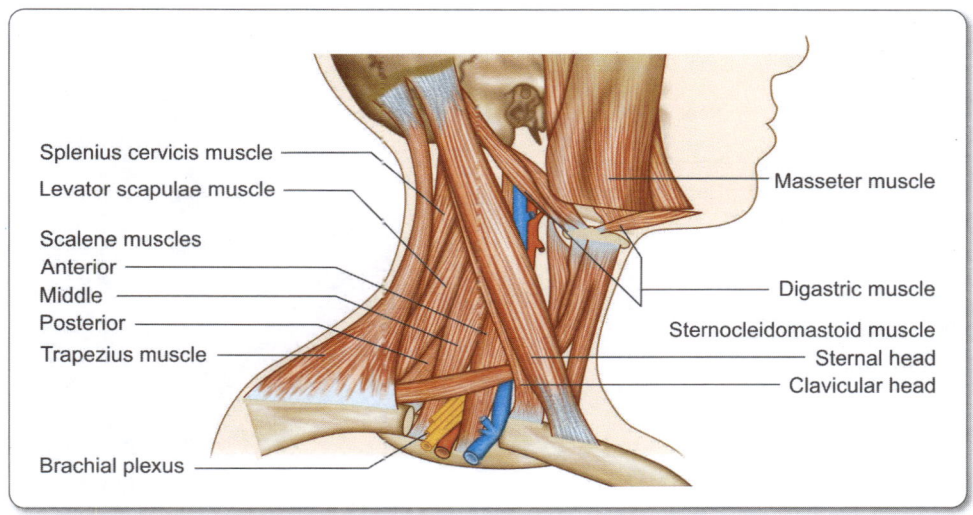

Fig. 7.3-2: Muscles that help in movement of head

TABLE 7.3-3: Origin, insertion, nerve supply and actions of muscles that move the head

Muscle	Origin	Insertion	Nerve supply	Actions
Sternocleid-omastoid	Anterior surface of sternum and upper surface of clavicle	Mastoid process of temporal bone	Accessory (CN XI) nerve	Pulls head to one side, pulls head toward chest, or raises sternum
Splenius capitis	Spinous processes of lower cervical and upper thoracic vertebrae	Mastoid process of temporal bone	Cervical spinal nerves	Rotates head, bends head to one side, or brings head into upright position
Semispinalis capitis	Processes of lower cervical and upper thoracic vertebrae	Occipital bone	Cervical spinal nerves	Extends head, bends head to one side, or rotates head
Longissimus capitis	Processes of lower cervical and upper thoracic vertebrae	Mastoid process of temporal bone	Cervical spinal nerves	Extends head, bends head to one side, or rotates head

Abbreviation: CN—Cranial nerve

- Muscles that move the forearm
- Muscles that move the wrist, hand and fingers.

Muscles that Move the Pectoral Girdle

Muscles that move the pectoral girdle are those which attach the scapulae to the trunk, humerus to the scapula and humerus to the chest wall. These muscles are responsible for upward, downward, forward and backward movements of the scapula. These include the following (Figs 7.3-3A and B):

- Trapezius
- Rhomboideus major
- Levator scapulae
- Serratus anterior
- Pectoralis minor.

Origin, Insertion, Nerve Supply and Actions

These are summarized in Table 7.3-4.

Muscles that Move the Upper Arm

Shoulder joint being multiaxis (ball and socket type) joint makes the upper arm freely movable part of the body. The muscles which attach the humerus with various regions of pectoral girdle, ribs and vertebral column are involved in the movements of upper arm. Depending upon their primary action, these muscles can be grouped as (Figs 7.3-5A and B):

- *Flexors* of upper arm, e.g., pectoralis major and coracobrachialis,
- *Extensors* of upper arm, e.g., teres major, latissimus dorsi.
- *Abductors* of upper arm, e.g., supraspinatus and deltoid.
- *Rotators* of upper arm, e.g., subscapularis, infraspinatus, and teres major.

Origin, Insertion, Nerve Supply and Actions

These are summarized in Table 7.3-5.

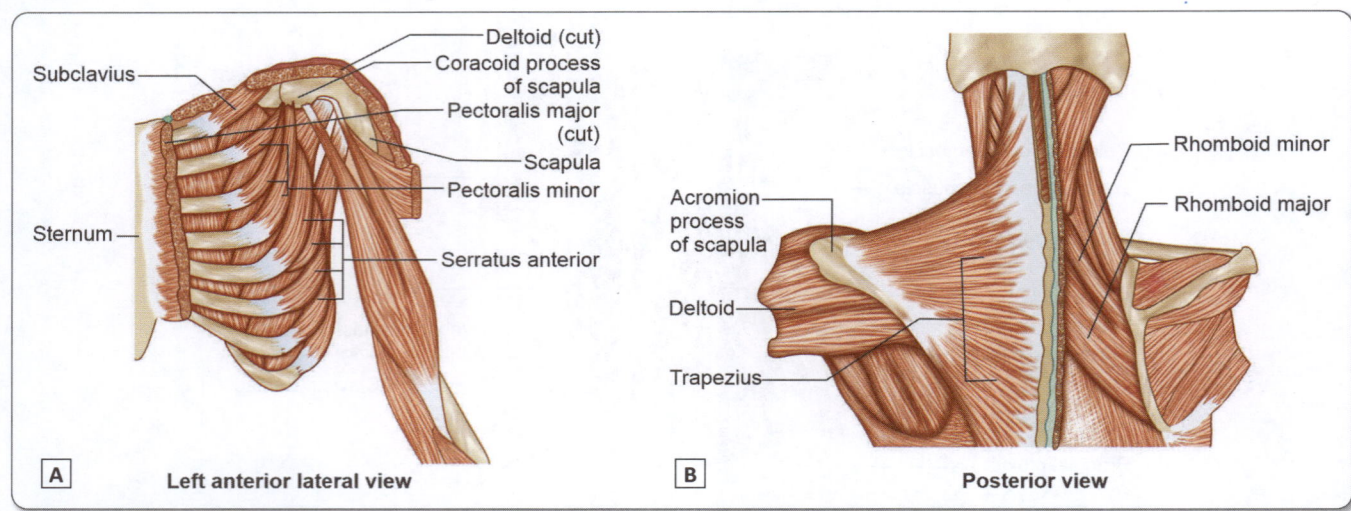

Figs 7.3-3A and B: Muscles of pectoral girdle

TABLE 7.3-4: Origin, insertion, nerve supply and actions of muscles that move the pectoral girdle

Muscle	Origin	Insertion	Nerve supply	Actions
Trapezius	Occipital bone and spines of cervical and thoracic vertebrae	Clavicle and spine and acromion process of scapula	Accessory (CN XI) nerve and cervical spinal nerve ($C_3 – C_5$)	Raises scapula, pulls scapula medially, or pulls scapula and shoulder downward
Rhomboideus major	Spines of upper thoracic vertebrae	Medial border of scapula	Dorsal scapular nerve	Raises and adducts scapula
Levator scapulae	Transverse processes of cervical vertebrae	Medial margin of scapula	Dorsal scapular nerve and cervical spinal nerve $C_3 – C_5$	Elevates scapula
Serratus anterior	Outer surfaces of upper ribs	Medial border of scapula	Long thoracic nerve	Pulls scapula anteriorly and downward
Pectoralis minor	Sternal ends of upper ribs	Coracoid process of scapula	Medial pectoral nerve	Pulls scapula forward and downward or raises ribs

Abbreviation: CN—Cranial nerve

IMPORTANT TO KNOW

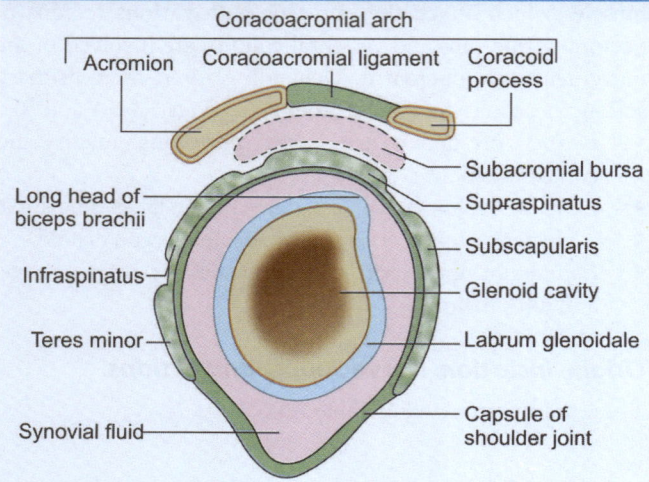

Fig. 7.3-4: Rotator cuff of shoulder

Rotator Cuff of Shoulder (Fig. 7.3-4):

- Fibrous sheath formed by the four flattened tendons which blend with the capsule of the shoulder joint and strengthen.
- Muscles which form the cuff are the subscapularis, the supraspinatus, the infraspinatus and the teres minor.
- Their tendons, while crossing the shoulder joint, become flattened and blend with each other on one hand, and with the capsule of the joint on the other hand, before reaching the points of insertion.
- Cuff gives strength to the capsule of the shoulder joint all around except inferiorly. This explains why dislocations of the humerus occur commonly in a anteroinferior direction.

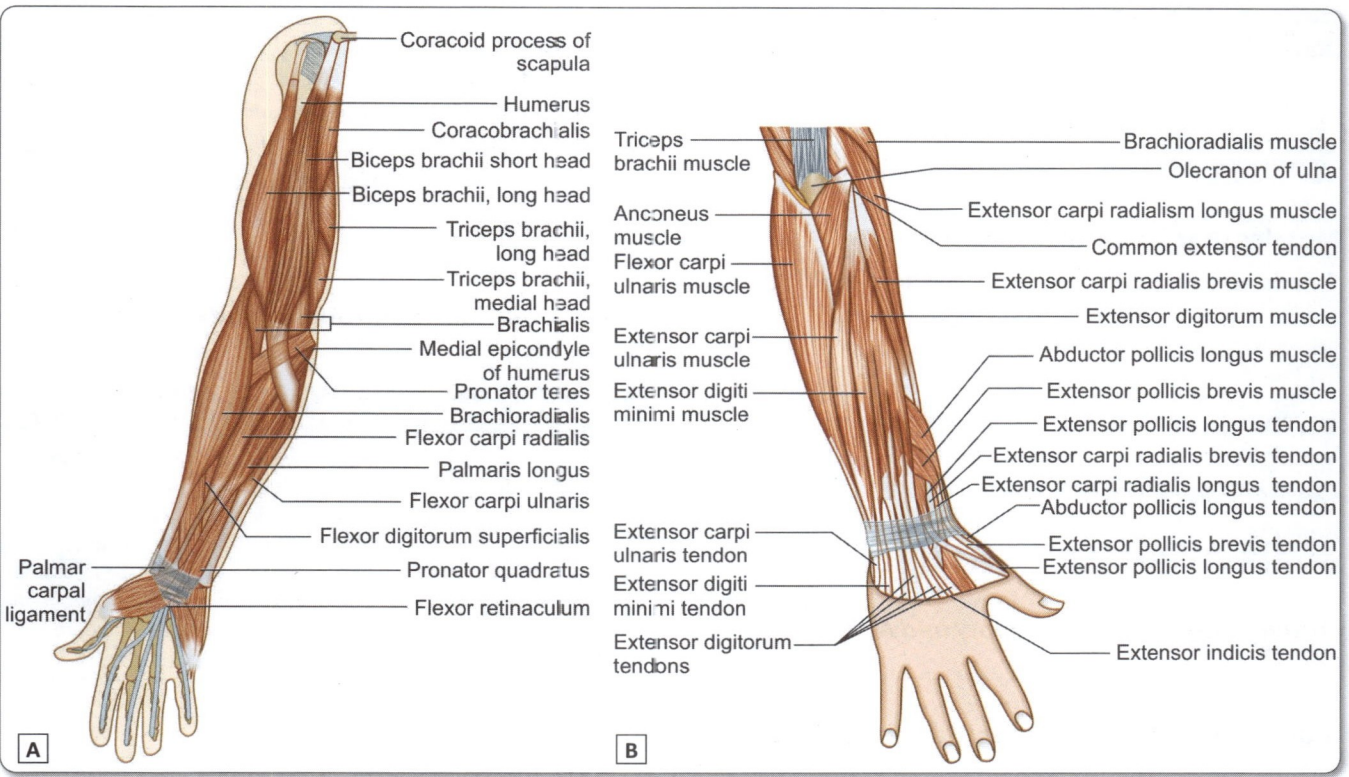

Figs 7.3-5A and B: Muscles of arm, forearm and hand

TABLE 7.3-5: Origin, insertion, nerve supply and actions of muscles that move the upper arm

Muscle	Origin	Insertion	Nerve supply	Actions
Flexors				
Coracobra-chialis	Coracoid process of scapula	Shaft of humerus	Musculocutaneous nerve	Flexes and adducts the upper arm
Pectoralis major	Clavicle, sternum, and costal cartilages of upper ribs	Intertubercular groove of humerus	Medial and lateral pectoral nerves	Pulls arm forward and across chest, rotates humerus, or adducts arm
Extensors				
Teres major	Lateral border of scapula	Intertubercular groove of humerus	Lower subscapular nerve	Extends humerus, or adducts and rotates arm medially
Latissimus dorsi	Spines of sacral, lumbar and lower thoracic vertebrae, iliac crest, and lower ribs	Intertubercular groove of humerus	Thoracodorsal nerve	Extends, adducts, and rotates humerus medially, or pulls the shoulder downward and back
Abductors				
Supraspinatus	Posterior surface of scapula	Greater tubercle of humerus	Suprascapular nerve	Abducts the upper arm
Deltoid	Acromion process and spine of scapula and the clavicle	Deltoid tuberosity of humerus	Axillary nerve	Abducts upper arm, extends humerus, or flexes humerus
Rotators				
Subscapularis	Anterior surface of scapula	Lesser tubercle of humerus	Upper and lower subscapular nerves	Rotates arm medially
Infraspinatus	Posterior surface of scapula	Greater tubercle of humerus	Suprascapular nerve	Rotates arm laterally
Teres minor	Lateral border of scapula	Greater tubercle of humerus	Axillary nerve	Rotates arm laterally

Muscles that Move the Forearm

Movers of the forearm are those muscles which attach the radius and ulna to the humerus or pectoral girdle. Depending upon their primary action these muscles can be grouped as below:

Flexors of forearm are biceps brachii, brachialis, and brachioradialis.

Extensor of forearm is only triceps brachii.

Rotators of forearm include supinator, pronator teres and pronator quadratus.

Origin, Insertion, Nerve Supply and Actions

These muscles are summarized in Table 7.3-6.

Muscles that Move the Wrist, Hand and Fingers

These muscles can be divided into two groups—flexors present on the arterior side of forearm and extensor present on the posterior side of the forearm. These muscles *arise* from the humerus, radius and ulna. The tendons of the flexor muscles in front and extensor muscles behind are inserted into the bases of the terminal phalanges of the digits. Slips are also given to the other phalanges. These muscles include the following:

Flexors include flexor carpi radialis, flexor carpi ulnaris, palmaris longus, and flexor digitorum profundus.

Extensors are extensor carpi radialis longus, extensor carpi radialis brevis, extensor carpi ulnaris and extensor digitorum.

Origin, Insertion, Nerve Supply and Actions

These are summarized in Table 7.3-7.

IMPORTANT TO KNOW

The thumb has separate muscles which, however, correspond to the main flexor and extensor groups in the forearm. Special muscles situated in the palm of hand also move the thumb and form the *thenar eminence* at the base of the thumb. The prominence on the ulnar side of the hand at the base of the little finger is called the *hypothenar eminence*. Arising between the metacarpal bones and inserted into the phalanges are the *lumbrical* and *interosseous* muscles.

MUSCLES OF TRUNK

Muscles of the trunk can be grouped as below:
- *Muscles of thorax*
- *Muscles of abdominal wall.*

TABLE 7.3-6: Origin, insertion, nerve supply and actions of muscles that move the forearm

Muscle	Origin	Insertion	Nerve supply	Actions
Flexors				
Biceps brachii	Coracoid process and tubercle above glenoid cavity of scapula	Radial tuberosity of radius	Musculocutaneous nerve	Flexes arm at elbow and rotates the hand laterally
Brachialis	Anterior shaft of humerus	Coronoid process of ulna	Musculocutaneous and radial nerves	Flexes arm at elbow
Brachioradialis	Distal lateral end of humerus	Lateral surface of radius above styloid process	Radial nerve	Flexes arm at elbow
Extensors				
Triceps brachii	Tubercle below glenoid cavity and lateral and medial surfaces of humerus	Olecranon process of ulna	Radial nerve	Extends arm at elbow
Anconeus	Lateral epicondyle of humerus	Olecranon and superior portion of shaft of ulna	Radial nerve	Extends forearm at elbow joint
Rotators				
Supinator	Lateral epicondyle of humerus and crest of ulna	Lateral surface of radius	Deep radial nerve	Rotates forearm laterally
Pronator teres	Medial epicondyle of humerus	Lateral surface of radius	Median nerve	Rotates arm medially
Pronator quadratus	Anterior distal end of ulna	Anterior distal end of radius	Median nerve	Rotates arm medially

TABLE 7.3-7: Origin, insertion, nerve supply and actions of muscles that move the wrist, hand and fingers

Muscle	Origin	Insertion	Nerve supply	Actions
Flexors				
Flexor carpi radialis	Medial epicondyle of humerus	Base of second and third metacarpals	Median nerve	Flexes and abducts wrist
Flexor carpi ulnaris	Medial epicondyle of humerus and olecranon process	Carpal and metacarpal bones	Ulnar nerve	Flexes and adducts wrist
Palmaris longus	Medial epicondyle of humerus	Fascia of palm	Median nerve	Flexes wrist
Flexor digitorum	Anterior surface of ulna	Bases of distal phalanges in fingers two through five	Median and ulnar nerves	Flexes distal joints of fingers
Extensors				
Extensor carpi radialis longus	Distal end of humerus	Base of second metacarpal	Radial nerve	Extends wrist and abducts hand
Extensor carpi radialis brevis	Lateral epicondyle of humerus	Base of second and third metacarpals	Radial nerve	Extends wrist and abducts hand
Extensor carpi ulnaris	Lateral epicondyle of humerus	Base of fifth metacarpal	Deep radial nerve	Extends and adducts wrist
Extensor digitorum	Lateral epicondyle of humerus	Posterior surface of phalanges in fingers two through five	Deep radial nerve	Extends fingers
Extensor digiti minimi	Lateral epicondyle of humerus	Tendon of extensor digitorum on fifth phalanx	Deep radial nerve	Extends proximal phalanx of little finger and hand of wrist joint

Muscles of Thorax

Muscles of Thoracic Wall (Fig. 7.3-6)

- Pectoralis major
- Pectoralis minor
- Serratus anterior
- Intercostal muscles.

Diaphragm

It is a large dome-shaped muscle separating the cavity of thorax from that of abdomen. It consists partly of muscle (around the circumference) and partly of membrane or flat tendon (in the center) (Fig. 7.3-7).

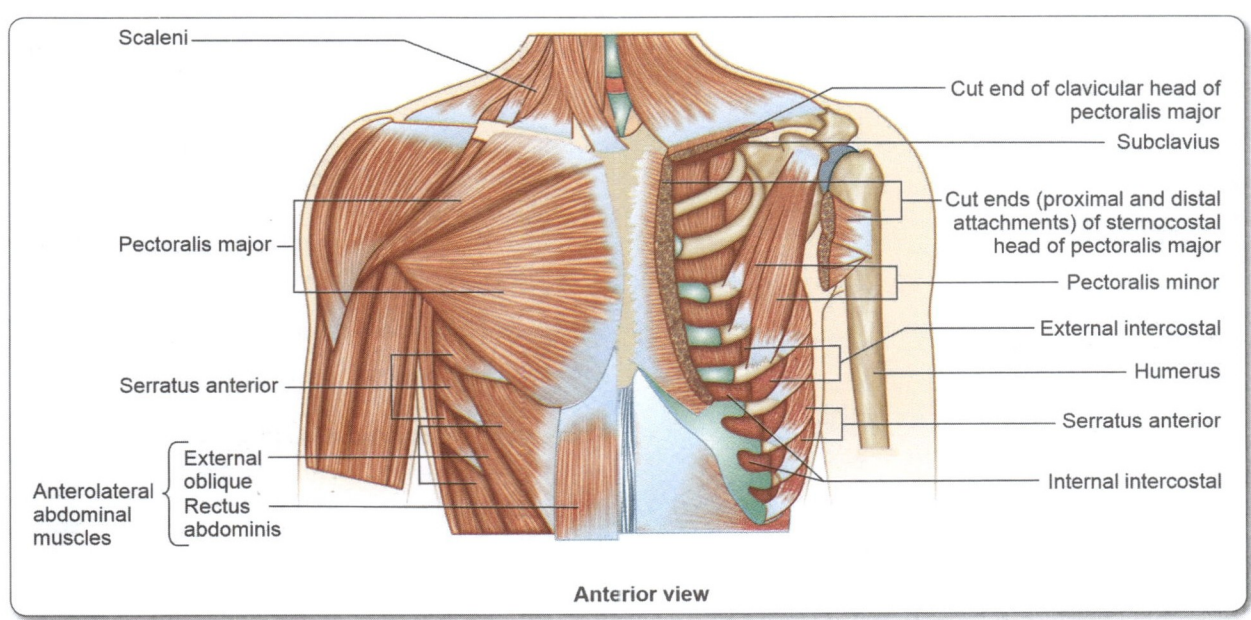

Anterior view

Fig. 7.3-6: Muscles of thoracic wall

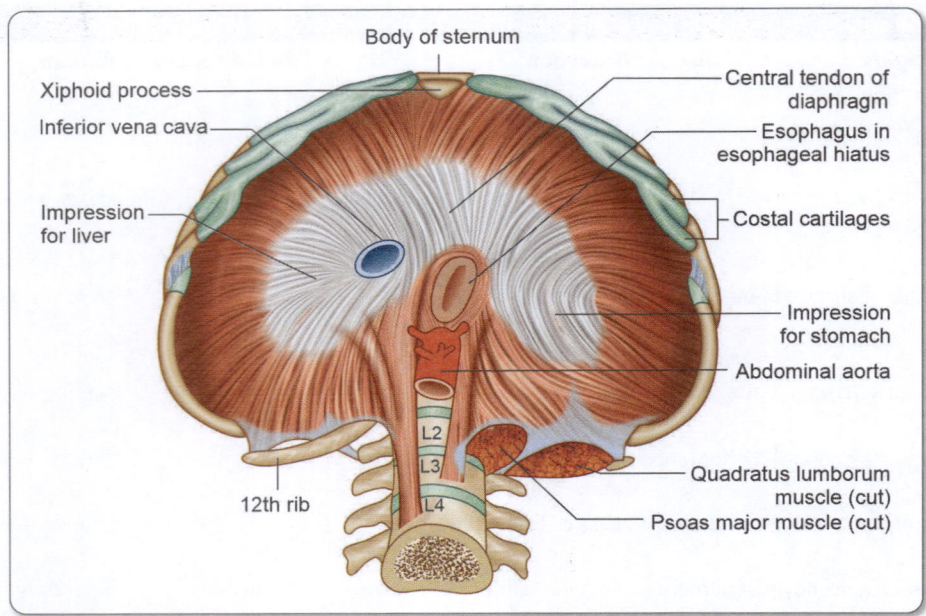

Fig. 7.3-7: Diagram showing under surface of diaphragm

Parts and Attachments

Sternal part is attached in front to the lower end of sternum.
Costal part is attached to the lower six ribs on either side.
Lumbar part is attached to the first 2 lumbar vertebrae by 2 slips called the crurae (legs) of the diaphragm.

Surfaces

Diaphragm has two surfaces:

Upper surface is related to the heart and pericardium in the center and to the pleura and base of lung on either side.

Under surface largely covered by peritoneum, is related on the right side and centrally to the upper surface of liver; and on the left side to the fundus of stomach and the spleen.

Openings

* For aorta in the midline
* For esophagus slightly to the left
* For inferior vena cava, slightly to the right.

Nerve supply and actions

The diaphragm is a very important muscle of respiration. It is supplied by *phrenic nerve* from the cervical plexus.

During inspiration, the muscle part of diaphragm contracts and it becomes flattened toward the abdomen; and thereby, helping to enlarge the size of thoracic cavity.

During expiration, the diaphragm relaxes and resumes its dome-shaped appearance.

Muscles of Abdominal Wall

Anterior Abdominal Wall

These include the following muscles (Fig. 7.3-8):

* Rectus abdominis
* External oblique
* Internal oblique
* Transverse abdominis

Salient features of the muscles of the anterior abdominal wall are:

* They connect the rib cage and vertebral column to the pelvic girdle.
* Linea alba, a tough connective tissue, which extends from the xiphoid process of the sternum to symphysis pubis, serves as an attachment for some of the abdominal wall muscles.
* Contraction of these muscles help in forceful expiration, defecation, urination, vomiting and childbirth.

Origin, insertion, nerve supply and actions

These are summarized in Table 7.3-8.

Posterior Abdominal Wall (Fig. 7.3-9)

Muscles of posterior abdominal wall include:

* Psoas muscle
* Iliacus muscle
* Quadratus lumborum.

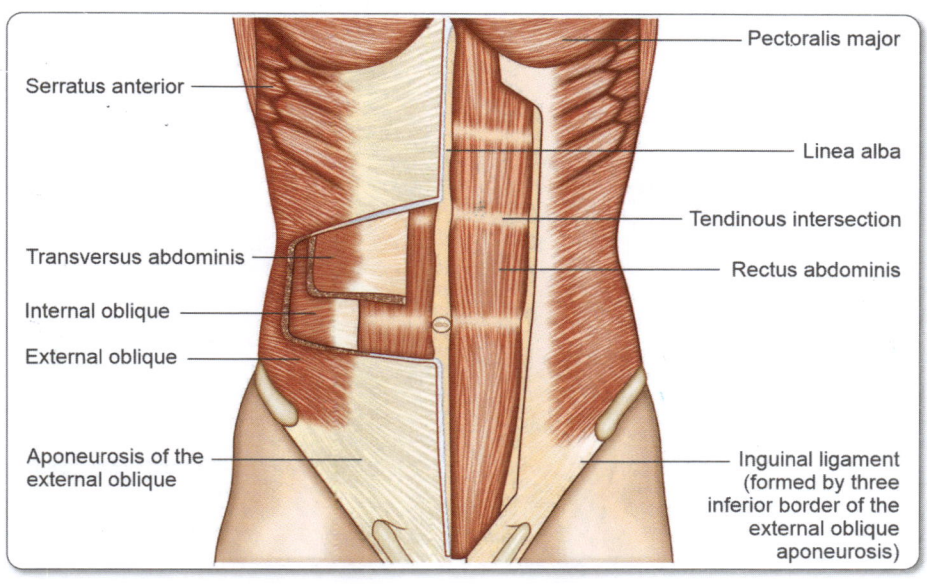

Fig. 7.3-8: Muscles of anterior abdominal wall

TABLE 7.3-8: Origin, insertion, nerve supply and actions of muscles of the abdominal wall

Muscle	Origin	Insertion	Nerve supply	Actions
Of anterior abdominal wall				
External oblique	Outer surfaces of lower ribs	Outer lip of iliac crest and linea alba	Thoracic spinal nerve T_7-T_{12} and iliohypogastric nerve	Tenses abdominal wall and compresses abdominal contents
Internal oblique	Crest of ilium	Cartilages of lower inguinal ligament ribs, linea alba, and crest of pubis	Thoracic spinal nerves T_8-T_{12}, iliohypogastric nerve and ilioinguinal nerve	Same as above
Transversus abdominis	Costal cartilages of lower ribs, processes of lumbar vertebrae, lip of iliac crest, and inguinal ligament	Linea alba and crest of pubis	Thoracic spinal nerves T_8-T_{12}, iliohypogastric nerve and ilioinguinal nerve	Same as above
Rectus abdominis	Crest of pubis and symphysis pubis	Xiphoid process of sternum and costal cartilages	Thoracic spinal nerve T_7-T_{12}	Same as above, also flexes vertebral column
Of posterior abdominal wall				
Psoas major	Transverse processes and bodies of lumbar vertebrae	With iliacus into lesser trochanter of femur	Lumbar spinal nerves L_2-L_3	Flexes thigh at hip joint
Iliacus	Iliac fossa of ilium	Lesser trochanter of femur	Femoral nerve	Flexes thigh
Qudratus femoris	Ischial tuberosity	Qudrate tubercle on posterior femur	Nerve to quadratus femoris	Laterally rotates and stabilizes hip joint

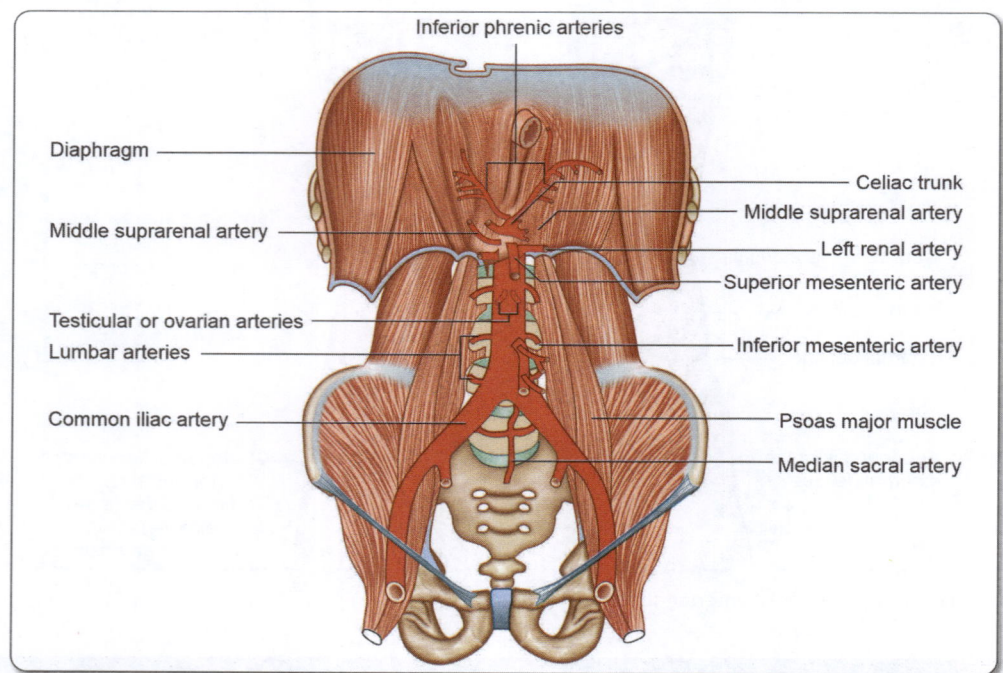

Fig. 7.3-9: Muscles of posterior abdominal wall

MUSCLES OF THE BACK

Muscles of the back include several group of muscles, which are placed on either side of the spine and extend the varying distances between the occiput above and the sacrum below.

Muscles of upper back extend the neck. These include:

- Splenius capitis
- Semispinalis capitis
- Longismus capitis.

Muscles of lower back, which straighten the spine, consist of three groups of muscles:

1. *Iliocostalis group* is laterally placed
2. *Longissimus group* is intermediately placed
3. *Spinalis group* is medially placed.
    Combined these muscles constitute the *erector spina.*

> ### NURSING IMPLICATIONS AND APPLICATIONS
>
> Gluteus medius is a common site for intramuscular injections. Generally the injection is given in the center of upper outer quadrant of gluteal (buttock) area to avoid damage to the sciatic nerve.

MUSCLES OF PELVIS AND PERINEUM

Muscles of Pelvis

They form the floor of the abdominal cavity, just as the diaphragm forms its roof. These include levator ani and coccygeus. The muscles of pelvic floor, together with the fasciae covering their internal and external surfaces are collectively referred to as the *pelvic diaphragm.*

Muscles of Perineum

The perineum is the entire outlet of pelvis. The muscles of pelvis include superficial transversus perinei, bulbospongiosus and ischiocavernosus. These muscles along with their fascia constitute the *urogenital diaphragm.*

Muscles of male and female pelvis and perineum are shown in figures 7.3-10A and B and their salient features are summarized in Table 7.3-9.

MUSCLES OF PELVIC GIRDLE AND LOWER LIMB

These can be divided into the following subgroups:

- Muscles that move the thigh
- Muscles that move the leg
- Muscles that move the ankle, foot and toes.

Muscles that Move the Thigh

Muscles that move the thigh are attached to the femur and to some part of the pelvic girdle. These can be divided into three groups:

1. *Flexors of thigh or muscles of anterior group* include psoas major and iliacus (Figs 7.3-11A to C). They primarily flex the thigh.

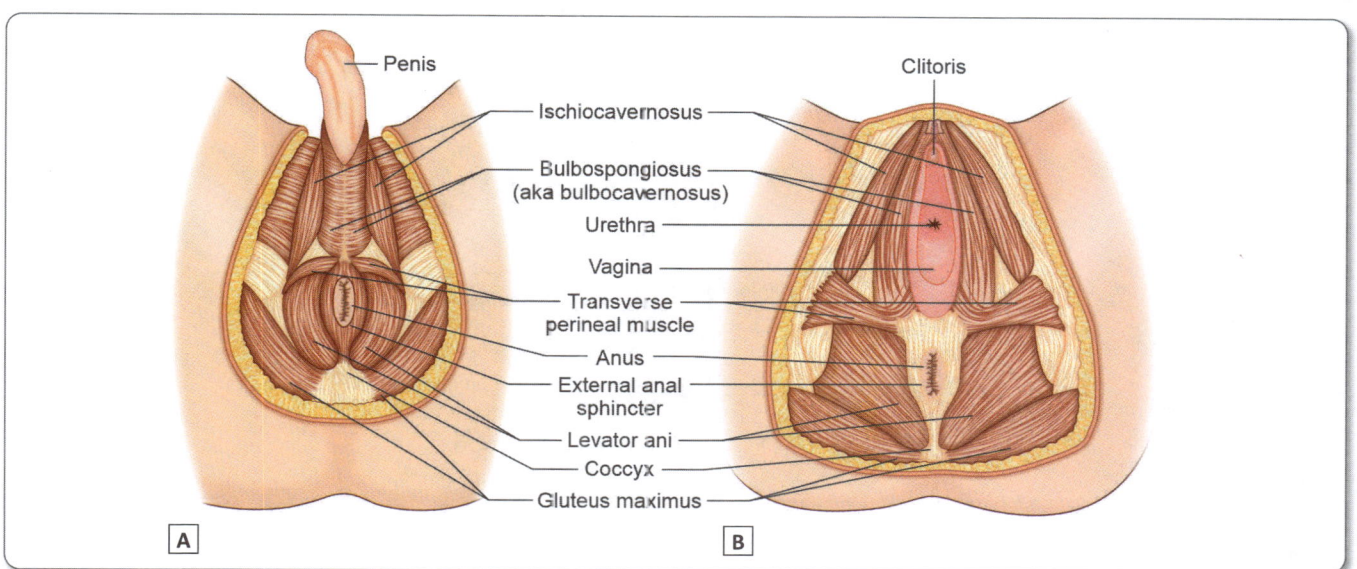

Figs 7.3-10A and B: Muscles of pelvis and perineum in males and females; A. Male perineal muscles: inferior view, B. Female perineal muscles: inferior view

TABLE 7.3-9: Origin, insertion, nerve supply and actions of muscles of the pelvic outlet

Muscle	Origin	Insertion	Nerve supply	Actions
Muscles of pelvic floor				
Levator ani	Pubic bone and ischial spine	Coccyx	Sacral spinal nerves S_1-S_4	Supports pelvic viscera, and provides sphincter-like action in anal canal and vagina
Coccygeus	Ischial spine	Sacrum and coccyx	Sacral spinal nerves S_1-S_4	Same as above
Superficial muscles of perineum				
Superficial transversus perinei	Ischial tuberosity	Central tendon	Perineal branch of pudendal nerve of the sacral plexus	Supports pelvic viscera
Bulbospongiosus	Central tendon	Males: Urogenital diaphragm and fascia of penis	Perineal branch of pudendal nerve of the sacral plexus	Males: Assists emptying urethra
		Females: Pubic arch and root of clitoris		Females: Constricts vagina
Ischiocavernosus	Ischial tuberosity	Pubic arch	Perineal branch of pudendal nerve of the sacral plexus	Same as above
Deep muscles of perineum				
Deep transversus perinei	Ischial rami	Perineal body of perineum	Perineal branch of pudendal nerve of the sacral plexus	Helps to expel last drop of urine
External urethral sphincter	Ischial and pubic rami	Median raphe in male and vaginal wall in female	Sacral spinal nerves S_4 and inferior rectal branch of pudendal nerve	Helps to expel last drop of urine
External anal sphincter	Anococcygeal ligament	Perineal body of perineum	Sacral spinal nerve S_4 and inferior rectal branch of pudendal nerve	Keep anal canal and anus close

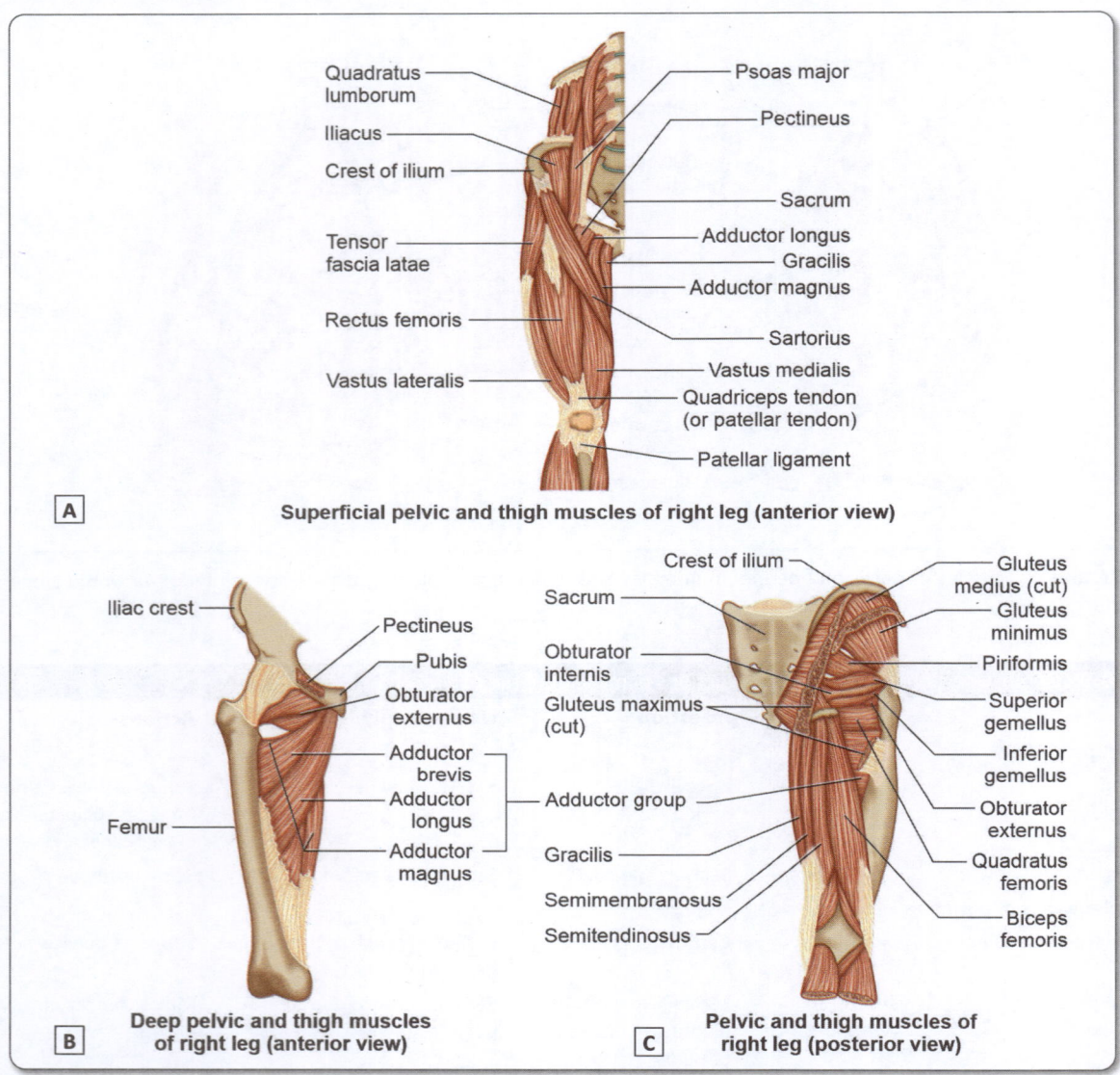

Figs 7.3-11A to C: Muscles that move the thigh

2. *Abductors of thigh or muscles of posterior group* also known as *muscles of the buttock* make up the rounded eminence of buttock. They include gluteus maximus, gluteus medius and gluteus minimus. These abductors rotate the thigh.

3. *Adductors of thigh* include adductor longus, adductor magnus, adductor brevis and gracilis.

Origin, Insertion, Nerve Supply and Actions

These are summarized in Table 7.3-10.

Muscles that Move the Leg

The muscles that move the leg connect the tibia and fibula to the femur or pelvic girdle. These are the muscles of thigh region which can be arranged in two groups:

1. *Anterior group muscle of thigh or extensors of leg* lie in front of the femur. These include rectus femoris, vastus lateralis, vastus medialis and vastus intermedius. These combined to constitute the *quadriceps femoris*.

2. *Posterior group muscles of thigh or flexors of leg* lie behind the femur. These include sartorius, biceps femoris semitendinosus, and semimembranosus. These combined to constitute the *hamstring* muscles.

Origin, Insertion, Nerve Supply and Actions

These are summarized in Table 7.3-11.

TABLE 7.3-10: Origin, insertion, nerve supply and actions of muscles that move the thigh

Muscle	Origin	Insertion	Nerve supply	Actions
Flexors				
Psoas major	Lumbar intervertebral	Lesser trochanter of femur, disks, bodies and transverse processes of lumbar vertebrae	Lumbar spinal nerves L_2-L_3	Flexes thigh
Iliacus	Iliac fossa of ileum	Lesser trochanter of femur	Femoral nerve	Flexes thigh
Gluteus maximus	Posterior surface of ileum	Posterior surface of sacrum and coccyx	Inferior gluteal femur and iliotibial tract	Extends leg at hip nerve
Abductors				
Gluteus medius	Lateral surface of ileum	Greater trochanter of femur	Superior gluteal nerve	Abducts and rotates thigh medially
Gluteus minimus	Lateral surface of ileum	Greater trochanter of femur	Superior gluteal nerve	Same as above
Tensor fasciae latae	Anterior iliac crest	Lateral condyle of tibia by fascia	Superior gluteal nerve	Abducts, flexes, and rotates thigh medially
Adductors				
Adductor longus	Pubic bone near symphysis pubis	Posterior surface of femur	Obturator nerve	Adducts, flexes, and rotates thigh laterally
Adductor brevis	Inferior ramus of pubis	Linea aspera of femur	Obturator nerve	Adducts, flexes and rotates thigh medially
Adductor magnus	Ischial tuberosity	Posterior surface of femur	Obturator and sciatic nerve	Adducts, extends, and rotates thigh medially
Gracilis	Lower edge of symphysis pubis	Medial surface of tibia	Obturator nerve	Adducts thigh, flexes and rotates leg at knee

TABLE 7.3-11: Origin, insertion, nerve supply and actions of muscles that move the lower leg

Muscle	Origin	Insertion	Nerve supply	Actions
Flexors (Hamstring group)				
Biceps femoris	Ischial tuberosity and posterior surface of femur	Head of fibula and lateral condyle of tibia	Tibial and common paroneal nerves from sciatic nerve	Flexes and rotates leg laterally and extends thigh
Semitendinosus	Ischial tuberosity	Medial surface of tibia	Tibial nerve	Flexes and rotates leg medially and extends thigh
Semimembranosus	Ischial tuberosity	Medial condyle of tibia	Tibial nerve	Flexes and rotates leg medially and extends thigh
Sartorius	Spine of ileum	Medial surface of tibia	Femoral nerve	Flexes leg and thigh, abducts thigh, rotates thigh laterally, and rotates leg medially
Extensors (Quadriceps femoris group)				
Rectus femoris	Spine of ileum and margin of acetabulum	Patella by common tendon which continues as patellar ligament to tibial tuberosity	Femoral nerve	Extends leg at knee
Vastus lateralis	Greater trochanter and posterior surface of femur	Lateral border of patella		
Vastus medialis	Medial surface of femur	Medial border of patella		
Vastus intermedius	Anterior and lateral surfaces of femur	Upper border of patella		

Muscles that Move the Ankle, Foot and Toes

The muscles located in lower leg region, attach the femur, tibia, and fibula to various bones of foot. These include (Table 7.3-12 and Figs 7.3-12A to C):

Dorsiflexors of foot. Tibialis anterior, peroneus tertius, and extensor digitorum longus.

Plantar flexors of foot. Gastrocnemius, soleus and flexor digitorum longus.

Invertor of foot. Tibialis posterior.

Evertor of foot. Proneus longus.

Small Muscles of Foot

There are a number of small muscles in foot similar to those in the hands, viz, short muscles in the sole which are attached to the big toe, *interosseous* and *lumbrical* muscles for the toes.

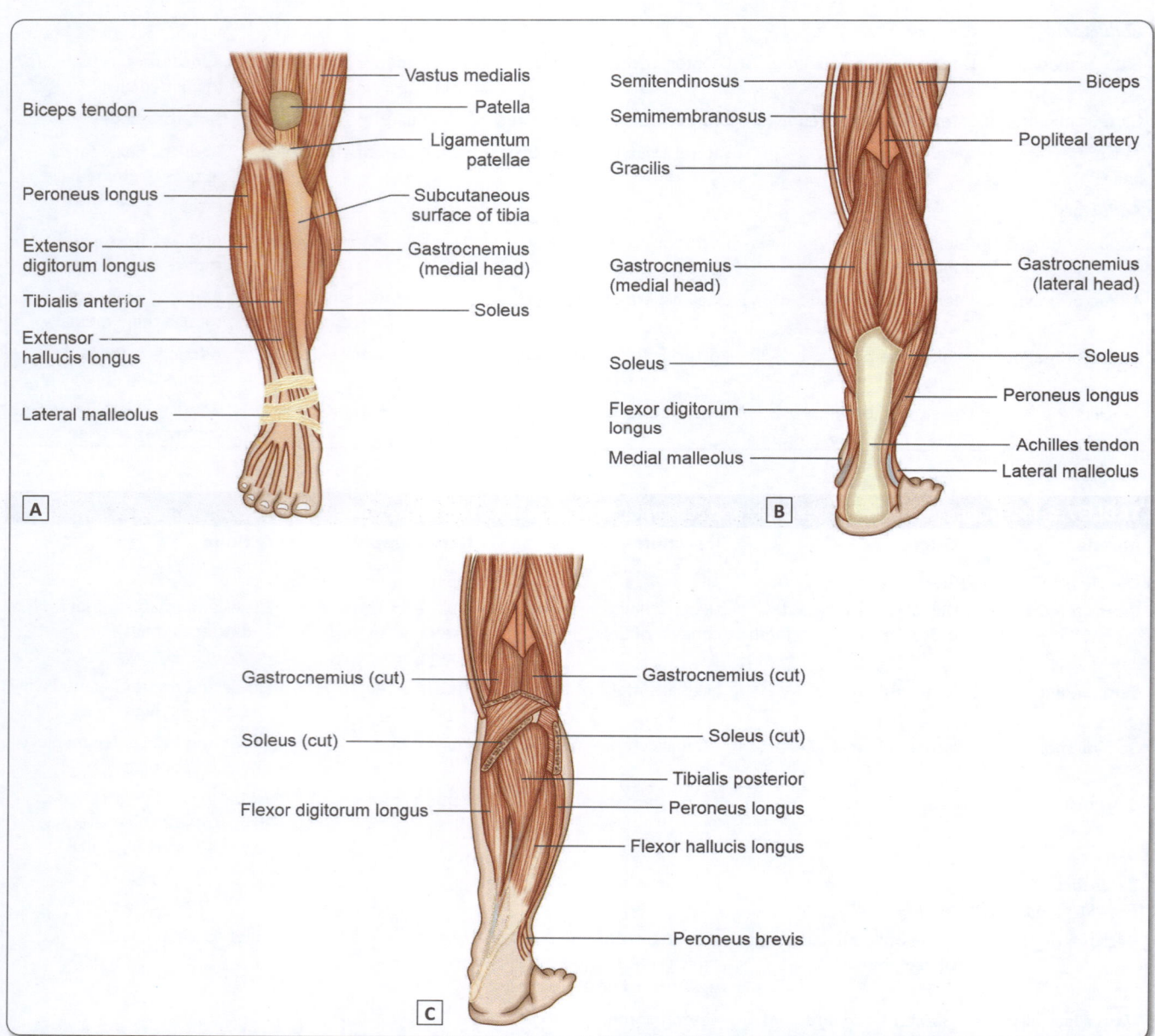

Figs 7.3-12A to C: Muscles of the leg region which move the ankle, foot and toes: A. Anterior view; B. Superficial posterior view; C. Deep posterior view

TABLE 7.3-12: Origin, insertion, nerve supply and actions of muscles that move the ankle, foot and toes

Muscle	Origin	Insertion	Nerve supply	Actions
Dorsiflexors				
Tibialis anterior	Lateral condyle and lateral surface of tibia	Tarsal bone (cuneiform) and first metatarsal	Deep fibular (peroneal) nerve	Dorsal flexion and inversion of foot
Fibularis (peroneus) tertius	Anterior surface of fibula	Dorsal surface of fifth metatarsal	Deep fibular (peroneal) nerve	Dorsal flexion and eversion of foot
Extensor digitorum longus	Lateral condyle of tibia and anterior surface of fibula	Dorsal surfaces of second and third phalanges of 4 lateral toes	Deep fibular (peroneal) nerve of toes	Dorsal flexion and eversion of foot and extension of toes
Plantar flexors				
Gastrocnemius	Lateral and medial condyles of femur	Posterior surface of calcaneus	Tibial nerve	Plantar flexion of foot and flexion of leg at knee
Soleus	Head and shaft of fibula and posterior surface of tibia	Posterior surface of calcaneus	Tibial nerve	Plantar flexion of foot
Flexor digitorum longus	Posterior surface of tibia	Distal phalanges of 4 lateral toes	Tibial nerve	Plantar flexion and inversion of foot and flexion of 4 lateral toes
Invertor of foot				
Tibialis Posterior	Lateral condyle and posterior surface of tibia and posterior surface of fibula	Tarsal and metatarsal bones	Tibial nerve	Plantar flexion and inversion of foot
Evertor of foot				
Fibularis (peroneus) longus	Lateral condyle of tibia and head and shaft of fibula	Tarsal and metatarsal bones	Superficial fibular (peroneal) nerve	Plantar flexion and eversion of foot; also supports arch
Fibularis (peroneus) brevis	Body of fibula	Base of fifth metatarsal	Superficial fibular (peroneal) nerve	

NURSING IMPLICATIONS AND APPLICATIONS

The middle third of vastus lateralis and anterior aspect of rectus femoris are common sites for intramuscular injections in very young children whose gluteal muscles are not very well developed.

CLINICAL ASPECTS

PARALYSIS

Loss of motor power (power of movements) in muscles is called paralysis. This causes inability of the muscles to contract. The root cause of paralysis can be of two types:
1. Damage to motor neural pathways
2. Inherent disease of muscles

In the type of paralysis caused by damage to motor neural pathways, either the upper or lower motor neuron might be the exact point of damage. In the case of upper motor neuron, spastic paralysis is caused which is accompanied by exaggerated tendon jerks. In the case of lower motor neurons, flaccid paralysis is caused in which there are no tendon jerks.

ASSESS YOURSELF

Short and Long Answer Questions

1. **Name the following groups of muscles and their nerve supply:**
   - Muscles of facial expression
   - Muscles of mastication
   - Muscles of shoulder girdle
2. **Name the followings:**
   - Muscles of thoracic wall
   - Muscles of abdominal wall
   - Muscles of upper limb
   - Muscles of lower limb
3. **Describe the clinical importance of:**
   - Diaphragm
   - Gluteal muscle
   - Deltoid
4. **Nerve supply of:**
   - Orbicularis oculi
   - Masseter muscle
   - Sternocleidomastoid

Multiple Choice Questions

1. **The main abductor of upper limb is:**
   a. Biceps brachii
   b. Pectoralis major
   c. Deltoid
   d. Lattimus dorsi

2. **The main action of biceps brachii and triceps brachii is;**
   a. Are synergists
   b. Are antagonists
   c. Both flex the forearm
   d. Both cause extension of forearm

3. **In normal breathing, the ribs are elevated by:**
   a. External intercostals
   b. Internal intercostals
   c. Diaphragm
   d. Rectus abdominis

4. **The thigh muscle that extends the leg is:**
   a. Sartorius
   b. Quadriceps femoris
   c. Hamstring
   d. Iliopsoas

5. **The rectus abdominis muscle is inserted into:**
   a. Xiphoid process
   b. 1-4 Ribs
   c. Linea alba
   d. Median raphae

6. **Which of the following is attached to the lateral surface of greater trochanter?**
   a. Gluteus maximus
   b. Gluteus medius
   c. Gluteus minimus
   d. Piriformis

7. **Which is the action of deltoid?**
   a. Abduction of shoulder
   b. Adduction of shoulder
   c. Flexion of neck
   d. Flexion of elbow

ANSWER KEY

| **1.** d | **2.** b | **3.** a | **4.** b | **5.** a | **6.** b | **7.** a |

Chapter

7.4 Neuromuscular Junction and Muscle Physiology

CHAPTER OUTLINE

Neuromuscular Junction
- Structure
- Neuromuscular Transmission

Muscle Physiology
- General Considerations
- Skeletal Muscles
- Process of Excitation-contraction Coupling
- Some Characteristics of the Skeletal Muscles in the Intact Body
- Smooth Muscle
- Cardiac Muscle

NEUROMUSCULAR JUNCTION

Neuromuscular junction refers to intimate contact of nerve endings with the muscle fibers to which they innervate. It is constituted by the following structures (Fig. 7.4-1).

STRUCTURE

Terminal Button

The axon of a neuron supplying a skeletal muscle loses its myelin sheath and divides into a number of fine branches, which end in small swellings (knobs) called *terminal buttons* or end feet, which form a neuromuscular junction, at the center of muscle fiber. The terminal knob contains large number of vesicles containing acetylcholine and mitochondria. The acetylcholine is synthesized by the mitochondria.

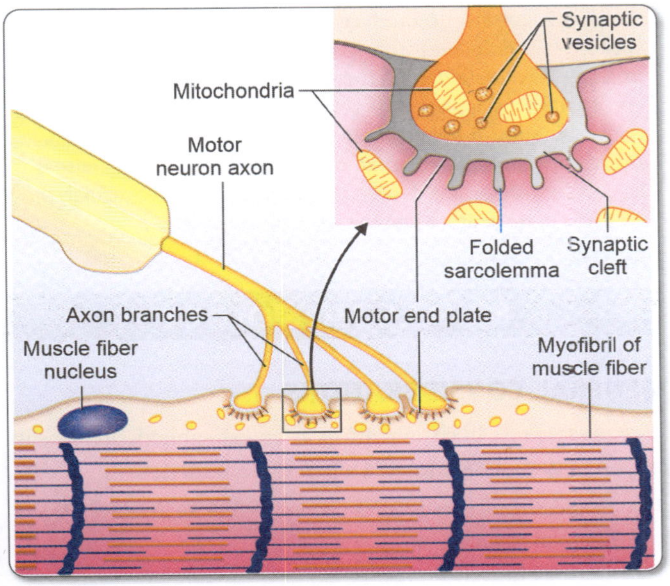

Fig. 7.4-1: Structure of neuromuscular junction; the axon of the neuron loses its myelin sheath and divides into fine branches; structure of terminal button and motor end plate

Presynaptic Membrane

This refers to the axonal membrane lining the *terminal buttons* of the nerve endings.

Synaptic Cleft

It is a 50–100 nm wide space between the presynaptic membrane and the postsynaptic membrane. It is filled by extracellular fluid with reticular fibers forming the matrix. It contains the enzyme cholinesterase, which can degrade acetylcholine.

Postsynaptic Membrane

This is the name given to the muscle fiber membrane (sarcolemma) in the region of neuromuscular junction. The muscle membrane in this region is thickened and depressed to form the *synaptic trough* in which the terminal button fits. This thickened portion of the muscle membrane is also called *motor end plate.* The postsynaptic membrane contains *receptor sites* for acetylcholine called the *nicotinic receptors.*

NEUROMUSCULAR TRANSMISSION

The skeletal muscle is stimulated only through its nerve. The neuromuscular junction transmits the impulses from the nerve to muscle. The *sequence of events* which causes transmission of impulse through neuromuscular junction are given below.

Release of Acetylcholine by the Nerve Terminals

When the nerve impulse (action potential) traveling in the nerve fiber (axon) reaches the terminal buttons, the voltage-gated Ca^{2+} channels present on the presynaptic membrane open up. Consequently the Ca^{2+} ions present in the extracellular fluid (ECF) of synaptic cleft enter the terminal buttons.

The elevated Ca^{2+} levels in the cytosol of terminal buttons trigger a marked increase in exocytosis of vesicles releasing acetylcholine in the synaptic cleft (Fig. 7.4-2).

Effect of Acetylcholine on the Postsynaptic Membrane

The acetylcholine so released diffuses in the synaptic cleft and binds to the nicotinic acetylcholine receptors located mainly on the junctional folds of the motor end plate (postsynaptic membrane) leading to opening up of the tubular channels.

Development of End Plate Potential

Due to opening of the acetylcholine-gated channels in the end plate membrane, a large number of Na^+ ions from the ECF enter inside the muscle fiber the following the electrochemical gradient.

When sodium ions enter inside, carrying with them large numbers of positive charges, depolarization occurs causing a local positive potential change inside the muscle fiber membrane called the *end plate potential.*

The end plate potential is nonpropagative but when a critical level of –60 mV is reached, it triggers the development of action potential in the muscle fiber and is conducted away from the end plate in both the directions along the muscle fibers thus, causing muscle contraction.

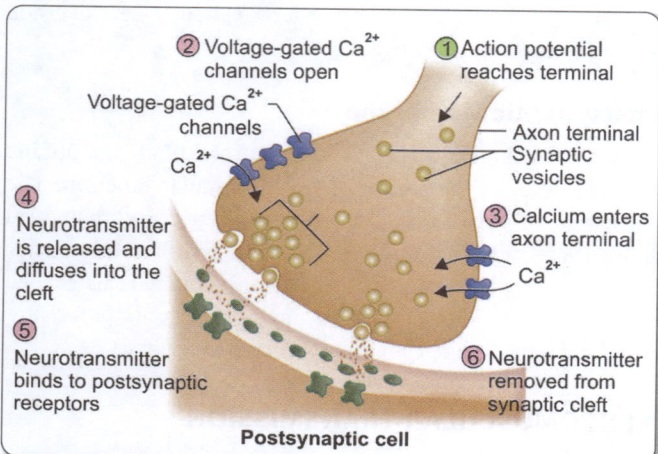

Fig. 7.4-2: Detailed structure of neuromuscular junction showing Ca^{2+} channels on presynaptic membrane and ACh receptors on postsynaptic membrane

Removal of Acetylcholine

The acetylcholine released in the synaptic cleft stays for short period and is removed within one millisecond by the enzyme acetylcholinesterase which is present in the matrix of synaptic cleft.

It is important to note that the rapid removal of acetylcholine prevents the repeated excitation of muscle fiber.

CLINICAL ASPECTS

DRUGS AFFECTING NEUROMUSCULAR JUNCTION

Neuromuscular Blockers

Neuromuscular blockers are the drugs that block transmission at the neuromuscular junction. Some of the common neuro-muscular blockers, which are commonly used in clinical practice and research are: Curare, succinylcholine and carbamylcholine, botulinum, etc.

Neuromuscular Stimulators

Drugs having acetylcholine-like action: Carbachol and nicotine are either not destroyed or are destroyed very slowly by the enzyme acetylcholinesterase.

Drugs that inactivate the enzyme cholinesterase (anticho-linesterase): The drugs like neostigmine and physostigmine stimulate the neuromuscular junction by inactivating the enzyme acetylcholinesterase.

DISORDER OF NEUROMUSCULAR JUNCTION

Myasthenia Gravis

Myasthenia is an autoimmune disease. In this disease, the antibodies are produced against the acetylcholine-gated channels (receptors) present on the motor end plate which destroy these channels. Thus, the acetylcholine released at the nerve terminal is not able to produce adequate end plate potential to excite the muscle fiber. This leads to extensive and progressive muscle weakness although the muscles are normal. Extraocular and eyelid muscles are affected first, followed by those of the neck and limbs. It affects females more than males and usually those between the age group of 20 and 40 years. If the disease is intense enough, the patient dies of paralysis, in particular, the paralysis of respiratory muscles.

MUSCLE PHYSIOLOGY

GENERAL CONSIDERATIONS

The muscle cell, like the neuron, is an excitable tissue, i.e., an action potential is generated when it is stimulated.

There are three different types of muscles in the body:

1. Skeletal muscles
2. Cardiac muscles
3. Smooth muscles.

Based on certain distinctive features, the muscles can be grouped as follows:

Striated versus Nonstriated Muscles

Striated muscle cells show large number of cross striations at regular intervals when seen under light microscope. Skeletal and cardiac muscles are striated.

Nonstriated muscle cells do not show any striations. Smooth muscles or the so-called plain muscles are non-striated.

Voluntary versus Involuntary Muscles

Voluntary muscles can be made to contract under our will to perform the movements, we desire. All skeletal muscles are voluntary muscles. These are supplied by somatic motor nerves.

Involuntary muscles activities cannot be controlled at will. Cardiac and all smooth muscles are involuntary muscles. These are innervated by autonomic nerves.

SKELETAL MUSCLES

The skeletal muscles, as the name indicates, are attached with the bones of the body skeleton and their contraction results in the body movements. The skeletal muscles constitute about 40% of the total body mass.

Structural Organization of Skeletal Muscle

Structurally, the skeletal muscle consists of a large number of muscle fibers and a connective tissue framework organized as (Figs 7.4-3A and B and Histology Plate 7.4-1):
- Each *muscle fiber* is surrounded by delicate connective tissue called *endomysium*.
- The muscle fibers are grouped into a number of bundles called *fasciculi*. Each fasciculus is surrounded by a sheath called *perimysium*.

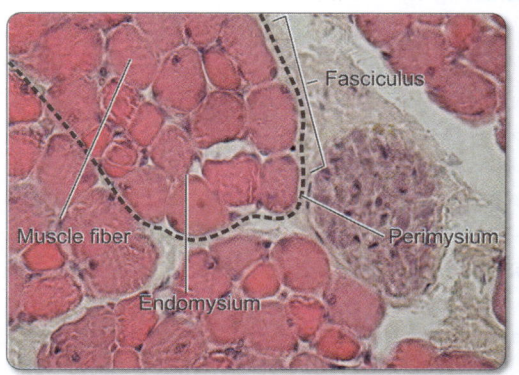

Histology Plate 7.4-1: Skeletal Muscle

Muscle fibers are managed in fasciculi. They are seen as irregularly round structures with peripheral nuclei. Each fascicle is surrounded by perimysium and each muscle fiber is surrounded by endomysium.

- All the fasciculi collectively form the *muscle belly*. The connective tissue that surrounds the entire muscle belly is called *epimysium*.
- At the junction of the muscle with its tendon, the fibers of endomysium, perimysium and epimysium become continuous with the fibers of the tendon.
- *Tendons* are fibrous terminal ends of the muscles made up of collagen fibers.

Structure of a Muscle Fiber

Each muscle fiber is basically a long (1–4 cm), cylindrical (10–100 μm in diameter) multinucleated cell. Its cell membrane is called *sarcolemma* and the cytoplasm is called *sarcoplasm*. The sarcoplasm contains number of *myofibrils*, which form the main structure of a muscle fiber. The sarcolemma along with

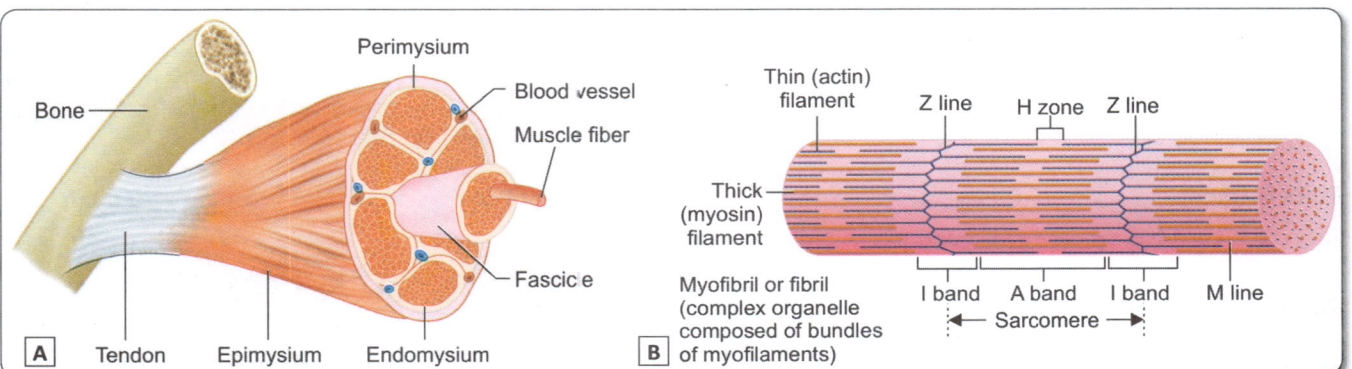

Figs 7.4-3A and B: Schematic diagram showing structural organization of skeletal muscle: A. Muscle belly; muscle fibers grouped into fasciculi; muscle fiber; B. Myofibril; and arrangement of thick and thin filaments

the sarcoplasmic reticulum form the so-called *sarcotubular system.*

Myofibril (Fig. 7.4-3B)

Each muscle fiber consists of a large number of myofibrils which are arranged parallel to each other and running along the entire length of the muscle fiber.

Each myofibril consists of many thick and thin filaments (myofilaments) made up of contractile proteins. Thick filaments are made up of myosin, while thin filaments are made of actin.

Striations of muscle fibers. The dark and light bands result from a difference in the refractive index of its different parts. The arrangement is as given below.

- The dark band is called *A band.* In the area of A band the thick (myosin) filaments line up the thin filaments.
- In the center of each A band, there is a lighter H zone where thin filaments do not overlap the thick filaments.
- In the center of each H zone is seen M line, which is more pronounced during muscle contraction.
- The light band is called *I band.* This area contains only thin (actin) filaments.
- Each I band is bisected by a narrow dark *Z line.* The portion of myofibril between two successive Z lines is called a *sarcomere.* Thus, a sarcomere includes ½ I band + A band + ½ I band and is about 2.5 μm in length at rest. The sarcomere is the structural and functional unit of the muscle fiber. During muscle contraction the sarcomere reduces in length to 1.5 μm and during stretching of the muscle, it increases in length to 3.5 μm.

Thick and Thin Filaments

The thick and thin filaments form the *contractile apparatus* of a striated muscle. These are made up of three types of proteins:

1. *Contractile proteins* are *myosin* and *actin* which interact to generate the contractile force in a muscle.
2. *Regulatory proteins* also called relaxation proteins include *tropomyosin* and *troponin.* These regulate the interaction between the myosin and actin.
3. *Anchoring proteins,* as the name indicates, anchor the different proteins to each other as well as to sarcolemma.

Thick filament

A thick filament is made up of hundreds of molecules of *myosin.*

Structure of myosin molecule. The myosin molecule is made up of 6 polypeptide chains, 2 heavy chains and 4 light chains. The 2 heavy chains form a double helix which constitutes the *tail* and *body* of the myosin molecule. The light chains form the

globular *head* of myosin molecule. The myosin molecule present in the skeletal muscle has two heads and is called *myosin-II* (Figs 7.4-4A and B).

Arrangement of myosin molecules in a thick filament. In a thick filament, half of the myosin molecules are oriented with their heads in one direction and the remaining half in opposite direction (Fig. 7.4-4C).

Thin filament

Each thin filament is made up of contractile protein molecules (actin) and two types of regulatory protein molecules (tropomyosin and troponin) (Fig. 7.4-5).

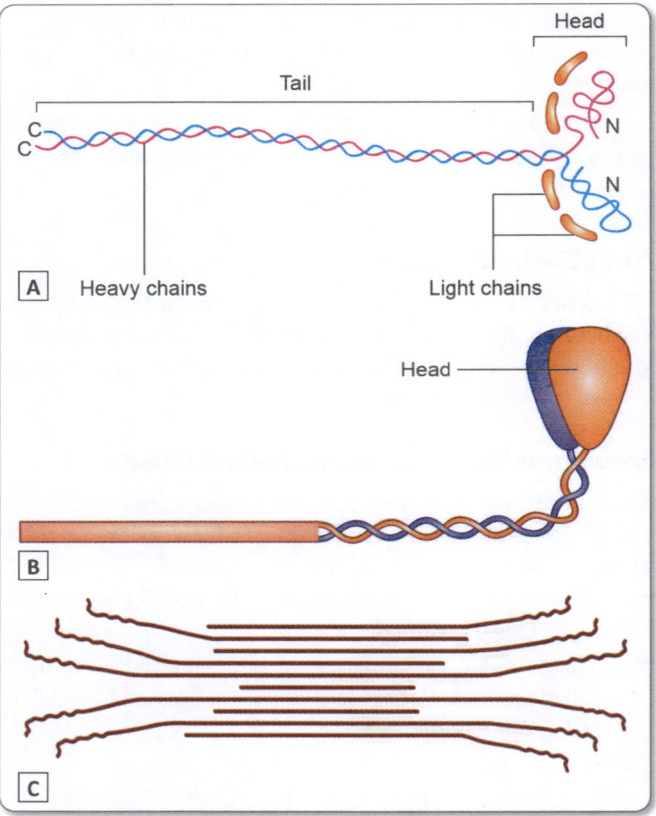

Figs 7.4-4A to C: Myosin molecules: A. Structure of myosin molecule; B. Molecule of myosin II (with two heads); C. Arrangement of myosin molecules in thick filament

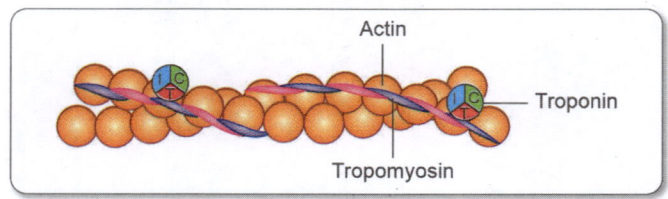

Fig. 7.4-5: Structure of a thin filament

Actin. About 300–400 actin molecules are present in each thin filament. The actin molecules form a long double helix consisting of two chains of globular units.

Tropomyosin. About 40–60 tropomyosin molecules are present in each thin filament. The tropomyosins are long filaments, which lie in the groove between the 2 chains of actin molecules. It covers the binding site of actin where myosin head comes in contact with actin, which prevents the interaction between actin and myosin filaments.

Troponin. Troponin molecules are small globular units located at intervals along the tropomyosin molecule. The troponin molecule has three subunits:

1. *Troponin-T* binds the other troponin components to tropomyosin.

2. *Troponin-I* prevents the interaction of myosin heads with active sites on actin.

3. *Troponin-C* contains binding site for Ca^{2+} that initiates muscle contraction.

Sarcotubular System

The sarcolemma (cell membrane of muscle cell) along with the sarcoplasmic reticulum (the endoplasmic reticulum of muscle cell) forms a highly specialized system called sarcotubular system. This plays an important role in the internal conduction of wave of depolarization within the muscle fiber. The sarcotubular system is primarily formed by a transverse tubular system (T-system) and a longitudinal sarcoplasmic reticulum (Fig. 7.4-6).

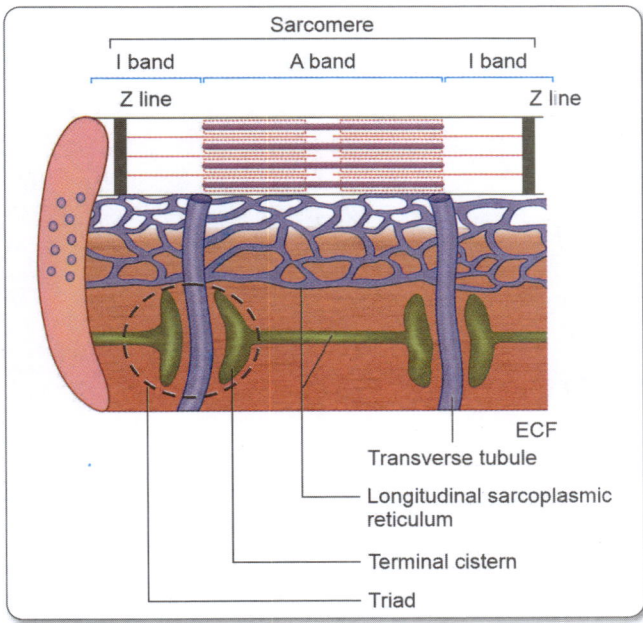

Fig. 7.4-6: Sarcotubular system showing transverse tubules and longitudinal sarcoplasmic reticulum

PROCESS OF EXCITATION-CONTRACTION COUPLING

The process by which depolarization of a muscle fiber initiates contraction is called excitation-contraction coupling. The sequence of events during this process are:

- Action potential initiated in the plasma membrane of a muscle fiber spreads rapidly on the surface as well as into the interior of the muscle fiber through the T-tubules.
- When the action potential reaches the tip of T-tubule, calcium ions diffuse into the cytoplasm. The concentration of Ca^{2+} in the intracellular fluid (ICF) is increased by some 2000 times.
- The Ca^{2+} ions get attached to troponin-C and start a chain of events, which produce contraction. Thus, the calcium ions act as linking or coupling material between the excitation and the contraction of the muscle.

Process of Muscle Contraction

Molecular basis of Muscle Contraction

AF Huxley and HE Huxley in 1954 put forward the *sliding theory* or *ratchet theory*. This theory explains that the sliding of filaments is brought about by a repeated cycle of formation of the *cross-bridges* between the head of myosin and actin molecules.

Initiation of cross-bridge cycling. During resting stage, troponin-I is lightly bound to actin and the tropomyosin molecules are located in the groove between the strands of actin filaments in such a way that they block the myosin-binding sites on actin (Fig. 7.4-7A). When activation takes place, the Ca^{2+} ions get attached to *troponin-C* subunit of the protein troponin. This causes the tropomyosin molecule to move laterally, uncovering the binding sites on the actin molecules for head of the myosin molecules. Thus, the cross-bridge cycle is switched on (initiated) by the lateral movement of tropomyosin (Fig. 7.4-7B and Fig. 7.4-8).

Changes Produced by Sliding of Thin Filaments over Thick Filaments During Muscle Contraction

Figure 7.4-9 shows the following changes produced by sliding of thin filaments over thick filaments during muscle contraction:

- The width of A band remains constant.
- H zone disappears.
- I band width decreases.
- The Z lines move closer.
- The sarcomere shortens.
- The actin filaments from the opposite end of the sarcomere approach each other and when the muscle shortening is marked, these filaments apparently overlap.

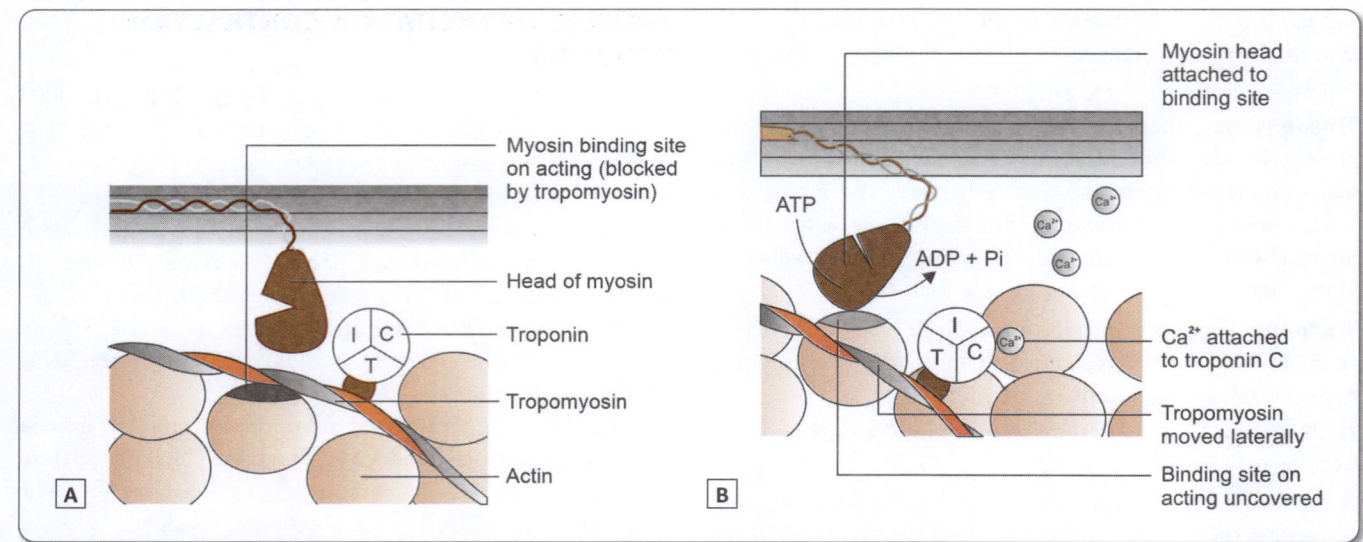

Figs 7.4-7A and B: Initiation of cross-bridge cycling: A. Resting state (myosin binding site on actin is covered by troponin-tropomyosin complex); B. On activation Ca^{2+} binds to troponin-C subunits resulting in conformational change and lateral displacement of tropomyosin (causing uncovering of binding site for myosin—head of myosin) on actin (initiation of cross-bridge cycle).

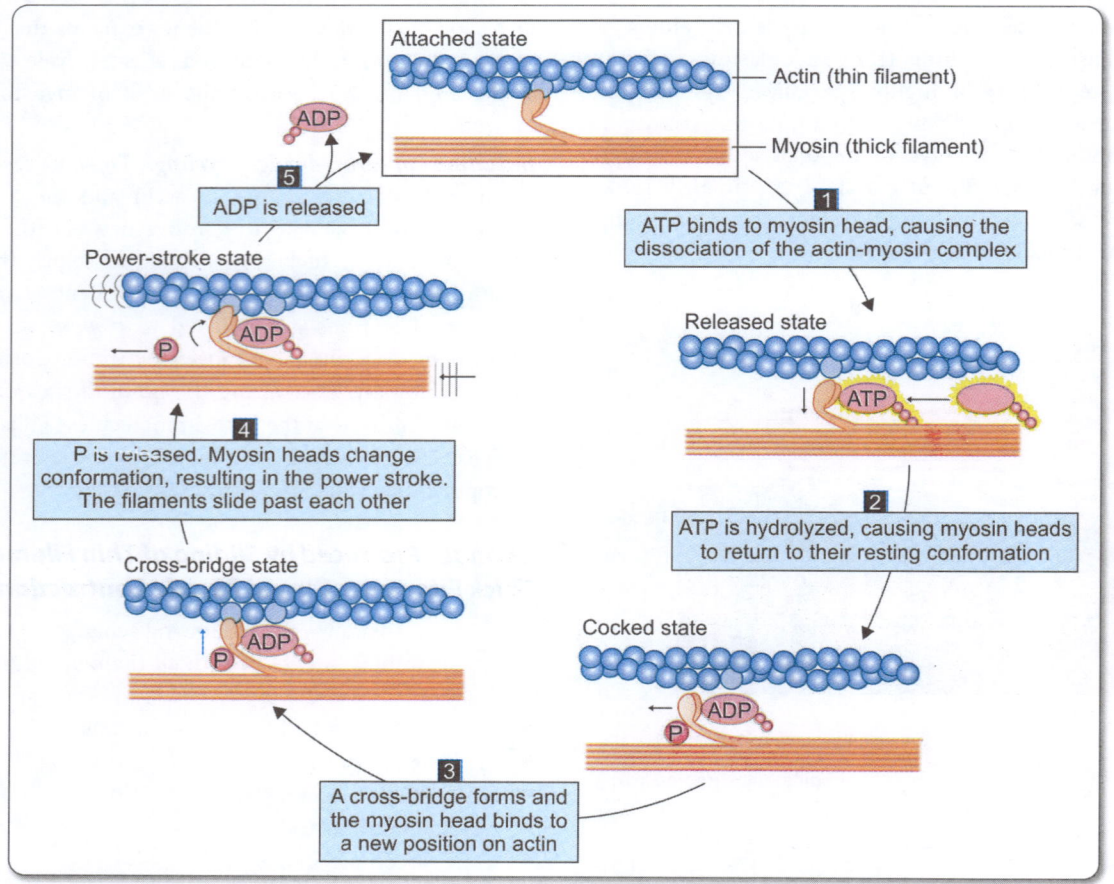

Fig. 7.4-8: Stages of cross-bridge cycling

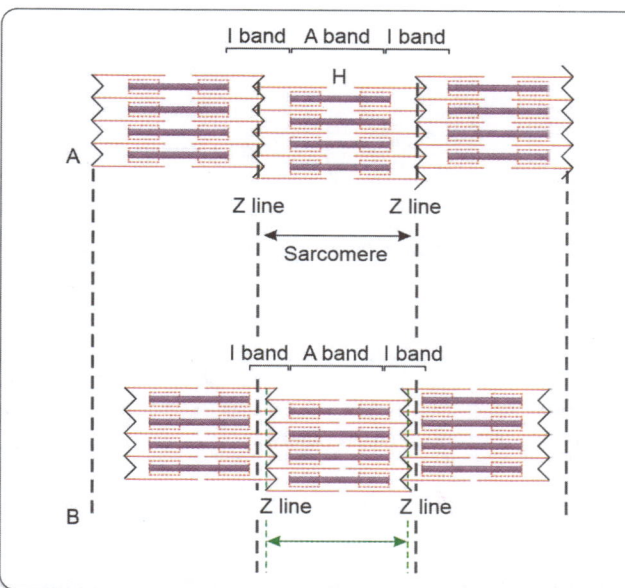

Fig. 7.4-9: Changes produced in a sarcomere by sliding of thin filament (actin) over thick filament (myosin) during muscle contraction: A. Relaxed state; B. Contracted stage

Muscle relaxation. Within a few milliseconds of the action potential, the calcium pump transports Ca^{2+} ions present in sarcoplasm during contraction back into the longitudinal portion of the sarcoplasmic reticulum.

Removal of calcium from troponin restores blocking action of troponin-tropomyosin complex. Myosin cross-bridge cycle closes and muscle relaxes.

NURSING IMPLICATIONS AND APPLICATIONS

Rigor mortis refers to shortening and rigidity of all the body muscles which occurs some hours after death. The rigidity occurs because of fixation of cross-bridges of myosin head to actin filaments due to loss of all the ATPs (which is normally required for detachment of cross-bridges of myosin heads from the actin filaments causing relaxation). The rigidity disappears after some hours due to destruction of the muscle proteins by enzymes released from the cellular lysosomes.

The appearance and disappearance of rigor mortis is used by the forensic experts in fixing the time of death.

Sequence of Events during Muscle Contraction and Relaxation when Stimulated by a Nerve

The events which occur during contraction and relaxation in a skeletal muscle, when excited by a nerve, are summarized sequence-wise in as follows:

Nerve Excitation

Stimulation of motor neuron

↓

Initiation of action potential in motor neuron's axon

Nerve Conduction

Propagation of action potential in the motor nerve

↓

Impulse reaching at nerve ending (at synaptic button)

Neuromuscular Transmission

Increased permeability of presynaptic membrane to Ca^{2+} ions

↓

Inflow of Ca^{2+} ions from ECF into the nerve terminals

↓

Release of ACh from the microvesicles present at the nerve terminal

↓

Diffusion of ACh into the synaptic cleft

↓

Binding of ACh to receptors on the motor end plate (Post-synaptic membrane)

↓

Opening of ACh-galed channels in the motor end membrane

↓

Entry of mainly Na^+ ions and to a lesser extent Ca^{2+} ions through these channels into the muscle fiber

↓

Development end-plate potential (EPP) Muscle excitation

↓

Muscle Excitation

Local EPP when reach a threshold magnitude, voltage-gated Na^+ channels are opened up at the site

↓

Generation of action potential (AP) in the muscle fiber by the end plate depolarization

Propagation of AP in muscle fiber along the surface and into the fiber along the T-tubules

↓

Excitation-contraction Coupling

Release of Ca^{2+} ions from terminal cistern

↓

Diffusion of Ca^{2+} ions into the sarcoplasm

↓

Binding of Ca^{2+} ions to troponin C

↓

Muscle Contraction (Molecular Theory)

Uncovering of binding sites for myosin on actin

↓

Cross-bridge formation between myosin head and actin

↓

Angular movement !of cross-bridges (power-stroke)

↓

Sliding of thin filaments over thick filaments

↓

Initiation of muscle contraction

↓

Muscle Relaxation

Active transport of Ca^{2+} into sarcoplasmic reticulun

↓

Decreased concentration of Ca^{2+} in sarcoplasm

↓

Removal of Ca^{2+} ions from troponin-C

↓

Cessation of cross-bridge cycling

↓

Relaxation of muscle fiber

Motor unit

Motor unit is the functional unit of muscle contraction in the intact body. It consists of the single motor neuron cell body, it's axon and the muscle fibers innervated by it (Fig. 7.4-10). The cell bodies of the motor neurons (a motor neuron) supplying

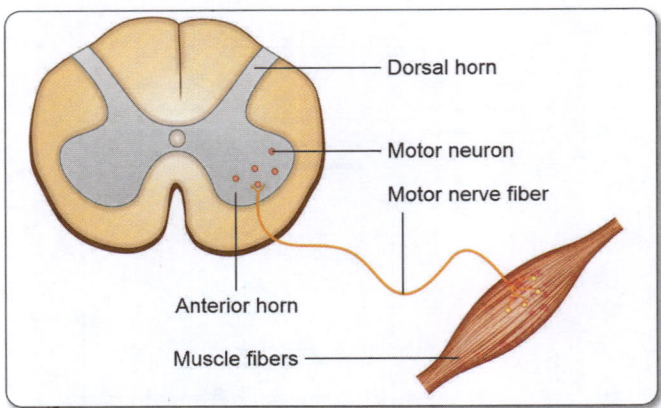

Fig. 7.4-10: Structure of a motor unit

the skeletal muscle fibers lie in the ventral horn of the spinal cord or the motor cranial nerve nuclei.

Type of motor units. Each motor neuron innervates only one type of muscle fibers. In other words, in a single motor unit the muscle fibers supplied by it are of the same type. Therefore, depending on the type of muscle fibers, the motor units are also of two types:

1. Type I (red or slow) motor units
2. Type II (white or fast) motor units. The characteristic features of each type of motor units are given in Table 7.4-1.

Contractile Response

Contractile response is the characteristic feature of a skeletal muscle. When stimulated, an action potential is developed in the muscle fiber, which is followed by the muscle contraction. The muscle contraction is manifested by either shortening (isotonic contraction) or development of tension (isometric contraction) or both. The contractile response can be studied in an isolated nerve–muscle preparation as single muscle twitch.

Isometric contraction

As the name indicates (iso = same, metric = measure, i.e., length), in this type of contraction, the length of muscle remains same but tension is developed in the muscle. Thus, there is no movement of the object. Since work done is the product of *force* and *distance*, therefore, in isometric contraction *no external work is done.*

Examples of isometric contraction of muscles

- Contraction of muscles, which help in maintaining posture against gravity
- Contraction of arm muscles when trying to push a wall.

TABLE 7.4-1: Characteristic features of type I and type II motor units

Characteristics	Motor unity	
	Type I	Type II
Muscle fiber type	The muscle fibers of type I motor units are slow, red (slow) and involved in tonic activity	The muscle fibers of type II motor unit are fast, white (fast) and involved in phasic activity
Axon diameter	Small	Large
Axon conduction velocity	Slow	Fast
Motor unit innervation ratio	High (120–160 muscle fibers/axon), e.g., postural muscles	Low (six muscle fibers/axon), e.g., extraocular muscles
Twitch duration	Long	Brief
Mitochondria number	High	Low
Metabolism	Aerobic, low glycolytic and high oxidative capacity	Anaerobic, high glycolytic and low oxidative capacity
Glycogen contents	Low	High
Myoglobin contents	High	Low

Isotonic contraction

As the name indicates (iso = same, and tonic = tone or tension), in this type of contraction, the tension in the muscle remains same, whereas its length decreases. Since the muscle length is shortened, so the *external work is done* in isotonic contraction.

Examples of Isotonic Muscle Contraction

- Contraction of leg muscles during walking and running
- Contractions of muscles while lifting a weight
- Contraction of muscles during flexion of arm.

SOME CHARACTERISTICS OF THE SKELETAL MUSCLES IN THE INTACT BODY

A. Muscle Tone

Muscle tone is the state of slight contraction with certain degree of vigor and tension. All the skeletal muscles exhibit muscle tone. However, it is more marked in the antigravity muscles, viz. extensors of the lower limbs, trunk muscles, and muscles of the neck.

Maintenance of Muscle Tone

Muscle tone is maintained by asynchronous discharge of impulses from gamma motor neurons in the anterior grey horn of the spinal cord concerned with the motor nerve supply of the muscles. The gamma motor neurons in turn are controlled by some higher centers in brain.

CLINICAL ASPECTS

Abnormalities of the muscle tone include:

- *Hypertonic state* or the spastic paralysis of the skeletal muscles occurs in upper motor neuron lesions. Spasticity results due to exaggerated activity of lower motor neurons the following or loss of inhibition activity of upper motor neurons.
- *Hypotonic state* or the flaccid paralysis of the muscles occurs in lower motor neuron lesions. The tone of the affected muscles is decreased or totally lost and ultimately the muscles undergo wasting.

B. Gradation of Force of Muscle Contraction in the Intact Body

For performing different kinds of work, e.g., picking up a pen from the table, or lifting 10 kg weight, same muscles are involved but on these different situations, muscles can generate different degree of power. This property of skeletal muscles is known as gradation of force of contraction. Gradation of muscle power in muscles is made possible by certain factors, which affect the force of contraction.

Recruitment of Motor Units

The force of contraction produced in a muscle depends upon the number of motor units recruited. When minimal activity is required, only a few motor units are recruited. With increasing effort, more and more motor units from the *motor neuron pool* of a muscle are recruited into activity. This phenomenon is called multiple motor unit summation.

Frequency of Nerve Impulses

The motor control system in the brain can vary the force of contraction by varying the frequency of nerve impulses stimulating the muscle. As the impulse frequency increases, its effects are summated (*wave summation*) and the muscle tension increases.

Synchronization of Impulses

At any one time, the motor units are in different phases of activity, i.e., some are contracting and others are relaxing. Due to algebraic summation, the muscle gives a steady but weak pull. With increasing synchronization of the motor units, the force of contraction increases.

C. Effect of Initial Length of Muscle Fiber

According to Starling's law, up to an optimal limit, the greater the initial length of the muscle fibers, greater is the force of contraction. This, however, is not the usual method of varying the force of contraction in the intact body.

Warming Up

Warming up is the term used in the parlor of sports persons for the exercises performed before actually participating in any game event. These pregame 'warm up' due to beneficial effects of the exercise increase the muscle performance when the person takes part in the actual event.

D. Muscle Fatigue

Fatigue is defined as failure of a muscle to maintain tension as a result of previous contractile activity due to repeated stimuli/activity. If the muscle is allowed to rest after the onset of fatigue, it recovers its ability to contract.

Therefore, the fatigue of most of the muscles that develop after prolonged general exercise such as marathon running, and competitive football match playing.

Onset and recovery of fatigue depends on:

- *Intensity and duration of exercise*
- *Type of muscle fibers:* Fast glycolytic fibers fatigue early and also recover rapidly from fatigue. Slow oxidative fibers do not fatigue early but they also require longer time of rest (up to 24 hours) for complete recovery.

Causes of fatigue are:

- Exhaustion of acetylcholine
- Accumulation of metabolites like lactic acid
- Lack of nutrition
- Lack of oxygen availability

E. Energy Source for Muscle Contraction

The muscle contraction requires lot of energy. The immediate source of energy is ATP and the ultimate source is the intermediary metabolism of carbohydrate and lipids.

Hydrolysis of ATP

The hydrolysis of ATP provides energy for muscle contraction. ATP stored in the muscle initiates the contractile activity but is consumed approximately within 3 seconds, all the ATP stored in the muscle cell is depleted. Thus, there is need for resynthesis of ATP.

Resynthesis of ATP

There are three ways in which muscle fiber can resynthesize ATP from ADP during contractile activity:

Phosphorylation of ADP by creatine phosphate. Immediately after the depletion of ATP stores of the muscle, ATP is regenerated using the energy released by the dephosphorylation of creatine phosphate reserves of the muscle fiber.

Creatine phosphate + ADP → Creatine + ATP

Glycolysis. After depletion of creatine phosphate reserves, the next important source of energy which is used to reconstitute both ATP and phosphocreatine is glycogen (previously stored in the muscle cell), by the process of glycolysis which can sustain muscle contraction for approximately 1 minute.

Oxidative metabolism. Oxidative metabolism, i.e., combining of oxygen with various cellular foodstuffs to liberate ATP is the final source of energy during muscle contraction. This source contributes more than 95% of all energy used by the muscles for sustained long-term contraction. Foodstuffs used in oxidative metabolism include fats, carbohydrates and proteins.

F. Oxygen Demand and Oxygen Consumption

Oxygen demand increases with the intensity of exercise, i.e., intensity of muscle contraction. It has been reported that in a sprint lasting for ½ min, the oxygen demand is around 20 L/min.

Oxygen consumption or oxygen utilization is the volume of oxygen which has been actually consumed during the exercise. The maximum amount of oxygen that can be consumed by a person while performing severe exercise is irrespective of the demand (VO_2 max). A world class sprinter is expected to have a VO_2 max around 75 mL/kg/min (approximately 4 L/min).

CLINICAL ASPECTS

COMMON DISORDERS OF SKELETAL MUSCLES

Muscular dystrophy: Muscular dystrophy is a syndrome, which occurs due to genetic mutation and is characterized by progressive muscle weakness.

Myotonia: Myotonia is a disorder which occurs due to abnormalities of the sodium and chloride channels caused by abnormal genes on chromosomes 7, 17 or 19. It is characterized by an abnormally prolonged muscle relaxation after voluntary contraction.

Fibrillation and denervation hypersensitivity: The denervation of skeletal muscles in lower motor neuron lesions causes flaccid paralysis of the muscle, fibrillation and denervation hypersensitivity.

- *Fibrillation* is characterized by fine, irregular contractions of individual muscle fibers.
- *Denervation hypersensitivity* refers to when the muscle becomes highly sensitive to acetylcholine.

ELECTROMYOGRAPHY

Electromyography refers to the technique of recording the total electrical activity of the motor nerve and the muscle under study. The machine used to record the said electrical activity is called *electromyograph* and the record obtained is called the *electromyogram.*

NURSING IMPLICATIONS AND APPLICATIONS

Oxygen Debt

- During intense exercise, the maximum oxygen consumed is much less than the oxygen demand. So, the energy requirement is met with by the anaerobic pathway. After the period of exercise, extra O_2 is consumed to remove the excess lactate collected due to anaerobic glucose breakdown, replenish the ATP and phosphoryl creatine store. This amount of extra oxygen consumed is called O_2 debt.
- To avoid excessive O_2 debt early in the race to prevent too much anaerobic metabolism and accumulation of lactic acid which hamper the efficiency.

SMOOTH MUSCLE

Functional Anatomy and Organization

Smooth muscles (nonstriated muscles), as the name indicates, are characterized by absence of the typical cross-striated pattern seen in the skeletal muscles. Because of their spontaneous activity or activity through the autonomic nervous system, they are also called involuntary muscles.

Arrangement of smooth muscle fibers. The smooth muscle cells are long fusiform in shape and are aggregated to form bundles or fasciculi. The fasciculi are aggregated to form layers of variable thickness. Thus, smooth muscles exist either in sheet or bundles of fibers. In each layer, the cells are so

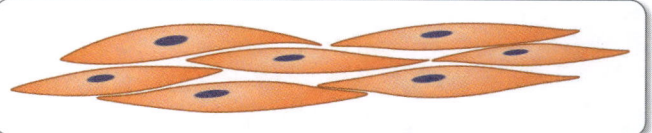

Fig. 7.4-11: Arrangement of smooth muscle fibers

arranged that thick central part of one cell is opposite to the thin tapering ends of adjoining cells (Fig. 7.4-11).

Types of Smooth Muscles

Smooth muscles are of two types: single-unit and multiunit smooth muscles.

1. *Single-unit smooth muscles* (Fig. 7.4-12): Single-unit smooth muscles are also called visceral smooth muscles because they are present in the walls of hollow viscera such as gastrointestinal tract, uterus, ureters, urinary bladder and respiratory tract.

2. *Multiunit smooth muscles.* Multiunit smooth muscles, as the name indicates, are made up of multiple individual units without interconnecting bridges, i.e., nonsyncytial in character. These are located in most blood vessels, epididymis, vas deferens, iris, ciliary body and piloerector muscles.

Innervation and Neuromuscular Junction of Smooth Muscles

Nerve supply. Smooth muscles are innervated by the autonomic nerves, both sympathetic as well as parasympathetic. The two have opposite effects. In some organs, sympathetic stimulation causes contraction and parasympathetic stimulation causes relaxation of smooth muscles. However, in some other organs a reverse action is seen.

Neuromuscular junction. The postganglionic nerve fibers, as approach the smooth muscles, branch extensively and come in close contact with large number of smooth muscle fibers (Fig. 7.4-13). The neuronal network so formed has a beaded appearance due to the large enlargements called varicosities. These varicosities contain the chemical neurotransmitter (acetylcholine or nor-epinephrine)

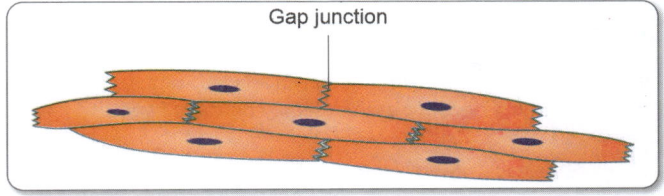

Fig. 7.4-12: Single-unit smooth muscle fiber showing gap junctions between two adjacent cells

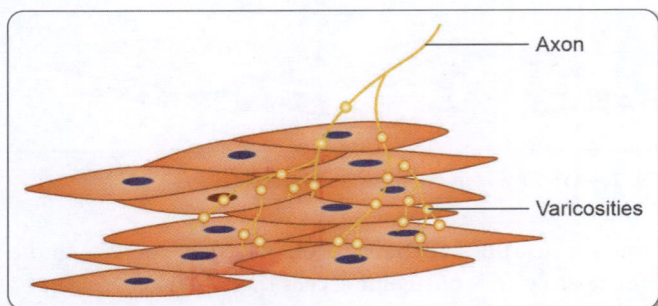

Fig. 7.4-13: The nerve supplying to smooth muscle showing varicosities (beaded appearance)

Structure of Smooth Muscle Fiber

Each smooth muscle fiber is a long spindle-shaped cell (myocyte) having a broad central part and tapering ends (Fig. 7.4-14A). The length of smooth muscle fiber is highly variable (15–500 μm) depending on the organ in which they are present. For example,

- Digestive tract fibers are 30–40 μm long and 5 μm in diameter.
- Fibers in blood vessels are 15–20 μm long and 2–3 μm in diameter.
- Fibers in uterus are 300 μm long and 10 μm in diameter.

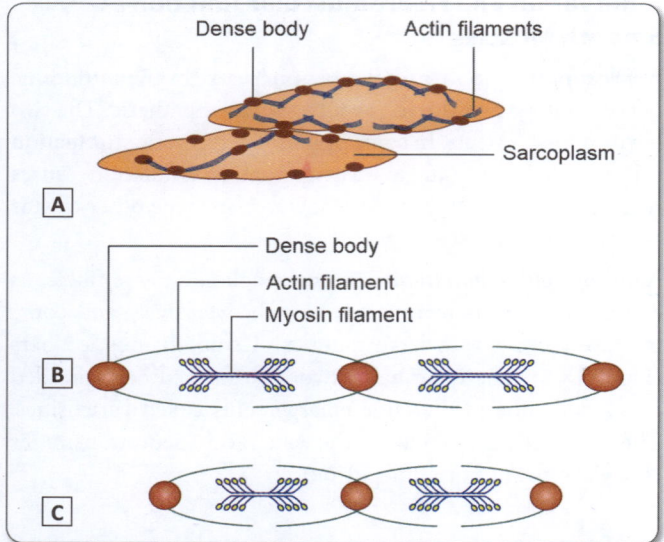

Figs 7.4-14A to C: Structure of smooth muscle: A. Arrangement of thin (actin filaments attached to dense bodies) and thick (myosin) filaments; B. Position of dense bodies in relaxed state; C. The dense bodies are drawn closer to each other in contracted state.

Salient Features of Structure of a Smooth Muscle Fiber

Plasma membrane which binds the smooth muscle is surrounded by an external lamina. Adjacent smooth muscle cells communicate through gap junctions.

Nucleus is oval or elongated and lies in the central part of the cell. *Sarcoplasm*, in addition to a single nucleus, contains other cell organelles like mitochondria (source of energy), a Golgi complex, some granular endoplasmic reticulum and free ribosomes. Apart from these, sarcoplasm also contains myofibrils and intermediate filaments. *Sarcoplasmic Reticulum (SR)*, similar to that in skeletal muscle, is present, but is not as developed.

Myofibrils are made of contractile proteins, the myosin and actin filaments (Fig. 7.4-14B).

The salient differences from the skeletal muscle are given as follows:

- The sarcotubular system is not well developed in smooth muscles.
- Smooth muscles contain relatively less **thick filaments** and more thin filaments.
- Z line is not well defined in smooth muscles.
- Myosin is chemically different from that seen in **skeletal** muscles. It binds to action only if its light chain is phosphorylated. Thus, phosphorylation of myosin is necessary for the contraction of smooth muscles.
- Thin actin filaments are also different from those in skeletal muscle due to absence of the troponin protein molecules.
- Dense bodies attached to the cell membrane and scattered all over the body of the fibers. The actin filaments are attached to these dense bodies. In between the actin filaments, the thick myosin filaments are situated.

There are cross bridges between actin and myosin, which help in sliding mechanism of muscle contraction. When the muscle contracts then the points on the cell membrane, where dense bodies are attached, are drawn closer to each other. This converts an oblongated smooth muscle in one that is oval (Fig. 7.4-14C).

Process of Excitability and Contractility

Process of muscle excitation: Process of muscle excitation basically includes the electrical activity in smooth muscles, which differs in a multiunit smooth muscle than that in a single-unit muscle.

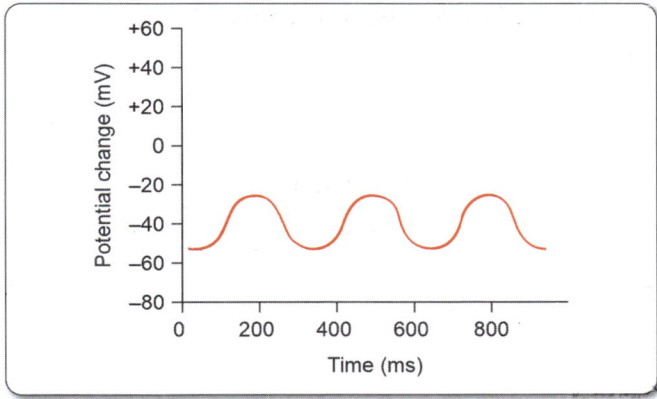

Fig. 7.4-15: Resting membrane potential (fluctuating type) in visceral smooth muscle

Electrical Activity in Single-Unit (Visceral) Smooth Muscles

The resting membrane potential (RMP) in a visceral smooth muscle ranges between –50 mV and –75 mV. The peculiarity of the resting membrane potential is its unstability, i.e., there is no true resting value rather it keeps on oscillating between –55 mV and –35 mV (Fig. 7.4-15). These oscillations in the RMP occur due to superimposition by the pacemaker potentials, which, in turn, occur due to rhythmic changes in either Ca²⁺ channel permeability and/or the activity of Na⁺– K⁺ pump state.

Action potential. When depolarization reaches threshold potential, an action potential is generated which is transmitted to the adjacent muscle cells through the gap junction. Three types of action potentials are known to occur in the visceral smooth muscle fibers, viz. Spike potential, spikepotential superimposed over pacemaker potential and action potential with plateau (Figs 7.4-16A to C).

Process of Excitation–Contraction Coupling

It occurs when the smooth muscle is excited through sarcolemmal depolarization. Due to depolarization of the membrane, the voltage-gated Ca²⁺ channels present on it are opened and the Ca²⁺ ions from the ECF move into the sarcoplasm. These Ca²⁺ ions, in turn, stimulate the release of more Ca²⁺ from the SR.

Process of smooth muscle contraction

The molecular mechanism of a smooth muscle contraction by cross-bridge cycling and sliding of filaments is similar to the skeletal muscle. However, the smooth muscle does not contain the regulatory protein tropomyosin and troponin, so its regulation is different. In smooth muscle, one of the light chains of the myosin filament located in the neck region serves the function of tropomyosin, and thus is called the regulatory chain of myosin. Similarly, the Ca²⁺ binding protein calmodulin plays the role of troponin. *Characteristics of smooth muscle contraction.* Certain characteristic features of smooth muscle contraction are as follows:

Plasticity. A smooth muscle exhibits the property of plasticity, i.e., it can readjust its resting length (the length at which a muscle generates maximum active tension). Thus, when smooth muscle is passively stretched, it first exerts increased tension, which gradually reduces to prestretch level (even when the stretch is maintained).

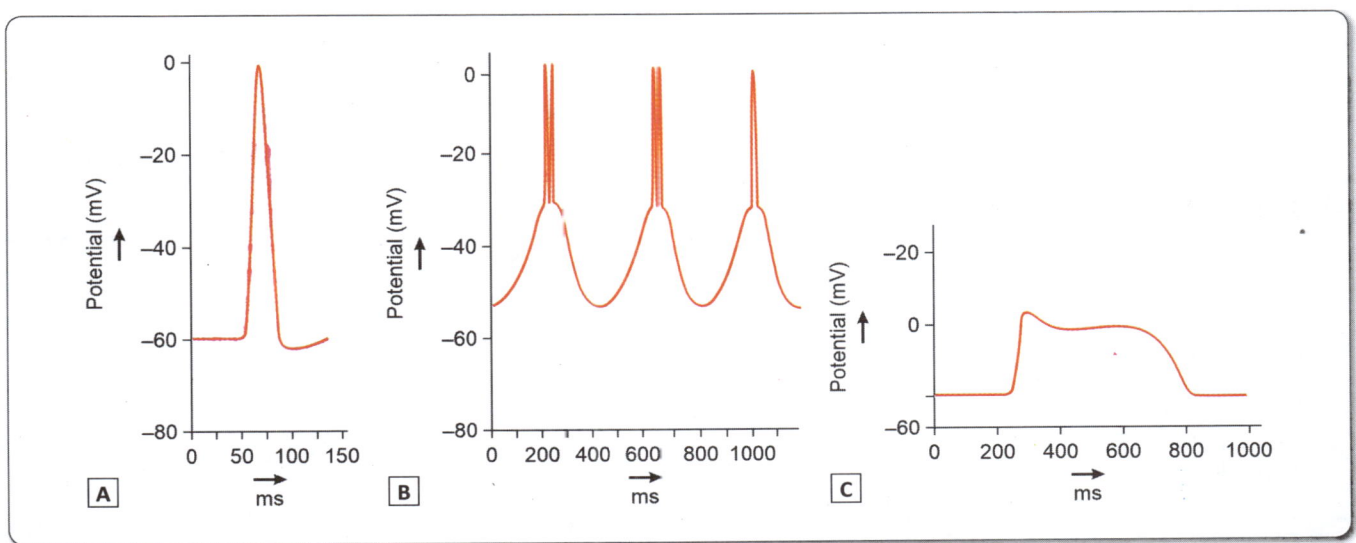

Figs 7.4-16A to C: Three types of action potentials recorded from smooth muscles: A. Spike potential; B. Spike potential superimposed over slow wave potentials; C. Action potential with plateau.

Latch phenomenon. Latch phenomenon is another characteristic exhibited by smooth muscles. It refers to the mechanism by which a smooth muscle can maintain a high tension without actively contracting. This phenomenon allows long term maintenance of tone in many smooth muscle organs.

CARDIAC MUSCLE
Functional Anatomy

- Structural organization of cardiac muscle
- Structure of a cardiac muscle fiber
- Sarcotubular system

Process of Excitability and Contractility

- Electrical potentials in cardiac muscle
- Excitation–contraction coupling phenomenon
- Process of cardiac muscle contraction

Properties of Cardiac Muscle

- Automaticity
- Rhythmicity
- Conductivity
- Excitability
- Contractility

Functional anatomy and physiology of cardiac muscle is discussed in Chapter 4.2 see page 198.

ASSESS YOURSELF

Short and Long Answer Questions

1. Draw a labeled diagram of structure of neuromuscular junction.
2. Briefly describe:
   - Sequence of events during excitation contraction coupling in skeletal muscle
   - Types of smooth muscles
   - Innervation and neuromuscular junction of smooth muscles
3. Differentiate between:
   - Isotonic and Isometric contraction
   - Type I and Type II motor units
4. Write notes on:
   - End plate potential
   - Myasthenia gravis
   - Sarcomere
   - Sarcotubular system
   - Fatigue phenomenon
   - Plasticity property in smooth muscle

Multiple Choice Questions

1. The basic structural and functional unit of skeletal muscle is:
   a. Myofibril
   b. Fasciculus
   c. Sarcomere
   d. Muscle fiber
2. True statement for neuromuscular junction is:
   a. Vesicles of presynaptic terminal contain Na⁺
   b. Vesicles of presynaptic terminal contain acetylcholine
   c. Released neurotransmitter cause influx of Ca^{2+} in presynaptic terminal
   d. Presynaptic terminal possess nicotinic receptors
3. During sliding mechanism, the energy is provided by:
   a. ATP
   b. ADP
   c. Glucose
   d. Lactic acid
4. The end plate potential is generated at:
   a. Presynaptic terminal
   b. Postsynaptic terminal
   c. Synaptic cleft
   d. Sarcotubular system
5. Which of the following is a neuromuscular blocker:
   a. Acetylcholine
   b. Cholinesterase
   c. Curare
   d. Physostigmine
6. In skeletal muscle, the Z line lies in the center of:
   a. H zone
   b. I band
   c. A band
   d. None of these
7. In skeletal muscle, the regulatory protein is:
   a. Actin
   b. Myosin
   c. Tropomyosin
   d. Nebulin
8. An example of isometric contraction is:
   a. Pushing of the wall
   b. Lifting of weight
   c. Walking
   d. Flexion of arm
9. Which is not the characteristic feature of Type II motor unit?
   a. Involved in tonic activity
   b. Has high glycolytic activity
   c. Also called white muscle fiber
   d. Involved in phasic activity
10. Rigor mortis occurs due to:
    a. Lack of Ca^{2+}
    b. Lack of ATP
    c. Proteolysis of muscle proteins
    d. Oxygen debt

ANSWER KEY

1. c	2. b	3. a	4. b	5. c	6. b	7. c	8. a
9. a	10. b						

Section
VIII

Renal System

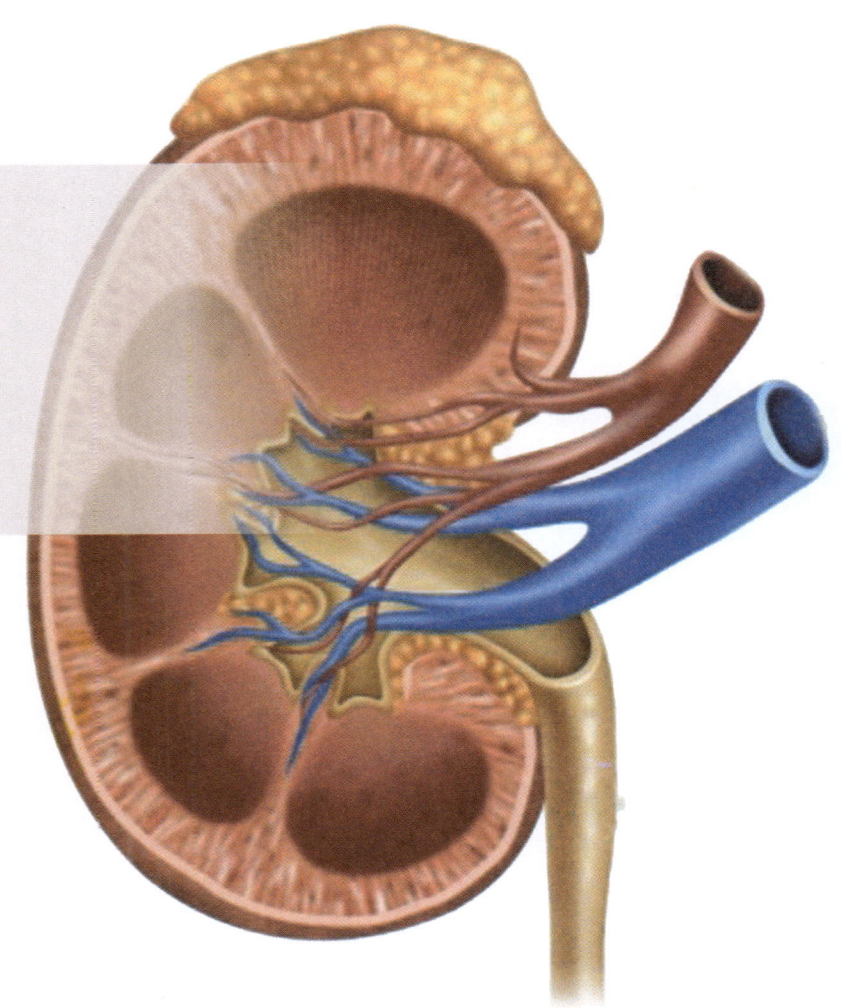

Section Outline

Anatomy and Physiology of Urinary System

ANATOMY OF URINARY SYSTEM

INTRODUCTION

Literally, the word "excretion" means elimination of any matter from the body of an organism. The organs which are involved in the process of excretion include:

- *Kidneys*, which excrete water and water-soluble waste products
- *Lungs*, which excrete carbon dioxide, water vapors and other volatile substances such as acetone
- *Skin*, which excretes water and salts mainly in the form of sweat
- *Gastrointestinal tract*, which excretes feces (excreta).

However, *sensu stricto*, the term "excretion" refers to elimination of principal products of metabolism except carbon dioxide. The principal products of metabolism, other than carbon dioxide, are ammonia, urea, uric acid, creatinine, various pigments and inorganic salts.

Excretory organs: Thus, in strictest sense, kidneys are the excretory organs. Together with a pair of ureters and a urinary bladder, kidneys constitute the excretory system (Fig. 8.1-1).

KIDNEYS

External Features

Gross anatomical features of a human kidney are illustrated in Figure. 8.1-1.

Location

The kidneys are bean-shaped organs that lie retroperitoneally on the posterior abdominal wall, one on each side of the

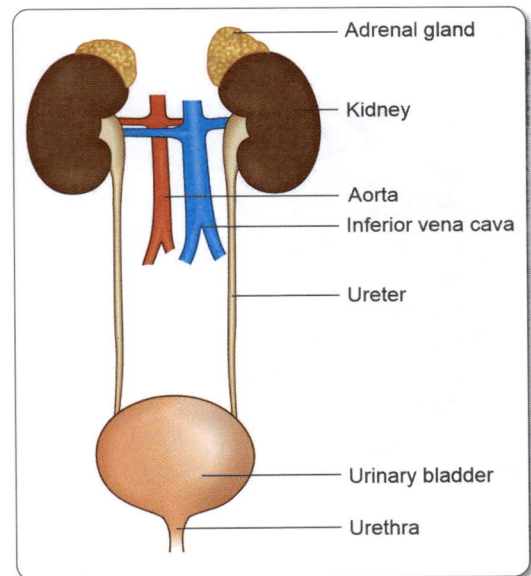

Fig. 8.1-1: The urinary organs

vertebral column at the level of T_{12} to L_1 vertebrae. The right kidney lies slightly inferior to the left kidney.

Size and Weight

During life, the kidneys are reddish-brown in color. Each kidney in an adult human weighs about 150 g and measures approximately 10 cm in length, 5 cm in width and 2.5 cm in thickness.

Renal Hilum and Sinus

The renal hilum is a vertical cleft present on the **concave** medial margin. It is the entrance to space within the **kidney—**

the renal sinus. Through renal hilum the renal artery enters, and the renal vein and renal pelvis leave the renal sinus. The *renal sinus* is thus occupied by the renal pelvis, calyces, vessels, nerves, and a variable amount of fat.

Renal Pelvis and Calyces

The renal pelvis is the flattened, funnel-shaped expansion of the superior end of ureter. Within the renal sinus, the pelvis divides into two (or three) parts called *major calyces*. Each major calyx divides into a number of *minor calyces*. The end of each minor calyx is shaped like a cup into which fits a projection of kidney tissue called renal papilla (the apex of renal pyramid).

Gross Internal Structure

Gross internal structure of the kidney, as seen in coronal section through the organ, exhibits that kidney tissue consists of an outer region called the cortex and an inner region called the medulla (Fig. 8.1-2).

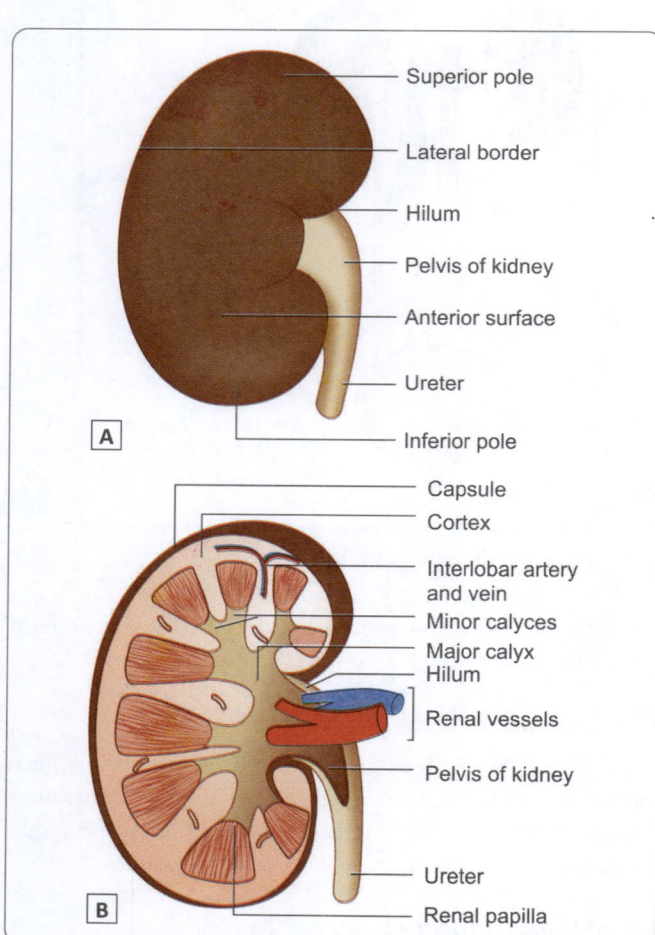

Figs 8.1-2A and B: Anatomical features of human kidney

Medulla

It is made up of triangular areas of renal tissues, that are called the renal pyramids. Pyramids are 4–14 in number and separated from each other by cortical columns of Bertin. Each pyramid has a base directed toward the cortex; and an apex (or renal papilla) which is directed toward the renal pelvis and fits into the minor calyx. The medulla can be subdivided into two parts:

1. **Outer medulla**, that is further subdivided into the outer stripe and the inner stripe.

2. **Inner medulla** is also called papillary zone.

Cortex

The renal cortex can be divided into two parts which are continuous with each other:

Cortical arches or cortical lobules refer to the tissue lying between the bases of pyramids and surface of the kidney.

Renal columns refer to the cortical tissue that lies in between the pyramids.

Lobe of kidney. Each pyramid, surrounded by a shell of cortex, constitutes a lobe of the kidney.

Coverings. The kidney is covered by three coverings from outside to inside; these are:

- *Pararenal fat* forms the cushion for the kidney.
- *Renal fascia* is also called false capsule having two layers; anterior and posterior. Superiorly it covers the suprarenal gland.
- *Perinephric fat* is also called middle fatty capsule. It acts as a shock absorber and keeps the kidneys in position.
- *Fibrous capsule* or true capsule is the innermost covering of the kidney.

Structure of Kidney

Microscopic Structure

Microscopically, the cortex and medulla of the kidney are composed of nephrons, blood vessels, lymphatics, and nerves (Histology Plate 8.1-1).

Nephron

Nephron is a structural and functional unit of the kidney. Each kidney contains approximately 1.2 million nephrons. Each nephron is capable of forming urine.

Structure of the nephron

A nephron consists of two major parts (Fig. 8.1-3):
1. Renal corpuscle
2. Renal tubule.

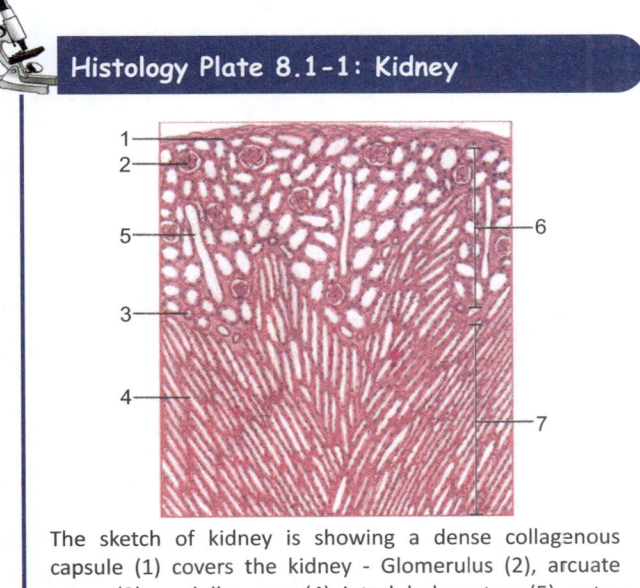

Histology Plate 8.1-1: Kidney

The sketch of kidney is showing a dense collagenous capsule (1) covers the kidney - Glomerulus (2), arcuate artery (3), medullary rays (4), interlobular artery (5), outer cortex (6) and inner medulla (7)

Renal corpuscle

Renal corpuscle or malpighian corpuscle is a rounded structure comprising glomerulus surrounded by glomerular capsule (Fig. 8.1-4A).

Glomerulus. Glomerulus refers to a rounded tuft of anastomosing capillaries. Blood enters the glomerulus through an *afferent arteriole* and leaves it through an *efferent arteriole* (note that the efferent vessel is an arteriole, and not a venule).

Glomerular capsule. Glomerular capsule, also known as Bowman's capsule, encloses the glomerulus and is formed of two layers: The inner layer covers the glomerular capillaries and is called *visceral layer*; and the outer layer is called *parietal layer*. In fact, the Bowman's capsule represents the cup-shaped blind beginning of the renal tubule. Space between the visceral and parietal layer of the capsule (called Bowman's space or urinary space) is continuous with the lumen of the renal tubule.

Ultrastructure of glomerular membrane. Glomerular membrane refers to the membrane that separates blood of glomerular capillaries from the fluid present in the Bowman's space. It is also called *filtration barrier* and consists of three major layers (Fig. 8.1-4B):

1. Capillary endothelium
2. Basement membrane
3. Bowman's visceral epithelium or the inner layer of Bowman's capsule which forms the third layer of glomerular membrane, is formed by special cells called *podocytes*.

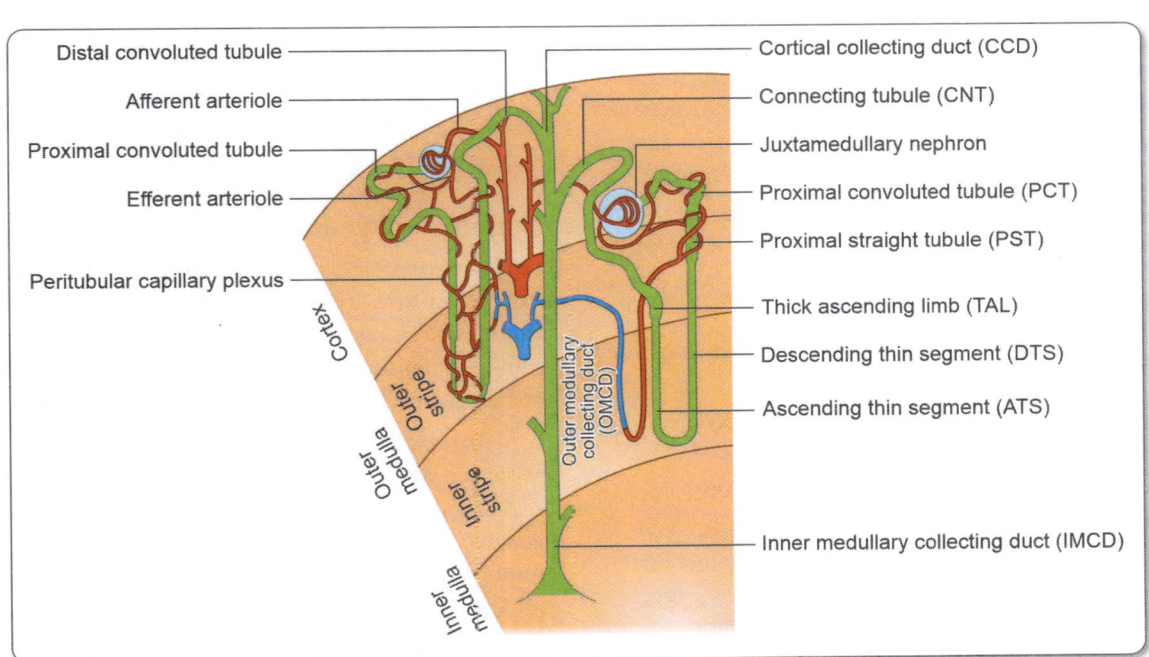

Fig. 8.1-3: Parts of a typical nephron. Organization of cortical and juxtamedullary nephrons showing different parts. Note the differences between two types of nephrons

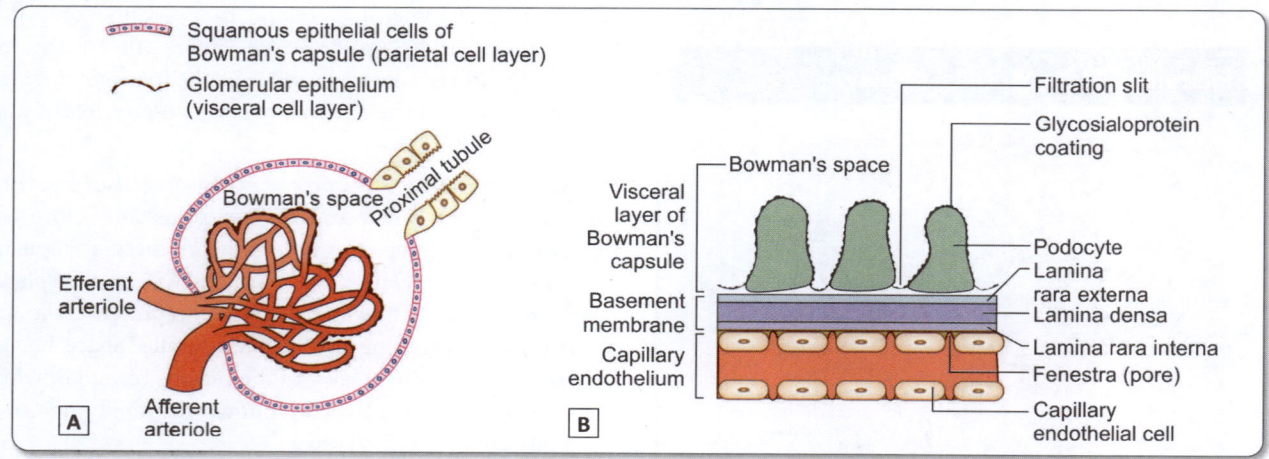

Figs 8.1-4A and B: Structure of A. Glomerulus; B. Glomerular membrane

Renal tubule

Renal tubule is a long complicated tubule that is divisible into the following main parts (Fig. 8.1-3):

Proximal tubule. The proximal tubule initially forms several coils, *proximal convoluted tubule* (PCT), followed by a straight segment, *proximal straight tubule* (PST) or *pars recta* that descends toward the medulla.

Intermediate tubule or loop of Henle that consists of:
- *Descending thin segment* (DTS)
- *Ascending thin segment* (ATS)
- *Thick ascending limb* (TAL)

In *juxtamedullary nephrons*, the DTS joins ATS to form the hair-pin band (loop). Near the end of TAL, the nephron passes between its afferent and efferent arterioles. This short segment of the thick ascending limb is called the *macula densa*.

Distal convoluted tubule. It begins at a short distance beyond the macula densa and extends to a point in the cortex where the connecting tubules (CNT) of two or more nephrons join to form the cortical collecting ducts.

Collecting duct. The collecting duct is divisible into three parts:

1. *Cortical collecting duct* (CCD), i.e., the portion present in the cortex

2. *Outer medullary collecting duct* (OMCD), i.e., the portion present in the outer medulla

3. *Inner medullary collecting duct* (IMCD), i.e., the portion present in the inner medulla. Several IMCDs coalesce together before finally opening at the tip of the renal papilla.

Characteristics of epithelium lining the renal tubule

The epithelium lining the different segments of renal tubule has some special characteristic features which are suited to perform specific transport functions.

Type of cells. The cells lining the renal tubule are mostly cuboidal except in the thin segment where these are flat or squamous type.

Cortical collecting duct is composed of two cell types:

1. Principal cells
2. Intercalated cells

Inner medullary collecting duct is composed of a single layer of cells that have poorly developed apical and basolateral surfaces and a few mitochondria.

Types of nephrons

There are two types of nephrons: cortical (superficial) and juxtamedullary. Differences between the cortical and juxtamedullary nephrons are depicted in Table 8.1-1.

Juxtaglomerular Apparatus

Juxtaglomerular apparatus as the name indicates (juxta – near) refers to a collection of specialized cells located very near to the glomerulus. It forms the major component of renin-angiotensin-aldosterone system. The juxtaglomerular apparatus comprises three types of cells (Fig. 8.1-5):

1. *Juxtaglomerular cells.* Juxtaglomerular (JG) cells are specialized *myoepithelial* (modified vascular smooth muscle) cells located in the media of the *afferent arteriole* in the region of juxtaglomerular apparatus. They act as *baroreceptors* (tension receptors) and respond to changes in the transmural pressure gradient between the afferent arterioles and the interstitium.

2. *Macula densa cells.* Macula densa cells refer to the specialized renal tubular epithelial cells of a short segment of the thick ascending limb of loop of Henle which passes between the afferent and efferent arterioles supplying its glomerulus of origin. They act as *chemoreceptors* and are

TABLE 8.1-1: Differences between cortical and juxtamedullary nephrons

Feature	Cortical nephron	Juxtamedullary Nephrons
Location of glomerulus	Upper region of cortex	Near the junction of cortex and medulla
Percentage of total nephron	85%	15%
Size of glomeruli	Small	Larger
Size of loop of Henle	Small, extend up to the outer layer of medulla	Large, extend deep into the medulla
Descending limb of loop of Henle comprises	Thin segment	Thin segment
Ascending limb of loop of Henle comprises	Thin segment	Thin segment
Efferent arterioles	Have a large diameter and break up into peritubular capillaries	Have a small diameter and continues as vasa recta
Rate of filtration	Slow	High
Major function	Excretion of waste products in urine	Concentration of urine by the counter current system

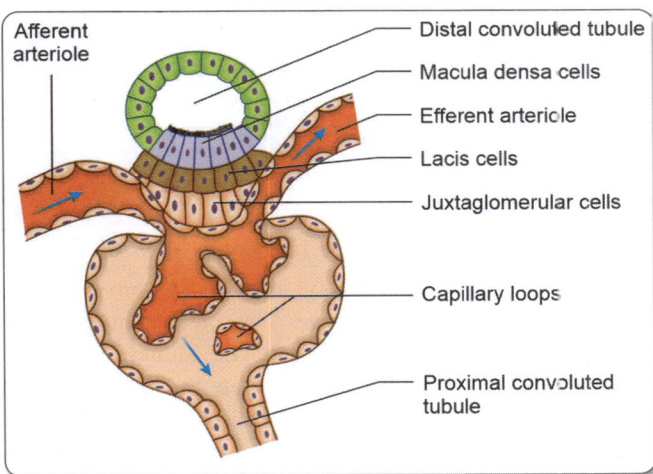

Fig. 8.1-5: Juxtaglomerular apparatus

stimulated by decreased NaCl concentration, thereby causing increased renin release.

3. Mesangial cells. Mesangial cells or *lacis* cells are the interstitial cells of the juxtaglomerular apparatus. Functionally, these cells possibly relay the signals from macula densa to granular cells after modulating the signals. In this way, a decreased intraluminal Na^+ load, Cl^- load, or both in the region of macula densa stimulates the juxtaglomerular cells to secrete renin.

Renal Blood Vessels

Arrangement of Arterial Vessels (Renal Artery and its Branches) in the Kidney (Fig. 8.1-6)

Renal artery (one for each kidney), a major branch from the aorta, divides into a number of lobular arteries at the hilum of kidney.

Lobular artery (one for each pyramid) divides into two or more interlobar arteries.

Interlobar arteries enter the tissue of the renal columns and run toward the surface of kidney. Reaching the level of the bases of the pyramids, the interlobar arteries divide into arcuate arteries.

Arcuate arteries run at right angles to the parent interlobar arteries. They lie parallel to the renal surface at the junction of pyramid and cortex. They give a series of interlobular arteries.

Interlobular arteries run through the cortex at right angles to the renal surface to end in a subcapsular plexus. It has been held that interlobular arteries divide the renal cortex into small lobules. Each interlobular artery gives off a series of afferent arterioles.

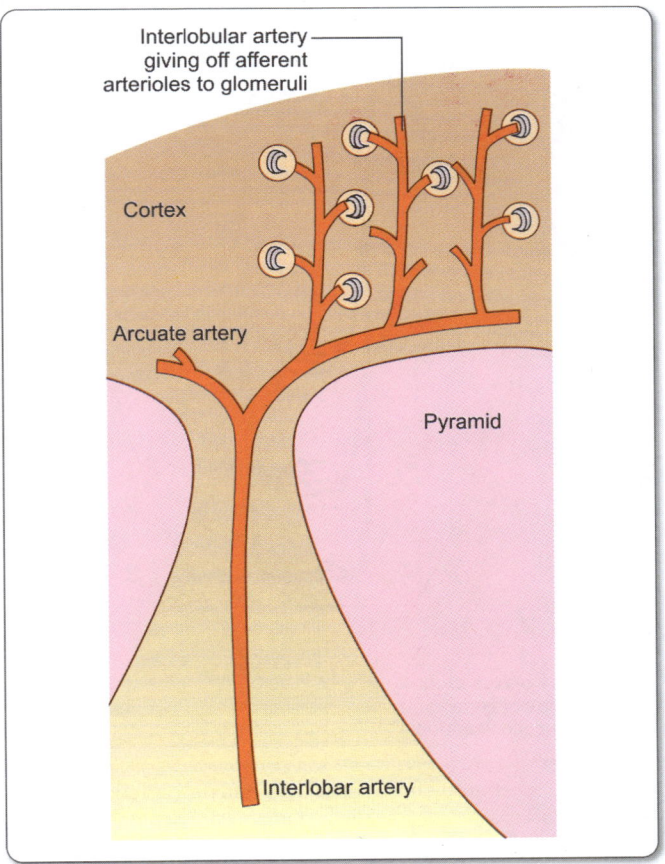

Fig. 8.1-6: Scheme to show arrangement of arteries within the kidney

Afferent arterioles. Each afferent arteriole enters the Bowman's capsule and divides into a rounded tuft of anastomosing capillaries called *glomerulus.* The glomerular capillaries join to form the efferent arteriole.

Efferent arterioles leaving the glomeruli of two types of nephrons exhibit different behavior:

1. *Efferent arterioles arising from the cortical nephrons* divide into *peritubular capillaries* that surround the proximal and distal convoluted tubule forming a rich meshwork of microvessels. These capillaries drain into interlobular veins.

2. *Efferent arterioles arising from the juxtamedullary nephrons* give rise to *vasa recta.* The *vasa recta* descend with the long loops of Henle into renal medulla and return to the area of the glomerulus, and drain into interlobular or arcuate vein.

Side branches arising from the vasta recta form capillary network at different levels along the loop of Henle (Fig. 8.1-7).

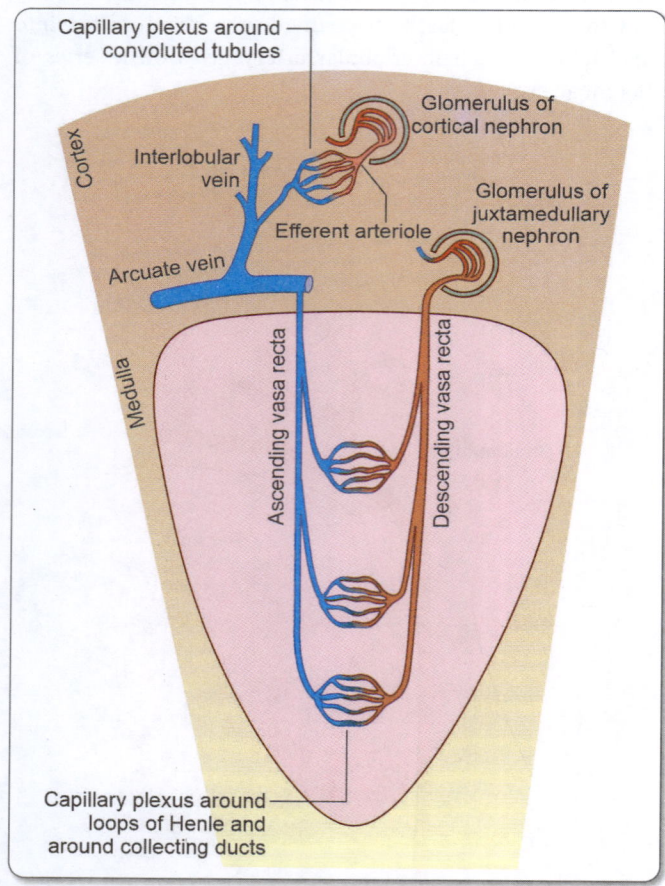

Fig. 8.1-7: Scheme to show behavior of efferent arterioles arising from the glomeruli of cortical and juxtamedullary nephrons

Arrangement of Venous Vessels (Renal Veins)

The pattern of renal venous system is similar to that found in the end arterial system, except for the presence of multiple anastomoses between veins at all levels of the venous circulation. The corresponding veins which run parallel to the arterial vessels are the interlobular veins, the arcuate veins, the interlobar veins, and the renal veins which exit the kidney at hilus.

CLINICAL ASPECTS

Anomalies of kidney. Congenital anomalies that occur due to developmental defects are:
- *Agenesis* (failure of development of kidney). It may be unilateral or bilateral. In bilateral agenesis, the baby cannot survive. However, the only treatment is renal transplantation.
- *Horseshoe kidney* occurs when lower ends of two kidneys fuse.
- *Ectopic Kidney* refers when kidney is placed at some other place.

Infections of kidney are mainly:
- Glomerulonephritis
- Tuberculosis

Nerve Supply

The kidneys are innervated by autonomic nervous system.

Sympathetic fibers are derived from T_{10} to L_1 segments of spinal cord and

Parasympathetic fibers from vagus nerve.

Functions of Kidneys

The kidneys serve several major functions:

Excretory function. The kidneys excrete a number of end products of metabolism in urine. Thus, formation of urine is the major function of kidneys. The kidneys eliminate these substances from the body at a rate that matches their production. In addition to the metabolic wastes, the kidneys also excrete foreign substances from the body, such as drugs, pesticides, and other chemicals ingested in food.

Regulation of water and inorganic ion balance. Control of volume of body fluids and their inorganic ion balance is an important homeostatic role of kidneys.

Regulation of acid-base balance. Kidneys, in co-ordination with lungs, liver and buffers in the body, play a role in regulation of acid-base balance.

Hormonal function. As an endocrine gland, kidneys produce and secrete renin, calcitriol, and erythropoietin.

- The angle between the lower border of the 12th rib and the outer border of the erector spinae is known as the *renal angle*. It overlies the lower part of the kidney. Tenderness in the kidney is elicited by applying pressure over this angle, with the thumb.
- Blood from a ruptured kidney or pus in a perinephric abscess first distends the renal fascia, then forces its way within the renal fascia downward into the pelvis. It cannot cross to opposite side because of the fascial septum and midline attachment of the renal fascia.
- The common manifestations of a kidney disease are renal edema and hypertension. Raised blood urea indicates suppressed kidney function and renal failure.

URETERS, URINARY BLADDER AND URETHRA

Ureters

The ureters (right and left) are long tubes which convey the urine from the renal pelvis to urinary bladder (Fig. 8.1-1). Each ureter is about 25–30 cm long and about 4–5 mm in diameter.

Parts

For the purpose of description only, the ureter can be divided into three parts:

1. *Abdominal part.* Extends from the renal pelvis to the brim of bony pelvis (Fig. 8.1-8). This part of the ureter lies behind the peritoneum in front of the psoas muscle along the posterior abdominal wall.

2. *Pelvic part.* At the brim of pelvis, the ureter crosses the upper end of the external iliac artery and vein, and comes to lie on the lateral wall of pelvis (Figs 8.1-8 and 8.1-9). Finally it leaves the pelvis wall and runs forward to reach the urinary bladder.

3. *Intracystic part.* It is a small part of the ureter which passes obliquely through the posterior wall of urinary bladder (Fig. 8.1-10). Because of this oblique intracystic course of the ureter, when urine accumulates and the pressure in the bladder rises, the ureters are compressed and the openings occluded. This prevents reflux of urine into the ureters (toward the kidneys) as the bladder fills and also during micturition, when pressure increases due to contraction of the muscular wall of the bladder.

Structure

The wall of ureter consists of three coats (Fig. 8.1-11):

1. *Outer fibrous coat* of the ureter becomes continuous with the fibrous capsule of the kidney.

2. *Middle muscular coat* consists of an inner longitudinal layer and an outer circular layer of smooth muscle.

3. *Inner mucous coat* consists of the lining transitional epithelium and the underlying connective tissue.

Function

The ureters propel the urine from the kidneys into the urinary bladder by peristaltic contractions of the smooth muscular coat.

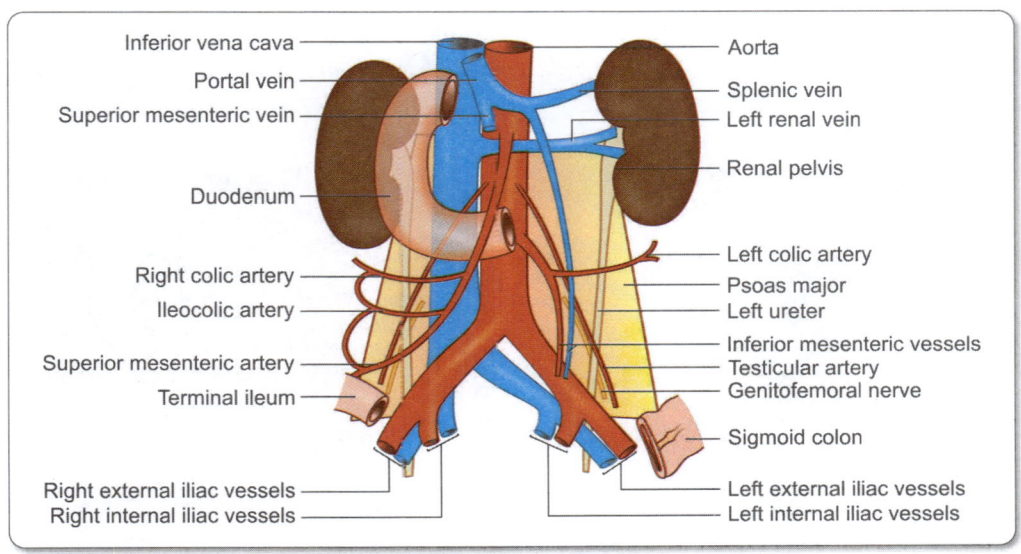

Fig. 8.1-8: Relations of abdominal part of ureter

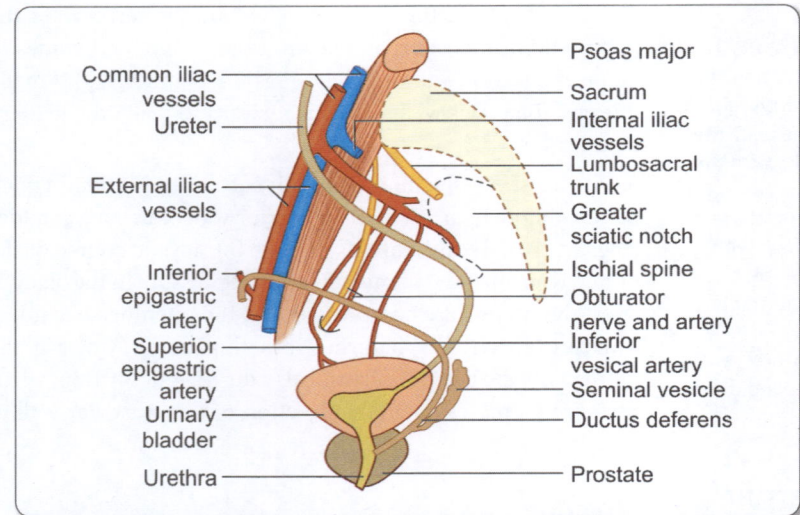

Fig. 8.1-9: Diagrammatic depiction of course and relations of pelvic part of ureter

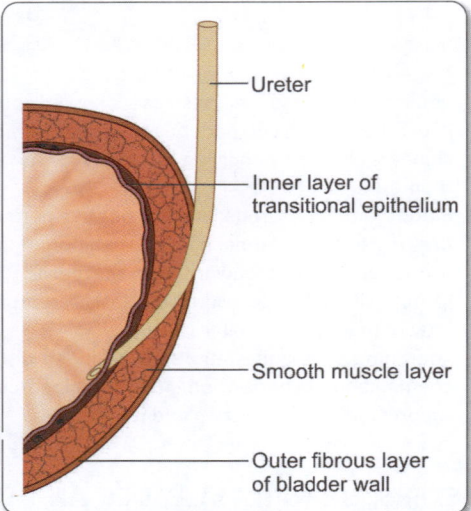

Fig. 8.1-10: Intracystic part of ureter

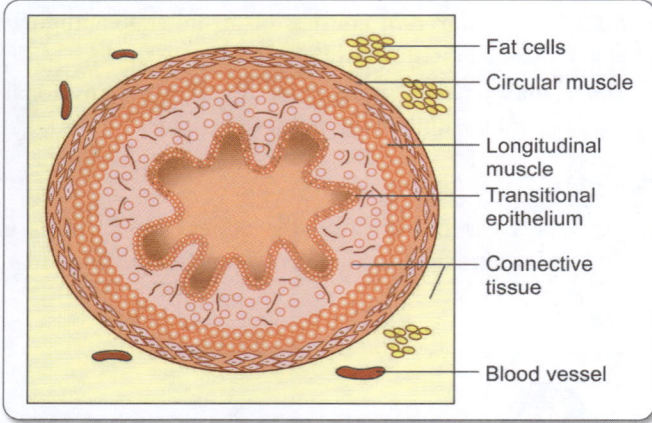

Fig. 8.1-11: Microscopic structure of ureter

Urinary Bladder and Urethra

Gross Anatomy of Urinary Bladder

Location. The urinary bladder, a hollow muscular viscus, is a temporary reservoir for urine. It is situated in the pelvic cavity behind the pubis, in front of the rectum in the male and in front of the anterior wall of the vagina and the neck of the uterus in the females. It is a freely movable organ but is held in position by folds of peritoneum and fascia (Figs 8.1-12A and B).

External Features. The main body of empty bladder is pyramidal, having an apex and a base. The lowest part of the bladder is called neck, which continues as urethra.

Interior of the Bladder. In an empty bladder, the greater part of the mucosa shows irregular folds due to its loose attachments

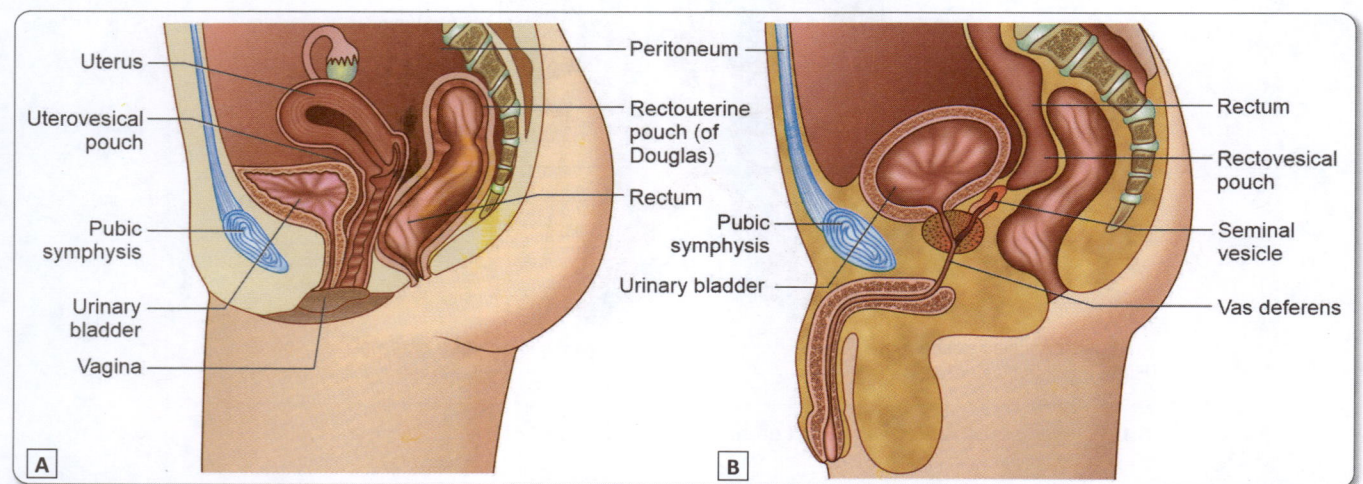

Figs 8.1-12A and B: Relations of urinary bladder in the pelvic cavity: A. Female pelvis; B. Male pelvis

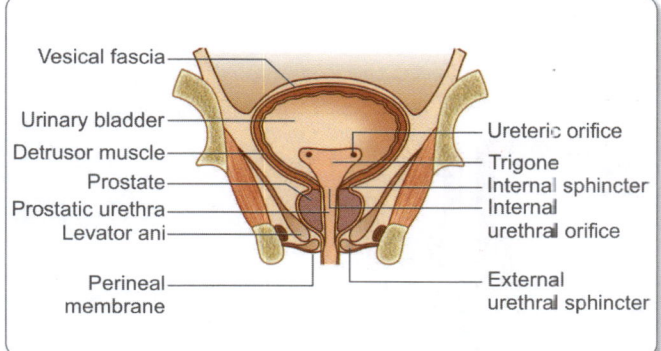

Fig. 8.1-13: Coronal section through the bladder and prostate to show the interior of the bladder, internal urethral sphincter and external urethral sphincter

to the muscular coat. The interior of the base (posterior surface) of the bladder presents a triangular area, the trigone where the mucosa is smooth due to its firm attachment (Fig. 8.1-13).

Internal urethral orifice is located at the apex (inferior angle) of the trigone. The ureters open into the bladder at superior angles of the trigone (Fig. 8.1-13). The ureters pierce the bladder wall obliquely, and this provides a valve-like action, which prevents the reverse flow of urine toward the kidneys as the bladder fills.

Structure of the Bladder

The wall of the urinary bladder consists of three layers: an outer serous layer, a thick coat of smooth muscle, and the inner mucous membrane (Histology Plate 8.1-2).

Mucous membrane is lined by transitional epithelium.

Muscular coat is formed by smooth muscle fibers which are arranged in three layers: inner longitudinal, middle circular and outer longitudinal. The fibers of outer layer, at the sides of bladder, are arranged obliquely and intersect one another. These fibers constitute the detrusor muscle. Contraction of this muscle coat is responsible for emptying of the bladder.

Serous coat is a reflection of the peritoneum and covers only the superior surface and the upper part of lateral surfaces of the bladder.

Urethra and its Sphincters

Urethra

Male urethra, about 20 cm in length, is divided into three parts: prostatic urethra (3 cm), membranous urethra (1.25 cm), and penile urethra (15.75 cm). Membranous urethra is surrounded by the external sphincter (Fig. 8.1-14).

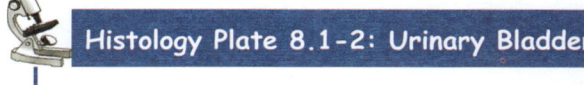
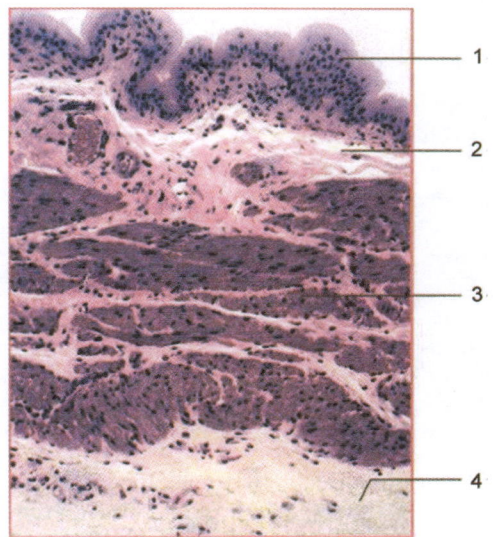

Histology Plate 8.1-2: Urinary Bladder

The photomicrograph of urinary bladder is shown. The urinary bladder in lined by transitional epithelium (1) and has thick muscle coat made of smooth muscle fibers (3) running in transverse, oblique and longitudinal directions. Lamina propria (2) and adventitia (4) are also seen.

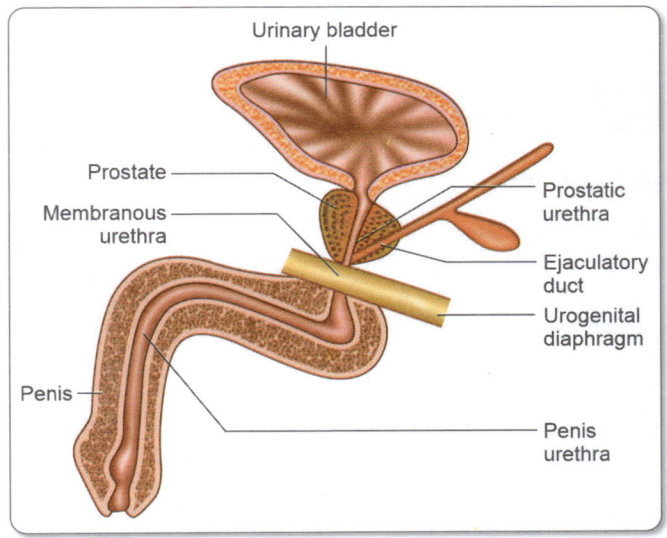

Fig. 8.1-14: Male urethra

Female urethra is about 3.8 cm long. It extends from the neck of the bladder to the external meatus. It traverses the external sphincter and lies immediately in front of the vagina.

Sphincters of the Urethra

Internal sphincter. The circular smooth muscle fibers in the area of the neck of bladder are thickened to form the internal sphincter (sphincter vesicae). The natural tone of the internal sphincter prevents emptying of the bladder until the pressure in the body of bladder rises above a threshold level.

External sphincter. Beyond the bladder neck, it is encircled by a ring of voluntary (skeletal type) muscle known as external sphincter of the bladder. The external sphincter provides voluntary control over micturition.

CLINICAL ASPECTS

Ureteric stone: A ureteric stone is liable to become impacted at one of the sites of normal constriction of the ureter, e.g., pelviureteric junction, brim of the pelvis and intravesical course. *Ureteric colic* occurs due to lodging of stone either in the pelvis or in the ureter. In this condition, there is sharp, stabbing pain in ureter.

Ectopic ureter: Single ureter and longer ureter insert more caudally and medially than normal one.

Ureteroceles: Cystic dilatation of the lower end of ureter.

Congenital anomalies like bifid ureter and double ureter on one side may be seen.

Ectopic vasicae is a congenital anomaly due to defect in development of anterior abdominal wall. In this condition the trigon area of bladder is exposed and ureteric opening is also seen.

Cystitis refers to infection of urinary bladder.

Rupture of urinary bladder sometimes occurs in fracture of pelvis.

PHYSIOLOGY OF URINARY SYSTEM

URINE FORMATION

The main function of the kidneys is to clear waste products from blood and excrete them in the urine. The kidneys accomplish their excretory function by formation of urine.

Three processes are involved in urine formation (Fig. 8.1-15):

1. Glomerular filtration
2. Tubular reabsorption
3. Tubular secretion

Glomerular Filtration

Glomerular filtration refers to the process of ultrafiltration of plasma from the glomerular capillaries into the Bowman's capsule.

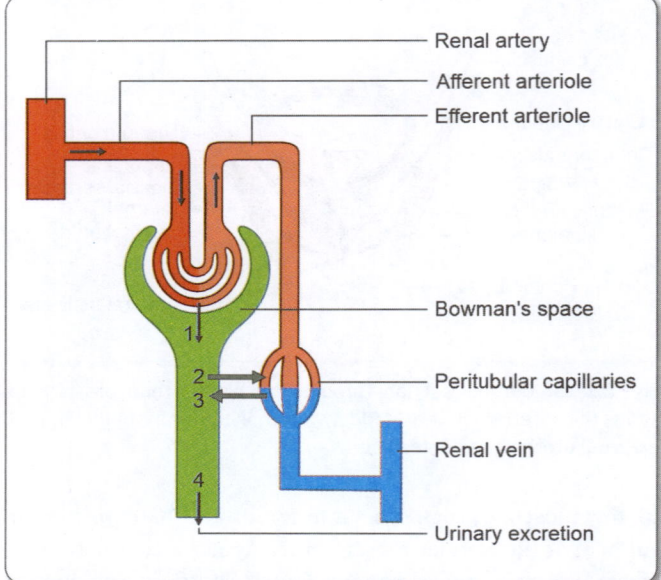

Fig. 8.1-15: Steps involved in the formation of urine: 1. Filtration; 2. Reabsorption; 3. Secretion; and 4. Excretion

Composition of Glomerular Filtrate

The unique characteristic features of the glomerular filtration membrane determine the composition of glomerular filtrate, in that it is like that of plasma except for absence of proteins (colloids) and cells. Filtration membrane permeability alteration in diseases, however, may alter diffusibility of colloids and cells. As a result, filtration of proteins is increased, and albumin appears in the urine in significant amount (*albuminuria* or *proteinuria*).

Dynamics of Glomerular Filtration

The forces which determine the bulk flow or ultrafiltration of protein-free plasma across the glomerular membrane are the same which determine formation of tissue fluid.

The glomerular filtration rate (GFR) will depend upon the balance of Starling forces (Fig. 8.1-16). According to Starling hypothesis, the GFR can be expressed as:

$$GFR = K_f [(P_{GC} - P_{BS}) - (\pi_{GC} - \pi_{BS})]$$

where:

GFR is the filtration across the glomerular membrane.

K_f or the filtration coefficient of the glomerular membrane.

P_{GC} is glomerular capillary hydrostatic pressure. Its normal value is about 45 mm Hg.

P_{BS} is the Bowman's space hydrostatic pressure. Its normal value is about 10 mm Hg.

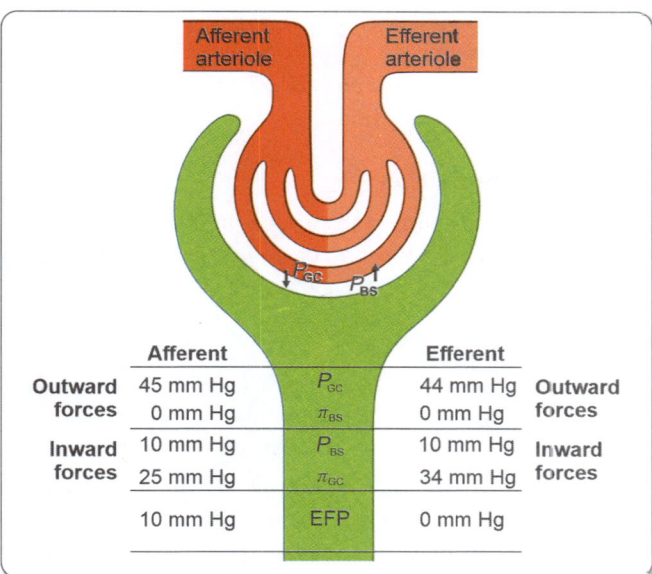

Fig. 8.1-16: Depiction of Starling forces across the glomerular filtration membrane.
Abbreviation: EFP, end filling detrusor pressure

π_{GC} is the glomerular capillary oncotic pressure. Its normal value is 25 mm Hg.

π_{BS} is the Bowman's space oncotic pressure. Its normal value is zero, because glomerular filtrate contains no proteins.

Effective filtration pressure is the net outward force and is calculated as the difference between the outwardly (i.e., P_{GC} and π_{BS}) and inwardly (P_{BS} and π_{GC}) directed forces (Fig. 8.1-16). Thus, under normal circumstances, we have
GFR = 12.5 (45–10) – (25–0) = 125 mL/min

Normal glomerular filtration rate (GFR): The normal GFR in an average-sized man is about 125 mL/min (range 90–140 mL/min). Thus, in 24 hours, 180 L of plasma is filtered. The values in women are 10% lower than those in men.

Factors Affecting Glomerular Filtration Rate

Filtration coefficient (K_f). Increased K_f raises GFR and decreased K_f reduces GFR as K_f is the product of permeability and filtration area of the glomerular capillary membrane.

Hydrostatic pressure in Bowman's space fluid (P_{BS}) opposes filtration and therefore, GFR is inversely related to it. It is increased in acute obstruction of urinary tract (e.g., a ureteric obstruction by stone).

Glomerular capillary hydrostatic pressure (P_{GC}). GFR is mainly dependent on arterial pressure, renal blood flow, afferent arteriolar resistance, and efferent arteriolar resistance.

Glomerular capillary oncotic pressure (π_{GC}). GFR is inversely proportional to π_{GC}. In hyperproteinemia and in hemoconcentration, the π_{GC} is raised leading to a decrease in GFR. Conversely in hypoproteinemia and hemodilution, the π_{GC} is reduced leading to increased GFR.

> **IMPORTANT TO KNOW**
>
> *Autoregulation of renal blood flow.* Kidney can regulate its blood flow in spite of changes in the systemic arterial pressure in the range of 80 mm Hg to 200 mm Hg. The RBF and thus, the GFR remain constant over a wide range of renal arterial pressure.

Tubular Reabsorption and Secretion

Out of the 180 L glomerular filtrate formed per day, about 1.5 L (i.e., <1%) per day is excreted as urine. Different segments of the renal tubule viz. proximal tubule, loop of Henle, distal tubule, and collecting duct determine the composition and volume of the urine by process of *selective reabsorption* of solutes and water and *selective secretion* of solutes.

Tubular reabsorption denotes the active transport of solutes and passive movement of water from the tubular lumen into peritubular capillaries. In other words, reabsorption is the removal of substances of nutritive value such as glucose, amino acids, electrolytes (Na^+, K^+, Cl^-, HCO_3^-) and vitamins from the glomerular filtrate. Small proteins and peptide hormones are reabsorbed in the proximal tubules by endocytosis.

Tubular secretion refers to the transport of solutes from the peritubular capillaries into the tubular lumen, i.e., it is the addition of a substance to the glomerular filtrate.

Active secretion of substances occurs into the tubular fluid with the help of certain non-selective carriers. The carrier which secretes para-aminohippuric (PAH) acid can also secrete uric acid, bile acids, oxalic acid, penicillin, probenecid, cephalothin and furosemide.

TRANSPORT ACROSS DIFFERENT SEGMENTS OF RENAL TUBULE

The substances transported across different segments of renal tubules are described below and enlisted in Table 8.1-2.

Transport across Proximal Tubule

The proximal tubule reabsorbs:

- Approximately 67% of the filtered water, Na^+, Cl^-, K^+ and other solutes
- Almost all the glucose and amino acids filtered by the glomerulus.

TABLE 8.1-2: Transport of substances across different segments of renal tubule

Reabsorption		Non-reabsorption	Secretion
Active	**Passive**		
Proximal tubule			
Na^+	Cl^-	Inulin	H^+
K^+	HCO_3^-	Creatinine	Water
Ca^{2+}	HPO_4^-	Sucrose	Penicillin
Mg^{2+}	Water	Mannitol	Sulfonamide
HPO_4^{2-}	Urea		Creatinine
SO_4^{2-}			
NO_3^-			
Glucose			
Amino acids			
Protein			
Urate			
Vitamins			
Acetoacetate			
β-hydroxybutyrate			
Henle's loop			
Na^+	Cl^-		
K^+	HCO_3^-		
Ca^{2+}	Water		
Distal tubule and collecting duct			
Na^+	Cl^-		K^+
Ca^{2+}	HCO_3^-		H^+
Mg^{2+}	Water		

The proximal tubule does not reabsorb inulin, creatinine, sucrose and mannitol.

The proximal tubule secretes H^+, PAH, urate, penicillin, sulphonamides, and creatinine.

Sodium Reabsorption

The process of sodium reabsorption in proximal tubule is *isosmotic*, i.e., the reabsorption of sodium and water is exactly proportional.

Mechanisms of Na^+ reabsorption

Na^+ is reabsorbed by *cotransport with H^+ or organic solutes (glucose, amino acids, phosphate and lactate)*. The Na^+ absorption is a two-step process (Figs 8.1-17A and B):

1. ***Across the basolateral membrane***, Na^+ moves against an electrochemical gradient *via* Na^+-K^+-ATPase pump, which pumps Na^+ into the paracellular spaces and lowers the intracellular Na^+ concentration.

2. ***Across the apical membrane***, the sodium moves down an electrochemical gradient as above. The entry of Na^+ is mediated by specific antiporter and symporter proteins, and not by diffusion through channels.

Water Reabsorption

Approximately 67% of the filtered water is absorbed in the proximal tubule by osmosis in response to a transtubular osmotic gradient established by the solute reabsorption (i.e., Na^+-Cl^-, Na^+-glucose, and so forth). The osmotic water absorption is termed *obligatory water absorption* as it cannot be changed according to the needs of the body.

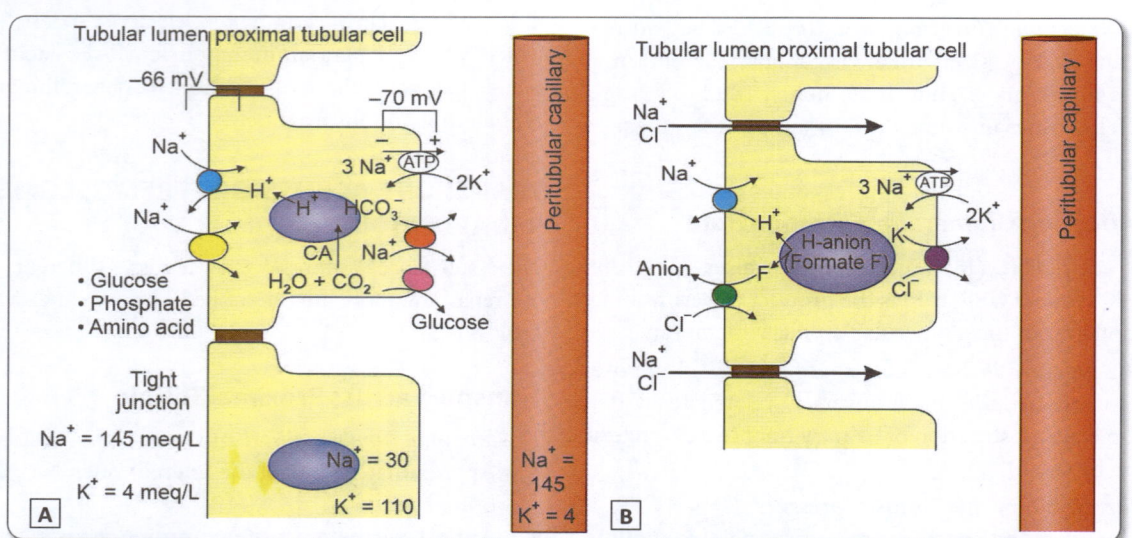

Figs 8.1-17A and B: Mechanism of reabsorption of sodium and other solutes in proximal tubule: A. Early proximal tubule; B. Late proximal tubule

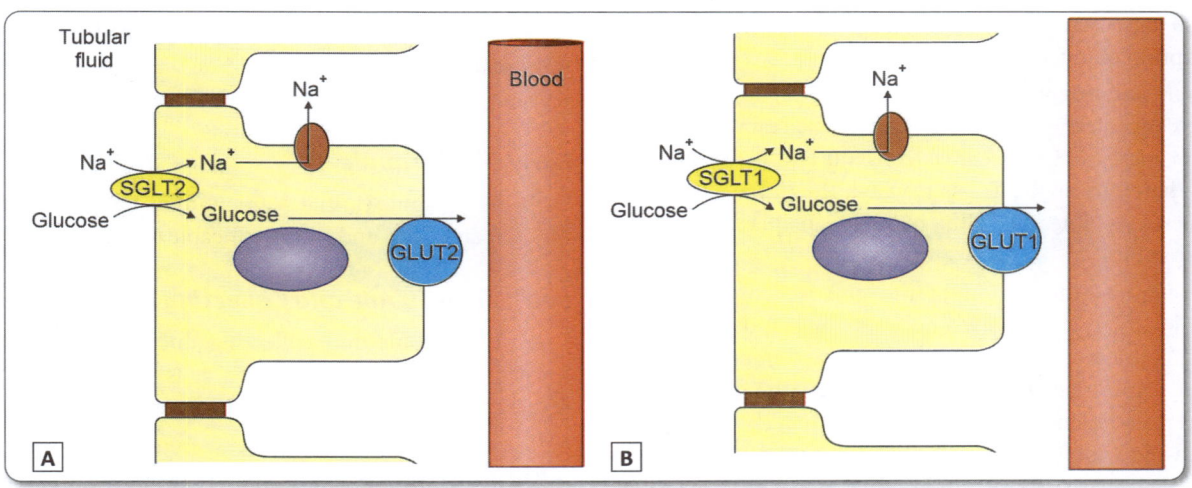

Figs 8.1-18A and B: Mechanism of glucose reabsorption in: A. Early proximal tubule; B. Late proximal tubule

Protein Reabsorption

Normally, only a small amount of proteins is filtered by the glomerulus (40 mg/L). However, because of high GFR (180 L/ day) the total amount of protein filtered per day is significant (180 L/day × 40 mg/L = 7.2 g/day). Normally, the proteins are completely taken into the cells of proximal tubules by the process of *endocytosis*. Once inside the cells, enzymes digest the proteins and peptides into their constituent amino acids which exit across the basolateral membrane and return to the blood in the peritubular capillaries.

When the amount of filtered proteins increases (due to disruption of glomerular filtration barrier in kidney diseases), the reabsorbing mechanisms saturate and the proteins may appear in the urine (*proteinuria*).

Glucose Reabsorption

Glucose is freely filtered into the glomerular filtrate. Filtration load of glucose increases in direct proportion to the plasma glucose concentration (P glucose).

Filtered load of glucose = GFR × P glucose (P_G).

Mechanism of tubular reabsorption

All the filtered glucose is completely reabsorbed into the proximal tubule by an active transport mechanism (Figs 8.1-18A and B):

Carrier mediated Na^+-glucose cotransport. Carrier protein located at the apical membrane in the proximal tubule reabsorbs glucose from tubular fluid into the blood.

- The carrier protein for glucose in early and late proximal tubule is called SGLT-2 and SGLT-1, respectively (SGLT = sodium-dependent glucose transporter).

Facilitated diffusion moves the glucose out of the cell through the basolateral membrane. The carrier for facilitated diffusion across the basolateral membrane in early and late proximal tubule is called GLUT-2 and GLUT-1, respectively (GLUT = glucose transporter).

Characteristics of glucose transport and glucose excretion

Glucose is reabsorbed by a transport maximum process, i.e., there are limited number of Na^+-glucose carriers. The characteristics of glucose transport and glucose excretion can be elicited from the glucose titration curve.

Glucose titration curve (Fig. 8.1-19) depicts that:

Filtered load increases with the plasma glucose concentration (P_G).

Renal threshold, i.e., the plasma glucose concentration at which glucose first appears in the urine (glycosuria) is about

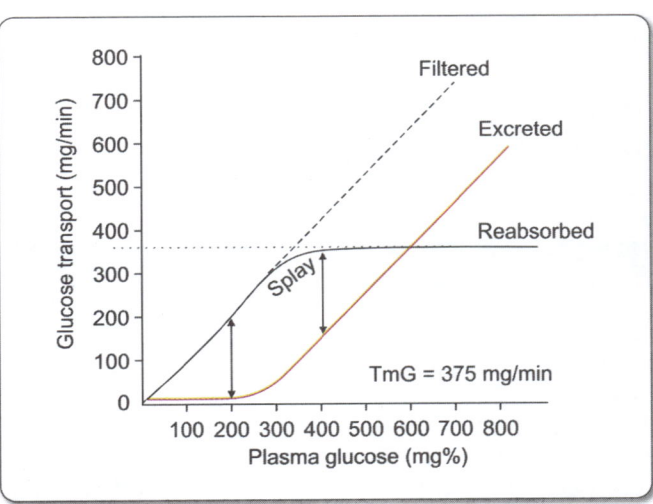

Fig. 8.1-19: Glucose titration curve (for details see text)

180–200 mg%. At plasma levels below renal threshold the reabsorption of glucose is complete (100%).

Transport maximum. As shown in Fig. 8.1-19, beyond plasma glucose concentration of 350 mg% (T_{mG}), the reabsorption rate does not increase, i.e., becomes constant and is independent of P_G. Therefore, as the T_{mG} is reached, the urinary excretion rate increases linearly with increase in plasma glucose concentration.

Splay refers to the region of the glucose curve between threshold and T_{mG}, i.e., between P_G 180 mg% and 350 mg%. It represents the excretion of glucose in urine before T_{mG} is fully achieved. Note that in the region of splay, the reabsorption curve is rounded indicating that though the reabsorption rate is increasing with increase in P_G, but reabsorption is less than filtration. Similarly, the excretion curve is also rounded in the region of splay, indicating that though the urinary excretion is increasing with increase in P_G, but there is no linear relation.

IMPORTANT TO KNOW

Causes of splay are:
- *Heterogeneity in glomerular size,* proximal tubular length, and number of carrier proteins for glucose reabsorption.
- *Variability in T_{mG} of the nephron.*

Transport across Loop of Henle

About 20% of filtered Na^+ and Cl^-, 15% of filtered water and cations such as K^+, Ca^{2+} and Mg^{2+} are reabsorbed in the loop of Henle. Reabsorption occurring in different parts of the loop of Henle is:

Thin Descending Limb of Loop of Henle

Water absorption occurs passively (because of hypertonic interstitial fluid) in this part of the loop of Henle. It is accompanied by diffusion of sodium ions from interstitial fluid into tubular lumen.

Thick Ascending Limb of Loop of Henle

This limb is impermeable to water but is involved in the reabsorption of 20% of the filtered Na^+, and Cl^- and other cations.

IMPORTANT TO KNOW

Thick ascending limb is impermeable to water. Thus, NaCl and other solutes are reabsorbed without water. As a result, tubular fluid Na^+ and tubular fluid osmolarity decreases to less than their concentration in plasma. This segment is, therefore, called the diluting segment. Further, Na^+ reabsorbed from this segment is the main driving force behind the counter-current multiplier system which concentrates Na^+ and urea in medullary interstitium.

Transport across Distal Tubules and Collecting Duct

Approximately 7% of the filtered NaCl, and about 8–17% of water is reabsorbed and K^+ and H^+ are secreted in these segments.

Early Distal Tubule

Early distal tubule (initial segment of distal tubule) reabsorbs Na^+, Cl^- and Ca^{2+}, and is impermeable to water.

Late Distal Tubule and Collecting Duct

Late distal tubule and collecting duct have two cell types (principal cells and intercalated cells) which perform both reabsorption and secretory functions:

Principal cells reabsorb Na^+ and secrete K^+.

Role of antidiuretic hormone. H_2O absorption occurs in response to the effect of antidiuretic hormone (ADH) on the principal cells. ADH increases H_2O permeability by directing the insertion of H_2O channels (aquaporins) in the luminal membrane. In the absence of ADH, the principal cells are virtually impermeable to water.

Role of aldosterone. Aldosterone by its effect on principal cell increases Na^+ reabsorption and increases K^+ secretion. About 2% of overall Na^+ absorption is affected by aldosterone (Fig. 8.1-20).

Intercalated cells reabsorb K^+ and secrete H^+

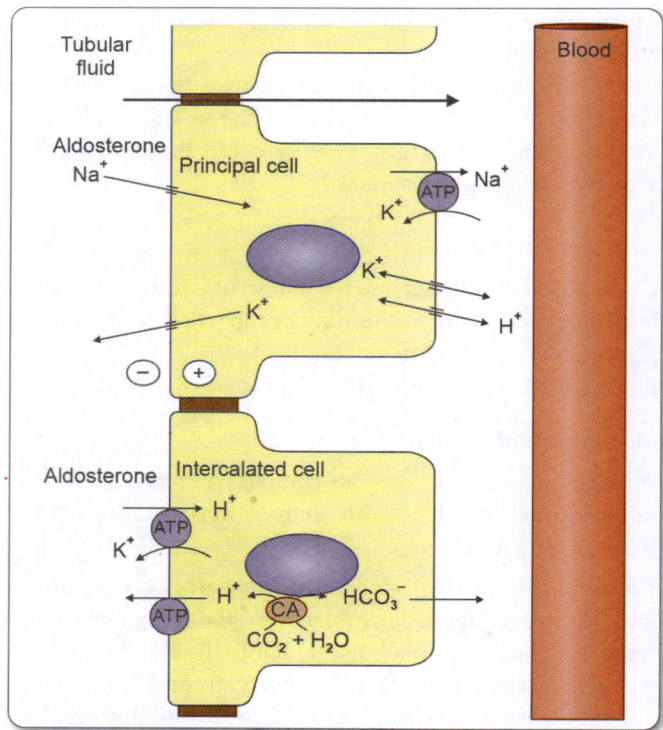

Fig. 8.1-20: Mechanism of transport in principal cells and intercalated cells of the late distal tubule and collecting duct.
Abbreviation: CA, carbonic anhydrase

Aldosterone also increases H⁺ secretion by intercalated cells by stimulating the H⁺-ATPase (in addition to its actions on the principal cells).

CONCENTRATION AND DILUTION OF URINE

The kidneys possess unique property of regulating the volume and osmolality of the urine by concentrating and diluting it as per needs of the body.

Purpose of Concentration and Dilution of Urine

The main purpose is to maintain the osmolality and volume of the body fluids within a narrow range which is accomplished by kidneys in concert with other systems by regulating the excretion of water and NaCl, respectively.

The kidney can produce urine with osmolality as low as 30 mOsm/kg H_2O to as high as 1400 mOsm/kg H_2O by changing the water excretion as high as 23.3 L/day to as low as 0.5 L/day, respectively.

Principal Factors

Principal factors responsible for mechanism of concentration and dilution of urine are:

- Antidiuretic hormones for details see page 418
- Hyperosmolality and osmolality gradient in medullary interstitium of kidneys.

Medullary Hyperosmolality and Medullary Gradient

The interstitial fluid of the medulla is critically important in concentrating the urine, because the osmotic pressure of this fluid provides the driving force for reabsorbing water from both the descending thin segment (DTS) and the collecting duct.

Normal osmolality of plasma and other body fluids is about 300 mOsm/kg H_2O. The interstitial fluid of the renal cortex has the same osmolality as that of plasma, and virtually all osmoles attributable to NaCl. The osmolality of the renal medulla is higher than the plasma (i.e., *hyperosmolar*) and that it goes on increasing progressively from about 300 mOsm/kg H_2O at corticomedullary junction to about 1200 mOsm/kg H_2O at papilla (medullary gradient) where a maximally concentrated urine is excreted (Fig. 8.1-21). This hyperosmolality and medullary gradient are generated, and maintained by the so-called countercurrent system.

Countercurrent System

A countercurrent system refers to a system in which the inflow runs parallel to, counter to, and in close proximity to the

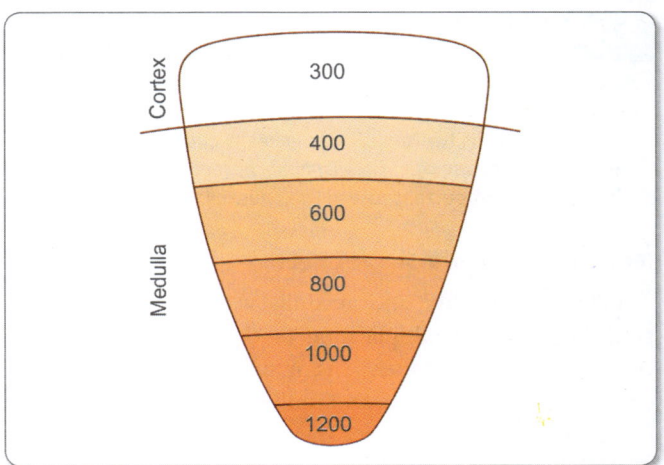

Fig. 8.1-21: Osmolality gradient of renal medullary interstitium (values are in mOsm/kg H_2O)

outflow for some distance. The countercurrent flow system is formed by U-shaped tubules.

In the kidney, the structures which form the counter- current system are the loop of Henle and the vasa recta. The countercurrent system of kidney consists of two components:

Countercurrent multiplier, which is formed by the operation of the loop of Henle and is responsible for production of hyperosmolality and a gradient in renal medulla.

Countercurrent exchanger which is formed by the operation of vasa recta and is responsible for maintenance of the medullary gradient and hyperosmolality.

Countercurrent Multipliers

The working of countercurrent multiplier, which operates in the loop of Henle and generates hyperosmolarity and medullary gradient, can be best understood by describing it as two processes:

1. Origin of single effect
2. Multiplication of the single effect

Origin of single effect in inner medulla

The origin of single effect for the development of medullary gradient and hyperosmolality occurs in the inner medullary interstitium due to:

- Passive transport of sodium ions from ascending thin segment into the interstitium
- Active transport of sodium from inner medullary collecting duct
- Diffusion of urea from the collecting duct into medullary interstitium.

Multiplication of the single effect

The hyperosmolality and medullary gradient are in fact generated by the multiplication of the single effect by the countercurrent multiplier. The main characteristics of the components of countercurrent multiplier which play a role in multiplication of single effect are:

- High permeability of descending thin segment to water.
- Impermeability to water and ability to actively absorb solutes by TAL.
- In renal medulla, all other tubular structures (except ascending limb) are in osmotic equilibrium. The descending limb, therefore, acquires the increased osmolality of the surrounding fluid. The effect is multiplied as new iso-osmolar filtrate arrives at the descending limb and forces the concentrated tubular contents toward the tip of loop of Henle (hair-pin band).

Countercurrent Exchanger

Vasa recta (the countercurrent exchanger). If the vasa recta would have been a straight blood vessel, the osmotic gradient in the medullary pyramid would not last long, as the Na^+ and urea in the interstitial spaces would have been removed by the circulation (Fig. 8.1-22). However, because of the hair-pin (U-shaped), anatomical arrangement of the vasa recta operates as countercurrent exchanger and retains these solutes in the medullary interstitium. Thus, the countercurrent exchanger formed by the vasa recta is responsible for the maintenance of the hyperosmolality medullary gradient generated by the countercurrent multiplier.

Mechanism of Urine Dilution and Concentration

Production of Diluted Urine

Conditions in which dilute urine is formed

Dilute urine is called *hyposmotic urine*, in which urine osmolality is less than blood osmolality. It is produced under the following circumstances:

- When circulating levels of ADH are low (e.g., after water drinking), central diabetes insipidus or
- When ADH is ineffective (e.g., nephrogenic diabetes insipidus.

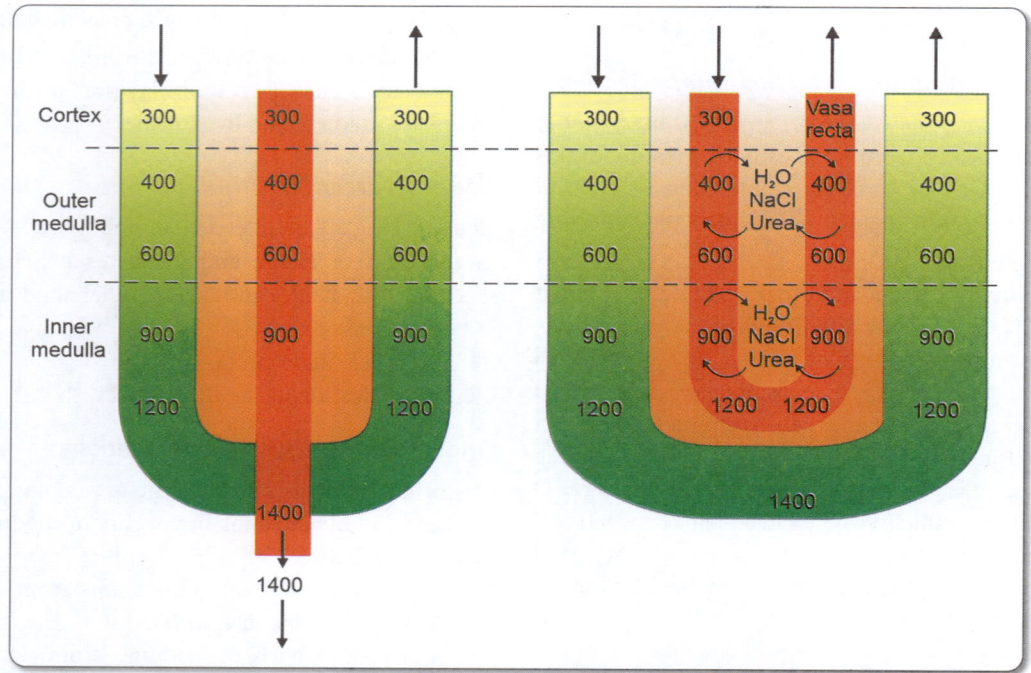

Fig. 8.1-22: Operation of vasa recta as countercurrent exchanger in the kidney: A. Effect on medullary osmolality if vasa recta would be straight tube; B. As vasa recta a 'U' shaped structure

Production of Concentrated Urine

Conditions in which concentrated urine is formed

Concentrated urine is also called *hyperosmotic urine*, in which urine osmolality is more than that of blood. It is produced when circulating ADH levels are high, e.g.,

- Water deprivation
- Hemorrhage
- Syndrome of inappropriate antidiuretic hormone, i.e., SIADH.

Urine Volume and Osmolality Changes in Response to Water Intake and Water Deprivation

Water Diuresis Versus Osmotic Diuresis

Water diuresis. Water diuresis refers to increased urinary output the following excessive intake of water or hypotonic solution.

Pathophysiology. It occurs due to the absence of ADH in the plasma.

Characteristic features:

- Water diuresis begins about 15 minutes after ingestion of water and reaches its maximum in 40 minutes.
- Urine output may be increased to 20 L/day.
- Urine formed is diluted, osmolality is always may be as low as 50 mOsm/kg H_2O.
- Specific gravity of urine is always below 1.010.

Osmotic diuresis. Osmotic diuresis refers to increased urine output because of an osmotic effect.

Pathophysiology. Presence of large quantities of unreabsorbed solutes in the proximal tubules exerts an appreciable osmotic effect. Osmotic diuresis may occur under the following circumstances:

- When the filtered load of naturally occurring substances such as Na^+, glucose, (e.g., in diabetes mellitus), urea, etc. exceeds the maximum capacity of the tubules to reabsorb (Tm).
- Following administration of compounds such as mannitol and related polysaccharides that are filtered but not reabsorbed.
- Following infusion of large amounts of sodium chloride and urea.

Characteristic features:

- Urine output may be >20 L/day, in spite of maximal ADH secretion.
- Urine osmolality is higher than 300 mOsm/kg H_2O.
- Urine specific gravity is more than 1.010.

Water Deprivation

Water deprivation is followed by a sequence of changes which are opposite to water diversis. As a consequence, urine volume is decreased but urine osmolality is increased.

ACIDIFICATION OF URINE

The pH of urine is variable depending upon the concentration of H^+ ions. Under normal circumstances, the pH of urine is acidic (~6.0). This clearly indicates that kidneys have contributed to the *acidification of urine*, when it is formed from the plasma (pH 7.4). In other words, H^+ ions generated in the body under the normal circumstances are eliminated by acidified urine. Thus, the role of kidneys in the maintenance of acid-base balance of the body (blood pH) is highly significant.

The kidneys regulate the blood pH by three main mechanisms:

1. Reabsorption of the filtered HCO_3^-
2. Generation of $NaHCO_3^-$ of the alkali reserve of the body
3. Excretion of acid in the form of titrable acid and ammonium ions.

All these mechanisms are accomplished through process of H^+ secretion by the nephron.

Hydrogen Ion Secretion

The tubular cells of proximal tubule, distal tubule, and collecting ducts are capable of secreting H^+. The kidney is the only organ which can eliminate the fixed acids by active secretion of H^+.

Mechanism of H^+ Secretion by Proximal Tubule

Steps involved are (Fig. 8.1-23):

Formation of carbonic acid. Carbonic acid (H_2CO_3) is first formed in the cells of proximal tubules from CO_2 and H_2O by a reaction that is catalyzed by the intracellular *carbonic anhydrase*.

Dissociation of carbonic acid (H_2CO_3) then occurs in H^+ and HCO_3^-.

Secretion of H^+ into the lumen occurs *via* Na^+-H^+ exchange mechanism in the luminal membrane by Na^+-H^+-antiporter (Figs 8.1-23A and B).

The secreted H^+, in the lumen, combines with the filtered HCO_3^- and helps its reabsorption (as described below). Therefore, this process does not result in net secretion of H^+. HCO_3^- *formed in the cell* (from dissociation of H_2CO_3) diffuses into the interstitial fluid. Thus, for each H^+ secreted, one Na^+ ion and one HCO_3^- ion enter the interstitial fluid. The latter adds up to the alkali reserve of the body.

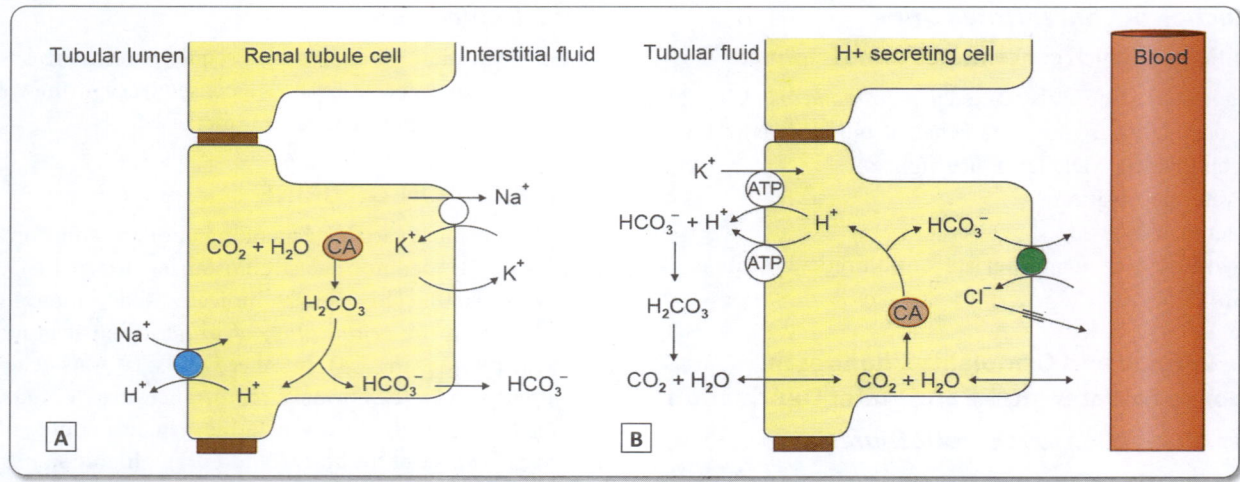

Figs 8.1-23A and B: Cellular mechanism for secretion of H$^+$ by A. Proximal tubular cell; B. Intercalated cells of late tubule

Mechanism of H$^+$ secretion by distal tubules and collecting ducts. In the distal tubule and collecting ducts, H$^+$ secretion occurs independent of Na$^+$.

- H$^+$ and K$^+$-ATPase are responsible for secretion of some of the H$^+$ coupled with reabsorption of K$^+$ in these parts of renal tubules.

Fate of H$^+$ secreted in the renal tubule. The secretion of H$^+$ in the renal tubule can continue only if the H$^+$ is immediately buffered in the luminal fluid.

- In proximal tubule, the secreted H$^+$ is buffered by the filtered HCO$_3^-$ (i.e., consumed in reabsorption of filtered HCO$_3^-$, vide infra)
- In distal tubule and connecting ducts, the secreted H$^+$ ions are buffered by Na$_2$HPO$_4$ and NH$_3$ and are excreted as titrable acid and ammonium ion (NH$_4^+$, vide infra).

Reabsorption of Filtered HCO$_3^-$

Proximal tubule reabsorbs approximately 80% of the filtered HCO$_3^-$.

Loop of Henle reabsorbs 15% of the filtered HCO$_3^-$, mainly in the region of thick ascending limb (TAL).

Generation of New HCO$_3^-$

As discussed above, the kidneys play an important role in the maintenance of acid-base balance of the body by completely reabsorbing the filtered HCO$_3^-$. However, in reality, HCO$_3^-$ reabsorption alone does not replenish the HCO$_3^-$ lost during the titration of non-volatile acids which are daily added to the plasma from the diet and produced by metabolism. Therefore,

to maintain acid-base balance, the kidneys replace this lost HCO$_3^-$ with new HCO$_3^-$ by the following processes:

- Excretion of H$^+$ as titrable acid
- Excretion of H$^+$ as NH$_4^+$

Excretion of H$^+$ as Titrable Acid

Excretion of H$^+$ as titrable acid refers to the excretion of secreted H$^+$ along with the primary urinary buffer, the dibasic phosphate (HPO$_4^{-2}$). This reaction occurs in the distal tubules and collecting ducts (Fig. 8.1-24).

As a result of H$^+$ excretion in the form of titrable acid, the pH of urine is progressively decreased (from 7.4, that of blood). The *acidification of the urine* may lower its pH to a minimum of 4.5.

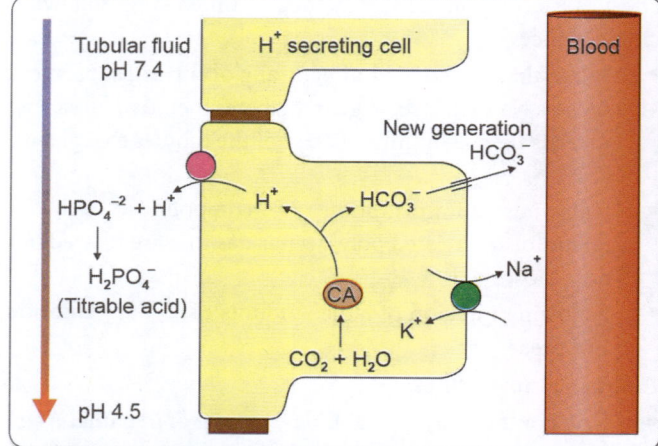

Fig. 8.1-24: Mechanism for excretion of H$^+$ as titrable acid and synthesis of new HCO$_3^-$

Excretion of H⁺ as Ammonium Ion

Excretion of H^+ as NH_4^+ is another mechanism of excretion of secreted H^+ and formation of new HCO_3^-. The amount of H^+ excreted as NH_4^+ depends upon both the amount of NH_3 synthesized by renal cells and the urine pH. *NH_4^+ is a major urine acid.* It is estimated that about half to two-third of body acid load is eliminated in the form of NH_4^+ ions. The process by which the kidneys excrete NH_4^+ is complex.

PHYSIOLOGY OF MICTURITION

Micturition is the process by which urinary bladder empties when filled. Before discussing the physiological events in micturition, it will be worthwhile to revise anatomy and innervation of urinary bladder for details see page 410.

INNERVATION OF THE URINARY BLADDER (FIG. 8.1-25)

Motor Innervation

Parasympathetic innervation. The parasympathetic efferent fibers (nervi erigentes) are derived from the second, third and fourth sacral segments (mainly S_2 and S_3). These fibers carry motor impulses to the urinary bladder causing contraction of detrusor muscle and emptying of the bladder. These fibers are inhibitory to the internal sphincter.

Sympathetic innervation. These nerves arise in the 11th thoracic to the second lumbar segments (T_{11} to L_2). These fibers are said to be inhibitory to detrusor muscle and motor to the sphincter vesicae.

Somatic motor innervation. The somatic pudendal nerve (S_2, S_3 and S_4) supplies the external sphincter which is voluntary.

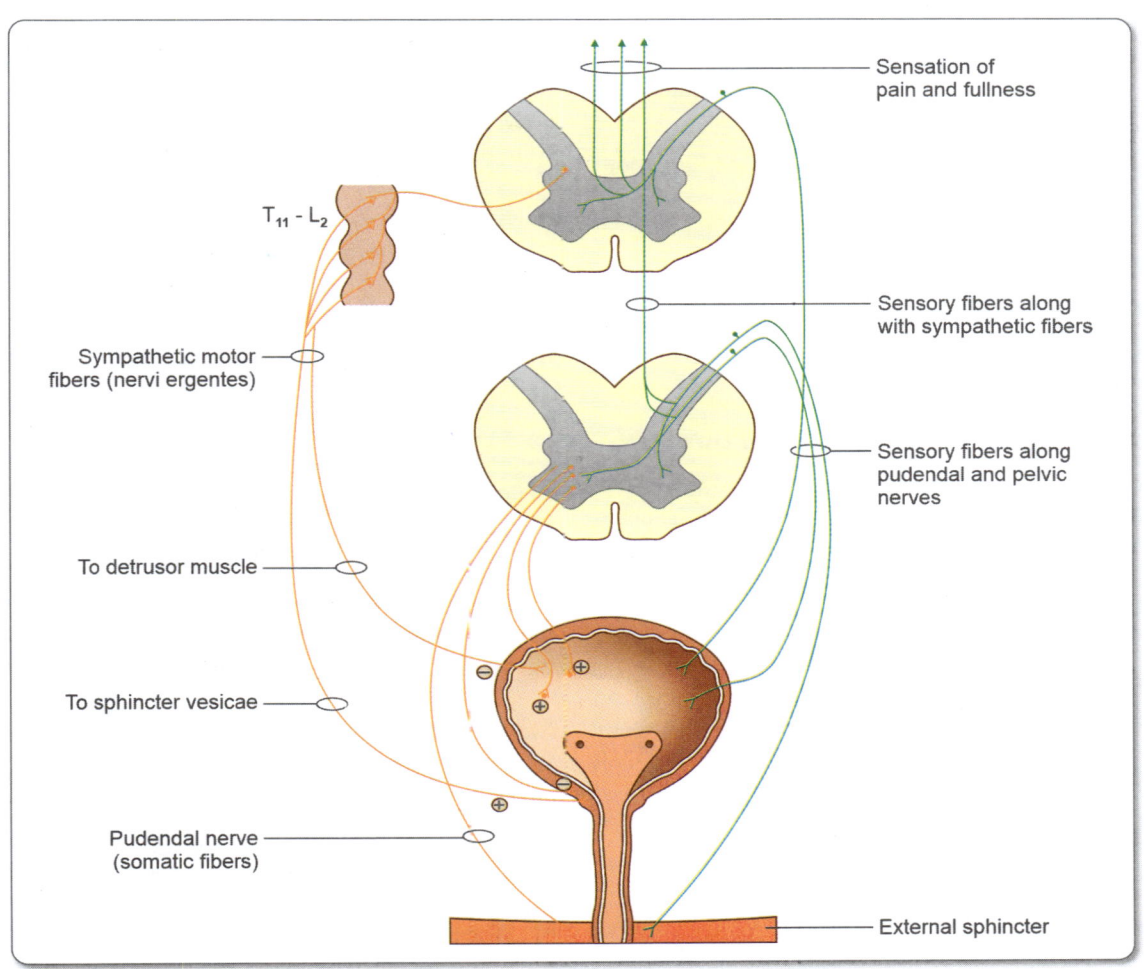

Fig. 8.1-25: Innervation of urinary bladder

Sensory Innervation

Sensation of bladder distension. Afferents from the detrusor stretch receptors travel to the spinal cord via the pelvic splanchnic nerve (nervi erigentes). From the region of the bladder neck and trigone, the afferents travel via the hypogastric plexus to spinal cord segments T_{11} to L_2.

In the spinal cord, the fibers of awareness of bladder distension run in the posterior column (fasciculus gracilis) to reach the spinal, pontine and suprapontine micturition centers.

Sensation of bladder pain. The pain fibers are stimulated by excessive distension or spasm of the bladder wall, or by stone, inflammation or malignant disease irritating the bladder. The pain fibers run predominantly in the hypogastric plexus but are also present in the nervi erigentes.

In the spinal cord, the fibers carrying pain sensation run in the lateral spinothalamic tract.

Urethral sensations. Including sensation of imminent voiding associated with maximal bladder filling, reach the spinal cord via the pudendal nerve.

In the spinal cord, fibers carrying urethral sensations travel in the dorsal column.

The main physiological events in the process of micturition are:

- Filling of urinary bladder
- Emptying of urinary bladder

FILLING OF URINARY BLADDER

Transport of Urine into Urinary Bladder through Ureters

As urine collects in the renal pelvis, the pressure in the pelvis increases and initiates a peristaltic contraction beginning in the pelvis and spreading along the ureter to force urine toward the bladder.

Capacity of the Bladder

Physiological capacity of the bladder varies with age, being 20–50 mL at birth, about 200 mL at 1 year, and can be as high as 600 mL in young adult males. In all cases, the physiological capacity is about twice that at which the first desire to void is felt.

EMPTYING OF THE BLADDER

Emptying of the bladder is basically a reflex action called the micturition reflex, which is controlled by supraspinal centers and is assisted by contraction of perineal and abdominal muscles.

Micturition Reflex

Initiation. Micturition reflex is initiated by stimulation of the stretch receptors located in the wall of urinary bladder.

Stimulus. Filling of bladder by 300–400 mL of urine in adults constitutes adequate stimulus for the micturition reflex to occur.

Afferents. The afferents from the stretch receptors in the detrusor muscle and urethra travel along the pelvic splanchnic nerves and enter the spinal cord through dorsal roots to S_2, S_3 and S_4 segments to reach the sacral micturition center (Fig. 8.1-26).

Sacral micturition center is formed by the sacral detrusor nucleus and sacral pudendal nucleus.

Efferents. Efferents arising from the sacral detrusor nucleus are the preganglionic parasympathetic fibers which relay in the ganglia near or within bladder and urethra (Fig. 8.1-26). The postganglionic parasympathetic fibers are excitatory to the detrusor muscle and inhibitory to the internal sphincter.

Response. Once micturition reflex is initiated, it is self-regenerative, i.e., initial contraction of the bladder wall further activates the receptors to increase sensory impulses (afferents) from the bladder and urethra which cause further increase in reflex contraction of detrusor muscle of the bladder. The cycle thus keeps on repeating itself again and again until the bladder has reached a strong degree of contraction.

Voluntary Control of Micturition

Role of Supraspinal Centers

The micturition reflex is fundamentally a *spinal reflex* facilitated and inhibited by higher brain centers (*supraspinal centers*) and, like defecation, is subjected to voluntary facilitation and inhibition. In infants and young children, micturition is purely a reflex action. *Voluntary control* is gradually acquired as a learned ability of the toilet training.

Supraspinal control centers which control the micturition reflex (a completely automatic cord reflex) include the pontine micturition center (PMC) and suprapontine centers.

Role of Perineal and Abdominal Muscles in Micturition

Certain muscular movements, which aid the emptying of bladder, but are not the essential component of micturition process are:

- At the onset of micturition, the levator ani and perineal muscles are relaxed
- The diaphragm descends
- The abdominal muscles contract, accelerating the flow of urine by raising intra-abdominal pressure which in turn secondarily increases the intravesical pressure, thereby increasing the flow of urine.

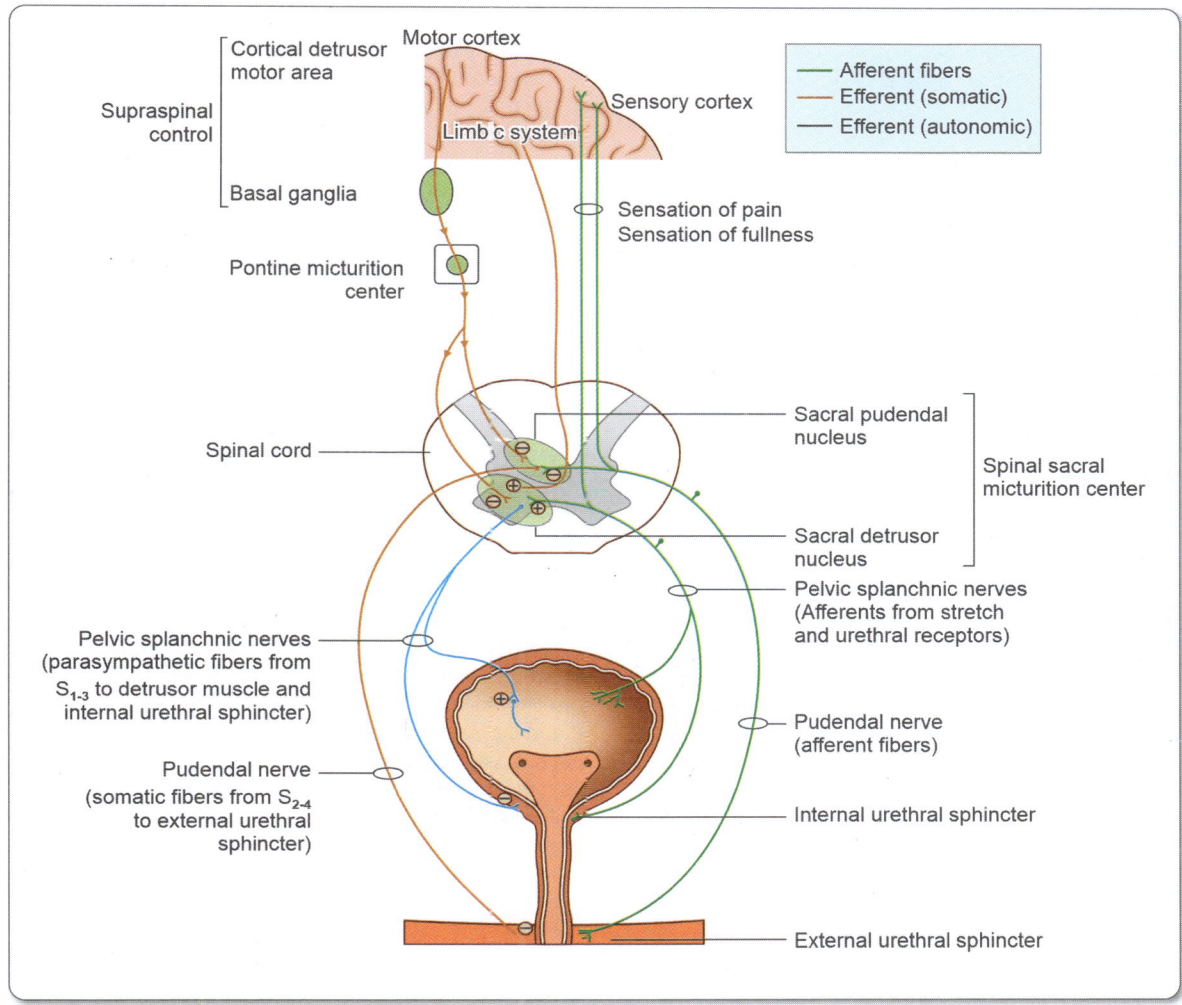

Fig. 8.1-26: Pathway and supraspinal control of micturition reflex

CLINICAL ASPECTS

PATHOPHYSIOLOGY OF COMMON RENAL DISORDERS

The applied aspects of common renal disorders which need some elaboration are:

- Common urinary symptoms
- Renal failure

Common Urinary Symptoms

Polyuria, nocturia and urinary frequency: Normal urine output per day is 800–2500 mL. Therefore, a reasonable criterion to satisfy the definition of polyuria is excretion of 3.0 L of urine daily, provided the patient is not on high fluid diet.

Nocturia means excessive amount of urine passed at night.

Urinary frequency means the increase in the number of times the patient goes for urination. Polyuria is differentiated from increased frequency by measuring the 24-hour urine output.

Dysuria and urgency of micturition: *Dysuria* refers to pain or burning during micturition. *Urgency of micturition* is the exaggerated sense or urge to micturate. It is due to either irritative or inflammatory disorders of urinary bladder. This is often associated with increased frequency of urination.

Incontinence: This refers to inability to retain urine in the bladder. It results from neurological or mechanical disorders of the complicated system that controls normal micturition.

Enuresis refers to the involuntary passage of urine at night or during sleep. It is also called night bedwetting or nocturnal enuresis. It is normal in children up to 2–3 years of age. In some children, it continues for long.

Oliguria refers to urine output less than 500 mL/day in an average adult. It invariably occurs in acute on chronic renal failure or acute renal failure.

Contd...

Anuria is said to occur when patient does not pass any urine or passes less than 50 mL of urine/day. In physiological sense, the term "anuria" means less formation or absence of formation of urine by the kidney.

Renal Failure

Renal failure refers to the deterioration of renal functions resulting in decline in glomerular filtration rate (GFR) and rise in urea and non-nitrogenous substances in the blood. It is of two types:

Acute renal failure: Acute renal failure refers to a sudden decrease in GFR, associated with a rapid rise in blood urea.

Common causes of acute renal failure are:

- Severe hemorrhage
- Shock
- Acute glomerulonephritis
- Urinary tract obstruction

Chronic renal failure refers to slow insidious deterioration of kidney functions resulting in uremia.

Common causes of chronic renal failure are mainly due to kidney diseases: polycystic kidney, pyelonephritis.

RENAL FUNCTION TESTS

Renal function tests are carried out to assess the functional capacity of the kidneys. Renal function tests can be divided into the following groups:

- Analysis of urine
- Analysis of blood
- Renal clearance tests
- Tests for tubular functions
- Radiology and renal imaging
- Renal biopsy

Analysis of Urine

Analysis of urine can be performed for volume, specific gravity, osmolality, pH, abnormal constituents, microscopic examination, and bacteriological finding.

Volume: Normal urine output per day is 800–2500 mL. Abnormalities of urine volume include: polyuria, oliguria and anuria.

Color: The normal light yellow color of the urine is due to the presence of urochrome pigment (a compound of urobilin and urobilinogen with peptide). On standing, the color deepens due to oxidation of urobilinogen into urobilin. Abnormalities of urine color include:

- *Brownish yellow*, due to the presence of conjugated bilirubin in patients with hepatic and post-hepatic jaundice.
- *Cloudy appearance* is seen in strongly alkaline urine due to precipitation of calcium phosphate, and due to precipitation of urates.
- *Frothy appearance* is indicative of proteinuria.
- *Red-dark brown* tinge of urine is seen in porphyria.

Osmolality and specific gravity: Normal urinary osmolality varies from 50 mOsm/kg to 1200 mOsm/kg and specific gravity from 1.003 to 1.030, depending upon the state of hydration of the body. If the early morning urine sample after an overnight fast has an osmolality of >600 mOsm/kg H_2O (and sp. gravity >1.018), then the patient has a normal urine concentrating ability. Certain abnormalities are:

- Fixed urinary osmolality of 300 mOsm/kg H_2O (sp. gr. 1.010) is an evidence of fairly advanced urinary failure.
- Persistently low urinary osmolality (less than 100 mOsm/kg H_2O) even after eight hours of fluid deprivation is diagnostic of diabetes insipidus.

Urine pH: Normal pH of urine varies from 4.5 to 8.0. Urine is normally slightly acidic, except for a short post-prandial alkaline tide. Intake of high protein non-vegetarian diet shifts the urinary pH toward acidic side, while vegetarian diet shifts it toward alkaline side.

Chemical analysis for abnormal urinary constituents may reveal:

Proteinuria: Normally, up to 150 mg of proteins are excreted daily in urine. Excretion of >150 mg/day of protein is called proteinuria. It occurs in the following conditions:

- In congestive heart failure
- After prolonged standing
- Renal diseases and in toxemia of pregnancy.

Glycosuria refers to the presence of glucose in the urine. Glycosuria may be due to diabetes mellitus, renal disorders (renal glycosuria), GIT disorders (alimentary glycosuria). Other sugars like galactose and fructose may also be present in urine in certain inborn errors of metabolism.

Ketonuria refers to the presence of ketone bodies (acetoacetic acid, β-hydroxybutyric acid, and acetone) in the urine. Ketonuria occurs in patients suffering from ketosis due to severe diabetes mellitus or prolonged starvation.

Bilirubinuria refers to the appearance of bilirubin in the urine in patients with elevated conjugated bilirubin levels, in hepatic or post-hepatic jaundice. Normally, 1–3.5 mg of urobilinogen is excreted daily in the urine. Its excessive excretion in the urine is one of the characteristic features of hemolytic jaundice.

Hemoglobinuria, i.e., presence of hemoglobin in the urine, indicates intravascular hemolysis, as seen in black-water fever due to falciparum malarial infection.

Hematuria, i.e., presence of blood in the urine is seen in acute glomerulonephritis, and renal stone disease.

Microscopic examination: Examination of a centrifuged sediment of urine may show casts, cells and crystals.

Casts are proteinaceous plugs formed by coagulation of Tamm-Horsfall protein within the renal tubules and washed out by the flow of tubular fluid.

Crystals are usually present in normal urine and thus, have no pathological significance. Commonly seen are crystals of calcium oxalate, calcium phosphate, calcium-ammonium-magnesium phosphate (triple phosphate) or uric acid.

Cells found on microscopic examination may be RBCs, leucocytes, tubular epithelial cells, and squamous epithelial cells.

Bacteriological examination of urine: The mid-stream sample of urine is examined for pus cells and bacteria. Bacteriuria and pyuria indicate urinary tract infection.

Analysis of Blood

Estimation of blood levels of the substances that are excreted by the kidneys throw some light on the functional status of kidney, although these tests are less sensitive than clearance tests.

Blood urea level (normal 20–40 mg%) is an index of glomerular function. The blood urea levels begin to rise after about 50% glomerular damage has occurred.

Contd...

Plasma creatinine concentration (normal 0.6–1.5 mg%) is more reliable than blood urea, as the latter is subjected to variations by dietary proteins, hydration, and tissue breakdown.

Serum protein levels (Normal: total protein, 6.7–8 g%; albumin, 3–5 g%; globulins, 2–3 g%; and A/G ratio, 1.7:1) are reduced if there is significant proteinuria with renal failure. In nephrotic syndrome, the albumin levels decrease and globulin levels increase, leading to reversal of A/G ratio.

Serum cholesterol levels (normal 150–200 mg%) are increased in nephrotic syndrome.

Serum electrolyte levels (normal: Na^+, 152 mEq/L; K^+, 5 mEq/L; Ca^{2+}, 9–11 mg%; PO_4^{3-}, 3–4.5 mg%; SO_4^{2-}, 0.5–1.5 mEq/L; and Mg^{2+}, 1.5–2.5 mEq/L) are of value in a variety of renal disorders. For example, chronic renal failure is mostly accompanied by high potassium and phosphate but low sodium and calcium levels in blood.

Renal Clearance Tests

The renal clearance can be defined as the volume of plasma that is cleared of a substance in one minute by excretion of the substance in the urine. It is a 'virtual volume'. The unit of renal clearance (C) is mL/min, and is calculated from the following formula:

$$C = \frac{UV}{P}$$

where C = renal clearance, U = urine concentration of the substance. V = rate of flow of urine, and P = plasma concentration of the substance.

Renal clearance as kidney function test: Renal clearance of a substance is correlated more directly with the status of kidney function. It shows a deviation from normal (earlier) in the course of renal damage.

Renal clearance tests, therefore, can be employed to assess the different functions of a nephron, e.g.,

- To assess glomerular filtration
- To assess tubular secretory capacity
- To assess renal plasma flow (RPF) and renal blood flow (RBF).

Tests for Tubular Functions

The reabsorptive and secretory functions of renal tubules can be tested by the following tests:

- Urine concentration test
- Urine dilution test
- Urine acidification test
- Other methods of study of tubular function

Radiology and Renal Imaging

Though not, strictly speaking, kidney function tests but are quite useful investigations in present day clinical practice to assess anatomical and physiological abnormalities of the kidneys.

Plain radiograph of abdomen is useful in detecting calcium containing (radiopaque) renal stones.

Intravenous pyelography (IVP) is performed by injecting a radiopaque dye like urografin intravenously and taking radiographs of the abdomen at short intervals (1, 5, 10, and 30 minutes) (Fig. 8.1-27).

Ultrasonography is a quick, noninvasive, inexpensive and harmless method to evaluate size, shape, position of kidney and to detect tumor, stones, cysts, etc. of the kidneys, ureter, prostate and urinary bladder.

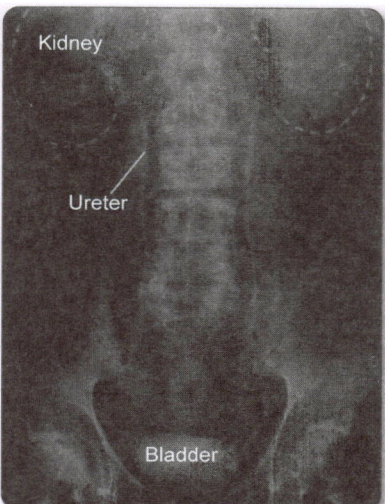

Fig. 8.1-27: Intravenous pyelogram

Computed tomography (CT) is performed to detect abnormalities in and around the kidneys as mentioned above in ultrasonography.

Radionuclide studies are carried out by injecting radioactive compounds which are concentrated and excreted by the kidneys. Radioactivity of the kidneys is recorded by gamma camera.

Renal Biopsy

Renal biopsy is performed percutaneously with the help of needle. The biopsy specimen is subjected to light, electron and immunofluorescence microscopic studies. This technique has increased knowledge and better understanding of glomerular and tubular diseases.

DIALYSIS AND RENAL TRANSPLANTATION

Dialysis

The term "dialysis" in physiological sense refers to the diffusion of solutes from an area of higher concentration to an area of lower concentration through a semipermeable membrane. This principle has been used to dialyze the blood of patients with renal failure especially those developing uremia.

Uremia develops when >75% of nephrons are damaged and is characterized by:

- Accumulation of nitrogenous waste products in the blood
- Metabolic acidosis
- Hyperkalemia

Types of dialysis: By dialysis the dissolved crystalloids of the plasma pass through a semipermeable membrane so that their levels are brought down to lower levels. The two types of dialysis procedures are available:

1. Hemodialysis or artificial kidney
2. Peritoneal dialysis

Renal Transplantation

Renal transplantation is the final answer to all the problems in cases of chronic renal failure. It reverses metabolic and excretory abnormalities.

NURSING IMPLICATIONS AND APPLICATIONS

Urinary catheterization: In some conditions, patient is unable to pass urine, therefore, catheterization is done, i.e., passing a catheter (tube) through urethra into the urinary bladder. A nurse should learn and know the procedure of catheterization both in males and females by taking all aseptic precautionary measures and to avoid injury to the urethra, ureter and urinary bladder.

ASSESS YOURSELF

Short and Long Answer Questions

1. **Discuss briefly:**
   - Structure of kidney
   - Functions of kidney
   - Structure of urinary bladder
   - Innervation of urinary bladder
   - Juxtaglomerular apparatus
   - Mechanism of urine formation
   - Dynamics of glomerular filtration
   - Mechanism of urine formation

2. **Write briefly:**
   - Factors affecting glomerular filtration
   - Concentration and dilution of urine by renal tubules

3. **Write notes on:**
   - Countercurrent system
   - Acidification of urine
   - Vasa recta
   - Glycosuria
   - Renal failure
   - Artificial kidney

4. **Describe the following:**
   - Renal function tests
   - Physiology of micturition
   - Micturition reflex

Multiple Choice Questions

1. **The kidneys are located at:**
   a. T12 – L1 Vertebrae   b. T12 – L2 Vertebrae
   c. T12 –L3 Vertebrae   d. T12 –L4 Vertebrae

2. **The upper part of ureter is:**
   a. Hilum   b. Renal sinus
   c. Renal pelvis   d. Major calyx

3. **The true statement for capsule of the kidney is:**
   a. Formed by perinephric fat
   b. Formed by paranephric fat
   c. Consists of renal fascia
   d. It is a fibrous tissue

4. **The ascending thin segment is part of:**
   a. Proximal tubule
   b. Loop of Henle
   c. Distal convoluted tubule
   d. Collecting duct

5. **Podocytes are present in which layer of glomerular membrane?**
   a. Basement membrane
   b. Capillary endothelium
   c. Inner layer of Bowman's capsule
   d. Parietal layer of Bowman's capsule

6. **The principal cells are present in which segment of the nephron?**
   a. Proximal tubule
   b. Distal convoluted tubule
   c. Thick ascending limb of loop of Henle
   d. Collecting duct

7. **The true statement for Macula densa cells:**
   a. Respond to pressure gradient between efferent and afferent arterioles
   b. Stimulated by increased concentration of NaCl in the tubular fluid
   c. Are modified cells of tunica media of afferent arteriole
   d. Are epithelial cells of ascending limb of loop of Henle

8. **The arcuate arteries of kidney:**
   a. Divide into interlobular arteries
   b. Run in the renal columns
   c. Lie parallel to the renal surface
   d. Is one for each renal pyramid

9. **The normal glomerular filtration rate is:**
   a. 25 mL/min   b. 50 mL/min
   c. 100 mL/min   d. 125 mL/min

10. **The mucous membrane of urinary bladder is lined by:**
    a. Simple columnar epithelium
    b. Stratified columnar epithelium
    c. Transitional epithelium
    d. Squamous epithelium

11. **The carrier for reabsorption of glucose from tubular lumen into the cell is:**
    a. SGLT-1
    b. SGLT-2
    c. GLUT-1
    d. GLUT-2

12. **Sodium reabsorption by the proximal tubule is:**
    a. 40%
    b. 50%
    c. 60%
    d. 67%

13. **The diluting segment of the nephron is:**
    a. Descending limb of loop of Henle
    b. Ascending limb of loop of Henle
    c. Distal convoluted tubule
    d. Collecting duct

14. **Tubular maximum for glucose is:**
    a. 180 mg/dL
    b. 200 mg/dL
    c. 300 mg/dL
    d. 350 mg/dL

15. **Water diuresis occurs in:**
    a. Diabetes insipidus
    b. Diabetes mellitus
    c. Hemorrhage
    d. Water deprivation

16. **The osmolality of urine more than 300 mOSm /kg H_2O occurs in:**
    a. Diabetes insipidus
    b. Excessive water drinking
    c. Water deprivation
    d. Hypopituitarism

ANSWER KEY

1. a	2. c	3. d	4. b	5. c	6. d	7. d	8. c
9. d	10. a	11. b	12. d	13. b	14. d	15. a	16. c

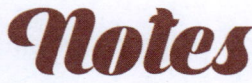

Physiology of Acid-Base Balance

GENERAL CONSIDERATIONS

ACIDS AND BASES

Acid refers to a substance that acts as proton (H^+) donor, while base refers to a substance that accepts proton (H^+). Examples of a few acids and their corresponding bases are:

Acid	Base
HCl	$H^+ + Cl^-$
H_2CO_3	$H^+ + HCO_3^-$

Alkalies refer to metallic hydroxides, e.g., sodium hydroxide (NaOH) and potassium hydroxide (KOH). These compounds do not directly satisfy the criteria of bases. However, they dissociate to form metallic ion and OH^- which being the base accepts H^+ ions. Therefore, for all practical purposes, alkalies are considered bases.

Strong acid and bases. Acid or base having strong tendency to dissociate into ions is called strong acid or strong base; and the acid or base having weak tendency to dissociate into ions is called weak acid or weak base. In general, a strong acid has a weak base, while a weak acid has a strong base. For example, strong acid hydrochloric acid (HCl) has weak base Cl^-, and weak acid hydrocyanic acid (HCN) has a strong base CN^-.

Ampholytes refer to the substances that can act both as acids and bases. Water is the best example of ampholyte.

CONCEPT OF PH AND H⁺ CONCENTRATION

H⁺ ion Concentration

The acidic or basic nature of a solution is measured by H^+ ion concentration. Since the concentration of H^+ ions in biological fluids is exceedingly low, the conventional units such as mEq/L or moles/L, etc. Therefore,

pH is the term suggested to express H^+ ion concentration. pH is defined as the negative logarithm of H^+ concentration.

$$pH = -\log [H^+]$$

It is important to note that pH and (H^+) are inversely related. For example, pH of plasma with an H^+ ion concentration of 0.00004 mEq/L is 7.4, while pH of HCl with H^+ ion concentration of 150 mEq/L is 0.8.

Neutral pH, acidic pH and alkaline pH. Pure water has an equal concentration of H^+ and OH^- ions, i.e., 10^{-7} M each. Thus, pure water has pH of 7 which is neutral. Therefore, solutions with pH less than 7 are considered acidic and those with more than 7 are considered alkaline.

H⁺ Concentration and pH of Biologic Fluids

The H^+ concentration and pH of some biologic fluids is depicted in Table 8.2-1.

MAINTENANCE OF BLOOD pH

GENERAL CONSIDERATIONS

Blood and Plasma pH

- The term "blood pH" always refers to plasma pH.
- Normal plasma pH is 7.4 (H^+ concentration ~40 mEq/L).
- Plasma pH compatible with life varies from 7.7 to 6.9 (H^+ concentration is 20–120 mEq/L).
- Normally, the pH of extracellular fluid (ECF) is maintained between a narrow range of 7.35 and 7.45.

TABLE 8.2-1: H⁺ concentration and pH of biologic fluids			
Fluid	**H⁺ concentration**		
	mEq/L	**mol/L**	**pH**
Pure water	100	1×10^{-7}	7.0
Blood			
Normal mean	40	3.98×10^{-8}	7.4
Normal range	44–36	4.36×10^{-8} to 3.6×10^{-7}	7.36–7.44
Acidosis (severe)	126	1.26×10^{-7}	6.9
Alkalosis (severe)	20	2.00×10^{-8}	7.7
Cerebrospinal fluid	44–36	4.36×10^{-8} 3.6×10^{-7}	7.36–7.44
Gastric juice (pure)	100,000,000	1×10^{-1}	1.0
Pancreatic juice	10	1×10^{-8}	8.0
Urine			
Normal average	1000	1×10^{-6}	6.0
Maximum acidity	31,600	3.16×10^{-5}	4.5
Maximum alkalinity	10	1×10^{-8}	6.0
Intracellular fluid (ICF)	158	1.58×10^{-7}	6.8

Dietary and Metabolic Production of Acids and Bases

The daily consumed diet contains many acids and alkalies. In addition, cellular metabolism produces a number of acidic and alkaline substances that have an impact on the body pH.

Acid production by the body

The metabolic activities of the body are accompanied by production of two types of acids:

1. **Volatile acids.** CO_2 is a volatile acid produced from the aerobic metabolism of cells. It is also major end product in oxidation of carbohydrates, fats and amino acids. CO_2 accounts for over 12,000 mEq/L of H⁺ per day. It is considered acid, because CO_2 combines with H_2O [by a reaction catalyzed by carbonic anhydrase, i.e., (CA)] to form weak acid H_2CO_3, (carbonic acid) which dissociates into H⁺ and HCO_3^- by the following reaction:

$$CO_2 + H_2O \rightleftharpoons H_2CO_3 \rightleftharpoons H^+ + HCO_3^-$$

It is called volatile because it is a gas, and under normal circumstances, almost all the CO_2 is excreted by lungs.

2. **Nonvolatile acids.** They are also called fixed acids and contribute about 50–100 mEq H⁺ per day, depending upon the diet.

These include:
- Sulfuric acid
- Phosphoric acid
- Hydrochloric acid
- Organic acids like lactic acid, acetic acid and β-hydroxybutyric acid
- Uric acid produced in metabolism of nucleoproteins.

Production of bases by the body

Under normal circumstances, a negligible amount of bases is formed in the body, because
- HCO_3^- produced by the metabolism of organic anions (e.g., citrate) offsets non-volatile acid production to some degree.
- *Ammonia* produced in the amino acid metabolism is converted to urea; hence, its contribution as a base in the body is insignificant.

DEFENSES AGAINST CHANGES IN H⁺ CONCENTRATION

There are three lines of defense to regulate the body's acid-base balance and maintain the blood pH (around 7.4):

1. **Buffer systems of body fluid.** These:
- Form first line of defense
- Act instantaneously in ECF
- Immediately combine with H⁺ to prevent changes in H⁺ concentration and form a temporary measure to control changes in H⁺ concentration.

2. **Respiratory mechanism** to regulate acid-base balance:
- Forms the second line of defense
- Acts within a few minutes
- Acts via respiratory center to regulate removal of CO_2 (and therefore H_2CO_3)
- Forms a short-term measure to regulate changes in H⁺ concentration.

3. **Renal mechanism** to regulate acid-base balance:
- Forms third line of defense
- Takes days or weeks
- Slow, but most powerful and effective in regulating pH
- Acts by reabsorbing filtered HCO_3^-, generating new HCO_3^- and excreting H⁺ as titrable acid and ammonium ion
- Provides a permanent solution to acid-base balance.

Buffer System: Primary Defense

A buffer is a solution, consisting of a weak acid and its salt with strong base, that prevents a change in pH when H⁺ ions are added to or removed from a solution. It must be borne in mind that a buffer cannot remove H⁺ ions from the body. It temporarily acts as a shock absorbant to reduce the free H⁺ ions. The H⁺ ions have to be ultimately eliminated by the renal mechanism.

When acid is added to a buffer solution, its H⁺ ion concentration is increased and the reaction is forced toward right leading to an increase in undissociated molecules, therefore, increase in H⁺ concentration is less.

When base is added to buffer, reaction shifts toward left; more H⁺ ions are released from the buffer to combine with base, thereby limiting the decrease in H⁺ concentration.

Henderson-Hasselbalch Equation

This equation is used to calculate the pH in a buffer system can be derived as:

The general equation for a buffer is

$$HA \rightleftharpoons H^+ + A^-$$

A^- represents any anion from a buffer (i.e., H⁺ acceptor) and *HA* represents the undissociated acid from a buffer (i.e., H⁺ donor). By the law of mass action, at equilibrium

$$K = \frac{[H^+][A^-]}{[HA]} \qquad ...(1)$$

(K = Dissociation constant of the acid HA)

The equation, to represent free H⁺ ion in a solution, can be rewritten as:

$$[H^+] = K = \frac{[HA]}{[A^-]} \qquad ...(2)$$

we know that $pH = \log \dfrac{1}{[H^+]}$

By taking the reciprocals and logarithms (for log, multiplication becomes addition).

$$\log \frac{1}{[H^+]} = \log \frac{1}{K} + \log \frac{[A^-]}{[HA]} \qquad ...(3)$$

As $\log \dfrac{1}{K} = pK$, equation (3) may be rewritten as:

$$pH = pK + \log \frac{[A^-]}{[HA]}$$

From this equation, it is evident that buffering capacity of a buffer system is greatest when the amount of anions [A⁻] and undissociated acid [HA] is same, i.e.,

$$\frac{[A^-]}{[HA]} = 1, \text{ or } \log \frac{A^-}{HA}$$

Thus, pH = pK. Therefore, most effective buffers in the body are those with pK close to the pH in which they operate.

Classification of the Buffer Systems

Buffer systems in the body can be classified by different methods:

Bicarbonate versus non-bicarbonate buffers

Bicarbonate buffer forms 53% of the buffering in the whole body. Out of it:

- Plasma HCO_3^- contributes 35%
- Erythrocyte HCO_3^- contributes 18%.

Non-bicarbonate buffers form remaining 47% of the buffering in the whole body. With a contribution from:

- Hemoglobin and oxyhemoglobin   35%
- Plasma proteins   7%
- Organic phosphate   3%
- Inorganic phosphate   2%

Extracellular versus intracellular buffers

Extracellular buffers include:

Bicarbonate (HCO_3^-) is the major extracellular buffer, which is produced from CO_2 and H_2O.

Phosphate is a minor extracellular buffer. Phosphate is most important as urinary buffer; excretion of H⁺ as $H_2PO_4^-$ is called titrable acid.

Plasma proteins form the non-bicarbonate buffer in the blood which is responsible for 7% of the total buffering of blood.

Hemoglobin, though found intracellularly, is more conventionally regarded as part of extracellular system (as described later).

Intracellular buffers

Organic phosphate, e.g., adenosine monophosphate (AMP), adenosine diphosphate (ADP), adenosine triphosphate (ATP), and 2, 3-diphosphoglycerate (DPG).

Proteins of the skeletal muscles.

HCO_3^- present in intracellular fluid of skeletal and cardiac muscles.

Major Buffer Systems of the Body

The major buffer systems involved in the maintenance of body pH are:

- Bicarbonate buffer
- Phosphate buffer
- Protein buffer

Bicarbonate buffer system

The carbonic acid-sodium bicarbonate (H_2CO_3-$NaHCO_3$) is the most predominant buffer system of the extracellular fluid;

particularly the plasma H_2CO_3 in the body is formed by CO_2 and H_2O:

$$CO_2 + H_2O \xrightarrow[\text{anhydrase}]{\text{carbonic}} H_2CO_3$$

This reaction is catalyzed by the enzyme carbonic anhydrase, which is present in the RBCs, walls of the lungs, alveoli, and epithelial cells of renal tubules.

Dynamics of bicarbonate buffer system

Carbonic acid dissociates into hydrogen and bicarbonate ions:

$$H_2CO_3 \rightleftharpoons H^+ + HCO_3^-$$

According to Henderson-Hasselbalch equation for this system:

$$pH = pK = \log \frac{[HCO_3^-]}{[H_2CO_3]} \qquad (1)$$

The pK of this system (6.1) is still low relative to the pH of the blood (7.4), but the system is one of the most effective buffer systems in the body because the amount of dissolved CO_2 is controlled by respiration, and plasma concentration of HCO_3^- is regulated by the kidney. Therefore, pH of ECF can be precisely controlled.

Phosphate buffer system
Inorganic orthophosphate buffer system

Inorganic orthophosphate buffer system is formed by sodium dihydrogen phosphate and disodium hydrogen phosphate ($NaH_2PO_4 \sim Na_3HPO_4$), which exist at a plasma pH of 7.4 in a concentration ratio of 1:4.

IMPORTANT TO KNOW

Sites of operation of $NaH_2PO_4 - Na_2HPO_4$ buffer

In ECF (plasma and interstitial fluid), the $HPO_4^{2-}/H_2PO_4^-$ buffer exists in small concentration (0.66 mmol/L) and thus, contributes little to the buffering capacity of plasma.

In intracellular fluid (ICF), the $HPO_4^{2-}/H_2PO_4^-$ forms an important buffer pair because:
- Its concentration in ICF is high (6 mmol/L), and
- Its pK (6.8) is much closer to pH of ICF (6.9).

In renal tubules, the $HPO_4^{2-}/H_2PO_4^-$ forms an effective extracellular buffer because:
- Phosphate becomes greatly concentrated in the tubular fluid due to reabsorption of H_2O, and
- pH of tubular fluid and urine is more acidic than the pH of ECF, i.e., it is close to pK of phosphate buffer.

The $HPO_4^{2-}/H_2PO_4^-$ system is a major elimination route for H^+ *via* the urine.

Organic Phosphate Buffer System

Organic phosphates such as AMP, ADP, ATP and 2, 3-diphosphoglycerate (2, 3-DPG) exist in quantitatively significant amount in ICF (8.4 mmol/L), giving this compartment the capacity to effectively buffer both non-carbonic and carbonic acids, as well as alkali.

Protein buffer system

The protein buffer system of the blood is constituted by the plasma proteins and hemoglobin combinedly.

Plasma proteins buffer system

Plasma proteins buffer system accounts for 15% of the buffering capacity of the whole blood. Plasma proteins are effective buffers because both their free carboxyl and free amino groups dissociate:

$$RCOOH \rightleftharpoons RCOO^- + H^+;$$

$$pH = pK^1 RCOOH + \log \frac{[RCOO^-]}{[RCOOH]}$$

$$RNH_3^+ \rightleftharpoons RNH_2^+ + H^+;$$

$$pH = pK^1 RNH_3 + \log (RNH_2)/(RNH_3)$$

Because of their amphoteric nature, plasma proteins can combine with acids and bases as:

In acidic pH, the NH_2 group of the proteins acts as base and accepts proton and is converted to NH_3.

In alkaline pH, the –COOH group of the proteins acts as acid and can donate a proton and thus, becomes COO^-.

At normal pH of blood, proteins act as acids and combine with cations (mainly sodium).

Hemoglobin buffer system

Hemoglobin buffer system (Hb/HHb and $HbO_2^-/HHbO_2$) accounts for 35% of the total buffering capacity of the whole blood. It mainly buffers the fixed acids, besides being involved in the transport of gases (O_2 and CO_2).

Deoxyhemoglobin (Hb) is better buffer than oxyhe-moglobin (HbO_2), because the imidazole groups of Hb dissociate less than those of HbO_2, making Hb a weaker acid.

Respiratory Mechanism for pH Regulation

Second line of defense against acid-base disorders is formed by the respiratory mechanism, which provides a short-term but rapid control. It acts *via* respiratory center, located in the medulla to regulate removal of CO_2 and therefore, carbonic acid (H_2CO_3) concentration in the blood.

Role of Respiratory Centers

Respiratory centers are influenced by both CO_2 as well as H^+ concentration through central and peripheral chemoreceptors.

Respiratory response occurs in response to metabolic acid-base disorders only and consists of:

Hyperventilation. It occurs in response to metabolic acidosis and results in lowering of pCO_2 to match the decreased HCO_3^-.

Hypoventilation occurs in response to metabolic alkalosis and results in raising the pCO_2 to match the increased HCO_3^-.

Renal Mechanisms for pH Regulation

The kidneys regulate blood pH by three main mechanisms:

1. Reabsorption of filtered HCO_3^-
2. Excretion of acid in the form of titrable acid and ammonium ions
3. Generation of new HCO_3^-

For details see Chapter 8.1 page 420

CLINICAL ASPECTS

ACID-BASE DISORDERS

Acidosis refers to decline in blood pH

Alkalosis refers to rise in blood pH. As described above, our body has been provided with an efficient system for the maintenance of acid-base equilibrium with a result that the pH of blood is almost constant (7.4). The blood pH compatible to life is 6.9–7.7, beyond which life cannot exist.

Simple Acid-base Disorders

The physiological aspects of simple acid-base disorders are summarized in Table 8.2-2 and described as follows:

Metabolic Acidosis

Physiological disturbance that produces metabolic acidosis is either increased net nonvolatile acid load or loss of base (HCO_3^-).

Primary disturbance in metabolic acidosis is *decreased plasma HCO_3^-* producing a *low plasma pH*.

Causes of metabolic acidosis include:
- Diabetic ketoacidosis.
- Lactic acidosis in hypoxia.
- Diarrhea (GI loss of HCO_3^-).
- Chronic renal failure (failure to excrete H^+ as titrable acid and NH_4).

Compensatory mechanisms. When metabolic acidosis is produced by non-renal factors, the respiratory and renal compensatory mechanisms tend to minimize the change in pH of blood. In renal failure, only respiratory compensation is possible.

Metabolic Alkalosis

Physiological disturbance that produces metabolic alkalosis is either addition of non-volatile alkali or loss of H^+ from the body.

Primary disturbance in metabolic alkalosis is *increased plasma HCO_3^-* producing a high plasma pH.

Causes of metabolic alkalosis include:
- Hemorrhage,
- Vomiting (H^+ is lost from the stomach), and

- Hyperaldosteronism (increased H^+ secretion by distal tubule).

Compensatory Mechanisms

Respiratory compensation: Increased pH (or decreased H^+) inhibits the respiratory center through peripheral chemoreceptors and produces *hypoventilation* which in turn elevates pCO_2 and thus, normalizes plasma pH.

Renal compensation for metabolic alkalosis consists of:
- *Decreased H^+ secretion* by the renal tubules, and
- *Increased HCO_3^- excretion*.

Respiratory Acidosis

Primary disturbance in respiratory acidosis is *increased pCO_2*, which by mass action causes an increase in H^+ and thus, lowers the blood pH.

Causes: The pCO_2 is increased due to decreased gas exchange across the alveoli because of the following causes:
- *Inadequate ventilation* (Airway obstruction).
- *Impaired gas diffusion*.

Compensatory mechanism: There is no respiratory compensation for respiratory acidosis, only renal compensation is there.

Respiratory Alkalosis

Primary disturbance in respiratory alkalosis is decreased pCO_2 associated with low H^+ and thus, an elevated plasma pH.

Causes. The pCO_2 is decreased due to increased gas exchange in the lungs because of increased ventilation.

Compensatory Mechanisms

There is no respiratory compensation for respiratory alkalosis.

Renal compensation. Decreased pCO_2 causes a deficit of H^+ in the renal cells for secretion which leads to:
- Decreased excretion of H^+ as titrable acid and NH_4^+,
- Decreased reabsorption of new HCO_3^-, and
- Decreased reabsorption of the filtered HCO_3^-.

TABLE 8.2-2: Summary of characteristics of simple acid-base disorders

Disorder	Primary disturbance	Arterial plasma			Buffering	Defense mechanism	
		pH (Normal 7.35-7.45)	HCO$_3^-$ (mEq/L) (Normal 22–28)	pCO$_2$ (mm Hg) (Normal 35–45)		Respiratory compensation	Renal compensation
Metabolic acidosis	↓Plasma HCO$_3^-$	↓ (7.28)	↓ (18)	→ (40)	ECF & ICF	Hyperventilation (↓pCO$_2$)	↑H$^+$ excretion ↑New HCO$_3^-$ reabsorption
Metabolic alkalosis	↑Plasma HCO$_3^-$	↑ (7.5)	↑ (30)	→ (40)	ECF & ICF	Hypoventilation (↑pCO$_2$)	↓H$^+$ excretion ↓New HCO$_3^-$ reabsorption
Respiratory acidosis	↑pCO$_2$	↓ (7.34)	↑ (28)	↑ (48)	ICF	None	↑H$^+$ excretion ↑New HCO$_3^-$ reabsorption
Respiratory alkalosis	↓pCO$_2$	↑ (7.53)	↓ (22)	↓ (27)	ICF	None	↓H$^+$ excretion ↓New HCO$_3^-$ reabsorption

ICF: Intracellular fluid; ECF: extracellular fluid; ↑ increased; ↓ decreased; → normal

ASSESS YOURSELF

Short and Long Answer Questions

1. Describe the renal mechanism of pH regulation.
2. Discuss in brief the body buffer system.
3. Write notes on:
   - Metabolic acidosis
   - Metabolic alkalosis

Multiple Choice Questions

1. **Plasma pH not compatible with life is:**
   a. 7.4   b. 7.5
   c. 7.0   d. 6.5
2. **Which of the following is a volatile acid?**
   a. Lactic acid   b. Hydrochloric acid
   c. Carbon dioxide   d. Uric acid

3. **Which of the following is first line buffer?**
   a. Bicarbonate buffer   b. Phosphate buffer
   c. Protein buffer   d. Hemoglobin
4. **The total buffering capacity of bicarbonate buffer is:**
   a. 7%   b. 18%
   c. 35%   d. 53%
5. **In which condition metabolic acidosis occurs?**
   a. Hypoventilation
   b. Vomiting
   c. Diabetes
   d. Impaired diffusion capacity of lungs
6. **Metabolic acidosis is compensated by:**
   a. Hypoventilation
   b. Hyperventilation
   c. Decreased renal excretion of H$^+$
   d. None of these

ANSWER KEY

1. d   **2.** c   **3.** a   **4.** d   **5.** d   **6.** b

Section
IX

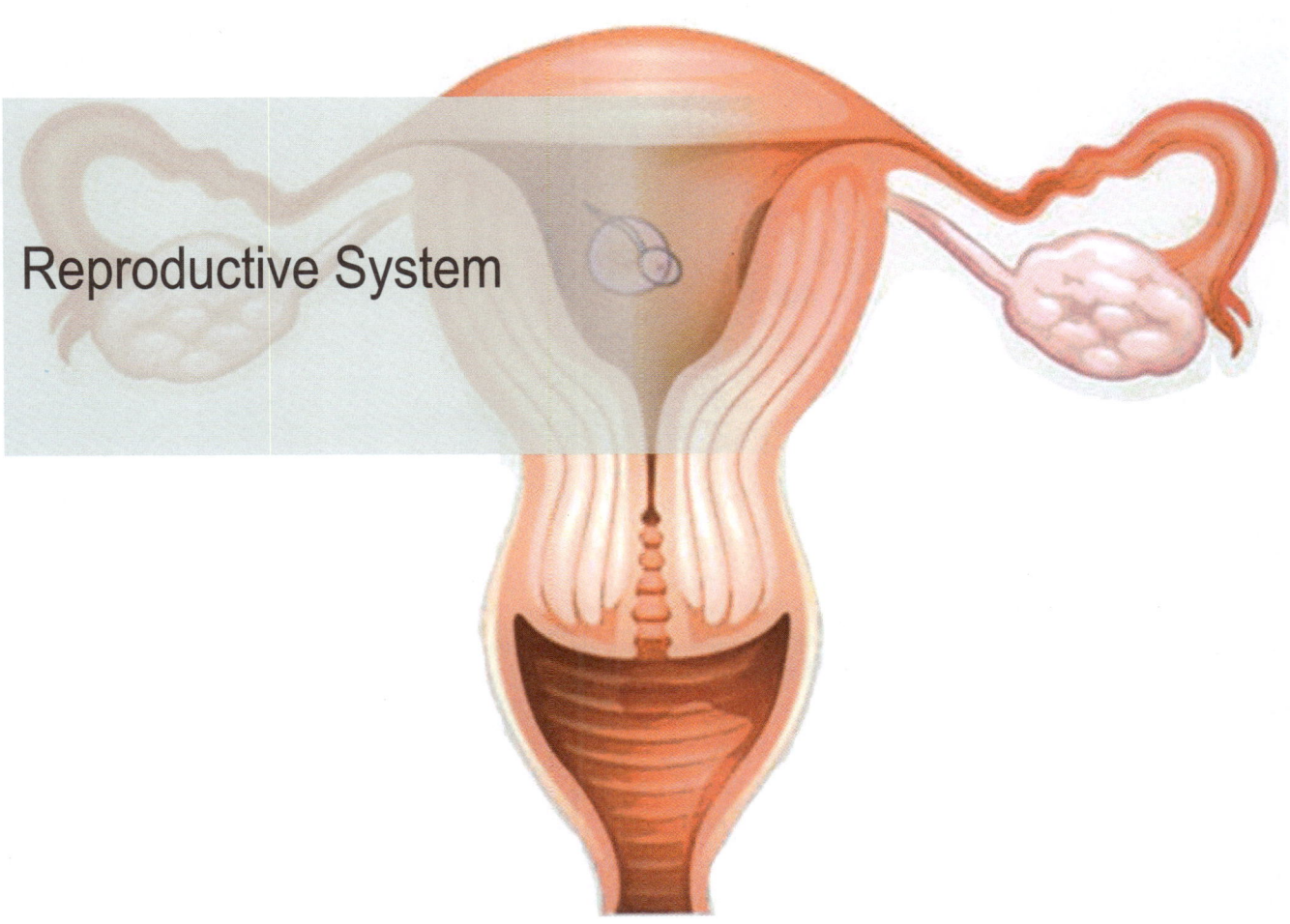

Reproductive System

Section Outline

Male and Female Reproductive System

SEXUAL GROWTH AND DEVELOPMENT

PREPUBERTAL SEXUAL GROWTH AND DEVELOPMENT

Reproduction is a multidimensional subject with physiological, biochemical, genetic, psychological, emotional, social, economic, moral and many other aspects. The physiology of reproductive system begins with sexual growth which involves two processes:
1. Sex determination
2. Sex differentiation

Sex Determination

Sex determination, also known as genetic differentiation, refers to the genotype of the fetus, whether male or female. The genotype is determined by the presence of sex chromosomes, hence also known as *chromosomal sex differentiation*.

Human Chromosomes

Each cell (except ovum and sperm) in a normal adult male and female possesses 46 chromosomes (44 autosomes + 2 sex chromosomes) usually arranged in an arbitrary pattern (karyotype). The sex chromosomes are called X and Y chromosomes.
- *The females* possess 44 autosomes plus two X chromosomes (44 + XX).
- *The males* possess 44 autosomes plus one X chromosome and one Y chromosome (44 + XY).

Human Gametes

The mature male gametes are called sperms and mature female gametes are called ova. During gametogenesis, there occurs meiosis (*reduction division*); therefore the mature sperm and ovum contain half the number of chromosomes, i.e., 23 (22 autosomes + one sex chromosome). This is called *haploid* number.
- Since, the primitive female germ cells (*oogonia*) from which mature ova are formed contain 44 + XX chromosomes, so each ovum will contain 22 + X chromosomes (Fig. 9.1-1).
- The primitive male germ cells (spermatogonia) from which mature sperms are formed contain 44 + XY chromosomes, so half of the normal sperms will contain 22 + X and other half will have 22 + Y chromosomes (Fig. 9.1-1).

Genetic sex determination of the embryo occurs during fertilization, i.e., penetration of the ovum by the sperm as:
- When an ovum (22 + X) is fertilized by a sperm containing 22 + X chromosomes, the resultant zygote's chromosomal pattern will be 44 + XX (*female genotype*).
- When an ovum (22 + X) is fertilized by a sperm containing 22 + Y chromosomes, the resultant zygote's chromosomal pattern will be 44 + XY (*male genotype*).

Sex Differentiation

After fertilization, the normal sex differentiation in the embryo proceeds sequentially. The stages of sex differentiation are:
- Gonadal differentiation
- Genital differentiation
- Psychological differentiation.

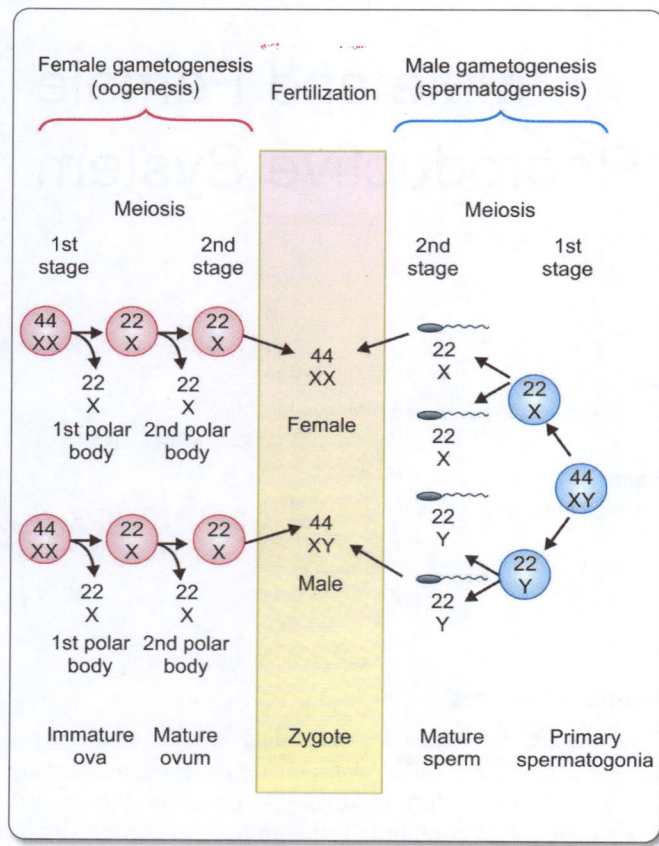

Fig. 9.1-1: Basis of genetic sex determination

Gonadal Differentiation

Gonadal differentiation or *gonadogenesis* refers to formation of gonads, i.e., testes in males and ovaries in females. Gonadal sex differentiation is dependent on the genotype of the embryo.

Testicular differentiation

In genetic male (44 + XY) embryo, the bipotential gonads begin to differentiate into testes at approximately 6th week. The Y chromosome plays key role in the process of testicular differentiation.

The gene responsible for testicular differentiation is called SRY gene (sex-determining region of Y-chromosome). The SRY gene encodes the *testis determining factor* (TDF), which triggers the testicular differentiation.

Ovarian differentiation

In genetic female (44 + XX) embryo, by about 10th week of gestation, ovarian differentiation occurs in the absence of testis determining factor (TDF). The ovaries develop on each side from the cortical region of the bipotential gonad.

Genital Differentiation

Genital sex differentiation, also known as *phenotypic sex* differentiation, refers to the differentiation of internal, and external genitalia.

Differentiation of internal genitalia

The primordia of internal genitalia are a paired set of Wolffian (male) ducts and a paired set of Müllerian (female) ducts. By 7th week of gestation, the embryo has both male and female primordial ducts (Fig. 9.1-2A).

Differentiation of male internal genitalia

In the genetic male fetus (44 + XY) with functioning testes (Fig. 9.1-2B), the testosterone secreted by the Leydig cells stimulates the Wolffian ducts to form the epididymis, vas deferens and seminal vesicles. The Mullerian inhibiting substance (MIS) (encoded by gene present on Y chromosome) causes regression of the Mullerian ducts by apoptosis.

Differentiation of female internal genitalia (Fig. 9.1-2C)

In the genetic female fetus (44 + XX), in the absence of MIS, the female ducts (Müllerian ducts) proliferate and form oviduct (uterine tubes), uterus and upper two-thirds of vagina. In the absence of testosterone Wolffian ducts degenerate.

Differentiation of external genitalia

The external genitalia in both sexes develop from *common anlagen*, which are the urogenital sinus, the genital sinus, the genital tubercle, the genital swelling, and the genital (urethral) folds (Figs 9.1-3A to C). The external genitalia derived from the common anlagen in male and female are shown in Table 9.1-1.

Psychological Differentiation

Psychological sex differentiation refers to normal sexual behavior in adult male and female. It is determined by the effect of androgens on the development of brain in the embryonic stage.

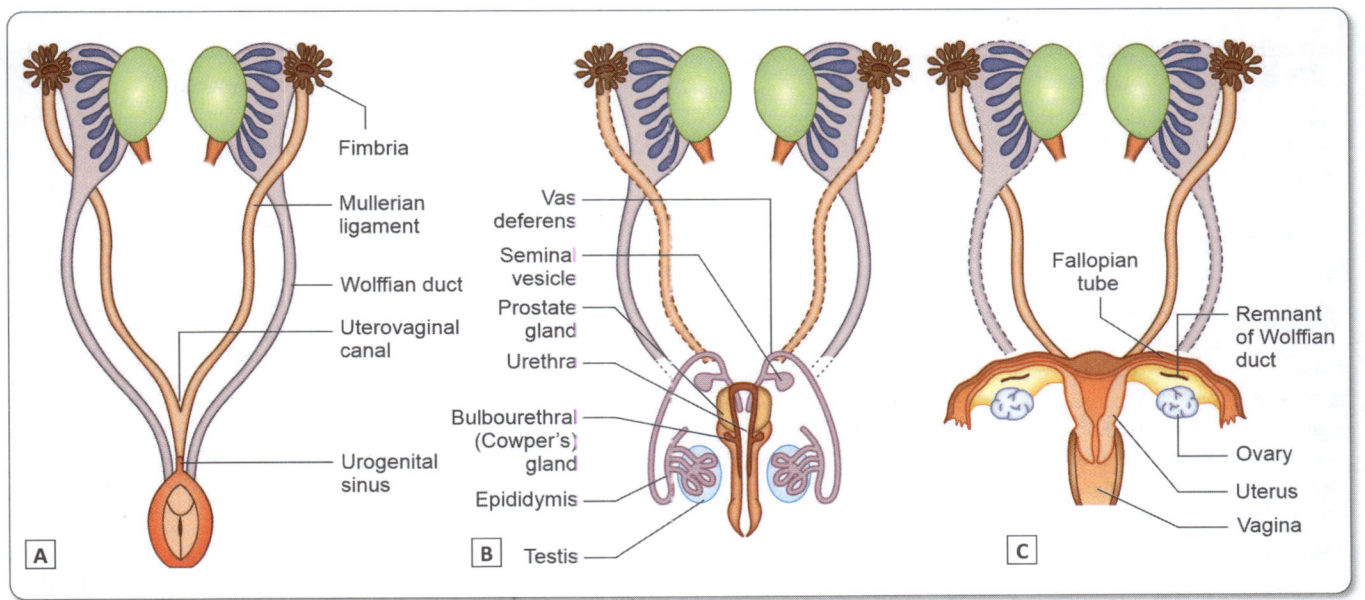

Figs 9.1-2A to C: Development of male and female genitalia from primordial genital ducts. A. Primordia of internal genitalia; B. Male genitalia; C. Female genitalia

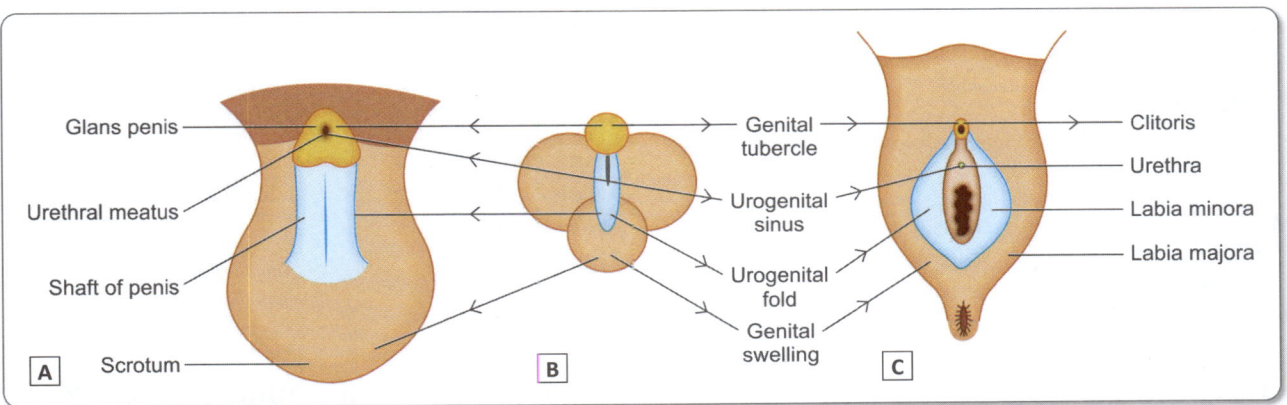

Figs 9.1-3A to C: Differentiation of male and female external genitalia from common anlagen. A. Male; B. Common anlagen; C. Female

TABLE 9.1-1: The male and female external genitalia derived from the common anlagen		
Anlagen part	**Male derivative**	**Female derivative**
Urogenital sinus	Prostate and prostatic urethra	Urethra
Urethral fold	Penile urethra and shaft of penis	Labia minora
Genital swelling	Scrotum	Labia majora
Genital tubercle	Glans penis	Clitoris

Disorders of Sexual Development

Abnormalities of sexual development occur due to:
- Defect in sex chromosomes leading to genetic abnormalities
- Hormonal abnormalities leading to defect in gonadal and genital differentiation.

Chromosomal Abnormalities

Trisomy

Chromosomal abnormalities usually arise during gametogenesis due to *nondisjunction* of sex chromosomes. The presence of extra X or Y chromosome (trisomy) gives rise to many syndromes associated with abnormal development, mental retardation and abnormal growth. For example, individual with XXY pattern of chromosomes (*Klinefelter syndrome*) is an abnormal male due to presence of Y chromosome. It is the most common sex chromosome disorder and has an incidence of 1 in 500 males.

Monosomy

It is absence of either X or Y chromosome, e.g., *Turner's syndrome* includes patient's chromosomal pattern (karyotype) as 44 + XO. As Y chromosome is absent, hence patient is phenotypically female. There is ovarian dysgenesis because of XO karyotype. Puberty is delayed. Other important associated feature is mental retardation.

Hormonal Abnormalities

Pseudohermaphroditism

- The most common developmental disorders due to hormonal abnormalities is pseudohermaphroditism, which means individual having genotype (gonads) of one sex (either testes or ovaries) and genitalia of other sex. It occurs in 2 forms:
  1. Female pseudohermaphroditism, and
  2. Male pseudohermaphroditism.

True Hermaphroditism

- It is a very rare condition, in which gonads of both sexes are present (an ovary on one side and testis on other side), thus resulting in numerous variations in phenotypic (internal and external genitalia) differentiation.

PUBERTY AND ADOLESCENCE

INTRODUCTION

Puberty and adolescence are the phases of growth between childhood and adulthood.

Puberty refers to the stage of gonadal development and maturation to the point where reproduction is possible for the first time.

Adolescence refers to the period of sudden spurt of physical growth between childhood and adulthood.

Since these two phases (adolescence and puberty) of growth are overlapping, the terms are interchangeable. The total period of growth spurt ranges between 3 and 5 years. It starts from the age of 8 years. The average age of onset of puberty is 12 years in girls and 14 years in boys.

COMPONENTS OF PUBERTY

The two principal components of puberty are sudden spurt of physical growth, and appearance of secondary sex characters.

Sudden Spurt of Physical Growth

During sudden spurt of physical growth there is increase in height, muscle mass and muscle strength of an individual. The height increases by 7–12 cm in boys and about 6–11 cm in girls. The increase in height is mainly of the trunk part rather than of limbs.

The muscle mass and muscle strength also increase in both the sexes but the increase is far greater in boys as compared to girls.

Appearance of Secondary Sex Characters

Stages of development of secondary sex characters. The sequence of events of puberty which occurs in 3–5 years period have been discussed in 5 stages (Table 9.1-2).

Types of secondary sex characters. The secondary sex characters are almost fully developed by the stage 5 of the puberty both in males and females. These can be grouped as (Table 9.1-3):
- Structural
- Functional
- Psychological

HORMONAL CHANGES DURING PUBERTY

Besides ovaries and testes, other endocrinal glands (adrenal, thyroid and anterior pituitary), also grow in size and their activity increases at the onset of puberty. The hormonal changes noticed at the time of puberty are:

Gonadotropins. In both sexes the levels of *gonadotropins*—follicular stimulating hormone (FSH) and luteinizing hormone (LH) secreted from *anterior pituitary gland*—rise slowly from birth of the child up to pre-adolescent age, but at the time of puberty (early teenage) their levels suddenly increase. In prepubertal stage the gonadrotropin secretion is not under the check of gonadal hormones (estrogen and testosterone).

Adrenal androgens. There is increase in the secretion of adrenal androgens at puberty. The onset of this stage of increase or activation is called adrenarche.

TABLE 9.1-2: Sequence of events during puberty in male and female

| Stage of puberty | In females | | In males | |
	Bone age in years	Characteristics	Bone age in years	Characteristics
Stage 1	Up to 7½	Pre-adolescent age	7½ years	Pre-adolescent age
Stage 2	10½	Appearance of breast buds (thelarche)	12	Genital development begins (enlargement of testis)
Stage 3	11½	• Axillary and pubic hair appear (pubarche) • Enlargement of breast (elevation) • Sudden increase in height (height spurt)	14	• Axillary and pubic hairs start appearing • Enlargement of penis
Stage 4	13	• Menstruation starts (menarche) • Breast areola begins to elevate and project	15	• Further growth of testis, penis and genitalia • Sudden increase in height (height spurt)
Stage 5	14	• Adult genitalia • Secondary sex characters	16½	• Adult genitalia • Secondary sex characters

TABLE 9.1-3: Secondary sex characters in female and male

Group	In female	In male
Structural:		
• Body configuration	Narrow shoulders, broad hips (broad pelvis) Thighs converge Arms diverge (wide carrying angle)	Shoulders are broader than pelvis
• Skin	Skin is smooth and light	Skin is thick, dark and oily (sebaceous glands' secretion thickens and predisposing to acne)

• Hair growth on:
  ▪ Body
  ▪ Face
  ▪ Scalp
  ▪ Pubic region
	Body hair fine and scanty
	—
	Thick growth, frontal hairline rounded
	Concave
		• Body hair rough and dark
		• Moustaches and beard appear
		• Frontal hairline indented at the side
		• Convex and extends toward umbilicus (triangle with apex up)

• Muscularity	Muscles are soft (+)	Muscle bulk and strength is far greater (+++)
• Subcutaneous fat	Female distribution of fat due to deposition of fat in breast and hips which gives characteristic curves and contours to the body	
• Genitalia and accessory sex organs	**Adult type:** • Clitoris increases in size, labia majora and minora get enlarged • Breasts are developed • Uterus and vaginal growth increases and their activity starts	**Adult type:** • Penis and scrotum increase in size and become pigmented, scrotal skin thickens and rugal folds appear • Prostate, seminal vesicles, bulbourethral glands enlarge and their secretion begins
Functional		
• Voice	No change (remains soft and shrill)	Larynx enlarges and vocal cords get thickened, therefore, voice becomes loud, bass (low-pitched), deep and breaks
• Basal metabolic rate (BMR)	Lower	5–10% higher than female
• RBC count and Hb concentration	Lower	Higher
• Menstrual cycle	Begins	Absent
Psychological	Girls are more emotional, shy, introvert and sexually attracted toward males	Behavior is more aggressive, extrovert, competitive, and interested in opposite sex

Functions subserved by adrenal androgens at puberty are:
- Growth of pubic and axillary hair in both sexes
- Growth of muscle mass and its strength.

Growth hormone. Normally from birth up to prepubertal stage the growth hormone secretion is intermittent (a few peaks every 24 hours) but at the time of puberty, though basal level of growth hormone does not rise, there is increase in the frequency and amplitude of the peaks. It is responsible for generalized growth spurt at adolescence.

Thyroid gland secretions (thyroxine) also increase during puberty. Thyroxine is necessary for normal growth and development.

Gonadal hormones (sex hormones). There is slow increase in secretion of sex hormones in children between the age of 7 and 10 years. But, there is rapid rise in estrogen secretion (in girls) and testosterone in boys in early teenage.

CLINICAL ASPECTS

Disorders of Puberty

Disorders of puberty are related to the time of its onset, e.g.
- Early onset of puberty (precocious puberty)
- Late onset of puberty (delayed or absent puberty).

Precocious Puberty

Precocious puberty refers to onset of puberty in a child before 8 years of age. It is more commonly seen in girls. There is early development of secondary sex characters and gametogenesis also starts earlier.

Delayed or Absent Puberty

Puberty is considered to be pathologically delayed in case of female, if menarche does not occur by 17 years of age, or in case of male, testicular development and maturation fails to occur by the age of 20 years.

Delayed puberty is more commonly observed in boys than in girls. Delayed or absent puberty is a matter of great concern when it occurs in the following conditions:

Failure of hypothalamus/pituitary to secrete gonadotropins, as in panhypopituitarism.

Primary gonadal failure: It refers to developmental failure or gonadal dysgenesis which occurs in Klinefelter's syndrome in males and Turner's syndrome in females.

MALE REPRODUCTIVE SYSTEM

ANATOMY OF MALE REPRODUCTIVE SYSTEM

Internal and External Genitalia

The male reproductive system comprises the internal and external genital organs which can be functionally organized as (Fig. 9.1-4).

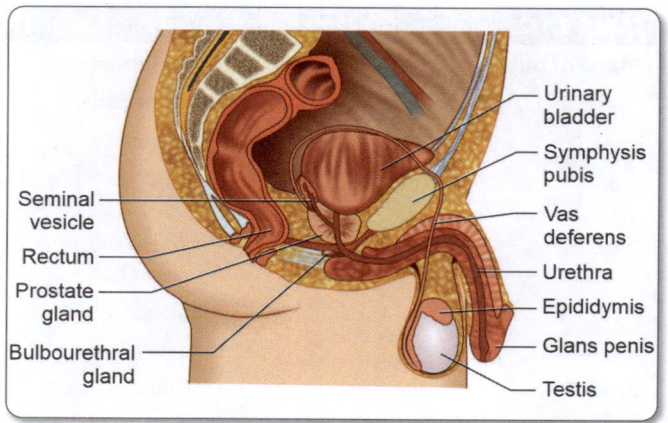

Fig. 9.1-4: Male reproductive system

Gonads or Primary Male Sex Glands

Gonads or primary male sex glands are a pair of testes. The main functions of the testes are to produce sperms and secrete testosterone (male sex hormone).

Accessory Sex Glands of Male Reproductive System

Seminal vesicles

Seminal vesicles are two lobulated glands situated on either side of the prostate between the urinary bladder and rectum.
- They secrete a thick alkaline fluid that mixes with the sperms as they pass into the ejaculatory ducts and urethra.
- The duct of each seminal vesicle joins the ductus deferens to form the ejaculatory duct.

Bulbourethral (cowper's) glands

Bulbourethral (Cowper's) glands are two pea-sized glands situated on either side of the membranous portion of the urethra a little inferior to the prostate gland. The secretion of these glands precedes ejaculation and adds lubricating and protective mucus to the semen.

Prostate gland

Prostate gland is the largest accessory gland of the male reproductive system. It is located immediately inferior to the bladder and internal urethral orifice. It surrounds the first portion of the urethra, known as the *prostatic urethra* (Fig. 9.1-5).

Lobes. The prostate consists of five lobes: two (right and left) lateral lobes, an anterior lobe, a posterior lobe and a median lobe.

Structure. The prostate is covered by a dense fibrous capsule and consists of glandular units surrounded by fibromuscular tissue that contracts during ejaculation. The glandular tissue

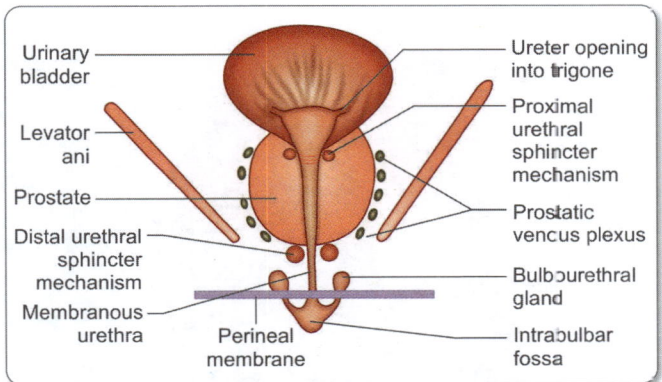

Fig. 9.1-5: Prostate and some related structures as seen in a coronal section

consists of tubules which communicate with the urethra by minute orifices.

Functions. It secretes a thin milky fluid which forms 30% the volume of semen and enhances spermatic motility.

Ducts of Male Reproductive System

Epididymis

It is formed by minute convolutions of the duct of the epididymis, so tightly compacted that they appear solid.

- The efferent duct transports the sperm from the rete testis to the epididymis where they are stored. The sperms can remain viable for a month in the epididymis.
- Secretions of epididymis provide nourishment to the spermatozoa and help them to mature.
- Non-motile spermatozoa become motile after passing through epididymis.

Ductus deferens or vas deferens

It is the continuation of the tail of epididymis. It ends by joining to the duct of seminal vesicle. It serves as a secondary storehouse for spermatozoa which will be released at the time of ejaculation.

Ejaculatory ducts

Each ejaculatory duct is a slender tube that arises by the union of the ductus deferens with the duct of seminal vesicle. The ejaculatory ducts open as minute slit-like opening into the prostatic urethra.

Urethra

The male urethra is a muscular tube (18–20 cm long) that conveys urine from the internal urethral orifice of the urinary bladder to the external urethral orifice at the tip of the glans penis. The urethra also provides an exit for semen (sperms and glandular secretions). The male urethra is divisible into three parts (Fig. 9.1-4):

1. *Prostatic urethra* is embedded within the prostate gland. It is about 3 cm long and extends from the internal urethral orifice to the urogenital diaphragm.

2. *Membranous part* is about 1.5 cm long and it passes through the deep perineal space. It is surrounded by the sphincter urethrae externus.

3. *Penile part* of urethra runs through the bulb and corpus spongiosum and is about 15 cm long.

Supporting Structures of Male Reproductive System

Spermatic cord

It suspends the testes in the scrotum and contains structures that pass through the inguinal canal to and from the testis, viz. ductus deferens, vessels and nerves of the testis.

Scrotum

It is a cutaneous fibromuscular sac (can be considered an outpouching of the lower part of the anterior abdominal wall) which houses testes, epididymis, and the lower ends of the spermatic cords. The smooth muscle layer of the scrotum that is covered by a thin layer of skin disposed in folds or rugae is called the dartos muscle.

The scrotum maintains the temperature lower than the normal body temperature (about 32°C), which is necessary for normal spermatogenesis.

Penis

It is the male copulatory organ and the common outlet for urine and semen.

Parts. Penis can be divided into three parts: root, body and glans penis. The glans penis contains external urethral orifice (meatus) and the sensory end organs that are stimulated during sexual intercourse. The glans penis is covered by prepuce or foreskin formed by the loose skin.

Structure. It is composed of three cylindrical bodies of erectile cavernous tissue—the corpora cavernosa and corpus spongiosum, which are bound together by fibrous strands and covered with skin.

TESTES

Gross Anatomy

Location. The testes are ovoid bodies suspended by spermatic cords into the scrotum.

Weight. In an adult male, the average weight of each testis is 25 g (range 10–40 g). Weight of testis decreases in old age.

Coverings. Each testis, from interior to exterior, is covered by the following three layers (Fig. 9.1-6A):

1. *Tunica vasculosa.* It is the innermost covering made up of loose connective tissue rich in blood vessels.

2. *Tunica albuginea.* It is also called capsule of the testis consisting of closely packed collagen fibers intermingling with many elastic fibers.

3. *Tunica vaginalis* is the outermost covering composed of mesothelial cells.

Blood Supply

The arterial blood supply to the testes is by testicular arteries (arise from abdominal aorta).

The venous blood is drained by testicular veins emerging from testes and epididymis and join to form a venous network (pampiniform plexus) consisting of 8–12 veins.

Lymphatic drainage of the testes to lumbar (lateral aortic) and preaortic lymph nodes.

IMPORTANT TO KNOW

Blood Testis Barrier

The tight junctions of Sertoli cells form the permeability barrier within the seminiferous epithelium is called Blood-Testis Barrier. The significance of blood testis barrier:

- Limits the transport of many substances from blood to the seminiferous lumen.
- Maintains germ cells at privileged location because mature sperm cells are highly immunogenic, so when entered into the circulation produce antibodies against sperm cells.
- Prevents byproducts of gametogenesis into the blood (This is the reason, why autoimmune reactions do not occur)

Nerves (innervation) of the testes. The autonomic nerves of the testes arise as testicular plexus of nerves on the testicular artery, which contain vagal *parasympathetic fibers* and *sympathetic fibers* from T_7 segment of the spinal cord.

Structure of Testis

Each testis is divided into many lobules by the fibrous septa which project from the mediastinal testis into the tunica albuginea. Each lobule is roughly conical in shape (Fig. 9.1-6A). Each lobule of the testis consists of:

- Seminiferous tubular compartment
- Interstitial compartment.

Seminiferous tubular compartment

The seminiferous tubular compartment of each lobule of the testis contains about 2–3 seminiferous tubules. The seminiferous tubules constitute about 80–90% of the testicular volume.

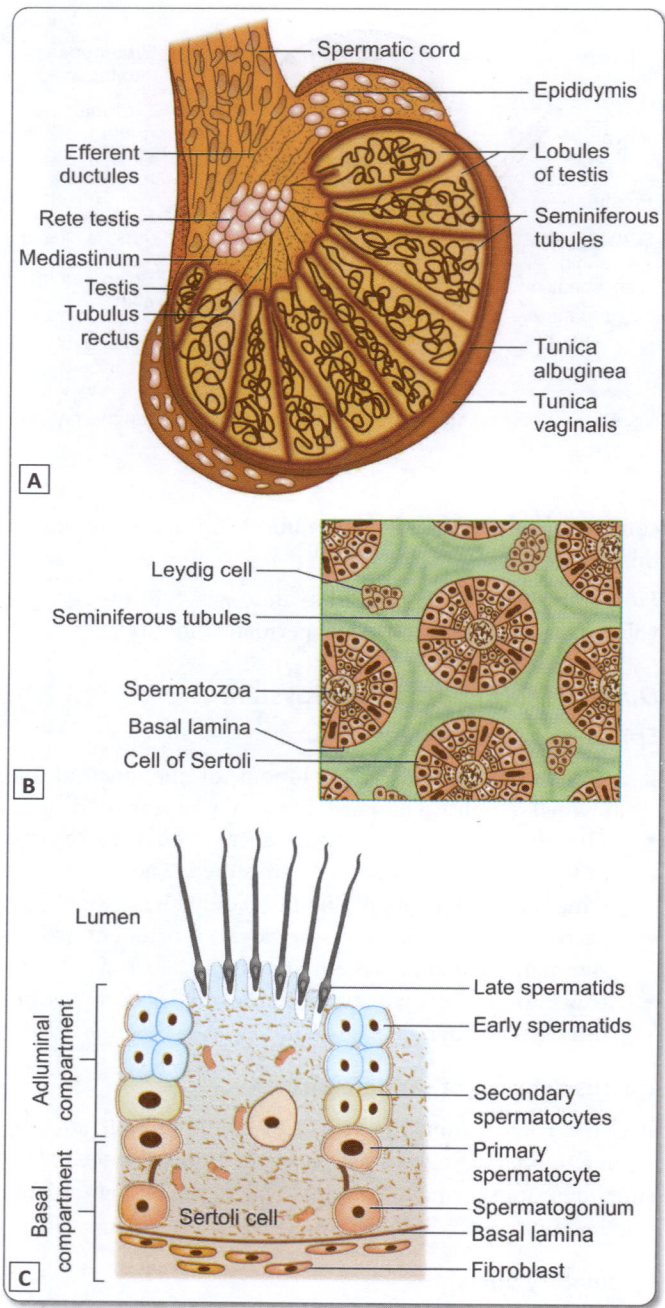

Figs 9.1-6A to C: Structure of testis. A. Lateral view showing the cut section of testis, epididymis and distal part of spermatic cord; B. Histology of testis; C. Detailed structure of seminiferous tubule

Each seminiferous tubule is about 80 cm long and 150 µm in diameter. It consists of two parts: the convoluted part and the straight part. The convoluted part forms the loops and continues as two straight ends. Near the apex of the lobules the straight ends join one another to form 20–30 larger straight tubules (tubule recti). The straight tubules pass through the fibrous tissue of mediastinal testis and unite to form a network called rete testis. At the upper end of each testis the rete testis gives off 10–20 efferent ductules which continue into the head of epididymis (Fig. 9.1-6A).

Histological structure of seminiferous tubule

Histologically, the wall of seminiferous tubules comprises of three layers (Fig. 9.1-6B):

1. Outer capsule or tunica propria. It consists of fibroelastic connective tissue containing few muscle-like cells (myoid cell). The contraction of myoid cells help in movement of spermatozoa along the wall of the seminiferous tubules.

2. Basement membrane (basal lamina). It is a thin homogenous lamina lying next to the tunica propria.

3. Epithelial layer of the seminiferous tubules. This is complex stratified epithelium. The epithelium contains mainly two types of cells Histology Plate 9.1-1:

a. Spermatogenic cells lie in-between the Sertoli cells. These are arranged in an orderly manner in 4–8 layers.

b. Sertoli cells are supporting cells. The functions attributed to Sertoli cells are:

- Physical support and nutrition
- Phagocytic function
- Maintain blood-testis barrier
- Secrete hormones and substances e.g. inhibin, androgen-binding protein (ABP) and Mullerian duct inhibitory factor (MIF).

Histology Plate 9.1-1: Seminiferous Tubule

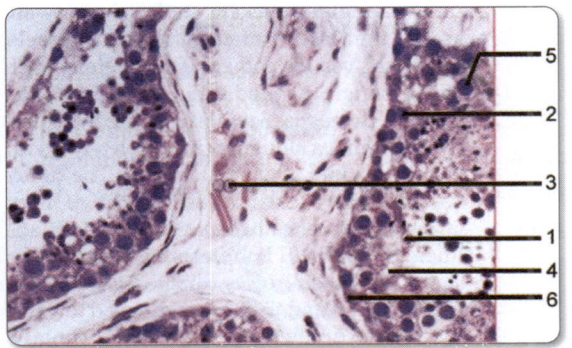

Photomicrograph of seminiferous tubule has been shown. Both spermatogenic and sertoli cells (6) are seen. Spermatogenic cells are: Spermatogonia (2) Spermatocyte (5) and spermatids (1) In-between the seminiferous tubules (4) lie interstitial cells of leydig (3).

Interstitial compartment

The interstitial spaces between the seminiferous tubules constitute about 10–20% volume of the testis. The interstitial compartment of each lobule is filled by loose connective tissue containing:

- *Blood vessels*
- *Lymphatics*

Leydig cells. The Leydig cells or the so called interstitial cells are present in groups. They have endocrine function of secretion of male sex hormone (testosterone).

Physiological Functions of Testes

The two principal functions of testes are:

1. Gametogenic function (spermatogenesis)
2. Endocrine function

Spermatogenesis

Spermatogenesis refers to the process of formation of spermatozoa from the primitive germ cells (spermatogonia).

Phases of spermatogenesis

The phases of spermatogenesis are as follows (Fig. 9.1-7):

Phase of mitotic division of spermatogonia. Each spermatogonium divides mitotically 5 times to form 32 spermatogonia.

Phase of formation of primary spermatocytes by mitotic division. The 32 spermatogonia (44 + X + Y) undergo mitosis to form 64 primary spermatocytes (44 + X + Y). Primary spermatocytes are large cells with large nucleus having diploid number of chromosomes (2n).

Phase of formation of secondary spermatocyte by meiotic division. Each primary spermatocyte undergoes meiotic division:

- After first reduction division (meiosis), the 64 tetraploid primary spermatocytes (4n) are converted into 128 primary spermatocytes with diploid number of chromosomes (2n).
- The 128 primary spermatocytes (meiosis) to form 256 secondary spermatocytes having haploid number of chromosomes (n), i.e., either 22 + X or 22 + Y. Therefore, 50% of sperms will have X chromosome and other 50% will have Y chromosome.

Phase of formation of spermatid. Each secondary spermatocyte divides mitotically to give rise to two spermatids. Thus, a total of 512 spermatids are formed from a single spermatogonium.

Phase of formation of spermatozoon (spermiogenesis). The spermatids do not divide further but undergo morphological changes to form sperms or spermatozoa.

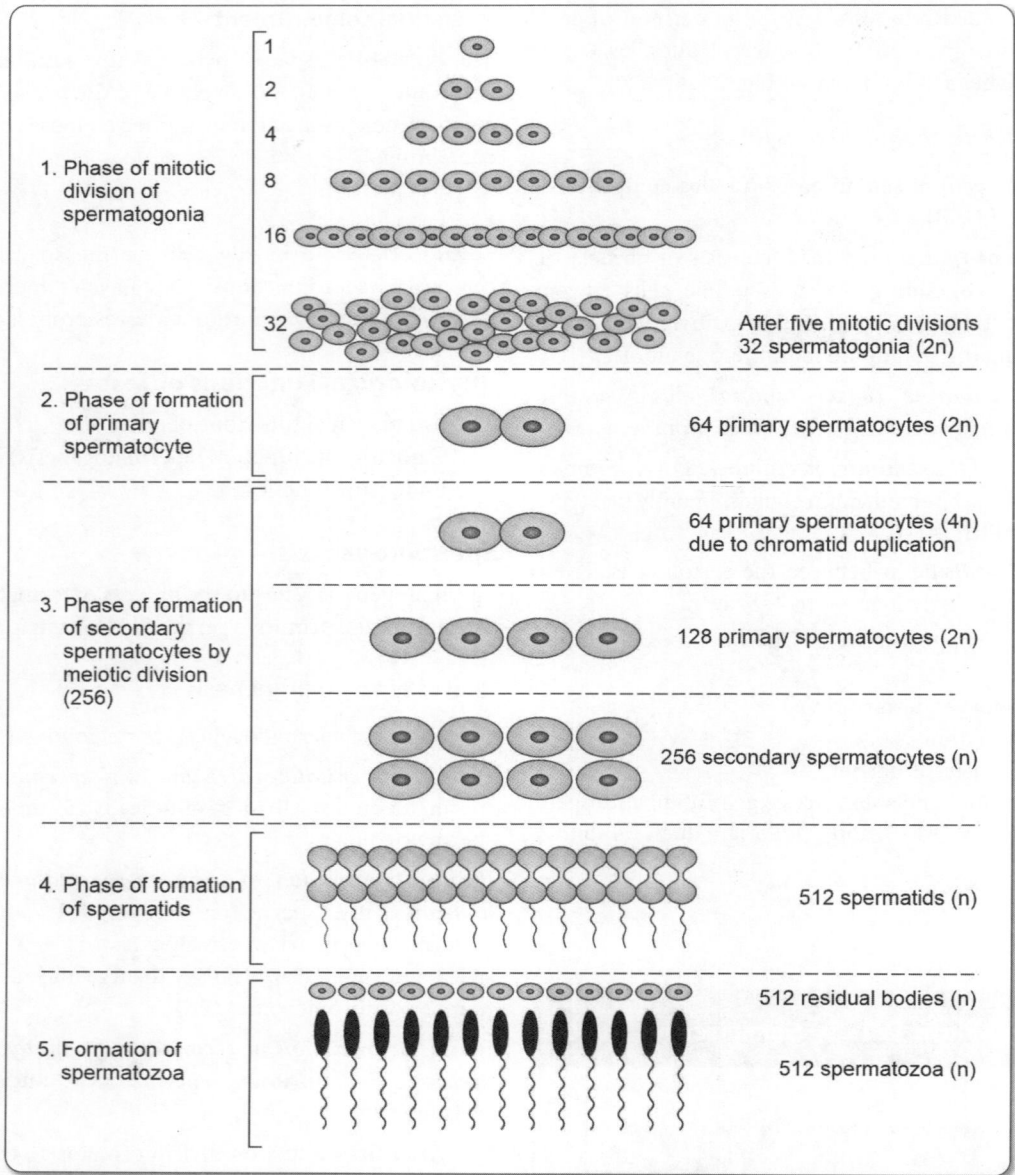

Fig. 9.1-7: Phases of spermatogenesis

Structure of spermatozoon

A fully formed spermatozoon is about 55–65 μm in length. It comprises the following parts (Fig. 9.1-8):

Head. The head is about 4–5 μm long, flattened from anterior to posterior. It is oval when seen from the front. It is surrounded by acrosome.

Acrosome is a thick cap-like structure which covers the anterior two-third part of the head. It contains a number of enzymes (hyaluronidase, proteolytic enzymes and acid phosphatase) which help the sperm in penetrating ovum during fertilization.

Neck. It is a narrow constricted part. It contains a funnel-shaped basal body and a spherical centriole.

Tail of the sperm is the motile portion and is also called the flagellum. It can be divided into three parts:

1. Middle piece
2. Principal piece
3. End piece.

Storage of spermatozoa

About 120 million sperms are formed each day. A small quantity of them is stored in the epididymis but most of

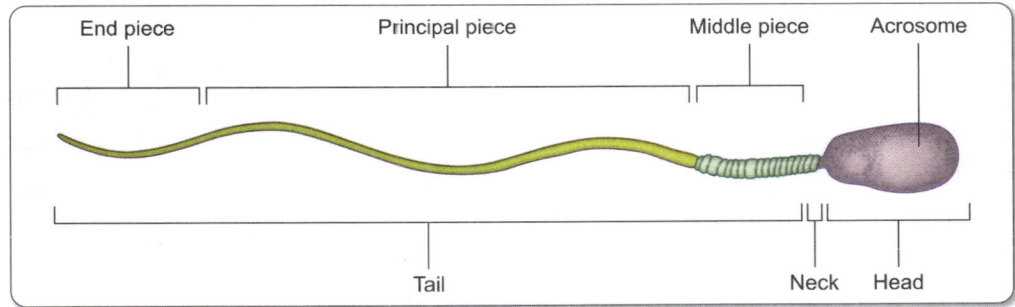

Fig. 9.1-8: Structure of mature human spermatozoon

them are stored in vas deferens and ampulla of vas deferens. They can remain stored maintaining their fertility for about a month.

Maturation and capacitation of spermatozoa

Role of epididymis. Epididymis is the site of extra testicular maturation of spermatozoa. When the sperms arrive in the epididymis they are non-motile and acquire some motility only after passing through the epididymis.

Role of seminal vesicles and prostate gland. The secretions of seminal vesicles and the prostate have a stimulating effect on sperm motility, but the spermatozoa become fully motile only after ejaculation.

Role of female genital tract. Spermatozoa acquire ability to fertilize the ovum only after they have been in the female genital tract for some time (1–10 hours). This final step in their maturation is called capacitation.

Semen

Semen or the seminal fluid refers to the fluid ejaculated during the orgasm at the time of male sexual act.

Characteristic features of semen

Volume. The average volume of semen per ejaculation is 2.5–3.5 mL after an abstinence of 2 days. Volume of semen decreases with repeated ejaculations.

Appearance of semen is milky due to prostatic secretions.

Specific gravity is about 1.028.

Reaction is alkaline with a pH of 7.5. The alkalinity is due to prostatic secretions. The alkaline semen brings the vaginal pH from 3.5–4 to 6–6.5, the pH at which sperms show optimum motility.

Nature of the semen when ejaculated is liquid but soon it coagulates in vitro or in the vagina, and finally undergoes secondary liquefaction after about 15–30 minutes.

Components of semen

The semen comprises the following components:

- Spermatozoa
- Secretions of seminal vesicles
- Secretion of prostate gland
- Secretion of bulbourethral gland

Endocrine Functions of Testes (Androgenes)

Testes secrete the following androgens (male sex hormones):

Testosterone. The most important testicular hormone is testosterone secreted by Leydig cells.

- A normal man secretes 4–9 mg of testosterone daily. Plasma testosterone level in adult males is about 0.65 µg%. More than 98% of secreted testosterone is bound to plasma proteins; and a very small percentage of the plasma testosterone is unbound. The free fraction alone is physiologically active in the target tissues.

Androstenedione is an important steroid precursor for blood estrogens in men. It is secreted by the testes at a rate of about 2.5 mg/day.

Dihydrotestosterone (DHT) is another important androgen present in the blood. Only 20% of the plasma DHT is formed in the testes by the action of 5-α-reductase (from the Sertoli cells) on the testosterone (secreted by Leydig cells). About 80% of the plasma DHT is derived from the peripheral conversion of testosterone.

Functions of androgens

(i) Functions of androgens in fetal period (in utero)

The testosterone is secreted by the fetal testes at about 2nd to 4th month of embryonic life. The functions of androgens in fetal period are:

Effect on sex differentiation in fetus. Genital differentiation is affected by testosterones.

Effect on descent of testes. The testes developed in the abdominal cavity are pushed into the scrotum through inguinal canal just before birth. Testosterone is necessary for this descent of testes.

(ii) Functions of androgens at puberty

Effects on external genitalia. Testosterone causes pubertal enlargement of penis. Scrotum increases in size and becomes pigmented. Rugal folds appear in scrotal skin.

Effect on accessory sex organs. Testosterone (with or without DHT) causes enlargement of seminal vesicles. DHT promotes growth of prostate and stimulates prostatic secretions.

Development of male secondary sexual characters in males is due to this hormone.

Effects on psyche. Psychological differentiation. A brief exposure of fetal hypothalamus to androgens (from its own testes) during early embryonic period causes male pattern of sexual behavior during puberty.

- *Aggressive behavior:* Testosterone produces aggressive behavior and interest in the opposite sex.

Anabolic and general growth promoting effects are. Testosterone causes nitrogen retention in the body and causes accelerated growth of the body and skeletal muscles in particular.

(iii) Functions of androgens in adults

Hair growth: Androgenic patterns of hair growth are maintained. With increasing age, male baldness may be initiated.

Psyche: Behavioral attitudes and sexual potency are maintained in postpubertal adults.

Bone: Bone loss and osteoporosis are prevented by the androgens in adult males.

Spermatogenesis is maintained in adulthood by testosterone along with FSH.

Hematopoiesis: Testosterone stimulates erythropoiesis. Therefore, it accounts for the greater hemoglobin concentration and RBC count in males.

Effects on circulating and stored body fats: Testosterone increases circulating levels of low density lipoprotein (LDL) cholesterol and decreases plasma high density lipoprotein (HDL) cholesterol.

Regulation of gonadotropin secretion. Androgen suppression of luteinizing hormone releasing hormone (LHRH) and luteinizing hormone (LH) by negative feedback effect.

Control of Testicular Functions

The two main functions of testes, viz. spermatogenesis and secretion of testosterone are controlled by the hypothalamic-hypophyseal-testicular axis.

Control of Spermatogenesis

The hypothalamic-hypophyseal-testicular (seminiferous tubular) axis controlling the spermatogenesis is as follows: (Fig. 9.1-9):

Stimulatory control

Role of hypothalamus. At puberty there is a pulsatile release (8–14 pulses per day) of gonadotropin releasing hormone (GnRH) from the *hypothalamus.* The GnRH stimulates anterior pituitary to secrete LH and FSH.

Role of anterior pituitary. The anterior pituitary controls spermatogenesis through the gonadotropic hormones (FSH and LH) and growth hormones.

Role of follicular stimulating hormone (FSH). FSH stimulates cells of Sertoli which help in conversion of spermatids to sperms. FSH indirectly affects testosterone synthesis by increasing the number of LH receptors on the Leydig cells.

Role of LH [also called interstitial cell stimulating hormone, (ICSH)]. The LH stimulates Leydig cells to cause testosterone secretion. The testosterone is required for normal spermatogenesis.

Role of growth hormone. Growth hormone specifically promotes early division of the spermatogonia themselves. In its absence, as in pituitary dwarfs, spermatogenesis is severely deficient or absent.

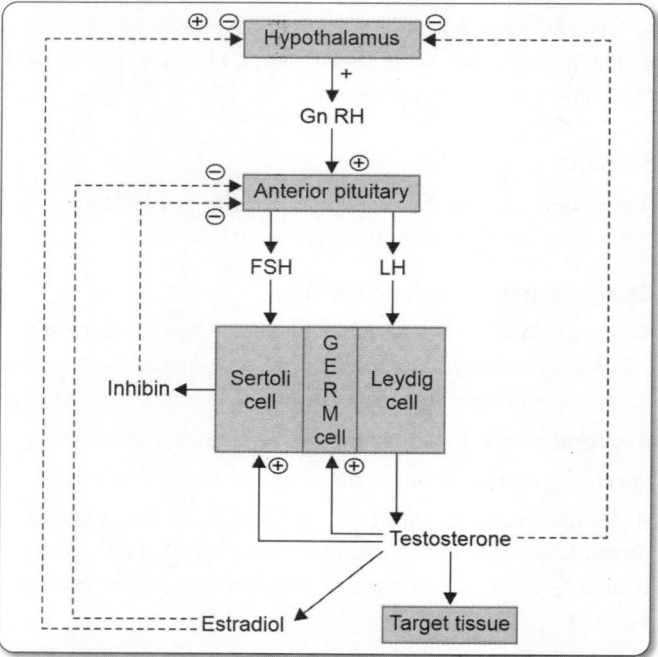

Fig. 9.1-9: Stimulatory and feedback inhibitory control of spermatogenesis

Abbreviations: GnRH, gonadotropin releasing hormone; FSH, follicle stimulating hormone; LH, luteinizing hormone

Role of testicular hormones. The testosterone acts on both Sertoli cells and germ cells and thus maintains spermatogenesis.

Feedback inhibitory control

The rapid speed of spermatogenesis is controlled by the following negative feedback mechanisms (Fig. 9.1-9):

Inhibin secreted by Sertoli cells acts directly on the anterior pituitary and inhibits the secretion of FSH.

Testosterone and estradiol inhibit LH secretion by negative feedback mechanism.

Control of Testosterone Secretion

In fetus

During fetal life, human chorionic gonadotropin (hCG) secreted by placenta stimulates the development of Leydig cells in the testes of fetus and causes testosterone secretion.

In adults

Stimulatory control

The hypothalamic-hypophyseal-testicular (Leydig cell) axis controls the secretion of testosterone in adults as (Fig. 9.1-10):

Hypothalamus produces gonadotropin releasing hormone (GnRH) which stimulates anterior pituitary to secrete FSH and LH.

Anterior pituitary controls secretion of testosterone (steroidogenesis) primarily through LH.

Leydig cells of testes have LH receptors located on their plasma membrane. LH binds to these receptors to activate

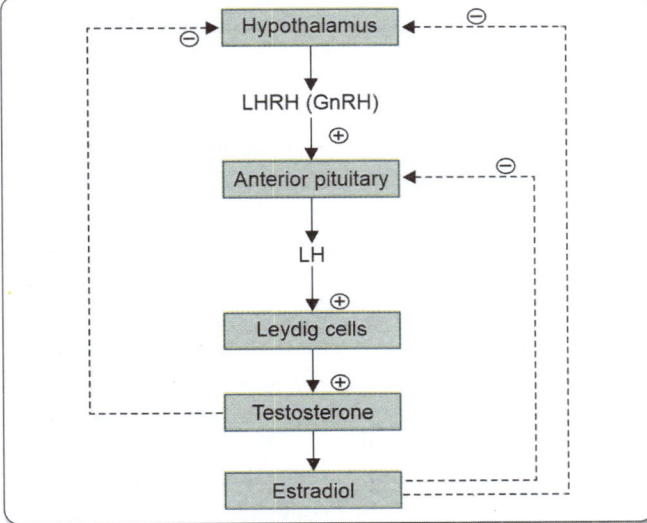

Fig. 9.1-10: Stimulatory and feedback inhibitory control of secretion of testosterone LHRH; luteinizing hormone releasing hormone;

Abbreviations: GnRH, gonadotropin releasing hormone; LH, luteinizing hormone

cyclic adenosine monophosphate (AMP) synthesis, which triggers testosterone synthesis and its secretion.

Feedback inhibitory control

Plasma testosterone level is maintained at a constant level by a feedback control exerted by testosterone and estradiol independently to control LH (Fig. 9.1-10).

CLINICAL ASPECTS

Some of the important clinical aspects in relation to male reproductive physiology, are:
- Cryptorchidism
- Hypogonadism in males
- Hypergonadism in males

Cryptorchidism

The testes develop in relation to the lumbar region of the posterior abdominal wall. During fetal life, they gradually descend to the scrotum by the end of the eighth month of gestation. *Cryptorchidism* refers to a condition in which the descent of the testes may fail to occur or may be incomplete.

Characteristic Features of Cryptorchidism are:
- The undescended testes may lie in the lumbar region, in the iliac fossa, in the inguinal canal, or in the upper part of scrotum.
- Spermatogenesis often fails to occur in cryptorchidism (due to high temperature of the abdominal cavity) resulting in sterility.

Hypogonadism in Males

Causes: Hypogonadism in males results from absent or deficient testicular functions which may occur in the following conditions:
- Congenital non-functioning of testes
- Underdeveloped testes
- Cryptorchidism (undescended testes)
- Extirpation of testes
- Absence of androgen receptors in testes.

Effects of male hypogonadism depend upon whether the testicular deficiency occurs before or after puberty.

Before puberty hypogonadism leads to permanent sterility, underdevelopment of external genitalia, underdevelopment of secondary sexual characters, and abnormal bone growth.

Hypogonadism *after the onset of puberty leads* to atrophy of accessory sex organs.

Hypergonadism in Males

Hypergonadism in males results from excessive secretion of male sex hormones (androgens) as occurs in tumors of Leydig cell. It is characterized by:
- Rapid growth of musculature and bones.
- But, the height is less due to early closure of epiphysis.
- There is excessive development of sex organs and secondary sexual characters at an early age.
- The tumors can also secrete estrogenic hormones which can cause overgrowth of breasts (gynecomastia).

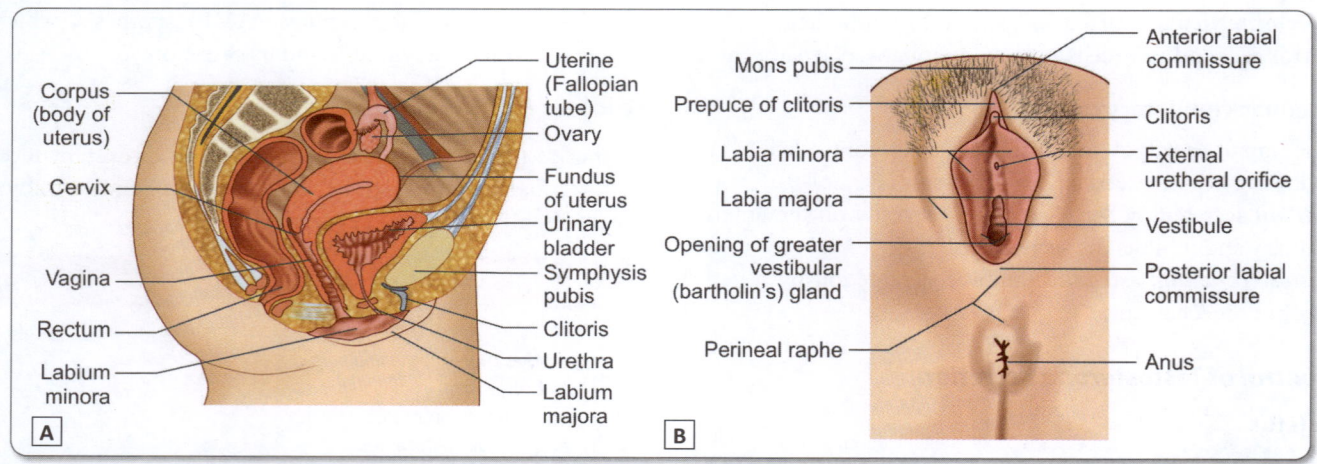

Figs 9.1-11A and B: Female reproductive organs. A. Lateral view showing position of internal reproductive organs in relation to pelvic viscera; B. Female external genitalia

FEMALE REPRODUCTIVE SYSTEM

ANATOMY OF FEMALE REPRODUCTIVE SYSTEM

The female reproductive system comprises internal and external genitalia which can be organized as (Figs 9.1-11A and B):

Primary sex organs or ovaries. The primary sex organs are a pair of ovaries which correspond with testes in males. The main functions of ovaries are:
- To produce ova
- To secrete female sex hormones.

Accessory sex organs. The accessory sex organs of females include internal genital organs and external genitalia.

Female Internal Genitalia

The internal genital organs include uterus, fallopian tubes, and vagina.

Uterus

Uterus is a hollow, thick-walled pear-shaped muscular organ, situated in the pelvic cavity between the urinary bladder and rectum. It can be divided into two parts (Fig. 9.1-12):

1. *Body of the uterus.* It forms upper 2/3rd part of the uterus. Its lower limit is marked by a constriction which corresponds to narrowing of uterine cavity at *internal os.* Body of the uterus can be divided into two parts:

a. *Fundus* is the rounded part of the body that lies superior to the openings of the fallopian tubes.

b. *Isthmus* is the relatively constricted region of the body (approximately 1 cm long) just above the cervix.

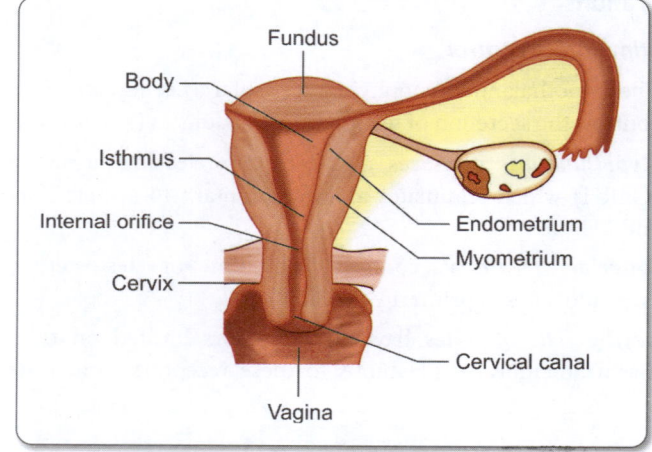

Fig. 9.1-12: Parts of uterus

2. *Cervix of the uterus.* It is the cylindrical lower part which protrudes into the uppermost vagina. It is approximately 2.5 cm long in an adult nonpregnant woman. Its cavity extends from the *internal os* to *external os* which opens into the vagina.

Structure of uterus

The wall of body of uterus consists of three layers (Fig. 9.1-13).

1. *Perimetrium* is the external serosal layer. It is derived from the peritoneum and covers the superior part of the uterus.

2. *Myometrium* is the middle muscular layer comprising bundles of smooth muscles amongst which there is connective tissue. Myometrium is about 2 cm thick.

3. *Endometrium* is inner layer of uterus which consists of epithelial lining and the stroma (Fig. 9.1-14):

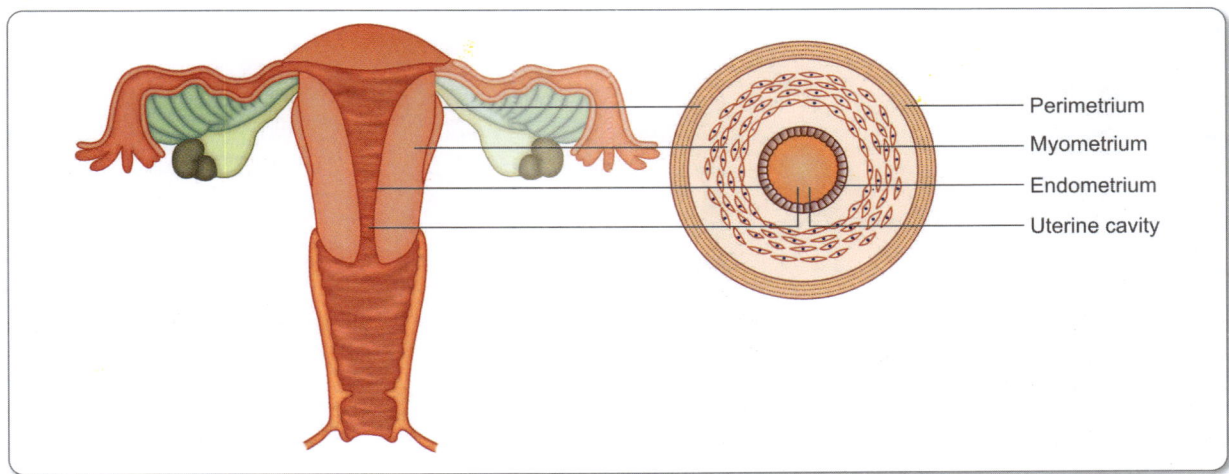

Fig. 9.1-13: Histological structure of the body of uterus

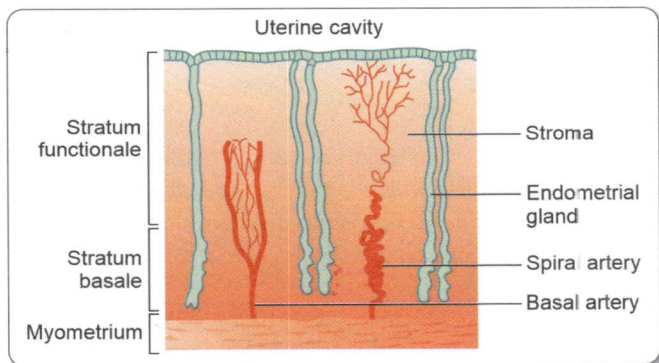

Fig. 9.1-14: Histological structure of the endometrium

- *Epithelial lining* is made up of columnar cells.
- *Stroma* of the endometrium is highly cellular and contains numerous blood vessels and numerous simple tubular uterine glands which are lined by columnar epithelium.

Functional divisions of endometrium. Functionally, the endometrium of body of uterus can be divided into two strata:

1. Stratum functionale includes superficial 2/3rd thickness of endometrium which undergoes monthly cyclic changes in preparation for the implantation of fertilized ovum and is shed during menstruation. This portion of endometrium is supplied by long and spiral (coiled) arteries.

2. Stratum basale is the deeper 1/3rd layer of endometrium. It does not participate in cyclic changes but functions as regenerative layer. This part of endometrium is supplied by short and straight *basal arteries.*

Structure of cervix

The structure of cervix of the uterus is somewhat different from that of the body.

Perimetrium is the outermost serous layer.

Myometrium layer of the cervix is much less muscular as compared to body of uterus, and contains more connective tissue. During childbirth, when the myometrium of body of uterus contracts, the myometrium of cervix dilates, consequently the cervical canal becomes large enough for the fetal head to pass through.

Endocervix refers to the innermost mucosal layer of cervix in contrast to endometrium of the body of uterus. Endocervix is not shed at the time of menstruation. Endocervix consists of:

Epithelium. The mucous membrane of the upper two-thirds of cervical canal is lined by *ciliated columnar epithelium*, but its lower one-third epithelium is nonciliated columnar. Near the external os the canal is lined by stratified squamous epithelium.

NURSING IMPLICATIONS AND APPLICATIONS

Cervical cancer. In women, cervical cancer is very common and is a major cause of the morbidity.
- *Pap smear test*. For early detection, Pap smear test should be done once in every three years, after the age of 30 years in every woman.
- *HPV Vaccine*. For primary prevention of cervical cancer, HPV vaccination of young girls, at the age of 9 years to be advised.

Stroma. The stroma of the cervix is less cellular than that of body of uterus.

Ligaments of uterus

Ligaments are fibrous cords covered with mesothelium and peritoneal folds. These assist in holding the internal reproductive organs in normal position and in anchoring them to the wall and floor of the pelvis. The ligaments of uterus are (Figs 9.1-15A and B):

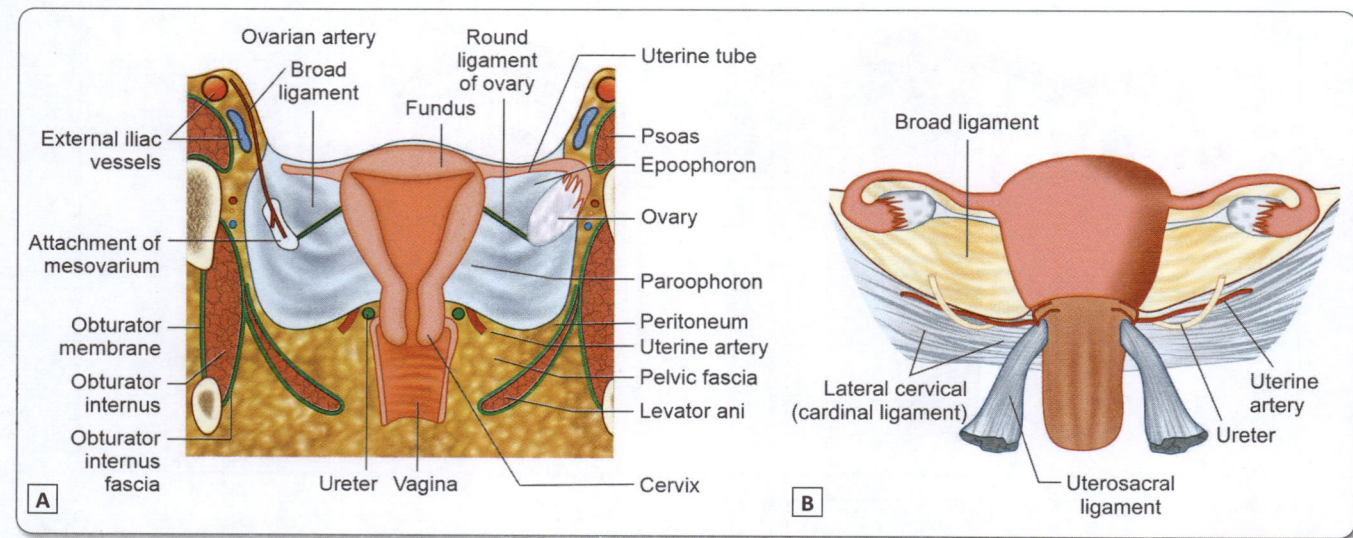

Figs 9.1-15A and B: Schematic section to show the relation of female reproductive organs (A) and ligaments of uterus (B)

Broad ligaments are wide peritoneal folds that stretch from the side of the uterus to the side wall and floor of the pelvis on each side.

Round ligaments of uterus are flattened fibrous cords that extend from the lateral borders of the uterus within the broad ligaments to the connective tissue and skin of the labia majora after passing through the inguinal canals of their respective sides. They help to hold the fundus forward in a slightly anteflexed position.

Uterosacral ligaments are peritoneal folds that pass from the cervix to the sacrum, and are extending on each side of rectum.

Cardinal ligaments are enveloping band of fascia that surround the uterine blood vessels as they pass to the vagina and cervix from the lateral pelvis.

Anterior ligament is the sheath of peritoneum that extends from the urinary bladder to uterus. It does not provide support to the viscera.

Posterior ligament is the fold of peritoneum reflected from the anterior surface of rectum upon the posterior surface of vagina and uterus. It also does not provide any support to the pelvic floor or viscera.

NURSING IMPLICATIONS AND APPLICATIONS

Uterus prolapse. The uterus is held in position by the support provided by various ligaments. However, due to certain reasons the support gets weakened, leading to downward displacement of uterus called uterus prolapse.

Fallopian Tubes

Each fallopian tube (also known as uterine tube) is approximately 10 cm in length and 8 mm in diameter. It has a medial or *uterine end* which is attached to and opens into the uterus and a *lateral end* opens into peritoneal cavity near the ovary.

Parts

Each fallopian tube can be divided into four parts (Fig. 9.1-16):

1. *Uterine or interstitial part* is the most medial part which passes through the thick uterine wall.
2. *Isthmus* is the relatively narrow and thick-walled part which is just next to the uterine part. It is about 2.5 cm in length.
3. *Ampulla* is the next thin-walled and dilated part of the uterine tube. It is the largest part (7 cm) of uterine tube.

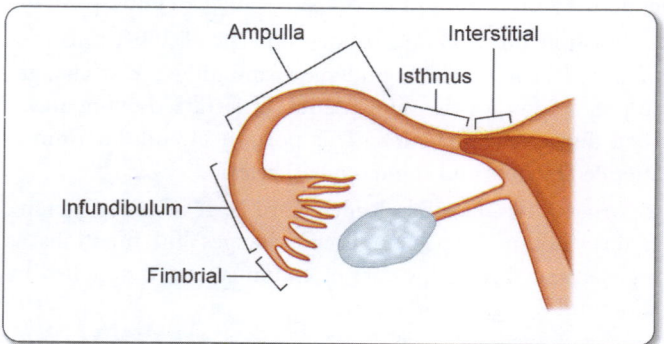

Figs 9.1-16: Fallopian tube

4. *Infundibulum* refers to the funnel-shaped lateral end of the tube. It is prolonged into a number of finger-like processes known as fimbria. One fimbria is longer than rest of the fimbriae and is attached to the outer pole of ovary.

Structure

Fallopian tubes consist of same three coats as of the uterus, viz. endometrium, myometrium and perimetrium.

Functions

The uterine tubes convey ova, shed by the ovaries, to the uterus. Secretions present in the tubes provide nutrition, oxygen, and other requirements for ova and spermatozoa passing through the tube. Fertilization takes place in the ampulla and the fertilized ovum travels toward the uterus through the tube.

NURSING IMPLICATIONS AND APPLICATIONS

Infertility in woman may occur due to blockage of fallopian tubes. The patency of uterine tubes can be determined by:
Hysterosalpingography (HSG) *is* a X-ray procedure that is used to view interior of the uterus and fallopian tubes. Radio-opaque dye is injected through vagina into the uterus and patency of fallopian tubes is visualized.
Sonosalpingography. In this procedure, normal saline is injected through vagina and flow of saline into the fallopian tubes is visualized by ultrasound.
Ectopic tubal pregnancy occurs when there is partial blockage of fallopian tubes due to infection. Therefore, fertilized ovum (zygote stage) may not be able to pass into the uterus and gets implanted into the mucosa of the fallopian tube. Ampulla is the common site of ectopic tubal pregnancy.

Vagina

The vagina is a musculomembranous tube (about 8–10 cm long) located anterior to the rectum and posterior to urethra and urinary bladder. Its upper end surrounds the lower part of cervix and forms vaginal recesses around it. These recesses are known as the anterior, posterior and lateral fornices. Its lower end, i.e., vaginal orifice, opens into the vestibule of vagina (the cleft between the labia minora).

Structure

The wall of vagina consists of a mucous membrane, a muscle coat, and an outer fibrous coat or adventitia.

Functions. The vagina serves the following functions:
- It serves as the excretory duct for menstrual fluid.
- It forms the inferior part of pelvic (birth) canal.
- It receives the penis and ejaculates during sexual intercourse.

Female External Genitalia

The external genital organs include mons pubis, labia majora, labia minora, clitoris, vestibule of vagina, bulbs of vestibule and greater vestibular glands (Fig. 9.1-11B).

The synonymous terms vulva and pudendum include all these parts.

Mons pubis is the rounded, fatty prominence anterior to the pubic symphysis, pubic tubercle, and superior pubic rami.

Labia majora are prominent folds of skin that bound the *pudendal cleft* and thus indirectly provide protection for urethral and vaginal orifices which open into this cleft.

Labia minora are folds of fat-free, hairless, pinkish skin. They are enclosed in the pudendal cleft and surround the *vestibule of vagina*. They have a core of spongy connective tissue containing erectile tissue and many small blood vessels.

Clitoris is an erectile organ located where the labia minora meet anteriorly. The clitoris is analogous to male penis, but unlike the penis, the clitoris is not functionally related to the urethra or to urination. It functions solely as an organ of sexual arousal.

Vestibule is the space between the labia minora that contains the opening of urethra, vagina, and ducts of greater and lesser vestibular glands. The vaginal orifice is surrounded by a thin fold of mucous membrane called *hymen* which is usually ruptured after first intercourse or otherwise. After childbirth, only a few remnants of the *hymen or hymenal caruncles* (tags) are visible.

Bulbs of the vestibule are paired masses of erectile tissue which lie along the sides of vaginal orifice under cover of bulbospongiosus muscles. These are homologous with the bulb of the penis and corpus spongiosum.

Vestibular glands include a pair each of greater vestibular and lesser vestibular glands. These glands secrete mucus into the vestibule during arousal.

NURSING IMPLICATIONS AND APPLICATIONS

Imperforation of hymen. Sometimes hymen is without opening (imperforated hymen). In such cases, when menarche starts, the menstrual blood is collected into the vagina leading to hematocolpos. Surgical intervention is required to drain the collected blood from vagina.

OVARIES

Gross Anatomy

A pair of ovaries is located (one on each side) behind and below the fallopian tubes. The ovaries are ovoid glands with a combined weight of 10–20 g during reproductive years, which

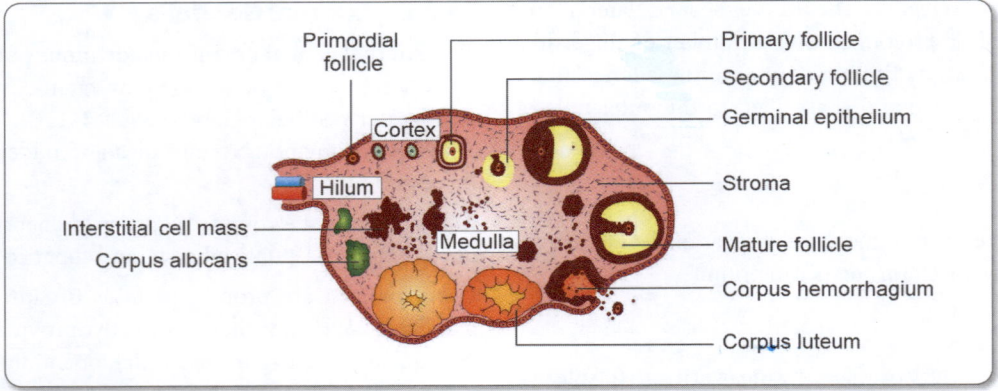

Fig. 9.1-17: Schematic diagram of the histology of ovary depicting various stages of development of follicles and corpus luteum

decreases with increasing age. Each ovary is about 3–5 cm in length and is attached to the uterus by the broad ligament and round ligament of ovary.

Structure

Histologically, each ovary consists of the following parts (Fig. 9.1-17):

Germinal epithelium. Germinal epithelium refers to the epithelium lining the outer surface of ovary and consists of a single layer of cuboidal cells. The term germinal epithelium is a misnomer, as it does not produce germ cells.

Cortex. The cortex is the outer thick main part of the substance of the ovary. It consists of the following tissues:
- *Tunica albuginea*
- *Stroma*
- *Ovarian follicles*

Medulla. The medulla is the inner small part of the substance of ovary. It consists of connective tissue in which numerous blood vessels (mostly veins), smooth muscles and elastic fibers are present.

Hilum. The hilum refers to the area where ovary attaches to mesentery. It is the site for entry of blood vessels and lymphatics.

Physiological Functions of Ovaries

The two principal functions of ovaries are:
1. Gametogenic function, i.e., oogenesis
2. Endocrine function, i.e., secretion of female hormones called ovarian hormones.

Oogenesis

Fetal oogenesis

Oogenesis refers to the process of formation of ova from the primitive germ cells.

Primitive germ cells. When the bipotential gonads differentiate into ovaries in genetic female (44 + XX) embryo by 10th week of gestation, the primitive germ cells increase in number by mitosis to form oogonia.

Oogonia are the stem cells from which ova are derived. The oogonia proliferate by mitosis to form primary oocytes.

Primary oocytes, formed from the oogonia, enter a prolonged prophase (*diplotene stage*) of the first meiotic division and remain in this state until ovulation occurs after puberty.

Primordial follicles. The *diploid primary oocytes* become enveloped by single layer of flat granulosa cells and in this form are called *primordial follicles.*

Pubertal oogenesis

After puberty, the oogenesis or formation of ovum occurs in a highly cyclic fashion, once every 28 days till menopause.

Every month, in each ovary, more than one primordial follicles start undergoing maturation process but only one reaches maturity and the rest undergo atresia at different stages of development. Thus throughout the whole normal reproductive life of about 30 years (from 13 to 42 years) about 450 ova are expelled and the remainder degenerate.

The different stages of maturation of primordial follicle into graafian follicle (*folliculogenesis*) (Figs 9.1-18A to E) are:

Primordial follicles are the fundamental reproductive units of ovary. At the time of puberty both ovaries contain about 3,00,000 primordial follicles (Fig. 9.1-18A).
- Each primordial follicle consists of the primary oocyte in prophase of the first meiotic division surrounded by a single layer of spindle-shaped (flat) cells called the granulosa cells.

Primary follicle. The primary follicle is formed when the primordial follicle undergoes the following developmental changes (Fig. 9.1-18B):

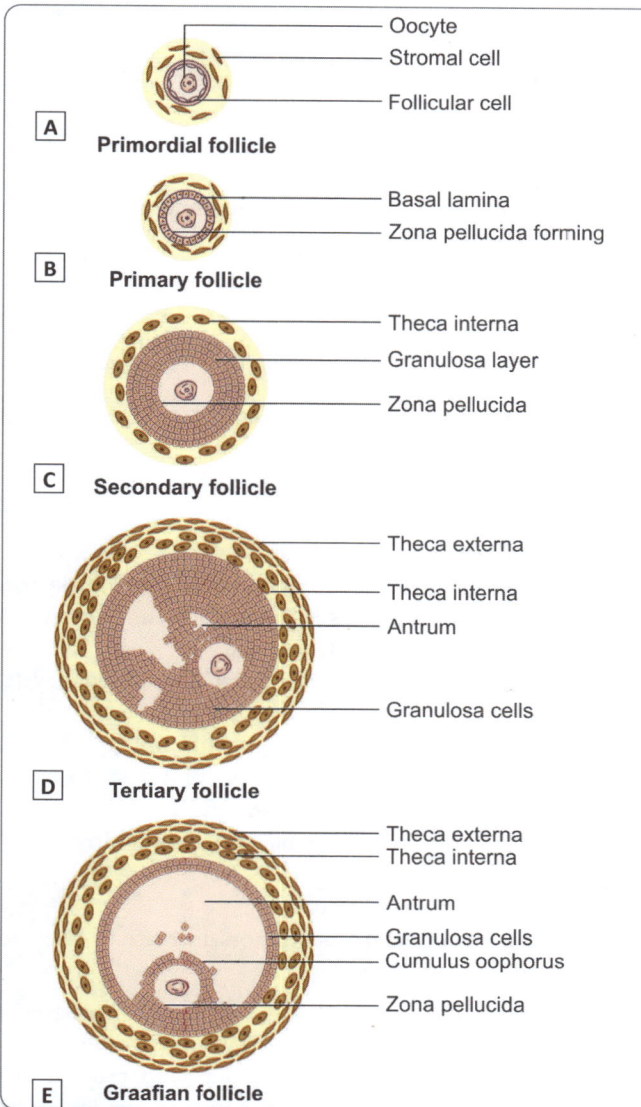

Figs 9.1-18A to E: Phases of folliculogenesis

- *Granulosa cells* become columnar and undergo mitotic division to form a multilayered stratum granulosum.
- *Oocyte enlarges*
- *Zona pellucida*, a homogeneous membrane, appears.

Secondary follicle is formed from the primary follicle when the following changes occur (Fig. 9.1-18C) Histology Plate 9.1-2:
- *Granulosa cells* undergo further proliferation.
- *Oocyte* further increases in size up to 100 μ. Its nucleus becomes larger.
- *Theca folliculi* or follicular sheath is formed outside the basal lamina from the spindle-shaped cells from the stroma of cortex in ovary. The theca folliculi consist of

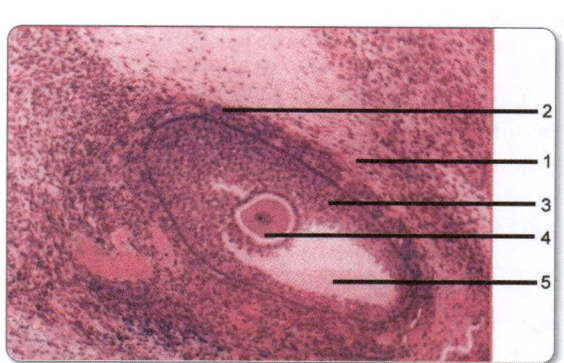

Histology Plate 9.1-2: Secondary Follicle

Photomicrograph of secondary follicle has been shown. Eccentric oocyte (4) and large fluid filled antrum (5) are seen. Oocyte is surrounded by granulosa cells (3). Theca folliculi differentiate in theca interna (2) and theca externa (1)

an inner rim of secretory cells called *theca interna* and an outer rim of thickly packed fibers and spindle-shaped cells called *theca externa*.

Tertiary follicle is characterized by the following features:
- *Formation of antrum.* The granulosa cells start secreting follicular fluid this causes cavity to be formed in the stratum granulosum (cavitation), which is called antrum or follicular cavity. The fluid filled in the antrum is called liquor folliculi which also contains estrogen (Fig. 9.1-17D).

Graafian (antral) follicle is fully matured follicle characterized by following features (Fig. 9.1-17E)
- Markedly increase in size (2–5 mm).
- Antrum becomes larges
- Theca interna becomes more prominent
- Formation of secondary oocyte occurs just prior to ovulation

Endocrine Function of Ovaries

The endocrine function of the ovaries is to produce female sex hormones which include:
- Estrogens
- Progesterone.

Estrogens

Estrogens are C-18 steroids. The naturally occurring estrogens include:

Estradiol. It is the principal and physiologically most potent estrogen. Ovarian estradiol accounts for more than 90% of the circulating estrogens.

Estrone. It is a weak ovarian estrogen.

Estriol. It is the degradation product of estradiol and estrone. It is the weakest of all naturally occurring estrogens.

Synthesis, plasma levels, and transport of estrogens

Sites

In the normal female, estrogens are mainly secreted by theca interna and granulosa cells of the ovarian follicles. A small quantity is also produced by adrenal cortex, breast, some areas of brain, placenta (during pregnancy), and by Sertoli cells (in males).

Plasma levels

In a normal adult woman the plasma levels of estrogen vary in different phases of ovarian cycle (Figs 9.1-19A to E). As shown in Fig. 9.1-19D, there are two peaks of estrogen secretion. The first occurs just before the ovulation (12–13th day of sexual cycle) and is called *estrogen surge*, and

the second peak occurs in the mid luteal phase. The secretion rate of estrogen in different phases is:

- In early follicular phase   :   36 μg/day
- Just before ovulation   :   380 μg/day
- During mid-luteal phase   :   250 μg/day.

After menopause estrogen level falls to minimum of 50 μg/day.

Functions of estrogens

The functions of estrogen for descriptive purposes can be grouped as reproductive actions and other actions.

(i) Reproductive actions

At puberty. At puberty estradiol is secreted in larger amounts which causes the following changes:

1. Growth and development of genital organs.
- *Ovaries* increase in size and complete ovarian cycles start.
- *Fallopian tubes* become functional.
- *Uterus.* It enlarges in size, endometrium gets thickened, the rhythmic cyclic changes (proliferative and secretory) occur with onset of menstrual cycle.
- *Cervix* also enlarges and with onset of menstrual cycle, endocervix undergoes cyclic changes.
- *Vagina* increases in size. Its epithelial lining increases in height (from 2–3 layer cuboidal epithelium to 10–12 layers cornified squamous epithelium).
- *External genitalia.* the following changes occur in external genitalia:
    - Increase in size of clitoris
    - Labia majora and labia minora increase in size and get widened.

2. Appearance of secondary sex characters: *Estrogen is* responsible for appearance of secondary sex characters:
- *In an adult woman.* Estrogens along with progesterone regulate the ovarian cycle, menstrual cycle and cyclic changes in cervix, vagina and fallopian tubes in non-pregnant state.
    - It plays an important role in the maintenance of pregnancy.
    - It is important for breast development.

(ii) Other actions

The other functions of estrogens include:

Effects on bones. Estradiol accelerates the linear growth of bones at puberty.

Effects on metabolism. Estrogens cause positive nitrogen balance, and fat deposition in subcutaneous tissues, in the breasts and the thighs.

Water and electrolyte balance. Estrogens, like other steroids in general, cause salt and water retention in the body and produce premenstrual tension in some women.

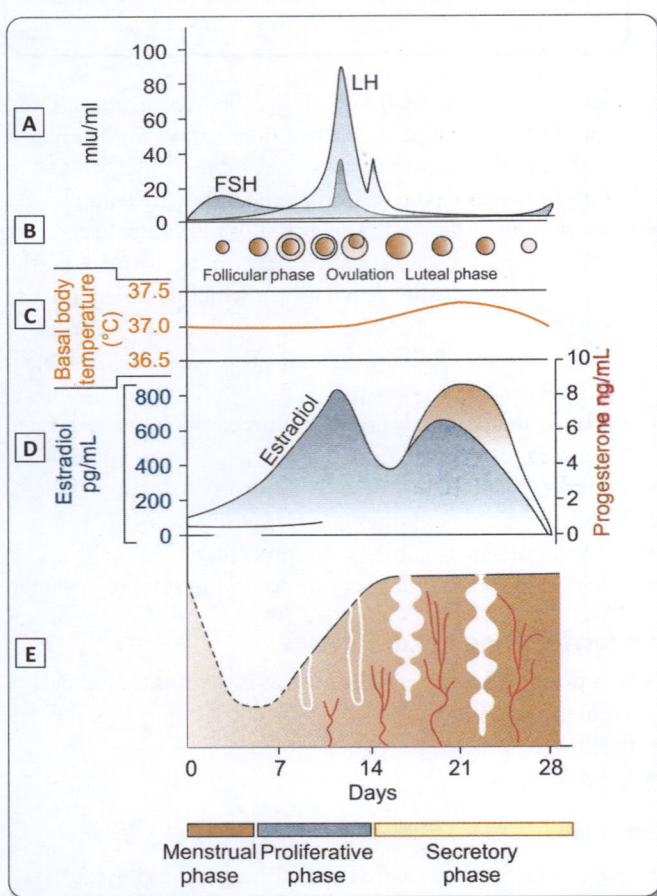

Figs 9.1-19A to E: Correlation of plasma concentration of gonadotropins (FSH and LH). A. Ovarian cycle changes; B. Basal body temperature; C. Ovarian hormones; D. Endometrial changes; E. During female sexual cycle

Effects on vasculature. In general estrogens have vasodilator and antivasoconstrictor effects.

Effects on CNS. Estrogens are responsible for estrus behavior in animals and also increase the libido in human females.

Effects on skin. Estrogens make the skin soft and more vascular. It makes the sebaceous gland secretions thin. Therefore, synthetic estrogens are used as a part of treatment in acne.

Progesterone

In a normal adult nonpregnant woman progesterone is mainly secreted by corpus luteum and during pregnancy by the placenta. A small amount is also secreted by adrenal cortex.

Plasma levels

In a normal adult woman the plasma levels of progesterone vary with different phases of sexual cycle (Fig. 9.1-19D).

Throughout the sexual cycle the levels of progesterone are higher than the estrogens.

During pregnancy the levels of progesterone further rise.

After menopause. Progesterone levels fall to its minimum (0.2 ng/mL) or even not detectable.

Functions of progesterone

The physiological actions of progesterone can be grouped as reproductive actions and other actions.

(i) Reproductive actions

Reproductive actions are mainly on the reproductive organs primed by estrogens and these include:

Action on uterus. The progesterone is responsible for secretory phase of the endometrial cycle and prepares the endometrium to receive the zygote.

- *Uterine motility:* Progesterone decreases the uterine motility.

Endocervix. The cervical secretions become thick and viscid, and ferning pattern disappears.

Vagina. Vaginal epithelium becomes thickened, cornified and infiltrated with leucocytes.

Fallopian tubes. Progesterone increases the epithelial cell secretions rich in nutritive materials to provide nutrition to shedded ovum, incoming sperm or to zygote if fertilization occurs.

Breast. Progesterone causes lobular and alveolar growth of breast.

During pregnancy the main function of progesterone is to maintain the pregnancy.

(ii) Other actions

The other systemic effects of progesterone are:

Thermogenic effect. Progesterone is known as a thermogenic steroid. It increases the basal body temperature by 0.5°C in postovulatory phase (Fig. 9.1-19C).

Effect on CNS. Progesterone alters the secretion and release of various neurotransmitters in the hypothalamus and other areas of the brain and thereby decreases the appetite, and produces *somnolence.*

Effect on respiration. Progesterone increases the sensitivity of the respiratory center to carbon dioxide stimulation. Due to this fact the partial pressure of CO_2 in arterial blood ($pACO_2$) is slightly less in women during luteal phase of sexual cycle.

Effect on fat metabolism. Progesterone (particularly C-19 progesterone) decreases the serum HDL. Thus, it acts as a proatherogenic agent.

Other ovarian hormones

Besides female sex steroids (estrogen and progesterone) ovaries also secrete peptide hormones which are:

Inhibin. It inhibits the FSH release.

Activin. Its action is to activate FSH secretion from anterior pituitary.

Relaxin is a polypeptide hormone produced by corpus luteum and other sites include uterus placenta and mammary glands and in males from the prostate gland. Its main role is during pregnancy as it relaxes pubic symphysis and pelvic joints, softens and dilates the uterine cervix and facilitates delivery.

FEMALE SEXUAL CYCLE

The sexual life-span of a female can be divided into three periods:

1. Birth to puberty. During this period primary and accessory female sex organs remain quiescent.

2. Puberty to menopause. With the onset of puberty the female sexual cycle starts, which repeats every 28 days. The occurrence of first menstrual cycle is called *menarche.* The permanent stoppage of menstrual cycle is called *menopause,* which occurs at the age of about 45–50 years. The period between menarche and menopause is called *reproductive period.* During this period females have rhythmical sexual cycles.

3. Postmenopausal period extends after menopause (45 to 50 years) to rest of the life. During this period the female sexual cycle ceases.

Female sexual cycle refers to monthly rhythmic sexual cycle occurring in females during the normal reproductive period.

Components of human female sexual cycle. During each female sexual cycle, rhythmical changes occur in ovaries and accessory sex organs—uterus, cervix and vagina.

Duration of female sexual cycle is usually 28 days. But under physiological conditions it may vary between 20 to 40 days. Traditionally, first day of the menstrual bleeding is taken as the 1st day of female sexual cycle.

Ovarian Cycle

Ovarian cycle refers to rhythmic changes occurring in ovaries during each female sexual cycle of about 28 days. During each cycle a single mature ovum is released from the ovary. The ovarian cycle can be divided into three phases:

1. Preovulatory phase or follicular phase
2. Ovulation
3. Postovulatory phase or luteal phase.

Preovulatory Phase

Preovulatory or follicular phase of the ovarian cycle extends from the 5th day of the cycle till the time of ovulation (which takes place at about 14th day of the cycle). Thus, this phase generally lasts for 8–9 days (but may vary from 10 to 25 days).

- Changes in the ovary during this phase are mostly under the influence of follicle stimulating hormone (FSH) and luteinizing hormone (LH) from the anterior pituitary.
- During this phase of each cycle, some 10–15 primordial follicles start maturing, but only one follicle matures fully and the rest undergo atresia (atrophy) at different stages of development (Fig. 9.1-19B). The process of maturation of follicle is called folliculogenesis (*see page 454*).

Ovulation

Ovulation refers to release of secondary oocyte from the ovary (following rupture of Graafian follicle) into the peritoneal cavity (Fig. 9.1-19B). It usually occurs 14 days after the onset of menstruation.

Postovulatory Phase

Postovulatory phase is also called luteal phase of ovarian cycle (about 14 days). This phase is characterized by the following events (Fig. 9.1-19B):

Formation of corpus luteum. The following ovulation, the outer wall of the Graafian follicle collapses and promptly fills with blood forming the so called corpus hemeorrhagicum. Soon, the granulosa cells and theca cells of the follicle lining begin to proliferate, and the clotted blood is rapidly replaced with yellowish lipid-rich *luteal cells.* This process is called *luteinization* and the total mass of the cells is now called *corpus luteum.* LH is responsible for luteinization.

Formation of corpus albicans. If no fertilization and pregnancy occur, the corpus luteum begins to involute (regress) after 24th day of the sexual cycle and is eventually replaced by a whitish scar tissue, called the corpus albicans.

Corpus luteum of pregnancy. However, if the ovum released is fertilized and pregnancy occurs, then the corpus luteum formed during postovulatory phase persists and serves as the major source of estrogen and progesterone till the 3rd month of pregnancy when the placenta takes over its endocrine function.

Endometrial Cycle

Endometrial cycle refers to the cyclic changes occurring in the endometrium during active reproductive period (menarche to menopause) in females leading to recurrent monthly bleeding per vaginum (menstruation). These cyclic changes in the endometrium are brought about by the cyclic production of estrogens and progesterone by the ovaries.

The endometrial cycle of 28 days can be divided into three phases (Fig. 9.1-19E):

1. Menstrual phase (1st–5th day)
2. Proliferative phase (6th–14th day)
3. Secretory phase (15th–28th day).

For the purpose of better understanding, the menstrual phase is described after proliferative and secretory phases.

Proliferative Phase

Extent of proliferative phase of endometrial cycle is from day 6th–14th day. It follows the phase of menstruation, after which only a thin basal layer of original endometrium is left.

Hormone responsible for changes in the endometrium during this phase is estrogen secreted by the developing graafian follicle in the ovary. The proliferative phase of endometrial cycle coincides with the follicular phase of ovarian cycle.

Changes in endometrium, which occur during proliferative phase, are (Histology plate 9.1-3):

- Thickness of endometrium, which is <1 mm at the end of menstrual phase, increases to 3–4 mm at the end of the proliferative phase.

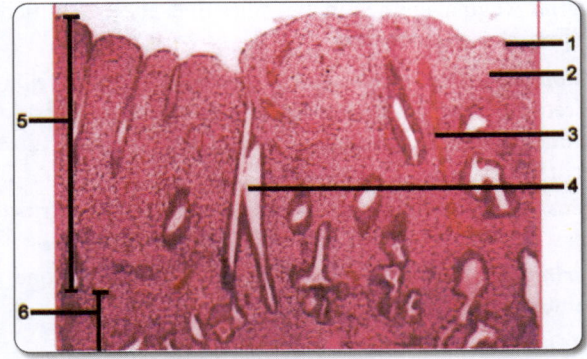

Histology Plate 9.1-3: Endometrium Proliferative Phase

Photomicrograph of proliferative phase of endometrium is shown showing straight uterine glands (4) with a narrow lumen. Simple columnar epithelium (1), lamina propria (2), coiled artery (3) functionalis layer (5) and basalis layer (6) are also seen.

- Angiogenesis in the stratum functionale leads to proliferation of blood vessels which become the spiral arterioles that profuse the stratum functionale.
- Endometrial glands are stimulated to grow. The glands contain glycogen but they are nonsecretory.

Secretory Phase

Extent of secretory phase (also known as postovulatory phase of endometrial cycle) is from day 15th to 28th day.

Hormones responsible for changes in the endometrium during this phase are both estrogen and progesterone secreted by the *corpus luteum* formed after ovulation. Thus, the secretory phase of endometrial cycle coincides with the luteal phase of ovarian cycle.

Changes in the endometrium, which occur during this phase, are:

Elongation and coiling of endometrial mucous glands. These glands become prominent corkscrew-shaped secretory and secrete thick viscous fluid containing glycogen.

Blood supply of endometrium further increases as progesterone promotes spiraling of blood vessels.

Thickness of endometrium increases to 5–6 mm at the end of secretory phase. Thus the thickened endometrium with large amounts of nutrients is ready to provide appropriate conditions for implantation of ovum during this phase.

If fertilization does not occur and there is no pregnancy, the corpus luteum in the ovary involutes to form corpus albicans and on day 26th of the menstrual cycle the levels of estrogen and progesterone fall suddenly and mark the end of secretory phase of endometrial cycle.

Menstrual Phase

The menstrual phase of endometrial cycle is also called bleeding phase. The average duration of this phase is 3–5 days. About 24 hours before the end of menstrual cycle, there is sharp decline in the plasma levels of estrogen and progesterone, which is responsible for menstrual bleeding. During menstrual phase about 2/3rd of the superficial endometrium is sloughed off and only a thin basal layer (2 mm thick) is left behind.

- *Average amount of blood loss during each* menstrual cycle is 30 mL.
- *Menstrual blood immediately gets clotted inside the uterine cavity but soon gets liquefied* by fibrolysins present in endometrial debris.
- *Endometrial debris* contains necrosed sloughed off tissue, blood, serous fluid and a large amount of prostaglandins and fibrolysins.

Cyclic Changes in Cervix

The mucosal lining of cervix (endocervix) also shows certain cyclic changes during sexual cycle. These are:

During menstruation phase the mucosa of cervix does not undergo desquamation (shedding off) like that of endometrium.

During proliferative phase (estrogen phase) the secretions of the mucosal cells of endocervix become thin, watery and alkaline. At the time of ovulation, the cervical mucus is thinnest and its elasticity is maximum. It can be stretched like a long, thin elastic thread up to 8–12 cm (spinnbarkeit effect). The mucus also produces a characteristic fern-like pattern when a drop of mucus is spread on the glass slide and allowed to dry (*Fern test*) (Fig. 9.1-20A).

This characteristic nature of cervical mucus favors the transport of sperms in the female genital tract and makes the conditions favorable for fertilization.

During secretory phase, under the influence of progesterone, cervical secretions decrease in quantity and become thick, tenacious and cellular, and fern pattern is not seen (Fig. 9.1-20B). These changes make a plug and prevent the entry of sperm through cervical canal.

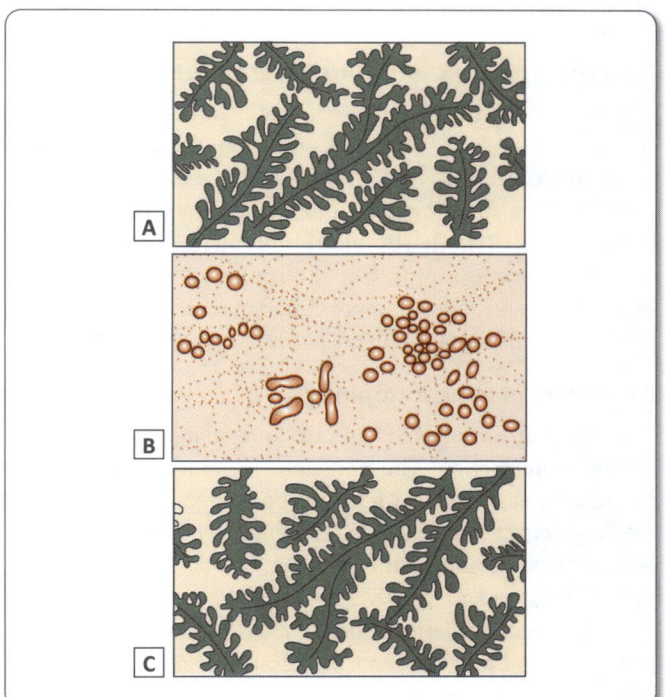

Figs 9.1-20A to C: Characteristics of cervical mucus as seen on smear examination during various phases of normal menstrual cycle. A. On 14th day (typical fern pattern); B. On 21st day (fern pattern disappears); C. 1st day of an anovulatory cycle (fern pattern persists)

Fern test: The fern pattern of cervical mucus in proliferative phase and its disappearance in secretory phase is indicative of ovulatory cycle, whereas persistence of fern pattern throughout the cycle indicates anovulatory cycle (Fig. 9.1-20C).

Cyclic Changes in Vagina

In proliferative phase, vaginal epithelium becomes thickened (by adding up more and more layers of epithelium) and cornified.

In secretory phase, under the influence of progesterone, vaginal epithelium proliferates and gets infiltrated with leucocytes and the vaginal secretions become thick and viscid.

Other Changes during Sexual Cycle

Hormonal oscillations during sexual cycle though mainly affect ovaries, uterus, cervix and vagina, some changes have also been observed in the fallopian tubes, breast and in the body weight.

Hormonal Control of Female Sexual Cycle

The hypothalamo-hypophyseal-gonadal axis regulates the cyclic changes occurring during female sexual cycle. The role of each component of the axis is (Fig. 9.1-21):

Role of Hypothalamus and Anterior Pituitary

Hypothalamus regulates the secretions of gonadotropins (both FSH and LH) through the gonadotropin releasing hormone (GnRH). The gonadotropin releasing hormone (GnRH) is also known as luteinizing hormone releasing hormone (LHRH). It stimulates the anterior pituitary cells to release gonadotropins. Gonadotropins in turn regulate the ovarian cycle, i.e., formation of Graafian follicles (folliculosis), ovulation and formation of corpus luteum.

Regulation of gonadotropins

The secretion of both FSH and LH is regulated by:

Gonadal hormones. The gonadal hormones (estrogen and progesterone) regulate gonadotropin secretion by their feedback effect (Fig. 9.1-21). Depending on relative plasma level of these hormones the effect may be positive or negative, or both positive and negative.

The feedback effect (positive or negative) of ovarian hormones is brought about by its action either directly on anterior pituitary or through the hypothalamus (Fig. 9.1-21).

Oral contraceptives are the preparations containing high concentration of estrogen and progesterone. These drugs inhibit gonadotropin release by negative feedback effect and prevent ovulation.

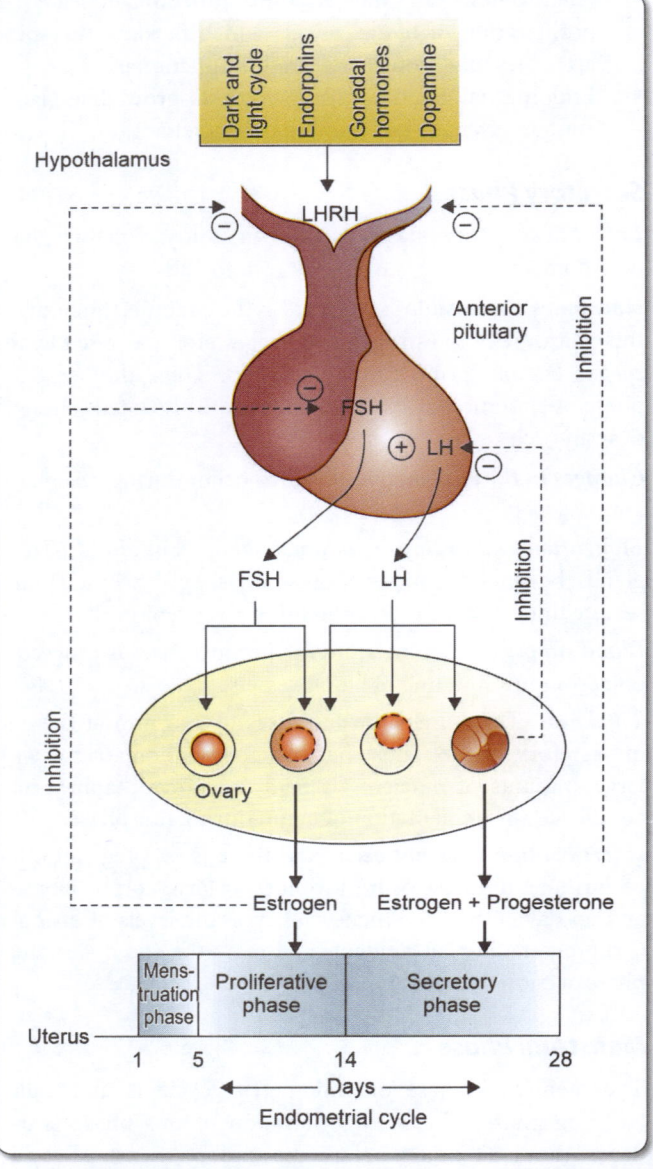

Fig. 9.1-21: Hypothalamo-hypophyseal-ovarian axis regulating the female sexual cycle through positive and negative feedback mechanisms

Abbreviations: LHRH, luteinizing hormone releasing hormone; FSH, follicle stimulating hormone; LH, luteinizing hormone

Prolactin. It is a mammotropic hormone secreted from anterior pituitary during lactation. It inhibits GnRh release and thus lowers the basal secretion of FSH and LH (cause for lactation amenorrhea).

Activin. It is structurally quite similar to inhibin (secreted from ovary). It is synthesized in the cells of anterior pituitary. It stimulates the synthesis and release of FSH by autocrine and paracrine actions.

Role of Ovaries

Ovaries play an important role in regulation of ovarian cycle and endometrial cycle by secreting gonadal hormones (estrogen and progesterone).

CLINICAL ASPECTS

ABNORMALITIES OF FEMALE SEXUAL CYCLE

The abnormalities of female sexual cycle are grouped as:
- Abnormalities of ovarian functions
- Abnormalities of menstruation.

A. Abnormalities of Ovarian Functions

Hypogonadism (hyposecretion of ovarian hormones) means less than normal secretions by the ovaries. It occurs when the ovaries are poorly developed or absent since birth or genetically become abnormal and nonfunctional. Hypogonadism results in female eunuchoidism.

Ovariectomy: When ovaries are removed surgically in a sexually mature female. It leads to the following effects:
- Atrophy of genital apparatus (i.e., uterus, vagina and external genitalia)
- *Stoppage of menstruation.*

B. Abnormalities of Menstruation

Anovulatory cycles means that menstrual cycles occur at normal intervals, but ovulation does not occur. Anovulatory cycles are the normal entity up to 1–2 years after the menarche and few years before menopause. Anovulatory cycles in the fertile period of womanhood is the main cause of female infertility.

Amenorrhea: The term amenorrhea refers to absence of menstrual bleeding or periods. It is of two types:
i. *Primary amenorrhea* means menstrual bleeding has never occurred and this condition is because of failure of sexual maturation.
ii. *Secondary amenorrhea* means cessation of menstrual cycles in a woman who previously had normal and regular cycles. Pregnancy is the most common cause of secondary amenorrhea. Other conditions which result in secondary amenorrhea are emotional disturbances, environmental changes, hypothalamic and pituitary disorders and certain systemic diseases.

Hypomenorrhea: The term refers to scanty menstruation.

Menorrhea: It refers to abnormally profuse bleeding during normal regular cycles.

Metrorrhagia: This condition refers to occurrence of uterine bleeding in-between the periods.

Oligomenorrhea means infrequent and reduced frequency of menstruation.

Dysmenorrhea is the term related to discomfort during menstruation (or painful menstruation).

Premenstrual syndrome (PMS): About 7–10 days before the end of cycle some women experience symptoms like irritability, lack of concentration, feeling of depression, heaviness, headache and constipation which is called premenstrual syndrome.

PHYSIOLOGY OF PREGNANCY

Physiology of pregnancy is mainly concerned with maternal adaptations to provide ideal atmosphere for fertilization, nutrition to the growing fetus, and safe child-birth. The physiology of pregnancy can be discussed under the following headings:
- Fertilization and implantation
- Formation of placenta and its functions
- Physiological changes during pregnancy

Fertilization and Implantation

Fertilization

Fertilization refers to fusion of male and female gametes (i.e., spermatozoon and ovum). It takes place in the middle segment (ampulla) of the fallopian tube. It involves the following events:

Transport of gametes. Before fertilization, the ovum and sperms reach the ampulla for fertilization.

Sperm capacitation. Sperm capacitation refers to the process that makes a sperm to fertilize an ovum. Sperm capacitation occurs due to removal of certain factors, which normally remain quiescent in male genital tract.

Fusion of gametes. The fusion of ovum and sperm occurs by penetration of sperm through ovum coverings due to acrosomal reaction which involves release of acrosin (protease enzyme) from anterior membrane of acrosome of the sperm. Only one sperm can enter into the oocyte, and further entry of sperms is prevented by the activation of ovum.

Implantation

Implantation of a fertilized ovum involves the following steps:

Formation of blastocyst. The fertilized ovum starts dividing immediately and is called morula (16-cell stage) and blastocyst (100-cell stage).

Transportation of blastocyst in uterine cavity. In next 3–4 days blastocyst is transported into the cavity of the uterus.

Implantation of blastocyst in the endometrium. The blastocyst then erodes and burrows into the endometrium (implantation) (Figs 9.1-22A and B). The blastocyst goes deeper and deeper into the uterus mucosa till whole of it lies within the endometrium.

Decidual reaction. After implantation the endometrium is called decidua. The stroma cells of endometrium get enlarged, become vacuolated and filled with glycogen and lipids. These cells are called decidual cells. The stored glycogen and lipids are the source of nutrition for the embryo till placenta takes up this function. Therefore this change in stroma cell is called decidual reaction.

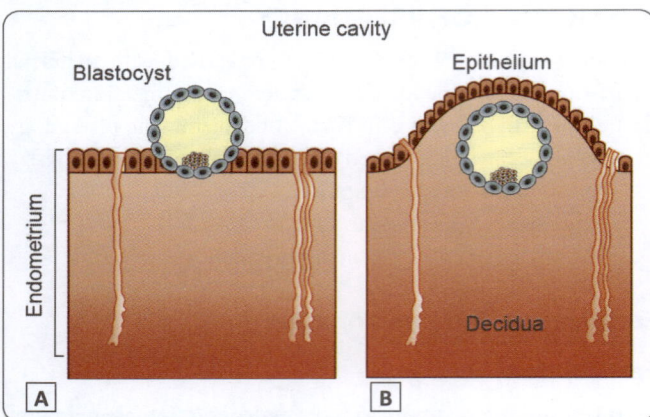

Figs 9.1-22A and B: A. Implantation of blastocyst in the endometrium; B. Decidual reaction

Placenta and Pregnancy Tests

Placenta

Placenta is a temporary organ formed during pregnancy. It is an important link between the mother and the fetus.

- When fully formed, the placenta is a disc-shaped structure, has a diameter of 15–20 cm and weighs about 500 g.
- After birth of the baby, the placenta is shed off along with the decidua.

Placental membrane

The maternal and fetal blood do not mix with each other. They are separated by a placental membrane, made up of the layers of the wall of the villus. From the fetal side these are (Fig. 9.1-23):

- Endothelium of fetal blood vessels and its basement membrane
- Surrounding mesenchymal tissue (connective tissue)
- Cytotrophoblast and its basement membrane
- Syncytiotrophoblast.

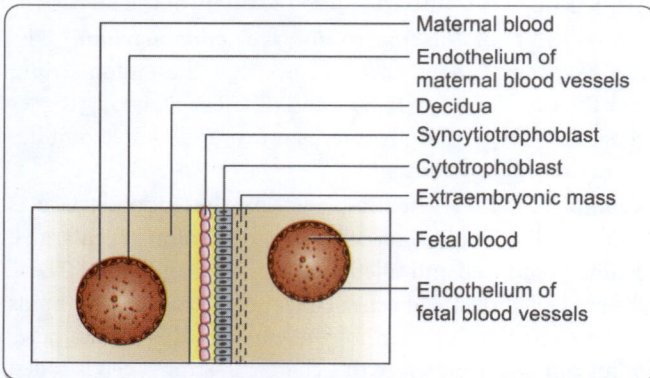

Maternal blood
Endothelium of maternal blood vessels
Decidua
Syncytiotrophoblast
Cytotrophoblast
Extraembryonic mass
Fetal blood
Endothelium of fetal blood vessels

Fig. 9.1-23: Structure of placental membrane

Functions of placenta

The fully functional placenta develops by the end of third month (12 weeks) of pregnancy. Placenta serves mainly three functions:

- Hormone secretion (endocrinal functions of placenta)
- Transport of substances between mother and fetus
- Protection of the fetus.

Hormone secretion

The syncytiotrophoblast of the placenta serves as an endocrine gland. The hormones secreted by the placenta are:

- Human chorionic gonadotropins (hCG)
- Human chorionic somatomammotropins (hCS)
- Human chorionic thyrotropin (hCT)
- Placental progesterone
- Placental estrogens
- Relaxin.

Human chorionic gonadotropins:

Human chorionic gonadotropin (hCG) is a polypeptide hormone. It is secreted by syncytiotrophoblast soon after fertilization. After fertilization it is detected in the maternal blood as early as 6–8 days after conception, and reaches its peak between 60–90 days of gestation. After this the concentration falls to a very low level and just before labor its level falls to zero. Its approximate peak value in human maternal blood during normal pregnancy is 5 mg/mL.

Physiological effects of hCG. Its actions are similar to LH of anterior pituitary hence also called second *luteotropic hormone*. It maintains the functions of the corpus luteum up to 7 weeks after conception until fetoplacental unit is able to synthesize its own estrogen and progesterone.

> **IMPORTANT TO KNOW**
>
> **Clinical Importance (Application) of hCG:**
>
> The presence of hCG in the urine forms the basis of all the pregnancy tests. hCG appears in the urine as early as 10 days after gestation with 99% accuracy.
>
> If fetus dies early then hCG disappears from the blood as well as from the urine.

Human chorionic somatomammotropin:

The syncytiotrophoblast cells of placenta also secrete a large amount of human chorionic somatomammotropin. It functions as maternal growth hormone of pregnancy, causes deposition of protein in the tissues, and brings about nitrogen, calcium and potassium retention.

Human chorionic thyrotropin:

The physiological role of this substance is not very clear.

Placental progesterone:

Plasma concentration. During pregnancy plasma concentration of progesterone rises steadily throughout gestation reaching a maximum plateau at 30–40 weeks of gestation. Just before the onset of labor its level decreases.

Physiological effects of placental progesterone include:

- It helps to preserve the pregnancy by promoting the growth of endometrium. It converts secretory endometrium of luteal phase of menstrual cycle to decidua during pregnancy.
- Progesterone has a marked inhibitory effect on the contractions of uterus.
- It causes development of alveolar system of mother's breast.

Placental estrogens:

Plasma concentration. Like progesterone, plasma estrogen (estriol) concentration rises throughout the gestation. Its peak value (14 ng/mL) and secretory curve parallels that of progesterone and maximum *plateau* is reached at 30–40 weeks of gestation.

The plasma concentration of estriol reflects the functional status of fetoplacental maternal unit activity.

Physiological effects of estrogen include:

- It causes growth and development of maternal reproductive organs. Uterus increases in size—weight, length and volume—both by hypertrophy and stretching of myometrium).
- Estrogen stimulates development of lactiferous ductal system in mammary glands.
- Just before term, estrogen to progesterone ratio increases and uterus is dominated by estrogen.

Other placental hormones:

A number of other substances which are secreted from placenta are:

- Corticotropin releasing hormone (CRH)
- β endorphins
- α MSH.

Transport of substances between the mother and the fetus

Transport of nutrients. The nutritive materials which are transported from mother's blood into the fetus are glucose, fats, amino acids, calcium and inorganic phosphates, potassium, sodium and chloride ions. Substances with molecular weight <1000 can cross readily by simple diffusion.

Excretion of waste products through placenta. Excretory products, especially urea, uric acid and creatinines, etc., formed in the fetus are transported into the mother's blood and then excreted by mother's kidneys. Thus placenta also acts as fetal kidney.

Diffusion of respiratory gases:

Oxygen transport. Dissolved oxygen from the maternal sinuses of placenta diffuses into the fetal blood.

Transport of CO_2. CO_2 from fetus is eliminated only through placenta. Thus placenta acts as fetal lungs.

Transport of antibodies. Maternal immunoglobulins are transferred into the fetus and are responsible for innate immunity.

Rh agglutinins are easily transported as compared to ABO agglutinins; that is why the effects of Rh incompatibility are more severe.

Transport of harmful substances. Certain viruses and many drugs (like nicotine and barbiturates) can easily cross the placental barrier and may produce harmful effect on the fetus. Therefore, as far as possible one should avoid these drugs and smoking during pregnancy.

Protection of the fetus

Placenta protects the fetus in many ways:

- It acts as a barrier for certain harmful substances
- It provides nutrition to the fetus
- Its hormonal secretion is responsible for proper growth of the fetus
- Placental progesterone decreases uterine contractions and thus protects the fetus from being expelled.

Pregnancy Tests

In an adult healthy woman amenorrhea is the first sign of pregnancy, but it occurs in many other conditions as well. Therefore, detection of early pregnancy is made possible by certain pregnancy tests. The pregnancy detection tests are based on presence of hCG in the urine of pregnant lady.

NURSING IMPLICATIONS AND APPLICATIONS

Gravindex test: Immunological pregnancy tests are based on the antigenic properties of HCG. The kit for this test consists of:

- Gravindex antigen (latex particles coated with HCG).
- Gravindex antibodies (serum containing antibodies against HCG) and a dark colored slide.

Procedure: This test is performed on the control and test samples of urine.

- Control sample. A drop of urine sample from non-pregnant subject (containing no HCG) is mixed with a drop of antiserum containing HCG antibodies.
- Then it is mixed with HCG-coated latex particles. There will be agglutination because urine of non-pregnant subject does not contain antigen; therefore, antibodies are not neutralized. Thus, occurrence of agglutination indicates no pregnancy or pregnancy test is negative.
- Test sample. A drop of urine of suspected pregnant lady (containing HCG) is mixed with a drop of antiserum (containing HCG antibodies). Then it is mixed with HCG-coated latex particles. There will be no agglutination because antibodies have been neutralized by the HCG present in the urine.
- Therefore, occurrence of no agglutination means positive pregnancy test.

Physiological Changes in Mother during Pregnancy

The normal average duration of pregnancy in human beings is 280 days (40 weeks) and is calculated from the first day of the last menstrual period, or 256–270 days from the time of ovulation. As the pregnancy progresses, various types of extra demands are imposed on the mother's body by the growing fetus, which are met with by certain adaptations in almost all the organ systems of the body. These physiological changes include:

Changes in Genital Organs

- To accommodate the growing fetus marked increase in the size of uterus takes place.
- Endocervix gets hypertrophied.
- Mammary glands show hyperplasia of ductal and alveolar tissue. The areola becomes pigmented and many sebaceous glands become prominent in the areola. Nipples also become larger and pigmented.

Weight Gain

A woman may gain total of 10–12 kg of weight during normal pregnancy, which is contributed by:
Fetus: 3 kg
Placenta and amniotic fluid: 1.5 kg
Uterus and breast enlargement: 1.0 kg
Increase in blood volume and interstitial fluid: 1.5 kg
Fat deposition: 3.5–4 kg.

PHYSIOLOGY OF PARTURITION

Parturition is the process by which baby is born. It may occur any time between 37th and 40th weeks of gestation. The uterine myometrium and cervix play an important role for this process.

Mechanics of Parturition

From the functional point of view mechanics of parturition mainly involves:
- Uterine contractions
- Cervical dilatation.

Uterine Contractions

The uterus, which remains quiescent during period of pregnancy, becomes progressively more and more excitable toward the end of pregnancy, until finally it begins strong rhythmical contractions with such a force that expel the fetus.

Control or regulation of uterine contractility

The exact cause of increased uterine activity is not known. It is attributed to increased myometrial excitability to oxytocin near term which occurs due to an increase in number of oxytocin receptors on the cells of the uterine smooth muscle during the final weeks of pregnancy and increased synthesis of contractile proteins in the myometrial cells.

Cervical Dilatation

Throughout pregnancy cervix remains as a rigid structure, but at the time of parturition certain structural and biochemical changes occur and the cervix becomes soft. This is known as *cervical ripening.* It allows the cervix to stretch when uterine contractions start.

Control of Parturition

The mechanisms responsible for onset of labor in human are still not understood exactly. The control of parturition includes the role of:
- Hormonal factors
- Mechanical factors.

Hormonal Factors

The hormonal changes that initiate the parturition and that cause increased excitability of uterine musculature are:

Activation of fetal hypothalamic-pituitary-adrenal axis. Resulting in an increase in ACTH secretion few days before parturition. ACTH causes fetal adrenal cortex to secrete a large amount of androgens.

The above changes lead to an altered estrogen-progesterone ratio.

Role of altered estrogen-progesterone ratio. The altered estrogen-progesterone ratio causes:
- An increase in release of oxytocin from maternal posterior pituitary
- An increase in number of oxytocin receptors in myometrium
- An increase in prostaglandin synthesis
- An increase in synthesis of myometrial contractile proteins.

Mechanical Factors

Mechanical factors that increase the contractility of uterus include:
Stretch of uterine musculature. As the pregnancy advances with growing fetus stretch increases leading to uterine contractility.

Positive feedback effect. Stretching and irritation of cervix is particularly important because of positive feedback effect through initiation of the reflex increase in uterine contractility. The positive feedback mechanism continues until the baby is expelled.

Role of Ferguson reflex. Once labor is started, the uterine contractions dilate the ripened cervix. The cervical dilatation in turn sets off signals in afferent nerves that increase oxytocin secretion from the posterior pituitary. This is called Ferguson reflex.

ANATOMY OF BREAST AND PHYSIOLOGY OF LACTATION

Anatomy of Breast

Breastfeeding is the characteristic feature of all the mammals, including human beings. It has evolved as the best method of nourishing the newborn. The mammary glands (the secondary sex organs) play an important role in lactation process.

Mammary glands are present in both the sexes; in males they remain rudimentary. In the female the breasts are small and immature and remain quiescent till puberty. At thelarche, i.e., at the time of puberty (9–11 years of age), before the start of menses, the breasts start developing and get enlarged. Thereafter, after the onset of menses (menarche) they grow and develop to their mature size under the influence of estrogen and progesterone.

Gross Appearance

The fully developed breast is a soft, rounded, elevated structure having central dark pigmented area (areola). The central part of areola, projected above the surface, is called nipple. The nipple is perforated at the tip by 15–20 minute openings of the lactiferous ducts.

Location and extent

Each breast covers nearly circular space anterior to the pectoralis muscles extending from the second to sixth ribs and from the sternum into the axilla.

Histological Structure

Each mammary gland is covered by overlying skin. Deep to skin the entire breast tissue lies in the superficial fascia (i.e., between skin and the deep fascia). The breast tissue consists of discrete masses of glandular tissue present in the connective tissue consisting of stroma and adipose tissue (Fig. 9.1-24 and Histology Plate 9.1-4).

The mammary glands consist of 15–20 lobes and each lobe has a number of lobules.

The glandular tissue mainly consists of alveoli having secretory cells.

The secretions from these cells are poured by apocrine manner and by exocytosis into the ducts (lactiferous ducts). About 15–20 ducts open at the summit of nipple, and just before opening lactiferous ducts show a dilatation called lactiferous sinus.

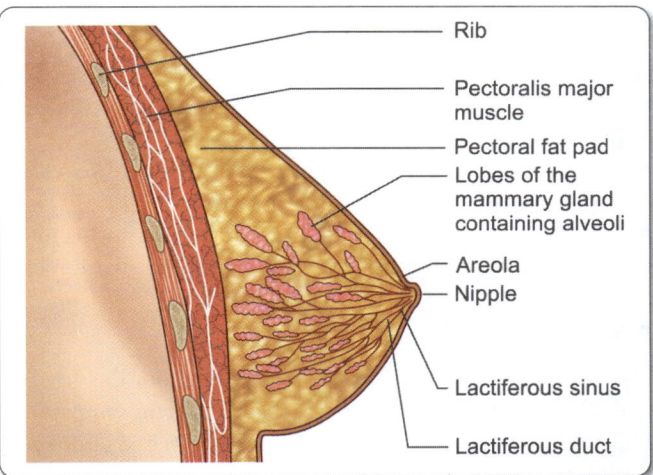

Fig. 9.1-24: Structure of mammary gland (breast)

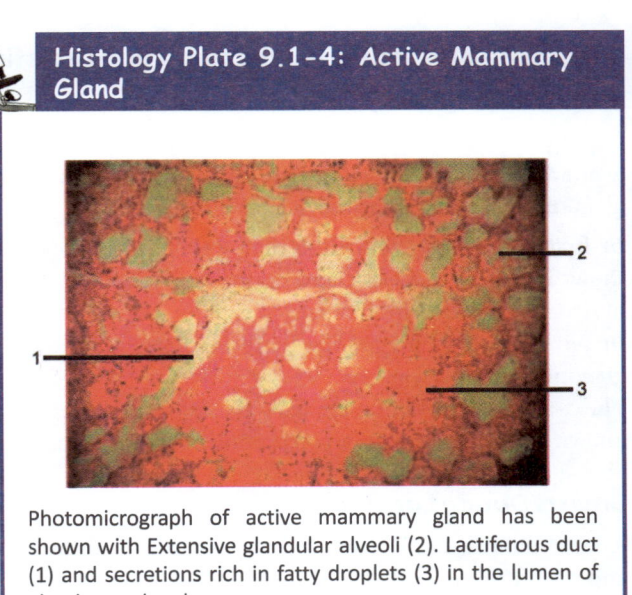

Histology Plate 9.1-4: Active Mammary Gland

Photomicrograph of active mammary gland has been shown with Extensive glandular alveoli (2). Lactiferous duct (1) and secretions rich in fatty droplets (3) in the lumen of glands are also shown.

Around the alveoli, ductules and lobules are present myoepithelial cells. They squeeze the contents and pour their secretions into the ductules.

Blood Supply, Lymphatic Drainage and Nerve Supply to the Breasts

Blood Supply

Arterial blood supply is by perforating branches of the internal thoracic artery and thoracic branches of axillary artery and intercostal arteries.

Venous drainage is along the veins corresponding to the arteries supplying the breasts.

Lymphatic Drainage

An understanding of the lymphatic drainage of the breast is of the greatest importance in relation to the malignant condition of the breast.

- Most of the lymphatics from the breast drain into *axillary lymph nodes.*
- Some lymphatics also drain into parasternal nodes, intercostal nodes, infraclavicular and supraclavicular nodes.

Nerve Supply

The nerve supply to the breasts is derived from the 4th, 5th and 6th thoracic spinal nerves which also contain sympathetic fibers. There are numerous somatic sensory nerve endings in the breasts, especially around the nipples. Touch receptors present in the areola region play role in suckling reflex during lactation period.

Changes in Breast during Pregnancy and Lactation

Breasts in Pregnancy

During pregnancy remarkable growth of both ductal and glandular systems occurs. It is only during first pregnancy that glandular tissue develops fully.

In first half of pregnancy the duct system proliferates and shows extensive sprouting and branching along with growth of stroma and deposition of fat.

In second half of pregnancy there is enormous growth of glandular tissue.

The extensive growth of mammary glands during pregnancy is known as *mammogenesis* or preparation of breast for lactation.

Breasts During Lactation

After childbirth the alveolar cells get enlarged and distended and start forming milk (lactogenesis).

Involution of breast. After a normal period of lactation (7–9 months), the alveolar epithelium undergoes apoptosis and glands revert to the prepregnant stage.

Control of Breast Development and Growth

Various hormones necessary for full growth and development of mammary glands at various stages are:

Estrogen. It is primarily responsible for ductal growth and fat deposition. It also causes thickening of nipples.

Progesterone. The development of glandular tissue mainly depends on progesterone. Both estrogen and progesterone work best with cooperation of hypo-thalamo-pituitary-adrenal cortex axis.

Other hormones including growth hormone, thyroxine, cortisol and insulin enhance overall growth and development of mammary glands at all stages.

Corpus luteal and placental hormones, particularly estrogen, progesterone, human chorionic somato-mammotropic hormone (HCS or HPL), are essential for further growth of breast during pregnancy.

Prolactin. It is another very important hormone for development of breasts during pregnancy and lactation. It acts on mammary gland tissue which has already grown under the influence of estrogen and progesterone.

Human Prolactin

Human prolactin is secreted by acidophilic cells of anterior pituitary gland. During pregnancy prolactin secretion starts rising from 8th weeks onward and peak value (200–400 ng/mL) is reached at term. The sources of prolactin during pregnancy are placenta, amniotic fluid and maternal anterior pituitary gland.

Physiological effects of prolactin

Breast growth. During pregnancy it increases the breast growth particularly of alveolar tissue in the form of alveolar distension, dilatation of mammary vessels, and formation of new capillaries.

Lactogenic effect. Prolactin acts on the alveolar epithelium and stimulates the secretory activity.

Suppression of ovarian cycle in nursing mothers. Prolactin inhibits the secretion of gonadotropin releasing hormone (GnRH) from hypothalamus. Therefore, gonadotropin (FSH and LH) secretion from anterior pituitary also decreases. Thus in nursing mothers due to low levels of gonadotropins the ovarian cyclic changes do not occur.

Physiology of Lactation

The physiology of lactation can be divided into four phases:
1. Preparation of breast for milk secretion (mammogenesis)
2. Synthesis and secretion of milk (lactogenesis)
3. Expulsion of milk (galactokinesis)
4. Maintenance of lactation (galactopoiesis).

Mammogenesis

During pregnancy. The breast develops fully and is prepared for milk secretion after delivery.

Lactogenesis

It is the initiation of lactation after childbirth. Immediately after the baby is born, sudden loss of estrogen and progesterone secretion by the placenta allows the lactogenic effect of prolactin.

Human Milk

Types of human milk

The nature and composition varies with postpartum period. Therefore, the human milk is of three types:
1. *Colostrum* is deep yellow-colored fluid secreted by the mammary glands during first few days of postpartum period.
2. *Transition milk or intermediate milk.* It is secreted from 6th day to 15th day of postpatrum period. The nature and composition of the secretion changes from colostrum to mature milk. Hence it is called transition milk.
3. *Mature milk* is formed from 15th day of postpartum onwards and continues during the whole lactation period (7–9 months).

Composition of human milk

Human milk contains 88.5% water and about 11.5% solids. The solids include both organic and inorganic constituents (Table. 9.1-4).

NURSING IMPLICATIONS AND APPLICATIONS

Human milk is a balanced diet as it contains first class proteins (caseinogen and lactalbumin), carbohydrates, fat, mineral salts and vitamins. Therefore, it is an ideal food for the baby. Therefore, the nurse should encourage the mothers for breast feeding and also guide them to take precautions while feeding the baby.

Expulsion of Milk or Galactokinesis

Though milk is secreted continuously into the alveoli of the breast, it does not flow continuously from alveoli into the duct

TABLE 9.1-4: Composition of colostrum, mature milk and cow's milk

Content/100 mL	Human colostrum	Human milk	Cow's milk
Water (g)	...	88	88
Lactose (g)	5.3	6.8	5.0
Proteins (g)	2.7	1.2	3.3
Fat (g)	2.9	3.8	3.1
Linoleic acid	...	8.3% of fat	1.65 of fat
Sodium (mg)	92	15	58
Postassium (mg)	55	55	1358
Chloride (mg)	117	43	103
Calcium (mg)	31	33	125
Magnesium (mg)	4	4	12
Phosphorus (mg)	14	15	100
Vitamin A (µg)	89	53	34
Thiamine (µg)	15	16	42
Riboflavin (µg)	30	43	157
Nicotinic acid (µg)	75	172	85
Ascorbic acid (mg)	4.4	4.3	1.6

system. It depends upon the suckling reflex and some local mechanisms acting within the breast.

Suckling reflex

It is a neuroendocrinal reflex. The characteristic features and mechanism of suckling reflex (Fig. 9.1-25) are:
- When baby suckles, the sensory nerve endings or receptors located in skin of areola and nipple get stimulated.
- The sensory impulses are transmitted to the hypothalamus through somatic nerves (from nipple and areola to spinal cord and then to hypothalamus). The activation of hypothalamus causes release of oxytocin and prolactin from pituitary gland.
- The oxytocin is carried to the breasts through blood, where it causes contraction of myoepithelial cells that surround the outer wall of the alveoli, thereby the milk is expressed from alveoli into the ducts. This process is called *milk ejection* or *milk expulsion* or *milk let down.*
- Another important observation is that suckling of one breast causes milk flow in the other breast also.
- Even stimuli such as sight, sound or crying of infant and thought of their infants also cause milk ejection, indicating the psychological component in the neuroendocrine reflex.

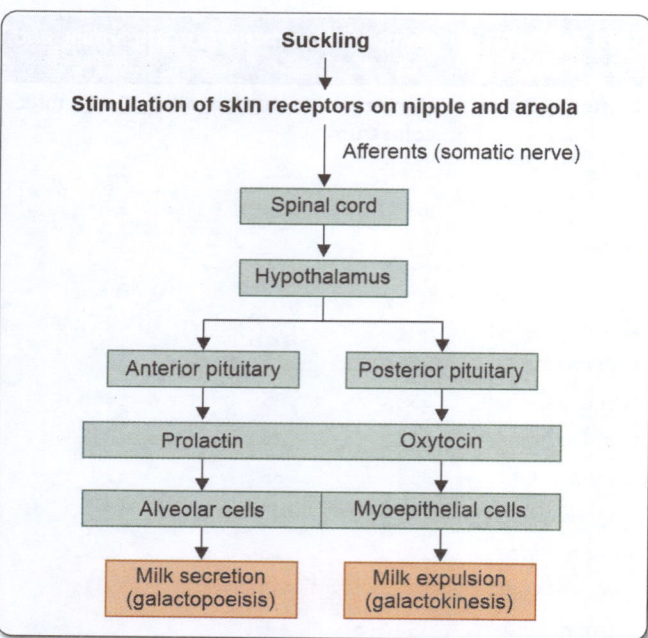

Fig. 9.1-25: Mechanism of suckling reflex

Maintenance of Milk Secretion or Galactopoiesis

Maintenance of milk secretion or galactopoiesis depends upon the surge in prolactin secretion. After few weeks of childbirth, prolactin level falls to its basal value, however, in nursing mothers neuroendocrine reflex causes 10–20 fold surge in prolactin secretion, that lasts for one hour. Each time when baby suckles, the impulses from nipple and areolar receptors are transmitted by somatic nerves up to the hypothalamus, which cause 1–20 fold surge in prolactin secretion.

The amount of milk production is related to infant's demand.

Importance of Lactation

Breastfeeding is being advocated all over the world because of its advantages both for the baby as well as for the mother.

Advantages of Breastfeeding to the Baby

Balanced diet. Human milk contains proteins, carbohydrates, fat, mineral salts (calcium and phosphorus) and vitamins. So, it is a natural balanced food for the newborn.

Protection against infections. Human milk has high count of lymphocytes, neutrophils and macrophages and high content of lysozymes and immunoglobulins. All these substances due to anti-infection property confer nonspecific as well as specific immunity.

Easily digestible. Human milk because of its digestive properties can be easily digested by the newborn babies.

Growth factors. Growth promoting factors, like epidermal growth factor, insulin and somatomedin-C, are present in the human milk.

Other advantages of breastfeeding to baby are:
- It is sterile, convenient to give at right temperature. It is inexpensive, and chances of allergy to breast milk are rare.

Advantages of Breastfeeding to the Mother

Lactational amenorrhea. Due to high plasma level of prolactin during lactation, there occurs suppression of FSH and LH. Therefore, after birth of the baby menstruation and ovulation do not start. The period of lactational amenorrhea is variable (3 months to 3 years). This is the natural way of contraception and birth spacing.

Involution of uterus. The oxytocin released during each session of breastfeeding also acts on the uterine myometrium, and helps it to involute during postpartum period. The proper involution of uterus protects it against infections.

Protection against breast engorgement. Breastfeeding does not allow the milk to stagnate, thus preventing the breast engorgement, which is a highly painful condition.

Protection against obesity. Body fat is used for milk synthesis, therefore, there are less chances of becoming obese after pregnancy.

Emotional bonding and psychological satisfaction is enhanced by breastfeeding.

Protection against cancer. Prolonged lactation provides protection against breast cancer.

NURSING IMPLICATIONS AND APPLICATIONS

Breast cancer is very common in females. The common signs and symptoms are:
- Blood stained discharge from the nipple
- Lump in the breast fixed to underlying tissue
- Retraction of overlying skin and nipple
- The skin becomes like an orange peel (Peau D' Orange)
- Enlargement of axillary lymph nodes

Early detection of breast cancer greatly increases the success rate of the treatment. A nurse should know how to palpate the breast for any lump.

Mammography is radiography of soft tissue for early detection of breast cancer. Therefore, regular mammography is advised to the women after the age of 50 years or even earlier.

ASSESS YOURSELF

Short and Long Answer Questions

1. **Describe briefly:**
   - Sex determination and sex differentiation.
   - Puberty, stages of puberty and control of onset of puberty.
   - Process of spermatogenesis and its control
   - Endocrinal functions of testes
   - Ovarian and endometrial changes during female sexual cycle
   - Hormonal control of female sexual cycle
   - Process of fertilization and implantation
   - Functions of placenta
   - Physiological changes in mother during pregnancy
   - Phases of lactation

2. **Write short notes on:**
   - Turner syndrome
   - Precocious puberty
   - Delayed puberty
   - Sertoli cells
   - Semen
   - Functions of prostate
   - Sperm capacitation
   - Blood–testis barrier
   - Cryptorchidism
   - Testosterone
   - Functions of estrogen
   - Functions of progesterone
   - Corpus luteum
   - Gonadotropins
   - Human chorionic gonadotropin
   - Immunological test of pregnancy
   - Placental membrane
   - Suckling reflex
   - Lactational amenorrhea

Multiple Choice Questions

1. **True about human chromosomes:**
   a. The female possesses 44 + XX
   b. The female possesses 44 + XY
   c. The male possesses 44 + XX
   d. The gametes possesses 22autosomes and 2 sex chromosomes

2. **In male embryo, testicular differentiation depends on:**
   a. XX chromosomes
   b. Sex determining factor
   c. Absence of Y chromosome
   d. SRY gene

3. **Differentiation of female internal genitalia depends on:**
   a. Absence of Mullerian ducts
   b. Presence of wolffian ducts
   c. Presence of Mullerian inhibitory substance
   d. Genetically embryo having 44+XX Chromosomes

4. **The true statement regarding epididymis:**
   a. In it sperms remain viable about a month
   b. Acts as secondary storehouse for sperms
   c. It is the largest accessory gland of male reproductive system
   d. Secretes thin milky fluid

5. **The statement not true for prostate is:**
   a. Its secretion constitutes 30% of the semen
   b. Acts as secondary storehouse for sperms
   c. Largest accessory gland of male reproductive system
   d. Its secretion increases the sperm motility

6. **Leydig cells are present in which of the following:**
   a. Epithelial layer of seminiferous tubules
   b. Lateral sides of sertoli cells
   c. Interstitial compartment of seminiferous tubules
   d. Scattered between the spermatogenic cells

7. **The sperms become motile in the:**
   a. Testis
   b. Epididymis
   c. Seminal vesicles
   d. Ejaculatory duct

8. **Which is not the function of testosterone:**
   a. Descent of testis
   b. Hair growth
   c. Stimulates erythropoiesis
   d. Increases sensitivity of respiratory center to CO_2

9. **The most important function of sertoli cells is:**
   a. Secretes testosterone
   b. Site for formation of sperms
   c. Maintains blood testes barrier
   d. Secretes enzyme hyaluronidase

10. **The milky appearance of semen is due to the secretion of:**
    a. Prostate gland
    b. Seminal vesicles
    c. Bulbourethral glands
    d. Sertoli cells

11. **The broad ligament extends from:**
    a. Lateral border of uterus to fallopian tubes
    b. Lateral border of uterus to labia majora
    c. Cervix to side of rectum
    d. Side of uterus to floor of pelvis

12. **Fertilization occurs in which part of the fallopian tube:**
    a. Infundibulum
    b. Isthmus
    c. Ampulla
    d. Interstitial part

13. **During oogenesis in which stage the number of chromosomes is 22 + X:**
    a. Primordial follicle
    b. Primary follicle
    c. Secondary follicle
    d. Graafian follicle

14. **Estrogen is secreted by:**
    a. Primary oocyte
    b. Theca interna cells
    c. Theca externa cells
    d. Zona pellucida

15. **The hormone that decreases Uterine motility is:**
    a. Estrogen
    b. Progesterone
    c. Inhibin
    d. Relaxin

16. **During which phase of menstrual cycle the cervical secretions become thin and watery:**
    a. Secretory phase
    b. Premenstrual phase
    c. Proliferative phase
    d. Pre-ovulatory phase

17. **The fern pattern of cervical secretion disappear due to:**
    a. Increased level of estrogen
    b. Decreased level of estrogen
    c. Increased level of progesterone
    d. Decreased level of progesterone

18. **Occurrence of bleeding in-between the periods is referred to as:**
    a. Dysmenorrhea
    b. Amenorrhea
    c. Metrorrhagia
    d. Menorrhea

19. **Gravindex pregnancy test is based on which hormone:**
    a. Human chorionic somatomammotropin
    b. Human chorionic gonadotropin
    c. Human chorionic thyrotropin
    d. Prolactin

20. **The action of oxytocin during lactation on breast is:**
    a. Mammogenesis
    b. Lactogenesis
    c. Galactokinesis
    d. Galactopoiesis

ANSWER KEY

1. a	2. d	3. d	4. a	5. b	6. c	7. b	8. d
9. c	10. a	11. d	12. c	13. c	14. b	15. b	16. d
17. c	18. c	19. b	20. c				

Contraception

INTRODUCTION

AIMS OF CONTRACEPTION

Contraception refers to prevention of pregnancy. The aims of contraception are:
- The main aim of contraception is family planning to check the enormous increase in population, which is the root cause of socioeconomic problems of poor and developing countries, like India.
- Certain contraceptive measures are important to prevent the sexually transmitted diseases, like AIDS.
- Contraceptives are also recommended on medical grounds to control the stress of pregnancy, labor and lactation in women suffering from heart diseases, etc.

METHODS OF CONTRACEPTION

They can be broadly grouped as:
- Spacing methods
- Terminal methods.

Both types of contraceptive measures are available for use by females as well as males, therefore, these can be described as:
- Contraceptive methods in females
- Contraceptive methods in males

CONTRACEPTIVE METHODS IN FEMALES

SPACING METHODS

The spacing methods increase the gap between two pregnancies. These include:

- Rhythm method
- Barrier methods
- Chemical methods
- Intrauterine contraceptive devices.

Rhythm Method

Rhythm method is also known as *calendar method* or *safe period method* or natural method. This method of contraception depends on the time of ovulation. In a woman having regular menstrual cycle, ovulation occurs on 14th day of the cycle. After ovulation, ovum remains viable for 48–72 hours. Similarly, after ejaculation, sperms remain alive for 24–48 hours. Thus, pregnancy occurs only if coitus is performed during this period. This is the period of high fertility and is called *dangerous period*.

Therefore, to avoid pregnancy, intercourse should be avoided in the dangerous period. Rest of the cycle, i.e., 5–6 days after bleeding phase of menstrual cycle and 5–6 days before the next cycle is the *safe period* (period of least fertility). This method of contraception is successful only if menstrual cycles are regular and woman knows the exact time of ovulation by keeping a record of basal body temperature.

Disadvantage

The disadvantage of this method is that it is the most unreliable method when the menstrual cycles are irregular and time of ovulation is variable.

Barrier Methods

Barrier methods of contraception prevent the meeting of ovum and sperms after coitus. These include:

Mechanical Barriers

The mechanical barriers used as contraceptive are diaphragm and cervical caps (Figs 9.2-1A to D).

Advantages

These devices are inexpensive and usually do not require any medical consultation.

Disadvantages

- Failures are quite common because chances of displacement of the device are very high.
- Some women get cervicitis (inflammation of cervix) and local irritation.

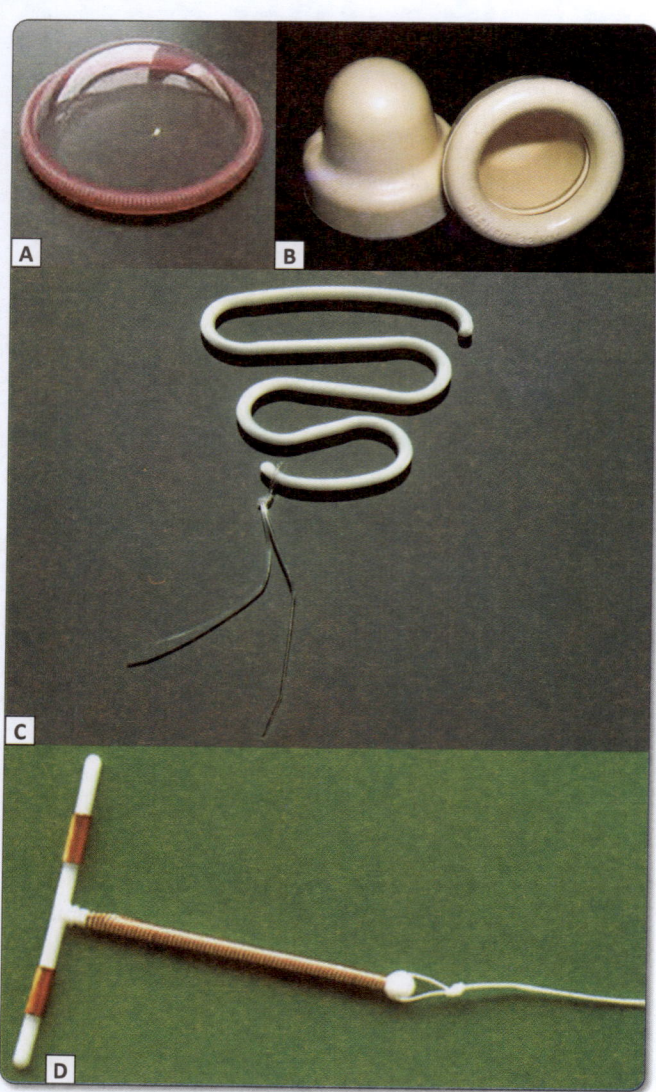

Figs 9.2-1A to D: Female contraceptive devices: A. Vaginal diaphragm; B. Cervical cap; C. Lippe's loop; D. Copper-T

Chemical Barriers

Chemical barriers refer to spermicidal agents which can destroy the sperms when applied in the female genital tract before coitus. The common sperimicidal agents used are Ricinoleic acid (oldest), Nanoxynol-9, and Octoxynol-3.

These spermicidal agents are available in various forms such as foam tablets, pastes, creams, jellies, and vaginal sponges. Vaginal sponge is a polyurethane sponge impregnated with nanoxynol-9. It is available by the trade name 'TODAY'.

Combined Methods

As mentioned above, mechanical barriers (diaphragm and cervical caps) along with spermicidal agents give good protection.

Chemical Methods

Chemical methods for contraception are used in various forms, like locally applied chemicals (in the form of cream, jellies, etc.) and taken as drugs (either orally or in injectable form or as implants).

Oral Contraceptives

Oral contraceptives are steroidal drugs, which are most widely used contraceptive measures by the women all over the globe. These are recommended in women of younger age group (up to 35 years). In general, oral contraceptives contain synthetic preparation of estrogen and progesterone and when taken orally they inhibit ovulation. The oral contraceptives are available in different types of pills:

- Combined pill (classical pill), e.g., MALA-N and MALA-D
- Sequential pill
- Minipill
- Postcoital (morning after) pill.

Depot Preparations

They are long-acting drugs and are highly effective. These are available in three forms:

- Injectable preparations
- Subdermal implants
- Vaginal rings.

Advantages

As depot preparations are long-acting drugs, therefore to avoid daily intake of oral pill, these preparations are preferred, and also, the contraceptive effectivity lasts for longer period.

Disadvantages

Sometimes they lead to sterility and alterations in menstrual bleeding pattern.

Intrauterine Contraceptive Devices

Intrauterine contraceptive devices (IUCDs) are inserted into the uterine cavity for long-term contraception. The devices are usually made up of inert materials like plastic, polythene and metal. These include:

Lippes Loop (Fig. 9.2-1C)

It is a serpentine or S-shaped device made up of plastic to which is attached a fine nylon tail. The plastic used is non-toxic and non-tissue reactive. A small amount of *barium sulphate* is also present in the plastic material to allow its radiographic observation. Lippes loop is available in different sizes.

Copper-T

Copper-T is the most commonly used IUCD in India. As the name indicates it is made up of copper and its shape resembles the letter T. Like Lippes loop it is also attached with a nylon thread (tail) (Fig. 9.2-1D).

Insertion. Most ideal time for its insertion is during menstruation or within 10 days of the beginning of menstruation, because the diameter of cervical cavity at this time is greater. It can also be inserted during first week after the delivery.

Mechanism of action. Copper-T prevents implantation and growth of fertilized ovum by evoking aseptic inflammation.

Advantage

- This method of contraception is quite safe, effective and reversible. IUCDs can be easily pulled out or removed when contraception is not required.
- Provides long-term contraception without adverse effects.

Disadvantage

- In some cases may cause heavy bleeding,
- The IUCD may come out accidently, when not inserted properly
- Risks of ectopic pregnancy are there.

TERMINAL METHODS

Terminal method of contraception means permanent sterilization, which can be achieved by the following methods.

Surgical Methods

Tubectomy

It is the permanent method of sterilization in female and is recommended only when the family is completed. In tubectomy operation, fallopian tubes are cut and then cut ends are ligated and buried as shown in Fig. 9.2-2.

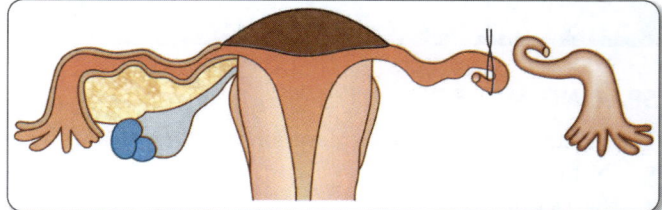

Fig. 9.2-2: Procedure of tubectomy (female sterilization)

Laparoscopic Occlusion

In this procedure, the fallopian tubes are occluded using silicon rubber bands, Fallope rings or Hulka-Clemens clips. This method is much quicker and simple and hospitalization is not required.

CLINICAL ASPECTS

Medical Termination of Pregnancy

Medical termination of pregnancy (MTP or abortion) is allowed under MTP Act, 1971. Medical Termination of Pregnancy Act has laid down the following criteria:
- Conditions in which pregnancy can be terminated
- The person who can do termination
- Place, where it should be performed.

Indications

Indications in which pregnancy can be terminated are:
- *Medical:* When continuation of pregnancy is hazardous to the mother.
- *Eugenic:* When there is substantial risk to the child if born from that pregnancy.
- *Humanitarian grounds:* When pregnancy is the result of rape.
- *Failure of contraceptive measure.*

Methods

Medical termination of pregnancy is possible only in first few months of pregnancy (from 7th week to beginning of second trimester). The following procedures have been employed depending upon the duration of pregnancy:
- *Dilatation and curettage (D and C):* In this procedure cervix is dilated with dilators and implanted ovum is removed by doing curettage of the endometrium.
- *Vacuum aspiration:* Like D and C, in this procedure cervix is dilated and then implanted ovum is removed (aspirated) by applying suction. This method is employed only up to 12 weeks of gestation.
- *Administration of prostaglandins:* In this method prostaglandins are administered into the vagina (intravaginally), which cause uterine contractions resulting in expulsion of the products of conception.

PREGNANCY VACCINES

Pregnancy vaccines are under experimental trial. These have not yet been tried on women.

CONTRACEPTIVE METHODS IN MALES

SPACING METHODS

The spacing methods of contraception used in males are:
- Natural method
- Barrier method
- Chemical methods.

Natural Method or Coitus Interruptus

It is the oldest method of voluntary fertility control. In this method male withdraws the penis before ejaculation into the vagina and tries to prevent deposition of semen into the vagina. This method needs practice and discipline. The failure rate is high because of the following reasons:
- Precoital secretions of the male may contain sperms and even a drop of semen is sufficient to cause pregnancy.
- Slightest mistake in timings of withdrawal may lead to deposition of certain amount of semen.

Barrier Methods

Condom

Condom is the most widely used barrier by the males all around the world. In India, it is known by its trade name *Nirodh* (Fig. 9.2-3). It consists of a fine latex sheath and is electronically tested.

Mechanism of action

Condom prevents deposition of semen into the vagina thus does not allow the sperms and the ovum to meet.

Advantages
- They are easily available, safe and inexpensive.
- Their use does not require any medical supervision.
- They also provide protection against sexually transmitted diseases.

Disadvantages
- It may slip off or tear off during coitus due to its incorrect use.
- It interferes with sexual sensations.

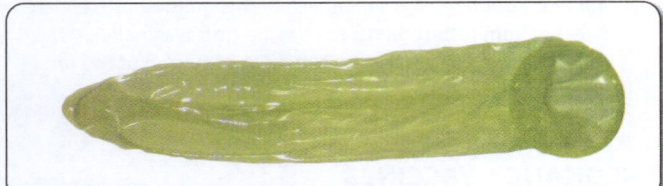

Fig. 9.2-3: Condom

Chemical Methods

Antispermatogenic drugs which inhibit spermatogenesis have been available. These include:

Male pill (Gossypol)

Hormonal preparations: Various hormonal preparations, which can be used as contraceptive measures in males are testosterone, such as testosterone with danazol (17α-ethyl testosterone), and cyproterone acetate.

Tripterygium wilfordii is a special type of wine which reduces the sperm count (mechanism of action is not yet known).

Calcium channel blockers. Calcium channel blockers (e.g. nifedipine) block the Ca^{2+} channels on the cell membrane of the sperms. As a result, the sperm membrane becomes rigid and loaded with cholesterol. The rigid membrane of sperm prevents its binding to the zona pellucida of the ovum.

TERMINAL METHODS

The permanent methods employed for sterilization in males are:
- Vasectomy
- Vas occlusion using no scalpel technique.

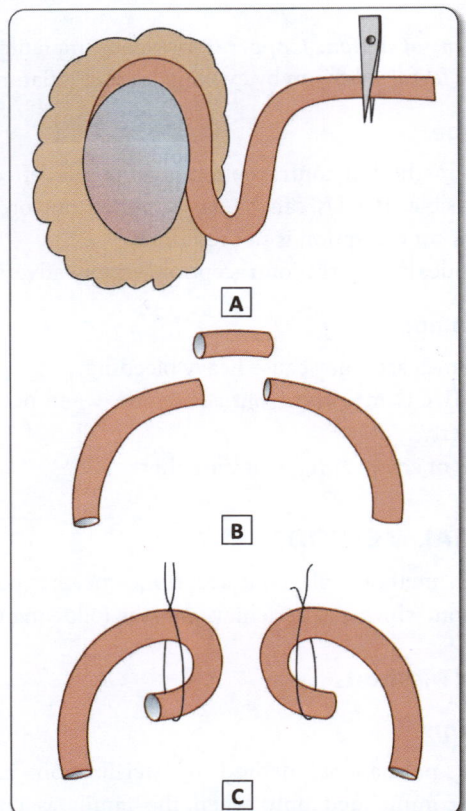

Figs 9.2-4A to C: Procedure of vasectomy (male sterilization)

Vasectomy

It is a simple operation in which about one cm piece of vas deferens is removed after clamping. Then both the ends are ligated and sutured so that they face away from each other (Fig. 9.2-4). This procedure reduces the risk of recanalization later on.

Advantages of vasectomy are that it is simpler, faster, less expensive procedure, and no hospitalization is required. It is 100% effective.

NURSING IMPLICATIONS AND APPLICATIONS

Postoperative instructions. Subjects should be advised to follow certain instructions postoperatively. Immediately after vasectomy he is not sterile because the sperms already formed are stored. After about 30 ejaculations, semen becomes free from sperms. Therefore, he must use contraceptive measure (condom) postoperatively before he becomes azoospermic.

No Scalpel Vas Occlusion

It is a newer technique, which is quite safe, convenient and is acceptable to males. In it an elastomer is injected into the vas deferens, it get hardened *in situ* within 20 mintues and plug the vas (occlude it). It is an easy procedure, and reversal is possible with 100% efficacy.

ASSESS YOURSELF

Short and Long Answer Questions

1. **Describe briefly:**
   - Methods of contraception in males.
   - Methods of contraception in females.
2. **Write notes on:**
   - Mechanism of action of oral contraceptive pills
   - Safe period
   - Medical termination of pregnancy

Multiple Choice Questions

1. **Which of the following is the safe period:**
   a. 5 to 6 days after ovulation
   b. 14th day of menstrual cycle
   c. 24–48 hours after ovulation
   d. 48–72 hours after ovulation

2. **The chemical method of contraception most effective in women:**
   a. Chemical foam tablets   b. Vaginal sponge
   c. Vaginal creams   d. Oral tablets
3. **Copper-T acts as contraceptive by preventing:**
   a. Fusion of gametes   b. Implantation
   c. Ovulation   d. Motility of sperms
4. **The statement not true for condom:**
   a. Prevents fusion of gametes
   b. Provides protection against sexually transmitted diseases
   c. Acts as anti-spermatogenic
   d. Consists of fine latex sheath
5. **The best method of contraception in young males:**
   a. Vasectomy
   b. Vas occlusion
   c. Calcium channel blockers
   d. Condom

ANSWER KEY

1. a   **2.** d   **3.** b   **4.** c   **5.** d

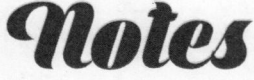
Notes

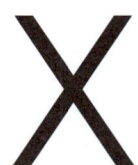

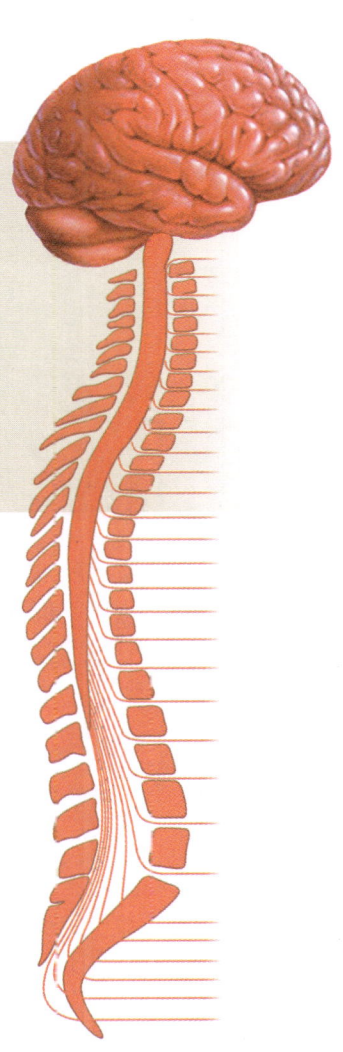

Nervous System

Organization of Nervous System and Nerve Physiology

ORGANIZATION OF NERVOUS SYSTEM

Nervous system acts as a control network within the body. The functional units of the nervous system are called *neurons*, which are responsible for the reception and response to changes in the internal and external environment. It is estimated that the human nervous system is composed of more than 100 billion neurons, which are linked together in a highly intricate manner. Thus, the various parts of the nervous system are interconnected, but for convenience of description the nervous system can be divided anatomically and functionally into different divisions.

ANATOMICAL DIVISIONS OF THE NERVOUS SYSTEM

The nervous system is broadly classified into two divisions: The central nervous system and the peripheral nervous system (Figs 10.1-1 and 10.1-2).

1. *Central nervous system (CNS)*, which occupies the central axis of the body, includes brain and spinal cord.
2. *Peripheral nervous system (PNS)* is the part of nervous system, which lies outside the central nervous system. The PNS consists of peripheral nerves and the ganglia associated with them. Peripheral nerves attached to the brain are called *cranial nerves* (12 pairs), and

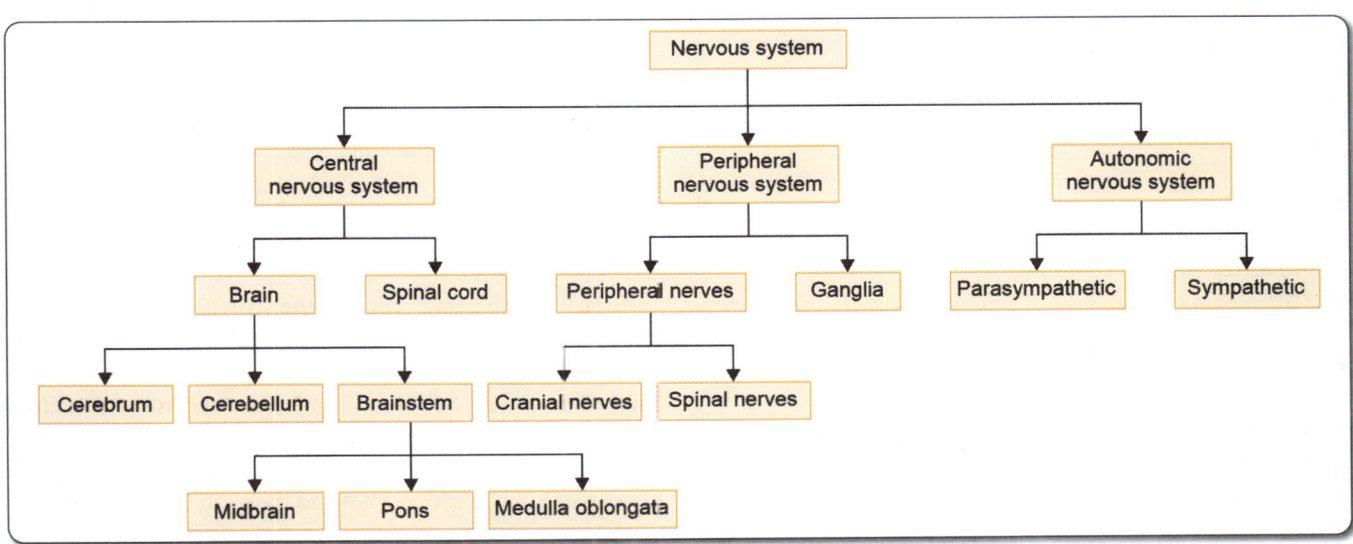

Fig. 10.1-1: Divisions of nervous system

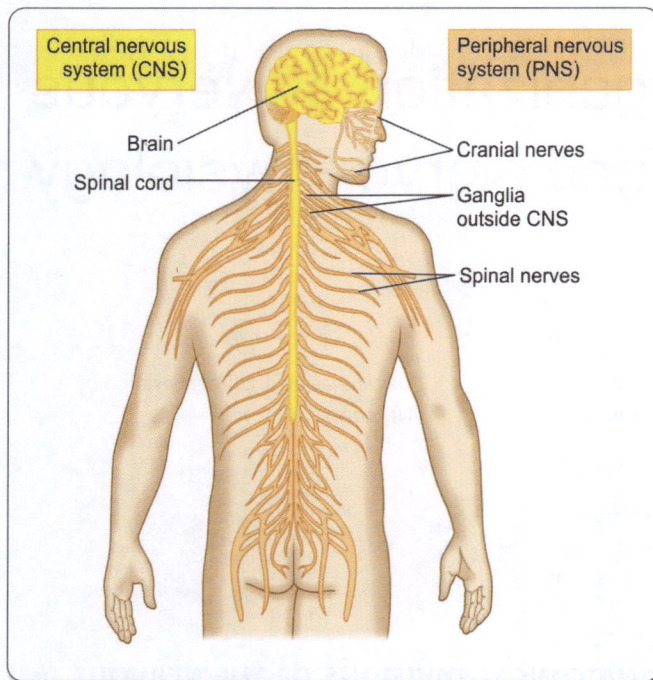

Central nervous system (CNS)

Peripheral nervous system (PNS)

Brain

Spinal cord

Cranial nerves

Ganglia outside CNS

Spinal nerves

Fig. 10.1-2: Components of central and peripheral nervous system

those attached with spinal cord are called *spinal nerves* (31 pairs).

FUNCTIONAL DIVISIONS OF THE NERVOUS SYSTEM

Functionally, nervous system can be divided into two parts:

Somatic Nervous System

Somatic nervous system has two divisions:

1. *Sensory division* of the somatic nervous system collects the information about the changes that take place in the external environment and interprets the meaning of these changes. The sensory division of the somatic nervous system consists of:

- *Sensory receptors* that receive stimulus from the external environment. The stimulus may be mechanical, chemical, thermal, auditory or visual.
- *Afferent neurons* that carry impulses from the receptors to the brain and spinal cord.
- *Parts of the brain* that primarily deal with the processing of information.

2. *Motor division* of the somatic nervous system executes appropriate actions with the help of skeletal muscles in response to changes in external environment detected by *the*

sensory division. It also coordinates the actions of different skeletal muscles of the body.

Motor division of the somatic nervous system consists of neurons that carry signals away from the brain and spinal cord to the skeletal muscles. Somatic nervous system is under voluntary control.

Autonomic Nervous System

The word autonomous is taken from the Greek words, the 'autos' meaning self and the 'nomos' meaning control. Thus, autonomic nervous system (ANS) is an involuntary system.

Divisions of ANS

The ANS has two main divisions:
1. Sympathetic nervous system
2. Parasympathetic nervous system, each having a central and a peripheral component.

The ANS collects the information about the changes that take place in the internal environment (i.e., internal viscera), interprets these changes, and guides the action and gets the plan executed with the help of smooth muscles of viscera, cardiac muscles and secretory epithelium of glandular tissues (which are effector organs of ANS). In other words, the ANS is responsible for activities of the organs of digestion, circulation, excretion, respiration and reproduction, as well as of adrenal medulla, sweat, salivary and lacrimal glands. It also controls the activities of smooth muscles of iris, ciliary body and arrectores pilorum.

NERVOUS TISSUE

CELLS OF NERVOUS TISSUE

The nervous tissue forming the nervous system is composed of:
- *Neurons*, the functional cells
- *Neuroglia*, the supporting cells.

Neuron

Structure

Neurons, or the nerve cells, are the structural and functional units of the nervous system. Neurons vary considerably in size, shape and other features. However, most of them have some major features in common. The basic structure of a neuron is best studied in a spinal motor neuron. A neuron primarily consists of the cell body and processes called *neurites,* which are of two kinds, the dendrites and the axon (Fig. 10.1-3).

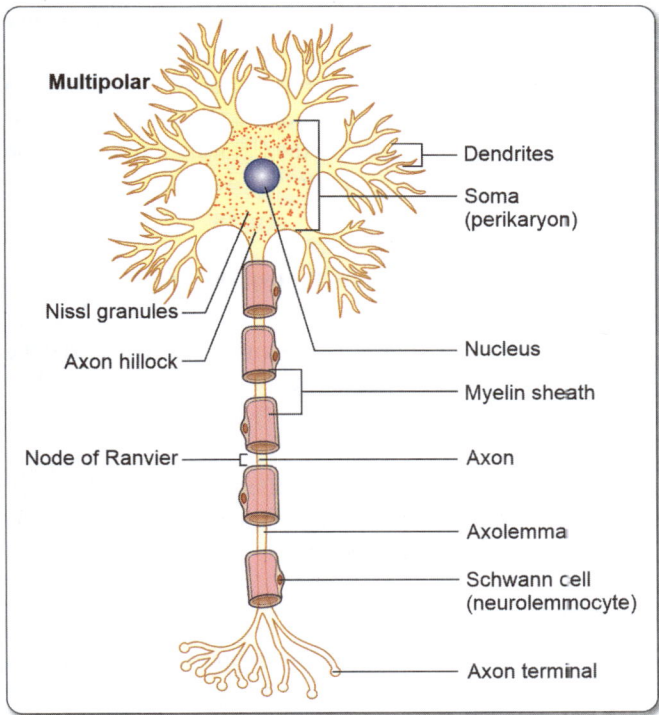

Fig. 10.1-3: Structure of a typical neuron

Cell body

The cell body of a neuron is also called the *soma* or *perikaryon* and may be round, stellate, pyramidal or fusiform in shape. Like any other cell, it consists of a mass of cytoplasm with all its principal constituents surrounded by a cell membrane. The cell body contains a large nucleus with one or two nucleoli but there is no centrosome. In addition to the general features of a typical cell, the cytoplasm of a neuron has the following distinctive characteristics (Fig. 10.1-3):

IMPORTANT TO KNOW

The absence of centrosome indicates that the neuron has lost ability for division. Thus, neurons once destroyed are replaced by neuroglia only.

Nissl granules/bodies. These are basophilic granules, seem to be composed of rough surfaced endoplasmic reticulum. The presence of abundant granular endoplasmic reticulum is an indication of the high level of protein synthesis in neurons.
Neurofibrillae. The presence of a network of neurofibrillae in the cytoplasm of the neuron is another distinctive feature. These consist of microfilaments and microtubules.

APPLIED ASPECTS

In certain degenerative disease like Alzheimer's disease, the neurofilament protein gets altered, resulting in the formation of *neurofibrillary tangles.*

Pigment granules. They are seen in some neurons. For example, neuromelanin is present in the neurons of substantia nigra. Aging neurons contain a pigment lipofuscin.

Dendrites

The dendrites are multiple small branched processes. Dendrites contain Nissl bodies and neurofibers. Dendrites are the *receptive processes* of the neuron receiving signals from other neurons via their synapses with axon terminals.

Axon

The axon is the single longer process of the nerve cell. It varies in length from a few microns to a meter.

- It arises from the conical extension of the cell body called *axon hillock,* which is devoid of Nissl bodies.
- The part of the axon between the axon hillock and the beginning of myelin sheath is called the *initial segment.*
- In the axon, the cell membrane continues as *axolemma* and the cytoplasm as *axoplasm.*
- The axon terminates by dividing into a number of branches, each ending in a number of *synaptic knobs* also known as *terminal buttons* or axon telodendria.
- Synaptic knobs contain microvesicles in which chemical neurotransmitters are stored.
- *Myelin sheath* is present around the axons in the so called myelinated nerve fibers (Fig. 10.1-4). Myelin sheath which consists of protein-lipid complex is produced by glial cells called *Schwann cells* which encircle the axon forming around it a thin sleeve. Each Schwann cell provides the myelin sheath for a short segment of the axon.
- At the junction of any 2 such segments, there is a short gap, i.e., periodic 1 μm constrictions at about 1 mm distance. These gaps are the *nodes of Ranvier.* There are some axons which are devoid of myelin sheath.

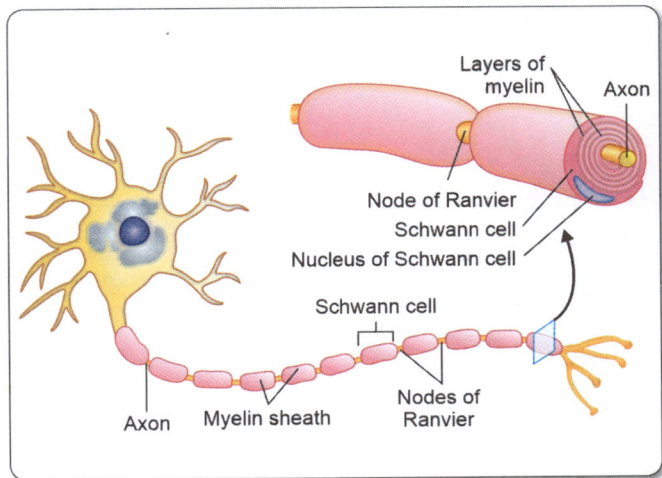

Fig. 10.1-4: Structure of a myelinated neuron

Axons perform the specialized function of conducting impulses away from the cell body. They transmit propagated impulses (all or none transmission).

Myelination of axons increases the speed of conduction, but greatly increases their diameter.

NURSING IMPLICATIONS AND APPLICATIONS

Multiple sclerosis (MS) is a demyelinating disease involving white matter of central nervous system. Currently it is considered to be an autoimmune disease.

Manifestations depend on area of CNS involved and severity of the disease. The commonest signs and symptoms include:

- Limb weakness, numbness, fatigue and tremors.
- Pain in back
- Impaired coordination of voluntary movements
- Vision loss may occurs due to optic neuritis

Types of Neurons

Neurons have been variously classified as:

Depending upon the number of poles

Depending upon the number of poles (from which processes arise), neurons are divided into unipolar, bipolar and multipolar.

Unipolar neurons have a single pole, from which both the processes, axon and dendrite, arise (Fig. 10.1-5A). True unipolar cells are present only in embryonic stage in human being. However, the primary sensory neurons (neurons conveying impulses from a sensory receptor to spinal cord) are *pseudounipolar* (Fig. 10.1-5B).

Bipolar neurons have two poles, one for axon and other for dendrite (Fig. 10.1-5C). Bipolar neurons are found in the

vestibular and cochlear ganglia, and in the nasal olfactory epithelium, and as bipolar cells in the retina.

Multipolar neurons have many poles. One of the poles gives rise to axon and all others to dendrites (Fig. 10.1-5D). Most vertebrate neurons, especially in the CNS, are multipolar. The dendrites branch profusely to form the dendritic tree.

Depending upon the functions

Depending upon the functions, the neurons are of two types—motor and sensory.

Motor neurons, also known as efferent nerve cells, carry the motor impulses from CNS to the peripheral effector organs like muscles, glands and blood vessels. These neurons have very long axon and short dendrites.

Sensory neurons, also known as afferent nerve cells, carry sensory impulses from periphery to the CNS. These neurons have short axon and long dendrites.

Neuroglia

Neuroglia or the glial cells are the supporting cells present within the brain and spinal cord. They are numerous, about 10 times more than the neurons. Glial cells may be divided into two major categories (Figs 10.1-6A to D):

Macroglia

Macroglia or large glial cells are ectodermal in origin. These are of two types:

1. Astrocytes. These are small star-shaped cells that give off a number of processes which frequently end in expansions in relation to blood vessels and in relation to the surface of brain. *Fibrous astrocytes* (Fig. 10.1-6A) are seen mainly in the white matter and *protoplasmic astrocytes* in the grey matter.

2. Oligodendrocytes. Oligodendrocytes have rounded or pear-shaped bodies with scanty processes (Fig. 10.1-6B). These cells provide myelin sheath to nerve fibers that lie within the brain and spinal cord. Oligodendrocytes gives off multiple processes which form myelin sheath on many neighboring axons.

Microglia

Microglia or the small glial cells are mesodermal in origin. These are the smallest neuroglial cells having flattened cell body and short processes (Fig. 10.1-6C). They are more numerous in grey matter than in white matter. These act as phagocytes and become active after damage to nervous tissue by trauma or disease.

Ependymal Cells

Are specialized cells which cover the choroidal plexuses located in the cerebral ventricles (Fig. 10.1-6D).

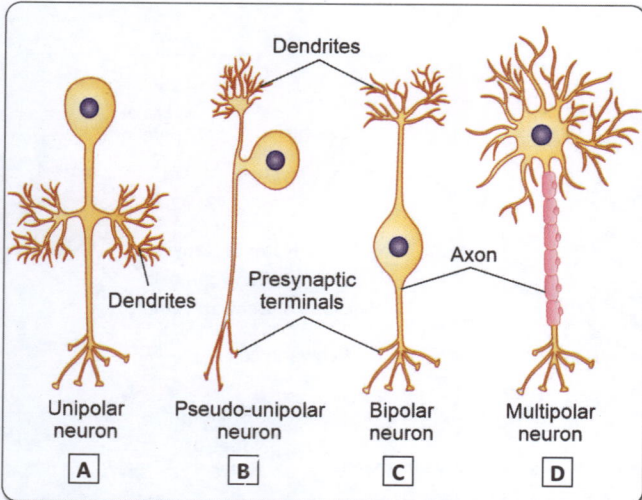

Figs 10.1-5A to D: Different types of neurons

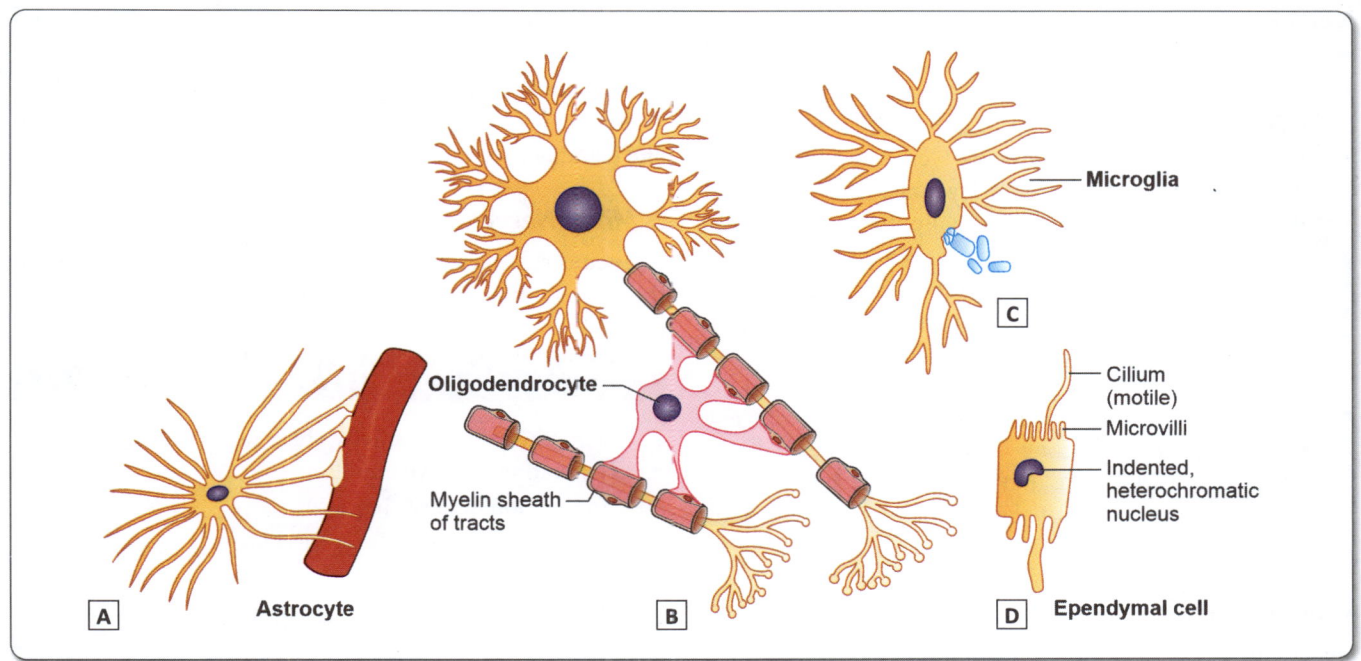

Figs 10.1-6A to D: Different types of glial cells: A. Astrocyte; B. Oligodendrocyte; C. Microglia, D. Ependymal cell

GREY VERSUS WHITE MATTER

The nervous tissue mass in general is organized into grey and white matter.

Grey Matter

Grey matter comprises the cell bodies of neurons and many of their processes (excluding axons). It is found in the outer layer of cortex and other parts of brain and in the core of spinal cord.

The grey matter also composes the ganglion, nucleus, center and unmyelinated nerve fibers.

White Matter

White matter, found in the brain, spinal cord, and nerves, is made up of the long axons of the neurons. It contains both myelinated and nonmyelinated fibers. However, the preponderance of myelinated fibers gives it a creamy color, hence, the name.

GANGLION, NUCLEUS AND CENTER

Ganglion

It is an aggregation of neuronal cell bodies located outside the central nervous system. For example:

Dorsal root ganglia. These are composed of cell bodies of the visceral and somatic sensory nerves.

Sympathetic and parasympathetic ganglia of the autonomic nervous system contain the cell bodies of postganglionic visceral efferent nerves.

Nucleus

Nucleus refers to an aggregation of the neuronal cell bodies located inside the central nervous system (brain and spinal cord). The axons (fibers) of the neurons forming nuclei either form a *nerve* (in peripheral nervous system) or a *tract* within the brain or spinal cord. For example:

Facial nucleus. The axons of the cell bodies forming facial nucleus form the facial nerve.

Nucleus gracilis. The axons of the neurons forming nucleus gracilis form the tract inside the central nervous system.

Center

Center refers to a group of neurons and synapses regulating certain function. A center may be located in a nucleus, or ganglion or any other mass of grey matter. Thus, center refers to a functional entity, while the nucleus and ganglion are anatomical entities. Examples of centers include respiratory control center, and vasomotor center located in medulla oblongata.

NERVE

A compact bundle of axons located outside the CNS is called a nerve. In a nerve, the axons are arranged in different bundles called fasciculi (Fig. 10.1-7).

- Each axon or the nerve fiber is covered by *endoneurium* which is bounded internally by basal lamina around the Schwann cells and externally by the relatively impermeable inner basal lamina of the perineurium.
- Each fasciculus is covered by *perineurium.* The cells of perineurium are tightly adherent and act as a barrier to passage of particulate traces, dye molecules or toxins into the endoneurium.
- The whole nerve is covered by *epineurium* which is a tubular sheath formed by areolar membrane. It limits the extent to which the nerve can be stretched by body movements or external pressure, thereby protecting the fragile axons inside the nerve.

Types of Nerves

Depending upon the type of nerve impulse transmission, the nerves are of three types:

1. Sensory Nerves

They consist of peripheral processes of the neurons which extend up to sensory receptors in the skin. These fibers pass on sensory information to the spinal cord and brain.

2. Motor Nerves

Consist of the axons which originate in the brain, spinal cord and autonomic ganglia. They transmit impulses to the effector organs, i.e., muscles and glands. Motor nerves are of two types:

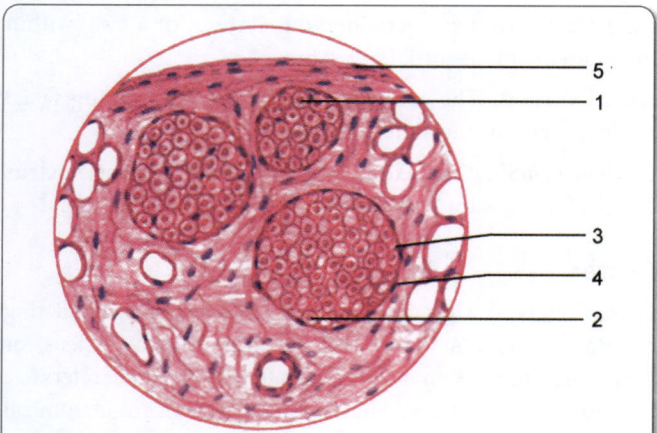

Fig. 10.1-7: Cross-section of a peripheral nerve. 1. Myelinated nerve fibers; 2. Axons of nerve fibers; 3. Endoneurium; 4. Epineurium and 5. Myelin sheath

1. *Somatic motor nerves.* These are involved in voluntary and reflex skeletal muscle contraction.

2. *Autonomic nerves (sympathetic and parasympathetic).* These are involved in cardiac and smooth muscle contraction and glandular secretion.

3. Mixed Nerves

They consist of sensory as well as motor fibers enclosed within the same sheath of connective tissue.

NERVE PHYSIOLOGY

The main physiological activity of the nerve fiber are:
- Generation of nerve impulse
- Conduction of nerve impulse
- Transmission of impulse at the synapse.

GENERATION OF NERVE IMPULSE

Excitability

Excitability is that property of the nerve fiber by virtue of which it responds by generating a nerve signal (electrical impulses or the so called action potentials) when it is stimulated by a suitable stimulus which may be mechanical, thermal, chemical or electrical. In experimental studies, electrical stimulus is more frequently employed since its strength and frequency can be accurately controlled.

Resting Membrane Potential

As shown in Fig. 10.1-8A, when two electrodes are placed on the surface of a nerve fiber and connected to a cathode ray oscilloscope (CRO), no potential difference is observed. However, if one of the microelectrodes is inserted inside the nerve fiber (Fig. 10.1-8B), a steady potential difference of –70 mV (inside negative) is observed on the cathode ray oscilloscope (CRO). This is resting membrane potential (RMP) and indicates the resting state of cell also called *state of polarization* (*See* page 485).

Action Potential

The *action potential* may be defined as the brief sequence of changes, which occur in the resting membrane potential when stimulated by a threshold stimulus. When the stimulus is subminimal or subthreshold, it does not produce action potential, but does produce some changes in the RMP. There is slight depolarization for about 7 mV which cannot be propagated, since propagation occurs only if the depolarization reaches a firing level of 15 mV (–55 mV). Once

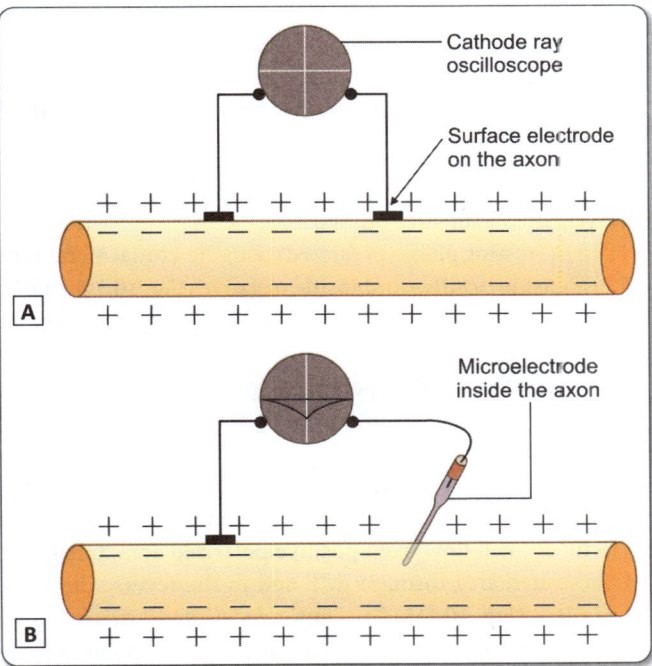

Figs 10.1-8A and B: Recording of resting membrane potential

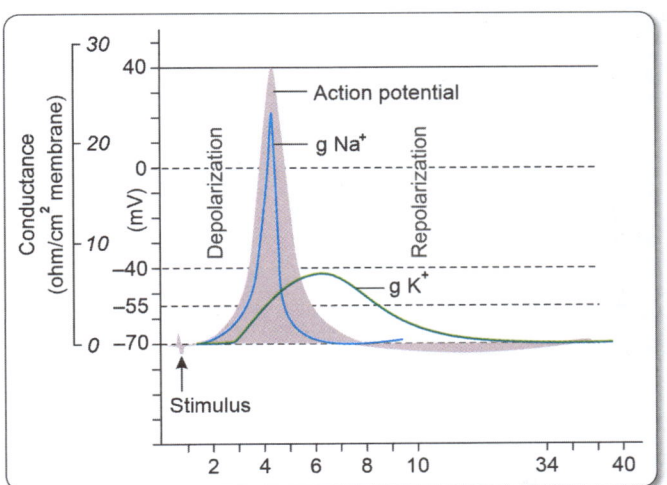

Fig. 10.1-9: Changes in g Na+ and g K+ conductance during action potential

the firing level is reached, there occurs action potential, i.e., there occurs abrupt depolarization with propagation (action potential). The adequate strength of stimulus necessary for producing the action potential in a nerve fiber is known as *threshold* or *minimal stimulus.*

Phases of action potential

The action potential basically occurs in two phases: depolarization and repolarization. When the nerve is stimulated, the polarized state (–70 mV) is altered, i.e., RMP is abolished and the interior of the nerve becomes positive (+35 mV) as compared to the exterior. This is called *depolarization phase.* Within no time, there occurs a reversal to the nearly original potential and this second phase of action potential is called *repolarization phase.*

Ionic basis of action potential

The development of action potential was studied by Hodgkin and Huxley using the *voltage clamp technique.* According to *Hodgkin-Huxley theory,* the sequence of events are (Fig. 10.1-9):

Polarization phase. Resting membrane potential (–70 mV) is due to distribution of more cations outside the cell membrane and more anions inside the cell membrane. At this point, though Na+ are more in ECF but they cannot enter the cell due to the impermeability of the membrane.

Depolarization phase. When threshold stimulus is applied to the cell membrane, at the point of stimulation the permeability

of the membrane for Na+ ions increases. There occurs a rapid influx of Na+ ions into the cell. This rapid entry of Na+ leads to depolarization.

Repolarization phase. Repolarization occurs due to decrease in further Na+ influx and K+ efflux through the voltage-gated K+ channels which open later than Na+ channels but remain activated for prolonged period.

Decrease in Na+ influx and efflux of K+ causes net transfer of positive charge out of the cell that serves to complete the repolarization.

Main Characteristics of Nerve Excitability

All or none response

A single nerve fiber always obeys 'all or none law', that is:

- *When a stimulus of subthreshold intensity* is applied to the axon, then no action potential is produced (*none response*);
- A response in the form of spike of action potential is observed when the stimulus is of threshold intensity; and
- There occurs no further increase in the magnitude of action potential when the strength of stimulus is more than the threshold level (*all response*).

This all or none relationship observed between the strength of stimulus and the response achieved is known as 'All or None Law'.

Refractory period

Refractory period refers to the period the following action potential (produced by a threshold stimulus) during which a nerve fiber either does not respond or responds subnormally to a stimulus of threshold intensity or greater than threshold intensity. It is of two types (Fig. 10.1-10):

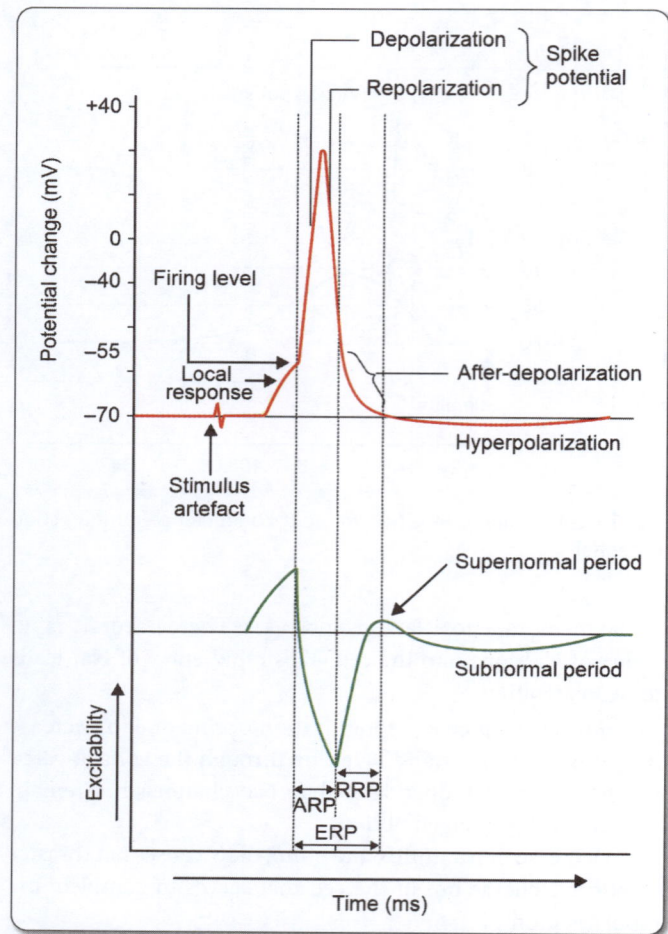

Fig. 10.1-10: Membrane excitability during different phases of action potential

Abbreviation: ARP; absolute refractory period, RRP; relative refractory period; ERP, effective refractory period.

1. *Absolute refractory period (ARP).* It is a short period the following action potential during which second stimulus, no matter how strong it may be, cannot evoke any response (another action potential). In other words, during absolute refractory period the nerve fiber completely loses its excitability.

2. *Relative refractory period (RRP).* It is a short period during which the nerve fiber shows response if the strength of stimulus is more than normal.

Conduction of Nerve Impulse

Conductivity refers to propagation of nerve impulse (action potential) in the form of a wave of depolarization through the nerve fiber. Normally, in the body, the action potential is transmitted through nerve fiber in one direction. Mechanism of

conduction of action potential along an unmyelinated nerve fiber and a myelinated nerve fiber is described below.

Propagation of Action Potential in an Unmyelinated Axon

The steps of propagation of action potential along an unmyelinated axon are summarized:

- In the resting phase (polarized state) the axonal membrane is outside positive and inside negative (Fig. 10.1-11A).
- When an unmyelinated axon is stimulated at one site by a threshold stimulus, there occurs action potential at that site, i.e., that site is depolarized. In other words, at that site outside membrane becomes negative and inside positive (reversal of polarity) but the neighboring areas until now remain in polarized state (Fig. 10.1-11B).
- As ECF and ICF are both conductive to electricity, a current will flow from positive polarized area to negative activated area through ECF and in the reverse direction in ICF (Fig. 10.1-11C). Thus, a *local circuit current* flows between the resting polarized site to the depolarized site of the membrane (current sink).
- This circular current flow depolarizes the neighboring area of the membrane up to firing level and a new action potential is produced which in turn depolarizes the neighboring area ahead. Thus, due to successive depolarization of the neighboring area, the action potential is propagated along the entire length of the axon (Figs 10.1-11D, E and F).

Propagation of Action Potential in a Myelinated Axon

The myelinated nerve fibers have a wrapping of myelin sheath with gaps at regular intervals which are devoid of myelin sheath (nodes of Ranvier). The axonal membrane in the naked area (nodes of Ranvier) bears densely packed ion channels. The myelin sheath acts as an insulator and does not allow the current flow. Therefore, in myelinated nerve fibers the *local circuit of current flow* only occurs from one node of Ranvier to the adjacent node (Figs 10.1-12A and B). That is, the impulse (action potential) jumps from one node of Ranvier to next. This is known as *saltatory conduction*. Since the impulse jumps from one node to other, the speed of conduction in myelinated fibers is much rapid (50–100 times faster) than the unmyelinated fiber.

Orthodromic Versus Antidromic Conduction

Normally, the action potential is propagated in one direction. That is, usually the nerve impulse from the receptors or

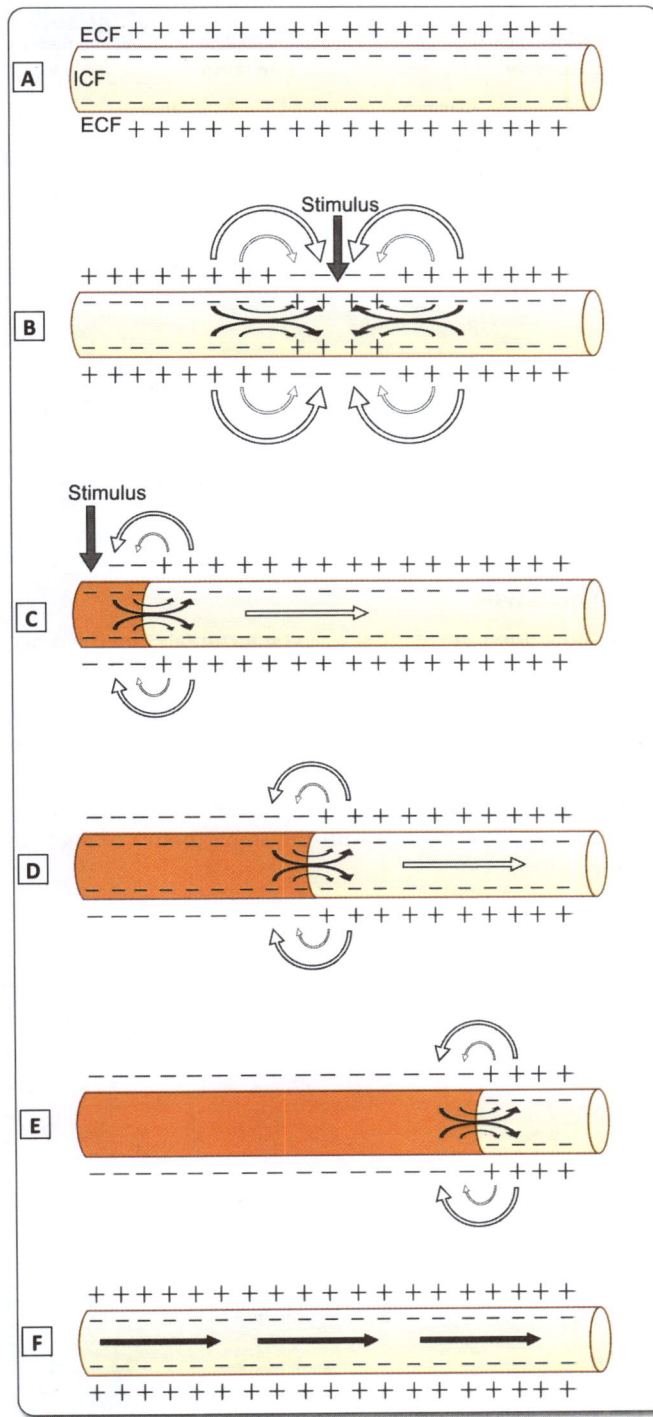

Figs 10.1-11A to F: Electronic conduction of impulse in an unmyelinated nerve fiber: A. Resting phase (polarized state); B. Conduction of impulse in both directions when stimulus applied at the middle of nerve fiber; C. When stimulus applied at one end of the nerve fiber; D. and E. Propagation of impulse in one direction along the nerve fiber; and F. Repolarization (occurs in same direction)

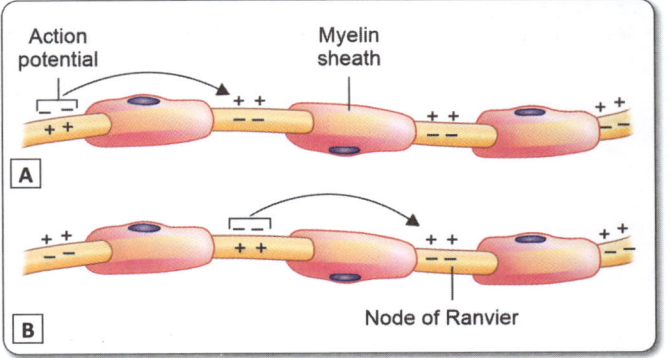

Figs 10.1-12A and B: Saltatory conduction along a myelinated nerve fiber

synaptic junctions travels along the entire length of axon to their termination. This type of conduction is called *orthodromic conduction*. The conduction of nerve impulse in the opposite direction, as seen in the sensory nerve supplying the blood vessels, is called *antidromic conduction*.

Factors Affecting Conduction Velocity

The velocity of conduction in nerve fibers varies from as little as 0.25 m/s in very small unmyelinated fibers to as high as 100 m/s in very large myelinated fibers. In general, the factors affecting conduction velocity are:

Temperature. A decrease in temperature delays conduction, i.e., slows down the conduction velocity.

Axon diameter affects the conduction velocity through the *resistance offered by the axoplasm* (R_i) to the flow of axoplasmic current. If the diameter of the axon is greater, the axoplasmic resistance (R_i) is lesser and hence, the velocity of conduction is higher.

Myelination increases conduction velocity by its the following effects:

- By increasing the axon diameter
- By the saltatory conduction produced due to its insulating effect (as discussed above).

Conduction Velocity and Nerve Fiber Types

Various schemes for classification of nerve fibers on the basis of their diameter and their conduction velocity have been proposed:

Letter classification of Erlanger and Gasser. This is the best known classification based on the diameter and conduction velocity of nerve fibers. The nerve fibers have been classified into type A, B and C. Their salient features are summarized in Table 10.1-1.

TABLE 10.1-1: Salient features of type A, B and C nerve fibers

Fiber type		Myelinated/ non-myelinated	Fiber diameter (μm)	Conduction velocity (m/sec)	Function	
					Efferent	**Afferent**
A	α	Myelinated	12–20	70–120	Somatic motor	Proprioception
	β	Myelinated	5–12	30–70	—	Touch pressure
	γ	Myelinated	3–6	15–30	Motor to muscle spindles	—
	δ	Myelinated	2–5	12–30	—	Pain, cold, touch
B	–	Myelinated	<3	3–15	Preganglionic autonomic	—
C	–	Non-myelinated	0.4–1.2	0.5–2	Postganglionic autonomic	Pain, temperature some mechano reception reflex responses

TABLE 10.1-2: Numerical vis-a-vis letter classification of sensory nerve fibers

Types of nerve fiber		Origin
Numerical classification	**Letter classification**	
Ia	Aα	Muscle spindle (annulospiral endings)
Ib	Aα	Golgi tendon organ
II	Aβ	Muscle spindle (flower spray endings), touch and pressure
III	Aδ	Pain and cold receptors, some touch receptors
IV	C	Pain, temperature and other receptors

Numerical classification. Some physiologists have classified sensory nerve fibers by a numerical system into type Ia, Ib, II, III and IV. A comparison of the numerical classification and the letter classification is shown in Table 10.1-2.

TRANSMISSION OF NERVE IMPULSE AT THE SYNAPSE (SYNAPTIC TRANSMISSION)

Synapse

Definition

The synapse is the anatomic site where the nerve cells communicate among themselves. There is no anatomical connection or continuity between different neurons. They are connected only functionally. So, synapse is the functional junction between two neurons.

Types of Synapses

Anatomical types

Depending upon the manner an axon terminates on the other neurons, the synapses can be of the following types:

Axodendritic synapse (Fig. 10.1-13A) is the synapse between axon of a neuron with dendrite of another neuron. It is the most common type of synapse.

Axosomatic synapse (Fig. 10.1-13B) refers to the synapse between axon of a neuron with the soma (body) of another neuron.

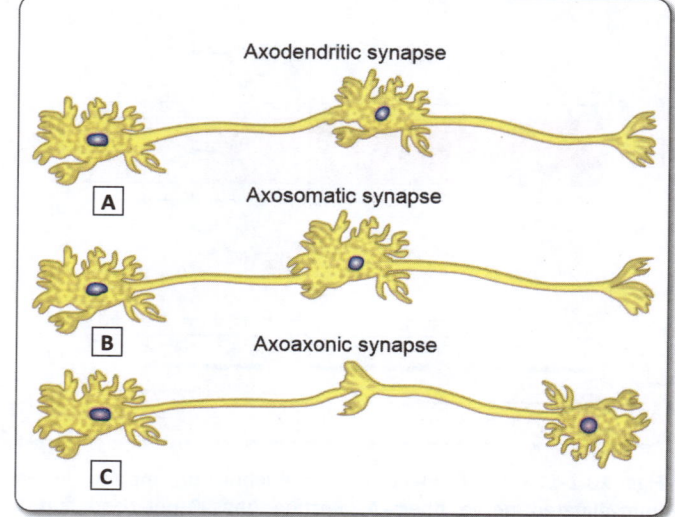

Figs 10.1-13A to C: Types of synapses

Axoaxonic synapse (Fig. 10.1-13C) is the synapse between axon of a neuron with axon of another neuron.

In some parts of the brain (e.g., thalamus), some synapses are seen in which the presynaptic element is dendrite instead of an axon. Such synapses may be *dendroaxonic* or *dendrodendritic*.

Physiological types

Depending upon the process of transmission of impulse, the synapses can be classified as:

Chemical synapses are those in which transmission is carried out by *neurotransmitter*. Most synapses in human nervous system are of this type.

Electrical synapses are those in which transmission occurs through gap junctions. Transmission at electrical synapses is essentially an electrotonic conduction between two neurons.

Electrical transmission is seen in a few locations (e.g., within the retina and olfactory bulb) in human nervous system.

Conjoint synapse refers to a synapse where both the chemical and electrical transmission coexist.

Chemical Synapse

Structure

A typical chemical synapse between the axon of one neuron and dendrite of other neuron exhibits the following characteristics (Fig. 10.1-14):

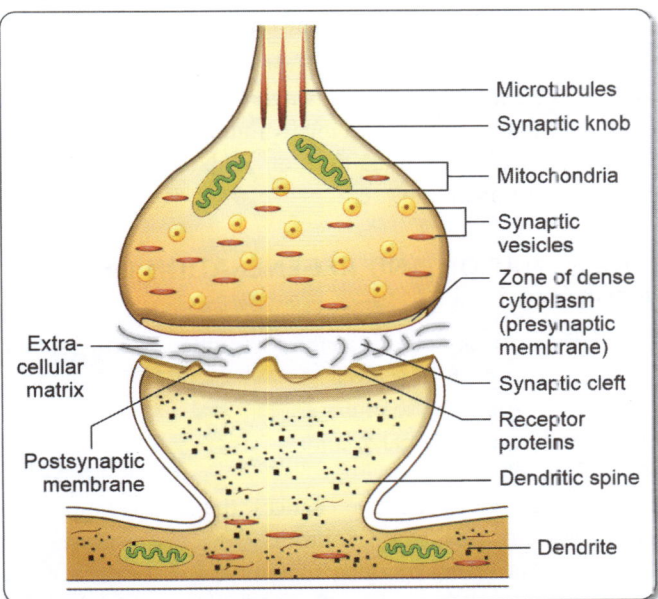

Fig. 10.1-14: Structure of a chemical synapse

Synaptic knob or button. As the axon of neuron approaches the synapse, it loses the myelin sheath and divides into a number of fine branches which end in small swellings called the synaptic knobs or synaptic buttons.

Presynaptic membrane refers to the axonal membrane lining the synaptic knobs.

Synaptic cleft is a small gap (20–40 nm wide) between the pre- and postsynaptic membranes.

Postsynaptic process is the name given to the region of receiving neuron (e.g., dendritic spine), where the synaptic knob synapses.

Postsynaptic membrane is the membrane lining the postsynaptic process.

Process of synaptic transmission

The sequence of events which occur during chemical synaptic transmission are:

Release of neurotransmitter

- When the nerve impulse (action potential [AP]) travelling in a nerve fiber (axon) reaches the nerve terminal (synaptic knobs), there occurs depolarization of the presynaptic terminal.
- As a result of depolarization, neurotransmitter than diffuses across the synaptic cleft and binds to the postsynaptic receptors.

Development of excitatory postsynaptic potential (EPSP) and inhibitory postsynaptic potential (IPSP)

Binding of the neurotransmitter to the postsynaptic receptors causes:
- Depolarization of the postsynaptic membrane, which is produced by the excitatory neurotransmitters. The most common excitatory neurotransmitter within the CNS is *glutamate.*
- Inhibitory postsynaptic potential (IPSP), i.e., hyperpolarization of the postsynaptic membrane, is produced by the inhibitory neurotransmitters released in the synaptic cleft. The most common inhibitory neurotransmitters within the CNS are glycine and γ-aminobutyric acid (GABA).

Inactivation of neurotransmitter from the synaptic cleft

The neurotransmitter released in the synaptic cleft from the presynaptic terminal is soon inactivated in one of the following three ways:
- Diffusion of the transmitter out of the cleft
- Enzymatic degradation of the transmitter, e.g., dissociation of acetylcholine by acetylcholinesterase

- Active transport back into the presynaptic terminal (transmitter re-uptake), e.g., active re-uptake of norepinephrine at sympathetic postganglionic nerve endings.

Development of action potential

The development of AP from EPSP can be considered to happen in the following two steps:

1. Generation of the initial segment spike
2. Generation of propagated signals, i.e., AP

Generation of initial segment spike. The potential spreads passively to the initial segment, and a threshold level of about 6–10 mV results in a spike potential called the *initial* spike (IS) is generated.

Generation of propagated signals, i.e., Action potential. The initial spike once initiated; it itself produces a further depolarization of 30–40 mV in turn, triggers the generation of the AP spike. Once generated, the AP travels peripherally in the axon as a nerve impulse.

Neurotransmitters

Neurotransmitters are the chemical substances which are responsible for transmission of an impulse through a synapse.

Neuromediators or neurohormones are chemical substances which are synthesized in neurons and poured into the blood stream through terminals resembling synapses in structure.

Neuromodulators are the chemical substances, which are associated with synapses but do not influence synaptic transmission directly.

Physiologically neurotransmitters can be divided into two groups:

1. *Excitatory neurotransmitters* can cause an action potential (if the target cell is another neuron), contraction (if the target cell is a muscle), or secretion (if the target cell is a gland).

In the CNS, the excitatory neurotransmitters produce a depolarization of the postsynaptic membrane called the excitatory postsynaptic potential (EPSP). The most common excitatory neurotransmitter within the CNS is glutamate. Other excitatory neurotransmitters are acetylcholine, aspartic acid, etc.

2. *Inhibitory neurotransmitters* reduce or block the activity of the postsynaptic cell. They produce a hyperpolarization of the postsynaptic membrane called the inhibitory postsynaptic potential (IPSP). The most common inhibitory neurotransmitters within the CNS are *glycine* or *gamma-aminobutyric acid* (GABA). Other inhibitory neurotransmitters include dopamine.

Properties and Significance of Synaptic Transmission

Some characteristic features of synaptic transmission as are follows:

One-way Conduction

The chemical synapse allows only one-way conduction of an impulse, i.e., from the presynaptic to the postsynaptic neuron and never in the opposite direction. This is called the *law of dynamic polarity or Bell-Magendie law*.

Significance. The synapses act like a valve and are responsible for the orderly conduction of impulse in one direction only.

Synaptic Delay

Synaptic delay refers to a time lapse, which occurs between the arrival of nerve impulse at the presynaptic terminal and its passage to the postsynaptic membrane.

Cause of synaptic delay include the time taken for the neurotransmitter to release and to act on postsynaptic membrane.

Significance. The synaptic delay is one of the causes for the latent period of the reflex activity.

Convergence and Divergence

Convergence at chemical synapse refers to the phenomenon of termination of signals from many sources, i.e., many presynaptic neurons on a single postsynaptic neuron. Information coming from the large number of presynaptic neurons is integrated to decide the onward effect.

Divergence. One presynaptic neuron may terminate on many postsynaptic neurons. Thus, a single impulse is contrverted into a number of impulses going to a number of postsynaptic neurons, this causes magnification and therefore helps in amplification of an impulse.

DEGENERATION AND REGENERATION OF NEURONS

When the axon of neuron is injured, a series of degenerative changes are seen at three levels:

- In the axon distal to injury
- In the axon proximal to injury
- In the cell body

Along with the degenerative changes, the reparative process (regeneration) also starts soon, if the circumstances are favorable. The effects of injury to a nerve and the occurrence of regenerative changes thereafter will depend on the degree and type of damage.

Stage of Degeneration

The degenerative changes which occur in the part of axon distal to the site of injury are referred to as an anterograde degeneration or Wallerian degeneration (after the discoverer A. Waller, 1862). The degenerative changes occurring in the neuron proximal to the injury are referred to as retrograde degeneration

Changes in the part of axon distal to injury. The degenerative changes start within few hours of injury and continue for about 3 months and include the following (Fig. 10.1-15):

Axis cylinder becomes swollen and irregular in shape within a few hours of injury. After a few days, it breaks up into small fragments, the neurofibrils within it break down into granular debris and are seen in the space occupied by the axis cylinder

Changes in the cell body of neuron: The changes in cell body of injured neuron start within 48 hours and continue up to 15–20 days. The changes are:

- Nissl substances undergo disintegration and dissolution (chromatolysis).
- Golgi apparatus, mitochondria and neurofibrils are fragmented and eventually disappear.
- Cell body draws in more fluid, enlarges and becomes spherical.
- Nucleus is displaced to the periphery (toward cell membrane). Sometimes the nucleus is extruded out of the cell, in which case the neuron atrophies and finally disappears completely.

Stage of Regeneration

The stage of regeneration starts within 4 days of injury but becomes more active after 30 days, and may take several months to a year for complete recovery.

Factors Affecting Regeneration

- Regeneration occurs more rapidly when a nerve is crushed than when it is severed and the cut ends are separated.
- Chances of regeneration of a cut nerve are considerably increased if the two cut ends are near each other (gap does not exceed 3 mm) and remain in the same line.
- Presence of neurilemma is a must for regeneration to occur. Therefore, axons in the CNS once degenerated never regenerate as these nerve fibers have no neurilemma.
- Presence of nucleus in the neuron cell body is also must for regeneration to occur. If it is extruded, the neuron is atrophied and the regeneration does not occur.

Regenerative Changes

1. *Formation of axis cylinder* from the proximal cut end of the axon elongates and gives out fibrils up to 100 in number in all directions. These branches grow into the connective tissue at the site of injury in an effort to reach the distal cut end of the nerve fiber (Fig. 10.1-15).

- Entry of fibrils into endoneural tube. Strands of the Schwann cells from the distal cut end of axon guide the regenerating fibrils to enter their axon endoneural tube, and once the fibril enters the endoneural tube, it grows rapidly within it. The axonal fibrils that fail to enter one of the tubes degenerate.
- Stage of Active Growth. The axonal fibril growing through the endoneural tube enlarges and establishes contact with an appropriate peripheral end organ. The new axon formed in this way is devoid of myelin sheath (Fig. 10.1-15). The process of regeneration up to this stage takes about 3 months.

Myelination. The myelin sheath is then formed slowly by the cells of Schwann. The myelination is completed in 1 year.

2. *Changes in the cell body of neuron:*

- Nissl granules followed by the Golgi apparatus appear in the cell body.
- The cell loses excess fluid and regains its normal size.
- The nucleus occupies the center

The above changes in some of the neurons start within 20 days of injury and are completed in 80 days. The functional (physiological) recovery, however, occurs after a long period.

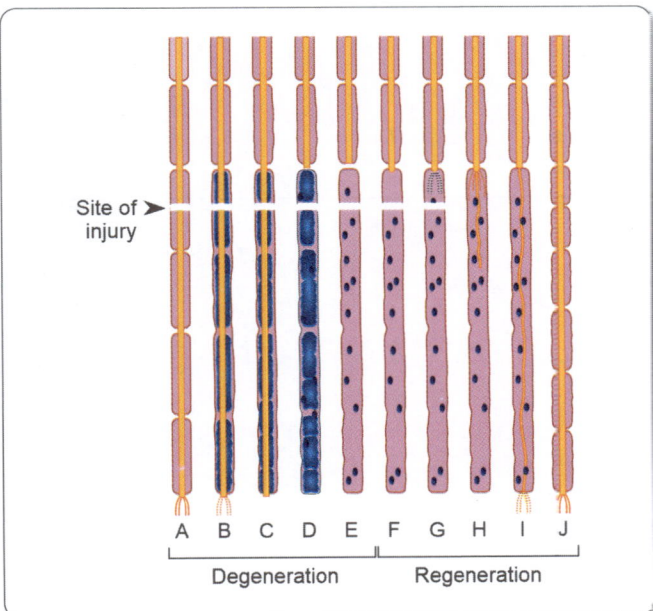

Site of injury →

A B C D E F G H I J

Degeneration · Regeneration

Fig. 10.1-15: Degenerative changes (Wallerian degeneration) in a distal part of a nerve fiber after injury (A–E) and subsequent regenerative changes (F–J)

ASSESS YOURSELF

Short and Long Answer Questions

1. With the help of flow diagram describe the organization of nervous system.
2. Describe the structure of neuron.
3. How is the nerve impulse conducted in myelinated and nonmyelinated nerve fibers?
4. Discuss the sequence of events during chemical synaptic transmission.
5. Define a neurotransmitter. Give classification of neurotransmitters.
6. Write notes on the following:
   - Basis of classification of nerve fibers
   - Wallerian degeneration
   - Phases of action potential
   - Functions of acetylcholine as a neurotransmitter.

Multiple Choice Questions

1. Not true for cell body of a neuron:
   a. Contains Nissl granules
   b. Nucleus contains nucleoli and centrosome
   c. Synthesizes neurotransmitter
   d. Its axon arises from axon hillock
2. Which of the following belongs to microglia?
   a. Asterocytes   b. Oligodendrocytes
   c. Ependymal cells   d. Schwann cells

3. Which of the following is white matter component?
   a. Myelinated nerve fibers
   b. Dorsal root ganglia
   c. Facial nucleus
   d. Core of spinal cord
4. The depolarization phase of action potential is due to:
   a. Influx of Na^+ b. Influx of K^+
   c. Influx of Ca^{2+} d. Efflux of K^+
5. Which is the excitatory neurotransmitter?
   a. Glycine   b. Dopamine
   c. Glutamate   d. Gamma-aminobutyric acid
6. The resting membrane potential of a nerve fiber is:
   a. −70 mV   b. −55 mV
   c. 0 mV   d. +35 mV
7. The diameter of Aα fiber:
   a. <3 μm   b. 3–6 μm
   c. 5–12 μm   d. >12 μm
8. The conduction velocity of α fibers is:
   a. 3–15 m/sec
   b. 12–30 m/sec
   c. 30–70 m/sec
   d. 70–120 m/sec
9. Post synaptic potential is generated by:
   a. Glycine
   b. GABA
   c. Dopamine
   d. Glutamate

ANSWER KEY

1. b   2. c   3. a   4. a   5. c   6. a   7. d   8. d
9. d

Central Nervous System

CHAPTER OUTLINE

THE BRAIN

The central nervous system (CNS) consists of the brain and the spinal cord (Figs 10.2-1A and B). The brain is the largest and most complex mass of nervous tissue in the body. It is contained in cranial cavity and weighs about 1380 g in the adult male and about 1250 g in the adult female.

PARTS OF BRAIN

The brain has three parts:

1. *Forebrain* (prosencephalon) comprises:
- Cerebral hemispheres (telencephalon)
- Diencephalon (thalamus plus hypothalamus)

2. *Midbrain* (mesencephalon)

3. *Hindbrain* (rhombencephalon) comprises:
- Pons
- Medulla oblongata
- Cerebellum.

Spinal cord traced upward becomes medulla oblongata. Above the medulla, a broad bridge, the pons, connects the two hemispheres of the cerebellum, which lie behind the pons and medulla. The midbrain connects the forebrain with hindbrain.

Medulla oblongata, pons and midbrain together constitute the *brain stem*.

CEREBRUM

External Features

Cerebrum consists of two cerebral hemispheres which are separated from each other in the upper part by a median longitudinal fissure in which the *falx cerebri* (a fold of dura mater) invaginates. In the lower part, the two cerebral hemispheres are connected by the largest white commissure called *corpus callosum*.

Sulci and Gyri

The surface of cerebral hemisphere is covered by a thin layer (2–4 mm thick) of grey matter called the cerebral cortex. The entire surface of cerebral hemisphere is folded with intervening grooves of fissures. The folds or convolutions are called gyri, and the intervening fissures are called sulci.

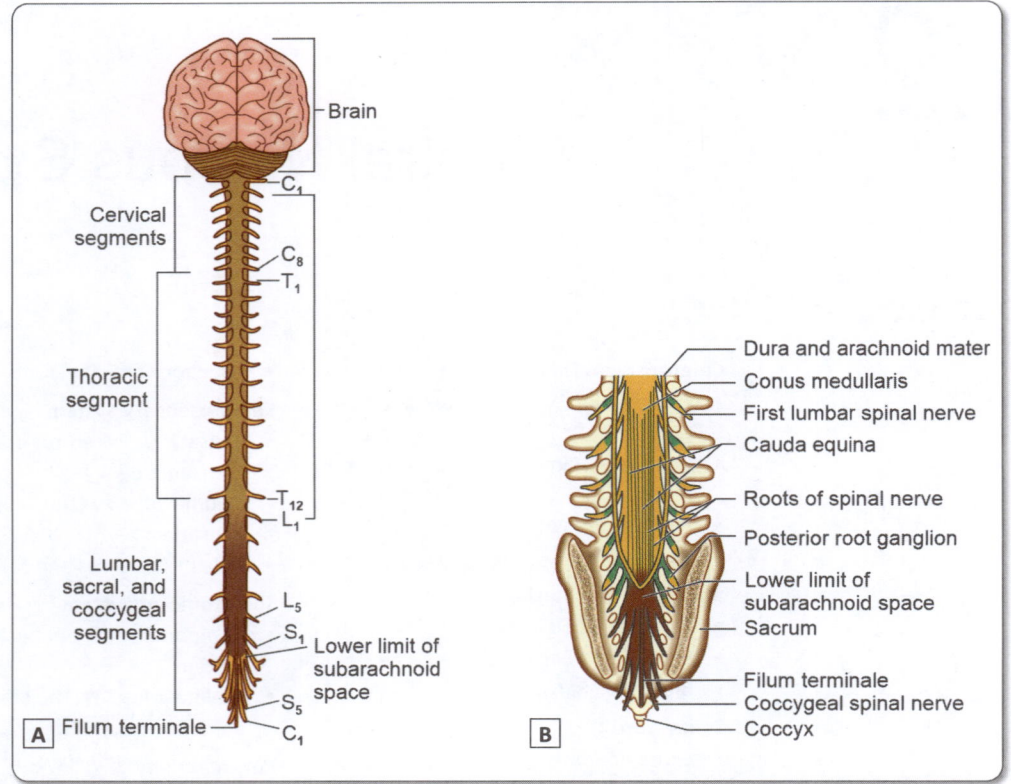

Figs 10.2-1A and B: A. Diagrammatic depiction of parts of central nervous system; B. Filum terminale

The cerebral cortex follows the contour of the sulci and gyri of the hemisphere. As a result of the folding of the cerebral surface, the cerebral cortex acquires a much larger surface area (about 2200 cm²).

Lobes and Functional Areas

Each cerebral hemisphere is divided into four lobes (Figs 10.2-2A to C):

(i) Frontal Lobe

The frontal lobe lies in front of the central sulcus and above the posterior ramus of the lateral sulcus (Figs 10.2-3A and B). It forms about one-third of cortical surface. On the basis of functions, the frontal lobe is subdivided into two main areas:

(a) Precentral cortex

Precentral cortex refers to posterior part of the frontal lobe that includes lip of central sulcus, precentral gyrus, and posterior part of superior, middle and inferior frontal gyri. The precentral cortex is also called excitomotor area of cortex.

Nowadays the motor cortex and sensory cortex are together known as *sensorimotor cortex*. The precentral cortex includes the following important areas:

Primary motor area (area 4). It lies in the precentral gyrus extending into the paracentral lobule on the medial surface. Different parts of the contralateral half of the body are represented separately in more or less inverted order. Those parts of the body which carry out the most skilled movements, e.g., the fingers and thumb have the largest areas of cortical representation. The body is represented upside down (however, face is not represented in inverted manner) (Figs 10.2-4A and B).

Functions. It is concerned with initiation of voluntary movements of the contralateral half of the body and initiation of speech.

Premotor Area

Premotor area lies anterior to the primary motor area and includes Brodmann's areas 6, 8, 44 and 45.

Area 6. It abuts on the primary motor cortex both above and behind. Cells from this area contribute fibers to pyramidal tracts. Topographical organization of this area is roughly the same as that of primary motor cortex.

Area 8. It is also called frontal eye field. It lies anterior to area 6. It is concerned with control of eye movements.

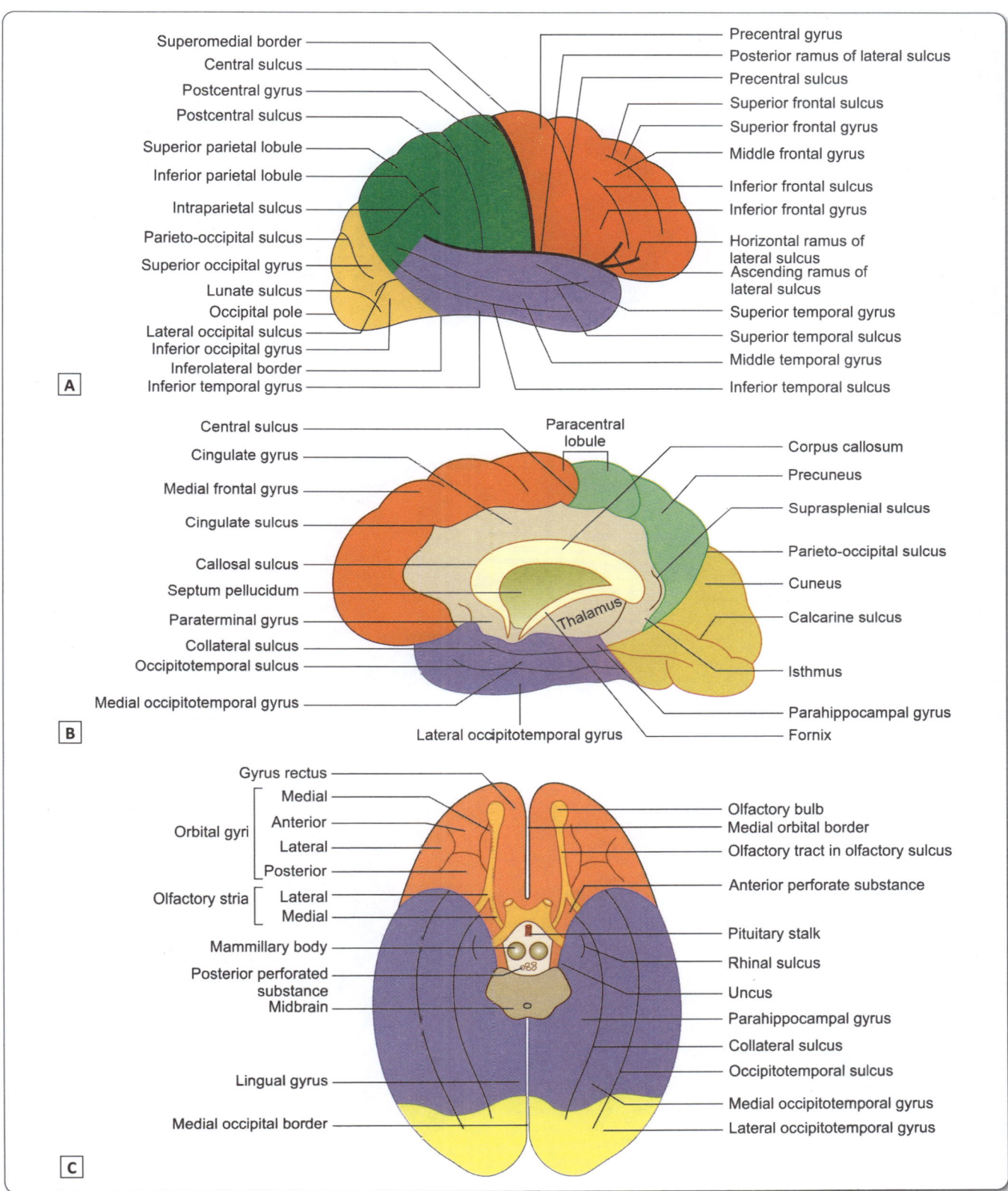

Figs 10.2-2A to C: Right cerebral hemisphere showing lobes, sulci, and gyri: A. Superolateral surface; B. Medial surface; C. Inferior surface

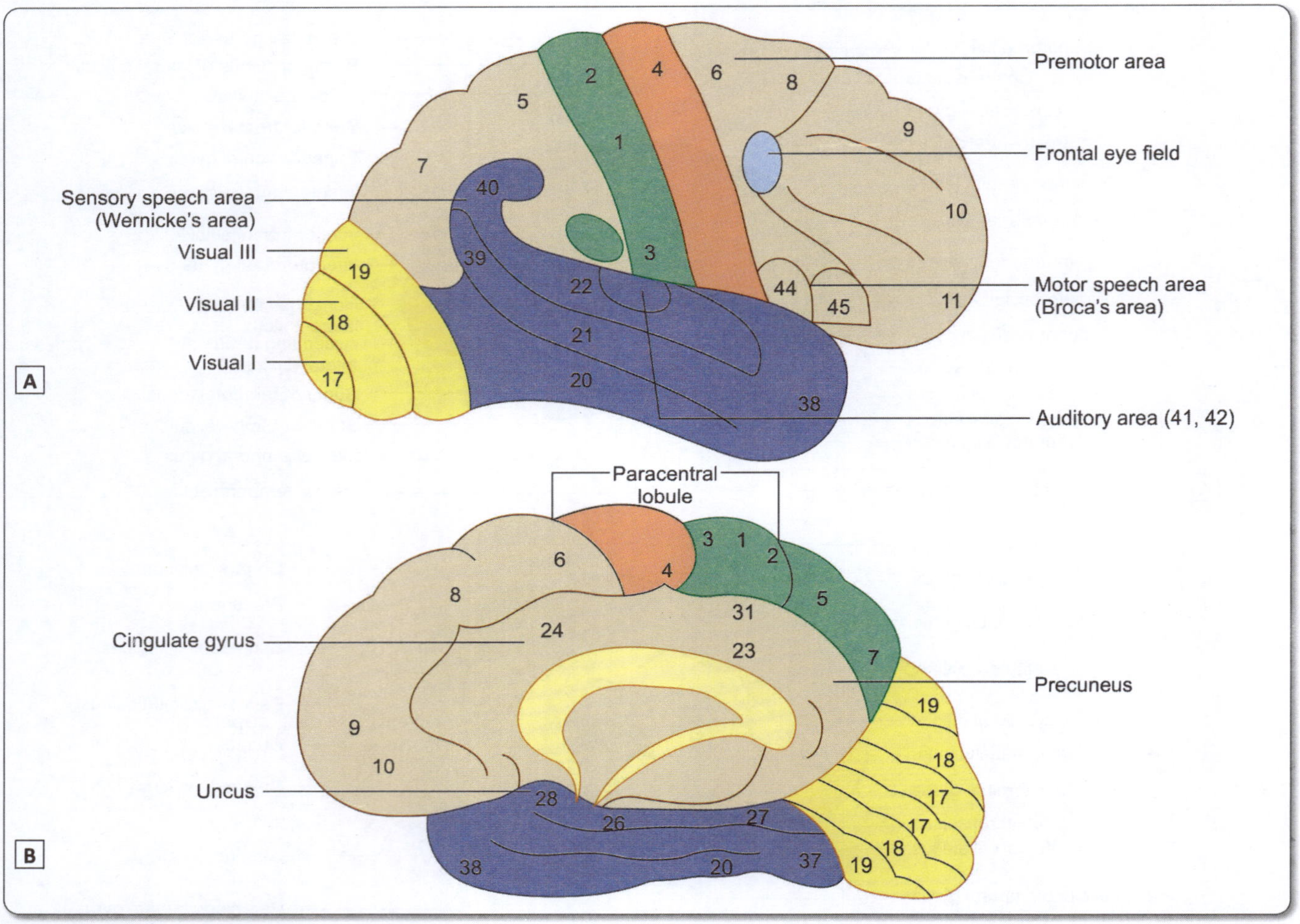

A

Premotor area

Frontal eye field

Sensory speech area
(Wernicke's area)

Visual III

Visual II

Visual I

Motor speech area
(Broca's area)

Auditory area (41, 42)

5

2

4

6

8

1

9

7

40

10

39

19

22

3

18

21

44

45

11

17

20

38

B

Paracentral
lobule

Cingulate gyrus

Precuneus

Uncus

6

3 1 2

4

5

8

31

24

23

7

9

19

10

18

28

17

26

27

17

38

20

37

19

18

Figs 10.2-3A and B: Function of brain: A. Superolateral surface; B. Medial surface

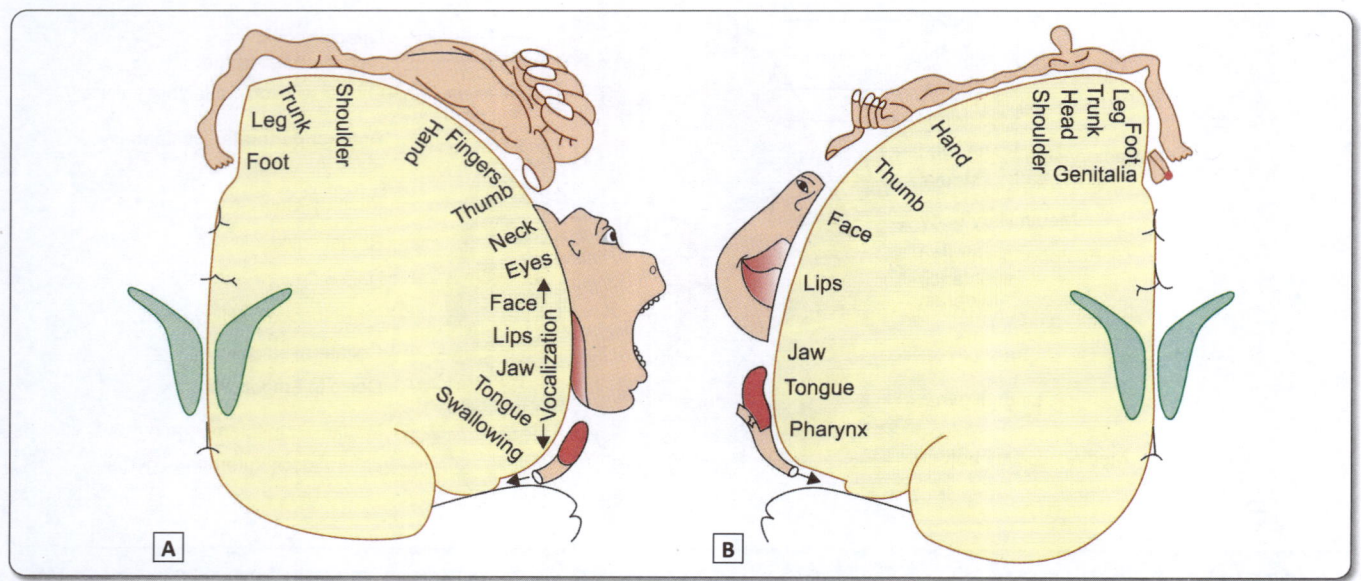

Figs 10.2-4A and B: Topographic representation (homunculus) of motor: A. Sensory; B. Areas in cerebral cortex

Area 44 and 45 or Broca's motor speech area. It is special region of premotor cortex situated in inferior frontal gyrus.

Functions. This area, especially in dominated hemisphere (left hemisphere in right-handed person), is concerned with movements of those structures which are responsible for the production of voice and articulation of speech.

Supplementary motor area

(b) Prefrontal cortex

Location. Prefrontal cortex also called prefrontal lobe or orbitofrontal cortex is the anterior part of frontal lobe lying anterior to area 8 and 44.

Major areas. Prefrontal cortex has different Brodmann's areas such as 9 to 14, 23, 24, 29, 32 and 44 to 47.

Functions

Preforontal cortex is mainly responsible for the following functions:
* Center for planned actions.
* Center for higher functions like emotions, learning, memory and scoial behavior.
* Control of intellectual activities; for example, planing of future, keep the track of bits of many information etc.

(ii) Parietal Lobe

Parietal lobe lies between the central sulcus and parieto-occipital sulcus and upper part of first imaginary line.

Areas of parietal lobe

Primary sensory area (First somatic sensory area):

Location. The first somatic sensory area (SI) occupies the posterior wall of the central sulcus, the postcentral gyrus and the postcentral part of the paracentral lobule.

Major areas. It includes Brodmann's area 3, 1 and 2.

Topographical organization. The primary sensory cortex receives sensory inputs from the opposite half of the body. The representation of the body within this area is similar to that already noted in primary motor cortex.

Secondary sensory area

Secondary sensory area, also called second somatic sensory area (SII), is situated in postcentral gyrus below the area of face of first somatic sensory area. Most of it is buried in the superior wall of the sylvian fissure (lateral cerebral sulcus).

Topographical representation. The secondary sensory (SII) area receives sensory impulses from primary sensory area (SI) as well as from thalamus directly. Like SI, the SII area also manifests a dermatomal (point-to-point) sequence of representation (although there is more overlap). Thus, the body is represented twice in the somatic sensory cortex, i.e., in area SI as well as in area SII.

Sensory association areas

The sensory association areas include area 5 and 7. The area 40 is higher association area.

(iii) Temporal Lobe

Temporal lobe lies below the posterior ramus of lateral sulcus and its continuation the second imaginary line.

Areas of temporal lobe

The major areas in the temporal lobe are:

Primary auditory area

Primary auditory area, also called audio sensory area, includes Brodmann's area 41 and 42 and forms the center for hearing.

Functions. This area perceives the nerve impulses as sound, i.e., auditory information such as loudness, pitch, source and direction of sound.

Auditory association area

Auditory association area corresponds to Brodmann's areas 22, 21 and 20.

Area 22, also called Wernicke's area, is a sensory speech center situated in the posterior part of superior temporal gyrus behind the area 41 and 42, in the categorical hemisphere, i.e., dominant hemisphere.

Functions. It is concerned with:
* Interpretation of the meaning of what is heard
* Comprehension of spoken language and the formation of ideas that are to be articulated in speech.

Areas 21 and 20. Are located in the middle and inferior temporal gyrus, respectively.

Functions. These areas receive impulses from primary area and are concerned with interpretation and integration of auditory impulses.

CLINICAL ASPECTS

Lesions of 22, 21 and 20 areas impair auditory, short-term memory without impairing visual memory.

(iv) Occipital Lobe

Occipital lobe lies behind the parieto-occipital sulcus and its continuation down an imaginary line.

Areas of occipital lobe

Occipital lobe is mostly formed of sensory and association areas. It contains visual cortex having three areas:

Primary visual cortex is also called striate area (area 17). It lies on the medial surface of the occipital lobe in and near the calcarine sulcus occupying parts of lingual gyrus and cuneus.

Peristriate area, also called visual association area (area 18), lies in the walls of lunate sulcus.

Parastriate area (area 19) is also a visual association area. It lies in the cortex in front of the lunate sulcus.

Functions:

- *Primary visual area (area 17)* is concerned with perception of visual impulses.
- *Visual association areas* (area 18 and area 19) are concerned with interpretation of visual impulses. These are involved in the recognition and identification of objects in the light of past experience.
- *Occipital eye field area* (area 19) is concerned with the movements of eyeball.

Summary of Cortical Functional Areas

Classically, cortical functional areas are subdivided into the following areas:

Motor areas include:

- Primary motor area (Brodmann's area 4)
- Premotor area (area 6)
- Frontal eye field (area 8)
- Supplementary motor area.

Sensory areas include:

- Primary somesthetic areas (area 3, 1 and 2).
- Secondary (supplementary) somesthetic area.
- Somesthetic association areas (area 5, 7 and higher association area 40).

Auditory areas include:

- Primary auditory area (area 41) or auditory area I
- Auditory association area (area 42) or auditory area II
- Higher auditory association area (area 22).

Visual areas include:

- Primary visual area (area 17) or visuol striate area of visual area I
- Visual association area 18 (peristriate area)
- Visual association area 19 (parastriate area).

Speech areas include:

- *Motor speech area* comprises:
  - Anterior area (Broca's area) or areas 44, 45
  - Superior area.
- *Sensory speech areas* comprise:
  - Area 39 (or reading center)
  - Area 40
  - Area 22 (Wernicke's area)

Smell area is: Area 28

Gustatory area is: Area 43.

Interior of Cerebrum

The interior of each cerebrum, below the thick layer of grey matter (cerebral cortex), consists of:

- *Basal ganglia*, the masses of grey matter, and
- *White matter* of cerebrum (Fig. 10.2-5).

Basal Ganglia

Components

The basal ganglia are subcortical areas of grey matter (nuclear masses). They are so named as they develop in the basal part of the cerebral hemisphere. The basal ganglia together comprise the *corpus striatum* which is divided almost completely by the fibers of internal capsule into two parts:

1. *Caudate nucleus* (medial part)
2. *Lenticular nucleus* (lateral part), which is further subdivided into two parts:
   a. Putamen (an outer part)
   b. Globus pallidus (the inner part).

Connections

There are connections between the individual members of the basal ganglia and between them and cerebral cortex, the thalamus and the reticular formation of brain stem.

Functions of Basal Ganglia

Control of voluntary motor activity

Basal ganglia control the voluntary movements, which are initiated by the motor cortex. The role of basal ganglia in controlling voluntary motor activity includes the following:

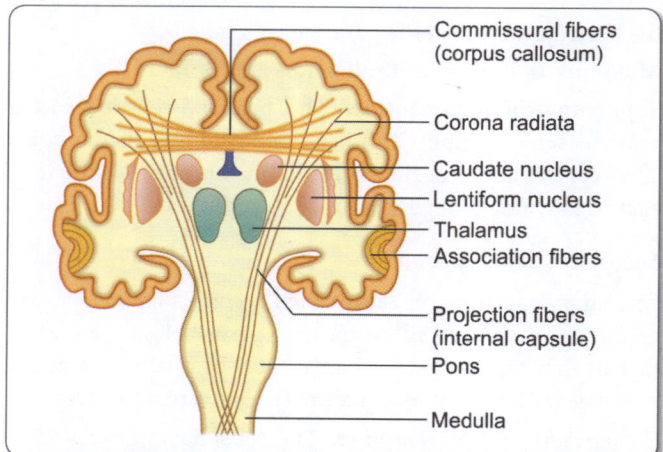

Fig. 10.2-5: Frontal view of coronal section of cerebrum showing basal ganglia and white matter in the interior

Cognitive control of motor activity. The basal ganglia, like the cerebellum, are involved in the planning and programming of the movement.

Timing and scaling of the intensity of movements. Two important capabilities of brain in controlling the movements are as follows:

- Timing of the movements, i.e., how rapidly the movements should be performed.
- Scaling of the intensity of movements, i.e., how large the movement should be.

Subconscious execution of some movements

Basal ganglia subconsciously execute some movements. Examples of movements executed subconsciously at the level of basal ganglia are as follows:

- Swinging of arm while walking
- Crude movement of facial expression that accompany emotions
- Movements of limbs while swimming

- Control of clutch and brake while driving (constant attention is required during initial stages; however, they are carried out subconsciously by basal ganglia as they become routine)

IMPORTANT TO KNOW

By subconscious control of activities, the basal ganglia relieve cortex from routine acts so that cortex can be free to plan its actions.

Control of reflex muscular activity: The basal ganglia exert an inhibitory effect on spinal reflexes and regulate the activity of muscles which maintain posture.

Control of Muscle Tone: Muscle spindles and the motor neurons of spinal cord (which are responsible for maintaining the tone of the muscles) are controlled by basal ganglia, especially substantia nigra.

Role in arousal mechanism: Globus pallidus and red nucleus are involved in the arousal mechanism because of their connections with reticular formation.

NURSING IMPLICATIONS AND APPLICATIONS

Disorders of Basal Ganglia

Parkinson disease: Parkinson disease, also called paralysis agitans or shaking palsy, was first described by James Parkinson in 1817. Parkinson disease occurs in elderly people due to a steady loss of dopamine and dopamine receptors in the basal ganglia in normal individuals, with aging.

Signs and symptoms: The patient is unable to initiate the voluntary movements (akinesia) or the voluntary movements are decreased (hypokinesia).

Manifestations of akinesia or hypokinesia include the following:

- Delayed motor initiative
- Slow performance of voluntary movements (bradykinesia)
- Mask-like facial expression due to decrease in movements of facial muscles
- Absence of normal associated movements, e.g., swinging of arms during walking, shuffling or festinant-type gait, in which the patient is bent forward and walks quickly with short steps as, if trying to catch up the center of gravity or preventing himself or herself from falling

- Retropulsion, i.e., when a walking patient is suddenly pulled backwards, he begins to walk backward and is unable to stop.

Rigidity: It refers to an increase in tone of the muscles. Characteristic features of rigidity occurring in Parkinson disease are as follows:

- Due to rigidity, the posture becomes that of flexion attitude in which the back is flexed, arms are abducted and flexed, and the knees are bent (Fig. 10.2-6).
- In advanced cases, the rigidity may increase to such an extent that a statue-like appearance is produced with complete absence of movements.

Tremors: Tremors (i.e., involuntary rhythmic oscillatory movements of the distal parts of limbs and head) seen in Parkinson disease have the following characteristics:

- The tremors are present at rest, but disappear during activity.
- Frequency of tremors ranges from four to six times per second.
- It is frequently seen as frill-rolling movements of the hand.
- Tremors are suppressed during sleep and exaggerated by stress, anxiety and excitement.

White Matter of Cerebrum

Passing through, between and around the subcortical masses of grey matter of cerebrum, are tracts of white fibers. The white fibers of cerebrum are of three types (Fig. 10.2-5):

Association fibers. Association fibers connect the different gyri of the same hemisphere:

Commissural fibers. Commissural fibers connect the corresponding parts of two cerebral hemispheres with each other. There are five bundles of commissural fibers.

1. Corpus callosum
2. Anterior commissure
3. Posterior commissure

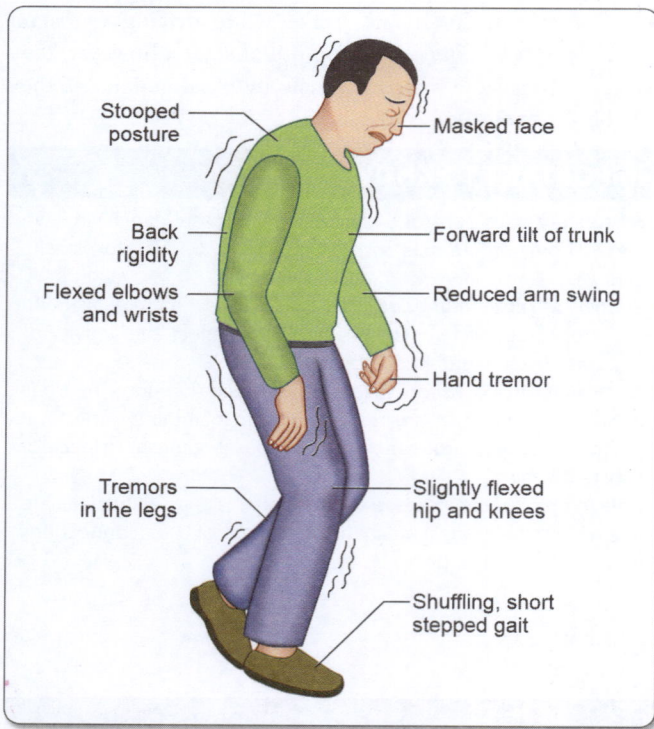

Fig. 10.2-6: Parkinson's disease symptoms

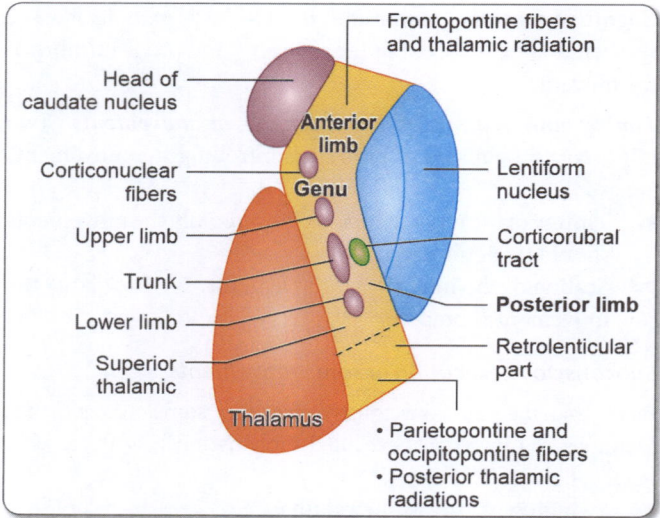

Fig. 10.2-7: Parts of internal capsule: disposition of motor fibers and thalamic radiations passing through it.

4. Habenular commissure
5. Hippocampal commissure.

Projection fibers. Projection fibers connect the cerebral hemispheres with other parts of CNS, e.g., thalamus, brain stem and spinal cord. Projection fibers include the afferent and efferent tracts contained in corona radiata and internal capsule.

Corona radiata. Corona radiata (fountain of fibers) refers to that part of projection fibers that radiates from the upper end of internal capsule to cerebral cortex. It contains both the ascending and descending fibers.

Internal capsule. Internal capsule is a thick curved band of projection fibers (ascending and descending) that occupy the space between the thalamus and caudate nucleus medially, and the lentiform nucleus laterally. Superiorly, it fans out as corona radiata and inferiorly, the fibers descend into the crus cerebri. The internal capsule can be divided into the following parts Fig. 10.2-7:

- Anterior limb
- Genu
- Posterior limb
- Retrolenticular of caudal part
- Sublentiform part.

DIENCEPHALON

The diencephalon consists of:

- Thalamus
- Hypothalamus.

THALAMUS

Gross Anatomy

The thalamus is a large ovoid structure placed immediately lateral to the third ventricle (Figs 10.2-8 and 10.2-9).

Posterior end (or pole) is expanded and is called pulvinar.

Dorsal or superior surface of the thalamus is convex and forms the part of floor of the central part of lateral ventricle (Fig. 10.2-9).

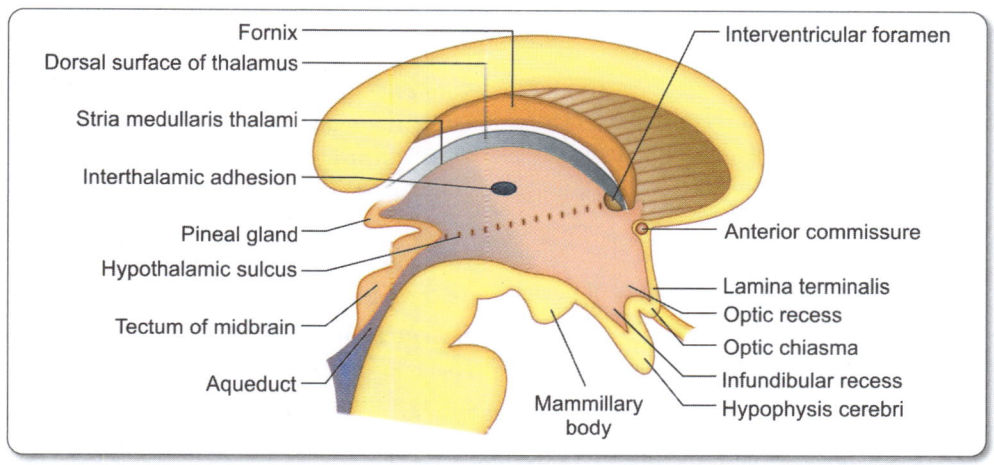

Fig. 10.2-8: Median section through the brain showing medial surface of thalamus and hypothalamus

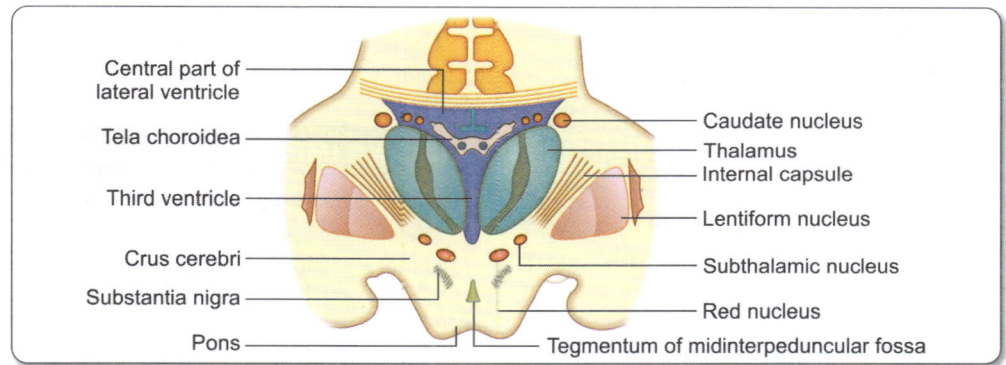

Fig. 10.2-9: Coronal section through the brain passing through the basilar part of pons showing the relations of ventral surface of thalamus and subthalamic structures

Medial surface forms the greater part of the lateral wall of third ventricle and is lined by ependyma. The medial surfaces of the two thalami are connected by a short bar of grey matter called the *interthalamic adhesion*. Inferiorly, the medial surface is separated from the hypothalamus by *hypothalamic sulcus* (Fig. 10.2-8).

Lateral surface of thalamus is related to the posterior limbs of internal capsule.

Internal Structure

Like other parts of brain, thalamus consists of grey matter (mainly) and white matter (Fig. 10.2-10).

White Matter

White matter is scanty in thalamus and includes:

Stratum zonale, a thin layer of white matter covering the superior surface of thalamus.

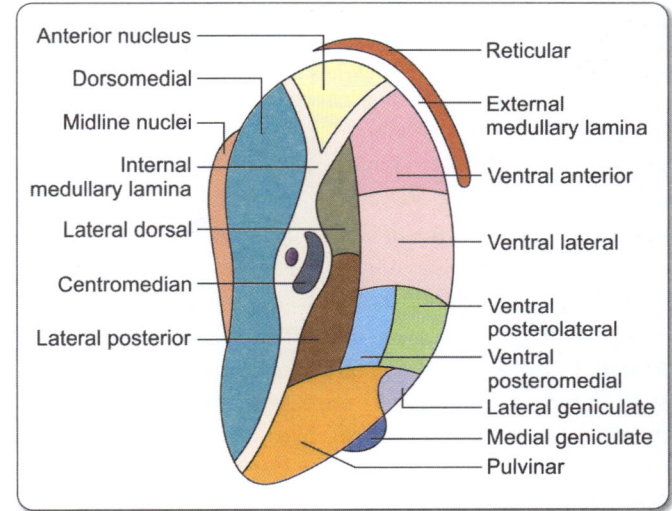

Fig. 10.2-10: Horizontal section of right thalamus (superior aspect) white matter and grey matter showing nuclear subdivisions

External medullary lamina is a thin layer of white matter covering the lateral surface of thalamus. It consists of thalamocortical and corticothalamic fibers.

Internal medullary lamina is a Y-shaped sheet of white matter placed vertically in the grey matter of thalamus. It consists mainly of internuclear thalamic connections.

Grey Matter

Grey matter of thalamus is divided into three masses of nuclei by the Y-shaped internal medullary lamina.

- Anterior group of nuclei
- Lateral group of nuclei
- Medial group of nuclei.

Functionally, the thalamic nuclei can be grouped under two divisions:

1. Non-specific projection nuclei
2. Specific projection nuclei.

Functions and Connections

Various functions of thalamus along with the connections through which these functions are mediated are summarized below:

1. Sensory relay center. Almost all the sensory impulses (except olfactory) reach the thalamic nuclei, which relay them to the cerebral cortex by thalamic radiations (ascending thalamocortical system). Because of this, thalamus is usually considered the *head ganglion* of all the sensory system.

2. Center for integration of sensory impulses. The thalamus also forms a major center for integration and modification of peripheral sensory impulses before the impulses are projected to specific areas of cerebral cortex. Because of this, thalamus is usually considered as a *functional gateway* of cerebral cortex.

3. Crude center for perception of sensations. Thalamus also acts as a crude center for sense perception. Pain sensation is perceived in the thalamus itself. Whether a sensation is pleasant or unpleasant and agreeable or disagreeable, is the function of thalamus.

4. Center for integration of motor function. Thalamus receives the output from the basal ganglia and the cerebellum before projecting it to the motor cortex, thereby helping in integration of motor functions by unconscious regulation of muscle tone.

5. Role in arousal and alertness reaction. Majority of non-specific ascending impulses from RAS are relayed to thalamus before proceeding to cortex. Through these fibers the thalamus is involved in controlling the level of consciousness and maintaining state of alertness and wakefulness.

6. Role in emotional aspect of behavior. Because of intimate connections between thalamus and frontal cortex and hypothalamus, the thalamus is involved in subjective feeling of various emotions.

7. Role in language. Thalamus is also concerned with language (speech) function. Integration between different cortical parts by subcortical connections in the thalamus helps to achieve speech.

8. Role in synchronization of electroencephalogram. Thalamus also plays an important role in the genesis of synchronization of electroencephalogram (EEG).

9. Center for integration of visceral and somatic function. Thalamus receives somatic as well as autonomic sensations, and is also connected with hypothalamus. Because of this it also acts as a center for integration of visceral and somatic functions.

10. Center for sexual sensations. Thalamus also acts as a center for perception of sexual sensations.

11. Center for reflex activity. All the sensory fibers relay in thalamus, so it forms the center for many reflex activities.

NURSING IMPLICATIONS AND APPLICATIONS

Thalamic Syndrome

The thalamic syndrome is a disturbance of emotional responses to sensory experience characterized by symptoms and signs which occur on the opposite side of the body. These include:

Astereognosis occurs due to loss of tactile localization, tactile discrimination and stereognosis.

Thalamic over-reaction, i.e., the threshold for pain, touch and temperature is decreased and the sensations become exaggerated and disagreeable.

- Ataxia, decreased muscle tone and profound muscular weakness.
- Involuntary movements.

HYPOTHALAMUS

The hypothalamus is a bilateral diencephalic diffuse nuclear mass situated below the thalamus. It is the most important organ of integration in the homeostatic control of internal environment.

Subdivisions and Nuclei of Hypothalamus

For convenience of description, the hypothalamus can be divided as:

From medial to lateral into two zones:

1. Medial zone
2. Lateral zone.

From anterior to posterior, the hypothalamic nuclear mass is arranged in four regions (Fig. 10.2-11):

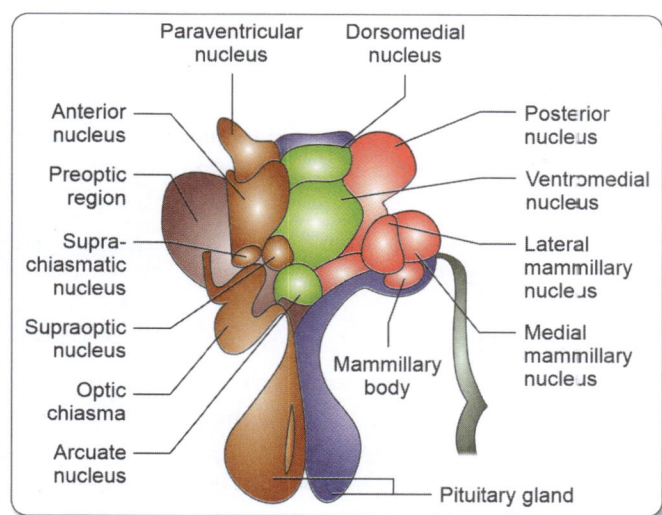

Fig. 10.2-11: Nuclei of hypothalamus
1. Preoptic region
2. Supraoptic region
3. Tuberal region
4. Mammillary region.

Connections of Hypothalamus

The hypothalamus serves as the main integrator of the autonomic nervous system and is concerned with visceral functions, and is, therefore, connected to other areas having a similar function. These include the various parts of the limbic system, the reticular formation, and autonomic centers in the brain stem and spinal cord.

Apart from its neural connections, the hypothalamus also acts by releasing secretions into the blood stream, and into the CSF.

Functions of Hypothalamus

Autonomic functions subserved by the hypothalamus are:

Cardiovascular regulation, through cardiovascular control centers in the reticular regions of medulla and pons.

Regulation of peristaltic and secretomotor functions of alimentary tract.

Endocrinal Functions

Control of anterior pituitary. Hypothalamus does the following functions through the releasing hormones:
- Controls the metabolism by controlling thyroid gland. For details see page 270
- Through its influence over adrenal cortex, controls the metabolism of different foodstuffs and maintains electrolyte balance. For details see page 278

- Keeps the gonads inhibited till the physical growth is complete. After physical growth is complete this inhibition is removed so that gonads start functioning and gametes are produced (propagation of species). For details see page 440
- Controls the formation of milk by the breasts by controlling prolactin secretion. For details see page 466.

Regulation of posterior pituitary functions. Neural control of posterior pituitary with the secretion of antidiuretic hormone (ADH) in regulation of water balance by controlling water excretion by kidneys. For details see page 262

Regulation of uterine contractility and regulation of milk ejection from the breast. Oxytocin secretion increases the contractility of uterus especially at end of the pregnancy and thus, helps during parturition. It also contracts the myoepithelial cells that surround the alveoli of breast and cause milk ejection. When the baby suckles the breast, signals from nipple to hypothalamus cause reflex oxytocin release which causes expulsion of milk through nipples. For details see page 467

Control of Circadian Rhythm (Biological Clock)

Circadian rhythm refers to rhythmic fluctuations in certain physiological parameters of the body. These are called circadian rhythms because they often show 24-hour cycles (circadian—around a day). *Common rhythmic variations* in homeostatic regulatory mechanism are:
- Rhythmic secretion of ACTH (see page 280)
- Rhythmic secretion of growth hormone (see page 263)
- Rhythmic secretion of melatonin (see page 291)
- Sleep-wake cycles (see page 291)
- Body temperature rhythm (see page 305)
- Rhythmic gonadotropin secretion (see page 460).

Regulation of Food Intake

Two centers namely, the *feeding center* and *the satiety center.* Normally, the feeding center is always active and its activity is inhibited by satiety center after food intake.

Regulation of Sexual Behavior and Reproduction

In animals, hypothalamus plays an important role in maintaining the sexual functions, especially in females. A decorticate female animal will have regular estrous cycle provided the hypothalamus is intact.

Emotional and Instinctual Behavior

The emotional and instinctual behavior is mainly regulated by limbic cortex. The two centers in hypothalamus involved in such a behavior and emotional changes are called *reward center* and *punishment center.*

Regulation of Body Temperature

The hypothalamus acts as principal integrating center for heat regulation. By adjusting a balance between heat production and heat loss, it helps to maintain body temperature at 37°C. Hypothalamus accomplishes this function by two centers: *heat loss center*, and *heat gain center*.

Regulation of Water Balance

Regulates water balance of the body by two mechanisms:
1. *Through thirst center* by controlling water intake, and
2. *Through osmoreceptors* in supraoptic nucleus by controlling water loss.

CLINICAL ASPECTS

Disturbances in hypothalamic lesions include:

- Autonomic disturbances
- Disturbances of body temperature regulation
- Sleep disturbances due to lesions in mammillary body and anterior hypothalamus
- Endocrine abnormalities, e.g., hypogonadism, and hypothyroidism
- Disturbance in sexual functions due to involvement of mid-hypothalamus
- Disturbance of body water balance due to damage to supraoptic nuclei or infundibular stalk, characterized by excessive thirst and polyuria
- Emotional disturbances leading to sham rage due to lesions in ventromedial and posterolateral parts.

BRAIN STEM

The brain stem consists (from below upward) of the medulla oblongata, pons and midbrain (Fig. 10.2-12A).

MEDULLA OBLONGATA

The medulla oblongata is conical in shape and connects the pons above and to the spinal cord below.

External Features

Surface of Medulla Exhibits (Fig. 10.2-12B)

Median fissure, present in the center of anterior surface of medulla, is continuous below with the anterior median fissure of spinal cord.

Pyramids are two swellings, one each present on either side of median fissure. These are composed of bundles of nerve fibers that originate in large nerve cells in the precentral gyrus of the cerebral cortex.

Olives are oval-shaped elevations, present one on each side just posterior to the pyramids. These are produced by the underlying olivary nuclei.

Inferior cerebellar peduncles, which connect the medulla to cerebellum, are present behind the olives.

Gracilis and cuneatus tubercles (produced by the medially placed underlying nucleus gracilis and nucleus cuneatus, respectively) are present on the posterior surface of the inferior part of the medulla oblongata.

Cranial nerves 9th, 10th, 11th and 12th emerge from the surface of medulla.

Internal Structure

The main features of the internal structure of the medulla oblongata are most easily reviewed by examining cross-sections at the following levels:

- The level of pyramidal decussation (Fig. 10.2-13A)
- Transverse section at the level of sensory decussation (Fig. 10.2-13B).

Functions

Pathway for ascending and descending tracts. The medulla oblongata forms the main pathway for the ascending and descending tracts of spinal cord.

House of vital centers. The medulla oblongata houses many important centers which control the vital functions of the body:

Respiratory centers (inspiratory and expiratory) control the normal rhythmic respiration

Vasomotor and cardiac centers control the blood pressure and functions of heart and vascular system

Deglutition center controls the pharyngeal and esophageal phase of deglutition

Vomiting center is responsible for inducing vomiting in disorders of gastrointestinal tract

Superior and inferior salivary nuclei, located in the medulla, control the salivary secretion.

Cranial nerve nuclei located in the medulla control the following functions:

Twelfth cranial (hypoglossal) nerve controls the movements of tongue

Eleventh cranial (accessory) nerve controls the movements of shoulder

Tenth cranial (vagus) nerve controls the functions of important viscera a viz, heart, lungs and gastrointestinal tract.

Eighth cranial nerve controls the auditory function (cochlear division of the nerve has the relay in medulla oblongata) and vestibular function (medial and inferior vestibular nuclei extend through much of the medulla).

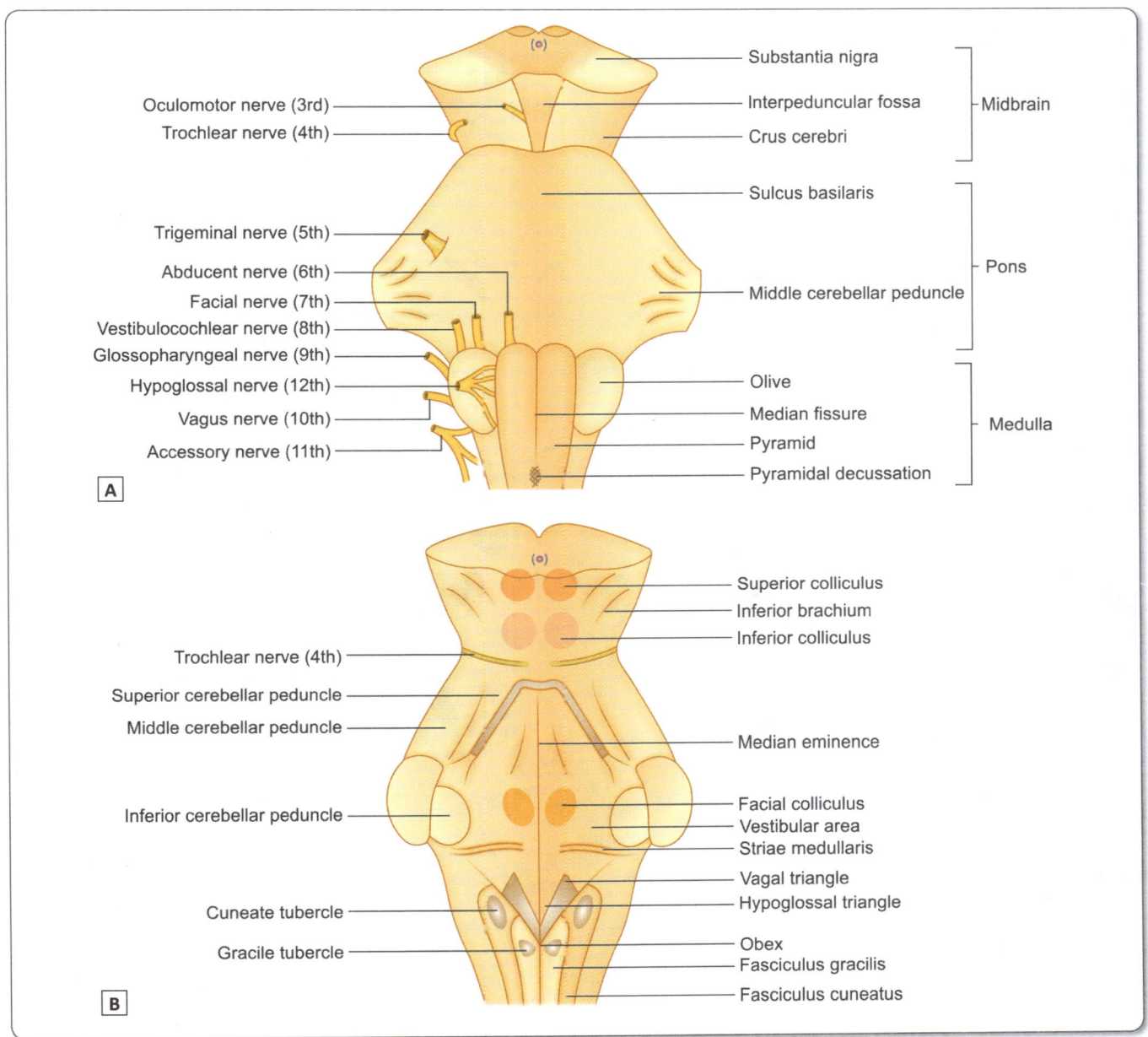

Figs 10.2-12A and B: Gross anatomy of brain stem: A. Ventral aspect; B. Dorsal aspect

PONS

The pons is situated on the anterior surface of the cerebellum below the midbrain and above the medulla oblongata.

Internal Structure

Internally pons is divisible into two parts (Fig. 10.2-14):

Ventral (Basilar) Part of the Pons Contains

Transverse fibers, laterally form the middle cerebellar peduncle.
Vertical fibers, present in the pons, are of two types:
  1. *Corticopontine fibers*
  2. *Corticospinal fibers*
Pontine nuclei are the groups of neurons which are scattered amongst the nerve fibers.

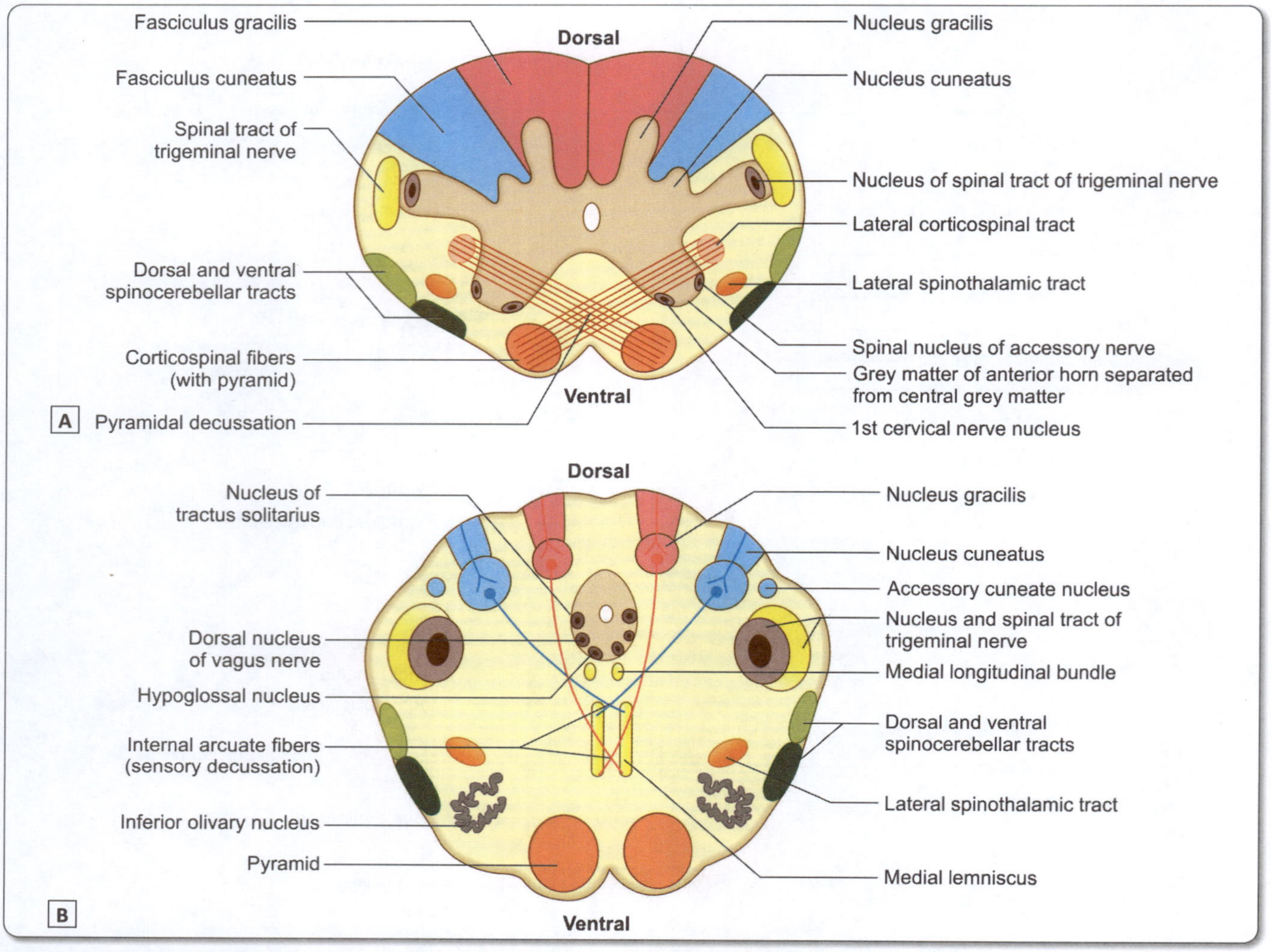

Fasciculus gracilis

Fasciculus cuneatus

Spinal tract of trigeminal nerve

Dorsal and ventral spinocerebellar tracts

Corticospinal fibers (with pyramid)

A Pyramidal decussation

Dorsal

Ventral

Nucleus gracilis

Nucleus cuneatus

Nucleus of spinal tract of trigeminal nerve

Lateral corticospinal tract

Lateral spinothalamic tract

Spinal nucleus of accessory nerve

Grey matter of anterior horn separated from central grey matter

1st cervical nerve nucleus

Dorsal

Nucleus of tractus solitarius

Dorsal nucleus of vagus nerve

Hypoglossal nucleus

Internal arcuate fibers (sensory decussation)

Inferior olivary nucleus

Pyramid

B

Ventral

Nucleus gracilis

Nucleus cuneatus

Accessory cuneate nucleus

Nucleus and spinal tract of trigeminal nerve

Medial longitudinal bundle

Dorsal and ventral spinocerebellar tracts

Lateral spinothalamic tract

Medial lemniscus

Figs 10.2-13A and B: Main features of internal structure of medulla oblongata exhibited by transverse section at the level of: A. Pyramidal decussation; B. Sensory decussation

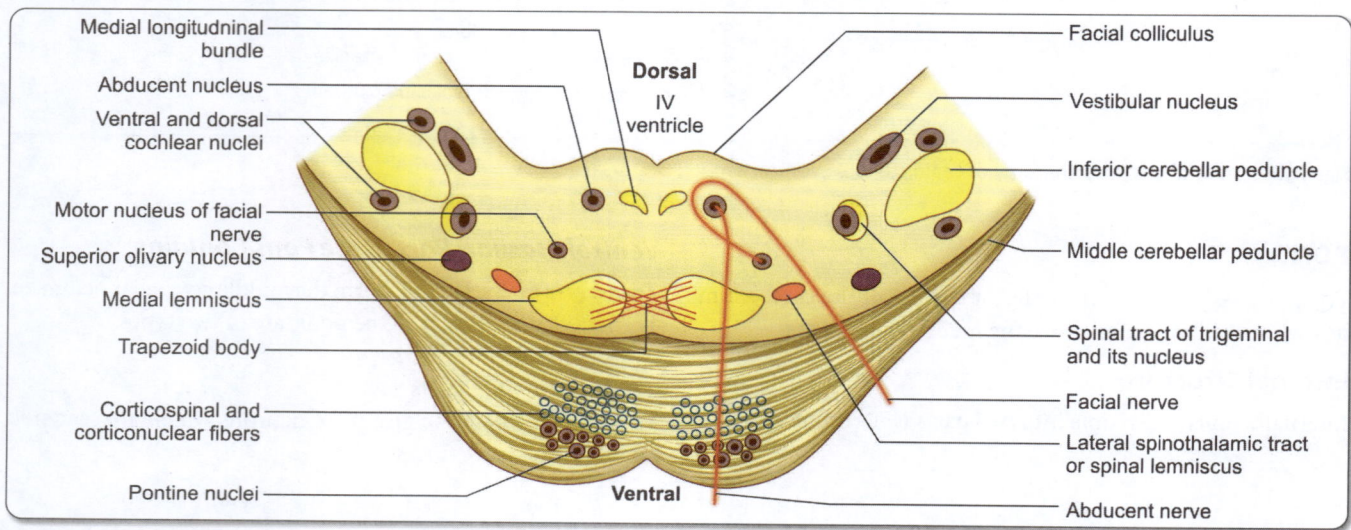

Medial longitudnninal bundle

Abducent nucleus

Ventral and dorsal cochlear nuclei

Motor nucleus of facial nerve

Superior olivary nucleus

Medial lemniscus

Trapezoid body

Corticospinal and corticonuclear fibers

Pontine nuclei

Dorsal

IV ventricle

Ventral

Facial colliculus

Vestibular nucleus

Inferior cerebellar peduncle

Middle cerebellar peduncle

Spinal tract of trigeminal and its nucleus

Facial nerve

Lateral spinothalamic tract or spinal lemniscus

Abducent nerve

Fig. 10.2-14: Internal structure of pons

Dorsal (Tegmental) Part of Pons

- Decussations of trapezoid body
- Nuclei of 5th, 6th, 7th and 8th cranial nerves
- Pontine reticular formation
- A number of descending and ascending tracts.

The most prominent ascending tracts are the four lemnisci: (i) medial, (ii) trigeminal, (iii) spinal, (iv) lateral.

Functions

Pons subserves the following functions:

- Connecting pathway between cerebral cortex and cerebellum.
- Pathway for ascending and descending tracts of spinal cord and medulla oblongata.
- Joining station for medial lemniscus with fibers of 5th, 7th, 9th and 10th cranial nerves.
- Contains pneumotaxic and apneustic centers for regulation of respiration.

MIDBRAIN

The midbrain is a narrow part of the brain that connects forebrain to hindbrain.

Posterior surface of midbrain exhibits:

Superior colliculi, two rounded swellings, one on each side of midline.

Inferior colliculi, two rounded swellings, one on each side of the midline located below the superior colliculi.

Internal Structure

Internally for convenience of description, the midbrain can be divided into two parts (Fig. 10.2-15):

1. **Tectum.** It consists of superior and inferior colliculi.
2. **Cerebral peduncles.** Each cerebral peduncle, in turn, consists of three parts, which from anterior to posterior side are:

Crus cerebri (or Basis Pedunculi)

It consists of large mass of vertically running descending fibers from cerebral cortex which include frontopontine fibers, corticospinal and corticonuclear fibers and temporopontine, parietopontine and occipitopontine fibers (occupying the lateral one-sixth of crus).

Substantia nigra is a mass of pigmented grey matter (therefore, appears dark in color).

Tegmentum of the two sides is continuous across the midline. It contains the following important masses of grey matter and nerve fibers:

- Red nucleus
- Nuclei of 3rd, 4th and 5th cranial nerves
- Reticular formation of midbrain
- Fiber bundles of the tegmentum
- Three decussations.

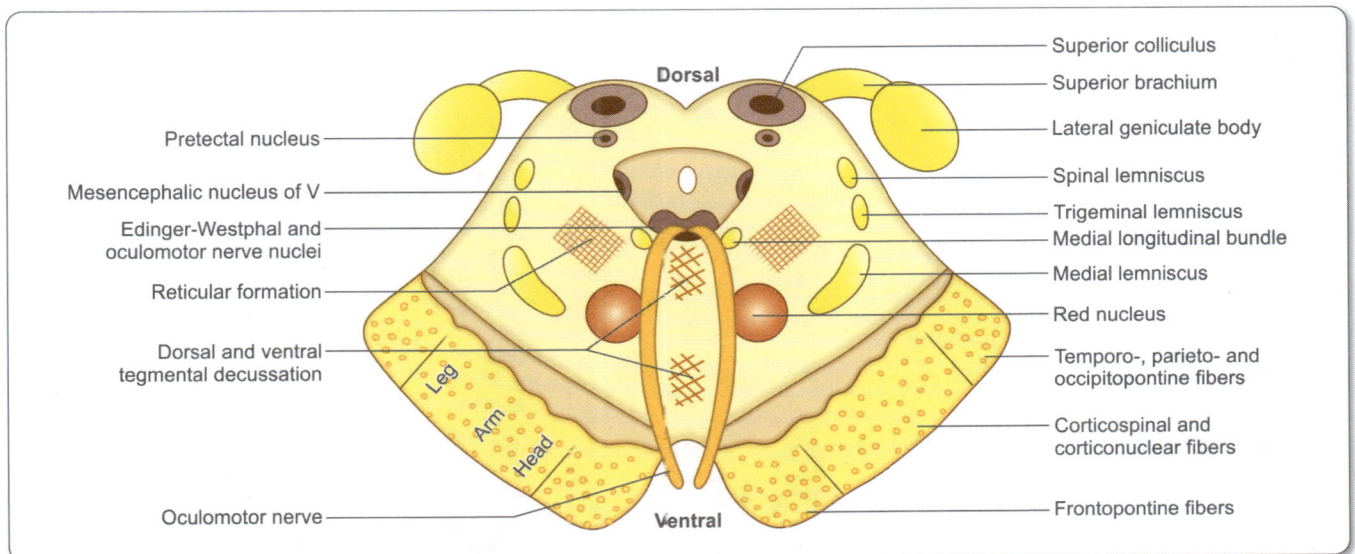

Fig. 10.2-15: Internal structure of midbrain exhibited by transverse section at the level of superior colliculi

CEREBELLUM

GROSS ANATOMY

Cerebellum, the largest part of hindbrain, consists of two lateral parts called the *cerebellar hemispheres* connected in the midline by a narrow central region called the *vermis*.

The cerebellum is thrown into numerous transverse folds called folia. The surface of the cerebellum presents three main fissures (Figs 10.2-16A and B):

1. *Primary fissure* is V-shaped, with open being forward. It forms the posterior limit of the anterior lobe.

2. *Horizontal fissure* separates the superior surface of the cerebellum from its inferior surface.

3. *Posterolateral fissure* is situated anteriorly on the inferior surface of the cerebellar hemisphere and separates the posterior lobe from the flocculonodular lobe.

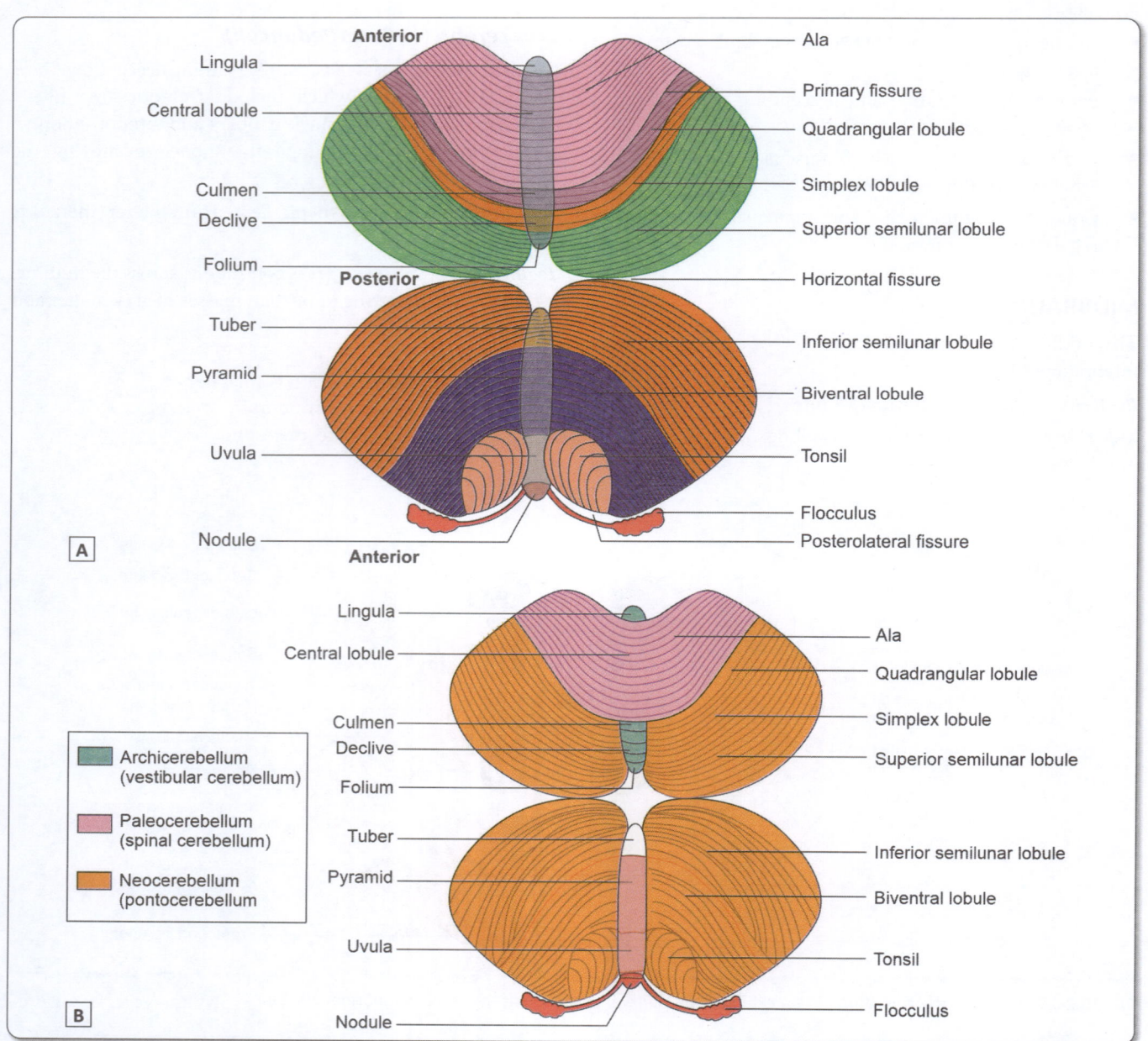

Figs 10.2-16A and B: Gross anatomy of cerebellum: A. Lobes and morphological subdivision of cerebellum; B. Functional subdivision of cerebellum

TABLE. 10.2-1: Lobes of cerebellum and parts of vermis and hemisphere forming them

Lobes of cerebellum	Part of vermis	Part of hemisphere
Anterior lobe	Lingula	No lateral projection
	Central lobule	Alae
	Culmen	Anterior quadrangular lobule
Primary fissure		
Posterior lobe	Declive	Posterior quadrangular lobule
	Folium	Superior semilunar lobule
Horizontal fissure		
	Tuber	Inferior semilunar lobule
	Pyramis	Biventral lobule
	Uvula	Tonsil
Posterolateral fissure		
Flocculo-nodular lobe	Nodule	Flocculus

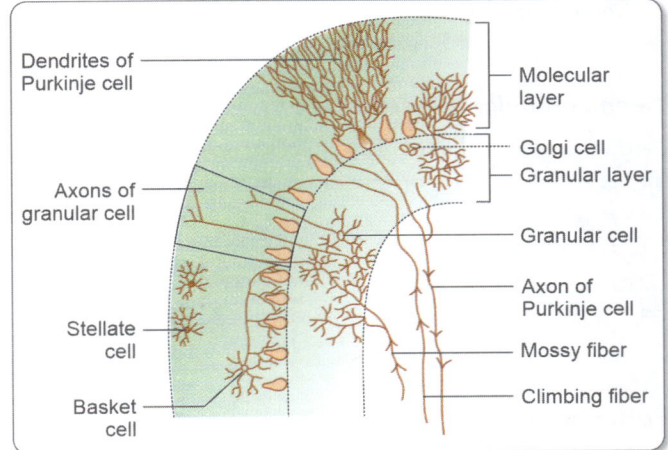

Fig. 10.2-17: Histology of cerebellar cortex

Vermis

Vermis is so named because it resembles a worm which is bent on itself to form a complete circle. It consists of the following parts: lingula, central lobule, culmen, declive, folium, tuber, pyramis, uvula and nodule (Table. 10.2-1).

Anatomical Divisions

Anatomically the cerebellum has been divided into three lobes.

1. *Anterior lobe* is that part of cerebellum which lies in front of the primary fissure on the superior surface.

2. *Posterior lobe* is that part of cerebellum which lies between the primary fissure and posterolateral fissure.

3. *Flocculonodular lobe* is that part of the cerebellum which lies anterior to the posterolateral fissure on the inferior surface. It consists of:

Nodule, which is rostral part of the vermis, and

Floculli, which are irregular shaped masses attached to nodule on each side. They are almost completely separated from the rest of cerebellum.

Histological Structure

Histologically, cerebellum consists of (Fig. 10.2-17):
- Cerebellar cortex (outer grey matter layer)
- White matter (formed by afferent and efferent nerve fibers of cerebellum) forming medullary core
- Deep cerebellar nuclei (masses of grey matter embedded in the medullary core).

Cerebellar Cortex

Microscopically the grey matter of cerebellar cortex consists of five main types of neurons (stellate cells, basket cells, Purkinje cells, granule cells and Golgi cells) which are arranged in three layers:

1. *Molecular layer* (most superficial) is composed of two types of neurons (stellate and basket cells) and unmyelinated nerve fibers.

2. *Purkinje cell layer.* It is composed of a single layer of large flask-shaped Purkinje cells and dendrites of Purkinje cells.

3. *Granule cell layer* consists of granule and Golgi cells, with their processes, and sensory mossy fibers with their synaptic glomeruli.

White Matter of Cerebellum

The cerebellar cortex, i.e., outer grey matter surrounds inner medullary core of white matter (an arrangement opposite to what is seen in spinal cord). White matter is formed by both afferent and efferent fibers. These fibers can be classified in three groups:

1. *Projection fibers* of the cerebellum leave or enter the cerebellum. These are arranged in three bundles:

a. *Inferior cerebellar peduncle* consists of fibers connecting cerebellum with medulla

b. *Middle cerebellar peduncle* contains the fibers which connect cerebellum with pons

c. *Superior cerebellar peduncle* which connects the cerebellum with midbrain.

2. *Association fibers* connect different regions of the same cerebellar hemisphere.

3. *Commissural fibers* connect the areas of two halves of cerebellar cortex with each other.

Deep Cerebellar Nuclei

Within the white matter of medullary core of cerebellum are embedded four pairs of masses of grey matter called deep cerebellar nuclei.

1. *Dentate nucleus*
2. *Emboliform nucleus*
3. *Globossus nucleus*
4. *Fastigial nucleus*

Functions of Cerebellum

Control of Body Posture and Equilibrium

Vestibulocerebellum which includes flocculonodular lobe as its principal component and nucleus fastigii (as its effector nucleus) and vermal region of the cerebellum are concerned with control of body posture and equilibrium.

Control of Muscle Tone and Stretch Reflexes

Spinocerebellum regulates the postural reflexes by modifying muscle tone. It facilitates the gamma motor neurons in the spinal cord. The γ motor neurons reflexly modify the activity of α motor neurons and thus, regulate the muscle tone. Thus, cerebellum forms an important site of linkage of α-γ systems responsible for muscle tone.

Control of Voluntary Movements

Cerebellum is not able to initiate any motor activity, but coordinates movements initiated by the motor cortex.

Control of movements by cerebellum includes regulation of time, rate, range (extent), force and direction of muscular activity.

Other Functions of Cerebellum

Recent studies have shown the importance of the cerebellum as:

Influence on autonomic system. It has been postulated that the cerebellum may influence autonomic functions and thus, respiratory, cardiovascular, pupillary and urinary bladder responses.

Influence on conduction in ascending sensory pathway. May be exerted by the cerebellum through the reticular formation and thalamus.

Control of eyeball movements. The oculomotor, trochlear and abducens nuclei which supply extraocular muscles of eye movements are brought under the cerebellar control through

vestibular nuclei. Medial longitudinal fasciculus is involved in these connections.

CLINICAL ASPECTS

Cerebellar Lesions

Common signs observed in patients with cerebellar dysfunction due to lesions of cerebellum are:

Disturbances in tone and posture include:

Atonia or hypotonia: Hypotonia refers to reduction and atonia to loss of tone in muscles. It occurs due to reduction of the facilitatory neocerebellar output to the descending inhibitory reticular formation.

Attitude changes: Trunk is bent with concavity toward the affected side; this is because the weight of the body is thrown on the unaffected leg.

Deviation movement: The arm held straight out in front of the body deviates laterally when the eyes are closed. In bilateral lesions both arms deviate.

Effect on deep reflexes: The deep or tendon reflexes become weak and pendular.

Disturbances in equilibrium: The patient suffering from disturbance of equilibrium walks on a wide base, sways from side to side (drunken-like gait), and is unable to maintain the upright posture due to involvement of vestibular system.

Disturbances in movements include:

Ataxia, i.e., lack of coordination of movements, is the hallmark of cerebellar disorder.

Intention tremors become evident during purposeful movements, and diminish or disappear with rest. These tremors become more marked as the hand approaches the object, i.e., are observed at the end of movement and are coarse, oscillating, to and fro and rhythmic.

Nystagmus refers to regular and rhythmic to and fro involuntary oscillatory movements of the eyes, occurring due to incoordination of extraocular muscles.

Dysarthria or scanning speech occurs due to incoordination of various muscles and structures involved in speech.

MENINGES AND CAVITIES

MENINGES

The brain is enclosed within the cranial cavity by three concentric connective tissue layers: pia mater, arachnoid mater and dura mater, which constitute the meninges of the brain (Fig. 10.2-18).

Pia Mater

Pia mater, covering closely and continuously the external surface of the brain, is a thin and highly vascular membrane. Folds of pia mater enclose tufts of capillaries called choroid plexuses to form tela choroidea in relation to ventricles of brain.

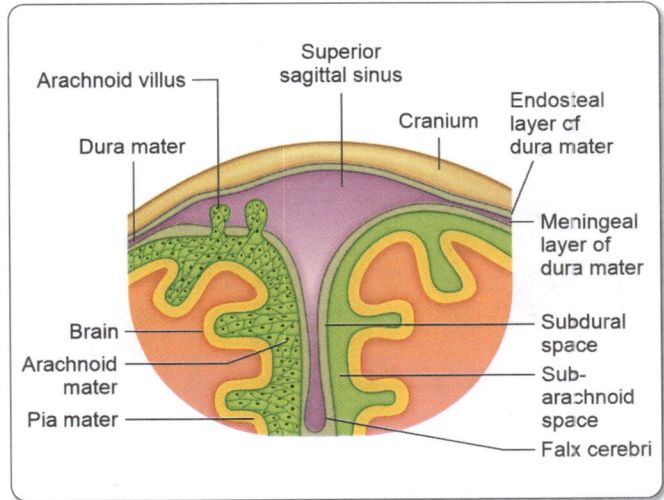

Fig. 10.2-18: Meninges of brain

Arachnoid Mater

Arachnoid mater is connected to the pia mater by many filamentous fibers. Subarachnoid space between these two layers is filled with cerebrospinal fluid (CSF).

Dura Mater

Dura mater is composed of two layers: outer endosteal and inner meningeal. These are fused except where folds form (e.g., falx cerebri) or venous sinuses (e.g., superior sagittal sinus) are enclosed between them. *Subdural space* separates the dura mater from arachnoid mater. The arachnoid mater has minute protrusions (*arachnoid villi*), which pass through fenestrae in the dura mater and project into the venous sinuses to allow escape of CSF into venous sinuses.

CAVITIES OF THE BRAIN

The interior of the brain has cavities (ventricles) containing cerebrospinal fluid are:

Lateral Ventricle (Fig. 10.2-19)

Lateral ventricles: Right and left two lateral ventricles are situated within each cerebral hemisphere. Each ventricle is C shaped having central part with three extensions called anterior, posterior and inferior horns (Fig. 10.2-19).

- *Anterior horn* extends into the frontal lobe
- *Posterior horn* extends into the occipital lobe
- *Inferior horn* extends into the temporal lobe

The lateral ventricles are connected to the third ventricle through interventricular foramina called *Foramen of Munro.*

Third Ventricle (Fig. 10.2-20)

Third ventricle is a slit like cavity between two thalami (Fig. 10.2-20) has anterior and posterior walls, floor and roof. The relations of third ventricle are shown in Fig. 10.2-21 and Table 10.2-2. Inferiorly it continues into cerebral aqueduct (aqueduct of Sylvius), which connects it to the fourth ventricle.

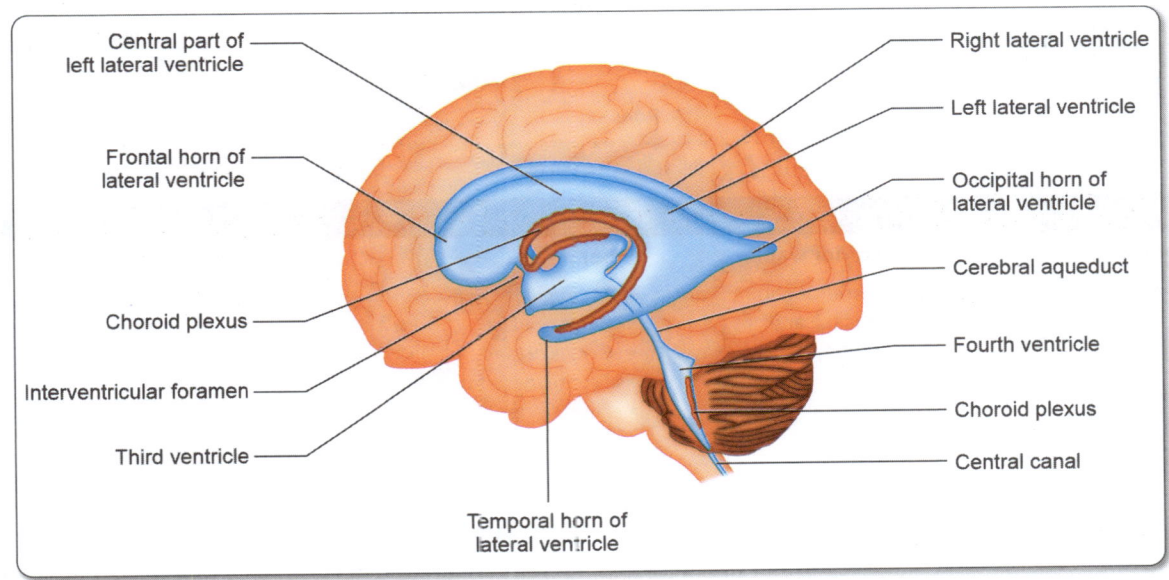

Fig. 10.2-19: Parts of lateral ventricle

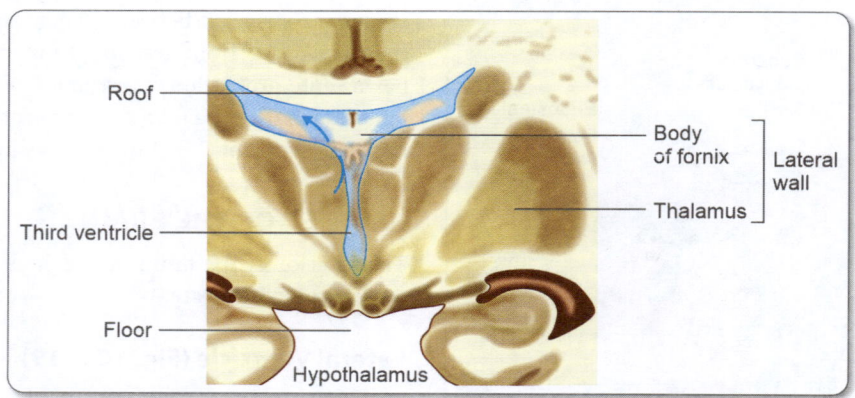

Fig. 10.2-20: Third ventricle

Relations of Third Ventricle (Fig. 10.2-21) and Table 10.2-2

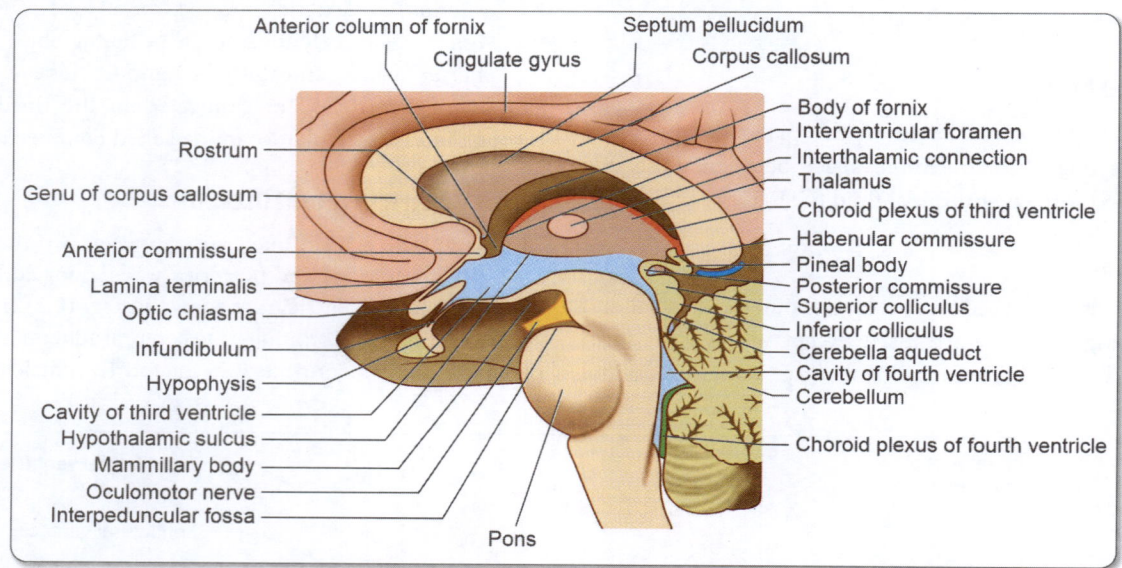

Fig. 10.2-21: Relations of third ventricle

TABLE 10.2-2: Relations of third ventricle			
Anterior wall	**Posterior wall**	**Floor**	**Lateral wall**
• Anterior commissure • Anterior column of fornix • Lamina terminalis	• Posterior commissure • Pineal gland	• Mammillary body • Infundibulum • Optic chiasma • Tuber cinereum • Posterior perforated substance • Tegmentum of midbrain	• Thalamus • Hypothalamus

Fourth Ventricle

It is the rhomboid (diamond) shaped cavity of hindbrain behind the lower part of pons and upper part of medulla.

Boundaries

Fourth ventricle and its relations are shown in Fig. 10.2-22 and Table 10.2-3.

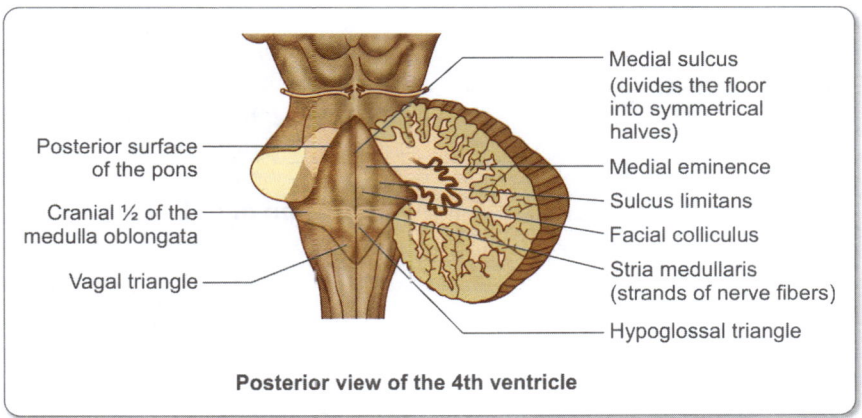

Posterior view of the 4th ventricle

Fig. 10.2-22: Boundaries of fourth ventricle

TABLE 10.2-3: Relations of fourth ventricle		
Lateral wall	**Roof**	**Floor**
• Above and laterally—superior cerebellar peduncle • Below and laterally—inferior cerebellar peduncle	• Superior and inferior medullary velum • Tela choroidea containing choroid plexus	• Rhomboidal shaped floor • Vestibular area containing vestibular nucleus lies lateral to sulcus limitans • Facial colliculus—facial nerve fibers (facial nerve nucleus) looping over abducens nucleus • Hypoglossal triangle overlying hypoglossal nucleus • Vagal triangle contains dorsal motor nucleus of vagus • Locus coeruleus—containing melanin pigment (substantia ferruginea) • Area postrema—chemoreceptor trigger zone

CEREBROSPINAL FLUID

Cerebrospinal fluid (CSF) cushions the brain and along with blood-brain barrier, the buffering function of neuroglia, and regulation of CNS circulation controls the extracellular environment of neurons. Within the substance of brain in the *ventricular system*, there are series of spaces filled with CSF.

COMPOSITION, VOLUME AND PRESSURE OF CSF

Composition of CSF

The extracellular fluid within the CNS communicates directly with the CSF. Thus, the composition of CSF indicates the composition of the extracellular environment of the neurons in the brain and spinal cord. The composition of CSF vis-a-vis blood is depicted in Table 10.2-4. The CSF differs from blood in having a lower concentration of K^+, glucose, and protein and a higher concentration of Na^+ and Cl^-. CSF normally lacks blood cells. The increased concentration of Na^+ and

TABLE 10.2-4: Composition of CSF vis-a-vis blood		
Constituent	**Lumbar CSF**	**Blood**
Na^+ (mEq/L)	148	136–145
K^+ (mEq/L)	2.9	3.5–5
Cl^- (mEq/L)	120–130	100–106
Glucose (mg/dL)	50–75	70–100
Protein (mg/dL)	15–45	6.8×10^3
pH	7.3	7.4

Cl^- enables the CSF to be isotonic to blood, despite the much lower concentration of proteins in the CSF.

Volume and pressure of CSF

The cranial cavity contains about 140 mL CSF.

The volume of CSF within the cerebral ventricles is approximately 40 mL, and that in the subarachnoid space is about 100 mL. The pressure in the CSF column is about 120–180 mm H_2O when a person is recumbent. Rate of CSF formation (about 0.35 mL/minute) is independent of CSF pressure as well as systemic blood pressure.

FORMATION, CIRCULATION, AND ABSORPTION OF CSF

Formation of CSF

The CSF is mainly formed by the choroidal plexuses, which are covered by specialized ependymal cells. The *choroidal plexuses* are located in the cerebral ventricles (lateral, third and fourth). About 500 mL of CSF is secreted per day.

Circulation of CSF (Fig. 10.2-23)

Cerebrospinal fluid formed in the lateral ventricles passes through the interventricular foramina (of Monro) into the third ventricle. Thence, the fluid flows through the cerebral aqueduct (of Sylvius) into the fourth ventricle. From fourth ventricle, some CSF passes into the central canal of spinal cord, but most escapes into the subarachnoid space (surrounding the brain and spinal cord) through the median aperture

(foramen of Magendie) of fourth ventricle and the two lateral apertures of fourth ventricle (foramina of Luschka).

Subarachnoid cistern refers to the regions where subarachnoid space is distended to form pools of CSF. An example is the *lumbar cistern* which surrounds the lumbar and sacral spinal roots below the level of termination of spinal cord. The lumbar cistern is the target for lumbar puncture, a procedure used clinically to sample the CSF.

Absorption of CSF

A large part of CSF is removed by bulk flow through the valvular *arachnoid villi* into the dural venous sinuses in the cranium. Unlike rate of formation, the absorption rate of CSF is a direct function of the CSF pressure.

FUNCTIONS OF CSF

- *Protection to CNS* by acting as a 'water-jacket', as it absorbs shock in the event of blow
- *Removal of waste products* of brain metabolism
- *Regulates extracellular environment* for the neurons of central nervous system
- *Transports* hormones and hormone-releasing factors.

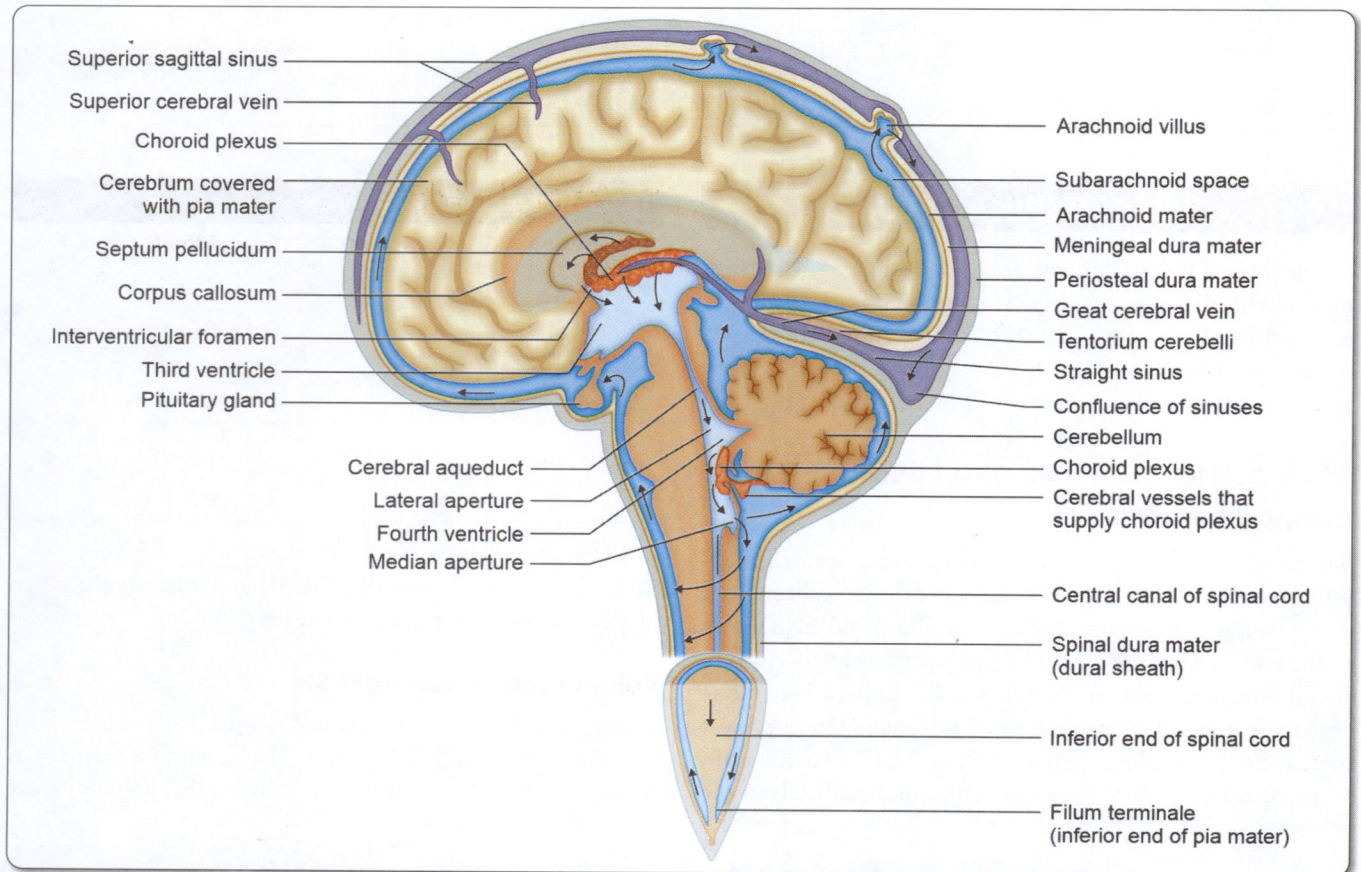

Fig. 10.2-23: Circulation of cerebrospinal fluid. Arrows indicate the direction of flow of cerebrospinal fluid

CLINICAL ASPECTS

Hydrocephalus (Figs 10.2-24A and B)

Hydrocephalus refers to an abnormal accumulation of CSF in the cranium.

Causes of hydrocephalus include:

- Obstruction to CSF circulation
- Excessive production of CSF
- Interference with absorption

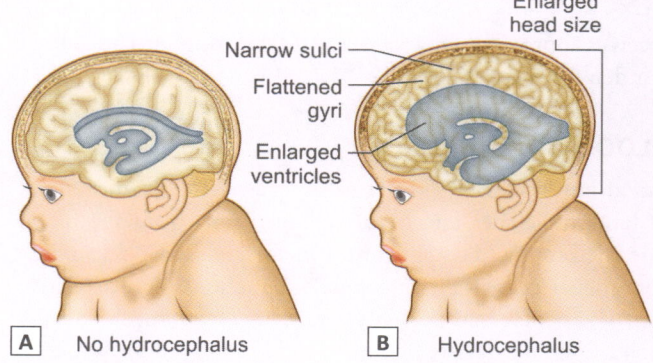

Figs 10.2-24A and B: A. Normal and B. Hydrocephalus

Lumbar and Cisternal Puncture

Lumbar Puncture

Lumbar puncture refers to tapping of CSF from lumbar cistern. CSF examination is required in many disorders of CNS. It is performed by inserting a needle in-between the L_2 and L_3 or L_3 and L_4 vertebrae (Fig. 10.2-25).

Cisternal Puncture

Cisternal puncture refers to tapping of CSF from cisterna magna. To do this, a needle is passed through the posterior atlanto-occipital membrane forward and upward to a depth of 4.5 cm from the surface.

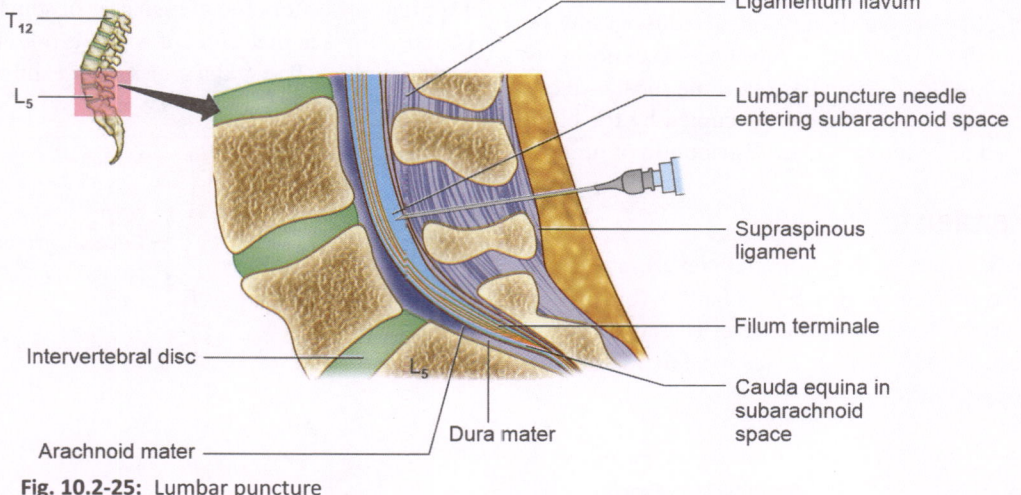

Fig. 10.2-25: Lumbar puncture

NURSING IMPLICATIONS AND APPLICATIONS

Hydrocephalus occurs at any age, but more frequently in infants. The signs and symptoms are:

- Headache
- Nausea and vomiting
- Sleepiness and dizziness
- Eyes foxed downwards
- Abnormal increase in head size is very common in infants (Fig. 10.2-24B)

CEREBRAL BLOOD FLOW, BLOOD-BRAIN BARRIER AND BLOOD-CSF BARRIER

Functioning of the brain is closely related to the level of cerebral blood flow. Total cessation of blood flow to the brain causes unconsciousness within 5–10 seconds because of the decrease in oxygen delivery and the resultant cessation of metabolic activity.

CEREBRAL BLOOD FLOW

Cerebral normal cerebral blood flow in an adult averages 50–65 mL/100 g, or about 750–900 mL/min. Thus, the brain receives approximately 15% of the total resting cardiac output. For detail see pages 209, 188.

BLOOD-BRAIN BARRIER

Blood-brain barrier (Fig. 10.2-26) restricts the movement of large molecules and highly charged ions from the blood into the brain and spinal cord. It is formed by CNS capillary endothelial cells, their intercellular junctions, and a relative lack of vesicular transport. Most substances that must cross the blood-brain barrier are not lipid soluble and therefore cross by specific carrier-mediated transport system.

Some areas of the brain do not have a blood-brain barrier, e.g., posterior pituitary and circumventricular organs. The absence of blood-brain barrier in these regions is consistent with their physiological functions. These leaky regions are isolated from the rest of the brain by specialized ependymal cells called *tanycytes*.

Disruption of blood-brain barrier occurs in a variety of pathological situations such as brain tumors and bacterial meningitis, etc. This fact can be exploited radiologically by introducing into the circulation a substance that normally cannot penetrate the blood-brain barrier. If the substance can be imaged, its leakage into the region occupied by the brain tumor can be used to demonstrate the distribution of tumor.

BLOOD-CSF BARRIER

The capillaries that traverse the choroidal plexuses are freely permeable to plasma solutes. However, a barrier (blood-CSF barrier) exists at the level of epithelial cells that make up the choroid plexuses. This barrier is responsible for carrier-mediated active transport.

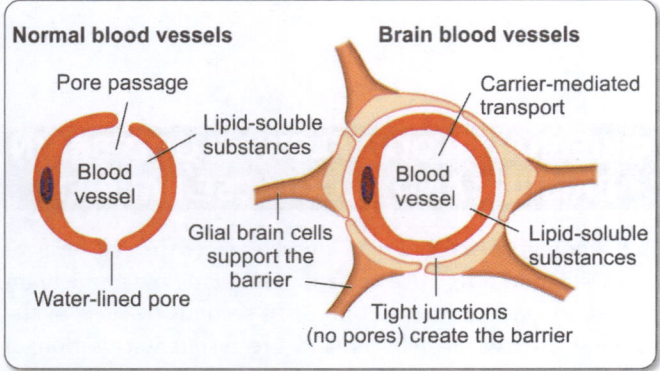

Fig. 10.2-26: Blood-brain barrier

SPINAL CORD

GROSS ANATOMY

- The spinal cord (Fig. 10.2-27) extends from the upper border of the first cervical vertebra to the lower border of the first lumbar vertebra.
- Its upper end becomes continuous with medulla oblongata and its lower end called *conus medullaris* becomes continuous with a fibrous cord called *filum terminale* (Fig. 10.2-1B).
- The spinal cord, like the brain, is surrounded by three meninges: (i) The dura mater, (ii) The arachnoid mater, (iii) The pia mater (Fig. 10.2-28).

INTERNAL STRUCTURE

As seen on cross-section (Fig. 10.2-29) the spinal cord presents inner grey matter and outer white matter. Grey matter is constituted by the nerve cell bodies, dendrites and parts of axons, while white matter is formed by the myelinated and unmyelinated nerve fibers.

Spinal Grey Matter

In transverse section, the grey matter of spinal cord forms an H-shaped mass in the center of which is present a canal called the spinal canal. The *spinal grey* matter exhibits the following parts:

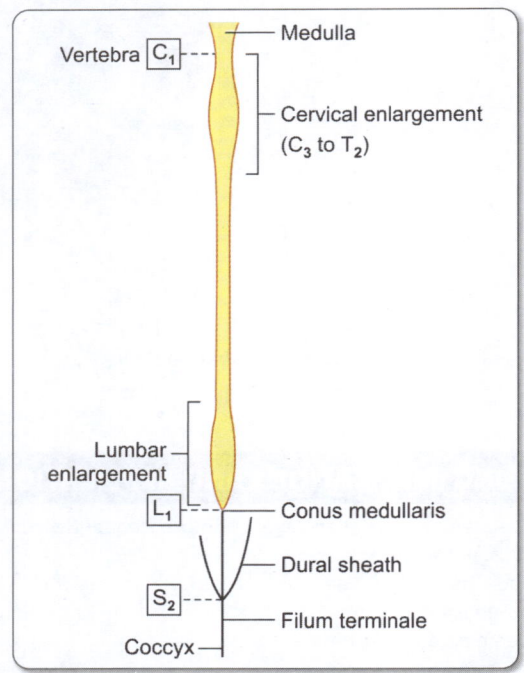

Fig. 10.2-27: Gross appearance of spinal cord and its relations with vertebrae

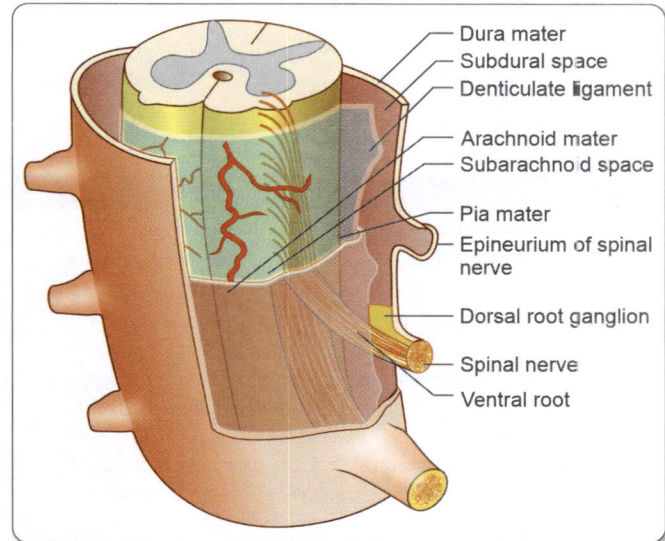

Fig. 10.2-28: Meninges of spinal cord

Dorsal horn or posterior grey column refers to the posterior horn-like projection of the H-shaped grey matter in each lateral half of the cord.

Ventral horn or anterior grey column refers to the anterior projection of the grey matter in each lateral half of the cord.

Lateral horn or intermediate horn or lateral column refers to small lateral projection between the ventral and dorsal grey columns, present in the thoracic segments and first two lumbar segments only.

Grey commissure is the part of the grey matter which connects the two (right and left) symmetrical halves of spinal grey matter across the midline. It is traversed by the central canal.

Neurons in Spinal Grey Matter

Neurons in ventral horn. The ventral horn neurons of spinal grey matter are involved in motor functions and send motor nerve fibers to the muscles and other effector organs.

Neurons in dorsal horn. The dorsal horn neurons of spinal grey matter are involved in sensory functions.

Neurons in the lateral horn. The lateral horn cells of spinal grey matter extend from T_1 to L_2 segments and from S_2 to S_4 segments of the spinal cord.

White Matter

White matter is formed by the nerve fibers which are arranged as ascending and descending tracts (described later). In general, the white matter of spinal cord is divided into right and left halves, in front by a deep *anterior median fissure*, and behind by the *posterior median septum*. In each half, the spinal white matter exhibits the following parts:

- Posterior funiculus or posterior white column
- Anterior funiculus or anterior white column
- Lateral funiculus
- Anterolateral funiculus
- Ventral (anterior) white commissure
- Dorsal (posterior) white commissure.

TRACTS OF SPINAL CORD

The tracts that transmit sensory impulses to the brain are termed ascending tracts and the tracts which are responsible for transmission of motor impulses from the brain to motor neurons reaching muscles and glands. There are numerous ascending and descending tracts in the spinal cord and brain stem.

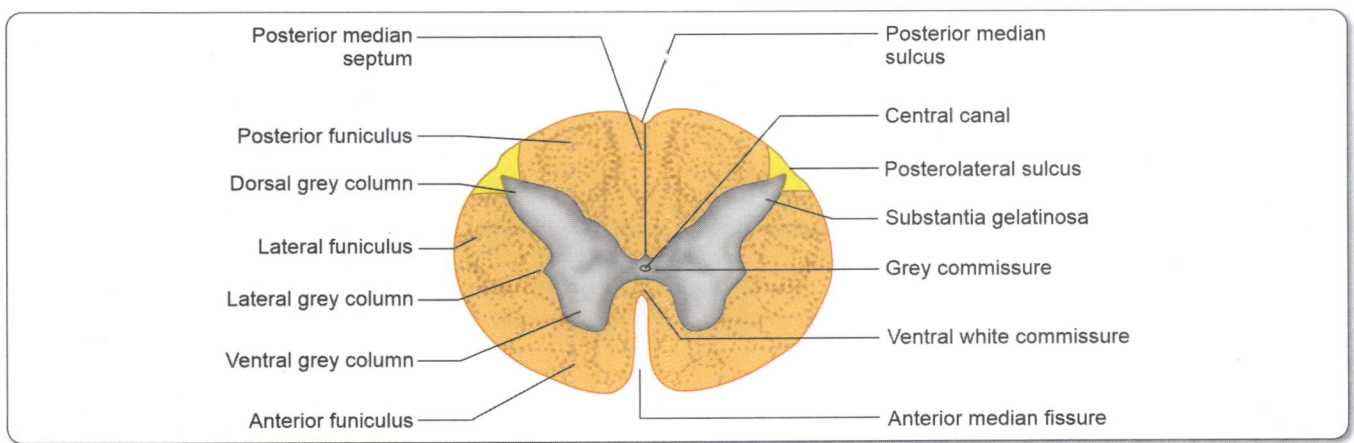

Fig. 10.2-29: Transverse section of spinal cord

Ascending tracts. Ascending tracts convey impulses arising in various parts of the body to different parts of the brain. The ascending tracts present in the spinal cord are summarized in Table 10.2-5

Descending tracts. The descending tracts concerned with the various motor activities of the body, and formed by the motor nerve fibers arising from the brain and descending into the spinal cord and brain stem are summarized in Table 10.2-6.

TABLE 10.2-5: Major ascending tracts in the spinal cord

Tract	Location	Origin*	Termination	Functions
Fasciculus gracilis and fasciculus cuneatus (tracts of Goll and Burdach)	Posterior white column of spinal cord.	Dorsal root ganglia of spinal nerves of the same side.	Nucleus gracilis and nucleus cuneatus in medulla of the soma e side	Joint sense, vibration sense, tow point discrimination, stereognosis, conscious kinesthesia.
Spinothalamic tracts • Lateral spinothalamic tract • Anterior spinothalamic tract	Lateral white column Anterior white column.	Posterior horn cells of spinal cord of opposite side Posterior horn cells of spinal cord of opposite side	Ventral posterolateral (VPL) nucleus of thalamus. Ventral posterolateral (VPL) nucleus of thalamus.	Carry pain and temperature from opposite side of the body. Carry light touch pressure, tickle ant itch sensation from opposite side of the body.
Spinotectal tract	Lateral white column.	Posterior horn cells of spinal cord of opposite side.	Superior colliculus of tectum of midbrain cerebellum.	Visuomotor reflexes *viz* head and eye movements toward the source of stimulation.
Spinocerebellar (anterior and posterior) tracts	Lateral white column (superficially)	Posterior horn cells of spinal cord of same side.		Unconscious kinesthesia (proprioception)

* Location of cell bodies of neurons from which the axons of tract arise.

TABLE 10.2-6: Major descending tracts of the spinal cord

Tract	Location	Origin*	Termination	Functions
Pyramidal tracts				
• Lateral corticospinal (crossed pyramidal) tract	Lateral white column of spinal cord	Primary motor cortex (area 4), premotor cortex (area 6) of the opposite cerebral hemisphere (*upper motor neurons*)	Anterior horn cells of the spinal cord (*lower motor neurons*)	Controls conscious skilled movements especially of hands (contraction of individual or small group of muscles particularly those which move hands, fingers, feet and toes)
• Anterior corticospinal (uncrossed pyramidal) tract	Anterior white column	Primary motor cortex (area 4), premotor cortex (area 6) of the opposite cerebral hemisphere (*upper motor neurons*)	Anterior horn cells of the spinal cord (*lower motor neurons*)	Same as that of lateral corticospinal tract
Extrapyramidal tracts				
• Rubrospinal tract	Lateral white column	Red nucleus of the opposite side located in midbrain	Anterior horn cells of the spinal cord	Unconscious coordination of movements (controls muscle tone and synergy)
• Vestibulospinal tract	Anterior white column	Vestibular nucleus	Anterior horn cells of the spinal cord	Unconscious maintenance of posture and balance
Reticulospinal tracts				
• Medial reticulospinal tract	Anterior white column	Reticular formation in medulla	Anterior horn cells of the spinal cord	Mainly responsible for inhibitory influence on the motor neurons to the skeletal muscles
• Lateral reticulospinal tract	Lateral white column	Reticular formation in midbrain, pons and medulla	Anterior horn cells of the spinal cord	Mainly responsible for facilitatory influence on the motor neurons to the skeletal muscles
Tectospinal tract	Anterior white column	Superior colliculus of the column opposite side	Cranial nerve nuclei in medulla and anterior horn cells of the upper spinal segments	Controls movements of head, neck and arms in response to the visual stimuli

*Location of cell bodies of neurons from which the axons of tract arise.

SPINAL SEGMENTS AND SPINAL NERVES

Spinal Segments

Spinal cord, though a continuous structure, can be considered to consist of 31 spinal segments, each giving attachment to rootlets of the ventral and dorsal root, of each spinal nerve (Fig. 10.2-30A). The 31 segments of spinal cord correspond symmetrically to 31 spinal nerves and are named as:

- *8 cervical segments* give attachment to 8 cervical nerves
- *12 thoracic segments* give attachment to 12 thoracic nerves
- *5 lumbar segments* give attachment to 5 lumbar nerves
- *5 sacral segments* give attachment to 5 sacral nerves
- *1 coccygeal segment* gives attachment to 1 coccygeal nerve.

Spinal Nerves

Each spinal nerve is a mixed nerve formed by union of two roots: (i) A dorsal (sensory) root, (ii) A ventral (motor) root (Fig. 10.2-30B).

Dorsal Nerve Root

The dorsal nerve root is formed by several rootlets. All sensory fibers reach the spinal cord through dorsal nerve roots. Each dorsal nerve root is marked by a swelling called dorsal nerve root ganglion or spinal ganglion. Dorsal root ganglion is composed of T-shaped unipolar neurons with peripheral and central processes.

Peripheral processes of dorsal root ganglion cells extend upto sensory receptors in the skin. The area of the skin supplied by a spinal nerve is called *dermatome*.

Central processes of dorsal root ganglion cells constitute the dorsal nerve root which is attached to spinal cord through various rootlets. Each rootlet just before entering the spinal cord divides into medial and lateral divisions.

Ventral Nerve Root

The ventral nerve root is composed of axons of motor neurons present in the ventral grey horn. The ventral root also contains the autonomic fibers originating from the lateral (intermediate) horn of the spinal grey matter.

FUNCTIONS OF SPINAL CORD

Sensory Functions

All the somatic afferent impulses enter the spinal cord through the dorsal nerve root as:

- The fibers mediating *thermal and pain sensations* enter the spinal cord through the lateral division of dorsal nerve root
- The fibers conveying all *other sensory impulses* and proprioceptive impulses (touch, deep pressure, joint sense and vibration sense) from muscles, tendons and joints enter the spinal cord through the medial division of the dorsal nerve root.

After entering the spinal cord, all the somatic sensations are conveyed to the brain (post-central gyrus) by ascending tracts.

Motor Functions

Spinal cord performs motor functions through the pyramidal tracts and extrapyramidal tracts. Motor functions served by spinal cord are:

- Control of tone and power of muscles
- Control of movement of muscles and joints

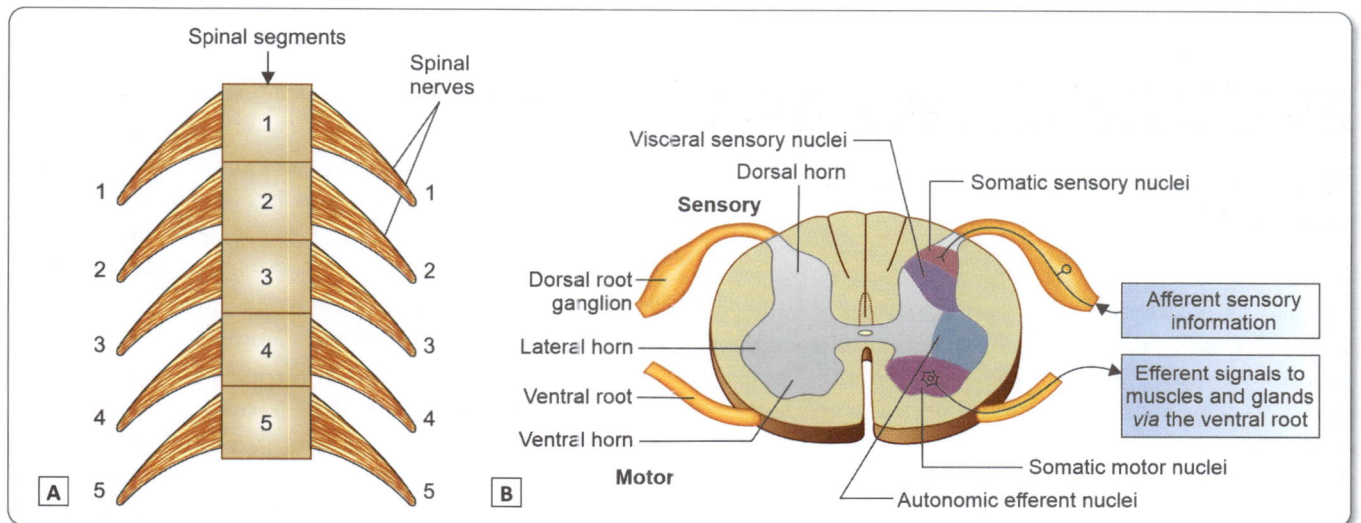

Figs 10.2-30A and B: Scheme to illustrate the concept of spinal segment and roots of spinal nerve

- Control of deep (tendon) reflexes
- Control of superficial reflexes.

Autonomic Functions

Visceral afferent impulses in spinal cord travel through dorsal nerve roots to lateral horns of T_1 to L_2 and S_2 to S_4 spinal segments.

Autonomic efferents traveling through spinal cord supply the visceral organs and control the activity of smooth muscles, heart, glands of gastrointestinal tract, sweat glands, and adrenals. The spinal cord also regulates the body temperature. In other words, spinal cord helps in maintaining the optimal internal environment of the body through its autonomic function.

CLINICAL ASPECTS

LESIONS OF SPINAL CORD

Complete Transection of Spinal Cord

The effects (symptoms and signs) produced by complete transection of the spinal cord occur in the following three stages:

1. *Stage of spinal shock:* Spinal shock refers to cessation of all the functions and activity below the level of the section immediately after injury. *Characteristic effects during shock* are summarized:

Motor effects include:

- *Paralysis of the muscles* below the level of section.
- Loss of tone in the paralyzed muscles. So, the muscles become atonic or flaccid. This is called state of flaccid paralysis.
- *Areflexia*, i.e., all the superficial and deep reflexes are markedly decreased or lost.

Sensory effects: All the sensations are lost below the level of transections.

Vasomotor effects: The sympathetic vasoconstrictor fibers leave the spinal cord between T_1 and L_2. Therefore, depending upon the site of lesion, the vasomotor effects produced are:

- Extremities are cold and blue (cyanotic).
- Skin becomes dry and scaly and bedsores may develop.

Visceral effects produced are:

- Retention of urine
- Constipation
- Penis becomes flaccid and erection becomes impossible.

2. *Stage of reflex activity:* After about 3 weeks period, depending largely upon the general health of the patient, the reflex activity begins to return to the isolated segments of spinal cord below the level of lesion. Various developments which take place are:

- Smooth muscles regain functional activity first of all.
- Sympathetic tone of the blood vessels is regained.
- Skeletal muscle tone then recovers slowly after 3 – 4 weeks.
- Reflex activity begins to return after few weeks of recovery of muscle tone.

3. *Stage of reflex failure:* The failure of reflex activity may occur when general condition of the patient starts deteriorating.

LOW MOTOR NEURON LESION (LMNL)

Refers to involvement of neurons of anterior horn of the spinal cord, therefore there is flacid paralysis of the involved muscle, loss of muscle power and areflexia (superficial and deep reflexes are lost) and Babiniskis's sign is negative (normal planter reflex, see page 531)

UPPER MOTOR NEURON LESION (UMNL)

Refers to involvement of neurons that influence actuality of LMN of the spinal cord, i.e., involvement of descending tracts (Pyramidal and extrapyramidal tracts)

In UMNL usually group of muscles are involved and there is spastic paralysis due to loss of inhibitory higher control.

- Superficial reflexes are lost but deep reflexes are exaggerated
- Babinski's sign is positive, i.e., on stoking the outer edge of sole of foot, with firm stimuli, there is dorsiflexion of great toes and fanning of small toes.

SOMATOSENSORY SYSTEM

SENSATIONS, RECEPTORS AND SENSORY TRANSDUCTION

Sensations

Sensory division of the human nervous system is concerned with collection of the information about outside world and changes occurring within the body itself. Sensation refers to conscious perception of sensory information reaching the brain. Sensations may be broadly classified into two groups:

1. *Special senses.* These include visual sensations, auditory sensations, gustatory (taste sensation), and olfactory (smell) sensations. These have been discussed in detail in Chapter 6.2.

2. *Somesthetic senses.* These, depending upon their point of origin, can be classified into three types:

a. *Exteroceptive sensations* also known as cutaneous sensations arise from the surface of the body and these include:

- Tactile sensation
- Pressure sensation
- Pain sensation
- Temperature sensation

b. *Visceral sensations* arise from the viscera, i.e., internal organs and are called visceral sensations.

c. *Proprioceptive and kinesthetic sensations* arise from the muscles, tendons and joints. These include:

- *Proprioceptive sensations:* These are concerned with the physical state of the body, i.e., the sense of position, tendon and muscle sensations, deep pressure and sense of equilibrium.

- *Kinesthetic sensations* or kinesthesia: It is the conscious recognition of rate of movement of different parts of the body. Kinesthetic sensations include both:
  - Conscious kinesthetic sensations, and
  - Unconscious kinesthetic sensations.

Receptors

Sensory receptors are specialized cells that receive stimuli from the external or internal environment and transduce these signals into neural signals. A *stimulus* is a change of environment of sufficient intensity to evoke a response in an organism.

Receptors for Cutaneous Sensations

Mechanoreceptors or receptors of touch, pressure and vibration sensation provide information about these stimuli to skin. In general, these receptors consist of an unmyelinated axon surrounded by lamellated connective tissue corpuscles. These include (Fig. 10.2-31):
- Pacinian corpuscles (pressure)
- Meissner's corpuscles (touch)
- Merkel's discs (touch)
- Ruffini's end organs (pressure)
- Hair end organs (touch)
- Krause's end bulbs (touch)
- Free nerve endings (pain, heat, cold)

Thermoreceptors. Thermoreceptors are responsible for detecting temperature sensation. Separate receptors exist for encoding warm and cold sensations and are called warm receptors and cold receptors respectively. Free nerve endings of unmyelinated C fibers form the *warm receptors* and that of *small myelinated Aδ fibers* form the *cold receptors*.

Location. Thermoreceptors are located in the skin of all parts of the body. However, density of thermoreceptors is greatest in the lips, moderate in the fingertips, and least in the skin of trunk.

Nociceptors. Nociceptors or pain receptors refer to special type of free nerve endings of:
- Aδ myelinated nerve fibers
- C unmyelinated nerve fibers.

Location. High density of pain receptors is present in the superficial layers of skin and in many deeper tissues like periosteum, joints, arterial wall and falx and tentorium in the cranium.

Receptors for Proprioceptive and Kinesthetic Sensations

The receptors concerned are called *proprioceptors* and include:
- Muscle spindle or stretch receptors
- Joint receptors located in the joint capsules and ligaments around the joints. Ruffini's end organs are the most important receptors for this function. A few pacinian corpuscles are also involved:
- Golgi tendon organ
- Vestibular receptors.

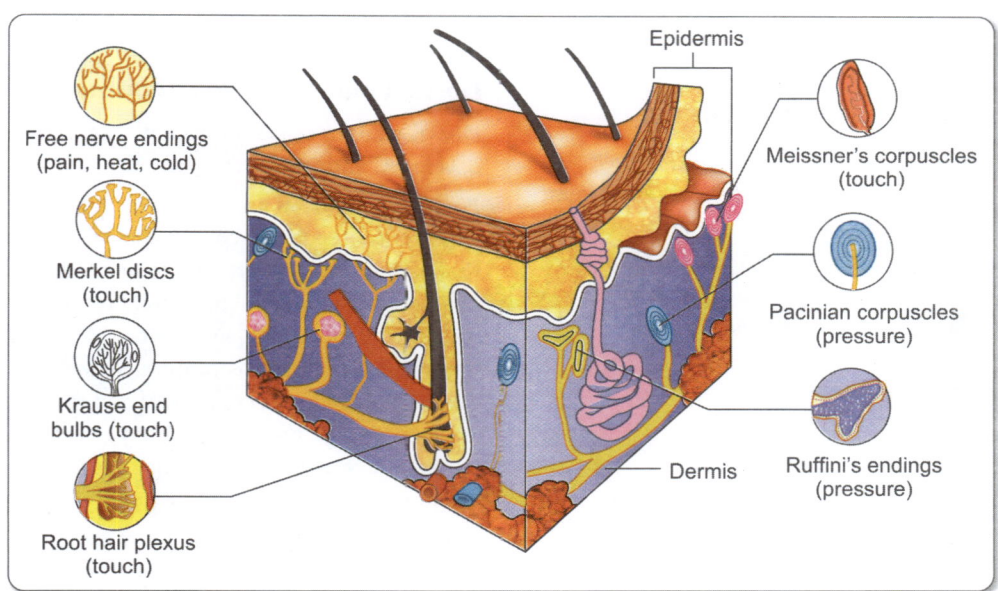

Fig. 10.2-31: Sensory receptors

Sensory Transduction

Sensory transduction refers to the phenomenon of transduction of environmental signals into neural signals by the receptors. Steps of sensory transduction are:

1. *Arrival of stimulus to receptor.* The stimulus arriving at the given sensory receptor may be in the form of:
   - *Mechanical force* causing depression of the skin which stimulates mechanoreceptors
   - *Cold* or *warm temperature* stimulating thermoreceptors.

2. *Production of receptor potential.* When a stimulus excites the receptor, it changes the potential across the membrane of the receptors. This change in the potential is called receptor or generator potential.

Mechanism of development of receptor potential. The change in membrane potential in a receptor is caused by a change in permeability of membrane of the unmyelinated terminals to Na^+. The resultant influx of Na^+ causes development of generator or receptor potential.

3. *Production of action potential in a sensory nerve.* The receptor potential developed in unmyelinated nerve ending (transducer region) depolarizes the sensory nerve at the first node of Ranvier (spike generator region) by electrotonic depolarization current sink action. When the receptor potential rises above the threshold level (i.e., above 10 mV), it brings the membrane potential of the first node of Ranvier to the firing level causing production of action potential, which is propagated in the nerve fiber (Fig. 10.2-32). Thus, the first node of Ranvier (spike generator region) converts the graded response of the receptor into action potential. Greater the magnitude of receptor potential, greater is the rate of discharge of action potentials in the nerve fiber.

NEURAL PATHWAY (TRANSMISSION OF SENSATIONS)

The transduced signals from the sensory receptor ultimately reach the thalamus and sensory cortex through the neural pathway. Pathways in somatosensory system are formed by a chain of three neurons, which constitute the spinal nerves, ascending sensory tracts and relay stations.

Ascending Sensory Tracts

The major ascending sensory tracts in the spinal cord have been grouped as:
- Dorsal (posterior) column sensory pathway
- Anterolateral sensory pathway
- Dorsolateral column sensory pathway.

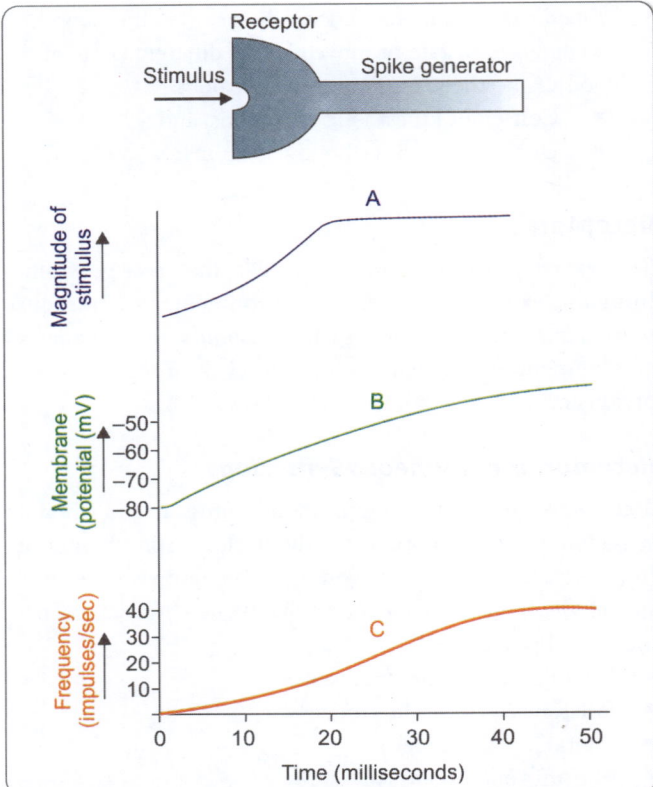

Fig. 10.2-32: Mechanism of development of generator potential and its relationship with intensity of stimulus: A. Stimulus to mechanoreceptors causes its deformation which opens up channels which are permeable to Na^+ causing membrane depolarization; B. The generator potential (receptor potential) follows the time course; C. The frequency of action potential. Note the magnitude of generator potential and frequency of action potential are proportionate to the magnitude of stimulus

Dorsal Column Sensory Pathway

Dorsal column sensory pathway (Fig. 10.2-33) in man is well developed and wholly myelinated.

First order neurons are formed by Aα (Ia), and Aβ (II) fibers which enter the spinal cord at medial division of dorsal nerve roots. These carry sensations of fine touch, tactile localization, two-point discrimination, vibration, pressure with intensity discrimination and sense of position and proprioception. These fibers run in the spinal cord through *dorsal column* as fasciculus gracilis and fasciculus cuneatus to end in the *nucleus gracilis* and *nucleus cuneatus*, respectively. Many fibers of the dorsal columns, on their way up, terminate or relay in the dorsal grey horn.

Second order neurons arise from the *nucleus gracilis* and *nucleus cuneatus* located in medulla oblongata. These decussate in the medulla as *internal arcuate fibers* and ascend

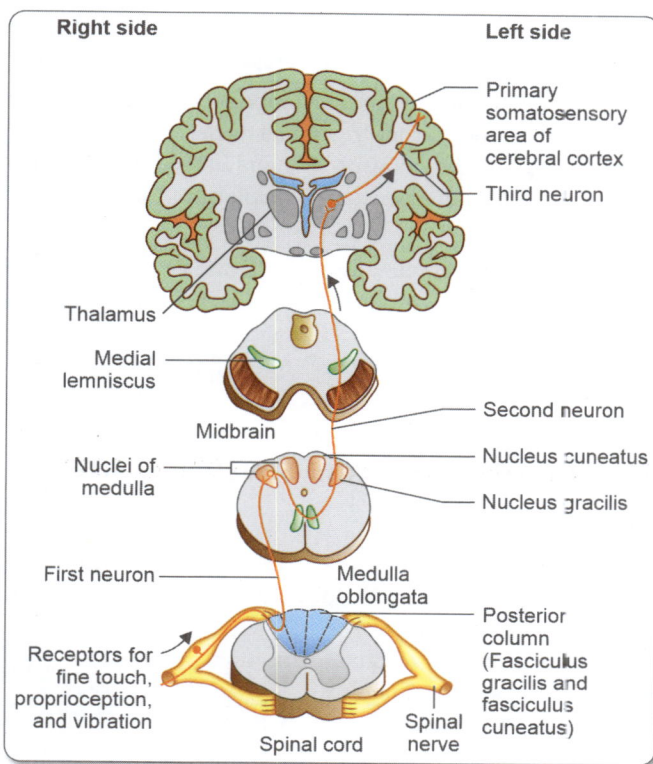

Fig. 10.2-33: Dorsal column sensory pathways. Fibers carrying touch, pressure and proprioceptive sensations are arranged as fasciculus gracilis and fasciculus cuneatus in dorsal column of spinal cord

up in the brain stem as medial lemniscus. The fibers of *medial lemniscus terminate* in the *ventroposterior lateral* (VPL) nucleus of thalamus.

Third order neurons are from the *VPL* of thalamus. These ascend to the sensory cortex through the thalamic radiations.

Anterolateral Sensory Pathway

First order neurons of anterolateral pathway are formed by Aδ (III) and (IV) fibers which enter the spinal cord as lateral division of the dorsal nerve root. These carry sensations of pain, temperature and crude touch. After entering the spinal cord these fibers separate into short ascending and descending branches. They finally terminate on the *nucleus proprius* of the spinal cord. Some sensory afferents end on the short interneurons in the *substantia gelatinosa* which connect them to nucleus proprius.

Second order neurons arise from the nucleus proprius and cross in the anterior commissure of the spinal cord to the opposite side in anterior and lateral white column in which they run upward to the brain as anterior and lateral spinothalamic tracts, respectively.

Anterior spinothalamic tract mainly carries sensation of crude touch, tickle, and itch, etc. Higher up in the brain stem, the anterior spinothalamic tract joins the medial lemniscus of thalamus.

Lateral spinothalamic tract consists of the fibers carrying pain and temperature sensation, and higher up in the brain stem is called the spinal lemniscus (Fig. 10.2-34).

Anterolateral pathways terminate in two areas:

- Throughout *reticular nuclei* of brain stem.
- Spinal and medial lemnisci terminate in the *ventrobasal complex* and *intralaminar* nuclei of thalamus.

Third order neurons arise from the ventrobasal complex of thalamus and carry tactile signals to the somatic sensory area of the cortex along with the fibers of dorsal column.

Dorsolateral Column Sensory Pathway

Dorsolateral column pathways carry proprioceptive impulses arising from the muscles and joint receptors of the lower part of the body to the cerebellum. Recent investigations have shown that touch may also reach the cerebellum through these pathways.

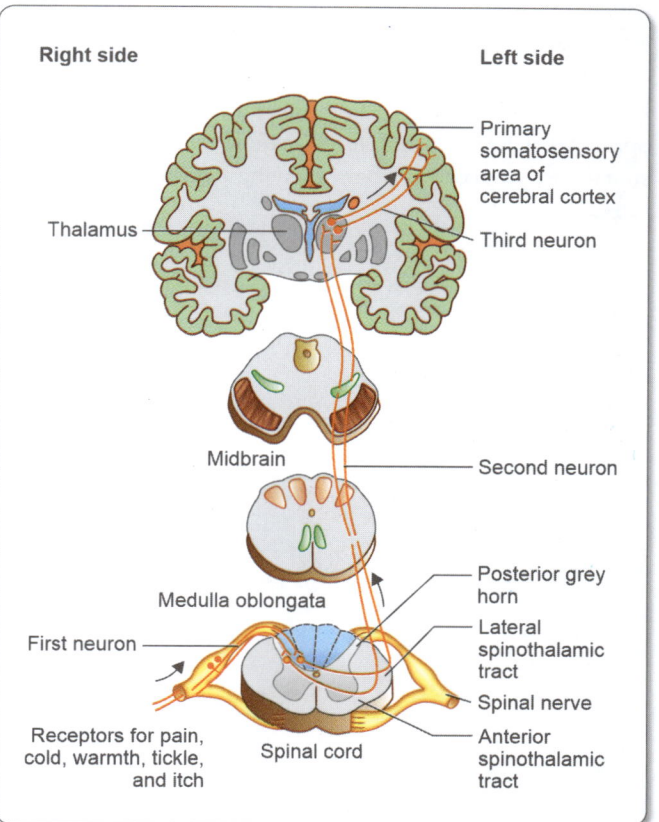

Fig. 10.2-34: Course of anterior and lateral spinothalamic tracts

First order neurons are located in the posterior root ganglia. Their peripheral processes receive impulses from muscle spindles, Golgi tendon organs and other proprioceptive receptors. Some fibers are related to end organs concerned with exteroceptive sensations (touch and pressure).

Second order neurons are located in the junctional area between the ventral and dorsal grey column in the lumbar and sacral segments of spinal cord. Their axons form the:

- Ventral spinocerebellar tract
- Dorsal spinocerebellar tract.

Pathway of Sensations from Face and Oral Cavity

The sensations of touch, pain and temperature from the face and oral cavity including teeth, and proprioceptive information from the jaw muscles are carried by trigeminal nerve.

First order neurons are located in the *trigeminal ganglion*, which is equivalent to dorsal nerve root ganglia in the spinal cord. The peripheral processes of these neurons form three divisions of the trigeminal nerve: (i) ophthalmic, (ii) maxillary, (iii) mandibular, which innervate different areas of the facial skin. The central processes of these neurons of trigeminal ganglia terminate in different components of trigeminal sensory nucleus as (Fig. 10.2-35):

Principal sensory trigeminal nucleus, located in the pons, receives fibers carrying *tactile* sensations.

Spinal nucleus is elongated and extends down to the upper spinal cord. It receives fibers carrying *pain* and *temperature* sensations.

Mesencephalic nucleus, which extends from the pons into midbrain, receives fibers carrying *proprioceptive* information.

Second order neurons are located in the above described three components of the sensory trigeminal nucleus. Axons of these neurons cross to the opposite side and ascend as *trigeminal lemniscus* to the ventroposterior medial (VPM) nucleus of thalamus.

Third order neurons are located in the VPM nucleus of thalamus. All the sensations reaching this nucleus are carried primarily to sensory area of cerebral cortex by fibers passing through the posterior limb of internal capsule (*superior thalamic radiations*).

ROLE OF THALAMUS AND SENSORY CORTEX

Thalamus

Third order neurons of sensory pathway are located in the *ventral posterior nucleus* of thalamus. Role of thalamus in sensory system is as below:

- Serves as *relay cortex* for all sensations
- *Integrates* sensory impulses
- Acts as *crude center* for sense perception.

Sensory Cortex

The sensory cortex includes primary sensory area, secondary sensory area and sensory association area located in parietal lobe.

Encoding: Recognition of Type of Sensation

As discussed above, the sensory receptors transduce all forms of sensory stimuli into a common type of neural signal, i.e., action potentials, which are carried by the peripheral nerves and sensory tracts in the spinal cord and brain stem to the sensory cortex. The question arises how does brain differentiate between the action potentials generated from a touch receptor and a pain receptor and interpret the sensation accordingly. It is believed that the sensory receptors themselves act as peripheral analyzers.

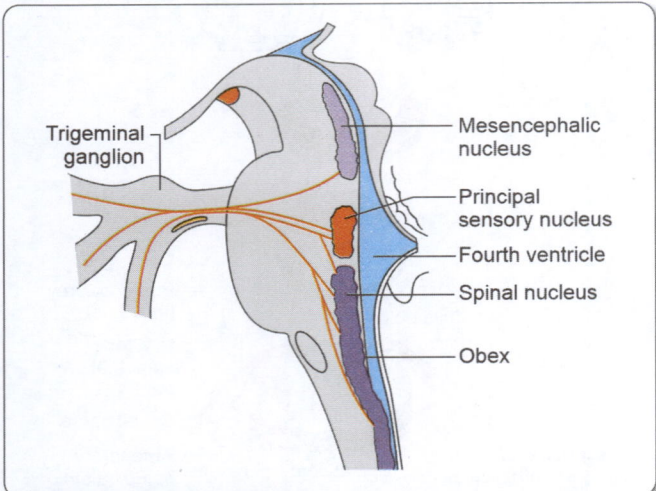

Fig. 10.2-35: Termination of central processes of trigeminal ganglion in three components of sensory nucleus of trigeminal nerve

- Trigeminal ganglion
- Mesencephalic nucleus
- Principal sensory nucleus
- Fourth ventricle
- Spinal nucleus
- Obex

SOMATOMOTOR SYSTEM

The execution, planning, coordination and adjustments of the movements of the body are under the influence of different parts of the nervous system which together constitute the somatic motor system, which is organized as three tier system consisting of highest level of motor control, middle level of motor control, and lowest level of motor control (Fig. 10.2-36).

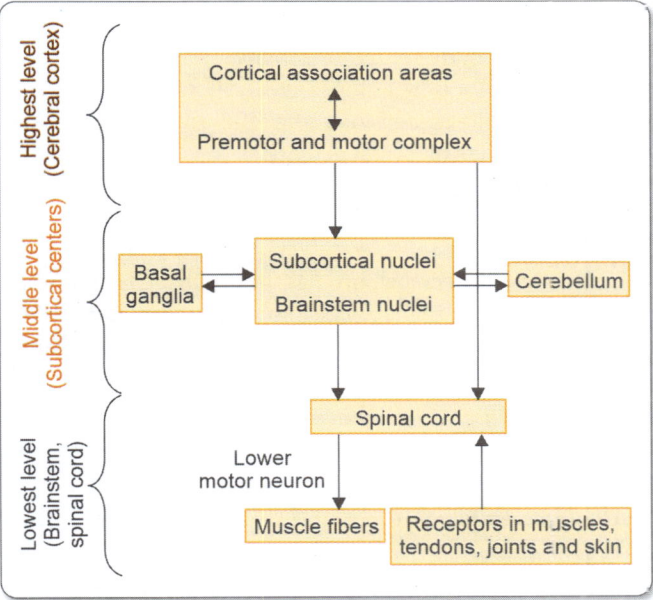

Fig. 10.2-36: Integration of highest, middle and lowest level of motor control system

Highest level of motor control involves activities of various areas of cerebral cortex. It is mainly concerned with generation of the idea of voluntary movements (motor plan) and issuing the motor commands for their execution.

Middle level of motor control involves activities of various subcortical centers such as basal ganglia, some brain stem nuclei and cerebellum. The middle level of motor control is concerned with developing and perfecting each motor program and subprogram for bringing out a motor act. It also supervises the implementation of motor program.

Lowest level of motor control is exerted by cranial nerve nuclei in brain stem and the spinal cord. The spinal cord contains the final common pathway through which a movement is executed.

Feedback signals to CNS from the proprioceptors in muscles, joints, skin and other sensory receptors are used to adjust the motor commands during somatic motor activity.

In view of the above background, the somatic motor control system is discussed in detail under the following headings:

- Components of somatic motor control system
- *Skeletal muscles:* The effector organ of somatic motor system
- Reflexes
- Regulation of posture and equilibrium.

COMPONENTS OF SOMATIC MOTOR CONTROL SYSTEM

Highest Level of Motor Control

The highest level of motor control is exerted through motor cortex and two major descending pathways emerging from the motor areas.

Motor Cortex

Areas of motor cortex include:
- *Primary motor cortex* (Brodmann's area 4)
- *Premotor cortex* (it includes Brodmann's area 6, 8, 44 and 45)
- *Supplementary motor cortex.*

Functional role of motor cortex in control of voluntary movements is
- *Supplementary motor cortex* is responsible for generating the idea for a movement.
- *Primary motor cortex* is responsible for execution of movement.
- *Premotor cortex* coordinates the voluntary activity.

Plasticity property of motor cortex

The motor system 'learns by doing', and performance improves with repetition. This involves synaptic plasticity. The motor cortex shows plasticity. This has been confirmed by PET and functional magnetic resonance imaging (fMRI) in intact experimental animals and humans.

Descending Motor Pathways from Motor Cortex

Pyramidal tracts

They include the tracts which are constituted by the axons that transmit motor signals directly from the cortex to spinal cord (*corticospinal tracts*) and cranial nerve nucleus (*corticobulbar tracts*). Corticospinal fibers are divided into two tracts (Fig. 10.2-37).

1. Lateral corticospinal tract is constituted by the 80% of fibers which cross the midline in the medullary pyramids. These fibers are responsible for making skilled precision movements (e.g., the muscles that move the fingers and hands and the muscles that produce speech) (*lateral motor system*).

2. Anterior corticospinal tract is formed by 20% uncrossed fibers which descend ipsilaterally in the ventral white column of the spinal cord. These fibers ultimately cross the midline but only at the level where they synapse. This pathway controls the axial (trunk muscles) and proximal limb muscles that

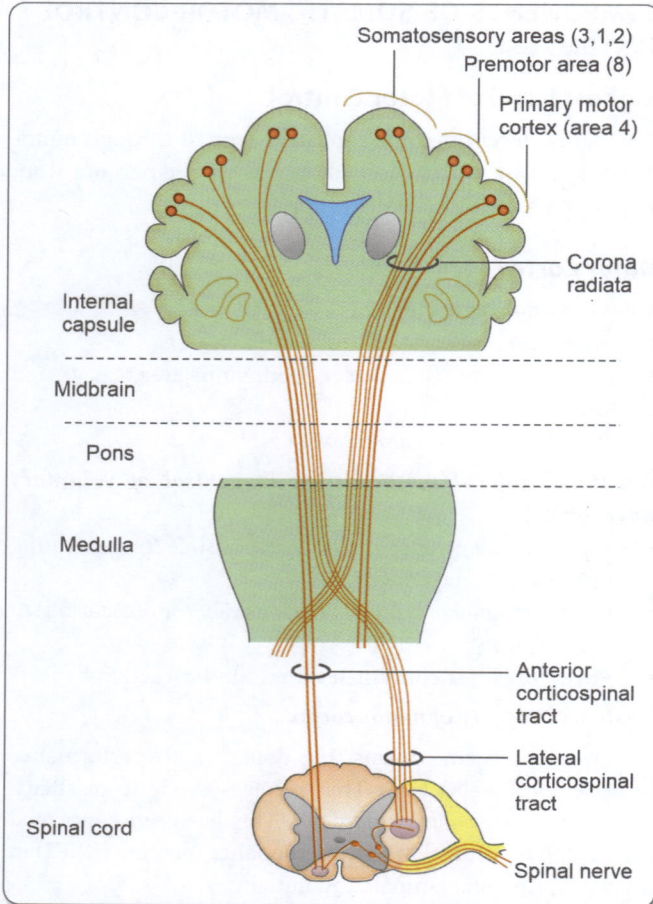

Fig. 10.2-37: Pathway of corticospinal (pyramidal) tracts

Role of basal ganglia in somatic motor activity

- Cognitive control of motor activity
- Timing and scaling of the intensity of movements
- Subconscious execution of some movements
- Control reflex muscular activity
- Control the muscle tone

Cerebellum

Functionally, the cerebellum has been divided into three divisions: (i) vestibulocerebellum, (ii) spinocerebellum (iii) corticocerebellum, which play important role in different motor activities.

Corticocerebellum is intimately associated with control of timing, rate, range (extent), duration, direction and strength of a movement.

Vestibulocerebellum is responsible for control of body posture and equilibrium.

Spinocerebellum controls the muscle tone and stretch reflex.

Brain Stem

Reticular formation and vestibular nuclei are important components of the motor control system present in the brain stem.

Reticular formation

The *motor control centers* within the reticular formation are a relay station for all descending motor commands, except those requiring the greatest precision, which are transferred directly from the cortex to spinal cord.

Vestibular nuclei

The vestibular system reflexes:
- Maintain tone in antigravity muscles
- Coordinate the adjustments made by the limbs and trunk to maintain balance
- Adjust the position of the eyes to maintain visual fixation when the position of head changes.

are concerned with posture and equilibrium (*medial motor system*).

Extrapyramidal tracts

Extrapyramidal pathways are chiefly concerned with regulation of muscle tone, posture and equilibrium.

Middle Level of Motor Control

The middle level of motor control specifies the postures and movements necessary to carry out the desired acts. It involves activities of basal ganglia, cerebellum and brain stem.

Basal Ganglia

Physiologically basal ganglia include corpus striatum (caudate nucleus and lenticular nucleus having two parts, e.g., putamen and globus pallidus), subthalamic nucleus and substantia nigra.

Lowest Level of Motor Control

The lowest level of motor control is exerted by motor nuclei of cranial nerves and spinal cord. The spinal cord contains the *final common pathway* through which a movement is executed.

Spinal Cord

Motor neurons of spinal cord present in ventral horn are:

Alpha motor neurons. These are responsible for contraction of muscles in upper limbs, trunk and lower part of the body.

Gamma motor neurons. These neurons innervate the intrafusal fibers of the muscle spindles and are responsible for maintenance of muscle tone.

Interneurons. The interneurons actually receive the bulk of synaptic input that reaches the spinal cord, either as incoming sensory information or signals descending from higher centers in the brain.

Renshaw cells. These are inhibitory neurons which play an important role in synaptic inhibition at the spinal cord.

Motor functions served by spinal cord are:
- Control of movement of muscles and joints
- Control of tone and power of muscles
- Control of deep (tendon) reflexes
- Control of superficial reflexes.

SKELETAL MUSCLES: THE EFFECTOR ORGAN OF SOMATIC MOTOR SYSTEM

The motor activity, be it in the form of walking, physical labor, skilled work like typing, performing surgical operations or even expression of thoughts and feelings through gesture or speech, is a result of highly co-ordinated movements produced by the skeletal muscles. The skeletal muscles, thus, form the effector organ of the somatic motor system. The physiology of skeletal muscle has been discussed on page 388. However, certain aspects which need elaboration of skeletal muscle as effector organ and are relevant to complete the study of somatic motor system are:
- Motor unit
- Muscle sensors (proprioceptors)
- Muscle tone

Motor Unit

The motor unit is the functional module used by the motor control system to carry out a movement. The movement produced by a skeletal muscle basically depends upon the pattern and ratio of discharge of motor neurons supplying the muscle. A *motor unit consists* of single motor neuron and the muscle fibers that it innervates *see page 394.*

Muscle Sensors

Muscle sensors refer to the proprioceptors present in the muscles, tendons of muscles, joints, ligaments and fasciae. Proprioceptors are the receptorst which give information about change in position of different parts of the body in space, especially joints or tension of muscles at any given moment. The muscle sensors are:
- Muscle spindle
- Golgi tendon organ
- Pacinian corpuscle
- Free nerve endings.

In addition to the above proprioceptors, the labyrinth also contains proprioceptors.

Muscle spindle are *stretch receptors* present in the skeletal muscles. Each skeletal muscle contains muscle spindles of variable number depending upon the task performed.

Golgi tendon organs are high threshold stretch receptors present in the tendons. They are supplied by group Ib afferent fibers and detect muscle tension.

Pacinian corpuscles are pressure receptors situated in fasciae throughout the muscles, tendons, joints and periosteum. They are supplied by *group II afferent fibers* and detect *vibration.*

Free nerve endings are basically pain receptors situated in the muscles, tendons, fasciae and joints. They are supplied by *group III and IV afferent fibers* and detect noxious stimuli.

Muscle Tone

Definition

Muscle tone is defined as resistance offered to active or passive stretch. In other words, muscle tone refers to sustained partial state of contraction of the muscle under resting condition, i.e., a state of partial tetanus. The muscle tone is present in all the muscles, but is well pronounced in the extensor muscles, i.e., antigravity muscles.

Basis of muscle tone

The muscle tone is purely a function of myotatic (stretch reflex), occurring due to low frequency and asynchronous discharge of γ motor neurons. The discharge is out of phase with each other which ultimately merges to produce contraction of the muscle smoothly.

NURSING IMPLICATIONS AND APPLICATIONS

Anomalies of muscle tone are hypotonia and hypertonia.
Hypotonia refers to decrease in muscle tone. The hypotonic or also called flaccid muscle offers little or no resistance to stretching. The muscles are generally hypotonic when the rate of γ efferent discharge is low, i.e., when stretch reflex becomes hypoactive.
Hypertonia refers to increase in muscle tone. The hypertonic or spastic muscle offers high resistance to stretch. The muscles are generally hypertonic when the rate of γ-efferent discharge is high, i.e., when stretch reflex becomes hyperactive. Hypertonia is of two types:
i. *Spasticity* refers to hypertonia which is confined to only one group of muscles. For example, lesions of internal capsule and upper motor neuron lesions produce spasticity.
ii. *Rigidity* refers to hypertonia which involves both groups of muscles, i.e., extensor as well as flexors equally. For example, lesions of basal ganglia produce rigidity.

REFLEX ACTIVITY

ANATOMICAL ASPECTS

A reflex is an involuntary response to a peripheral nervous stimulation. In other words, it is a mechanism by which sensory impulse is automatically converted into a motor effect through the involvement of CNS. It is a type of protective mechanism which tries to protect the body from irreparable damage.

Reflex Arc

The pathway for a reflex activity is called reflex arc. It consists of (Figs 10.2-38A and B):
- Afferent limb
- Center
- Efferent limb.

Afferent Limb

Afferent limb of each reflex arc consists of a receptor and an afferent or sensory nerve. *Afferent neuron* carries sensory input from the receptor to the center. The afferent neurons enter the CNS *via* the dorsal roots or cranial nerves and have their cell bodies in the dorsal root ganglia or in the homologous ganglia on the cranial nerves.

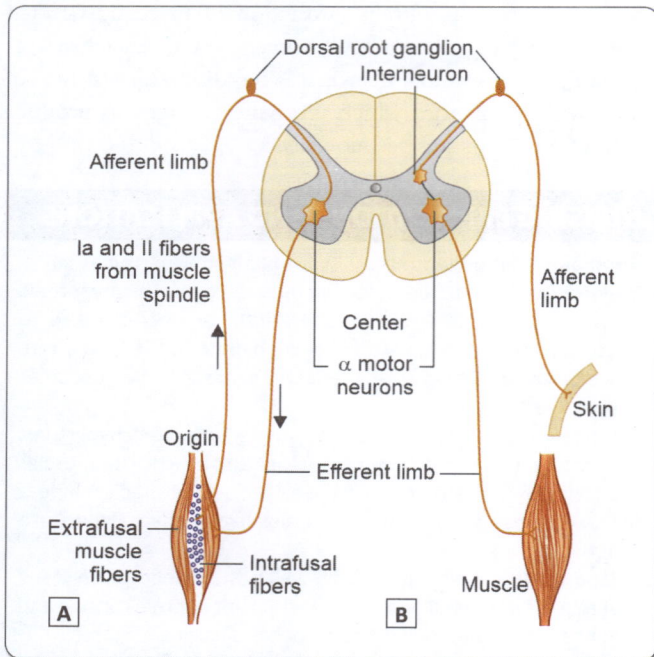

Figs 10.2-38A and B: Components of reflex arc in monosynaptic: A. Disynaptic; B. Reflexes

Center

This is the part of CNS (spinal cord or brain) where afferent limb ends and either synapses directly with efferent motor neuron or establishes connection with the efferent neuron *via* interneurons (internuncial or intercalated neurons).

Efferent Limb

Efferent limb of a reflex arc consists of an efferent or motor nerve and an effector organ.

Efferent nerve transmits motor impulses from the center to the effector organ.

Effector organ may be in the form of a muscle or a gland which shows the response to the stimulus.

SPINAL CORD REFLEXES

Spinal cord reflexes enhance the ability of the motor control system to produce a coordinated movement. According to the receptors from which they originate the spinal cord reflexes can be categorized into muscle reflexes and cutaneous reflexes.

Muscle reflexes. Two important reflexes which originate in muscles are:
- Stretch reflex
- Lengthening reaction or Golgi tendon reflex.

Cutaneous reflexes. The most important of the cutaneous reflexes is:
- Withdrawal (flexor) reflex.

Stretch Reflex

Stretch reflex, also known as myotatic, refers to reflex contraction of a muscle that is stretched. It is the best known monosynaptic reflex in the body. *Stimulus* that evokes the reflex response is 'stretch' to the muscle. *Stretch reflex is well developed in antigravity muscles such as extensor group of muscles of legs and flexor groups of muscles of arm. Examples of stretch reflexes* are knee jerk, ankle jerk, biceps jerk, and triceps jerk.

Reflex Arc of Stretch Reflex (Fig. 10.2-39)
Afferent limb

Afferent limb consists of receptor *muscle spindle* and *afferent nerve* fibers emerging from the muscle spindle which travel along the spinal nerve and enter the spinal cord through the dorsal root and send branches to α-motor neuron that goes to the muscle from which the Ia originated.

Structure of muscle spindle

Each muscle spindle consists of 3–10 small muscle fibers (called intrafusal muscle fibers) encapsulated in a thin connective

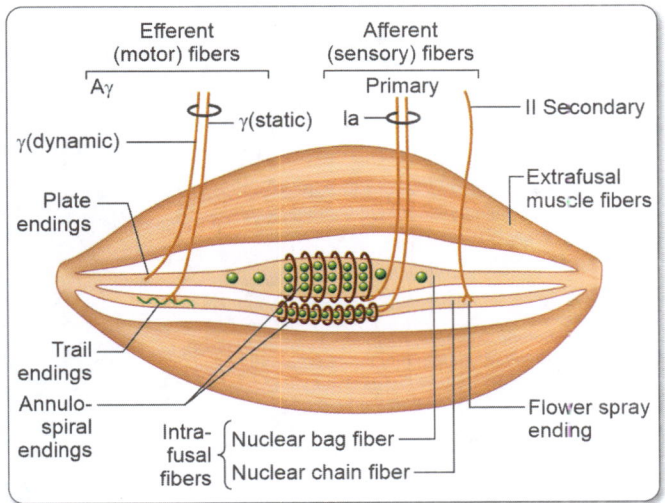

Fig. 10.2-39: Structure of a muscle spindle

tissue capsule containing fluid. The muscle spindles are present in-between and parallel to the extrafusal fibers. Either end of the muscle spindle is attached to the endomysium of the extrafusal muscle fibers. Intrafusal muscle fibers consist of a central noncontractile portion and are devoid of striations. The central part of each intrafusal fiber is the sensory portion. Intrafusal fibers are of the following two types:

1. Nuclear bag fibers
2. Nuclear chain fibers

Nerve supply of the muscle spindle

The muscle spindle is innervated by both sensory and motor nerve fibers.

1. Sensory nerve supply. The following are the two types of sensory fibers:

Group Ia fibers, also known as primary sensory endings, supplying central receptor portions of both nuclear bags as well as nuclear chain fibers. The primary endings are stimulated when the muscle spindle is stretched.

Type II fibers, also known as secondary sensory endings, innervate the receptor portion of mainly nuclear chain fibers. These nerve endings respond mainly to sustained stretch, therefore, measuring the muscle length.

2. Motor supply. The efferent fibers to the muscle spindle are called gamma fibers because their axons belong to the A group of fibers. The following are the two types of gamma fibers:

Dynamic gamma fibers primarily innervate the striated poles of nuclear bag fibers. These fibers increase the sensitivity of the Ia afferent fibers to stretch.

Static gamma fibers primarily innervate the striated poles of nuclear chain fibers. They increase the tonic activity in the Ia.

Center

Center for stretch reflex is the ventral grey horn area where the afferent nerve ends and synapses directly with the α-motor neuron. Thus, α-motor neuron is the final common pathway, serving as both integrating center and efferent pathway.

Efferent limb

Efferent nerve. The axons of α-motor neurons form the efferent nerve fibers which leave the spinal cord through the ventral root and supply the skeletal muscle fibers.

Effector organs. Both extensor and flexor muscles exhibit stretch reflexes.

Reciprocal Innervation in Stretch Reflex

The stretch reflex is characterized by reciprocal innervation, i.e., excitation of one group of muscles is associated with inhibition of the antagonistic group of muscles on the same side, allowing the agonist muscles to contract without interference. Reciprocal innervation is one of the important features of both flexor and extensor reflexes.

Functions of Stretch Reflex

- Role in maintaining muscle tone
- Role in maintaining posture
- Role in control of voluntary movement.

Golgi Tendon Reflex (Disynaptic Reflex)

The Golgi tendon reflex, also called 'inverse stretch reflex', is a disynaptic reflex. The receptors involved are the Golgi tendon organs.

Golgi Tendon Organs (Fig. 10.2-40)

Golgi tendon organs are high-threshold stretch receptors located in the tendons and musculo-aponeurotic junction. They are placed in series between the muscle fibers and the tendon, and are thus, stretched whenever the muscle contracts.

Nerve supply. The Golgi tendon organs are supplied by Ib type sensory nerve fibers.

Pathway and activity of reflex (Fig. 10.2-41). When a muscle contracts, the muscle tension increases. The Golgi tendon organ detects the muscle tension and sends impulses through afferent (group Ib) fibers, which enter the spinal cord through the dorsal root.

- In the spinal cord, the group Ib afferents stimulate the inhibitory inter-neurons.
- The inhibitory inter-neurons, in turn, release inhibitory mediator glycine, which inhibits-motor neurons and causes relaxation of the muscle that was originally contracted.

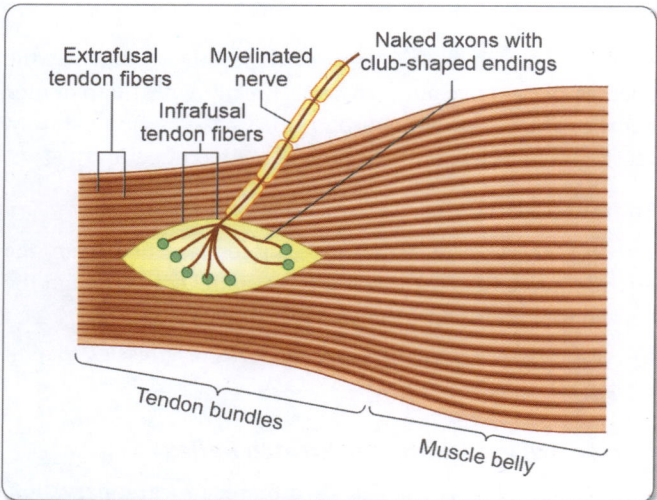

Fig. 10.2-40: Structure of Golgi tendon organ

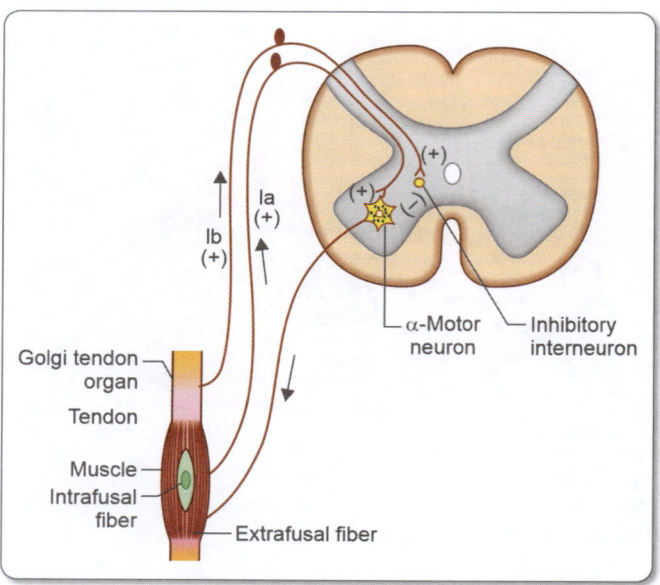

Fig. 10.2-41: Pathway of stretch and inverse stretch reflexes

- At the same time, due to reciprocal innervation, the antagonistic muscles are excited.

Physiological role or the functions of Golgi tendon reflex are:

- *Protective function:* Historically, this reflex has been described as a protective reflex in which a strong and potentially damaging muscle force reflexively inhibits the muscle, causing the muscle to lengthen instead of trying to maintain the force and risking damage.
- *Regulation of tension during normal muscle activity.*

CLINICAL ASPECTS

Clasp-knife reflex refers to an exaggerated form of the Golgi tendon reflex, which can occur with disease of the corticospinal tracts (hypertonicity or spasticity). For example, when the arm is hypertonic, the increased sensitivity of the muscle spindles in the extensor muscles (triceps) causes resistance to flexion of the arm. Eventually, tension in the triceps increases to the point at which it activates Golgi tendon reflex, causing triceps to relax and the arm to flex closed like a jack knife, hence, the name clasp-knife reflex. The physiological name for it is *lengthening reaction*, because it is the response of a spastic muscle to lengthening.

Withdrawal Reflex (Polysynaptic Reflex)

Definition

Withdrawal reflex, also known as flexor reflex, is a cutaneous reflex which occurs in response to nociceptive (pain) stimuli and is characterized by removal of a body part from painful stimulus.

Receptors

Receptors for withdrawal reflex are *nociceptors* located in free nerve endings of Aδ and C fibers.

Pathway (Reflex Arc) of Withdrawal Reflex (Fig. 10.2-42)

The pain fibers carrying impulses, upon entering the spinal cord, synapse on many interneurons. Some of these also convey information to CNS. Others form several reflex pathways.

- Some of the interneurons project onto α-motor neurons on the ipsilateral side and stimulate the flexors which withdraw the limbs.
- Some of the interneurons form inhibitory pathway and terminate on α-motor neurons supplying the extensor muscles on the ipsilateral side producing their relaxation. This is called reciprocal innervation which ensures that the flexion movement is not impeded by contraction of the extensors.
- Some of the interneurons cross to the opposite side of spinal cord and end on the α-motor neurons supplying the extensors on contralateral side. In case of need, this pathway produces extension of the opposite limbs (crossed extensor reflex).

Effector Organs

The effector organs of the withdrawal reflex are the skeletal muscles that cause withdrawal of the limb, i.e., flexor responses.

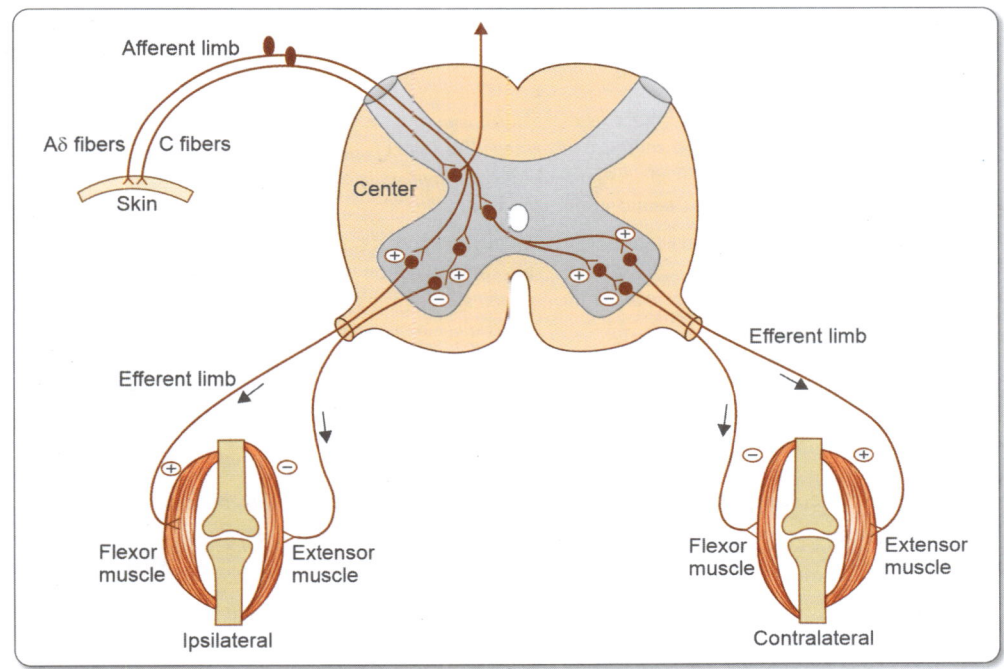

Fig. 10.2-42: Reflex arc of polysynaptic reflex (withdrawal reflex or crossed extensor reflex)

Clinical Reflexes

Clinically, the reflexes can be grouped as follows:

1. *Physiological reflexes* are further grouped as:

Superficial reflexes. These reflexes are initiated in response to stimulation of receptors on skin (cutaneous reflexes, e.g., plantar, abdominal, cremasteric, bulbocavernous) or mucous membranes (mucous membrane reflexes), e.g., corneal, conjunctival and palatal reflex. The superficial reflexes are summarized in Table 10.2-7)

Deep reflexes. These reflexes are basically stretch reflexes and are elicited on stroking a tendon, so called tendon reflexes (e.g.,

knee jerk, ankle jerk); the stretch reflex has been described in detail on page 532; however, the various clinically known stretch reflexes are summarized in Table 10.2-7

Visceral reflexes are elicited from the visceral organ, or at least one part of the reflex arc is formed by the autonomic nerve, e.g., carotid sinus reflex (see page 227) and micturition reflex (see page 422).

2. *Pathological reflexes.* The pathological reflexes are abnormal reflexes which are not found normally.

TABLE 10.2-7: Characteristic features of clinical reflexes			
Reflex	**Method to elicit**	**Response**	**Spinal segment/cranial nerve and center involved**
I. Superficial reflexes *(a) Cutaneous reflexes*			
1. Plantar reflex	Strike the outer aspect of the sole of the foot with a blunt object (e.g., key) and move toward the ball of small toes	Plantar flexion of the foot and toes (i.e., Babinski's negative). However in UMNL it becomes, positive (i.e., dorsiflexion of great toes and fanning out of other toes, see page 520) **Note:** Positive Babinski' sign is physiologically present below one year of age.	L_5 to S_1

Contd...

Reflex	Method to elicit	Response	Spinal segment/cranial nerve and center involved
2. Abdominal reflex	Lightly stimulate the wall of abdomen by stroking with key or some blunt object from out to inside (parallel to costal margin) in upper quadrants and (parallel to inguinal ligament) in lower quadrants of the abdomen	Contractions of the underlying abdominal muscle Note. The reflex is difficult to elicit in elderly individuals, obese persons and multipara	L_2 to S_{12}
3. Cremasteric	Stimulate the skin of upper and inner part of the reflex thigh	Pulling upward of scrotum and testicles due to contraction of cremasteric muscles; this reflex may not be elicited in elderly individuals	L_1 to L_2
4. Scapular reflex	Stroke the skin of interscapular region	Contraction of supraspinatus and infraspinatus muscles	C_5 to T_1
5. Anal reflex	Gently stimulate the skin of perianal region	Contraction of external and internal anal sphincters	S_2 to S_4
6. Bulbocavernous reflex	Gently pinch the dorsum of glans penis	Contraction of bulbocavernous muscle	S_3 to S_4
(b) Mucous membrane reflexes			
7. Corneal reflex	Touch the cornea with wisp of cotton from lateral aspect	Closure of eye of same and of opposite side	Afferents: Via ophthalmic division of (trigeminal) cranial nerve V Center: In the pons Efferents: Via facial nerve to orbicularis oculi muscle
8. Conjunctival reflex	Touch the conjunctiva with wisp of cotton	Closure of the eyes	Pathway is same as for corneal reflex
9. Palate reflex	Touch either side of posterior pharyngeal wall with a swab stick	The contraction of the palate	Afferents: Cranial nerve IX Center: Nucleus ambiguus Efferents: Cranial (vagus) nerve X
II. Deep reflexes (tendon reflexes)			
1. Knee jerk	The subject is in lying or in sitting position. Place the left hand under the knee (to be tested). Tap the tendon of the quadriceps midway between its origin and insertion with knee hammer	Observe the extension of knee due to contraction of quadriceps femoris muscle; sometimes, if unable to elicit, then apply reinforcement (Jendrassik's maneuver, for this ask the individual to pull the hands apart when flexed fingers are hooked together)	Femoral nerve (L_2, L_3 and L_1)
2. Ankle jerk	With foot slightly everted and dorsiflexed, strike on the tendo-Achilles	Plantar flexion of the foot occurs due to contraction of calf muscle elbow	S_1 and S_2
3. Triceps jerk	Keep the forearm of the subject to rest across his/her chest; then tap the triceps tendon with broader side of the patellar hammer	Contraction of triceps with extension of the elbow	C_6 and C_7
4. Biceps jerk	Keep the position of elbow at right angle with forearm and the forearm is semipronated; the examiner then places his/her thumb or index finger on the tendon of the biceps muscle and then strikes on the finger (kept on biceps tendon) with pateller hammer	Contraction of biceps with flexion of elbow	C_5 and C_6

Contd...

Reflex	Method to elicit	Response	Spinal segment/cranial nerve and center involved
5. Supinator	Tap the lower end of the radius at styloid process, keeping the position of same elbow as for biceps jerk	Supination of forearm and flexion of elbow	C_5 and C_6
6. Jaw jerk	Ask the subject to open the mouth slightly; then place one finger firmly be ow the lower lip and tap on the finger in a downward direction	Contraction of masseter muscle causes closure of the jaw	Afferent and efferents are carried by trigeminal nerve; center lies in the pons

ASSESS YOURSELF

Short and Long Answer Questions

1. **Describe briefly:**
   - Organization of central nervous system
   - The functional areas of cerebral lobes and their functions
   - The components of basal ganglia and its role in control of motor activity
   - The functions of thalamus
   - The role of hypothalamus in regulation of body temperature
   - Functions of medulla oblongata
   - The functional divisions of cerebellum and their functions
   - Sensory transduction
   - Components of the somatic motor control system.

2. **Define the following:**
   - Muscle tone
   - Reflex activity
   - Stretch reflex

3. **Differentiate between the following:**
   - Superficial and deep reflexes
   - Stretch reflex and inverse stretch reflex
   - Monosynaptic and polysynaptic reflex

4. **Write notes on:**
   - Parkinson disease
   - Cerebrospinal fluid
   - Functions of spinal cord
   - Plantar reflex

Multiple Choice Questions

1. **Primary motor area 4 is located in:**
   a. Frontal lobe
   b. Parietal lobe
   c. Occipital lobe
   d. Temporal lobe

2. **The Broca's motor speech area is:**
   a. Area 6
   b. Area 8
   c. Area 21 and 22
   d. Area 44 and 45

3. **True about primary auditory area is:**
   a. Present in frontal lobe
   b. Present in post-central gyrus
   c. It is Brodmann area 41 and 42
   d. It is Brodmann area 20, 21 and 22

4. **Caudate nucleus is component of:**
   a. Thalamus
   b. Hypothalamus
   c. Cerebellum
   d. Basal ganglia

5. **Which is the function of basal ganglia?**
   a. Control of voluntary movements
   b. Center for integration of sensory impulses
   c. Regulation of food intake
   d. Control of biological clock

6. **The inferior cerebellar peduncle connects cerebellum to:**
   a. Pons
   b. Midbrain
   c. Thalamus
   d. Medulla oblongata

7. **9th cranial nerve emerges from:**
   a. Midbrain
   b. Pons
   c. Medulla
   d. Cerebellum

8. **Which of the center is located in the medulla?**
   a. Deglutition center
   b. Feeding center
   c. Reward center
   d. Sleep center

9. **Superior and inferior salivary nuclei are situated in:**
   a. Thalamus
   b. Hypothalamus
   c. Midbrain
   d. Medulla oblongata

10. **The statement not true for Pons:**
    a. Is a connecting link between midbrain and medulla
    b. Contains nuclei of 6th cranial nerves
    c. Contains nuclei of 8th cranial nerves
    d. Contains vomiting center

11. **True about horizontal fissure of cerebellum:**
    a. Forms posterior limit of posterior lobe
    b. Separates superior surface of cerebellum from its inferior surface
    c. Separates anterior lobe from flocculonodular lobe
    d. Connected to pons through superior cerebellar peduncle

12. **Golgi cells are mainly present in which layer of cerebellar cortex:**
    a. Molecular layer
    b. Granular cell layer
    c. Purkinje cell layer
    d. None of these

13. **The fastigial nucleus of cerebellum is concerned with:**
    a. Control of muscle tone
    b. Control of voluntary movements
    c. Regulation of body posture and balance
    d. Autonomic functions

14. **The white matter of spinal cord mainly consists of:**
    a. Nerve cell bodies
    b. Dendrites
    c. Myelinated nerve fibers
    d. Part of the axons

15. **The number of cervical nerves is:**
    a. 12 pairs   b. 8 pairs
    c. 5 pairs   d. 1 pair

16. **The spinal ganglion is located on:**
    a. Dorsal root   b. Ventral root
    c. Rootlets   d. Medial division of rootlet

17. **Which is not the feature of spinal shock?**
    a. Flaccid paralysis   b. Areflexia
    c. Hyper-reflexia   d. Loss of sensations

18. **The receptors for pressure sensation are:**
    a. Krause end organs   b. Ruffini end organs
    c. Muscle spindles   d. Golgi tendon organs

19. **The main function of muscle spindles to detect:**
    a. Proprioceptive sensation
    b. Tectile sensation
    c. Thermal sensation
    d. Pain sensation

20. **During sensory transduction the site of propagated impulse is:**
    a. Cell body   b. Axon hillock
    c. First node of Ranvier d. Nerve terminal

21. **The second order neuron of dorsal column is located in:**
    a. Nucleus Gracilis
    b. Medial lemniscus
    c. Ventro-posterior nucleus of thalamus
    d. Nucleus proprius of spinal cord

22. **The anterolateral sensory pathway transmits:**
    a. Pain, temperature and fine touch
    b. Pain, temperature and crude touch
    c. Tectile localization
    d. Two points discrimination

23. **The trigeminal nucleus that receives tectile sensation from face:**
    a. Principal nucleus
    b. Mesencephalic nucleus
    c. Spinal nucleus
    d. None of these

24. **True statement for lateral cortico-spinal tract:**
    a. Crosses midline in the spinal cord
    b. Formed by 20% uncrossed fibers
    c. Controls movements of trunk muscles
    d. Controls movements of fingers and hand muscles

25. **Not true for vestibular nuclei:**
    a. Maintain tone of antigravity muscles
    b. Maintain balance by adjusting movements of hands and trunk
    c. Co-ordinate eye ball movements
    d. Cognitive control of motor activity

26. **The receptors for stretch reflex are:**
    a. Pacinian corpuscles
    b. Golgi tendon organs
    c. Muscle spindles
    d. Ruffini's end organs

27. **The type of nerve fibers for inverse stretch reflex:**
    a. Ia
    b. Ib
    c. III
    d. IV

28. **Type of withdrawal reflex:**
    a. Monosynaptic
    b. Disynaptic
    c. Polysynaptic
    d. None of these

ANSWER KEY

1. a	2. d	3. c	4. d	5. a	6. d	7. c	8. a
9. d	10. d	11. b	12. b	13. c	14. c	15. b	16. a
17. c	18. b	19. a	20. c	21. b	22. b	23. a	24. d
25. d	26. c	27. b	28. c				

Peripheral Nervous System

INTRODUCTION

The peripheral nervous system is that part of nervous system which lies outside the central nervous system (CNS). It consists of peripheral nerves and the ganglia associated with them. A peripheral nerve consists of the following three divisions:

1. Somatic sensory division
2. Somatic motor division
3. Autonomic division

Somatic system connects the CNS to the skin and skeletal muscles, while the autonomic fibers connect the CNS to visceral organs such as the heart, stomach, intestine, various glands and smooth muscles in the body. The peripheral nervous system includes:

1. Cranial nerves
2. Spinal nerves

CRANIAL NERVES

There are twelve pairs of cranial nerves which arise from the brain (Fig. 10.3-1). Some of them are sensory bringing impulses to the brain, others are motor, carrying impulses from the brain to periphery, while a few are mixed containing both motor and sensory fibers.

Cranial nerves are designated either by a number or a name. The numbers indicate the order in which the cranial nerves arise from the front to the back of brain, and the names which describe their nature and function. The highlights of all 12 cranial nerves are given in Table 10.3-1.

OLFACTORY NERVE

Each olfactory nerve consists of about 15–20 nerve filaments. It is a sensory nerve associated with sense of smell (For details, refer to chapter 6.2, page 329).

CLINICAL ASPECTS

Anosmia: Loss of olfactory fibers with aging.

Head injury: Olfactory bulbs may be torn away from olfactory nerves as these pass through fractured cribriform plate of ethmoid leading to anosmia. Such a fracture may also cause cerebrospinal fluid (CSF) rhinorrhea, i.e., CSF leakage through the nose.

OPTIC NERVE

The optic nerve is a sensory nerve associated with sense of vision (For details, refer to chapter 6.2, page 317).

CLINICAL ASPECTS

Lesion of Visual Pathway
- Lesion in retina leads to scotoma, that is certain points may become blind spots.
- Loss of vision in one half (left or right) of visual field is called hemianopia.
- Optic chiasma lesion, if central, will lead to bitemporal hemianopia, but if peripheral on both sides will lead to binasal hemianopia.

Papilledema: It results due to increased intracranial pressure. It leads to swelling of optic disc due to blockage of tributaries of the retinal veins.

Optic neuritis: Lesion of optic nerve that results in decrease of visual acuity. Optic disc appears pale and smaller. Methyl alcohol is a usual toxic chemical leading to blindness.

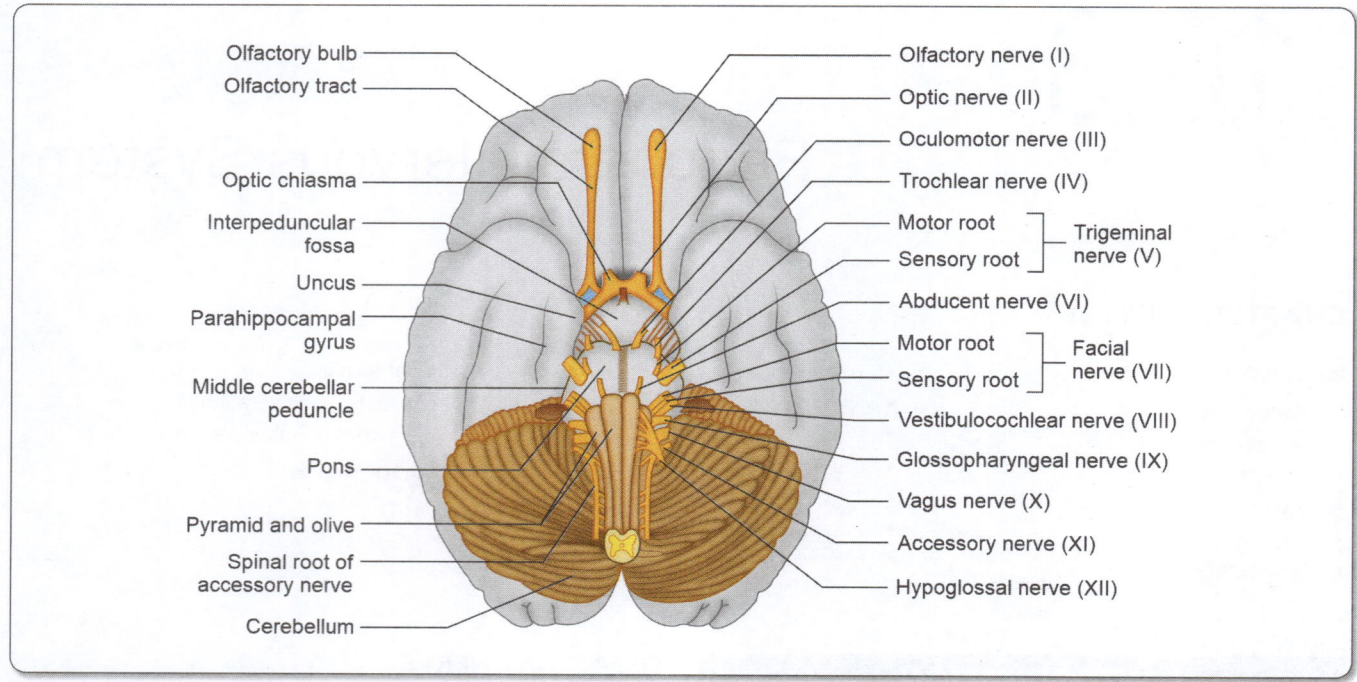

Fig. 10.3-1: Under surface of brain showing attachment of various cranial nerves

TABLE 10.3-1: Highlights of the cranial nerve

Number	Name	Nature	Important structure supplied
I	Olfactory nerve	Sensory	Nasal cavity (smell)
II	Optic nerve	Sensory	Eye (vision)
III	Oculomotor nerve	Motor	Ciliary muscle, sphincter pupillae and all extraocular muscles except superior oblique and lateral rectus
IV	Trochlear nerve	Motor	Superior oblique muscle
V	Trigeminal nerve	Mixed	Sensory: Face Motor: Muscles of mastication
VI	Abducens nerve	Motor	Lateral rectus muscle
VII	Facial nerve	Mixed	Muscles of face, posterior belly of digastric, stylohyoid, auricularis muscles and stapedius
VIII	Vestibulocochlear nerve	Sensory	Cochlear (balancing) vestibular (hearing)
IX	Glossopharyngeal nerve	Mixed	Taste—posterior 1/3 of tongue Sensory—tonsil, pharynx, middle ear Motor—stylopharyngeus, parotid gland
X	Vagus nerve	Mixed	Motor—heart, lungs, palate, pharynx, larynx, trachea, bronchi and gastrointestinal tract Sensory—heart, lungs, trachea, bronchi, larynx, pharynx, gastrointestinal tract and external ear
XI	Accessory nerve	Motor	Sternocleidomastoid and trapezius muscles Sternocleidomastoid and trapezius muscles
XII	Hypoglossal nerve	Motor	Tongue muscles strap muscles (C1, 2, 3 fibers)

NURSING IMPLICATIONS AND APPLICATIONS

In papilledema, lumbar puncture is contraindicated because a sudden decrease in pressure the following lumbar puncture may results in herniation of medulla oblongata or cerebellum through foramen megnum, which is a fatal condition.

OCULOMOTOR NERVE

Functional Components

The oculomotor nerve is entirely motor in function having three functional components:

1. Somatic efferent component is concerned with the movements of eyeball and supplies all the extraocular muscles except the lateral rectus and superior oblique.

2. General visceral efferent (parasympathetic) component of nerve is meant for accommodation and constriction of pupil. It supplies the ciliary muscle and sphincter pupillae muscle.

3. General somatic afferent component is associated with proprioceptive impulses from the extraocular muscles supplied. Thus, although the III nerve is a motor nerve, some sensory fibers are present.

Nucleus

The nuclear complex of the oculomotor nerve is situated in the midbrain (Fig. 10.3-2). It has two motor nuclei:

1. Main motor nucleus is composed of five subnuclei each supplying a muscle.

2. Accessory motor nucleus (Edinger-Westphal nucleus) sends preganglionic parasympathetic fibers along the other oculomotor fibers.

Course and Distribution

Each third nerve (Fig. 10.3-3) emerges from the midbrain, runs forward through the cavernous sinus. In the anterior part of cavernous sinus, it divides into superior and inferior divisions which enter the orbit through the middle part of superior oblique fissure (Fig. 10.3-4).

Superior division supplies the superior rectus and levator palpebral superioris muscle.

Inferior division divides into three branches:
1. Nerve to medial rectus
2. Nerve to inferior rectus
3. Nerve to inferior oblique, which gives off the *motor root* containing preganglionic parasympathetic fibers to *ciliary ganglion*.

CLINICAL ASPECTS

Complete and total paralysis of the third nerve results in:
- Ptosis, i.e., drooping of the upper eyelid
- Lateral squint
- Dilatation of the pupil
- Loss of accommodation
- Slight proptosis, i.e., forward projection of the eye
- Diplopia or double vision

A midbrain lesion causing contralateral hemiplegia and ipsilateral paralysis of the third nerve is known as *Weber's syndrome.*

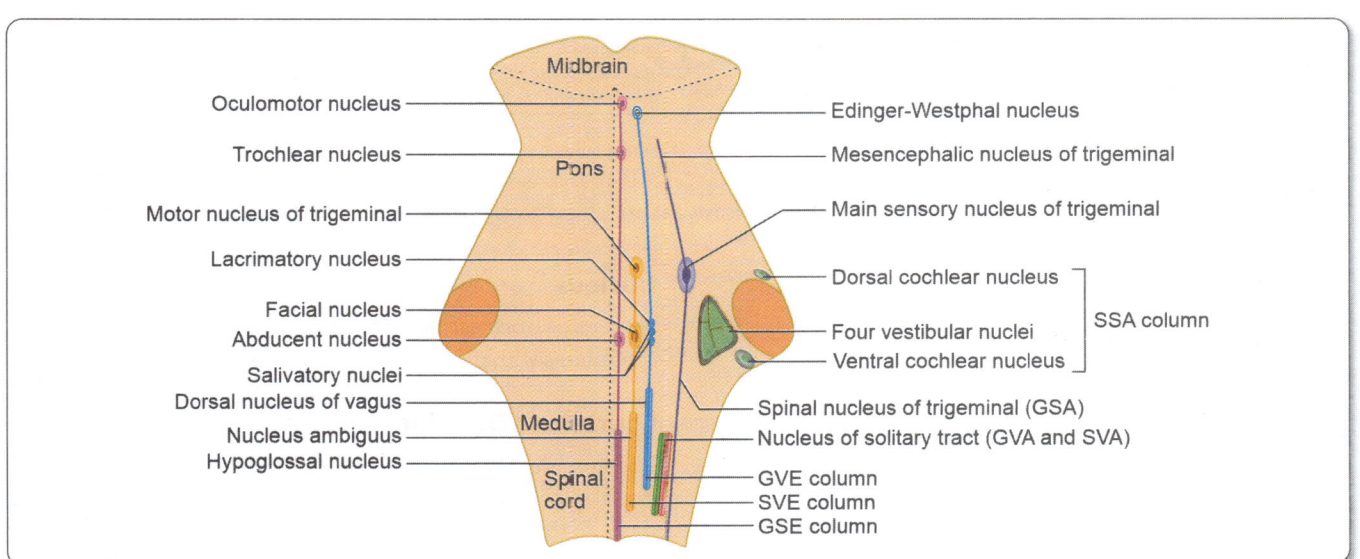

Fig. 10.3-2: Scheme to show the cranial nerve nuclei as projected on to the posterior surface of brain stem.
Abbreviations: SSA, special somatic afferent; GSA, general somatic afferent; GVA, general visceral afferent; SVA, special visceral afferent; GVE, general visceral efferent; SVE, special visceral efferent; GSE, general somatic efferent

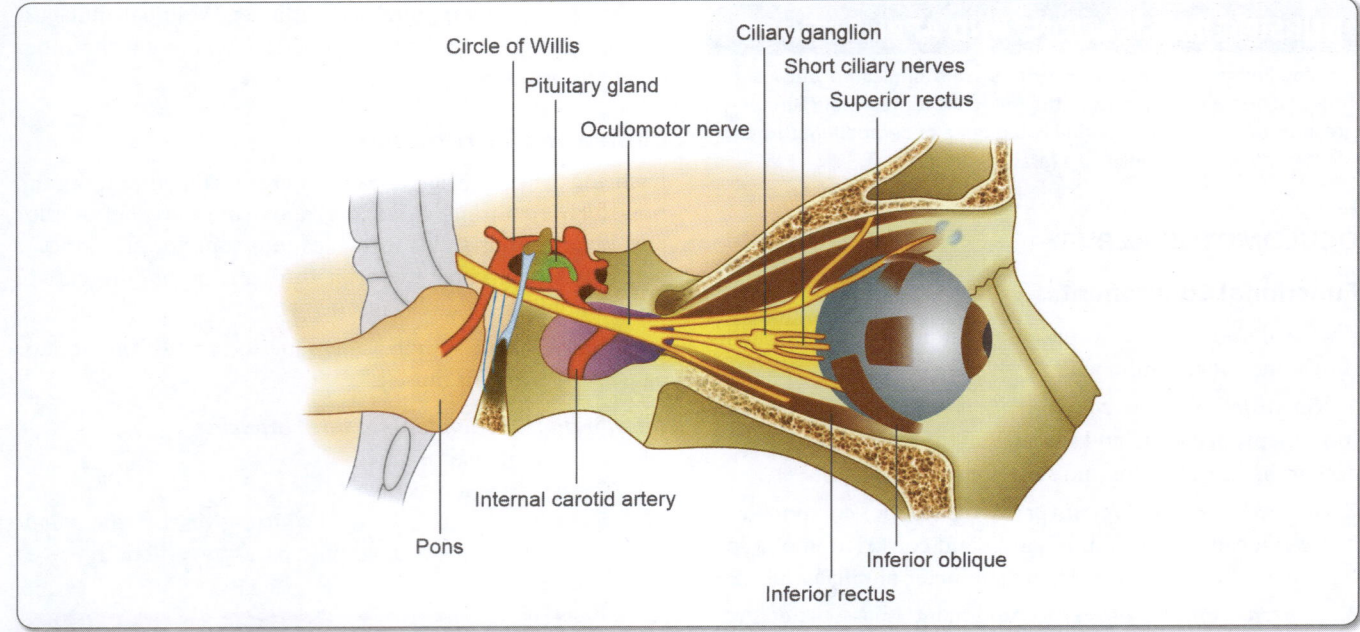

Fig. 10.3-3: The course of oculomotor nerve

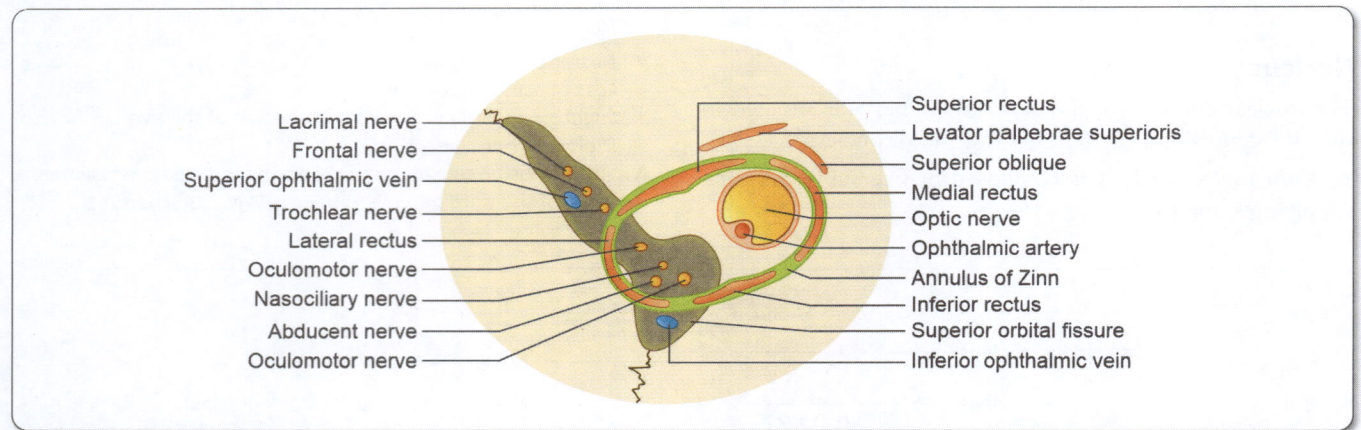

Fig. 10.3-4: Apical part of orbit showing origin of extraocular muscles and structures passing through superior oblique fissure and optic canal

TROCHLEAR NERVE

Functional Components

The trochlear nerve is entirely motor in function having two functional components:

1. *Somatic efferent* component is concerned with the movement of eyeball through the superior oblique muscle.

2. *General somatic afferent* component carries proprioceptive impulses from the superior oblique muscle. These impulses are relayed to the mesencephalic nucleus of the trigeminal nerve.

Nucleus

Nucleus of trochlear nerve is located in midbrain caudal to and continuous with third nerve nuclear complex (Fig. 10.3-2).

Course and Distribution

The trochlear nerve (Fig. 10.3-5), after emerging from the dorsal aspect of midbrain, winds around it and runs forward through the cavernous sinus. In the anterior part of cavernous sinus, it rises up, enters the orbit through the lateral part of superior oblique fissure (Fig. 10.3-4) and ends by supplying the superior oblique muscle.

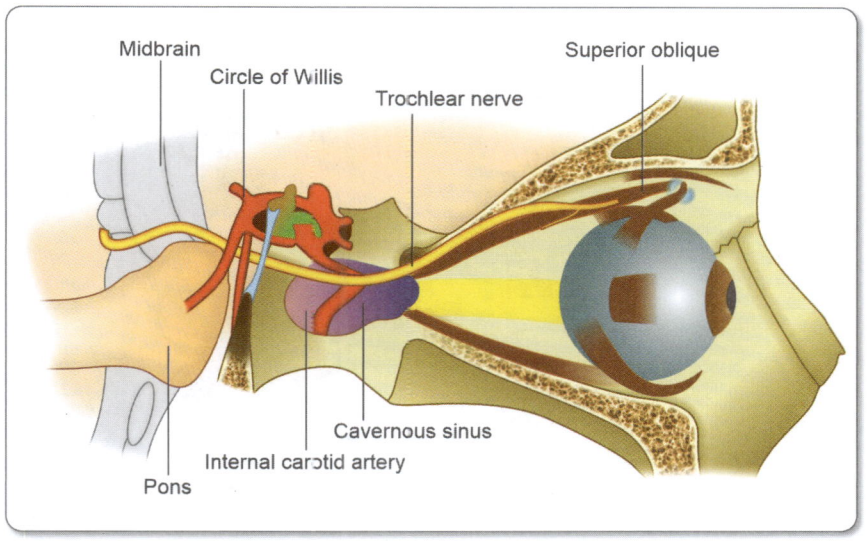

Fig. 10.3-5: Course of trochlear nerve

ABDUCENT NERVE

Sixth cranial nerve is described before fifth cranial nerve, as like third and fourth nerve, it also supplies extraocular muscle

Functional Components

The abducent nerve is small and entirely motor nerve having two functional components:

1. *Somatic efferent* component, for lateral movement of the eyeball.

2. *General somatic afferent,* component for proprioceptive impulses from the lateral rectus muscle. These impulses ultimately reach the mesencephalic nucleus of trigeminal nerve.

Nucleus

The abducens nucleus is situated in the lower part of pons, close to midline, beneath the floor of fourth ventricle. It lies in line with nuclei of fourth and third nerves above and with nucleus of hypoglossal nerve below (Fig. 10.3-2).

Course and Distribution

The abducent nerve emerges from the junction of pons and runs forwards, upwards and slightly laterally. At the sharp upper border of petrous temporal bone, the nerve bends forward at right angle and enters the cavernous sinus through its posterior wall (Fig. 10.3-6). In the cavernous sinus, the nerve runs forward and leaves the sinus to enter the orbit through the middle part of superior oblique fissure within the annulus of Zinn. In the orbit, the nerve runs forward and enters the ocular surface of the lateral rectus muscle (Fig. 10.3-6).

TRIGEMINAL NERVE

The trigeminal (fifth cranial) nerve is the largest cranial nerve and contains both sensory and motor fibers.

Nuclei

The trigeminal nerve has four nuclei (Fig. 10.3-2):

1. *Main sensory nucleus* lies in the upper part of pons.

2. *Spinal nucleus* extends from below the main sensory nucleus in the pons, through the whole length of the medulla oblongata into the upper two segments of the spinal cord.

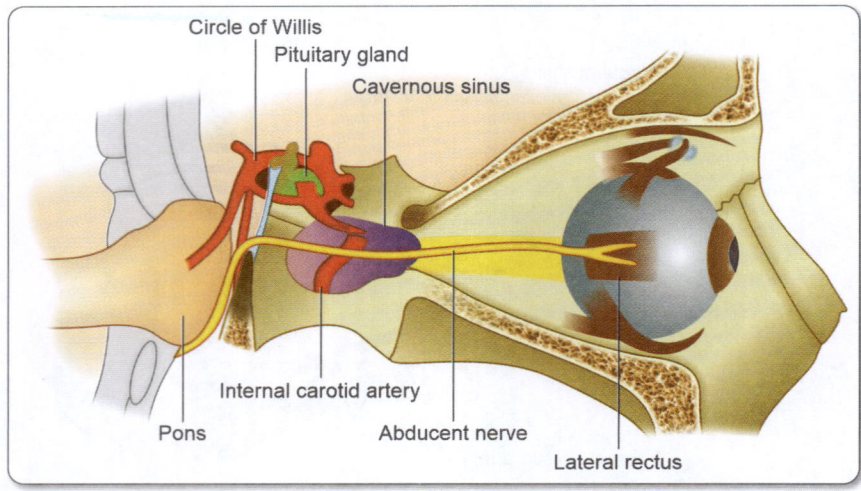

Fig. 10.3-6: Course of sixth cranial nerve

3. *Mesencephalic nucleus* extends from the midbrain down in the pons up to the main sensory nucleus.

4. *Motor nucleus* is situated in the upper part of pons medial to the main sensory nucleus.

Functional Components

Trigeminal nerve is a mixed nerve, having two functional components:

1. *General somatic afferent* component is constituted by sensory nuclei which receive the sensory fibers from trigeminal nerve as below:

- *Main sensory nucleus* receives fibers carrying sensations of touch and pressure.
- *Spinal nucleus* receives fibers carrying sensations of pain and temperature.
- *Mesencephalic nucleus* receives fibers carrying proprioceptive impulses from the facial and extraocular muscles and muscles of mastication.

2. *Branchial efferent (motor) component* for muscles of mastication and certain muscles in the floor of mouth.

Course and Distribution

The trigeminal nerve emerges from the anterior aspect of pons as a small motor root and large sensory root (Fig. 10.3-1). It passes forward and joins the trigeminal (gasserian) ganglion.

Trigeminal ganglion is the sensory ganglion of the fifth cranial nerve. It is homologous with the dorsal root ganglion of a spinal nerve.

Division of Trigeminal Nerve

It has three divisions (Fig. 10.3-7):

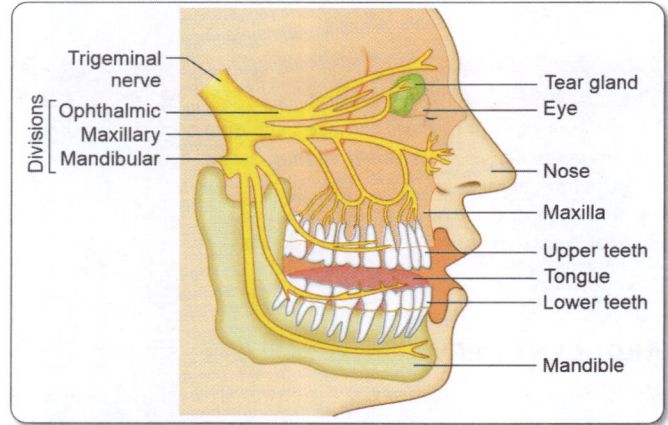

Fig. 10.3-7: Course of trigeminal nerve

1. *Ophthalmic division or nerve.* It consists of sensory fibers that bring impulses to the brain from the surface of eye, the lacrimal gland, skin of upper eyelid, forehead, and anterior part of scalp (Fig. 10.3-8). Main branches are lacrimal nerve, frontal nerve and nasociliary nerve.

2. *Maxillary division or nerve.* It is also a sensory nerve and consists of the fibers which bring impulses to the brain from the area of cheek, upper lip, upper gums, upper teeth and mucous lining of palate (Fig. 10.3-8). It ends by dividing into two terminal branches: infraorbital and zygomatic nerve.

3. *Mandibular nerve.* It is a mixed nerve formed by the union of two trunks—the large sensory and small motor.

Sensory trunk consists of the fibers which bring impulses from the lower lip, lower jaw, lower gums, lower teeth and skin of scalp behind the ear (Fig. 10.3-8).

Motor root supplies the muscles of mastication, tensor tympani muscles and certain muscles of the floor of mouth.

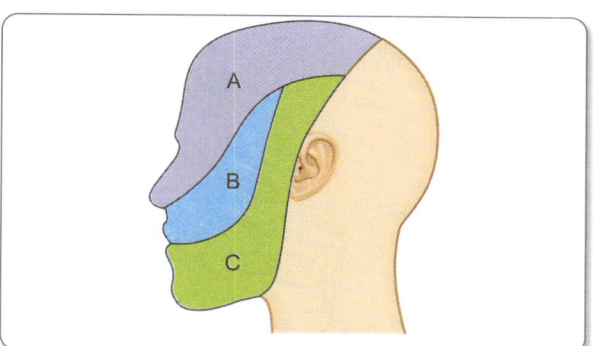

Fig. 10.3-8: Area of face and scalp supplied by 3 divisions of trigeminal nerve: A. Ophthalmic nerve; B. Maxillary nerve; C. Mandibular nerve

CLINICAL ASPECTS

Trigeminal neuralgia: Pain along the distribution of the nerve which is caused due to herpes zoster virus cause. The principal disease affecting sensory root of V nerve is characterized by attacks of severe pain in the area of distribution of maxillary or mandibular divisions. Maxillary nerve is most frequently involved.

NURSING IMPLICATIONS AND APPLICATIONS

Mandibular nerve block. For anesthetizing the branches of mandibular division of trigeminal nerve, the anesthetic agent is injected into the infra- temporal fossa through mandibular notch.
Infraclavicular nerve block. For infraclavicular nerve block, the injection is given around the mandibular fossa.
These blocks are commonly used in dental procedures.

FACIAL NERVE

Functional Components

The facial (seventh cranial) nerve is both a motor and sensory nerve. It consists of three functional components:

1. *Special visceral efferent* component for facial expression and elevation of hyoid bone.

2. *General visceral efferent* component is concerned with parasympathetic supply of the lacrimal gland, submandibular and sublingual salivary glands.

3. *Special visceral afferent* for taste sensation from the tongue.

4. *General somatic afferent* from the skin of external ear. These fibers end in spinal nucleus of trigeminal nerve.

Nuclei

The facial nerve has three nuclei.

1. *Main motor nucleus* is located deep in the pons. Special visceral efferent fibers arise from this nucleus. The part of

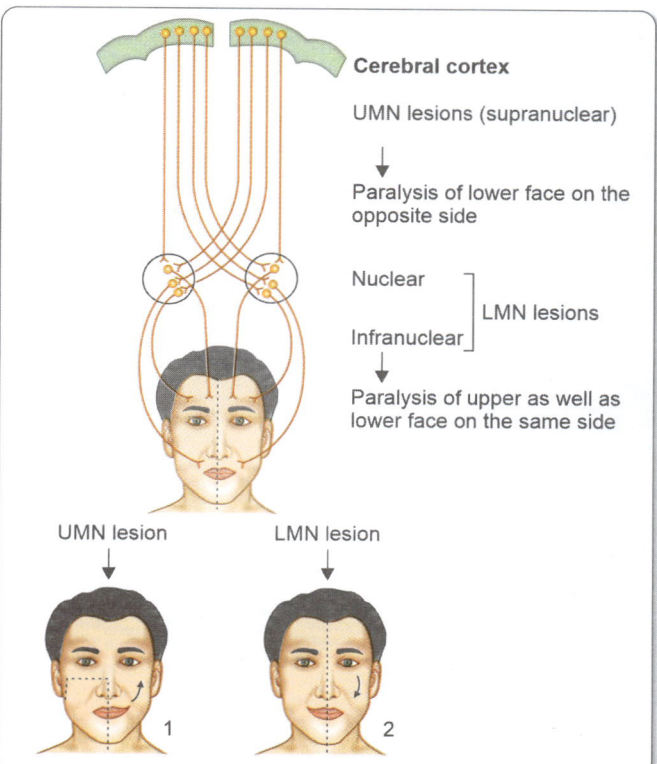

Fig. 10.3-9: Facial nerve nucleus, connections vis-a-vis supply to upper and lower part of face and facial expression defects associated with lesion of 1, upper motor neuron; and 2, lower motor neuron
Abbreviations: UMN, upper motor neuron; LMN, lower motor neuron

nucleus that supplies the muscles of upper part of face receives corticonuclear fibers from both cerebral hemispheres and that supplies to the lower part of face receives corticonuclear fibers from the opposite cerebral hemisphere only (Fig. 10.3-9).

2. *Parasympathetic nuclei* are:

Superior salivatory nucleus which sends preganglionic (general visceral) fibers for submaxillary and sublingual salivary glands.

Lacrimatory nucleus. It sends preganglionic (general visceral) fibers for innervation of the lacrimal gland.

3. *Sensory nucleus* is formed by the upper part of the *nucleus tractus solitarius* which belong to the special visceral efferent group. It receives afferent fibers carrying sensation of taste.

Course and Distribution

The two roots (motor and sensory) of facial nerve emerge from the junction of pons and medulla (Fig. 10.3-10). These roots then run laterally and forward and enter the internal *acoustic meatus*, where it joins to form single trunk. The *geniculate ganglion* associated with the nerve is formed by cell bodies of the *sensory neurons* carrying impulses from the skin of external ear.

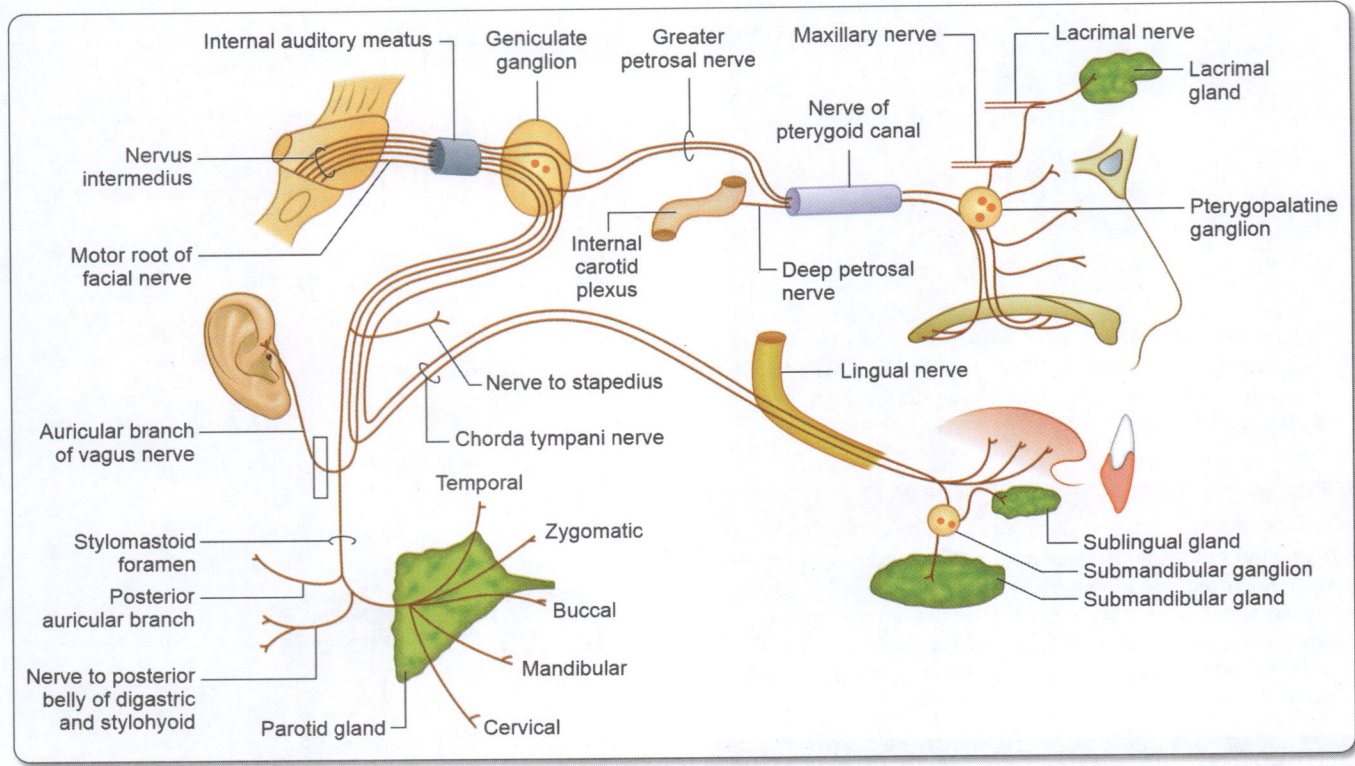

Fig. 10.3-10: The course and distribution of branches of facial nerve within the facial canal in the petrous part of temporal bone

Branches and course of the nerve within petrous part of temporal bone is shown in Figure 10.3-10 and its extracranial course and branches after emerging from the stylomastoid foramen are shown in Figure 10.3-11.

CLINICAL ASPECTS

Bell's palsy: Sudden paralysis of facial nerve at the stylomastoid foramen, results in asymmetry of corner of mouth, inability to close the eye, disappearance of nasolabial fold and loss of wrinkling of skin of forehead on the same side.

Lower motor neuron paralysis of VII nerve causes paralysis of ipsilateral half of face, i.e., both upper quadrant and lower quadrant of same side as the injury (Fig. 10.3-9).

Upper motor neuron paralysis of VII nerve results in paralysis of contralateral lower quadrant of face only (Fig. 10.3-9).

Crocodile tears syndrome: Lacrimation during eating occurs due to aberrant regeneration after trauma.

Ramsay-Hunt syndrome: Involvement of geniculate ganglia by herpes zoster results in this syndrome. It shows the following symptoms:

- Hyperacusis
- Loss of lacrimation
- Loss of sensation of taste in anterior two-thirds of tongue
- Bell's palsy and lack of salivation
- Vesicles on the auricle.

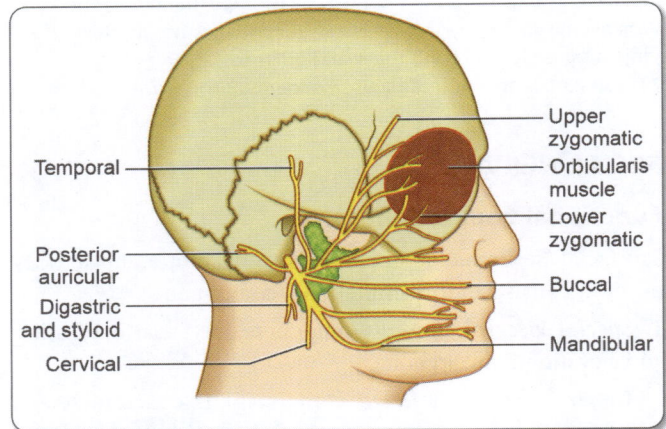

Fig. 10.3-11: Branches of facial nerve after emerging from the stylomastoid foramen

VESTIBULOCOCHLEAR NERVE

Functional Component and Nuclei

The vestibulocochlear nerve consists of two divisions, both made of *special somatic afferent fibers*. The sensory nuclei include:

1. Vestibular nuclei are four in number, which are situated partly in the medulla and partly in the pons, immediately beneath the lateral part of the floor of fourth ventricle (Fig. 10.3-2).

2. Cochlear nuclei are two in number, dorsal and ventral. They are located on the dorsal and ventral aspects of the inferior cerebellar peduncle, respectively in the upper part of the medulla (Fig. 10.3-2).

Course and Distribution

The vestibulocochlear nerve arises from the medulla (Fig. 10.3-1). It consists of two divisions:

1. Vestibular nerve consists of the central processes of bipolar neurons while cell bodies are located in the *vestibular ganglion* near the vestibule and semicircular canals of the ear. The peripheral processes of these neurons innervate the vestibular receptors in the semicircular ducts and saccule and utricle of the inner ear. These receptors are sensitive to changes in the position of head. The impulses they initiate pass into the cerebellum, where they are used in reflexes associated with the maintenance of equilibrium.

2. Cochlear nerve consists of the central processes of bipolar neurons of spiral ganglia. The peripheral processes of these neurons innervate the *organ of Corti* (hearing receptors). Impulses from the cochlear nerve pass through the pons and medulla oblongata on their way to temporal lobe (auditory cortex) for interpretation.

NURSING IMPLICATIONS AND APPLICATIONS

Injury to vestibulo-cochlear nerve causes the following symptom
- Ringing in the ears (Tinnitus)
- Giddiness or loss of balance (Vertigo)
- Hearing loss.

GLOSSOPHARYNGEAL NERVE

Functional Components and Nuclei

Glossopharyngeal nerve is a mixed nerve having the following nuclei and functional components (Fig. 10.3-12).

Special visceral (branchial) efferent (SVE) fibers arise from the *nucleus ambiguus*, which is elongated and not clearly defined [(hence the name ambiguous, nucleus that extends throughout the length of medulla Fig. 10.3-2)]. The special visceral efferent fibers arising from it supply only one muscle—the *stylopharyngeus*.

General visceral efferent (GVE) fibers, which arise from the *inferior salivatory nucleus*, is located in the pons, immediately caudal to superior salivatory nucleus and just above the upper end of the dorsal nucleus of vagus (Fig. 10.3-2).

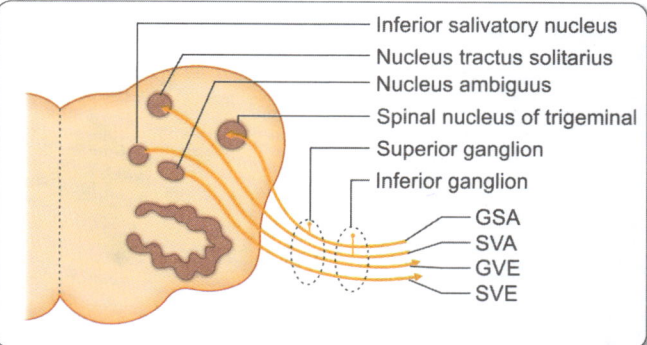

Fig. 10.3-12: Functional components and nuclei of IX (glossopharyngeal) nerve
Abbreviations: GSA, general somatic afferent; SVA, special visceral afferent; GVE, general visceral efferent; SVE, special visceral efferent

The preganglionic parasympathetic fibers arising from this nucleus relay in the *otic ganglion*; and the postganglionic fibers supply the parotid gland (Fig. 10.3-3).

General visceral afferent (GVA) component of the glossopharyngeal nerve is formed by sensory neurons located in the *superior ganglion* of glossopharyngeal nerve.

Peripheral processes of these neurons collect general sensations (touch, pain and temperature) from the posterior 1/3rd of the tongue, pharynx and carotid body.

Central processes of these neurons relay these sensations to the spinal nucleus of trigeminal nerve.

Special visceral afferent (SVA) component of ninth cranial nerve is formed by the sensory neurons located in the *inferior ganglion* of the nerve.

Peripheral processes of these neurons collect taste sensation from the posterior 1/3rd of tongue.

Central process of these neurons relay the taste sensation to the nucleus of tractus solitarius, located in the medulla (Fig. 10.3-2).

Course and Distribution

Glossopharyngeal nerve arises from the medulla (Fig. 10.3-1). Course and distribution of its fibers described above in the functional components is depicted in Figure 10.3-13.

CLINICAL ASPECTS

Lesion of glossopharyngeal nerve causes:
- Absence of secretions of parotid gland
- Absence of taste from posterior one-third of tongue and the circumvallate papillae
- Loss of pain sensations from tongue, tonsil, pharynx and soft palate.
- Gag reflex is absent.

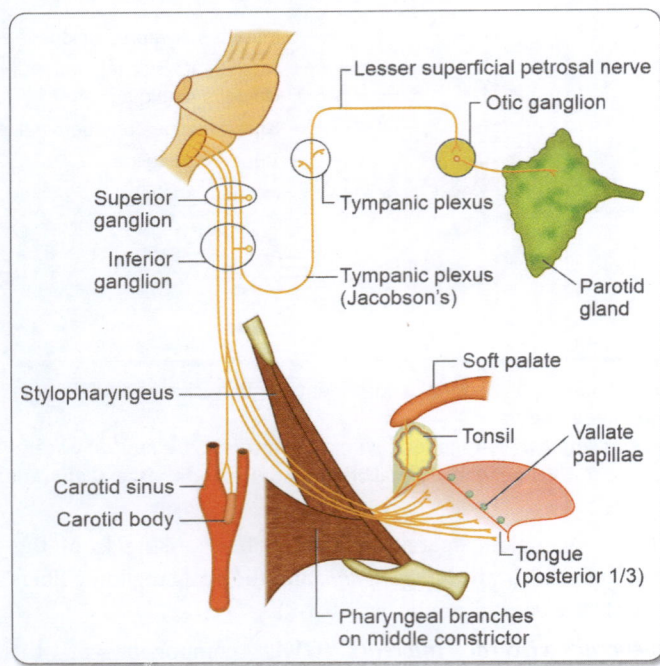

Fig. 10.3-13: Course and distribution of glossopharyngeal nerve

VAGUS NERVE

Functional Components and Nuclei

Vagus nerve is a *mixed nerve* having the following functional components and associated nuclei (Fig. 10.3-14):

Special visceral efferent (SVE) fibers arise from the *nucleus ambiguus* and supply muscles of pharynx and larynx.

General visceral efferent (GVE) fibers arise from the *dorsal nucleus of vagus* also called *motor nucleus of vagus*, which is elongated and extends in most of the length of medulla (Fig. 10.3-2).

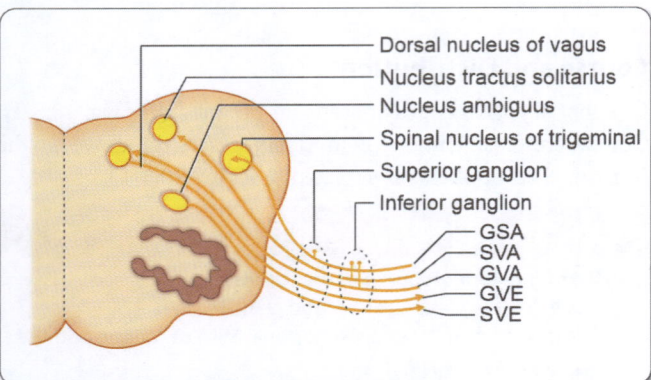

Fig. 10.3-14: Functional components and nuclei of vagus. *Abbreviations:* GSA, general somatic afferent; SVA, special visceral afferent; GVA, general visceral afferent; GVE, general visceral efferent; SVE, special visceral efferent

Preganglionic parasympathetic fibers arising from the dorsal vagus nucleus relay in the small ganglia situated close to or within the walls of viscera supplied.

Postganglionic parasympathetic fibers arising from the small ganglia supply the heart, lungs, GIT up to the junction of right 2/3rd and left 1/3rd of transverse colon (Fig. 10.3-2).

General visceral afferent (GVA) component of vagus nerve is formed by the sensory neurons located in *inferior ganglion of* the nerve.

Peripheral processes of these neurons collect sensations from the pharynx, trachea, esophagus and thoracic and abdominal viscera.

Central processes of these neurons convey the impulses to *nucleus tractus solitarius* and dorsal nucleus of vagus.

Special visceral afferent (SVA) component of the vagus nerve is formed by the sensory neurons located in the *inferior ganglion of the vagus nerve.*

Peripheral processes of these neurons bring taste sensations from the posterior-most part of the tongue and epiglottis.

Central processes of these neurons convey these impulses to the upper part of nucleus tractus solitarius.

General somatic afferent (GSA) component of the nerve is formed by the sensory neurons located in the *superior ganglion of the vagus nerve.*

Peripheral processes of these neurons collect general sensations from the skin of external ear.

Central processes of these neurons convey these impulses to the spinal nucleus of trigeminal nerve.

Course and Distribution

The vagus nerve originates from the medulla, and extends downward through the neck into the abdomen. Course and distribution of its various branches carrying different fibers described above in the functional components are shown in Figure 10.3-15.

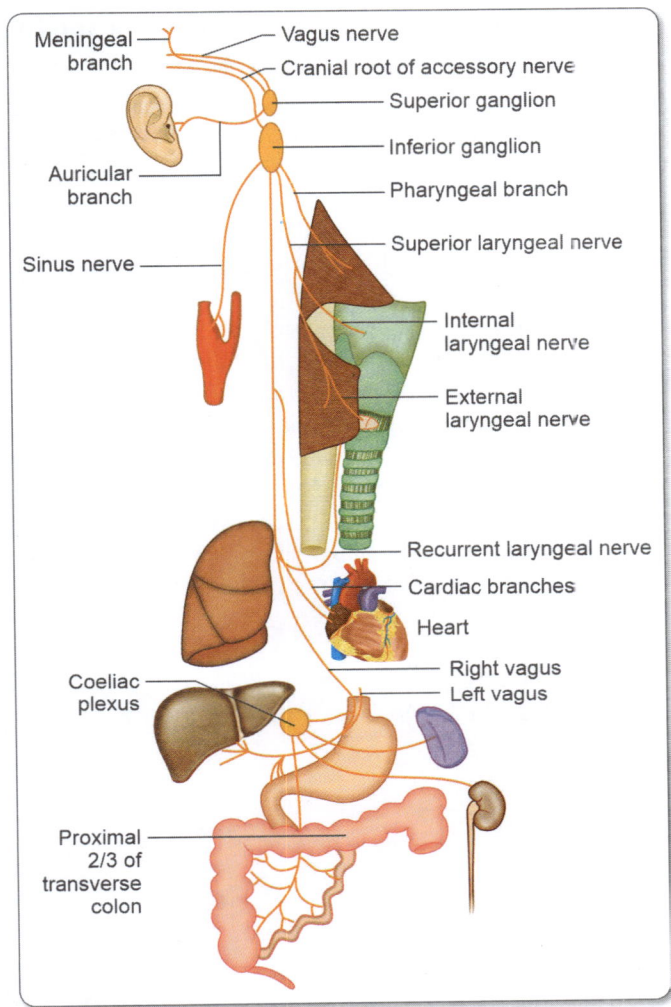

Fig. 10.3-15: Distribution of vagus nerve

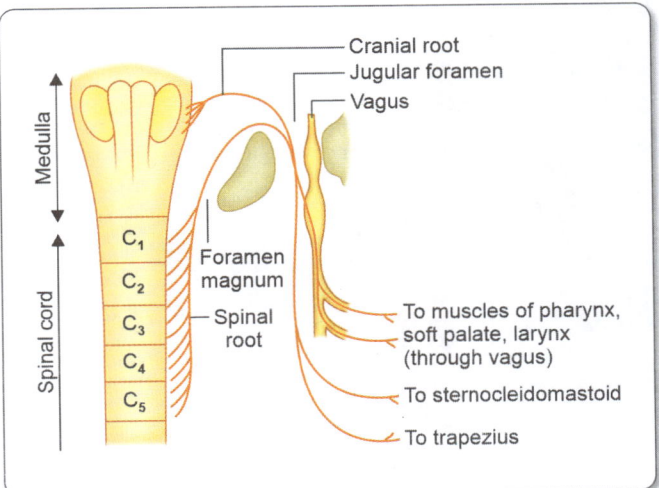

Fig. 10.3-16: Course and distribution of accessory nerve

Course and Distribution

The accessory nerve originates as two roots (Fig. 10.3-1):

1. *Cranial root* of the accessory nerve arises from the medulla and joins the vagus nerve. As mentioned above, it carries motor impulses to muscles of palate, larynx and pharynx (Fig. 10.3-16).

2. *Spinal root* of the nerve arises from the spinal cord and descends into the neck and supplies motor fibers to trapezius and sternocleidomastoid muscles(Fig. 10.3-16).

CLINICAL ASPECTS

Lesions of spinal root of accessory nerve cause drooping of the shoulder and inability to turn chin to opposite side.

ACCESSORY NERVE

Functional Components and Nuclei

Special visceral efferent (SVE) fibers arise from the *nucleus ambiguus* and form the *cranial root* of the nerve. These fibers are distributed through the vagus nerve to supply:

Muscles of palate except tensor palati which is supplied by mandibular division of trigeminal nerve.

Muscles of pharynx except stylopharyngeus which is supplied by the glossopharyngeal nerve.

Muscles of larynx.

General somatic efferent (GSE) component of the nerve is formed by the motor fibers arising from the *spinal nucleus of accessory nerve*, which is located in the lateral part of the anterior grey column of the upper five cervical spinal segments. These fibers form the *spinal root* of the nerve.

HYPOGLOSSAL NERVE

Functional Components and Nuclei

Hypoglossal nerve is a motor nerve having the following functional components and associated nuclei:

General somatic efferent (GSE) component is formed by the nerve fibers arising from the *hypoglossal nucleus*, which is an elongated column extending throughout the length of medulla oblongata in the paramedian plane (Fig. 10.3-2). These fibers supply all the intrinsic and extrinsic muscles of the tongue except the palatoglossus which is supplied by the cranial root of accessory nerve through the vagus nerve.

General somatic afferent (GSA) component is formed by the sensory fibers which carry proprioceptive impulses from muscles of the tongue. The location of the neurons of origin of these fibers is uncertain.

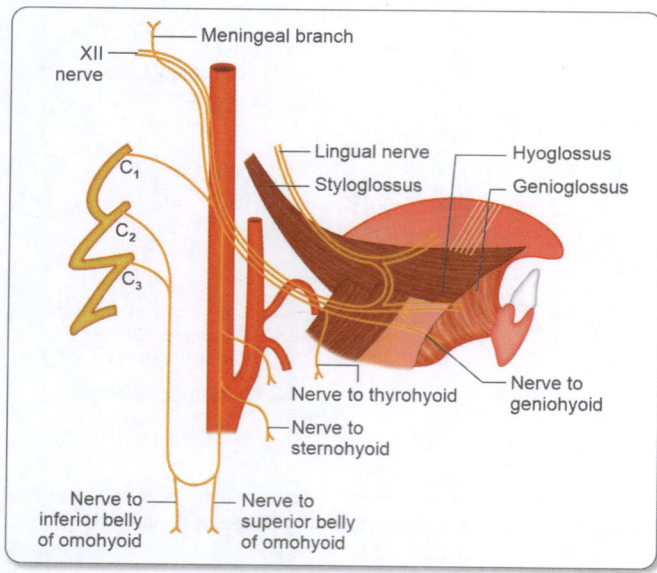

Fig. 10.3-17: Course and distribution of hypoglossal nerve

Course and Distribution

Hypoglossal nerve arises from the medulla by 10–15 rootlets (Fig. 10.3-1). It leaves the cranial cavity through the hypoglossal canal and extends downward in the neck up to the level of angle of mandible. Then it passes forward into the tongue and supplies the muscles that move the tongue in speaking, chewing, and swallowing. Course and distribution of nerve are depicted in Figure 10.3-17.

NURSING IMPLICATIONS AND APPLICATIONS

- The hypoglossal nerve is tested clinically by asking the patient to protrude his/her tongue. Normally, the tongue is protruded straight forwards. If the nerve is paralyzed, the tongue deviates to the paralyzed side.
- An infranuclear unilateral lesion of the hypoglossal nerve produces paralysis of the tongue on that side.

SPINAL NERVES

GENERAL CONSIDERATIONS

There are 31 pairs of spinal nerves which originate from the spinal cord. They are grouped together in five groups. Nerves belonging to different groups are named according to the regions of vertebral column with which they are associated. Various groups of spinal nerves are as below:

- Cervical nerves   :   8 pairs
- Thoracic nerves   :   12 pairs
- Lumbar nerves   :   5 pairs
- Sacral nerves   :   5 pairs
- Coccygeal nerves   :   1 pair.

Relationship with Vertebrae (Figs 10.3-18A and B)

- There are 8 cervical nerves and 7 cervical vertebrae. First seven cervical nerves lie above the numerically corresponding vertebrae. The 8th cervical nerve lies below 7th cervical vertebrae.
- The number of spinal nerves in *thoracic, lumbar* and *sacral* region corresponds to that of vertebrae, and each nerve lies below the numerically corresponding vertebrae, e.g., 8th thoracic nerve emerges from the vertebral column below the 8th thoracic vertebra.
- In the upper part of spinal cord, the spinal nerves pass outward nearly horizontally while those from the lower portion of spinal cord descend at sharp angles. This is because of the fact that in the adults the spinal cord ends at the level of 1st and 2nd lumbar vertebrae so, the lumbar, sacral and coccygeal nerves descend to their exit point in a bunch called *cauda equina* (because of its resemblance to horse's tail) (Fig. 10.3-18).

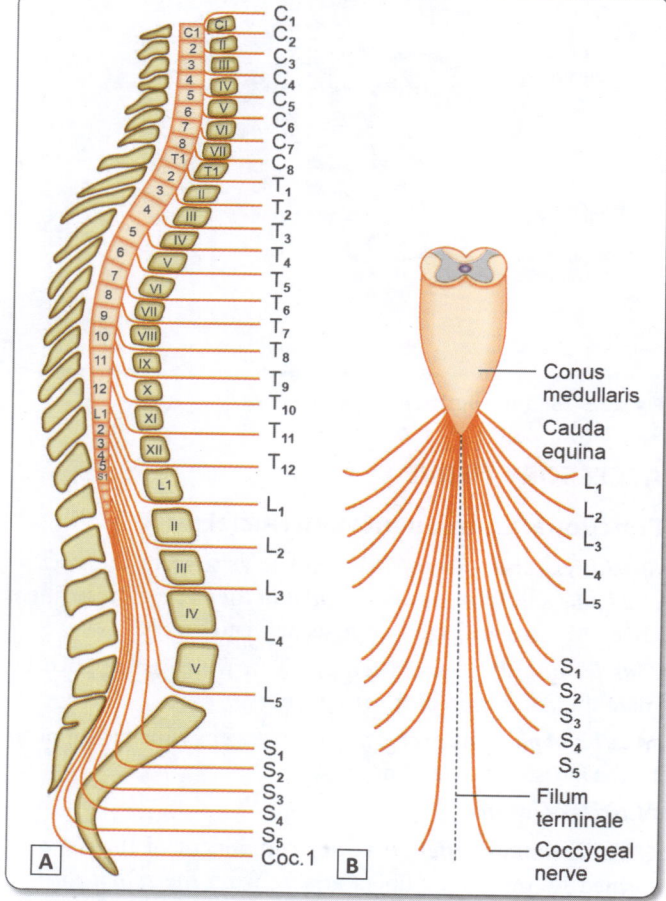

Figs 10.3-18A and B: A. Lateral view showing relationship of the spinal cord to the vertebral column. Note the site of origin of each spinal nerve in the cord and its point of exit from the vertebral column; B. Formation of cauda equina

Description of a Typical Spinal Nerve

A typical spinal nerve is a mixed nerve, i.e., it consists of sensory and motor nerve fibers.

Origin of Spinal Nerve

Each spinal nerve arises by two roots, a ventral root and a dorsal root from the spinal cord (Fig. 10.3-19).

Ventral root (motor root) consists of efferent fibers which are axons of the motor neurons present in the grey matter of anterior or ventral horn of the spinal cord. These convey motor impulses from the spinal cord to the periphery.

Dorsal root (sensory root) consists of the afferent fibers which carry impulses from the periphery to the spinal cord. The cell bodies of these fibers are located outside the spinal cord in a swelling on the dorsal root called the *dorsal root ganglion*. The dendrites of these sensory neurons conduct impulses inward from peripheral parts of the body, while their axons extend through the dorsal root into the spinal cord, where they form synapses with dendrites of other neurons.

The ventral and dorsal roots join to form the spinal nerve just before leaving the canal through the intervertebral foramen.

Course and Distribution of a Spinal Nerve

Immediately after emerging from the intervertebral foramen, each spinal nerve gives a recurrent meningeal branch and divides into posterior ramus and an anterior ramus each containing both sensory and motor fibers (Fig. 10.3-19):

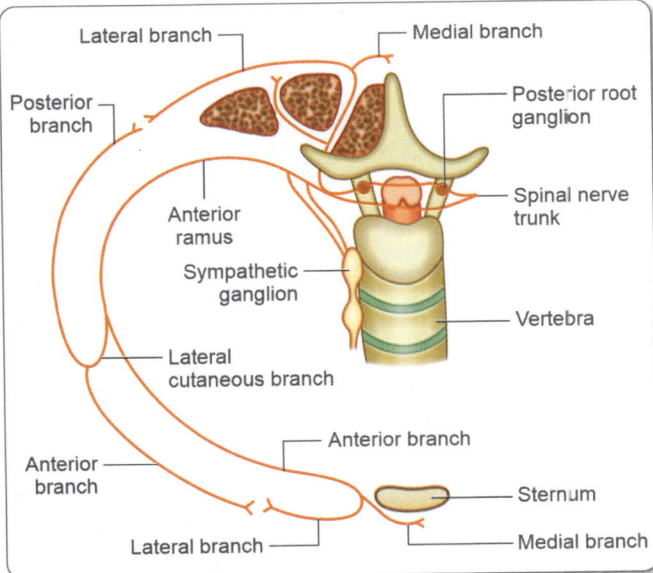

Fig. 10.3-19: Diagram of typical spinal nerve showing scheme of branching and relationship to spinal cord, sympathetic ganglion and vertebral column

Recurrent meningeal branch re-enters the vertebral canal to innervate the meninges.

Posterior ramus passes posteriorly around the vertebral column and supplies the muscles and skin of the back.

Anterior ramus is larger than the posterior ramus. It runs anteriorly to supply the skin and muscles over the anterolateral part of the body. In its initial course, the anterior ramus of 1st thoracic to 3rd lumbar spinal nerve is connected to a sympathetic ganglion by grey and white rami communicants (Fig. 10.3-19).

PLEXUSES OF SPINAL NERVES

The anterior rami of spinal nerves (except for thoracic nerves from T_3 to T_{11}) join together and/or branch to form a network of nerves known as nerve plexuses. In this way, the body structures get supply from more than one spinal nerve and, therefore, damage to one spinal nerve does not cause loss of function of a region.

There are five plexuses of mixed nerves formed on each side of the vertebral column. These include:

1. Cervical plexus
2. Brachial plexus
3. Lumbar plexus
4. Sacral plexus
5. Coccygeal plexus.

Dermatome

Dermatome refers to area of the skin supplied by a single segment of spinal cord. Thus, each spinal cord segment is related to the body in a segmental way by its spinal nerves (Fig. 10.3-20).

Cervical Plexus

The cervical plexuses lie deep in the neck on either side, opposite the 1st, 2nd, 3rd and 4th cervical vertebrae under cover of sternocleidomastoid muscle. The ventral rami of first four cervical (C_1, C_2, C_3 and C_4) nerves unite with each other to form the cervical plexus (Fig. 10.3-21).

Branches

Many branches arise from the cervical plexus.

Cutaneous branches are superficial, supply the skin of neck up to the level of sternum and back and side of head.

Muscular branches are deep and supply the muscles of neck.

Phrenic nerve (C_3, C_4, C_5) is the only motor supply to diaphragm.

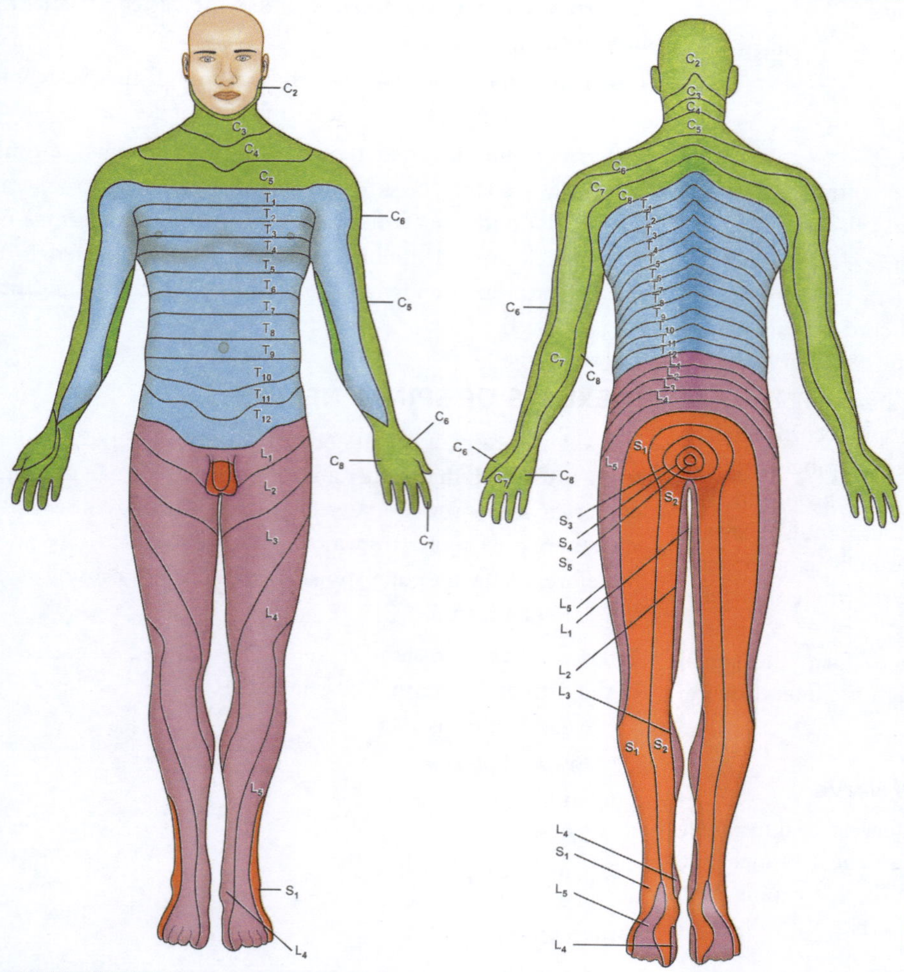

L$_1$, L$_2$, L$_3$, L$_4$	Anterior and inner surface of lower limbs
L$_4$, L$_5$, S$_1$	Foot
L$_4$	Medial side of great toe
S$_1$, S$_2$, L$_5$	Posterior and outer surface of lower limbs
S$_1$	Lateral margin of foot and little toe
S$_2$, S$_3$, S$_4$	Perineum
T$_{10}$	Level of umbilicus
T$_{12}$	Inguinal or groin regions
C$_5$	Clavicles
C$_5$, C$_6$, C$_7$	Lateral parts of upper limbs
C$_8$, T$_1$	Medial sides of the upper limbs
C$_6$	Thumb
C$_6$, C$_7$, C$_8$	Hand
C$_8$	Ring and little fingers
T$_4$	Level of nipples

Fig. 10.3-20: Dermatome distribution of body

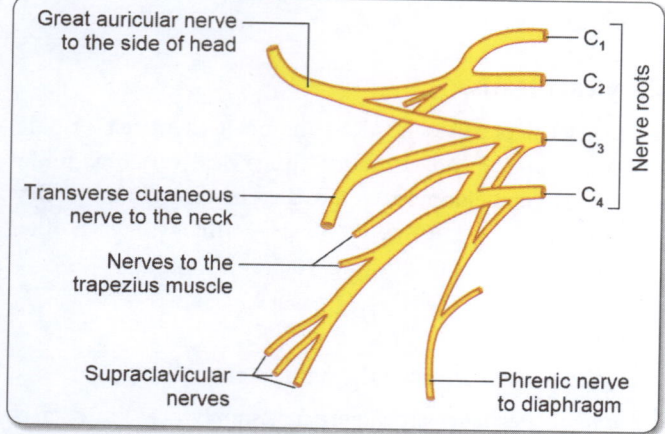

Fig. 10.3-21: The cervical plexus

Brachial Plexus

The brachial plexus is situated in the neck and shoulder above and behind the subclavian vessels and in the axilla. Its construction is as below (Fig. 10.3-22).

Roots are constituted by the anterior rami of lower four cervical nerves and a large part of first thoracic nerve (C$_5$ to C$_8$ and T$_1$).

Trunks are formed by union of roots:

Upper trunk is formed by union of roots of C$_5$ and C$_6$.

Middle trunk is formed by roots of C$_7$.

Lower trunk is formed by roots of C$_8$ and T$_1$.

Divisions. Each trunk divides into ventral and dorsal division (which ultimately supply the anterior and posterior aspects of limbs).

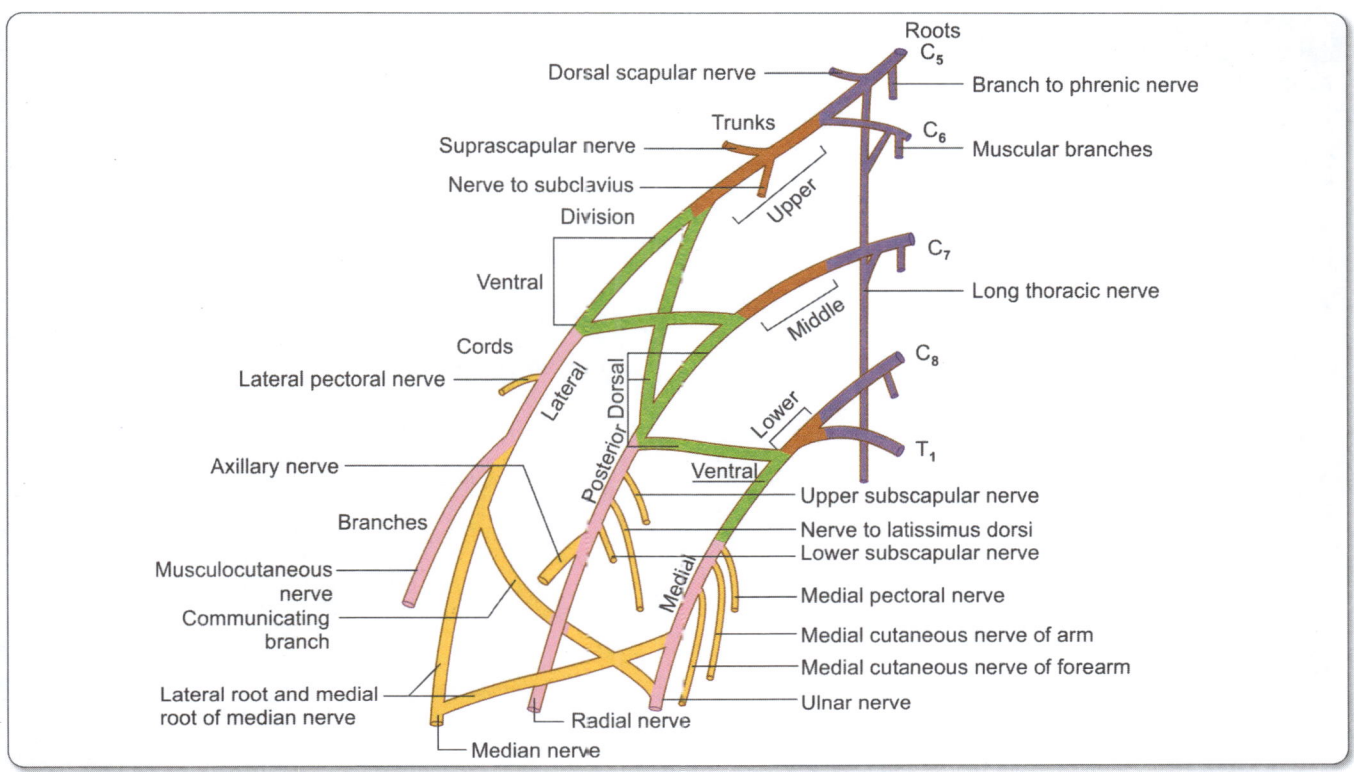

Fig. 10.3-22: The brachial plexus

Cords are formed by union of divisions:

Lateral cord is formed by union of ventral divisions of upper and middle trunks.

Medial cord is formed by the ventral division of the lower trunk.

Posterior cord is formed by union of dorsal divisions of all the three trunks.

Branches of brachial plexus are many and supply the skin and muscles of upper limbs and some of the chest muscles. The major branches of brachial plexus are (Figs 10.3-23A and B):

Axillary nerve (C_5, C_6), which supplies the deltoid muscle, shoulder joint and overlying skin.

Musculocutaneous nerve (C_5, C_6, C_7), which supplies muscles of the arms on the anterior side and skin of forearm.

Ulnar nerve (C_7, C_8, T_1) supplies muscles of the forearm and hands, and the skin of hands.

Median nerve (C_5, C_6, C_7, C_8, T_1) also called labourer's nerve supplies muscle of the forearm and hands, and skin of the hand.

Radial nerve (C_5, C_6, C_7, C_8, T_1) supplies muscles of the arm on the posterior aspect, and the skin of forearm and hands.

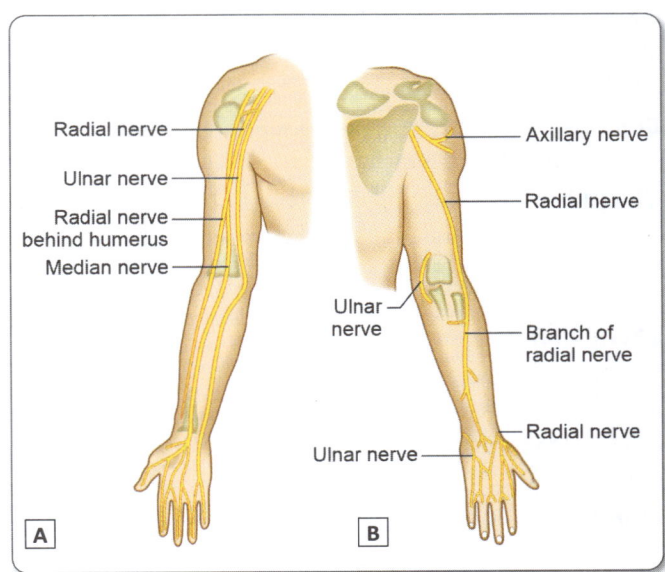

Figs 10.3-23A and B: Main nerves of arm: A. Anterior view; B. Posterior view

NURSING IMPLICATIONS AND APPLICATIONS

Axillary Nerve

Injury to axillary nerve occurs due to fracture of neck of the humerus resulting in paralysis of deltoid muscle. Therefore, the patient is unable to abduct the arm.

Intramuscular injection is usually given in the lower half of deltoid muscle to avoid injury to the axillary nerve.

Ulnar Nerve

- *In the elbow region,* the ulnar nerve is very superficial. A sharp tap behind the medial condyle of humerus bone causes its stimulation leading to pain and tingling sensation in the ring and little finger.
- Injury to ulnar nerve causes paralysis of intrinsic muscles of hand leading to claw hand.

Median Nerve

- *Carpal tunnel syndrome.* In the wrist region, the median nerve lies in a very narrow space called carpal tunnel. When this space gets reduced due to swelling or bony injury resulting in pain, tingling sensation and weakness of thumb and loss of sensations in lateral three and half of the fingers

Radial Nerve

- *Saturday night palsy.* Compression of radial nerve by placing outstretched arm on the armchair for long time. This happens usually in drunken condition (mostly on weekend, i.e., on Saturday person takes lot of drinks), hence known as Saturday night palsy.

Lumbar Plexus

The lumbar plexus is formed by the ventral rami of upper four lumbar (L_1, L_2, L_3 and L_4) nerves (Fig. 10.3-24). It is located in front of the transverse processes of lumbar vertebrae and behind the psoas major muscle.

Branches from the lumbar plexus supply mostly the muscles of thigh. The largest branches are:

Obturator nerve which supplies the adductor muscles of thigh

Femoral nerve is a motor and sensory nerve to the structures of thigh.

Sacral Plexus

The sacral plexus is formed by union of ventral rami of first four sacral nerves (S_1, S_2, S_3 and S_4), along with the lumbosacral trunk (derived from the few fibers of L_4 and all fibers of L_5) (Fig. 10.3-24).

Branches. Apart from the sciatic and pudendal nerves (main branches), sacral plexus gives off several branches that supply skin and muscles in the lower extremity (Fig. 10.3-25).

Sciatic nerve (L_4, L_5, S_1, S_2, S_3). It is the largest and longest nerve in the body. It passes downward into the buttock and descends into the thigh, where it divides into *tibial and*

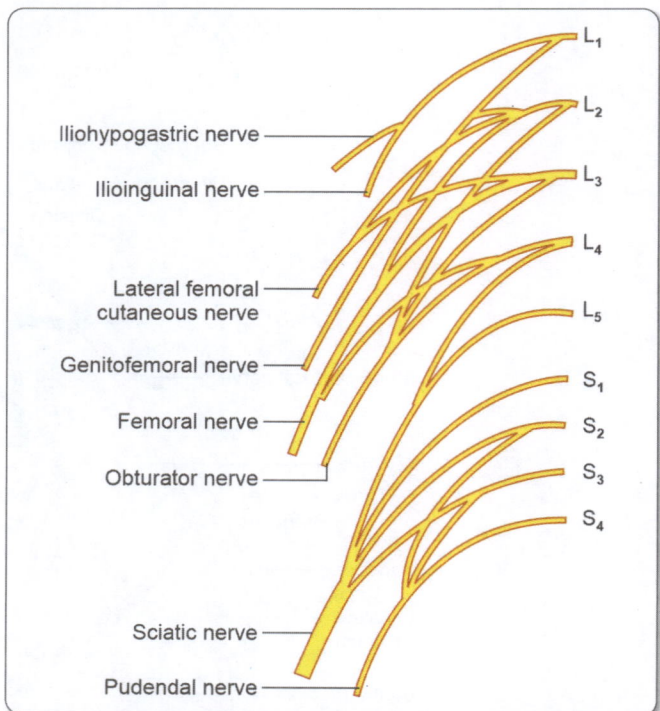

Fig. 10.3-24: Lumbar, sacral and coccygeal plexuses

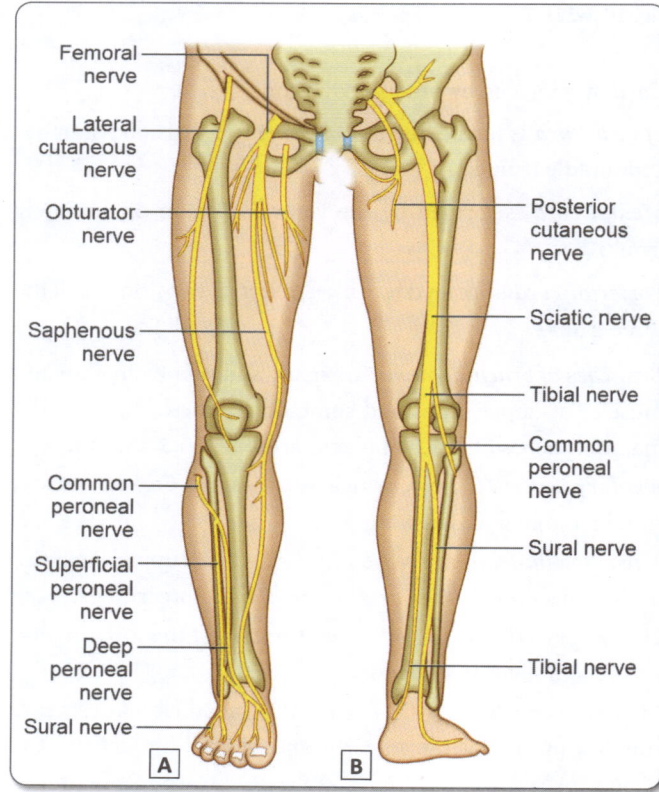

Figs 10.3-25A and B: Main nerves of the lower limb: A. Anterior view; B. Posterior view

common peroneal nerves. The many branches of these nerves supply skin and muscles of thigh, leg and foot.

Pudendal nerve *(S₂, S₃, S₄).* After arising from the sacral plexus it leaves the pelvis, enters the gluteal region and finally ends by dividing in the pudendal canal. It supplies structures in the perineum.

Coccygeal Plexus

Coccygeal plexus is a very small plexus. It is formed by the coccygeal nerve with a contribution from fourth and fifth sacral nerves (Fig. 10.3-24).

Branches from coccygeal plexus supply the skin in the region of coccyx, and some muscles of floor of pelvis.

NURSING IMPLICATIONS AND APPLICATIONS

Sleeping foot*.* After sitting for a long time the sciatic nerve get compressed against femur. Therefore, on standing for few minutes one feels uncomfortable and cannot move and feels pins and needles on the body (technically paresthesia), this is but soon is able to walk normally known as sleeping foot.

Sciatica refers as shooting pain along the distribution of branches of sciatic nerve. It occurs due to compression of sciatic nerve during inter vertebral disc prolapsed or in osteoarthritis

Intramuscular injection in gluteal region. Nurse should be very careful while injecting medicine intramuscularly in the gluteal region. To avoid injury to the sciatic nerve, the recommended site is upper outer quadrant of buttock.

Foot drop refers to difficulty in lifting the front part of the foot. It occurs due to weakness or paralysis of muscles involved in lifting of foot. The cause of foot drop is injury to peroneal nerve (branch of sciatic nerve).

Pudendal nerve block is a regional anesthetic technique to anesthetize the perineal muscles during obstetric procedures. The anesthetic drug (lignocaine) is injected near ischial spine through vaginal wall.

THORACIC NERVES

Ventral rami (anterior branches) of thoracic spinal nerves do not make any plexus. These branches pass as *intercostal nerves* out into the intercostal spaces to supply the intercostal muscles and upper abdominal muscles. They also receive sensory impulses from the skin of thorax and abdomen.

ASSESS YOURSELF

Short and Long Answer Questions

1. **Describe the origin and functions of the following cranial nerves:**
   - Fifth
   - Seventh
   - Tenth
2. **Draw diagram of:**
   - Cervical plexus
   - Brachial plexus
   - Sacral plexus
3. **Write notes on:**
   - Lumbar puncture
   - Branches of femoral nerve
   - Bell's palsy
   - Trigeminal neuralgia

Multiple Choice Questions

1. **The main function of first cranial nerve is:**
   a. Sense of pain   b. Sense of smell
   c. Sense of taste   d. Cough reflex
2. **Trochlear nerve innervates which extra-ocular muscle?**
   a. Superior rectus
   b. Superior oblique
   c. Lateral rectus
   d. Inferior oblique
3. **Which of the following is not innervated by oculomotor nerve?**
   a. Medial rectus
   b. Inferior rectus
   c. Lateral rectus
   d. Inferior oblique

4. **The somatic efferent component of abducent nerve causes:**
   a. Outward movement of eyeball
   b. Inward movement of eyeball
   c. Upward movement of eyeball
   d. Downward movement of eyeball

5. **Muscles of mastication are innervated by:**
   a. Ophthalmic division of trigeminal
   b. Maxillary division of trigeminal
   c. Mandibular division of trigeminal
   d. Facial nerve

6. **Bell's palsy occurs due to damage of:**
   a. Trigeminal nerve
   b. Facial nerve
   c. Hypoglossal nerve
   d. Glossopharyngeal nerve

7. **The cervical plexus branches which form phrenic nerve?**
   a. C_1, C_2 and C_3 b. C_2, C_3 and C_4
   c. C_3, C_4 and C_5 d. C_6, C_7 and C_8

8. **The middle trunk of brachial plexus is formed by union of roots of:**
   a. C_5 and C_6
   b. C_6 and C_7
   c. C_7
   d. C_7 and C_8

9. **Axillary nerve supplies to:**
   a. Deltoid muscle
   b. Muscles of anterior aspect of arm
   c. Skin of anterior aspect of arm
   d. Skin of posterior aspect of arm

10. **The lateral cord of brachial plexus is formed by union of:**
    a. Dorsal divisions of upper, middle and lower trunk
    b. Ventral divisions of lower trunk
    c. Ventral divisions of upper, middle and lower trunk
    d. Dorsal divisions of middle and lower trunk

ANSWER KEY

| 1. | b | 2. | b | 3. | c | 4. | a | 5. | c | 6. | b | 7. | c | 8. | c |
| 9. | a | 10. | c | | | | | | | | | | | | |

Autonomic Nervous System

ANATOMICAL CONSIDERATIONS

DIVISIONS OF AUTONOMIC NERVOUS SYSTEM

The word autonomous is taken from Greek words, the *autos* meaning 'self' and the *nomos* meaning 'control'. Thus, autonomic nervous system (ANS) is an involuntary system. Since it controls the vegetative functions, it is also called vegetative system.

ANS has two main divisions:

1. *Sympathetic division*, also called thoracolumbar division, consists of thoracic and lumbar chains of sympathetic ganglia.

2. *Parasympathetic division*, also called craniosacral division, consists of the ganglia associated with 3rd, 7th, 9th, and 10th cranial nerves.

GENERAL ORGANIZATION OF THE ANS

The ANS is organized as follows:

Autonomic Areas in the Cerebral Hemispheres

The autonomic areas controlling visceral functions located in the cerebral hemisphere are:

Higher Brain Centers

The higher brain centers such as the limbic cortex, parts of the cerebral cortex, can influence the activity of autonomic nervous system by sending signals to the hypothalamus and lower brain area.

Hypothalamus

Hypothalamus is the site of integration of somatic, autonomic and endocrine functions. Such an integration is essential for maintenance of homeostasis during stresses like extreme hot, extreme cold, stress of surgical operation, stress of injuries and hemorrhage and so on.

Since hypothalamus plays an important role in the regulation of autonomic activity, it has been called the main ganglion of the ANS. However, it is now known that the limbic cortex is equally important in the regulation of the ANS.

Autonomic Centers in the Brainstem

These are located in the reticular formation and in the general visceral nuclei of cranial nerves.

General Visceral Nuclei of Cranial Nerves

These include both general visceral afferent and efferent nuclei.

General visceral afferent (GVA) nucleus. It is represented by the *nucleus of solitary tract* present in the medulla. It receives fibers carrying general visceral sensations through the vagus and glossopharyngeal nerves. This nucleus plays an important role in reflex control of respiratory and cardiovascular functions.

Fibers of taste (special visceral afferents) carried by the facial, glossopharyngeal and vagus nerves end in the upper part of the nucleus of the solitary tract which is sometimes called *gustatory nucleus*.

According to some authorities, some general visceral afferents end in the dorsal vagal nucleus.

General visceral efferent (GVE) nuclei. These nuclei give origin to preganglionic fibers that constitute the cranial parasympathetic outflow. The general visceral efferent nuclei include:

Edinger-Westphal nucleus (of oculomotor nerve) situated in the midbrain

Salivary nucleus (superior and inferior) located in the pons

Dorsal nucleus of vagus present in the medulla.

Autonomic Centers in the Spinal Cord

These are located in the intermediolateral grey column of spinal cord at two levels:

1. Thoracolumbar outflow. Neurons present in the thoracic and upper two or three lumbar segments of spinal cord (T_1 to L_3) constitute the preganglionic neurons of sympathetic nervous system (thoracolumbar outflow).

2. Craniosacral outflow. Neurons present in the second, third and fourth sacral segments of spinal cord (S_2 to S_4) are the preganglionic neurons of the sacral part of parasympathetic system, which along with the cranial part constitute the craniosacral outflow.

Peripheral Part of Autonomic Nervous System

This is made up of all autonomic nerves and ganglia throughout the body. In fact, autonomic fibers are intimately related to different cranial and spinal nerves.

NEURONS OF ANS

Unlike in motor nerves, where a single motor neuron travels all the way from spinal cord or cranial nuclei to the muscle, the autonomic efferent pathway from the spinal cord or cranial nuclei is made of two neurons:

Preganglionic neurons. The cell body of the preganglionic neuron is located either in the brain stem or spinal cord. The axon of this visceral motor neuron projects as a thinly myelinated preganglionic fiber to an autonomic ganglion.

Postganglionic neuron. The body of the post-ganglionic neuron is located in the autonomic ganglion and sends an unmyelinated axon, the post-ganglionic fiber, to visceral effector cells.

In general, sympathetic ganglia are located close to the central nervous system, whereas parasympathetic ganglia are located close to the effector tissues. Therefore, sympathetic pathway has short preganglionic fibers and long postganglionic fibers, whereas parasympathetic pathway has long preganglionic fibers and short postganglionic fibers.

ANATOMY OF SYMPATHETIC NERVOUS SYSTEM

Sympathetic Preganglionic Neurons

The cell bodies of sympathetic preganglionic neurons are located in the intermediolateral horn of the spinal cord from level T_1 to L_2. The myelinated axons of these visceral motor neurons leave the spinal cord via the ventral root and then pass via the white rami communicantes to the paravertebral ganglia of the sympathetic trunk (Fig. 10.4-1). After reaching, the sympathetic trunk preganglionic fibers may pass to one of the following three destinations:

1. They may terminate in the ganglion at the level of entrance by synapsing with an excitor cell in the ganglion (Fig. 10.4-2).
2. They may travel up or down in the sympathetic trunk to terminate in the ganglia located at a higher or lower level (Fig. 10.4-2).
3. They may travel through the sympathetic trunk and exit without synapsing via splanchnic nerve and terminate in a prevertebral ganglion (Fig. 10.4-2).

Preganglionic fibers that innervate the adrenal medulla travel through the sympathetic trunk, exit without synapsing via greater splanchnic nerve and end directly on the cells of suprarenal medulla. These medullary cells may be regarded as modified sympathetic excitor cells that secrete epinephrine and norepinephrine into the blood stream. These secretory cells of the adrenal medulla are derived embryologically from nervous tissue and are analogous to postganglionic neurons.

Sympathetic Ganglia

Sympathetic ganglia are of three types:

1. Paravertebral ganglia. Paravertebral ganglia are arranged along the entire length of two sympathetic trunks (right and left placed on either side of vertebral column throughout its length). Paravertebral ganglia of sympathetic trunk are divided into:

Cervical ganglia. These are 3 in number: superior, middle and inferior.

Thoracic ganglia. These are 11–12 in number.

Lumbar ganglia. These are 4 in number.

In all, there are 22 or 23 ganglia on each trunk.

The inferior cervical ganglion and the first thoracic ganglion are often fused to form a large stellate ganglion.

The two sympathetic trunks end below by joining together to form a single ganglion, the *ganglion impar.*

2. Prevertebral or collateral ganglia. These are three in number (coeliac ganglion, inferior mesenteric ganglion and superior mesenteric ganglion).

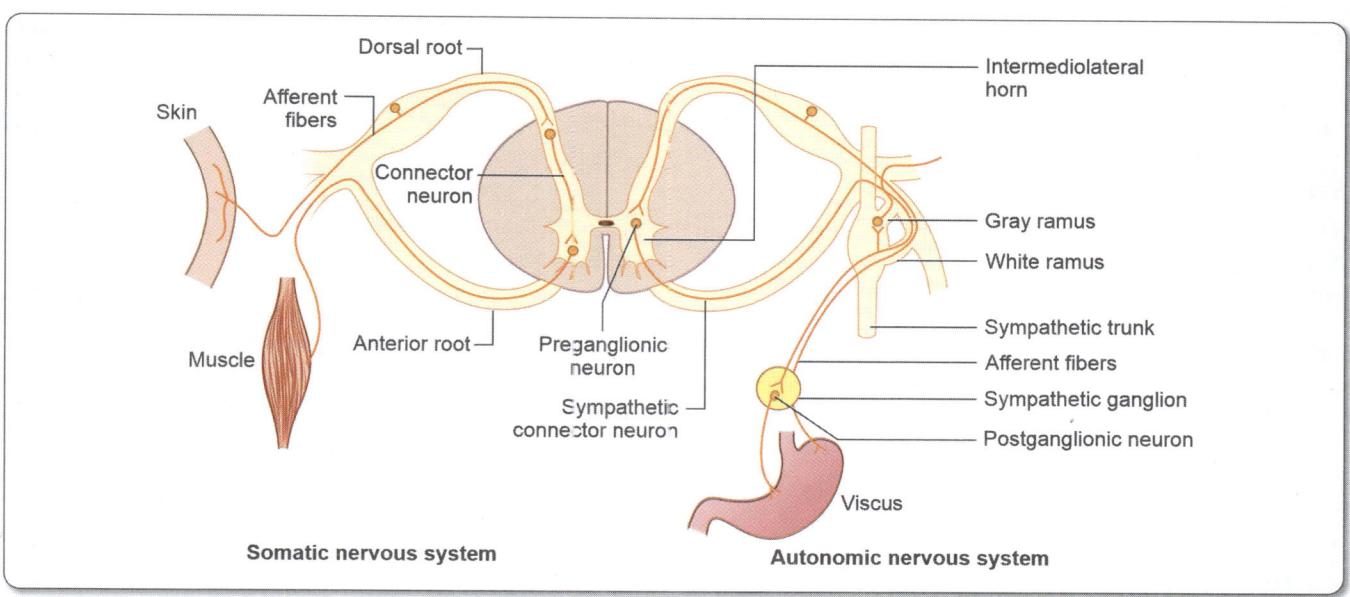

Fig. 10.4-1: General arrangement of somatic part of nervous system (on left) compared with autonomic part of nervous system (on right)

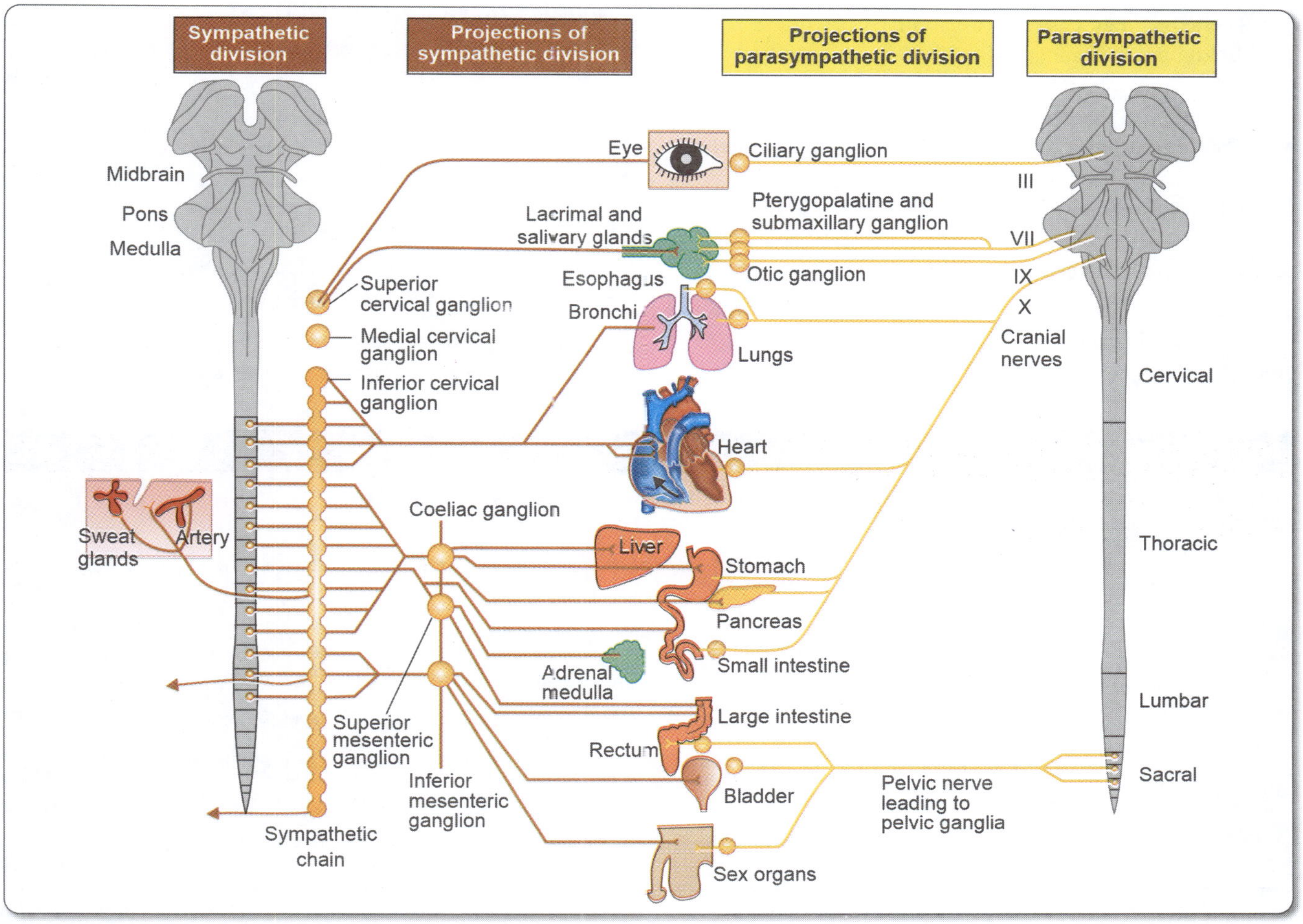

Fig. 10.4-2: Efferent part of autonomic nervous system: Sympathetic (on left) and parasympathetic (on right)

3. *Peripheral or terminal ganglia.* These are located within or close to structures innervated by them. Heart, bronchi, pancreas, and urinary bladder are innervated by the terminal ganglia.

Sympathetic Postganglionic Neurons

Sympathetic postganglionic neurons are located primarily in ganglia on the sympathetic trunks. Some are located in the prevertebral ganglia and the peripheral autonomic plexus (Figs 10.4-1 and 10.4-2). Axons arising from these neurons behave in one of the following ways:

- *The axons may pass through grey ramus communicantes* and re-enter ventral root to reach a spinal nerve. In the spinal nerve, the postganglionic fibers travel through its branches to innervate sweat glands and arrectores pilorum muscles of the skin in the region to which spinal nerve is distributed.
- *The axons may reach a cranial nerve* through a communicating branch and may be distributed through it as in the case of spinal nerve.
- The axons may pass into a vascular branch and may be distributed to branches of the vessel.
- Some fibers from these plexuses may pass to other structures in the neighborhood of the vessel.
- *The axons of postganglionic neurons arising* in sympathetic ganglia may travel through vascular branches and through autonomic plexus to reach some viscera (e.g., the heart).

Sympathetic Afferent Fibers

The afferent myelinated fibers travel from the viscera through the sympathetic ganglia without synapsing (Fig. 10.4-1). They enter the spinal nerve via the white rami communicantes and reach their cell bodies in the posterior root ganglia of the corresponding spinal nerve. The central axons then enter the spinal cord and may form the afferent component of a local reflex arc. Others may pass up to higher autonomic centers in the brain.

Distribution of Sympathetic Preganglionic Neurons and Postganglionic Fibers

The distribution of preganglionic neurons and postganglionic fibers is shown in Table 10.4-1 and Fig. 10.4-2.

ANATOMY OF PARASYMPATHETIC NERVOUS SYSTEM

Parasympathetic Preganglionic Neurons

The parasympathetic fibers form the *craniosacral outflow*, consisting of cranial parasympathetic outflow and sacral parasympathetic outflow.

Cranial Parasympathetic Outflow

The cell bodies of the neurons are located in the general visceral efferent nuclei. Cranial parasympathetic outflow can be further divided into:

- Midbrain or tectal outflow
- Bulbar outflow.

Midbrain or tectal outflow

The general visceral efferent nucleus associated with midbrain outflow is Edinger-Westphal nucleus.

Edinger-Westphal nucleus. It lies in the midbrain and is closely related to the oculomotor nucleus complex.

TABLE 10.4-1: Distribution of sympathetic preganglionic neurons and postganglionic fibers		
Segmental level of preganglionic neurons	**Area of distribution**	**Final distribution of postganglionic fibers**
T_1, T_2	Head and neck	Dilator pupillae muscle, superior and inferior, Muller's muscles of eyelids, blood vessels and sweat glands
T_3, T_4	Thoracic viscera	Heart, esophagus, trachea, bronchi and lungs
T_5 to T_9	Upper limb	Blood vessels, sweat glands and arrectores pilorum muscles
T_{10} to L_2	Lower limb	Blood vessels, sweat glands and arrectores pilorum muscles
T_6 to T_{12}	Upper abdominal viscera	Gastrointestinal tract, liver, spleen adrenal capsule, medulla, and urinary tract
L_1, L_2	Lower abdominal viscera	Bladder, uterus, fallopian tubes (or testes, vas deferens, seminal vesicles and prostate)
T_1 to T_{12}	Thoracic and abdominal parietes	Blood vessels, sweat glands and arrectores pilorum muscles

- *Preganglionic fibers* arising from Edinger-Westphal nucleus pass through oculomotor (3rd cranial) nerve and relay in ciliary ganglion.
- *Postganglionic fibers* arising in the ciliary ganglion pass through the short ciliary nerves and supply the sphincter pupillae and the ciliary muscle.

Bulbar outflow

The general visceral efferent nuclei associated with bulbar outflow are:

Superior salivary nucleus. Preganglionic fibers arising from superior salivary nucleus enter the facial (7th cranial) nerve and ultimately relay in *submandibular ganglion*. Postganglionic fibers pass to submandibular and sublingual salivary glands to which they are secretomotor.

Lacrimal nucleus of 7th cranial nerve sends preganglionic fibers to the *pterygopalatine* (spheno-palatine) ganglion. The postganglionic fibers reach the lacrimal gland to which they are secretomotor.

Inferior salivary nucleus sends preganglionic fibers into the glossopharyngeal (9th cranial) nerve. These fibers relay in the otic ganglion, from where the postganglionic fibers go to parotid gland to which they are secretomotor.

Dorsal (motor) nucleus of the vagus. About 75% of all parasympathetic fibers arise from dorsal nucleus.

Preganglionic fibers traveling in the vagus nerve end in ganglia (or nerve plexuses) closely related to the visceral organs such as heart, lungs, bronchi, esophagus, stomach, small intestine and large intestine up to two-thirds of transverse colon.

Postganglionic fibers arise in these ganglia, and run a short course to supply smooth muscles and glands in these organs.

Sacral Parasympathetic Outflow

Preganglionic fibers. Cell bodies of the preganglionic neurons, of sacral parasympathetic outflow, are located in the intermediolateral grey horn of second, third and fourth sacral segments (S_2, S_3 and S_4) of spinal cord (Fig. 10.4-2). Their axons form the preganglionic fibers which pass out through the ventral spinal root of corresponding nerves. These axons leave the spinal nerves to form the pelvic splanchnic nerves which end in the pelvic autonomic plexuses.

Postganglionic fibers. The postganglionic neurons are located in the pelvic autonomic plexuses close to or within the viscera. Their axons (postganglionic fibers) run a very short course to supply the concerned pelvic viscera. These fibers also supply the rectum, the sigmoid colon, the descending colon and the left one-third of transverse colon.

Parasympathetic Afferent Fibers

The afferent myelinated fibers travel from viscera to their cell bodies located either in the sensory ganglia of the cranial nerves or in the posterior root ganglia of the sacrospinal nerves. The central axons then enter the central nervous system and take part in the formation of local reflex arc, or pass to higher centers of the ANS.

PHYSIOLOGICAL CONSIDERATIONS

AUTONOMIC NEUROTRANSMITTERS AND RECEPTORS

Neurotransmitters of ANS

Parasympathetic Fibers

Preganglionic fibers. Acetylcholine.
Postganglionic fibers. Acetylcholine.

Sympathetic Fibers

Preganglionic fibers. Acetylcholine.
Postganglionic fibers:
- *Adrenergic fibers:* Norepinephrine (mainly), or epinephrine
- *Cholinergic fibers:* Acetylcholine (the post-ganglionic sympathetic cholinergic nerve fibers supplying sweat glands, blood vessels in heart and skeletal muscles).

Autonomic Receptors

The autonomic neurotransmitters (acetylcholine or norepinephrine) produce their effects on the organs by combining with specific protein molecules known as receptors, which are of the following types:

Cholinergic Receptors

On the basis of their pharmacologic properties, these are of two types:

1. *Nicotinic receptors.* These receptors are located in/at autonomic ganglia of sympathetic and para-sympathetic nervous system, neuromuscular junction, and adrenal medulla.

The receptors at these locations are similar but not identical.

Activation. Nicotinic receptors are activated by acetylcholine (ACh) and nicotine.

Effect. These receptors produce excitation.

Blockage. Ganglion blockers (e.g., hexa-methonium, trimethaphan) block the nicotinic receptors for ACh in the autonomic ganglia, but not at the neuromuscular junction.

2. *Muscarinic receptors.* These receptors are located in the heart, smooth muscles (except vascular smooth muscle) and glands.

Activation. These receptors are activated by acetylcholine (ACh) and muscarine.

Effects produced by their stimulation is:

- *Inhibitory in the heart*, e.g., decreased heart rate, and decreased conduction velocity in AV node.
- *Excitatory* in smooth muscle and glands (e.g., increased gastrointestinal motility and increased secretion).

Blockage. Muscarinic receptors for acetylcholine are blocked by atropine.

Adrenergic Receptors

On the basis of their pharmacologic properties, adrenergic receptors are of two types: *Alpha (α) adrenergic receptors* (which are of further two types: α_1 and α_2), and *Beta (β) adrenergic receptors* (which are of further three types: β_1, β_2 and β_3).

α_1 ***receptors*** are located on vascular smooth muscles of skin and splanchnic regions, gastrointestinal and bladder sphincters, and radial muscles of the iris.

Effect. These receptors produce excitation, e.g., contraction or constriction.

α_2 ***receptors*** are located in presynaptic nerve terminals, platelets, fat cells, and walls of the gastrointestinal tract.

Effect. Often produce inhibition (e.g., relaxation or dilatation).

β_1 ***receptors*** are located in the sinoatrial (SA) node, atrioventricular (AV) node, and ventricular muscles of the heart.

Effect. These receptors produce excitation (e.g., increased heart rate, increased conduction velocity and increased contractility).

β_2 ***receptors*** are located on vascular smooth muscle of skeletal muscle, bronchial smooth muscle, walls of the gastrointestinal tract and bladder.

Effect. These receptors produce relaxation (e.g., dilation of vascular smooth muscle, dilation of bronchioles, and relaxation of bladder wall).

β_3 ***receptors*** are located on the adipose tissue and cause lipolysis.

The type of adrenergic receptors present in various organs and the effects produced by their stimulation are depicted in Table 10.4-2.

FUNCTIONS OF AUTONOMIC NERVOUS SYSTEM: EFFECTS OF AUTONOMIC NERVE IMPULSES ON EFFECTOR ORGANS

General Principles

- ANS controls the various vegetative functions which are beyond voluntary control and thus plays an important role in maintaining the constant internal environment (homeostasis).
- Most of the visceral organs have dual innervation, i.e., are supplied by both sympathetic and parasympathetic divisions of ANS. The two divisions produce antagonistic effects on each organ and provide a very fine degree of control over the effector organ.
- Some of the visceral organs are innervated by one division of ANS only; e.g.,
    - *Uterus*, adrenal medulla and most of the arterioles are innervated by sympathetic division only.
    - *Glands of stomach and pancreas* are innervated by parasympathetic division only.
- In the case of sphincter's muscles, both adrenergic and cholinergic innervations are excitatory, but one supplies the constrictor component of the sphincter and other the dilator.
- *Effects of acetylcholine*, i.e., of localized cholinergic discharge are generally discrete and shortlasting, because ACh is rapidly removed from the nerve endings due to high concentration of acetylcholine esterase at cholinergic nerve endings.
- *Effects of norepinephrine* are more prolonged than ACh, as it spreads further. In the blood, epinephrine and dopamine come from the adrenal medulla, while norepinephrine diffuses from the adrenergic nerve endings.

Effects of Stimulation of Sympathetic and Parasympathetic Divisions of ANS

Responses of effector organs to autonomic nerve impulses are summarized in Table 10.4-2.

Differences between Sympathetic and Parasympathetic Systems

As summarized in Table 10.4-2, sympathetic and parasympathetic systems produce antagonistic effects on each organ of the body. The main differences between sympathetic and parasympathetic systems are depicted in Table 10.4-3.

TABLE 10.4-2: Responses of effector organs to sympathetic and parasympathetic stimulation

Effector organ	Parasympathetic effect	Sympathetic effect	
		Receptor type	**Response**
Eyes			
• Dilator pupillae muscle	—	α	Contraction (mydriasis)
• Sphincter pupillae muscle	Contraction (meiosis)	—	—
• Ciliary muscle	Contraction (produces accommodation for near vision)	β_2	Relaxes (flattens lens for far vision)
Heart			
• SA node	↓ Heart rate, vagal arrest	β_1 & β_2	↑ Heart rate
• Atria	↓ Contractility	β_1 & β_2	↑ Contractility
	↓ Conductivity		↑ Conductivity
• A-V node and conduction system	↓ Conduction velocity	β_1 & β_2	↑ Conduction velocity
• Ventricles	↓ Contractility	β_1 & β_2	↑ Contractility
Arterioles			
• Coronary		α_1 & α_2	Constriction
		β_2	Dilatation
• Cutaneous and mucosal	No supply	α_1 & α_2	Constriction
• Skeletal muscle	No supply	α_1	Constriction
		β_2	Dilatation
• Cerebral	Dilatation	α_1	Constriction
• Pulmonary	Dilatation	α_1	Constriction
		β_2	Dilatation
• Abdominal viscera	No supply	α_1	Constriction
• Renal	No supply	α_1 & α_2	Constriction
		β_1 & β_2	Dilatation
• Salivary glands	Dilatation	α_1 & α_2	Constriction
Systemic veins	No supply	α_1 & α_2	Constriction
		β_2	Dilatation
Lungs			
• Bronchial muscles	Contraction	β_2	Relaxation
		α_1	Inhibition
• Bronchial glands	Stimulation	β_2	Stimulation
Salivary glands	Stimulation (profuse watery secretion)	α_1	Stimulation (thick viscous secretion)
Stomach			
• Motility and tone	Increases	α_1, α_2, β_2	Decreases

Contd...

Effector organ	Parasympathetic effect	Sympathetic effect	
		Receptor type	Response
• Sphincters	Relaxation	α_1	Contraction
• Secretion	Stimulation	α_2	Inhibition
Gall bladder	Contraction	β_2	Relaxation
Liver	—	α_1, β_2	Glycogenolysis
Pancreas			
• Exocrine glands	Stimulates secretion	α_1	Inhibits secretion
• Endocrine glands	—	α_2	Inhibits insulin secretion
		β_2	Stimulates glucagon
Spleen capsule		α_1	Contraction
		β_2	Relaxation
Adrenal medulla	Secretion of epinephrine and norepinephrine		
Urinary bladder			
• Detrusor muscle	Contraction	β_2	Relaxation (usually)
• Sphincter	Relaxation	α_1	Contraction
Uterus	Variable	α_1	Contraction (pregnant)
		β_2	Relaxation (nonpregnant)
Male sex organ	Erection	α_1	Ejaculation
Lacrimal glands	Secretion		
Skin			
• Pilomotor muscle	—	α_1	Contraction (erection of hair)
• Sweat glands	Generalized (cholinergic sweating)	α_1	Localized (adrenergic) sweating
Nasopharyngeal glands	Secretion	—	—
Adipose tissue	—	$\alpha_1, \beta_1, \beta_3$	Lipolysis, release of free fatty acids
Juxtaglomerular cells	—	β_1	Increased renin secretion
Pineal gland	—	β_1	Increased melatonin synthesis and secretion
Skeletal muscles	—	β_2	Increased glycogenolysis
Basal metabolic rate	—	β_2	Increased
Mental activity	—		Increased

TABLE 10.4-3: Main differences between sympathetic and parasympathetic system

Feature	Sympathetic system	Parasympathetic system
Location	Cell bodies of preganglionic neurons are located in intermediolateral horn of T_1 to L_2 or L_3 spinal segments, so also called thoracolumbar outflow.	Cell bodies of preganglionic neurons are located in: • *Cranial nuclei* associated with 3rd, 7th, 9th and 10th cranial nerves (cranial outflow) • Intermediolateral horn of S_2 to S_4 spinal segments (sacral outflow). So, it is also called craniosacral outflow
Components and ganglia	• Components are consolidated. • Ganglia are linked up to form a chain.	• Components are isolated • Ganglia remain isolated
Preganglionic fibers	Are short, myelinated and end in paravertebral or prevertebral ganglia	Are long, myelinated and end on short postganglionic neurons located on or near the viscera
Postganglionic fibers	• Long • Nonmyelinated	• Short • Myelinated
Neurotransmitter • Preganglionic fibers • Postganglionic fibers	• Cholinergic • Mostly adrenergic	• Cholinergic • Cholinergic
Area of effect	Preganglionic fibers branch, enter several ganglia and transmit nerve impulse to many postganglionic fibers. So, sympathetic activity is spread over many segments.	Preganglionic fibers do not branch, each enters a single ganglion and transmits nerve impulses to a single postganglionic fiber. Therefore, parasympathetic activity is localized, i.e., target is usually a single organ or system.
Functions	Mass sympathetic discharge usually occurs in threatening situation, i.e., it prepares the individual to cope with the emergency. It causes flight or fight reactions characterized by: • Dilatation of pupil • Increased heart rate • Increased blood pressure (providing better perfusion of the vital organs and muscles) • Constriction of cutaneous arterioles (which limits blood loss from wounds, if any) • Increased alertness and arousal due to decreased threshold in the reticular formation • Increased blood glucose and free fatty acids levels (supplying more energy) Because of these actions sympathetic system is also sometimes called *catabolic nervous system*	Unlike sympathetic nervous system, the functions of parasympathetic system are discrete and each function is separately regulated. This system is concerned with vegetative aspect of day-to-day living. For example, its action favors: • Digestion and absorption of food, increased activity of intestinal musculature and increased gastric secretion and pyloric relaxation • Micturition • Pupillary constriction • Bradycardia. Since, parasympathetic system decreases the rate of metabolism, it is also called *anabolic nervous system*.

CLINICAL ASPECTS

AUTONOMIC FAILURE

Types. Autonomic failure is of two types:
1. **Primary autonomic failure** from unexplained (primary) autonomic neuronal degeneration.
2. **Secondary autonomic failure** occurs secondary to some general medical disorders. Diabetes mellitus is the most common cause of secondary autonomic dysfunction.

Features of autonomic failure (primary or secondary) are:
• *Cardiovascular features* include tachycardia and orthostatic hypotension.
• *Sudomotor features* are anhidrosis and heat intolerance.
• *Gastrointestinal features* include constipation, occasional diarrhea and dysphagia.
• *Urinary features* are nocturia, frequency, urgency, incontinence and retention of urine.

• *Reproductive* organ problems include erectile and ejaculation failure.
• *Ocular* features include miosis and enophthalmos.

HORNER'S SYNDROME

Horner's syndrome refers to ipsilateral *oculosympathetic paresis* due to any cause. Its common causes are Pancoast's tumor of the lung, malignancy of cervical lymph nodes pressing on the cervical sympathetic chain.

Clinical features of Horner's syndrome are:
• *Ptosis* (drooping down of upper eyelid) due to paralysis of Muller's muscle of upper eyelid.
• *Miosis* (small pupil) due to paralysis of dilator pupillae muscle.
• *Facial anhidrosis,* i.e., reduced sweating on the ipsilateral face and neck.

ASSESS YOURSELF

Short and Long Answer Questions

1. **Discuss briefly the organization of the autonomic nervous system.**
2. **Differentiate between:**
   - Activity of sympathetic and parasympathetic systems
   - Adrenergic and cholinergic receptors
   - Preganglionic and postganglionic fibers
   - Nicotinic and muscarinic receptors

Multiple Choice Questions

1. **Which of the following is not concerned with autonomic activity?**
   a. Temporal lobe of cerebrum
   b. Hypothalamus
   c. Limbic cortex
   d. Edinger Westphal nucleus
2. **For thoraco-lumbar outflow the neurons are present in:**
   a. T1 to L3 segments   b. T2 to L4 segments
   c. T3 to L5 segments   d. T4 to L6 segments
3. **Coeliac ganglion is a:**
   a. Paravertebral ganglion
   b. Prevertebral ganglion
   c. Perivertebral ganglion
   d. Terminal ganglion

4. **The preganglionic sympathetic neurons from spinal segments T1 and T2 innervate:**
   a. Heart
   b. Trachea
   c. Dilator pupillae muscle
   d. Bronchi
5. **Preganglionic parasympathetic fibers arising from superior salivary nucleus relay in:**
   a. Otic ganglion
   b. Submandibular ganglion
   c. Sphenopalatine ganglion
   d. Pterygopalatine ganglion
6. **The type of receptors present at autonomic ganglia are:**
   a. Nicotinic   b. Muscarinic
   c. α1   d. β1
7. **β2 adrenergic receptors are located at:**
   a. Ventricular muscles of heart
   b. Vascular smooth muscle of skeletal muscle
   c. Adipose tissue
   d. Adrenal medulla
8. **The muscarinic receptors are blocked by:**
   a. Hexamethonium
   b. Atropine
   c. B blockers
   d. Verapamil

ANSWER KEY

1. a   **2.** a   **3.** b   **4.** c   **5.** b   **6.** a   **7.** a   **8.** b

Index

S

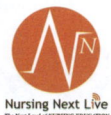
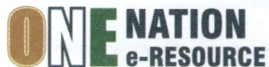
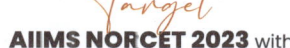
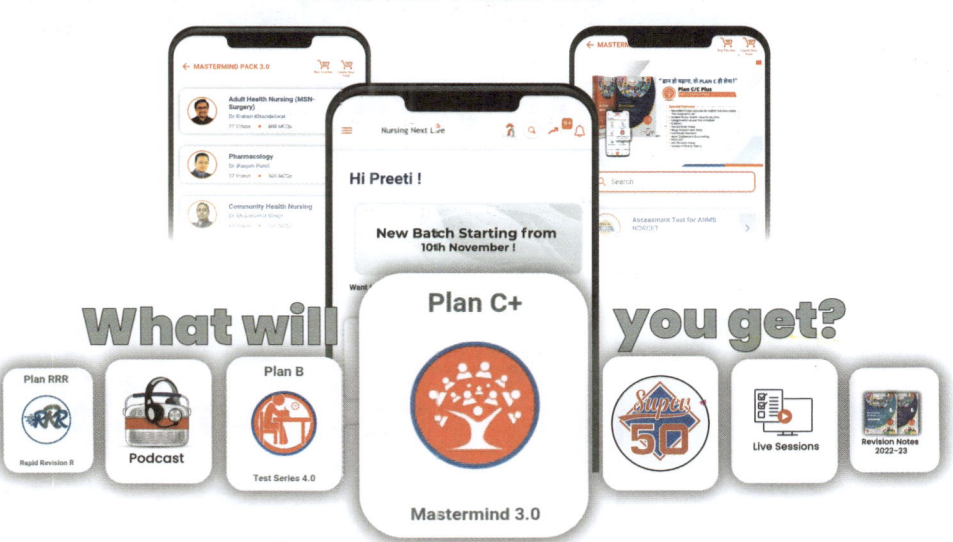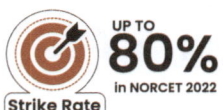 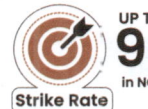 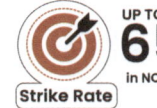
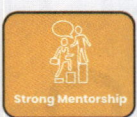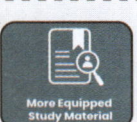
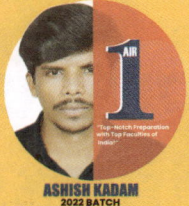
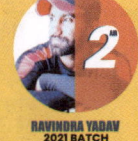

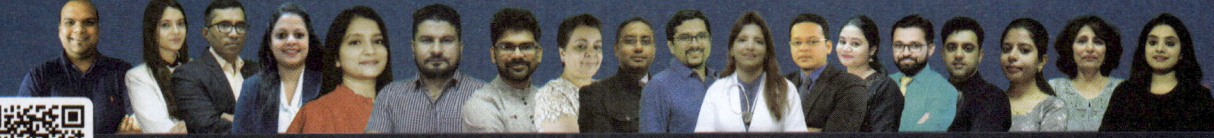

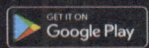
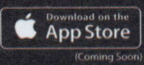

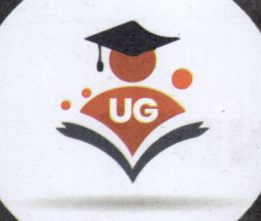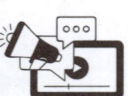
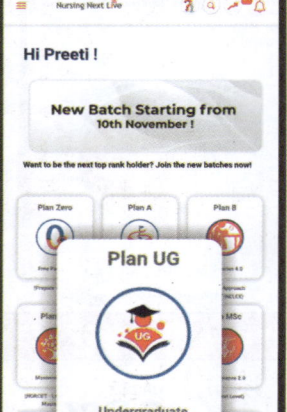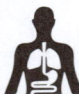
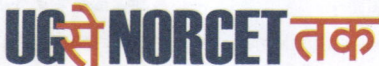
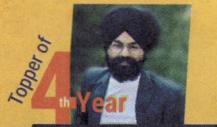
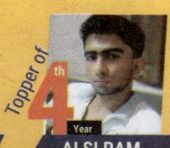
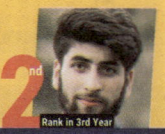
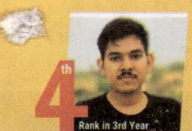
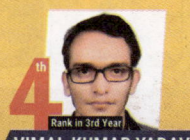
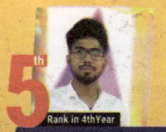

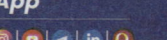
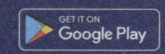
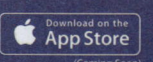